C. Seep
I1030099

ROY AND FRAUNFELDER'S CURRENT OCULAR THERAPY

SIXTH EDITION

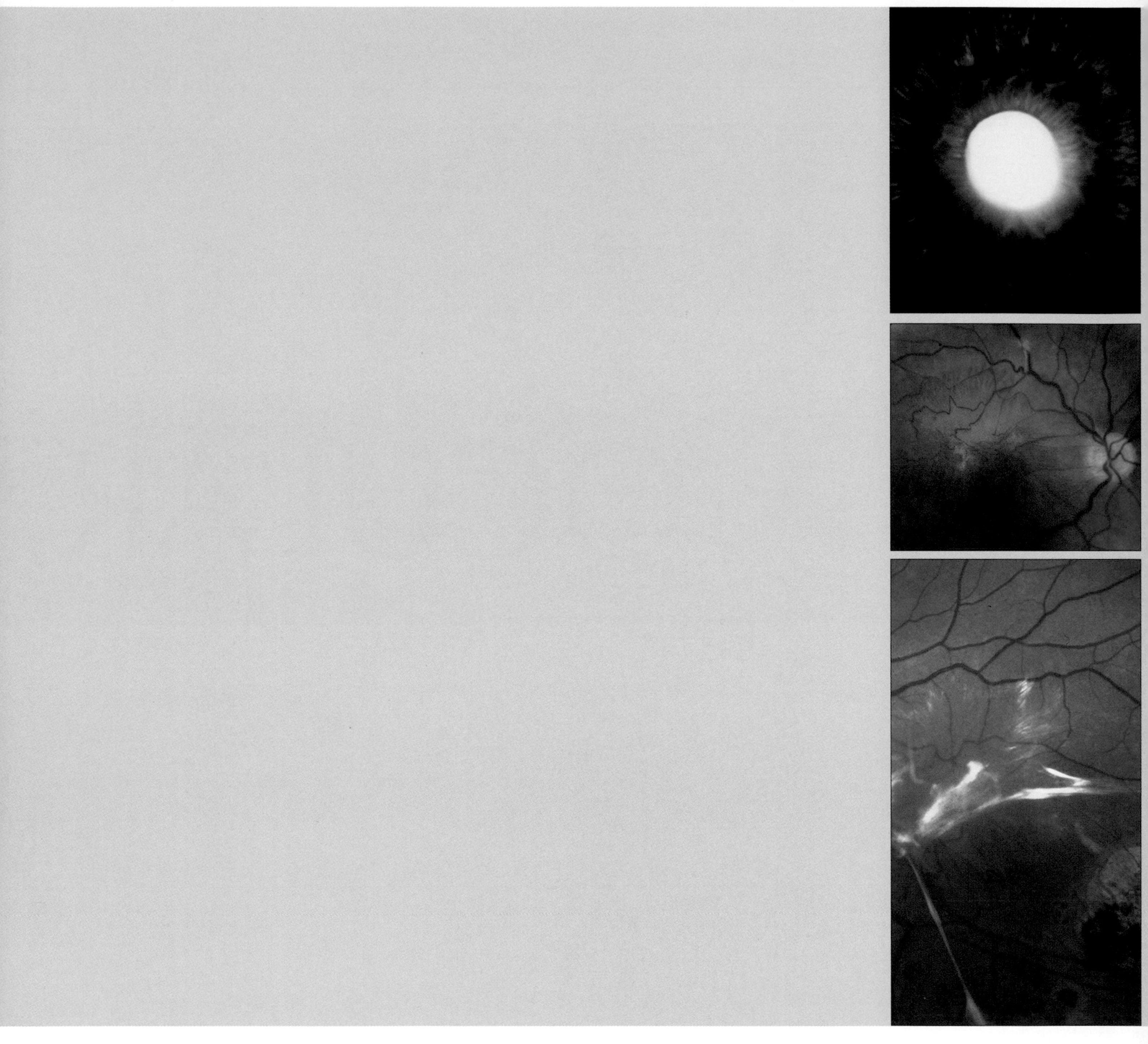

Commissioning Editor: Russell Gabbedy
Development Editor: Alexandra Mortimer
Project Manager: Alan Nicholson
Design Manager: Jayne Jones/Stewart Larking
Marketing Manager(s) (UK/USA): John Canelon/Lisa Damico

SIXTH EDITION

ROY AND FRAUNFELDER'S CURRENT OCULAR THERAPY

EDITED BY

F. Hampton Roy MD FACS

Medical Director
Hampton Roy Eye Center
Little Rock, Arkansas
USA

Frederick W. Fraunfelder MD

Associate Professor
Department of Ophthalmology
Oregon Health and Science University
Casey Eye Institute
Portland, Oregon
USA

Frederick T. Fraunfelder MD

Professor
Department of Ophthalmology
Oregon Health and Science University
Casey Eye Institute
Portland, Oregon
USA

ASSOCIATE EDITORS

Renee Tindall RN

Little Rock, Arkansas
USA

Bree Jensvold BS

Casey Eye Institute
Portland, Oregon
USA

SAUNDERS

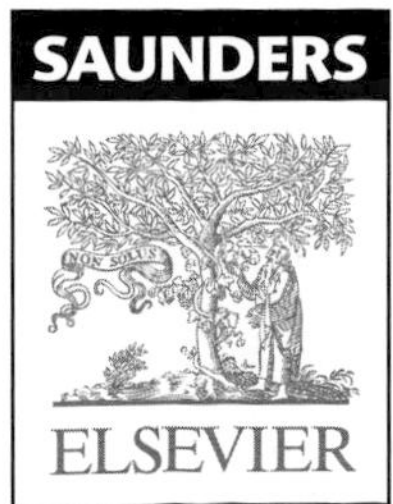

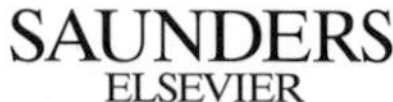

An imprint of Elsevier Inc.

First edition 1980
Second edition 1985
Third edition 1990
Fourth edition 1995
Fifth edition 2000
Sixth edition 2008

ISBN 978-1-4160-2447-7

British Library Cataloguing in Publication Data
A catalogue record for this book is available from the British Library

Library of Congress Cataloging in Publication Data
A catalog record for this book is available from the Library of Congress

Notice
Medical knowledge is constantly changing. Standard safety precautions must be followed, but as new research and clinical experience broaden our knowledge, changes in treatment and drug therapy may become necessary or appropriate. Readers are advised to check the most current product information provided by the manufacturer of each drug to be administered to verify the recommended dose, the method and duration of administration, and contraindications. It is the responsibility of the practitioner, relying on experience and knowledge of the patient, to determine dosages and the best treatment for each individual patient. Neither the Publisher nor the author assume any liability for any injury and/or damage to persons or property arising from this publication.
The Publisher

Printed in China
Last digit is the print number: 9 8 7 6 5 4 3 2 1

CONTENTS

14 MECHANICAL AND NONMECHANICAL INJURIES

15 UNCLASSIFIED DISEASES OR CONDITIONS

16 ANTERIOR CHAMBER

Contents

20 EXTRAOCULAR MUSCLES

21 EYELIDS

22 GLOBE

PREFACE

A text that has gone into its 6th edition has been well received by the medical profession.

This book is designed to be concise with a consistent format so that the clinician can focus on a specific area. In some instances the text can be photocopied and given to the patient as a reference. In this way, the time necessary to explain the problem to the patient may be significantly reduced.

This edition has had major modifications and embraces evidence-based medicine. Perhaps the biggest change in this edition is the addition of pictures. This allows the clinician to read about and actually see a picture of select disease entities.

The authors have been selected based on their expertise, their recent publications, and the methods of management based on the most recent clinical advances. The format includes the CPT codes for billing purposes, short description of the condition, etiology/incidence, course/prognosis, laboratory findings, differential diagnosis; prophylaxis, treatment (local and systemic, surgical or other), miscellaneous (names and addresses of support groups) and key references.

Although drug dosages and methods of administration have been scrutinized, it is important that each physician exercise his or her own judgment in the choice and use of a drug. The physician is advised to check the product information included in the drug's package insert before drug administration. New data and individual clinical situations can change the drug regimen.

We have had contributions from more than 400 authors throughout the world. In sincere gratitude for their time and effort, we have acknowledged them in the front of this book.

We wish to express our appreciation and pay special tribute to Renee Tindall and Bree Jensvold, who worked with diligence, devotion, and skill to create this book.

F. Hampton Roy
Frederick W. Fraunfelder
Frederick T. Fraunfelder

CONTRIBUTORS

Richard L. Abbott MD
Thomas W. Boyden, Endowed Chair in Ophthalmology
Health Science Clinical Professor
Research Associate, Francis I. Proctor Foundation
University of California, San Francisco
Beckman Vision Center
San Francisco CA
USA
14 Erysipelas

Natalie A. Afshari MD
Associate Professor of Ophthalmology
Cornea and Refractive Surgery
Duke University Eye Center
Duke University Medical Center
Durham NC
USA
209 Reis–Bucklers Corneal Dystrophy

Jaya Agrawal MS, DNB, MNAMS, FRCS
Consultant Ophthalmologist
T. P. Agrawal Institute of Ophthalmology
Meerut
Uttar Pradesh
India
58 Cysticercosis

Shishir Agrawal MS, DNB, FRCS, MRCOphth, FRF
Consultant Ophthalmologist
T. P. Agrawal Institute of Ophthalmology
Meerut
Uttar Pradesh
India
58 Cysticercosis

Trilok P. Agrawal MS
Consultant Ophthalmologist
T. P. Agrawal Institute of Ophthalmology
Meerut
Uttar Pradesh
India
58 Cysticercosis

Levent Akduman MD
Associate Professor of Ophthalmology
Department of Ophthalmology
St Louis University School of Medicine
St Louis MO
USA
82 Thalassemia

Esen K. Akpek MD
Associate Professor of Ophthalmology
Director, Ocular Surface Diseases and Dry Eye Clinic
Wilmer Eye Institute
Johns Hopkins Hospital
Baltimore MD
USA
347 Scleritis

Amal Al-Sayyed MD
Oculoplastics Fellow
University of Toronto Ophthalmology
Toronto East General Hospital
Toronto ON
Canada
41 Rabies

Thomas A. Albini MD
Fellow, Vitreoretinal Diseases and Surgery
Department of Ophthalmology
Baylor College of Medicine
Houston TX
USA
257 Fungal Endophthalmitis

Deborah M. Alcorn MD
Associate Professor of Ophthalmology and Pediatrics
Department of Ophthalmology and Pediatrics
Stanford University School of Medicine
Stanford CA
USA
67 Oculocerebrorenal Syndrome
70 Galactosemias

Amar Alwitry MD, MRCS, MRCSEd, MRCOphth, FRCOphth
Consultant Ophthalmologist
Derbyshire Royal Infirmary
Derby
UK
331 Central or Branch Retinal Artery Occlusion

Anouk Amzel MD, MPH
Assistant Professor of Pediatrics
Columbia University School of Medicine
New York NY
USA
17 Haemophilus influenzae

Nicole J. Anderson MD
Ophthalmologist
Mississippi Vision Correction Center, PLLC
Flowood MS
USA
208 Posterior Polymorphous Dystrophy

Ejaz A. Ansari BSc(Hons), MBBCh, FRCOphth, MD
Consultant Ophthalmic Surgeon
Eye, Ear and Mouth Unit
Maidstone Hospital
Maidstone Kent
UK
66 Hypovitaminosis

Andrew Antoszyk MD
Charlotte Eye Ear Nose and Throat Associates
Charlotte NC
USA
350 Persistent Hyperplastic Primary Vitreous

James H. Antoszyk MD
Charlotte Eye Ear Nose and Throat Associates
Charlotte NC
USA
350 Persistent Hyperplastic Primary Vitreous

James V. Aquavella MD
Professor of Ophthalmology
University of Rochester Eye Institute
Rochester NY
USA
200 Keratoconjunctivitis Sicca and Sjögren's Syndrome
296 Lacrimal Hyposecretion
348 Scleromalacia Perforans

Sumaira A. Arain MD
Research Fellow
Department of Ophthalmology
University of California
Sacramento CA
USA
236 Distichiasis

J. Fernando Arévalo MD
Director
Clínica Oftalmologica Centro Caracas
Caracas
Venezuela
57 Coenurosis

Guruswami Arunagiri MD, FRCSEd
Attending Physician
Department of Ophthalmology
Geisinger Medical Center
Danville PA
USA
188 Corneal Abrasions, Contusions, Lacerations and Perforations

Carlos W. Arzabe MD
Ophthalmic Surgeon
Hospital del Ojo
Santa Cruz
Bolivia
61 Ocular Toxocariasis

La-ongsri Atchaneeyasakul MD
Associate Professor
Department of Ophthalmology
Division of Pediatric Ophthalmology and Strabismus
Faculty of Medicine
Siriraj Hospital
Mahidol University
Bangkok
Thailand
76 Mucopolysaccharidosis IV
336 Gyrate Atrophy of the Choroid and Retina with Hyperornithinemia
338 Refsum's Disease

Huban Atilla MD
Associate Professor of Ophthalmology
Department of Ophthalmology
Pediatric Ophthalmology and Strabismus
Ankara University, Faculty of Medicine
Ankara
Turkey
113 Functional Amblyopia

Ümit Aykan MD
Assistant Professor
Department of Ophthalmology
GATA H. Pasa Training Hospital
Istanbul
Turkey
260 Exfoliation Syndrome

Brandon D. Ayres MD
Cornea Fellow
Wills Eye Hospital
Philadelphia PA
USA
201 Keratoconus

Juan J. Barbón MD
Consultant Ophthalmologist
Ophthalmology Department
Hospital San Agustín
Avilés-Asturias
Spain
87 Psoriasis

Kristi Bailey MD
Resident
Department of Ophthalmology
Oregon Health and Science University
Casey Eye Institute
Portland OR
USA
325 Orbital Cellulitis and Abscess
326 Orbital Graves' Disease

Frank G. Baloh MD
Lehigh Valley Eye Center
Allentown PA
USA
27 Molluscum Contagiosum

Irina S. Barequet MD
Lecturer in Ophthalmology
Goldschleger Eye Institute
Sheba Medical Center
Tel Aviv University Sackler Faculty of Medicine
Tel Hashomer
Israel
186 Bacterial Corneal Ulcers

André Barkhuizen MBBCh(Rand), MMed(UCT), FCP(SA), FACR
Associate Professor of Medicine and Staff Physician
Arthritis and Rheumatic Disease
Oregon Health and Science University and Portland VA Medical Center
Portland OR
USA
97 Systemic Lupus Erythematosus

Michael A. Bearn FRCOphth, BMedSci
Consultant Ophthalmologist
Dr Gray's Hospital
Elgin
Scotland
UK
295 Lacrimal Hypersecretion

Rubens Belfort Jr MD
Professor of Ophthalmology
Department of Ophthalmology
Federal University of São Paulo
São Paulo
Brazil
3 Acquired Immune Deficiency Syndrome

A. Robert Bellows MD
Boston Eye Surgery and Laser Center
Ophthalmic Consultants of Boston
Boston MA
USA
170 Choroidal Detachment

Audina M. Berrocal MD
Assistant Professor of Ophthalmology
Department of Ophthalmology
Bascom Palmer Eye Institute
University of Miami School of Medicine
Miami FL
USA
28 Moraxella

Marijke Wefers Bettink-Remeijer MD
Neuro-Ophthalmologist
Neuro-Ophthalmology Department
Rotterdam Eye Hospital
Netherlands
110 Cluster Headache

Anuja Bhandari MD, FRCOphth
Assistant Professor
Department of Ophthalmology
University of Washington
Seattle WA
USA
253 Trichiasis

M. Tariq Bhatti MD
Associate Professor
Departments of Ophthamology and Medicine (Division of Neurology)
Duke University Eye Center
Duke University Medical Center
Durham, NC
USA
80 Carotid Cavernous Fistula

Mark S. Blumenkranz MD
Professor and Chairman
Department of Ophthalmology
Stanford University School of Medicine
Stanford CA
USA
329 Acute Retinal Necrosis

Kostas G. Boboridis MD, PhD
Ophthalmic and Oculoplastic Surgeon
Ophthalmology Department
Aristotle University of Thessaloniki
Thessaloniki
Greece
237 Ectropion

James P. Bolling MD
Associate Professor and Chair
Department of Ophthalmology
Mayo Clinic
Jacksonville FL
USA
353 Vitreous Wick Syndrome

Vivien Boniuk MD, FRCS(C)
Director of Ophthalmology, Queens Hospital Center
Associate Professor of Ophthalmology
Albert Einstein College of Medicine
Long Island Jewish Medical Center
New York NY
USA
44 Rubella

Paul Jorge Botelho MD
Clinical Assistant Professor at Brown Medical School
Department of Surgery
Center for Sight
Fall River MA
USA
13 Epidemic Keratoconjunctivitis

Paul W. Brazis MD
Professor of Neurology
Department of Ophthalmology
Mayo Clinic, Jacksonville
Jacksonville FL
USA
106 Acquired Inflammatory Demyelinating Neuropathies

Fion D. Bremner BSc, MBBS, PhD, FRCOphth
Consultant Ophthalmic Surgeon and Consultant in Neuro-ophthalmology
Department of Neuro-ophthalmology
National Hospital for Neurology and Neurosurgery
London
UK
312 Congenital Pit of Optic Disc

Edward G. Buckley MD
Professor, Ophthalmology and Pediatrics
Department of Pediatric Ophthalmology & Strabismus & Neuro-ophthalmology
Duke University Eye Center
Durham NC
USA
220 Congenital Esotropia

John D. Bullock MD, MPH, MSc
Infectious Disease Epidemioligist
Clinical Professor of Community Health
Professor of Mathematics and Statistics
Emeritus Professor and Chair of Ophthalmology
Wright State University School of Medicine
Dayton OH
USA
32 Nocardiosis
171 Choroidal Folds

David Matthew Bushley MD
Cornea and Refractive Surgery
Duke University Eye Center
Duke University Medical Center
Durham NC
USA
209 Reis–Bucklers Corneal Dystrophy

Jorge Alberto F. Caldeira MD
Emeritus Professor of Ophthamology
Division of Ophthalmology
Faculdade de Medicina
University of São Paulo
Brazil
233 V-pattern Strabismus

Anne Carricajo PhD
Microbiologist
Department of Microbiology
Bellevue Hospital
Saint-Etienne
France
1 Acinetobacter

Gian Maria Cavallini MD
Associate Professor of Ophthalmology
Department of Ophthalmology
University of Modena and Reggio Emilia Medical School
Modena
Italy
313 Drug-induced Optic Atrophy

Matilda Frances Chan MD, PhD
Ophthalmology Resident
Department of Ophthalmology
University of Rochester Eye Institute
Rochester NY
USA
20 Infectious Mononucleosis

Damon B. Chandler MD
Fellow, Ophthalmic Plastic and Reconstructive Surgery
Scheie Eye Institute
University of Pennsylvania
Philadelphia PA
USA
29 Mucormycosis

H. Channa MD
Professor in Ophthalmology
Service d'Ophtalmologie
Hôpital Militaire d'Instruction Med V
Rabat
Morocco
131 Kaposi's Sarcoma

Devron H. Char MD
Director, The Tumori Foundation
San Francisco CA
Clinical Professor of Ophthalmology
Department of Ophthalmology
Stanford University School of Medicine
Palo Alto CA
USA
139 Metastatic Tumors to the Eye and Its Adnexa
142 Neuroblastoma

Steve Charles MD
Clinical Professor of Ophthalmology
Department of Ophthalmology
University of Tennessee College of Medicine
Memphis TN
USA
351 Proliferative Vitreoretinopathy

Teresa C. Chen MD
Assistant Professor of Ophthalmology
Harvard Medical School
Massachusetts Eye and Ear Infirmary
Glaucoma Service
Boston MA
USA
101 Weill–Marchesani Syndrome
269 Normal-tension Glaucoma (Low-tension Glaucoma)

Steven S. T. Ching MD
Professor of Ophthalmology
Department of Ophthalmology
University of Rochester
Rochester NY
USA
20 Infectious Mononucleosis

Christophe Chiquet MD, PhD
Associate Professor of Ophthalmology
Department of Ophthalmology
University Hospital Grenoble
Grenoble
France
157 Intraocular Foreign Body: Steel or Iron

Phillip Hyunchul Choo MD
Associate Professor of Clinical Ophthalmology
Department of Ophthalmology
University of California
Sacramento CA
USA
236 Distichiasis

Timothy Y. Chou MD
Corneal Specialist
Nassau University Medical Center, Cornea Division
Ophthalmic Consultants of Long Island
Rockville Center NY
USA
211 Superior Limbic Keratoconjunctivitis

Stephen P. Christiansen MD
Professor of Ophthalmology and Pediatrics
Director, Pediatric Ophththalmology and Adult Strabismus
Department of Ophthalmology
University of Minnesota
Minneapolis MN
USA
68 Tyrosinemia II
222 Convergence Insufficiency

Kelly D. Chung MD
Assistant Professor, Ophthalmology
Casey Eye Institute
Portland OR
USA
298 Adults Cataracts

George A. Cioffi MD
Chairman, Devers Eye Institute
Clinical Vice President of Ophthalmology
Legacy Health System and Professor of Ophthalmology
Oregon Health and Science University
Portland OR
USA
268 Malignant Glaucoma
282 Iris Bombé

Michael P. Clarke MBBChir, DO, FRCS, FRCOphth
Reader in Ophthalmology
University of Newcastle
Claremont Wing Eye Department
Royal Victoria Infirmary
Newcastle Upon Tyne
UK
218 Basic and Intermittent Exotropia

David K. Coats MD
Professor of Ophthalmology and Pediatrics
Baylor College of Medicine
Department of Pediatric Ophthalmology
Houston TX
USA
289 Congenital Anomalies of the Lacrimal System

Elisabeth J. Cohen MD
Director, Cornea Service
Wills Eye Institute
Professor of Ophthalmology
Jefferson Medical College
Philadelphia PA
USA
281 Iridocorneal-endothelial Syndrome

R. Max Conway MBBS, PhD, FRANZCO
Director
Sydney Ocular Oncology Center
University of Sydney
Sydney NSW
Australia
284 Iris Melanoma

Catherine Creuzot-Garcher MD, PhD
Head, Department of Ophthalmology
Professor
University of Burgundy
Dijon
France
111 Creutzfeldt–Jakob disease

Emmett T. Cunningham Jr MD, PhD, MPH
Director, The Uveitis Service
California Pacific Medical Center
San Francisco, CA
and Adjunct Clinical Professor
Department of Ophthalmology
Stanford University School of Medicine
Stanford CA
USA
24 Leptospirosis

Theodore H. Curtis MD
Fellow
Oregon Health and Science University
Casey Eye Institute
Portland OR
USA
52 Typhoid Fever
130 Juvenile Xanthogranuloma
229 Nystagmus

Roger A. Dailey MD, FACS
Professor of Ophthalmic Facial Plastic Surgery
Lester T. Jones Endowed Chair
Director, Oculofacial Plastic Surgery Division
Oregon Health and Science University
Casey Eye Institute
Portland OR
USA
148 Sebaceous Gland Carcinoma
238 Entropion
239 Epicanthus
244 Lagophthalmos
248 Marcus Gunn Syndrome
250 Orbital Fat Herniation
326 Orbital Graves' Disease

Richard M. Davis MD
Professor and Chair
Department of Ophthalmology
University of South Carolina School of Medicine
Columbia SC
USA
190 Corneal Mucous Plaques

Romain De Cock MBChB, FRCS, FRCOphth
Consultant Ophthalmologist
Ophthalmology Clinic
Queen Elizabeth the Queen Mother Hospital
Margate Kent
UK
182 Ligneous Conjunctivitis

Jan-Tjeerd H. N. de Faber MD
Pediatric Ophthalmologist
The Rotterdam Eye Hospital
Rotterdam
The Netherlands
109 Chronic Progressive External Ophthalmoplegia
110 Cluster Headache

Daniel de la Mano MD
Consultant Dermatologist
Dermatology Department
Hospital San Agustín
Avilés-Asturias
Spain
87 Psoriasis

Nick W. H. M. Dekkers MD, PhD
Formerly, Ophthalmologist
St Elizabeth Hospital
Tilburg
The Netherlands
45 Rubeola

Monte Anthony Del Monte MD
Skillman Professor of Pediatric Ophthalmology
Professor of Pediatrics and Communicable Diseases
Director of Pediatric Ophthalmology and Strabismus
WK Kellogg Eye Center and Mott Children's Hospital
University of Michigan
Ann Arbor MI
USA
105 Sturge–Weber Syndrome

David A. Della Rocca MD
New York Eye and Ear Infirmary
Department of Oculoplastics
St Luke's Roosevelt Hospital Center
Department of Ophthalmology
New York NY
USA
240 Eyelid Contusions, Lacerations and Avulsions

Robert C. Della Rocca MD, FACS
Chairman of Ophthalmology
St Luke's Roosevelt Hospital Center
Chief of Oculoplastic Surgery
The New York Eye and Ear Infirmary
New York NY
USA
240 Eyelid Contusions, Lacerations and Avulsions

Deepinder K. Dhaliwal MD
Associate Professor, Ophthalmology
Eye and Ear Institute
Pittsburgh PA
USA
39 Pseudomonas aeruginosa

Diana V. Do MD
Assistant Professor of Ophthalmology
Wilmer Eye Institute
Johns Hopkins University School of Medicine
Baltimore MD
USA
34 Ocular Histoplasmosis
99 Uveitis Associated with Juvenile Idiopathic Arthritis

Peter J. Dolman MD, FRCSC
Clinical Professor, Ophthalmology
UBC Eye Care Centre
Vancouver BC
Canada
323 Orbital Inflammatory Syndromes

Sean P. Donahue MD, PhD
Professor of Pediatric Ophthalmology and Adult Strabismus
Vanderbilt Eye Center
Vanderbilt University Medical Center
Nashville TN
USA
6 Bacillus Species Infections
33 Ocular Candidiasis

Eric D. Donnenfeld MD, FACS
Founding Partner, Ophthalmic Consultants of Long Island
Co-Director, Cornea Division
Manhattan Eye, Ear and Throat Hospital
New York NY
USA
211 Superior Limbic Keratoconjunctivitis

Graham Duguid MD, BMedBiol, FRCS
Consultant Ophthalmic Surgeon
Western Eye Hospital
London
UK
339 Retinal Detachment

Jay S. Duker MD
Director, New England Eye Center
Chairman and Professor of Ophthalmology
Tufts New England Medical Center
Tufts University School of Medicine
Boston MA
USA
308 Macular Hole

James P. Dunn Jr MD
Associate Professor of Ophthalmology
Director, Division of Ocular Immunology
The Wilmer Ophthalmological Institute
Baltimore MD
USA
310 Ankylosing Spondylitis and Reiter's Disease

Steven P. Dunn MD
Michigan Cornea Consultants
Southfield MI
USA
89 Amyloidosis

Hon-Vu Q. Duong MD
Attending Ophthamlogist
Westfield Eye Centre
Las Vegas NV
USA
81 Sickle Cell Disease
122 Basal Cell Carcinoma

Robert A. Egan MD
Assistant Professor of Ophthalmology, Neurology and Neurosurgery
Casey Eye Institute
Portland OR
USA
49 Tetanus
138 Meningioma

Michael D. Eichler MD
Staff Ophthalmologist
Eye Surgeons and Physicians, PA
St. Cloud Hospital
St. Cloud MN
USA
136 Lymphoid Tumors

Mays El-Dairi MD
Chief Resident
Department of Ophthamology
American University Beirut
Beirut
Lebanon
79 Hyperlipoproteinemia

Forrest J. Ellis MD
Assistant Professor of Pediatrics and Ophthalmology
Director, Pediatric Ophthalmology
Rainbow Babies and Children's Hospital
Case Western Reserve University School of Medicine
Cleveland OH
USA
221 Congenital Fibrosis of the Extraocular Muscles

Geoffrey Emerson MD, PhD
Resident
Department of Ophthalmology
The Wilmer Eye Institute
Baltimore MD
USA
334 Diffuse Unilateral Subacute Neuroretinitis

M. Vaughn Emerson MD
Fellow
Department of Ophthalmology
Oregon Health and Science University
Portland OR
USA
328 Acquired Retinoschisis
343 Subretinal Neovascular Membranes

Laura B. Enyedi MD
Assistant Professor of Ophthalmology and Pediatrics
Department of Ophthalmology
Duke University Eye Center
Durham NC
USA
220 Congenital Esotropia

Teodoro Evans MD
Vitreoretinal Fellow
Institute of Ocular Surgery
University of Costa Rica
San Jose
Costa Rica
57 Coenurosis

Julie Falardeau MD, FRCSC
Assistant Professor of Ophthalmology
Casey Eye Institute
Portland OR
USA
127 Ewing's Sarcoma
311 Compressive Optic Neuropathies

Bishara M. Faris MD, FACS
Lecturer on Ophthalmology, Harvard Faculty of Medicine
Clinical Professor of Ophthalmology
Department of Ophthalmology
Boston University School of Medicine
Westboro MA
USA
346 Scleral Staphylomas and Dehiscences

Marianne E. Feitl MD
Associate Professor of Ophthalmology and Visual Science
Department of Ophthalmology and Visual Science
University of Chicago Hospitals
Chicago
USA
266 Juvenile Glaucoma

Warren L. Felton III MD
Professor and Associate Chair of Clinical Activities
Department of Neurology
Associate Professor of Ophthalmology
Chair, Division of Neuro-Ophthalmology
Virginia Commonwealth University
Richmond VA
USA
129 Hodgkin's Disease

Stephen S. Feman MD, FACS
Davisson Professor of Ophthalmology
Department of Ophthalmology
St Louis University School of Medicine
St Louis MO
USA
82 The Thalassemias

Timothy J ffytche LVO, FRCS, FRCOphth
Consultant Ophthalmologist
Formerly, The London Clinic
Harley Street
London
UK
23 Leprosy

Christina J. Flaxel MD
Associate Professor of Ophthalmology
Casey Eye Institute
Portland OR
USA
340 Retinal Venous Obstruction

Rod Foroozan MD
Assistant Professor of Ophthalmology
Department of Ophthalmology
Baylor College of Medicine
Houston TX
USA
119 Tolosa–Hunt Syndrome

Allen Foster OBE, FRCS
Professor
Clinical Research Unit
London School of Hygiene and Tropical Medicine
London
UK
50 Trachoma

Frederick T. Fraunfelder MD
Professor
Department of Ophthalmology
Oregon Health and Science University
Portland OR
USA
153 Electrical Injury

Frederick W. Fraunfelder MD
Associate Professor
Department of Ophthalmology
Oregon Health and Science University
Portland OR
USA
124 Conjunctival or Corneal Intraepithelial Neoplasia and Squamous Cell Carcinoma
149 Squamous Cell Carcinoma
297 Uveoparotid Fever

H. Mackenzie Freeman MD
Associate Clinical Professor
Harvard University Faculty of Medicine
Retina Specialists of Boston
Boston MA
USA
346 Scleral Staphylomas and Dehiscences

Mitchell H. Friedlaender MD
Head, Division of Ophthalmology
Director, Scripps Clinic Laser Vision Center
La Jolla CA
USA
88 Urticaria and Hereditary Angioedema

Larry P. Frohman MD
Professor of Ophthalmology & Visual Sciences and Neurology & Neurosciences
Department of Ophthalmology
University of Medicine and Dentistry of New Jersey
New Jersey Medical School
Newark NJ
USA
96 Scleroderma

Wayne E. Fung MD
Clinical Professor of Ophthalmology
California Pacific Medical Center
Pacific Eye Associates
San Francisco CA
USA
306 Cystoid Macular Edema

Philippe Gain MD, PhD
Professor of Ophthalmology
Department of Ophthalmology
University Hospital
Saint-Etienne
France
1 Acinetobacter
157 Intraocular Foreign Body: Steel or Iron

Jaime R. Gaitan MD
Department of Ophthalmology
Bascom Palmer Eye Institute
University of Miami School of Medicine
Miami FL
USA
28 Moraxella

Stephen Gancher MD, FAAN
Adjunct Associate Professor
Department of Neurology
Oregon Health and Science University and Staff Neurologist
Kaiser Permanente
Portland OR
USA
118 Parkinson's Disease

Tim Gard MD
Clinical Instructor, Ophthalmology
Oregon Health and Science University
Hillsboro Eye Clinic
Hillsboro OR
USA
309 Solar Retinopathy

Devin M. Gattey MD
Assistant Professor of Ophthalmology
Casey Eye Institute
Oregon Health and Science University
Portland OR
USA
301 Dislocation of the Lens

Peter L. Gehlbach MD, PhD
Associate Professor of Ophthalmology
Wilmer Eye Institute
Johns Hopkins University School of Medicine
Baltimore MD
USA
156 Intraocular Foreign Body: Nonmagnetic, Chemically Inert

Mehdi Ghajarnia MD
Cornea Fellow
John A Moran Eye Center
Salt Lake City, UT
USA
39 Pseudomonas aeruginosa

Vinícius Coral Ghanem MD
Ophthalmologist
Sadalla Amin Ghanem Eye Hospital
Santa Catarina
Brazil
86 Ocular Rosacea

Amit Kumar Ghosh MD, FACP
Associate Professor of Medicine
Mayo Clinic College of Medicine
Rochester MN
USA
116 Multiple Sclerosis

Chandak Ghosh MD, MPH
Medical Consultant for Federal Policy
US Department of Health and Human Services
Health Resources and Services Administration
New York NY
USA
17 Haemophilus influenzae

Matthew Giegengack MD
Fellow
Casey Eye Institute
Portland OR
USA
273 Phacanaphylactic Endophthalmitis

Geoffrey Gladstone MD, FAACS
Clinical Professor of Ophthalmology
Michigan State University School of Medicine
Southfield, MI
USA
254 Xanthelasma

Daniel H. Gold MD, FRCOphth
Clinical Professor of Ophthalmology
University of Texas Medical Branch
Galveston TX
USA
and Visiting Lecturer
Tel Aviv University Sackler Medical School
Tel Aviv Sourasky Medical Center
Tel Aviv
Israel
95 Sarcoidosis

Richard L. Golub MD
Pediatric Ophthalmology Fellow
Storm Eye Institute / MUSC
Charleston SC
USA
227 Inferior Rectus Muscle Palsy

Dan S. Gombos MD, FACS
Associate Professor, Section of Ophthalmology
Department of Head & Neck Surgery
The University of Texas
MD Anderson Cancer Center
Houston TX
USA
304 Traumatic Cataract

George M. Gombos MD, FACS
Professor Emeritus
State University of New York
Health Science Center at Brooklyn
Chief, Section of Ophthalmology, Department of Surgery
New York Harbor Health Science Center – Brooklyn
Veterans Administration Hospital
Brooklyn NY
USA
304 Traumatic Cataract

William V. Good MD
Senior Scientist
Smith-Kettlewell Eye Research Institute
San Francisco CA
USA
183 Ophthalmia Neonatorum

Shawn Goodman MD
Ophthalmologist
Child Eye Care Associates
Lake Oswego OR
USA
224 Duane's Retraction Syndrome

John D. Gottsch MD
Margaret C. Mosher Professor of Ophthalmology
Wilmer Ophthalmological Institute
The Johns Hopkins Hospital
Baltimore MD
USA
13 Epidemic Keratoconjunctivitis

Srinivas Goverdhan MD, FRCS(Ed)
Specialist Registrar in Ophthalmology
Southampton Eye Unit
Southampton University Hospitals
Southampton
UK
84 Contact Dermatitis

Baird S. Grimson MD
Professor of Ophthalmology
Department of Ophthalmology
University of North Carolina
Chapel Hill NC
USA
120 Trigeminal Neuralgia

Adolfo Güemes MD
Professor of Ophthalmology
Consultores Oftalmológicos
Montevideo
Buenos Aires
Argentina
303 Microspherophakia

Roberto Guerra MD
Professor of Ophthalmology
Department of Ophthalmology
University of Modena and Reggio Emilia School of Medicine
Modena
Italy
313 Drug-induced Optic Atrophy

Julia A. Haller MD
Robert Bond Welch Professor of Opthalmology
Wilmer Ophthalmological Institute
Johns Hopkins Medical Institutions
Baltimore MD
USA
166 Intraocular Epithelial Cysts

Kristin M. Hammersmith MD
Instructor, Jefferson Medical College
Thomas Jefferson University
and Assistant Surgeon, Cornea Service
Wills Eye Hospital
and Director, Cornea Fellowship Program
Wills Eye Institute
Philadelphia PA
USA
210 Schnyder's Crystalline Corneal Dystrophy

Irvin L. Handelman MD
Retina Northwest
Portland OR
USA
352 Vitreous Hemorrhage

Roderick N. Hargrove MD
Assistant Professor of Ophthalmology
Department of Ophthalmology
University of Tennesse
Memphis TN
USA
123 Capillary Hemangioma

Michael S. Harney MD, MB, FRCSI(ORL)
Specialist Registrar in Otolaryngology
Department of Otolaryngology
RCSI Education and Research Centre
Beaumont Hospital
Dublin
Ireland
107 Bell's Palsy

Richard A. Harper MD
Associate Professor of Ophthalmology
Department of Ophthalmology
University of Arkansas for Medical Sciences
Little Rock AR
USA
158 Iris Lacerations, Iris Holes and Iridodialysis

Sarah R. Hatt DBO
Research Orthoptist
Ophthalmology Research
Mayo Clinic
Rochester MN
USA
218 Basic and Intermittent Exotropia

Barbara S. Hawkins PhD
Professor of Ophthalmology and Epidemiology
Wilmer Eye Institute, Clinical Trials and Biometry
Johns Hopkins University School of Medicine
Baltimore MD
USA
34 Ocular Histoplasmosis

Sohan S. Hayreh MD, MS, PhD, DSc, FRCS(Edin), FRCS(Eng), FRCOphth
Professor Emeritus of Ophthalmology and Director Ocular Vascular
Department of Ophthalmology and Visual Sciences
University of Iowa Hospitals and Clinics
Iowa City IA
USA
98 Giant Cell Arteritis

Arnd Heiligenhaus MD
Professor of Ophthalmology
Department of Ophthalmology
St. Franziskus Hospital
Münster
Germany
83 Atopic Dermatitis

Carsten Heinz MD
Department of Ophthalmology
St Franziskus Hospital
Münster
Germany
83 Atopic Dermatitis

Leon W. Herndon MD
Associate Professor of Ophthalmology
Duke University Eye Center
Durham NC
USA
261 Glaucoma Associated with Anterior Uveitis

Simon J. Hickman MA, PhD, MBBChir, MRCP
Consultant Neurologist and Neuro-Ophthalmologist
Department of Neurology
Royal Hallamshire Hospital
Sheffield
UK
314 Inflammatory Optic Neuropathies
316 Optic Neuritis

Koji Hirano MD, PhD
Professor
Department of Ophthalmology
Ban-Buntane Hotokukai Hospital
Fujita Health University
Nagoya
Japan
78 Fabry Disease

Edward J. Holland MD
Director, Cornea Services
Professor of Ophthalmology
University of Cincinnati
Cincinnati Eye Institute N.KY
Edgewood KY
USA
203 Macular Corneal Dystrophy

Gary N. Holland MD
Vernon O. Underwood Family Professor of Medicine
Chief, Cornea and Uveitis Division
Department of Ophthalmology
David Geffen School of Medicine at UCLA
Jules Stein Eye Institute
Los Angeles CA
USA
63 Toxoplasmosis

Eric R. Holz MD
Assistant Professor of Ophthalmology
Baylor College of Medicine
Houston TX
USA
256 Bacterial Endophthalmitis
257 Fungal Endophthalmitis

Sachiko Hommura MD, PhD
Assistant Professor
Department of Ophthalmology
University Hospital of Tsukuba
Ibaraki
Japan
173 Expulsive Hemorrhage

Jeffrey D. Horn MD
Assistant Professor of Ophthalmology
Department of Ophthalmology and Visual Sciences
Vanderbilt Eye Institute
Nashville TN
USA
7 Blastomycosis

Richard B. Hornick MD, MACP
Clinical Professor of Medicine
University of Florida School of Medicine and Florida State University School of Medicine
Orlando FL
USA
40 Q Fever

H. Dunbar Hoskins Jr MD
Executive Vice President
American Academy of Ophthalmology
San Francisco CA
USA
260 Exfoliation Syndrome

James W. Hung MD
Ophthalmic Consultants of Boston
Boston MA
USA
170 Choroidal Detachment

Brian A. Hunter MD
Ocular Pathology Fellow
Morgan Eye Center
University of Utah
Salt Lake City UT
USA
255 Anophthalmos

Krista A. Hunter MD
Pediatric Fellow
Department of Ophthalmology
Oregon Health and Science University
Casey Eye Institute
Portland OR
USA
226 Extraocular Muscle Lacerations
300 Congenital and Infantile Cataracts

Alex P. Hunyor MBBS, FRANZCO, FRACS
Vitreoretinal Surgeon
Sydney Eye Hospital
Sydney
Australia
307 Epimacular Proliferation
349Familial Exudative Vitreoretinopathy

Brian Hurwitz MD, FRCP, FRCGP
General Practitioner
and Professor of Medicine and the Arts
King's College London
London
UK
177 Bacterial Conjunctivitis

Thomas S. Hwang MD
Assistant Professor of Ophthalmology
Casey Eye Institute
Portland OR
USA
305 Age-related Macular Degeneration
330 Branch Retinal Vein Occlusion
335 Eales Disease

Robert A. Hyndiuk MD
Professor Emeritus
Department of Ophthalmology
Medical College of Wisconsin
Milwaukee WI
USA
46 Sporotrichosis

Ozge Ilhan-Sarac MD
Fellow in Ophthalomolgy
Ocular Surface Diseases and Dry Eye Clinic
The Wilmer Eye Institute
The John Hopkins School of Medicine
Baltimore MD
USA
347 Scleritis

Edsel Ing MD, FRCSC
Assistant Professor of Ophthalmology
University of Toronto Ophthalmology
Toronto East General Hospital
Toronto ON
Canada
41 Rabies

Masanori Ino-ue MD, PhD
Associate Director
Chairman in Ophthalmology
Kohnan Hospital
Kobe
Japan
287 Rubeosis Iridis

Carlos M. Isada MD
The Cleveland Clinic
Cleveland OH
USA
16 Gonococcal Ocular Disease

Saylin Iturriaga MD
Institute of Ocular Surgery
San José
Costa Rica
57 Coenurosis

Joseph D. Iuorno MD
Clinical Instructor
Department of Ophthalmology
University of Minnesota
Minneapolis MN
USA
198 Granular Corneal Dystrophy

Andrew G. Iwach MD
Associate Clinical Professor of Ophthalmology
University of California, San Francisco
Glaucoma Center of San Francisco
San Francisco CA
USA
260 Exfoliation Syndrome

Mohan N. Iyer MD
Fellow, Vitreoretinal Diseases and Surgery
Ophthalmology Department
Baylor College of Medicine
Houston TX
USA
256 Bacterial Endophthalmitis

Natalio J. Izquierdo MD
Associate Professor of Ophthalmology
Medical Sciences
University of Puerto Rico
San Juan
Puerto Rico
102 Down Syndrome

Lee M. Jampol MD
Louis Feinberg Professor and Chairman
Department of Ophthalmology
Northwestern University Medical School
Chicago IL
USA
162 Hypertension

Suzanne Johnston MD
Chief Resident
Eastern Virgina Medical School
Norfolk VA
USA
8 Brucellosis

Sibel Kadayifçilar MD
Professor of Ophthalmology
Department of Ophthalmology
Hacettepe University
Ankara
Turkey
94 Rheumatoid Arthritis

Ian H. Kaden MD
Morristown Memorial Hospital
Randolph NJ
USA
30 Mumps

Dieudonne Kaimbo Wa Kaimbo MD, PhD
Professor of Ophthalmology
Department of Ophthalmology
University of Kinshasa
Kinshasa
Democratic Republic of Congo
51 Tuberculosis

Rashmis Kapur MD
Resident in Ophthalmology
Department of Ophthalmology and Visual Sciences
University of Illinois at Chicago
Chicago IL
USA
189 Corneal Edema

Peter R. Kastl MD, PhD
Professor of Ophthalmology and Biochemistry
Department of Ophthalmology
Tulane University School of Medicine
New Orleans LA
USA
199 Juvenile Corneal Epithelial Dystrophy

Garyfallia Katsavounidou MS
Graduate Student
Department of Architecture and Design
Massachusetts Institute of Technology
Boston MA
USA
278 Aniridia

Ayat Kazerouni BS, BA
Back Office Supervisor
Ophthalomogy
Tayani Eye Institute
San Clemente CA
USA
46 Sporotrichosis

Michael Kazim MD
Clinical Professor of Ophthalmology and Surgery
Department of Ophthalmology
Columbia University
New York NY
USA
135 Lymphangioma

Sanjay R. Kedhar MD
Clinical Instructor of Ophthalmology
Division of Ocular Immunology
The Wilmer Eye Institute
Johns Hopkins School of Medicine
Baltimore MD
USA
310 Ankylosing Spondylitis and Reiter's Disease

Ronald V. Keech MD
Clinical Professor of Ophthalmology
Department of Ophthalmology
University of Iowa Hospitals & Clinics
Iowa City IA
USA
223 Dissociated Vertical Deviation

Robert C. Kersten MD
Professor of Clinical Ophthalmology
Department of Ophthalmology
University of Cincinnati
College of Medicine
Cincinnati OH
USA
140 Mucocele

Marshall P. Keys MD, PA
Ophthalmologist in Private Practice
Rockville MD
USA
112 Dyslexia

Sangeeta Khanna MD
Fellow, Neuro-Ophthalmology
Division of Ophthalmology
Case Western Reserve University
MetroHealth Medical Center
Cleveland OH
USA
47 Staphylococcus
73 Mucopolysaccharidosis II
74 Mucopolysacccharidosis III

Peng Tee Khaw PhD, FRCP, FRCS, FRCOphth, FIBiol, FRCPath, FMedSci
Professor of Glaucoma and Ocular Healing
Paediatric Glaucoma Unit
Moorfields Eye Hospital
London
UK
265 Primary Congenital Glaucoma

James L. Kinyoun MD
Professor of Ophthalmology
Department of Ophthalmology
University of Washington
Seattle WA
USA
100 Wegener Granulomatosis

Caitriona Kirwan MB, MRCOphth
Fellow, Department of Ophthalmology
Mater Private Hospital
Dublin
Ireland
137 Medulloepithelioma

Tero Kivelä MD, FEBO
Professor of Ophthalmology
Department of Ophthalmology
Helsinki University Central Hospital
Helsinki
Finland
146 Periocular Merkel Cell Carcinoma

Michael L. Klein MD
Professor of Ophthalmology
Director, Macular Degeneration Center
Casey Eye Institute
Portland OR
USA
305 Age-related Macular Degeneration
330 Branch Retinal Vein Occlusion
335 Eales Disease

Stephen A. Klotz MD
Professor of Medicine
Section of Infectious Diseases
University of Arizona
Tuscon AZ
USA
10 Coccidioidomycosis

John Ko MD, FACS
Clinical Assistant Professor
Department of Ophthalmology
Michigan Wayne State University Hospital
Detroit MI
and Clinical Instructor
William Beaumont Hospital
Loyal Oak MI
USA
240 Eyelid Contusions, Lacerations and Avulsions

Regis P. Kowalski MS, [M]ASCP
Associate Research Professor of Ophthalmology
Ophthalmic Microbiology
The Eye and Ear Institute
Pittsburgh PA
USA
39 Pseudomonas aeruginosa

Jay H. Krachmer MD
Professor; Head, Department of Ophthalmology
Department of Ophthalmology
University of Minnesota
Minneapolis MN
USA
89 Amyloidosis
198 Granular Corneal Dystrophy

Theodore Krupin MD
Professor of Ophthalmology
Northwestern University
Chicago IL
USA
266 Juvenile Glaucoma

Ferenc Kuhn MD, PhD
Associate Professor of Ophthalmology
Department of Ophthalmology
University of Alabama at Birmingham School of Medicine
and President , American Society of Ocular Trauma
Birmingham AL
USA
154 Management of Screral Ruptures and Lacerations

Abhaya Vivek Kulkarni MD, PhD, FRCSC
Consultant Neurosurgeon
Division of Neurosurgery
Hospital for Sick Children
Toronto, Ontario
Canada
125 Craniopharyngioma

Robert C. Kwun MD
Partner
Retina Associates of Utah
Salt Lake City UT
USA
169 Angioid Streaks

Peter R. Laibson MD
Professor of Ophthalmology
Jefferson Medical College
Thomas Jefferson University
and Director Emeritus, Cornea Service
Wills Eye Institute
Philadelphia PA
USA
193 Epithelial Basement Membrane Dystrophy
210 Schnyder's Crystalline Corneal Dystrophy

Rohit R. Lakhanpal MD
Clinical Assistant Professor of Ophthalmology and Visual Sciences
Vitreoretinal Surgery Service
Department of Ophthalmology
University of Maryland School of Medicine
Practice Partner
Eye Consultants of Maryland
Owings Mills MD
USA
257 Fungal Endophthalmitis

Byron L. Lam MD
Professor, Department of Ophthalmology
Bascom Palmer Eye Institute
Miami FL
USA
43 Rocky Mountain Spotted Fever
245 Lid Myokymia

Laurent Lamer MD, FRCS(c)
Associate Professor
Department of Ophthalmology
University of Montreal
Montreal, Quebec
Canada
31 Newcastle Disease

David P. Lawlor MD
Ophthalmologist
Private Practice
Newport VT
USA
302 Lenticonus and Lentiglobus

Andrew W. Lawton MD
Clinical Associate Professor of Ophthalmology
University of Tennessee, Memphis
Little Rock Eye Clinic
Little Rock AR
USA
317 Papilledema

Alan B. Leahey MD
Lehigh Valley Eye Center
Allentown PA
USA
27 Molluscum Contagiosum

Russell LeBoyer MD
Department of Ophthalmology
Baylor College of Medicine
Houston TX
USA
119 Tolosa–Hunt Syndrome

Andrew G. Lee MD
Professor of Ophthalmology, Neurology and Neurosurgery
University of Iowa Hospitals
Iowa City IA
USA
106 Acquired Inflammatory Demyelinating Neuropathies

Wen-Hsiang Lee MD, PhD
Clinical Fellow, Retina Division
Wilmer Ophthalmological Institute
Johns Hopkins University School of Medicine, Baltimore MD
and Assistant Professor of Clinical Ophthalmology
Vitreoretinal Service
Bascom Palmer Eye Institute
University of Miami School of Medicine
Miami, FL
USA
166 Intraocular Epithelial Cysts

William Barry Lee MD, FACS
Consultant
Eye Consultants of Atlanta
Piedmont Hospital
Atlanta GA
USA
160 Shaken Baby Syndrome
216 Accommodative Esotropia

Sharon S. Lehman MD
Clinical Assistant Professor of Ophthalmology and Pediatrics
Jefferson Medical College
Division Chief, Ophthalmology
A.I. duPont Hospital for Children
Wilmington DE
USA
85 Erythema Multiforme Major

Howard M. Leibowitz MD
Sherwood J. and H. Lorene Tarlow Professor of Ophthalmology
Chairman of the Department, Emeritus
Department of Ophthalmology
Boston University School of Medicine
Boston MA
USA
38 Proteus

James Leong MMed(OphthSc) MBBS(Hons)
Ophthalmology Regsitrar
Sydney Eye Hospital
Sydney NSW
Australia
37 Propionibacterium acnes

Alex V. Levin MD, MHSc, FAAP, FAAO, FRCSC
Associate Professor
Department of Pediatrics, Genetics & Ophthalmology & Vision Sciences Department
University of Toronto
Ontario, Toronto
Canada
77 Mucopolysaccharidosis VII

Leonard A. Levin MD, PhD
Canada Research Chair
Department of Ophthalmology
University of Montreal
Montreal, Canada
and Professor
Department of Ophthalmology and Visual Sciences
University of Wisconsin
Madison WI
USA
318 Traumatic Optic Neuropathy

Mark R. Levine MD, FACS
Clinical Professor of Ophthalmology
Case Western Reserve School of Medicine
Cleveland OH
USA
159 Orbital Implant Extrusion

Norman S. Levy MD, PhD
Director
Florida Ophthalmic Institute
Gainesville FL
USA
141 Neurilemoma

Thomas J. Liesegang MD
Professor of Ophthalmology
Mayo Clinic College of Medicine
Jacksonville FL
USA
53 Varicella and Herpes Zoster
280 Fuchs' Heterochromic Iridocyclitis

Lyndell L. Lim MBBS, FRANZCO
Mankiewicz-Zelkin Crock Fellow
Centre for Eye Research Australia
University of Melbourne
East Melbourne, Victoria
Australia
344 White Dot Syndromes

Linda H. Lin MD
Ophthalmologist, Glaucoma Specialist
Private Practice
Houston TX
USA
180 Filtering Blebs and Associated Problems

Richard D. Lisman MD, FACS
Clinical Professor of Ophthalmology
New York University School of Medicine
Surgeon Director, Manhattan Eye, Ear & Throat Hospital
New York NY
USA
321 External Orbital Fractures
322 Internal Orbital Fractures

David Litoff MD
Chief of Ophthalmology
Kaiser Permanente Colorado
Assistant Clinical Professor of Ophthalmology
University of Colorado
Boulder CO
USA
285 Iris Prolapse

James C. Liu MD, MBA
Chairman of Ophthalmology Department
Good Samaritan Hospital
San Jose CA
USA
187 Conjunctival, Corneal or Scleral Cysts

Evan Loft MD
Resident Physician in Ophthalmology
Emory Eye Center
Emory University
Atlanta GA
USA
235 Blepharoconjunctivitis

Ronald R. Lubritz MD, FACP
Clinical Professor of Medicine (Dermatology)
Tulane Medical Center New Orleans, LA
Hattiesburg Clinic
Hattiesburg MS
USA
121 Actinic and Seborrheic Keratosis

David C. W. Mabey DM, FRCP
Professor, Clinical Research Unit
London School of Hygiene & Tropical Medicine
London
UK
50 Trachoma

Ian A. Mackie MBChB, DO, FRCS, FCOphth
Consulting Ophthalmologist
Harley Street
London
UK
205 Neuroparalytic Keratitis

Srilakshmi Maguluri MD
Clinical Instructor and Retina Fellow
Department of Ophthalmology and Visual Sciences
Vanderbilt University Medical Center
Nashville TN
USA
33 Ocular Candidiasis

M. Maliki MD
Specialist in Anatomy Pathology
Department of Anatomy Pathology
Ibn Sina Hospital Rabat
Rabat
Morocco
131 Kaposi's Sarcoma

Nick Mamalis MD
Professor of Ophthalmology
John A Moran Eye Center
Department of Ophthalmology and Visual Sciences
University of Utah
Salt Lake City UT
USA
255 Anophthalmos

Mark J. Mannis MD, FACS
Professor and Chairman
Department of Ophthalmology
University of California, Davis
Sacramento CA
USA
86 Ocular Rosacea

Steven L. Mansberger MD, MPH
Associate Scientist, Devers Eye Institute
Legacy Health System
Adjunct Assistant Professor
Department of Ophthalmology
Clinical Assistant Scientist
Department of Public Health and Preventative Medicine
Oregon Health and Science University
Portland OR
USA
271 Ocular Hypotony

Ahmad M. Mansour MD
Clinical Professor
Department of Ophthalmology
AUB American University of Beirut
Beirut
Lebanon
79 Hyperlipoproteinemia

Alexandre S. Marcon MD
Director, Cornea Service and Medical Director
Santa Casa de Porto Alegre Eye Bank
Porto Alegre RS
Brazil
192 Detachment of Descemet's Membrane
203 Macular Corneal Dystrophy

Italo M. Marcon MD
Ophthalmologist in Chief
Santa Casa de Porto Alegre University Hospital
Professor of Ophthalmology
Faculdade Federal de Ciências Médicas — FFFCMPA
Porto Alegre RS
Brazil
192 Detachment of Descemet's Membrane
203 Macular Corneal Dystrophy

Peter B. Marsh MD
Kaiser Permanente
Clackamas Eye Care
Portland OR
USA
252 Seborrheic Blepharitis

Rookaya Mather MD, MBBCh, FRCS(C), DABO
Assistant Professor
Department of Ophthalmology
University of Western Ontario
London, Ontario
Canada
48 Streptococcus

William D. Mathers MD
Professor of Ophthalmology
Department of Ophthalmology
Oregon Health and Science University
Casey Eye Institute
Portland OR
USA
59 Demodicosis
62 Pediculosis and Phthiriasis

K. Matti Saari MD, MedScD, FEBO
Professor and Chairman
Department of Ophthalmology
Institute of Clinical Sciences
University of Turku
Tampere
Finland
54 Yersiniosis

Louise A. Mawn MD, FACS
Associate Professor of Ophthalmology and Neorological Surgery
Director, Ophthalmic Plastic and Reconstructive Surgery
Vanderbilt Eye Institute
Vanderbilt University Medical Centre
Nashville TN
USA
293 Lacrimal System Contusions and Lacerations

Penny J. McAllum FRANZCO
Formerly at Department of Ophthalmology
University of Auckland
Auckland
New Zealand
26 Microsporidial Infection

Rex M. McCallum MD
Professor of Medicine
Duke University School of Medicine
Durham NC
USA
91 Cogan Syndrome

Peter McCluskey MD, FRANZCO,FRACS
Professor of Ophthalmology
Department of Ophthalmology
Liverpool Hospital
Liverpool NSW
Australia
37 Propionibacterium acnes

Gregory J. McCormick MD
Fellow, Cornea and Refractive Surgery
University of Rochester Eye Institute
Rochester NY
USA
348 Scleromalacia Perforans

Steven A. McCormick MD
Director
Department of Pathology
The New York Eye and Ear Infirmary
New York NY
USA
249 Melanocytic Lesions of the Eyelids

James P. McCulley MD, FACS, FRCOphth
Professor and Chairman of Ophthalmology
Department of Ophthalmology
UT Southwestern Medical Center
Dallas TX
USA
150 Acid Burns

John G. McHenry MD, MPH
Associate Professor of Ophthalmology
Department of Ophthalmology
UT Southwestern Medical Center at Dallas
Dallas TX
USA
319 Vasculopathic Optic Neuropathies

Alan A. McNab MBBS, FRANZCO
Director, Orbital Plastic and Lacrimal Clinic
St Vincents Private Hospital
Fitzroy
Australia
134 Liposarcoma

Jared J. Mee MBBS
Ophthalmologist
Northern Hospital
Epping, Melbourne
Australia
117 Myasthenia Gravis

Douglas L. Meier MD
Ophthalmologist
Department of Ophthalmology
The Portland Clinic
Portland OR
USA
202 Lattice Corneal Dystrophy

David M. Meisler MD, FACS
Professor of Opthalmology
Cleveland Clinic Lerner College of Medicine
Cole Eye Institute
Cleveland OH
USA
16 Gonococcal Ocular Disease

Saul C. Merin MD
Professor of Ophthalmology
Department of Ophthalmology
Hadassah Hebrew University Medical Center
Jerusalem
Israel
341 Retinitis Pigmentosa

Dale R. Meyer MD
Director, Ophthalmic Plastic Surgery
Professor of Ophthalmology
Lions Eye Institute
Albany Medical Center
Albany NY
USA
246 Lid Retraction

Roger F. Meyer MD
Professor Emeritus of Ophthalmology
University of Michigan
Ann Arbor MI
USA
30 Mumps

Kevin S. Michels MD
Ophthalmology Resident
Department of Ophthalmology
Oregon Health and Science University
Portland OR
USA
243 Hordeolum

Tatyana Milman, MD, FAAO
Department of Pathology
Wills Eye Hospital
Thomas Jefferson University
Philadelphia PA
USA
249 Melanocytic Lesions of the Eyelids

Roni Mintz MD
Lecturer of Ophthalmology
WK Kellogg Eye Center
University of Michigan
Ann Arbor MI
USA
22 Koch–Weeks Bacillus

Chantal F Morel MD, FRCP(C)
Genetic Metabolic Fellow
Division of Clinical and Metabolic Genetics
The Hospital for Sick Children
Toronto, Ontario
Canada
77 Mucopolysaccharidosis VII

William R. Morris MD
Associate Professor of Ophthalmology
Department of Ophthalmology
University of Tennessee Health Science Center
Hamilton Eye Institute
Memphis TN
USA
194 Filamentary Keratitis

Mark L. Moster MD
Director, Neuro-Ophthalmology
Albert Einstein Medical Center
and Professor of Neurology, Thomas Jefferson University School of Medicine
and Instructor, Neuro-Ophthalmology, Wills Eye Hospital
Philadelphia PA
USA
29 Mucormycosis

John Mourani MD
Fellow in Infectious Diseases
Section of Infectious Diseases
University of Arizona
Tuscon AZ
USA
10 Coccidioidomycosis

Cristina Muccioli MD
Professor of Ophthalmology
Department of Ophthalmology
Federal University of São Paulo
São Paulo
Brazil
3 Acquired Immune Deficiency Syndrome

Raghu C. Mudumbai MD
Associate Professor
Residency Program Director
Department of Ophthalmology
University of Washington Medical Center
Seattle WA
USA
215 Abducens (Sixth Nerve) Paralysis
219 Brown's Syndrome
258 Angle Recession Glaucoma

Fernando H. Murillo-Lopez MD
Instructor
Department of Ophthalmology
Bolivian Ophthalmology Society
Bolivian National Institute of Ophthalmology
La Paz
Bolivia
71 Mucopolysaccharidosis IH
72 Mucopolysaccharidosis IH/S

Shoib Myint DO, FAACS
Departments of Ophthalmic and Facial Plastic Surgery
William Beaumont Eye Institute
Royal Oak MI
USA
254 Xanthelasma

Parveen K Nagra MD
Instructor of Ophthalmology
Cornea Service
Wills Eye Institute
Thomas Jefferson University
Philadelphia PA
USA
213 Thygeson's Superficial Punctate Keratopathy

A Naoumi MD
Professor in Ophthalmology
Service d'Ophtalmologie
Hôpital Militaire d'Instruction Med V
Rabat
Morocco
131 Kaposi's Sarcoma

John Nassif MD
Private Practice
Clearwater FL
USA
240 Eyelid Contusions, Lacerations and Avulsions

Michelle T. Nee MD
Clinical Fellow in Glaucoma
Department of Ophthalmology
University of California, San Francisco
San Francisco CA
USA
267 Lens-induced Glaucoma

Marcelo V. Netto MD
Cornea and Refractive Surgery Staff
Department of Ophthalmology
University of São Paulo
São Paulo
Brazil
204 Mooren's Ulcer

John D. Ng MD, MS, FACS
Associate Professor of Ophthalmology
Casey Eye Institute
Oregon Health and Science University
Portland OR
USA
148 Sebaceous Gland Carcinoma
239 Epicanthus
248 Marcus Gunn Syndrome
290 Dacryoadenitis
292 Epiphora

Hau T. Nguyen MD
Fellow
Devers Eye Institute
Portland OR
USA
268 Malignant Glaucoma

Quan Dong Nguyen MD, MSc
Assistant Professor of Ophthalmology
Diseases of the Retina and Vitreous, and Uveitis
Wilmer Eye Institute
Johns Hopkins Hospital
Baltimore MD
USA
99 Uveitis Associated with Juvenile Idiopathic Arthritis

Denis M. O'Day MD, FACS
Professor of Ophthalmology
Vanderbilt Eye Institute
Nashville TN
USA
6 Bacillus Species Infections
33 Ocular Candidiasis
197 Fungal Keratitis

A. Justin O'Day MBBS, FRANZCO
Associate Professor
Victoria Parade Eye Consultants
St Vincents Medical Centre
Fitzroy
Melbourne
Australia
117 Myasthenia Gravis

Henry S. O'Halloran MD, DOphth, FRCSI
Pediatric and Neuro-Ophthalmologist
Children's Hospital San Diego
San Diego CA
USA
160 Shaken Baby Syndrome
216 Accommodative Esotropia

Michael O'Keefe MB, FRCS, FRCOphth
Professor of Ophthalmology
Department of Ophthalmology
Mater Private Hospital
Dublin
Ireland
137 Medulloepithelioma

Fumiki Okamoto MD, PhD
Assistant Professor
University of Tsukuba
Ibaraki-ken
Japan
173 Expulsive Hemorrhage

Richard J. Olson MD
Associate Clinical Professor of Ophthalmology
Department of Ophthalmology
University of Iowa, Hospitals and Clinics
Iowa City IA
USA
223 Dissociated Vertical Deviation

James C. Orcutt MD, PhD
Department of Ophthalmology
University of Washington Medical Center
Seattle WA
USA
253 Trichiasis
324 Optic Foramen Fractures

Sema Oruc Dundar MD
Professor of Ophthalmology
Department of Ophthalmology
Adnan Menderes University
School of Medicine
Aydin
Turkey
286 Pars Planitis

Aaron Osbourne MD, MRCOphth
Specialist Registrar in Ophthalmology
Department of Ophthalmology
Eye, Ear, Nose and Throat Centre
Queens Medical Centre
Nottingham
UK
331 Central or Branch Retinal Artery Occlusion

Maristela Amaral Palazzi MD, PhD
Ophthalmologist
Department of Ophthalmology
Boldrini Children Center
Campinas
São Paulo
Brazil
145 Papilloma

Earl A. Palmer MD, FAAP
Professor of Ophthalmology and Pediatrics
Departments of Ophthalmology and Pediatrics
Casey Eye Institute
Portland OR
USA
342 Retinopathy of Prematurity

Maria Papadopoulos MBBS, FRACO
Consultant Ophthalmic Surgeon
Paediatric Glaucoma Unit
Moorfields Eye Hospital
London
UK
265 Primary Congenital Glaucoma

Jeffrey R. Parnell MD
Clinical Instructor of Ophthalmology
Department of Ophthalmology
Northwestern University Medical School
Retina Services of Illinois, LLC
Chicago IL
USA
162 Hypertension

Cameron F. Parsa MD
Assistant Professor of Ophthalmology
Johns Hopkins University School of Medicine
Wilmer Ophthalmological Institute
The Johns Hopkins Hospital
Baltimore MD
USA
104 Neurofibromatosis
143 Optic Gliomas
163 Papillorenal Syndrome
277 Accommodative Spasm

Sanjay V. Patel MD
Assistant Professor of Ophthalmology
Mayo Clinic College of Medicine
Rochester MN
USA
11 Dermatophytosis

Emily Patterson MD
Devers Eye Institute
Portland OR
USA
272 Open-angle Glaucoma
276 Primary Angle-closure Glaucoma

Scott D. Pendergast MD
Vitreoretinal Surgeon
Partner, Retina Associates of Cleveland Inc.
Beachwood OH
USA
172 Choroidal Ruptures

Henry D. Perry MD, FACS
Senior Founding Partner and Director, Cornea Division
Ophthalmic Consultants of Long Island and Clinical Associate Professor of Ophthalmology
Weill Cornell School of Medicine
New York NY
USA
211 Superior Limbic Keratoconjunctivitis

Keith Roberson Peters MD, ABR, CAQ VIR, CAQ NR
Associate Professor
Department of Radiology
University of Florida College of Medicine
Gainsville FL
USA
80 Carotid Cavernous Fistula

Stephanie M. Po MD
Chief
Department of Ophthalmology
Kaiser Permanente
Walnut Creek CA
USA
267 Lens-induced Glaucoma

Russell Pokroy MD
Senior Ophthalmologist
Department of Ophthalmology
Kaplan Medical Center
Rehovot
Israel
176 Allergic Conjunctivitis
185 Vernal Keratoconjunctivitis

Allen Michael Putterman MD
Professor of Ophthalmology
Chief, Oculoplastic Surgery
University of Illinois College of Medicine
Chairman, Department of Ophthalmology
Michael Reese Hospital and Medical Center
Chicago IL
USA
247 Madarosis

Rubén Queiro PhD
Consultant Rheumatologist
Rheumatology Division
University Hospital Central de Asturias
Oviedo
Spain
87 Psoriasis

Nastaran Rafiei MD
Wilmer Ophthalmogical Institute
Johns Hopkins University School of Medicine
Baltimore MD
USA
104 Neurofibromatosis Type 1

Bahram Rahmani MD, MPH
Assistant Professor of Ophthalmology
Department of Ophthalmology
Northwestern University
Division of Ophthalmology
Children's Memorial Hospital
Chicago IL
USA
168 Traumatic Hyphema

Christopher J Rapuano MD
Co-Director and Attending Surgeon, Cornea Service
Co-Director, Refractive Surgery Department
Wills Eye Institute
and Professor of Ophthalomology
Jefferson Medical College of Thomas Jefferson University
Philadelphia PA
USA
192 Detachment of Descemet's Membrane
201 Keratoconus

Karim Rasheed MD, MSc, MRCOphth
Medical Director
Sani Eye Center
Templeton CA
USA
206 Pellucid Marginal Degeneration

S. R. Rathinam MNAMS, PhD
Professor of Ophthalmology and Head,Uveitis Service
Aravind Eye Hospital and Post Graduate Institute of Ophthalmology
Madurai
India
24 Leptospirosis

Lawrence A. Raymond MD
Associate Professor of Clinical Ophthalmology
Retinal-Vitreous Surgeon
Cincinnati Eye Institute
Cincinnati OH
USA
56 Baylisascaris

Russell W. Read MD
Associate Professor
Ophthalmology and Pathology
University of Alabama at Birmingham
Birmingham AL
USA
164 Vogt–Koyanagi–Harada Disease

August Lafayette Reader III MD, FACS
Clinical Professor of Ophthalmology
California Pacific Medical Center
San Francisco CA
USA
114 Hysteria, Malingering and Anxiety States

Franco M. Recchia MD
Assistant Professor of Ophthalmology, Vitreo-retinal Surgery
Department of Ophthalmology and Visual Sciences
Vanderbilt University Medical Center
Nashville TN
USA
6 Bacillus Species Infections
33 Ocular Candidiasis

James J. Reidy MD, FACS
Associate Professor of Ophthalmology
State University of New York
School of Medicine and Biomedical Sciences
Buffalo NY
USA
42 Rhinosporidiosis

Adam C. Reynolds MD
Assistant Clinical Professor
Intermountain Eye Center
Boise ID
USA
180 Filtering Blebs and Associated Problems
270 Ocular Hypertension

Larry F. Rich MS, MD
Professor of Ophthalmology
Casey Eye Institute
Portland OR
USA
152 Conjunctival Lacerations and Contusions
184 Pterygium and Pseudopterygium

Robert Ritch MD
Professor of Clinical Ophthalmology
New York Medical College
Valhalla NY
USA
275 Plateau Iris

Richard M. Robb MD
Associated Professor of Harvard Medical School
Emeritus Chief of Ophthalmology, Department of Ophthalmology
Children's Hospital Boston
Boston MA
USA
126 Dermoid

Pierre-Yves Robert MD, PhD
Ophthalmologist
CHU Dupuytren
Limoges
France
1 Acinetobacter

Joseph E. Robertson Jr MD
Professor and Chairman
Department of Ophthalmology
Casey Eye Institute
Portland OR
USA
307 Epimacular Proliferation
349 Familial Exudative Vitreoretinopathy

Shiyoung Roh MD
Assistant Clinical Professor pf Ophthalmology
Department of Ophthalmology
Tufts University School of Medicine
Lahey Clinic
Peabody MA
USA
103 Angiomatosis Retinae

Jean-Paul Romanet MD
Professor of Ophthalmology
Department of Ophthalmology
Hôspital Michallon
Grenoble
France
157 Intraocular Foreign Body: Steel or Iron

Jack Rootman MD, FRCSC
Professor
Department of Ophthalmology & Visual Sciences
Faculty of Medicine
Eye Care Center
Vancouver BC
Canada
323 Orbital Inflammatory Syndromes

Barbara L. Roque MD
Ophthalmologist
EYE REPUBLIC Ophthalmology Clinic
Asian Hospital and Medical Center
Alabang Muntinlupa City
Philippines
133 Leiomyoma
178 Conjunctival Melanotic Lesions

Manolette R. Roque MD, MBA
Ophthalmologist
EYE REPUBLIC Ophthalmology Clinic
Asian Hospital and Medical Center
Alabang Muntinlupa City
Philippines
133 Leiomyoma
178 Conjunctival Melanotic Lesions

Arthur L. Rosenbaum MD
Professor of Ophthalmology
and Vice Chairman, Department of Ophthalmology
Chief, Pediatric Ophthalmology and Strabismus Division
Jules Stein Eye Institute
Los Angeles CA
USA
225 Esotropia-High Accommodative Convergence-to-Accommodation Ratio

James Todd Rosenbaum MD
Professor of Medicine, Ophthalmology and Cell Biology
Oregon Health and Science University
Casey Eye Institute
Portland OR
USA
97 Systemic Lupus Erythematosus

F. Hampton Roy MD, FACS
Medical Director
Hampton Roy Eye Center
Little Rock AR
USA
12 Diphtheria
18 Herpes Simplex
19 Inclusion Conjunctivitis
36 Pneumococcus
60 Echinococcosis
65 Inflammatory Bowel Disease
69 Diabetes
75 Mucopolysaccharidosis IV
92 Pseudoxanthoma Elasticum
108 Cerebral Palsy
132 Keratoacanthoma
147 Retinoblastoma
151 Alkaline Injury
161 Thermal Burns
165 Epithelial Ingrowth
167 Postoperative Flat Anterior Chamber
175 Sympathetic Ophthalmia
179 Corneal and Conjunctival Calcifications
191 Corneal Neovascularization
196 Fuchs' Dellen
217 Acquired Nonaccommodative Esotropia

Paul A. Rundle MBBS, FRCOphth
Consultant Ocular Oncologist
Department of Ophthalmology
Royal Hallamshire Hospital
Sheffield
UK
174 Malignant Melanoma of the Posterior Uvea

Alfredo A. Sadun MD, PhD
F Thornton Professor of Vision Research
University of Southern California
Department of Ophthalmology
Doheney Eye Institute
Los Angeles CA
USA
315 Ischemic Optic Neuropathies

Norman A. Saffra MD
Professor of Ophthalmology
Medical and Surgical Eyesite
Brooklyn NY
USA
128 Fibrosarcoma

Sarwat Salim MD, FACS
Assistant Professor
Department of Ophthalmology
Hamilton Eye Institute
University of Tennessee Medical Center at Memphis
Memphis TN
USA
258 Angle Recession Glaucoma

John R. Samples MA, MD
Glaucoma Consultant
Glaucoma Consultants & The Eye Clinic
Portland OR
USA
241 Facial Movement Disorders
259 Corticosteroid Induced Glaucoma
262 Glaucoma Associated with Elevated Venous Pressure

Alvina Pauline D Santiago MD
Clinical Associate Professor
University of the Philippines College of Medicine
and Chief, Section of Pediatric Ophthalmology, The Medical City
and Consultant in Pediatric Ophthalmology
St Luke's Medical Center
Quezon City
Philippines
225 Esotropia: High Accommodative Convergence-to-Accommodation Ratio

David A. Saperstein MD
Associate Professor of Ophthalmology
University of Washington
Seattle WA
USA
332 Central Serous Chorioretinopathy

Richard A. Saunders MD
Professor of Ophthalmology and Pediatrics
Department of Ophthalmology
MUSC, Storm Eye Institute
Charleston SC
USA
227 Inferior Rectus Muscle Palsy

James A. Savage MD
Nevada Eye and Ear
Henderson NV
USA
274 Pigmentary Dispersion Syndrome and Pigmentary Glaucoma

Tina A. Scheutele MD
Fellow in Vitreoretinal Surgery, New England Eye Center
Tufts University School of Medicine
Boston MA
USA
308 Macular Hole

Vivian Schiedler MD
Ophthalmic Plastic and Reconstructive Surgery Fellow
Department of Ophthalmology
University of Washington
Seattle WA
USA
324 Optic Foramen Fractures

Thomas K. Schlesinger MD, PhD
Department of Ophthalmology
Oregon Health and Science University
Portland OR
USA
340 Retinal Venous Obstruction

Abraham Schlossman MD, FACS
Formerly, Clinical Professor of Ophthalmology
New York University College of Medicine
New York NY
USA
264 Glaucomatocyclitic Crisis

Lee K. Schwartz MD
Consulant, Corneal External Disease
Department of Ophthalmology
California Pacific Medical Center
San Francisco CA
USA
242 Floppy Eyelid Syndrome

Ingrid U. Scott MD, MPH
Professor of Ophthalmology and Health Evaluation Sciences
Department of Ophthalmology
Penn State College of Medicine
Hershey PA
USA
35 Pharyngoconjunctival Fever

Jennifer Scruggs MD
Clinical Instructor of Ophthalmology
New York University School of Medicine
New York NY
USA
135 Lymphangioma
321 External Orbital Fractures
322 Internal Orbital Fractures

Ernesto I. Segal MD
Clinical Assistant Professor
University of Texas Medical Branch in Galveston
Boca Raton FL
USA
95 Sarcoidosis

Ismail A. Shalaby MD, PhD
Instructor in Ophthalmology
Jonas Friedenwald Eye Institute
Baltimore MD
USA
2 Acquired and Congenital Syphilis

Aziz Sheikh MSc, DCH, DRCOG, MD, FRCP, FRCGP
Professor of Primary Care Research and Development
Division of Community Health Sciences, GP Section
University of Edinburgh
Edinburgh
UK
177 Bacterial Conjunctivitis

John D. Sheppard MD, MMSc
Professor of Ophthalmology,
Microbiology and Molecular Biology
Eastern Virginia Medical School
Virginia Eye Consultants
Norfolk VA
USA
8 Brucellosis

Mark D. Sherman MD
Assistant Professor
Department of Ophthalmology
Loma Linda University School of Medicine
San Luis Obispo CA
USA
5 Aspergillosis

Carol L. Shields MD
Professor, Thomas Jefferson Medical College
Attending Surgeon and Associate Director
Wills Eye Hospital
Philadelphia PA
USA
144 Orbital Rhabdomyosarcoma
263 Glaucoma Associated with Intraocular Tumors

Jerry A. Shields MD
Director, Oncology Services
Wills Eye Hospital
Philadelphia PA
USA
144 Orbital Rhabdomyosarcoma
263 Glaucoma Associated with Intraocular Tumors

Amarpreet Singh MD
Fellow in Oculoplastic Surgery
Case Western Reserve University of School of Medicine
Cleveland OH
USA
159 Orbital Implant Extrusion

Christopher N. Singh MD
Resident
Department of Ophthalmology
University of Washington
Seattle WA
USA
219 Brown's Syndrome
332 Central Serous Chorioretinopathy

Eric L. Singman MD, PhD
Director
Neuro-Ophthalmology, Low Vision and Vision Rehabilitation
Family Eye Group
Lancaster PA
USA
115 Idiopathic Intracranial Hypertension and Pseudotumor Cerebri
288 Uveitis

Donna Siracuse-Lee MD
Physician in Ophthalmology
Medical and Surgical Eyesite
Brooklyn NY
USA
128 Fibrosarcoma

Aaron D. Smalley MD
Resident in Ophthalmology
Department of Ophthalmology
Penn State Milton S Hershey Medical Center
Hershey PA
USA
35 Pharyngoconjunctival Fever

Patricia W. Smith MD
Triangle Eye Physicians, PA
Raleigh NC
USA
166 Intraocular Epithelial Cysts

Anthony W. Solomon MBBS, PhD
Lecturer, Clinical Research Unit
London School of Hygiene & Tropical Medicine
London
UK
50 Trachoma

Hassane Souhail MD
Resident in Ophthalmology
Service d'Ophtalmologie
Hôpital Militaire d'Instruction Med V
Rabat
Morocco
131 Kaposi's Sarcoma

Daniel H. Spitzberg MD, FACS
Ophthalmologist, Uveitis Specialist
Ophthalmology
Whitson Eyecare
Indianapolis IN
USA
21 Influenza

Thomas C. Spoor MD, MS, FACS
Michigan Neuro-Ophthalmology
Grosse Point Farms MI
USA
319 Vasculopathic Optic Neuropathies

Robert L. Stamper MD
Professor of Ophthalmology
Director of the Glaucoma Service
Department of Ophthalmology
University of California, San Francisco
San Francisco CA
USA
267 Lens-induced Glaucoma

Walter J. Stark MD
Professor of Ophthalmology
Director of the Stark-Mosher Center for Cataract and Corneal Disorders
The Wilmer Eye Institute
The John Hopkins Hospital
Baltimore MD
USA
166 Intraocular Epithelial Cysts

Eric A. Steele MD
Assistant Professor of Ophthalmology
Casey Eye Institute
Oregon Health and Science University
Portland OR
USA
244 Lagophthalmos
250 Orbital Fat Herniation
251 Ptosis
294 Lacrimal Gland Tumors

Thomas L. Steinemann MD
Associate Professor of Ophthalmology
Division of Ophthalmology
Case Western Reserve University
MetroHealth Medical Center
Cleveland OH
USA
47 Staphylococcus
181 Giant Papillary Conjunctivitis
212 Terrien's Marginal Degeneration

Ann U. Stout MD
Assistant Professor of Ophthalmology
Casey Eye Institute
Portland OR
USA
214 A-pattern Strabismus
230 Oculomotor (Third Nerve) Paralysis
232 Superior Oblique (Fourth Nerve) Palsy

J. Timothy Stout MD, PhD
Director Retina Services
Devers Eye Institute and Casey Eye Institute
Legacy Health System
and Department of Ophthalmology
Oregon Health and Science University
Portland OR
USA
328 Acquired Retinoschisis

R. Doyle Stulting MD, PhD
Professor of Ophthalmology
Emory Eye Center
Emory University
Atlanta GA
USA
208 Posterior Polymorphous Dystrophy
235 Blepharoconjunctivitis

Alan Sugar MD
Professor of Ophthalmology and Visual Sciences
WK Kellogg Eye Center
University of Michigan
Ann Arbor MI
USA
11 Dermatophytosis
22 Koch–Weeks Bacillus

Joel Sugar MD
Professor of Ophthalmology
Department of Ophthalmology and Visual Sciences
University of Illinois at Chicago
Chicago IL
USA
189 Corneal Edema

Donny W. Suh MD
Clinical Assistant Professor
Department of Ophthalmology
University of Nebraska
West des Moines IA
USA
15 Escherichia coli

Eric B. Suhler MD, MPH
Chief of Ophthalmology
Portland VA Medical Center
and Assistant Professor of Ophthalmology
Co-Director, Uveitis Service
Casey Eye Institute
Oregon Health and Science University
Portland OR
USA
9 Cat-scratch disease
49 Tetanus
344 White Dot Syndromes

John H. Sullivan MD
Clinical Professor
Department of Ophthalmology
University of California San Francisco
San Francisco CA
USA
234 Blepharochalasis

John Everett Sutphin MD
Professor and Chair
Department of Ophthalmology
University of Kansas Medical Center
Kansas City KS
USA
55 Acanthamebiasis

Kenneth C. Swan MD
Formerly, Professor
Department of Ophthalmology
Oregon Health and Science University
Portland OR
USA
283 Iris Cysts

Khalid F. Tabbara MD, ABO, FRCOphth
Adjunct Professor of Ophthalmology
Johns Hopkins University School of Medicine
Baltimore MD
USA
and Medical Director
The Eye Center
Riyadh
Saudi Arabia
64 Trichinosis
207 Phlyctenulosis

Mandeep S. Tamber MD
Neurosurgery Fellow
Division of Neurosurgery
Hospital for Sick Children
Toronto, Ontario
Canada
125 Craniopharyngioma

Angelo P. Tanna MD
Director, Glaucoma Service
Department of Ophthalmology
Northwestern University Feinberg School of Medicine
Chicago IL
USA
266 Juvenile Glaucoma

Sinan Tatlipinar MD
Cinical Fellow
Retina Service
The Wilmer Eye Institute
The Johns Hopkins Hospital
Baltimore MD
USA
347 Scleritis

Ramin Tayani MD, MPH, FAAO
Medical Director
Tayani Eye Institute
San Clemente CA
USA
46 Sporotrichosis

Klaus D. Teichmann MD, FRCSC, FRACO, DiplABO
Senior Academic Consultant and Chief of Anterior Segment
King Khaled Eye Specialist Hospital
Riyadh
Kingdom of Saudi Arabia
327 Orbital Hemorrhages

Mark A. Terry MD
Director, Corneal Services
Devers Eye Institute
Scientific Director
Lions Vision Research Laboratory of Oregon
Portland OR
USA
195 Fuchs' Corneal Dystrophy

Clement Chee Yung Tham FRCS, FCOphth(HK)
Professor, Department of Ophthalmology and Visual Science
The Chinese University of Hong Kong
Queen Mary Hospital
Hong Kong SAR
China
275 Plateau Iris

A. Therzaz MD
Professor in Ophthalmology
Service d'Ophtalmologie
Hôpital Militaire d'Instruction Med V
Rabat
Morocco
131 Kaposi's Sarcoma

Gilles Thuret MD, PhD
Ophthalmologist
University Hospital
Saint-Etienne
France
1 Acinetobacter
157 Intraocular Foreign Body: Steel or Iron

Christopher Graham Tinley MBChB, MRCOphth
Ophthalmology Specialist Registrar
West of England Eye Unit
Royal Devon and Exeter NHS Foundation Trust
Exeter
UK
299 After-Cataracts

Andrea C. Tongue MD
Ophthalmologist
Child Eye Care Associates
Lake Oswego OR
USA
231 Superior Oblique Myokymia

Rodrigo J. Torres MD
Fellow
Devers Eye Institute
Portland OR
USA
282 Iris Bombé

Robert N. Tower MD
Assistant Professor, Ophthalmic Facial Plastic and Orbital Surgery
Department of Ophthalmology
University of Washington School of Medicine
Seattle WA
USA
238 Entropion
291 Dacryocystitis and Dacryolith

Elias I Traboulsi MD
Professor of Ophthalmology
Cleveland Clinic Lerner College of Medicine
Head, Department of Pediatric Ophthalmology and Strabismus
Cole Eye Institute
Cleveland OH
USA
73 Mucopolysaccharidosis II
74 Mucopolysacccharidosis III

Rupan Trikha MD
Ophthalmology Resident
Department of Ophthalmology
Geisinger Medical Center
Danville PA
USA
188 Corneal Abrasions, Contusions, Lacerations and Perforations

Brenda J. Tripathi PhD
Distinguished Professor of Pathology, Microbiology and Immunology
University of South Carolina School of Medicine
Columbia SC
USA
190 Corneal Mucous Plaques

Ramesh C. Tripathi MD, MS(Ophth), PhD, FACS, FICS, FRCOphth, FRCPath, FNASc(I)
Distinguished Professor of Ophthalmology
Department of Ophthalmology
University of South Carolina School of Medicine
Columbia SC
USA
190 Corneal Mucous Plaques

Ilknur Tugal-Tutkun MD
Professor of Ophthalmology
Department of Ophthalmology
Istanbul Faculty of Medicine
Istanbul University
Istanbul
Turkey
90 Behçet's Disease

Irene Tung MD
Resident
Baylor College of Medicine
Houston TX
USA
183 Ophthalmia Neonatorum

Judith A. M. Van Evendingen MD
Neuro-ophthalmologist
Rotterdam Eye Hospital
Rotterdam
The Netherlands
109 Chronic Progressive External Ophthalmoplegia

Jean D. Vaudaux MD
Department of Ophthalmology
Jules Gonin Eye Hospital
Lausanne
Switzerland
63 Toxoplasmosis

Niteen S Wairagkar MBBS, MD
Deputy Director
National Institute of Virology
Pune
India
4 Acute Hemorrhagic Conjunctivitis

Joseph D. Walrath MD
Resident
Edward S. Harkness Eye Institute
New York NY
USA
135 Lymphangioma

Rory McConn Walsh MD, MB, FRCSI(ORL)
Consultant Otolaryngologist and Senior Lecturer
Department of Otolaryngology
RCSI Education and Research Center
Beaumont Hospital
Dublin
Ireland
107 Bell's Palsy

David S. Walton MD
Clinical Professor of Ophthalmology
Harvard Medical School
Boston MA
USA
101 Weill–Marchesani Syndrome
278 Aniridia

Ronald E. Warwar MD
Clinical Assistant Professor
Department of Surgery
Wright State University School of Medicine
Dayton OH
USA
32 Nocardiosis
171 Choroidal Folds

Peter G. Watson MA, MBBChir, FRCS, FRCOphth, DO
Honorary Consultant Ophthalmic Surgeon
Addenbrooke's Hospital, Cambridge and Moorfields Eye Hospital
London
UK
93 Relapsing Polychondritis
345 Episcleritis

John J. Weiter MD, PhD
Associate Clinical Professor of Ophthalmology
Department of Ophthalmology
Harvard Medical School
Cambridge MA
USA
103 Angiomatosis Retinae

Richard G. Weleber MD
Professor of Ophthalmology and Molecular & Medical Genetics
Casey Eye Institute
Oregon Health and Science University
Portland OR
USA
76 Mucopolysaccharidosis IV
336 Gyrate Atrophy of the Choroid and Retina with Hyperornithinemia
338 Refsum's Disease

Fleming D. Wertz III MD, FACS
Consultant in Ophthalmology
Department of Ophthalmology
Lahey Clinic Northshore
Peabody MA
USA
155 Intraocular Foreign Body: Copper

Igor Westra MD, MSc
Assistant Clinical Professor
University of North Carolina, Chapel Hill
Retina of Coastal Carolina PLLC
Wilmington NC
USA
279 Ciliary Body Concussions and Lacerations

David T. Wheeler MD
Associate Professor of Ophthalmology and Pediatrics
Oregon Health and Science University
Casey Eye Institute
Portland OR
USA
52 Typhoid Fever
130 Juvenile Xanthogranuloma
229 Nystagmus
300 Congenital and Infantile Cataracts

Charles P. Wilkinson MD
Chairman, Department of Ophthalmology, Greater Baltimore Medical Center
Professor, Department of Ophthalmology
John Hopkins University
Baltimore MD
USA
337 Peripheral Retinal Breaks and Vitreoretinal Degenerative Disorders

David J. Wilson MD
Thiele-Petti Chair, Ophthalmology
Director, Eye Pathology Laboratory
Oregon Health and Science University
Casey Eye Institute
Portland OR
USA
271 Ocular Hypotony

M. Edward Wilson MD
Pierre G. Jenkins Professor and
Chairman
Department of Ophthalmology
and Director, Storm Eye Institute
Medical University of South Carolina
Charleston SC
USA
228 Monofixation Syndrome

Matthew W. Wilson MD, FACS
Associate Professor
Department of Opthalmology
University of Tennessee Health
Services Center
Memphis TN
USA
123 Capillary Hemangioma

Steven E Wilson MD
Professor of Ophthalmology
and Director of Corneal Research
Cole Eye Institute
The Cleveland Clinic
Cleveland OH
USA
204 Mooren's Ulcer

John L. Wobig MD
Formerly, Professor of Ophthalmology
Casey Eye Institute
Oregon Health and Science University
Portland OR
USA
292 Epiphoria

Terry D. Wood MD
Neuro-Ophthalmology Fellow
Casey Eye Institute
Oregon Health and Science University
Portland OR
USA
9 Cat-scratch disease
49 Tetanus
127 Ewing's Sarcoma
311 Compressive Optic Neuropathies

Lihteh Wu MD
Associate Surgeon
Institute of Ocular Surgery
San José
Costa Rica
57 Coenurosis
333 Coats' Disease

Ozgur Yalcinbayir MD
Visiting International Scholar
Department of Ophthalmology
St Louis University School of Medicine
St Louis MO
USA
82 Thalassemia

Howard Shann-Cherng Ying MD, PhD
Assistant Professor of Ophthalmology
Department of Ophthalmology
The John Hopkins University
Wilmer Eye Institute
Baltimore MD
USA
156 Intraocular Foreign Body: Nonmagnetic, Chemically Inert

Peter N. Youssef MD
Resident
Department of Ophthalmology
University of Washington Medical
Center
Seattle WA
USA
219 Brown's Syndrome
332 Central Serous Chorioretinopathy

Gerald W. Zaidman MD
Professor of Ophthalmology
Department of Ophthalmology
Westchester Medical Center
Valhalla NY
USA
25 Lyme Disease

DEDICATION

To

Michelle, Charles, Frederick, Kimberly, Robert, Nichols and Helena

---

Wendee, Mikayla, Jacob, Gracie-Anne and Sara-Jane

Yvonne, Yvette, Helene Jean, Nina, Rick and Nick

Neeli, Blake, Tyler, Trey, Cooper and Keetin

SECTION

1 Infectious Diseases

1 ACINETOBACTER 041.9

Gilles Thuret, MD, PhD
Saint-Etienne, France
Pierre-Yves Robert, MD, PhD
Limoges, France
Anne Carricajo, PhD
Saint-Etienne, France
Philippe Gain, MD, PhD
Saint-Etienne, France

Bacteria of the *Acinetobacter* genus are ubiquitous and may live in soil, water, plants and on the healthy skin of human beings and animals. *Acinetobacter* spp. are frequently isolated in wastewater and activated sludge from wastewater treatment. Some have emerged as important healthcare-associated pathogens in hospitals, but they are rarely involved in eye and annex infections. There is no pathognomonic clinical presentation of *Acinetobacter* ocular infection, therefore laboratory diagnosis is necessary for the choice of antibiotic treatment.

CLINICAL DIAGNOSIS

General considerations

Acinetobacter spp. belong to the usual cutaneous flora, especially in wet zones (groin, axilla, interdigital spaces) and are also isolated from the mouth, throat, trachea, nose, conjunctiva, bladder and rectum. Colonization and type of species differ between healthy and hospitalized patients. They can survive on inert surfaces or in dust for more than 8 days. The most frequently isolated are *Acinetobacter baumannii, A. lwoffii, A. haemolyticus, A. johnsonii, A. radioresistens, A. genomospecies* 3 and *A. genomospecies* 13 (Tjernberg and Ursing). *A. baumannii* is linked to many hospital acquired infections (up to 90% of all *Acinetobacter* hospital infection in some countries) including skin and wound infections, pneumonia, septicemia, urinary tract infection and meningitis. *A. lwoffi*, especially, is responsible for most cases of *Acinetobacter*-related meningitis. *Acinetobacter* spp. are responsible for nearly 10% of all nosocomial infections. Community-acquired infections, mainly pneumonia, generally happen in immunocompromised patients. Mortality and morbidity resulting from *A. baumannii* infection relate to the underlying cardiopulmonary and immune status of the host rather than the inherent virulence of the organism.

In ophthalmology

Acinetobacter species can colonize normal conjunctiva. They have been described in post mortem conjunctival flora and detected during corneal storage before graft. Conjunctival colonization seems not to be modified by frequent-replacement contact lenses. They have been described in various ocular infections but remain scarce.

Endophthalmitis

This most severe ocular infection due to *Acinetobacter* spp. has a rather chronic presentation. It can be postoperative, posttraumatic, endogenous or bleb-related.

Orbital abscess

Keratitis

Acinetobacter is the third most frequent bacteria involved in corneal ulcers and abscesses, after *Pseudomonas aeruginosa*, and staphylococci. Main risk factors are lagophthalmos, burns, and stay in an intensive care unit. *Acinetobacter* keratitis may present as crystalline keratopathy (although not pathognomonic), contact lens adverse effect. It results, very occasionally, in corneal perforation.

Purulent conjunctivitis (mono or polymicrobial)

Chronic blepharitis

Not categorically involved.

TAXONOMY AND LABORATORY DIAGNOSIS

Acinetobacter spp. are included in the *Moraxellaceae* family. The classification has been completely reorganized since 1986 and constantly enriched. Previously, names included *Achromobacter, Alcaligenes, Cytophaga, 'Diplococcus,' 'Bacterium,' 'Herellea,' 'Lingelsheimia,' 'Mima,' Micrococcus, Moraxella, Neisseria.* Thirty-two species have been isolated among which 17 received a published validated name. Only 10 of them have been held responsible for human infections.

Species belonging to the *Acinetobacter* genus are Gram-negative cocobacillary rods, not sporulated, sometimes encapsulated, non motile, non fermentative, strictly aerobic, catalase positive and oxidase-negative.

Bacterial growth is easily obtained on the usual broth — both rich and minimal salts media (trypticase soy broth, brain heart infusion). Incubation temperature must be between 30 to 35°C since some species do not grow at 37°C.

Diagnosis can also be achieved using universal polymerase chain reaction (PCR) amplifying a portion of the *16S rRNA* gene followed by direct sequencing of the resulting amplicon. This technique is particularly relevant for small ocular samples, including aqueous and vitreous taps.

TREATMENT

While colonization should not be treated, infection should. *Acinetobacter* spp. has a chromosomic beta-lactamase not inhibited by clavulanate, active against first generation cephalosporine but not against ticarcillin. Nevertheless, due to the importance of resistant strains, susceptibility testing is required for each clinically significant strain. Throughout the years multiresistant strains have emerged in hospitals. Some strains of *A. baumannii* are considered as the most resistant of all Gram-negative bacteria. Mechanisms of resistance are numerous:

- secretion of β-lactamases encoded either by the chromosome or by plasmids,
- acquisition of plasmids encoding resistance to aminosides,
- mutation of the DNA gyrase causing resistance to quinolones,
- transposon encoding resistance to chloramphenicol, etc.

Antibiotics

Aminoglycosides (with amikacin the most active one > tobramycin > gentamicin), *carbapenems* (meropenem, imipenem — but associated with the rapid and worrying development of resistance), and *fluoroquinolones* remain the mainstay of therapy.

Among *β-lactams*, although the carbapenems are still the most active antimicrobials against *Acinetobacter* species, carbapenems resistant strains have been reported in nosocomial outbreaks. *Acinetobacter* remains highly sensitive to other β-lactams: piperacillin/tazobactam, ticarcillin/clavulanate, ceftazidime, cefepime. Reappraisal of older compounds (e.g. polymyxin B, ampicillin/sulbactam) is necessary.

Regarding *fluoroquinolones*, novel third and fourth-generation fluoroquinolones demonstrate superior activity (×4 to ×16) when compared to ciprofloxacin: clinafloxacin > gatifloxacin > levofloxacin > trovafloxacin > gemifloxacin = moxifloxacin. They should be the first line drugs in the treatment of acinetobacter endophthalmitis (before ciprofloxacin) because of their good biodisponibility and intra ocular penetration.

Other antibiotics: trimethoprim-sulfamethoxazole are effective against most strains whereas chloramphenicol, tetracycline, macrolides have little and/or no activity against *Acinetobacter*.

Acinetobacter baumannii remains susceptible to antiseptics or disinfectants.

Specificity in ophthalmology

- Active antibiotics commercially available topically: polymyxin B, tobramycin, ciprofloxacin, levofloxacin*, moxifloxacin* (* in certain countries).
- Active antibiotic that can be prepared for topical use (fortified antibiotic): ceftazidime.
- Active antibiotic for intravitreous injection (endophthalmitis): ceftazidime.
- Severe corneal abscess may require fortified antibiotics (ceftazidime), surgical scraping (see Chapter 186).
- Endophthalmitis is an actual emergency and often require repeated intra vitreous injections, and often a vitrectomy (see Chapter 257 and Chapter 258).

REFERENCES

Gopal L, Ramaswamy AA, Madhavan HN, et al: Endophthalmitis caused by *Acinetobacter calcoaceticus*. A profile. Indian J Ophthalmol 51:335–340, 2003.

Heinemann B, Wisplinghoff H, Edmond M, et al: Comparative activities of ciprofloxacin, clinafloxacin, gatifloxacin, gemifloxacin, levofloxacin, moxifloxacin, and trovafloxacin against epidemiologically defined *Acinetobacter baumannii* strains. Antimicrob Agents Chemother 44:2211–2213, 2000.

Jain R, Danziger LH: Multidrug-resistant *Acinetobacter* infections: an emerging challenge to clinicians. Ann Pharmacother 38:1449–1459, 2004.

Kämpfer P, Tjernberg I, Ursing J: Numerical classification and identification of *Acinetobacter* genomic species. J Appl Bacteriol 75:259–268, 1993.

Kau HC, Tsai CC, Kao SC, et al: Corneal ulcer of the side port after phacoemulsification induced by *Acinetobacter baumannii*. J Cataract Refract Surg 28:895–897, 2002.

Kirwan JF, Potamitis T, el-Kasaby H, et al: Microbial keratitis in intensive care. BMJ 314:433–434, 1997.

Rudolph T, Welinder-Olsson C, Lind-Brandberg L, et al: *16S rDNA* PCR analysis of infectious keratitis: a case series. Acta Ophthalmol Scand 82:463–467, 2004.

Van Gelder RN: Applications of the polymerase chain reaction to diagnosis of ophthalmic disease. Surv Ophthalmol 46:248–258, 2001.

Van Looveren M, Goossens H: Antimicrobial resistance of *Acinetobacter* spp. in Europe. Clin Microbiol Infect 10:684–704, 2004.

2 ACQUIRED AND CONGENITAL SYPHILIS 095.8

Ismail A. Shalaby, MD, PhD
Baltimore, Maryland

Syphilis is a chronic systemic infection caused by the spirochete *Treponema pallidum*, for which humans are the only natural host. It has been known as a cause of ophthalmic disease for more than 100 years. Infections occurring through passage of the organism from an infected mother across the placenta to her fetus define congenital syphilis. Acquired syphilis is usually transmitted sexually. Although congenital and acquired syphilis are caused by the same organism and are treated in a qualitatively similar fashion, their clinical course and physical findings are sufficiently different to warrant separate discussions.

Acquired syphilis

ETIOLOGY/INCIDENCE

Acquired syphilis is a systemic disease that is caused by *T. pallidum* and that is usually transmitted through sexual contact, including vaginal, orogenital and anorectal intercourse. There have been rare cases of acquired syphilis occurring through nonsexual personal contact or from blood transfusion. Patients are most contagious during untreated primary and secondary syphilis, although patients with early latent syphilis can sometimes transmit disease. Infection does not confer immunity.

The number of new cases in syphilis in the United States declined after the introduction of penicillin. A dramatic rise in the number of new cases of syphilis among homosexual men occurred in the 1970s. Between 1981 and 1990, the incidence of primary and secondary syphilis increased from 13.7 to 20.3 per 100,000 persons. This increase, which primarily involved urban minorities, was attributed to various factors, including illegal drug use, trading sex for drugs, concurrent human immunodeficiency virus (HIV) infection, and decreased access to healthcare. Although by 2001 the national rate had fallen to 2.2 cases per 100,000, there was yet another rate increase in 2002 reaching 2.4 cases per 100,000. This increase occurred only in men, and in particularly among men who have sex with men (MSM). It is reported that a substantial number of MSM with syphilis report meeting anonymous partners in venues such as bathhouses and Internet chat rooms.

Syphilitic uveitis, the most common ocular manifestation of syphilis, occurs in about 5% of patients with syphilis and accounts for about 1% to 2% of all cases of uveitis.

COURSE/PROGNOSIS

Primary syphilis

T. pallidum penetrates intact mucous membranes at the site of sexual contact and causes an ulcerated papular lesion known as a chancre in 10 to 90 days (mean, 21 days), depending on the size of the inoculation. Multiple chancres are common, particularly in HIV-infected patients. Regional nontender lymphadenopathy appears within 1 week of onset of the chancre but is absent in chancres involving the anus, lower vulva and cervix, which drain to deep lymph nodes. Most chancres heal without scarring in 4 to 6 weeks, but lymphadenopathy may persist for months.

Secondary syphilis

This stage of infection is characterized by localized or diffuse mucocutaneous lesions and generalized nontender lymphadenopathy. A primary chancre may persist in 15% to 25% of patients. The frequently pruritic skin rash consists of macular, papular, papulosquamous, and occasionally pustular lesions or a combination of all patterns. Condylomata lata (broad, moist, pink or gray-white vegetations resulting from enlargement and erosion of papular lesions in moist intertriginous areas) are seen in 10% of patients and are highly infectious. Superficial painless mucosal erosions called mucous patches occur in as many as 15% of patients and involve the lips, oral mucosa, tongue, palate, vulva, vagina, and glans penis. Flu-like symptoms such as malaise, weight loss, anorexia, sore throat, headache, and fever occur in 50% of patients. Patchy, nonscarring alopecia may be present. Uveitis and the many other ocular manifestations usually occur in this stage (see later).

Latent syphilis

Latent syphilis is marked by immunity, the absence of clinical signs of infection, and an increased incidence of false-negative nontreponemal tests. One third of patients with untreated latent disease develop tertiary syphilis, usually 2 to 20 years after primary infection but much sooner in HIV-infected patients.

Tertiary (late) syphilis

Tertiary syphilis is the end result of a slowly progressive inflammatory disease that begins early after the *T. pallidum* infection. Manifestations include:

- central nervous system (CNS) infection in about 8% of patients (see Neurosyphilis),
- inflammatory lesions of the cardiovascular system (aortitis, aortic regurgitation, and saccular aneurysms) in about 10% of patients, and
- gummas (gummata), which are rubbery, granulomatous, nodular lesions that can involve the skin, skeletal system, mouth, respiratory tract, liver, stomach and CNS. Gummas of the skin are often painless and indolent and may heal spontaneously with scarring. Gummas of the skeletal system frequently involve the long bones of the legs and often present with focal pain and tenderness.

Neurosyphilis

Five patterns of syphilitic infection of the CNS are as follows:

1. Asymptomatic neurosyphilis: abnormal CSF findings only; frequently progresses to clinical neurosyphilis.
2. Acute meningitis: cranial nerves 7 and 8 most commonly involved.
3. Meningovasculitis: classic picture of meningovascular syphilis is a relatively young adult who presents with a stroke syndrome that was preceded by subacute symptoms of meningitis and encephalitis.
4. Parenchymatous neurosyphilis: tabes dorsalis and generalized paresis. Tabes dorsalis symptoms include ataxia, paresthesia, wide-based gait and foot drop, deep pain, impotence, bladder disturbance, Charcot's joints, and optic nerve atrophy. General paresis presents with widespread symptoms according to the mnemonic *paresis* (*p*ersonality, *a*ffect, *r*eflexes [hyperactive], *e*ye [Argyll Robertson pupils], *s*ensorium [illusions and delusions], *i*ntellect [dementia, orientation, and so on] and *s*peech).
5. Gummatous neurosyphilis.

DIAGNOSIS

Ocular manifestations

Ophthalmic signs and symptoms can be present at any stage of syphilis and can involve any ocular structure. Eye disease is most frequently found in secondary syphilis and with CNS infection.

Primary syphilis

Chancres can present, albeit rarely, on the conjunctiva or eyelid.

Secondary syphilis

Iridocyclitis (usually granulomatous) is the most common finding. Other manifestations include papulosquamous eyelid rash, alopecia of the eyebrows and eyelashes, dacryocystitis, dacryoadenitis, conjunctivitis, episcleritis, scleritis, iris papules, lens dislocation, interstitial keratitis, intermediate uveitis, posterior uveitis, panuveitis, cystoid macular edema, retinitis (including retinal necrosis), pseudoretinitis pigmentosa, retinal periphlebitis, placoid posterior chorioretinitis, neuroretinitis, choroiditis and choroidal neovascular membrane. Optic nerve involvement includes optic neuritis, optic perineuritis, papilledema and papillitis. HIV-infected patients have more severe and more bilateral disease. In one study, more than half of the patients had ocular complaints as the initial manifestation of syphilis, usually with concurrent maculopapular rash.

Late syphilis

Manifestations include the presence of gummas on the optic nerve, retina, extraocular muscles, sclera and iris. Ptosis, extraocular muscle weakness or palsy, pupillary abnormalities (Argyll Robertson pupils), optic nerve atrophy, retinal pigment hypertrophy and posterior pole/macular scars are other signs of late syphilis. Unexplained visual field defects may also be due to a late-stage syphilitic infection.

Neurosyphilis

Early CNS infections can present with iritis, iridocyclitis and other forms of uveitis. Late CNS disease causes pupillary abnormalities or optic atrophy. Ocular syphilis is more closely associated with cerebrospinal fluid (CSF) and neurologic abnormalities in HIV-positive than in HIV-negative patients. Acute syphilitic meningitis has occurred as early as 4 months after initial infection in HIV-infected patients.

Latent syphilis

This is defined as seroreactivity without other evidence of disease. Early latent syphilis is diagnosed in patients infected within the previous year by either a documented seroconversion, unequivacol symptoms of primary or secondary syphilis, or having had a sex partner documented to have primary, secondary or early latent syphilis.

Laboratory findings

Nontreponemal tests (Venereal Disease Research Laboratory [VDRL] and rapid plasma reagin [RPR]) are used to quantify antibodies against cardiolipin, and the titer may be used to assess the response to treatment. The titer is not proportional to the severity of disease; extremely high titers in HIV-infected patients may result from polyclonal B cell stimulation. Treponemal tests (fluorescent treponemal antibody absorption [FTA-ABS] and microhemagglutination-*Treponema pallidum* [MHA-TP]) are more specific but less quantifiable and the test remains positive after treatment. False-positive results can occur with either test; a weakly positive FTA-ABS often is a false positive. Because all positive nontreponemal tests require confirmation with a treponemal test and because 38% of patients with ocular syphilis had a negative VDRL in one study, it is recommended by many clinicians that both tests be ordered. All patients with syphilis should be tested for HIV infection.

Primary syphilis

Laboratory tests are negative for 1 to 2 weeks after infection, so diagnosis requires confirmation of treponemes in lesions by dark-field microscopy. Treponemal tests become positive earlier than nontreponemal tests.

Secondary syphilis

Both treponemal and nontreponemal tests are positive in nearly all cases.

Latent syphilis

Nontreponemal tests become negative in 99% of treated patients and 30% of untreated patients. Treponemal tests remain positive in 98% of treated and untreated patients. All patients who may have had syphilis for longer than 1 year should undergo lumbar puncture to look for evidence of neurosyphilis.

Tertiary syphilis

Laboratory tests are similar to those in latent syphilis. Organisms are rarely identified in gummas.

Neurosyphilis

Laboratory diagnosis and confirmation include a reactive serologic test plus a reactive VDRL in the CSF. However, neurosyphilis can be diagnosed if there is a positive serologic test with a negative VDRL, as long as there is elevated CSF protein or leukocyte count plus clinical signs or symptoms consistent with neurosyphilis in the absence of any other known cause for these abnormalities. Positive CSF serology and pleocytosis are found much more commonly in HIV-infected patients who have ocular syphilis than in HIV-negative patients who do not have ocular syphilis.

Differential diagnosis

- Uveitis: sarcoidosis.
- Necrotizing retinitis: herpetic retinitis, cytomegalovirus retinitis.
- False-positive serologic tests for syphilis: other spirochetal infections (e.g. Lyme disease), malaria, leptospirosis, leprosy, measles, tuberculosis, chronic liver disease, connective tissue disease and blood transfusions.

TREATMENT

Parenteral penicillin is the preferred treatment for all stages of syphilis. The route, dosage, and length of treatment depend on the stage of the infection. Treatment of HIV-infected patients is discussed separately. Below are the United States Center for Disease Control recommendations. For pregnant women and neonates, see Congenital syphilis.

Primary and secondary syphilis

- Penicillin G benzathine at 2.4 million units IM in a single dose.
- For *penicillin-allergic* (non pregnant) patients, doxycycline 100 mg PO b.i.d. or tetracycline 500 mg PO q.i.d. for 14 days.

Late latent syphilis, tertiary syphilis and syphilis of unknown duration

- Penicillin G benzathine at 2.4 million units IM weekly for 3 weeks.
- For *Penicillin-allergic* (non pregnant) patients are treated with doxycycline 100 mg PO b.i.d. or tetracycline 500 mg PO q.i.d. for 14 days for early latent and 28 days for late latent infection; data regarding the efficacy of non penicillin regimens are scarce.
- Treatment of latent syphilis is intended to prevent occurrence or progression of late complications.

Neurosyphilis and syphilitic eye disease

- Aqueous crystalline penicillin G 3.0 to 4.0 million units IV every 4 hours is administered for 10–14 days (total of 18–24 million units per day) (penicillin G benzathine does not achieve treponemicidal levels in the CSF).
- *Penicillin-allergic* (nonpregnant) patients are treated with doxycycline 100 mg PO b.i.d. or tetracycline 500 mg PO q.i.d. for 2 weeks for early latent and 4 weeks for late latent infection; data regarding the efficacy of nonpenicillin regimens are scarce.

Ocular disease

The ideal systemic regimen for ocular syphilis is not known. Many investigators recommend that all intraocular disease be treated as neurosyphilis, even if the CSF examination is normal. Topical corticosteroids (e.g. prednisolone acetate 1%) and cycloplegic agents should be used to relieve the symptoms of anterior uveitis and other anterior segment inflammations. The dose and frequency of corticosteroid drops should be titrated according to the extent of the inflammation and then tapered carefully to avoid recurrence.

HIV-infected patients

- Early syphilis can be treated as in HIV-negative patients.
- Because of reports of treatment failure in HIV-infected patients, some investigators recommend that all HIV-infected patients be treated with a regimen appropriate for neurosyphilis, regardless of the clinical stage of syphilis (aqueous penicillin G 4.0 million units IV every 4 hours for 10 days, followed by penicillin G benzathine 2.4 million units IM weekly for 3 weeks).
- Quantitative nontreponemal tests should be repeated at 1, 2, and 3 months after treatment and then every 3 months thereafter, until a satisfactory serologic response occurs.

Complications

The Jarisch–Herxheimer reaction is an acute self-limited systemic febrile reaction accompanied by headache, myalgia, tachycardia, hyperventilation, and mild hypotension that occurs within 1 to 2 hours and lasts 12 to 24 hours after any effective therapy for syphilis. It can occur in any stage of syphilis (10% to 25%) but is particularly common in secondary syphilis (70% to 90%). It may also induce early labor or cause fetal distress in pregnant women. This should not prevent or delay therapy; patients should be warned of this reaction before treatment. The Jarisch–Herxheimer reaction is self-limited and can be symptomatically treated with aspirin every 4 hours for 24 to 48 hours. Treatment with prednisone is warranted in cardiovascular syphilis and neurosyphilis because the reaction may be catastrophic in these patients.

Other antibiotic therapy

There have been reports about the possible efficacy of ceftriaxone, and azithromycin in infectious syphilis. The human clinical studies on ceftriaxone have been limited, and the initial positive reports with azithromycin have been followed by several reports on treatment failures. Therefore, neither therapy is generally recommended at this time.

Congenital syphilis

ETIOLOGY/INCIDENCE

The transmission of *T. pallidum* from an untreated or inadequately treated mother to her fetus may occur at any stage of pregnancy and is especially common in untreated primary or secondary syphilis. The lesions of congenital syphilis may become apparent anytime after the first trimester up to early adolescence. Congenital syphilis causes fetal or perinatal death in 10% to 40% of the infants affected.

The number of reported cases of congenital syphilis in the US rose between 1984 to 1991, reaching a peak of 100 cases per 100,000 live born infants. This increase paralleled the rise of primary and secondary syphilis, which were usually associated with the practice of trading sex for drugs. Fortunately, there has been a steady overall decline of incidence since then reaching a nadir of 11.2 cases per 100,000 live born infants in 2002. This parallels the decline in incidence of acquired infection in women.

COURSE/PROGNOSIS

Systemic findings

- Infants: hepatosplenomegaly, generalized vesicular or bullous skin rash, condylomata lata, rhinitis (snuffles), jaundice (syphilitic hepatitis), osteochondritis and bone fractures, pseudoparalysis and edema secondary to nephrotic syndrome.
- Older children: anterior bowing of the shins, frontal bossing, Clutton's joints, mulberry molars, saddle nose, rhagades and cardiovascular disease; widely spaced, peg-shaped teeth, eighth cranial nerve deafness and interstitial keratitis constitute Hutchinson's triad. Meningovascular syphilis with nerve deafness (secondary to eighth cranial nerve involvement) is more common than other forms of neurosyphilis.

Ophthalmic findings

- Bilateral interstitial keratitis is the classic and most common finding (10% of patients), occurring in persons 5 to 20 years of age. There is associated anterior uveitis, which is followed by endothelial edema leading to a generalized corneal edema. The cornea is then invaded by superficial and deep blood vessels from the periphery that appear to push a faint opacity in front of them. The blood vessels can form to meet a 'salmon patch' and the inflammation then subsides, leaving clear branching 'ghost vessels' around a translucent scar anterior to Descemet's membrane.
- Chorioretinitis appearing as a bilateral salt-and-pepper granularity of the fundus.
- Pseudoretinitis pigmentosa.
- Secondary glaucoma may develop due to chamber angle damage from the initial anterior segment inflammation.

DIAGNOSIS

Laboratory findings

- *Confirmed* congenital syphilis is defined by the Centers for Disease Control and Prevention as that occurring in an infant in whom *T. pallidum* is identified by dark-field microscopy.
- *Presumptive* congenital syphilis is defined as that occurring in an infant whose infected mother went untreated or was inadequately treated during pregnancy or an infant or a child who has a reactive treponemal test for syphilis plus (1) any evidence of congenital syphilis on physical examination, (2) evidence of congenital syphilis on long-bone radiographs, (3) a reactive CSF VDRL, (4) elevated CSF cell or protein count without other cause, (5) quantitative nontreponemal serologic titer 4-fold higher than the mother's titer (with both drawn at birth), or (6) reactive test for FTA-ABS-19S-IgM antibody.
- Serologic tests in both infants and mothers may be negative if the syphilis was acquired near the end of the pregnancy.
- Maternally acquired antibodies will decrease during the first year of life.

Differential diagnosis

- Other congenital infections (cytomegalovirus, rubella, toxoplasmosis), acquired syphilis (in cases of sexual abuse).

TREATMENT

Pregnant mothers

Regardless of the state of pregnancy, women should be treated with penicillin according to the dosage and schedules appropriate for the stage of acquired syphilis recommended for nonpregnant individuals. Penicillin-allergic patients (positive for skin reaction tests) should undergo desensitization. Tetracycline is not recommended for pregnant women because of the potential for adverse effects to the fetus. Erythromycin is discouraged except for individuals who have been proved to be allergic to penicillin who are not candidates for desensitization.

Neonates (younger than 4 weeks)

Aqueous crystalline penicillin G is preferred with the dosage based on chronologic rather than gestational age. The recommended dosage is 50,000 units/kg IV every 12 hours for the first week and then every 8 hours to complete a 10- to 14-day course. Some recommend procaine penicillin G at 50,000 units/kg IM daily for 10 days, but adequate CSF concentrations may not be achieved with this regimen. If more than 1 day of therapy is missed, the entire course should be restarted.

Infants

Because of the difficulty of establishing a diagnosis of neurosyphilis in infants older than 4 weeks, it is recommended that aqueous crystalline penicillin G be given at a dose of 50,000 units/kg IV every 6 hours over a 10- to 14-day period. This is the same treatment as for neurosyphilis. For asymptomatic infants whose mothers were adequately treated during pregnancy, treatment is not necessary if follow-up can be ensured. For asymptomatic neonates with adequately treated mothers whose follow-up cannot be ensured, many recommend treatment with benzathine penicillin G 50,000 units/kg IM in a single dose (although efficacy data are lacking).

Older children

Lumbar puncture should be performed to rule out neurosyphilis. If the CSF is abnormal, then the recommendation is to treat like neurosyphilis (i.e. aqueous crystalline penicillin G 50,000 units/kg IV every 6 hours for 10 to 14 days). The same treatment is given for children older than 1 year who have late or previously untreated congenital syphilis. If the CSF is normal, the CSF VDRL is negative, and there is minimal clinical manifestation of disease, some treat with only three doses of benzathine penicillin G 50,000 units/kg IM.

Ocular

Topical corticosteroids and cycloplegics can relieve the symptoms of anterior uveitis and interstitial keratitis. Subconjunctival corticosteroids have been administered to relieve recalcitrant anterior segment inflammation. Severe corneal opacification may require keratoplasty. Greater postoperative inflammation and graft rejection may result after such surgery even in an old interstitial keratitis, requiring a more frequent or stronger anti-inflammatory corticosteroid regimen.

Follow-up

The American Academy of Pediatrics recommends that follow-up for all infants be incorporated into routine newborn care at 1, 2, 4, 6, and 12 months. Serologic tests should be performed until the patients become nonreactive. Patients with persistent, stable, low titers should be considered for retreatment. Treated infants should be similarly followed, with a CSF examination at 6-month intervals until the patient becomes nonreactive. A reactive CSF VDRL test at 6 months is an indication for retreatment. All patients with neurosyphilis must be carefully monitored with periodic serologic testing, clinical evaluation at 6-month intervals, and repeat CSF examinations for at least 3 years. A thorough developmental evaluation should be done at age 2 on all children treated in infancy who are symptomatic at birth or had active congenital infection.

PREVENTION

The ultimate cure for congenital syphilis is its prevention. Comprehensive prenatal care starting early in pregnancy is essential to detect any infection in the pregnant mother and institute adequate treatment. Sexually transmitted disease programs and drug addiction programs institute prenatal outreach programs to identify and reach the at-risk individuals. Partners of infected women (or men) should be identified and contacted to reach an even greater at-risk population.

REFERENCES

Aldave AJ, King JA, Cunningham ET, Jr: Ocular syphilis. Curr Opin Ophthalmol 12:433–441, 2001.

Centers for Disease Control and Prevention: Congenital syphilis–United States, 2002. MMWR 53:716–719, 2004.

Centers for Disease Control and Prevention: Guidelines for the treatment of sexually transmitted diseases 2002. MMWR 51:1–78, 2002.

Centers for Disease Control and Prevention: Primary and secondary syphilis–United States, 2002: MMWR 52:1117–1120–1497, 2003.

Chen JC: Brief report: azithromycin treatment failures in syphilis infections–San Francisco, California, 2002–2003. Ann Emerg Med 44:232–233, 2004.

Golden MR, Marra CM, Holmes KK: Update on syphilis. Resurgence of an old problem. JAMA 290:1510–1514, 2003.

Lynn WA, Lightman S: Syphilis and HIV: a dangerous combination. Lancet Infectious Diseases 4:456–466, 2004.

Shalaby IA, Dunn JP, Semba RD, Jabs DA: Syphilitic uveitis in human immunodeficiency virus-infected patients. Arch Ophthalmol 115:469–473, 1997.

Sung L, MacDonald NE: Syphilis: a pediatric perspective. Pediatr Rev 19:17–22, 1997.

Zeltser R, Kurban AK: Syphilis. Clin Dermatol 22:461–468, 2004.

3 ACQUIRED IMMUNE DEFICIENCY SYNDROME (AIDS) 090.9

Cristina Muccioli, MD, MBA
São Paulo, Brazil
Rubens Belfort, Jr., MD, PhD, MBA
São Paulo, Brazil

DEFINITION/ETIOLOGY

The acquired immune deficiency syndrome (AIDS) was first recognized in USA in 1981 as a newly infectious disease that became a global pandemic with the most devastating morbidity rate. The causative agent, known as human immunodeficiency virus (HIV) was first identified in 1983 and serologic tests for HIV antibodies were available in 1985.

HIV is a member of the lentivirus family. There are two types of HIV: Type 1 (worldwide) and Type 2 (west Africa). HIV is a human retrovirus with RNA genome with reverse transcriptase enzyme.

Three routes of human transmission of HIV have been described: sexual, blood-borne and mother-infant.

COURSE/PROGNOSIS

HIV has the ability to cause an insidious and progressive deterioration of the host's immune function, leading to profound immunossupression. Central to the immunopathogenesis of the HIV is its interaction with the CD4 molecule in the helper/inducer subset of T-lymphocytes. As CD4 T-lymphocytes play a key role in the induction of most immunologic responses, HIV-induced damage of the CD4 T lymphocyte population results in the abolition of a wide range of immune functions, ultimately leading to extreme immunosupression manifested by opportunistic infections and neoplasms pathognomonic for AIDS.

EPIDEMIOLOGY

The AIDS pandemic enters its 24th year and the total number of people living with the human immunodeficiency virus (HIV) rose in 2004 to reach its highest level ever: an estimated 39.4 million (35.9 million–44.3 million) people are living with the virus. From this total, 4.9 million (4.3 million–6.4 million) people acquired HIV in 2004. The global AIDS epidemic killed 3.1 million (2.8 million–3.5 million) people in the past year.

The number of people living with HIV has been rising in every region, compared with two years ago, with the steepest increases occurring in East Asia, and in Eastern Europe and Central Asia. The number of people living with HIV in East Asia rose by almost 50% between 2002 and 2004, an increase that is attributable largely to China's swiftly growing epidemic. In Eastern Europe and Central Asia, there were 40% more people living with HIV in 2004 than in 2002. Accounting for much of that trend is Ukraine's resurgent epidemic and the ever-growing number of people living with HIV in the Russian Federation.

Sub-Saharan Africa remains by far the worst-affected region, with 25.4 million (23.4 million–28.4 million) people living with HIV at the end of 2004, compared to 24.1 million (22.5 million–27.3 million) in 2002. Just under two thirds (64%) of all people living with HIV are in sub-Saharan Africa, as are more than three quarters (76%) of all women living with HIV.

The epidemics in sub-Saharan Africa appear to be stabilizing generally, with HIV prevalence at around 7.4% for the entire region. But such a summary perspective hides important aspects. First, roughly stable HIV prevalence means more or less equal numbers of people are being newly infected with HIV and are dying of AIDS. Beneath the apparent constancy of steady prevalence levels lie devastating realities-especially in southern Africa, which accounts for one third of all AIDS deaths globally. Second, the epidemics in Africa are diverse, both in terms of their scale and the pace at which they are evolving. There is no single 'African' epidemic. Some urban parts of East Africa display modest declines in HIV prevalence among pregnant women, while in West and Central Africa prevalence levels have stayed roughly steady at lower levels than in the rest of sub-Saharan Africa. National HIV data, though, hide much higher levels of infection in parts of countries, as Nigeria illustrates. Southern Africa, unfortunately, offers only slight hints of possible future declines in HIV prevalence.

The AIDS epidemic is affecting women and girls in increasing numbers. Globally, just under half of all people living with HIV are female. Women and girls make up almost 57% of all people infected with HIV in sub-Saharan Africa, where a striking 76% of young people (aged 15–24 years) living with HIV are female. In most other regions, women and girls represent an increasing proportion of people living with HIV, compared with five years ago.

DIAGNOSIS

HIV-infected individuals whose CD4 T lymphocyte count is less than 200 cells/mL is classified as having AIDS. The presence of one of the specified indicator diseases (e.g. cytomegalovirus diseases, encephalopathy, candidiasis, etc.) is also diagnostic of AIDS, regardless of the CD4 T-lymphocyte count.

Clinical signs and symptoms

An infectious mononucleosis-like syndrome (recognized as acute retroviral syndrome), develop in more than 50% of HIV-infected persons. This is observed 3 to 6 weeks after exposure and resolves spontaneously.

Laboratory findings

Detectable antibody to HIV develops in the overwhelming majority of infected individuals within 6 months of exposure. The enzyme-linked immunosorbent assay (ELISA) is used for screening. Western blot, immunofluorescent antibody studies, p24 antigens determinations, qualitative DNA PCR studies, viral cultures and other techniques are used to evaluate suspected false-positive and false-negative test results.

Ophthalmologic disorders

Until potent antiretroviral therapy (ART) became available, the most common retinal manifestation of immunodeficiency in advanced AIDS was CMV retinitis.

Retinitis is the most common manifestation of CMV disease in adult individuals with AIDS. Before the era of potent antiretroviral therapy (ART), 16.5% to 34% of HIV-infected individuals eventually had reactivation of latent infection and development of clinically apparent CMV end-organ disease.

Epidemiologic data regarding AIDS and CMV retinitis changed dramatically following the introduction of potent antiretroviral drugs (ARV) in the late 1990s. Several classes of antiretroviral drugs are currently available, including nucleoside reverse-transcriptase inhibitors, non-nucleoside reverse transcriptase inhibitors, and protease inhibitors; the latter target viral proteases involved in the assembly of new viral particles rather than the viral genome. Any combination of three or more antiretroviral drugs, or a combination containing one protease inhibitor and one non-nucleoside reverse transcriptase inhibitor, are considered ART.

The use of ART has been associated with reduced HIV replication and an increase in CD4+ T-lymphocyte counts, as well as a marked increase in survival. A reduced incidence of opportunistic infections, and a drop in newly diagnosed cases of CMV retinitis by 55% to more than 90%, were also observed.

Most improvements in immune function seem to occur during the first year following initiation of ART and long-term immune reconstitution may not be complete. Moreover, community-based studies reveal that only a low proportion of patients actually end up with undetectable HIV blood levels after 14 months of HAART and that virological failure (manifested as recurrence of elevated HIV blood levels) may occur in up to 44% of patients treated with protease inhibitor within the first 6 months following initiation of therapy.

Despite advances in immune reconstitution from ART, CMV retinitis remains the leading cause of blindness among patients with AIDS.

Vision loss is common in patients with AIDS and CMV retinitis and may result from the agressiveness of the retinitis itself or from the retinal detachment. The rate of retinal detachment in patients with CMV retinitis may vary from 15 to 29%, according to the literature.

The diagnosis of CMV retinitis is based on the clinical appearence of the retinal lesions. Typically, in the AIDS patients not receiving ART, the disease appears as a yellow to white area of retinal necrosis with hemorrhage and edema that follows a vascular distribution.

The retinitis is necrotizing, with white-yellowish areas, hemorrhage to variable degrees and vasculitis. Anterior chamber and vitreous inflammation is usually mild without formation of posterior synechiae. Retinitis may be unilateral or bilateral, but cases presenting with unilateral disease have a high risk of second eye involvement, probably due to hematogenic dissemination. Spontaneous remission was extremely rare before ART.

Three patterns of CMV retinitis are described: classical or hemorrhagic, granular and frosted branch angiitis.

The first, classical, pattern of CMV retinitis, called hemorrhagic, is characterized by retinal areas with a granular, whitish and hemorrhagic aspect, usually with lesions close to the vascular arcades or to the optic nerve, and subretinal exudation. The retinal vessels in the necrotic area may be sheathed by vasculitis and consequently present retinal vascular, specially venous, occlusions. Central healing of the lesions occurs after necrosis, leading to atrophy of the retina and choroid.

The second pattern of retinitis is the granular or atypical. The retina shows granular focal infiltrates which increases linearly and slowly, leaving areas of retinal destruction with an atrophic retinal pigmentary epithelium allowing observation of details of the choroid. Retinal hemorrhages and vitreous cells usually are absent in this retinitis pattern.

The third pattern, more rarely observed, associated or not with the classical, hemorrhagic form is characterized by severe vasculitis, with intense sheathing shown by arteries and veins, resembling frosted branch angiitis.

Symptoms of CMV retinitis are often poor and may include floaters, light flashes, loss of central or peripheral visual field, and blurred vision. Asymptomatic retinitis can be detected by ophthalmologic screening of HIV-infected persons at high risk.

Because of the unspecific and poor visual symptoms, patients with HIV infection should be educated about the symptoms of CMV retinitis and advised to seek care in a timely manner after the onset of visual symptoms. Many experts recommend that patients at high risk should have ophthalmologic screening every 3 to 6 months depending on the CD4 count levels. In general, ophthalmologic examinations should be performed immediately before therapy is initiated, at the end of the induction (or reinduction) therapy, and monthly thereafter.

The recent availability of several new modalities of therapy for CMV retinitis provides a number of appropriate treatment options.

Since 1989, with the release of ganciclovir for endovenous use, the natural history of the disease changed. Foscarnet, in 1991, was approved for endovenous use and more recently, in 1996, another antiviral, cidofovir, was approved.

All are virostatic and, when applied endovenously, cause important side effects: neutropenia for ganciclovir and renal toxicity for foscarnet and cidofovir. Before the ART era, treatment with any of the drugs had to be given initially as an induction (twice a day) dose for 2 to 3 weeks and then, a maintenance (once a day) dose for the rest of the life of the patient, leading to a significant worsening in the quality of life.

Ganciclovir has poor oral bioavailability and oral ganciclovir, 3000 mg/day, is less effective than the IV form as a maintenance regimen but higher doses (4500 or 6000 mg/day) are approximately as effective as IV therapy.

A new drug named Valcyte (valganciclovir) that is a prodrug of ganciclovir was developed for the treatment of cytomegalovirus (CMV) retinitis in patients with AIDS. Oral valganciclovir 900 mg provides a daily exposure of ganciclovir comparable to that of intravenous ganciclovir 5 mg/kg. The most common adverse events related to valgancyclovir is neutropenia.

Local therapies (intraocular injections and intraocular implants) are efficient in CMV retinitis treatment. Indications include patients which are not able to receive intravenous therapy and as supplement in patients whose retinal disease is not completely controlled using maximum tolerated systemic medication. Maybe the best use for local therapy is in association with oral antivirals forms.

Intraocular injections of ganciclovir or foscarnet, weekly or twice-weekly through a small-gauge needle have appeared to slow the progression of retinitis in uncontrolled case series conducted primarily in patients who cannot tolerate systemic therapy or in whom retinitis had progressed despite attempts at systemic therapy.

The intravitreal ganciclovir implant is a pellet of ganciclovir to be implanted into the vitreous cavity without systemic absorption, drug interactions or side effects. This way for delivering drug into the eye could be more effective to better control of the retinitis. The majority of adverse events are retinal detachments; major intravitreous bleeding and rarely endophthalmitis.

The recent availability of ART are changing the incidence, clinical presentation, and course of CMV disease, at least temporarily.

The effectiveness of ART should not lull the medical community into the perception that CMV end-organ disease will disappear. Although the incidence of CMV retinitis are decreasing, patients may develop CMV disease prior to initiating antiretroviral therapy or before its full benefit is achieved (Figure 3.1.).

Differential diagnosis

Acute retinal necrosis

Acute retinal necrosis (ARN) syndrome represents a specific pattern of clinical presentations for certain herpes virus infections in the posterior segment of the eye. These include varicella zoster virus and herpes simplex virus 2. Patients with ARN usually complain of mild to moderate ocular or periorbital pain, foreign body sensation and red eye. Visual symptoms usually include hazy vision, floaters, and, rarely, decreased peripheral vision. Granulomatous keratic precipitates, cells, and

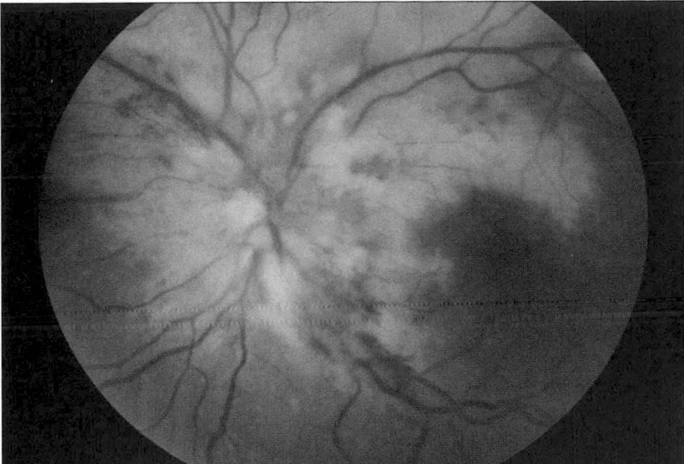

FIGURE 3.1 CMV retinitis (hemorrhagic pattern).

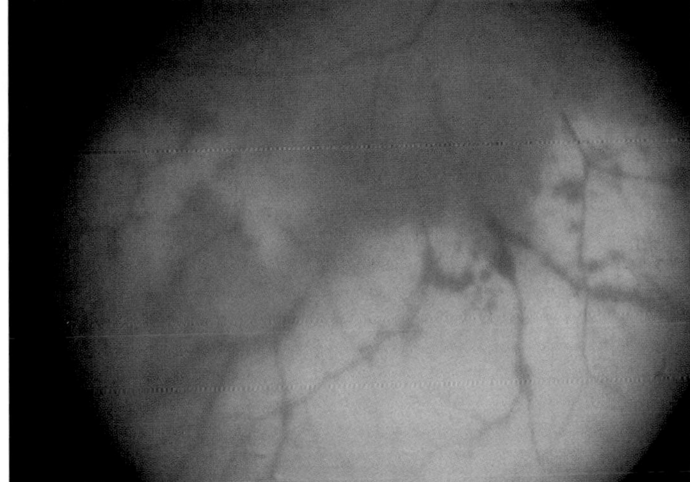

FIGURE 3.2 Acute retinal necrosis in AIDS.

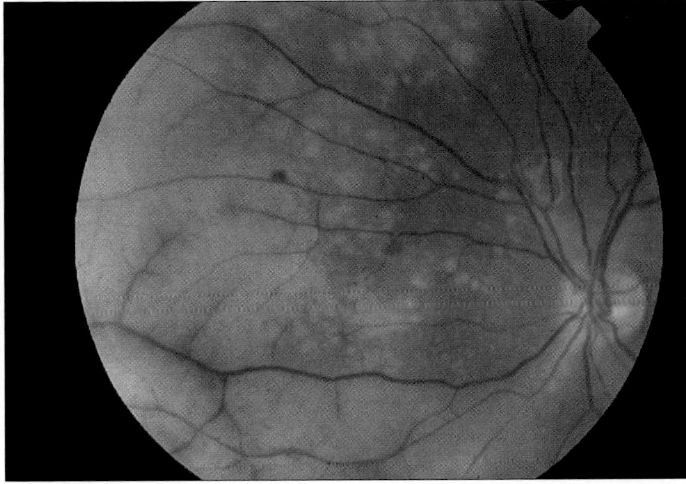

FIGURE 3.3 Progressive outer retinal necrosis.

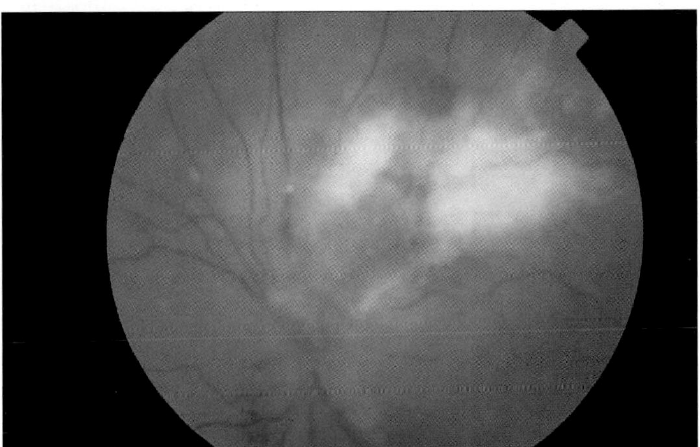

FIGURE 3.4 Toxoplasmic lesion in AIDS.

flare in the anterior chamber as well as elevated intraocular pressure and an increasing number of vitreous cells are observed.

The initial retinitis consists of the round or oval deep, yellow-white lesions at the level of the retinal pigment epithelium or deep retina in the postequitorial fundus, typically sparing the macula area. The retinitis may remain limited to less than one quadrant of involvement, may involve multiple peripheral quadrants of the retina, or may become confluent in the periphery. Vitritis increases, sometimes limiting visualization of the fundus in severe cases. An exsudative retinal detachment occasionally develops in the inferior periphery. Medical treatment of choice is IV aciclovir. Retinal detachment is the most common cause of vision loss in patients with ARN, occurring in 24 to 80% of the cases. If retinal detachment is present, vitrectomy with endolaser, internal drainage of subretinal fluid, air-fluid exchange and silicone oil tamponade are recommended (Figure 3.2.).

Progressive outer retinal necrosis (PORN) syndrome

Progressive outer retinal necrosis (PORN) syndrome is a form of the varicella zoster virus (VZV) chorioretinitis found almost exclusively in people with the acquired immunodeficiency syndrome (AIDS). This destructive infection has an extremely rapid course that may lead to no light perception in affected eyes within days or weeks. Attempts at its treatment have had limited success. Rhegmatogenous retinal detachments often occur after the development of atrophic retinal holes, and silicone oil temponade has been found to be the most successful reattachment procedure (Figure 3.3.).

Ocular toxoplasmosis

In HIV-infected patients, toxoplasmosis is the most common cause of non-viral central nervous system infection leading to toxoplasmic encephalitis. Ocular toxoplasmic lesions can be more severe and aggressive than the ones observed in immunocompetent individuals. Ocular toxoplasmosis occurs in 1–2% of patients with AIDS in the US and in 8–10% of AIDS patients in Brazil.

Toxoplasmic retinochoroiditis is a serious disorder in HIV-infected patients and in other immunosuppressed individuals such as cancer patients or organ transplant recipients. It is generally more severe than in immunocompetent patients, with a broader range of clinical features.

Ocular toxoplasmosis in immunosuppressed patients can be single lesions, multifocal lesions in one or both eyes, and broad areas of retinal necrosis.

Although the majority of reported cases in HIV-infected patients have been unilateral, it is not uncommon to see bilateral cases.

In cases with full-thickness necrosis, the retina appears to have a hard, 'indurated' appearance, with sharply demarcated borders. There is usually little retinal hemorrhage within the lesion itself.

A prominent inflammatory reaction in the vitreous body and anterior chamber has been described in several reports of HIV-associated ocular toxoplasmosis.

Lesions will continue to enlarge without treatment, which probably explains the fact that most reported patients have had extensive areas of retinal necrosis by the time diagnosis is made.

In most reported cases of ocular toxoplasmosis in immunosuppressed patients, there have not been pre-existing scars.

Infection of the iris with *T. gondii* has been reported in a patient with AIDS. (Figure 3.4.)

REFERENCES

Arruda RF, Muccioli C, Belfort R, Jr: Ophthalmological findings in HIV infected patients in the post-HAART (Highly Active Anti-retroviral Therapy) era, compared to the pre-HAART era. Rev Assoc Med Bras 50(2):148–152, 2004. Epub 2004 Jul 21.

Belfort R, Jr: The ophthalmologist and the global impact of the AIDS epidemic. LV Edward Jackson Memorial Lecture. Am J Ophthalmol 129(1):1–8, 2000.

Campo RE, Lalanne R, Tanner TJ, et al: Lopinavir/ritonavir maintenance monotherapy after successful viral suppression with standard highly active antiretroviral therapy in HIV-1-infected patients.

d'Arminio Monforte A, Sabin CA, Phillips A, et al: The Antiretroviral Therapy Cohort Collaboration. The changing incidence of AIDS events in patients receiving highly active antiretroviral therapy. Arch Intern Med 165(4):416–423, 2005.

Jabs DA, Van Natta ML, Thorne JE, et al: Studies of Ocular Complications of AIDS Research Group. Course of cytomegalovirus retinitis in the era of highly active antiretroviral therapy: 2. Second eye involvement and retinal detachment. Ophthalmology 111(12):2232–2239, 2004.

Jabs DA, Van Natta ML, Thorne JE, et al: Studies of Ocular Complications of AIDS Research Group. Course of cytomegalovirus retinitis in the era of highly active antiretroviral therapy: 1. Retinitis progression. Ophthalmology 111(12):2224–2231, 2004.

Jabs DA: AIDS and ophthalmology in 2004. Arch Ophthalmol 122(7):1040–1042, 2004.

Muccioli C, Belfort R, Jr: Treatment of cytomegalovirus retinitis with an intraocular sustained-release ganciclovir implant. Braz J Med Biol Res 33(7):779–789, 2000.

Nguyen QD, Kempen JH, Bolton SG, et al: Immune recovery uveitis in patients with AIDS and cytomegalovirus retinitis after highly active antiretroviral therapy. Am J Ophthalmol 129(5):634–639, 2000.

UNAIDS: 2004 Report on the global AIDS epidemic. Geneva, UNAIDS, 2004.

Vrabec TR: Posterior segment manifestations of HIV/AIDS. Surv Ophthalmol 49(2):131–157, 2004.

4 ACUTE HEMORRHAGIC CONJUNCTIVITIS 077.4

(Epidemic Hemorrhagic Conjunctivitis, Apollo 11 Disease)

Niteen S. Wairagkar, MD
Pune, India

Acute hemorrhagic conjunctivitis (AHC), also known as epidemic hemorrhagic conjunctivitis and Apollo 11 disease, is a relatively new disease entity. However, a similar eye disease occurring on ships was reported in 1819.

EPIDEMIOLOGY

First reported in 1969 in Ghana, AHC, spreading very fast across the continents, became pandemic in Africa, Southeast Asia, and Japan by the 1970s. Since then pandemics of AHC have been reported in 1981, 1986–1988, 1994–1996, and 2002–2003 from various countries. Though the magnitude of each outbreak could not be assessed properly, the 2003 outbreak in Puerto Rico reported 490,000 persons with conjunctivitis. A few infections (4–20%) may be asymptomatic. AHC, affecting all age groups, causes economic loss due to absenteeism. Outbreaks are reported with mass movement of populations (e.g. refugees, pilgrims, etc.). Overcrowding, low socioeconomic status and poor sanitation, favors the transmission of the disease.

ETIOLOGY

AHC is mainly caused by enterovirus-70 and coxsackie A 24 virus, though adenoviruses are also reported to be associated. Evolutionary analysis of EV-70 and CA24v, using the nucleotide sequence, indicates that the two viruses branched off from the prototype strain in 1984 in Taiwan. In 2002–2003 outbreaks of AHC, the virus strains were isolated from China, which on sequencing were identified as novel, unclassified human enteroviruses. Viruses responsible for AHC have been isolated from infected humans only with no animal reservoir being implicated. However, animals may play a role in maintaining the natural cycle during an interepidemic period.

DIAGNOSIS

Clinical signs and symptoms

After a short incubation period of 24 to 48 hours, patients experience an explosive onset of symptoms, like ocular irritation, foreign body sensation, and periorbital pain. Full-blown conjunctivitis involving both eyes develops within hours with lid edema, chemosis, seromucous discharge, photophobia, excessive lacrimation, and subconjunctival hemorrhages in bulbar and palpebral conjunctiva. Pre-auricular lymphadenopathy with variable tenderness is present. Moderate follicular hypertrophy, diffuse epithelial keratitis, a transient low-grade iritis may also be present. Mild corneal ulceration after an episode of AHC has also been reported. Systemic symptoms are rare. In some cases respiratory disturbances accompanied the eye signs. Neurological complications like facial palsy, cranial nerve involvement, lumbosacral radiculomyelitis, and polio-like motor paralysis have been reported after episodes of AHC. In a series of patients (21–55 years) in Taiwan, radicular pains and acute flaccid paralysis developed within 5–37 days after the onset of AHC. Permanent incapacitation due to paralysis and muscular atrophy in the affected proximal muscles of the lower limbs was the main sequela in severe cases. Involvement of the meninges, cranial nerves and the white matter of the cord were observed in a few patients. Mortality due to AHC has not been reported.

TREATMENT

Ocular

Topical broad-spectrum antibiotics, such as 10% sulfacetamide eye drops, four times daily, may be used to prevent secondary bacterial infection. Use of topical corticosteroids may predispose an already compromised cornea to develop microbial keratitis and such practice should be discouraged. In the majority of patients, infection is short in duration, self-limiting, and free of significant ocular sequelae.

PREVENTIVE MEASURES

AHC is transmitted mainly by infected eye-to-hand-to-eye contact. Fomites, contaminated instruments, public washing facilities and swimming pools may be implicated in transmission. Careful hand washing, sterilization of ophthalmic instruments, avoiding contact with infected patients may prevent the transmission.

COMMENTS

AHC is an extremely contagious, symptomatic and highly visible ocular disease that occurs in epidemics. Prolonged visual disability does not occur and patients recover with remarkably few sequelae. Because of the relatively benign course of the disease, over treatment with topical antibiotics and corticosteroids should be avoided.

REFERENCES

Asbell PA, de la Pena W, Harms D, et al: Acute hemorrhagic conjunctivitis in central America: first enterovirus epidemic in the western hemisphere. Ann Ophthalmol 17:205–209, 1985.

Centers for Disease Control and Prevention (CDC): Acute hemorrhagic conjunctivitis outbreak caused by coxsackievirus A24–Puerto Rico, 2003. Morb Mortal Wkly Rep 53(28):632–634, 2004.

Dalapathy S, Lily TK, Madhavan HN: Development and use of nested polymerase chain reaction for identification of adenovirus from conjunctivitis. J Clin Virol 11:77–84, 1998.

Dussart P, Cartet G, Huguet P, et al: Outbreak of acute hemorrhagic conjunctivitis in French Guiana and West Indies caused by coxsackievirus A24 variant: phylogenetic analysis reveals Asian import. J Med Virol 75(4):559–565, 2005.

Hung TP, Sung SM, Liang HC, et al: Radiculomyelitis following acute haemorrhagic conjunctivitis. Brain 99(4):771–790, 1976.

Kew OM, Nottay BK, Hatch MH, et al: Oligonucleotide fingerprint analysis of enterovirus 70 isolates from the 1980 to 1981 pandemic of acute hemorrhagic conjunctivitis: evidence for a close genetic relationship among Asian and American strains. Infect Immun 41(2):631–635, 1983.

Kono R: Apollo 11 disease or acute hemorrhagic conjunctivitis: a pandemic of a new enterovirus infection of the eyes. Am J Epidem 101(5):383–390, 1975.

Kono R, Miyamura K, Tajiri E, et al: Neurologic complications associated with acute hemorrhagic conjunctivitis virus infection and its serologic confirmation. J Infect Dis 129(5):590–593, 1974.

Lin KH, Takeda N, Miyamura K, et al: The nucleotide sequence of 3c proteinase region of the coxsackievirus A24 variant: comparison of the isolates in Taiwan in 1985–1988. Virus Genes 5:121–131, 1991.

Lu YY, Yan JY, Feng Q, et al: A novel enterovirus associated with acute hemorrhagic conjunctivitis. Complete genome data. NCBI-GenBank Accession numbers: AY876913, AY876912. Online. Available at: http://www.ncbi.nlm.nih.gov, 29 Apr 2005.

Park SW, Lee CS, Jang HC, et al: Rapid identification of the coxsackievirus A24 variant by molecular serotyping in an outbreak of acute hemorrhagic conjunctivitis. J Clin Microbiol 43(3):1069–1071, 2005.

Wadia NH, Irani PF, Katrak SM: Neurological complications of a new type of conjunctivitis. Lancet 1:350–352, 1973.

Wairagkar NS, Gogate SS, Labhsetwar AS: Investigation of an epidemic of acute haemorrhagic conjunctivitis in Pune, India. J Commun Dis 31(1):41–43, 1999.

5 ASPERGILLOSIS 117.3

Mark D. Sherman, MD

Anaheim Hills, California

Aspergillosis is a generic term indicating infection by a member of the saprophytic fungus *Aspergillus*. Approximately 21 of the 900 species and subspecies of *Aspergillus* have been associated with human disease. *Aspergillus* spp. are commonly isolated from soil, vegetation, grains, airway systems and decaying organic matter. The spectrum of human disease caused by *Aspergillus* spp. includes allergic reactions, colonization of debilitated tissue without invasion, invasive destruction of specific organs and disseminated disease. Infection most commonly results from inhalation of spores. The respiratory system is the most common site of infection. Disseminated aspergillosis may involve the skin, central nervous system, brain, kidney and bone. Less common manifestations of aspergillosis include otomycosis, corneal ulcers, endophthalmitis and naso-orbital disease.

ETIOLOGY/INCIDENCE

Aspergillus fungi can be found in most parts of the world. Aspergillosis is a major cause of fungal infection in both tropical and temperate climates. Infection is more common in individuals where contamination is more likely, such as with grain farmers and breeders of poultry. Orbital involvement is most commonly a result of spread from the paranasal sinuses. Corneal involvement requires direct inoculation such as occurs during ophthalmic surgery or occurs as a complication of contact lens wear or other local insult. Corneal involvement is more likely in individuals with compromised ocular defenses or pre-existing corneal disease. Keratomycosis caused by *Aspergillus* spp. accounts for almost 50% of all reported cases of oculomycosis. Endogenous *Aspergillus* endophthalmitis is associated with disseminated *Aspergillus*. Individuals at greatest risk are those who are intravenous drug abusers, immunosuppressed, or recipients of organ transplants. *Aspergillus* causes an occlusive vasculitis in the retina and choroid. Hyphae can penetrate the walls of the blood vessels to infect contiguous structures such as the vitreous and sclera.

COURSE/PROGNOSIS

The therapy of *Aspergillus* infections is often complicated by a delay in diagnosis, the previous use of corticosteroids and the long-term use of antifungal medications. Aspergillosis requires intensive and aggressive treatment. Orbital aspergillosis has a poor prognosis for maintaining useful vision and a poor prognosis for life. Despite extensive debridement and antifungal treatment, *Aspergillus* spp. can reappear in previously involved tissues, especially when vascular invasion has occurred. The prognosis for *Aspergillus* endophthalmitis is similarly poor. Successfully treated *Aspergillus* keratomycosis may require later penetrating keratoplasty for visual rehabilitation.

DIAGNOSIS

Clinical signs and symptoms (ocular and periocular)

Eyelid

Lid edema may occur in association with deeper orbital involvement. A local chronic ulcerative granuloma may occur with direct inoculation.

Conjunctive

Chemosis occurs with orbital involvement. Conjunctivitis may occur with *Aspergillus* canaliculitis.

Cornea

Aspergillus keratomycosis may present with a foreign body sensation, pain, redness and decreased vision. The eye is usually severely inflamed. There may be a central or paracentral corneal abscess, diffuse keratitis and satellite lesions. There commonly is an intense anterior chamber reaction with hypopyon.

Lacrimal system

Canaliculitis, dacryocystitis and dacryoadenitis can occur.

Sclera

Scleritis is rare but may progress to perforation.

Orbit

Patients may present with slowly progressive, unilateral proptosis with or without pain. Later signs include decreased vision and changes in ocular motility. An orbital granuloma or abscess may form. Optic atrophy due to vascular compromise in the orbital apex has been reported.

Uveal tract

Multifocal choroiditis associated with vitreous cells and retinal vasculitis can occur.

Endophthalmitis

Patients may present with decreased vision, pain, and photophobia. Clinical signs include anterior chamber cells, hypopyon, vitreous cells or snowball opacities, serous or exudative retinal detachment, posterior ischemic optic neuropathy and central retinal artery occlusion.

Laboratory findings

- *Aspergillus* keratitis: six to eight scrapings with a Kimura spatula from the bed of the infection are needed for culture.
- In cases of suspected intraocular *Aspergillus*, intravitreal and anterior chamber aspirates should be concentrated by the use of a filter or by centrifugation before plating.
- Orbital biopsy material should be plated soon after collection because *Aspergillus* is a ubiquitous organism and false-positive results could occur if the specimen remains unnecessarily exposed.
- Gram's, Giemsa, and GMS stains are better than KOH stains for detecting the branching septated hyphae that are typical of *Aspergillus* spp.
- Either Sabouraud's media (Emmon's modification) or blood agar will usually be positive within 48 hours.
- Blood cultures are routinely negative, even in fulminant cases.

Differential diagnosis

- Fungal infection: *Candida, Fusarium, Mucor, Coccidioides, Blastomyces* and others depending on geographic location and risk factors.
- Bacterial infection: orbital cellulitis, subperiosteal abscess, syphilis, *M. tuberculosis*, or atypical mycobacteria.
- Orbital inflammatory disease: orbital pseudotumor, Graves' ophthalmopathy, sarcoidosis, Wegener's granulomatosis, idiopathic sclerosing orbititis, polyarteritis nodosa, other collagen-vascular disorders.
- Neoplasm: metastases, lacrimal gland tumor, lymphoma, leukemia.
- Vascular disease: carotid-cavernous fistula, cavernous sinus thrombosis, varix.

TREATMENT

Systemic

- Systemic treatment should be prescribed in coordination with consultation from an infectious disease subspecialist.
- Amphotericin B (0.5 to 1.5 mg/kg/day) has been the mainstay of systemic therapy for disseminated aspergillosis. Amphotericin B has substantial and varied toxicity, which can limit its use. Newer therapies are now becoming available.
- Itraconazole (200 to 600 mg/day) has been reported to show effectiveness in some cases in which amphotericin B failed.
- The combination of amphotericin B with flucytosine (100 to 200 mg/kg/day) or rifampin (600 mg b.i.d.) has been reported to improve the clinical response.
- Other azole antifungal agents (fluconazole, miconazole, ketoconazole) have shown less effectiveness in the treatment of aspergillosis.
- The use of systemic steroids is controversial. They may be necessary in cases of visual loss and proptosis but should not be used until effective antifungal therapy has been started.

Local

- Natamycin (5% suspension) is the only commercially available topical formulation for the treatment of ocular aspergillosis (keratomycosis). It is effective for superficial corneal infections but less effective for deep stromal infection.
- Topical amphotericin B (0.05% to 0.15% eyedrops prepared from the intravenous formulation) can be used for cases of deeper keratomycosis or cases refractory to natamycin.
- Subconjunctival injection of amphotericin B (1 mg) has been described but may be associated with significant local toxicity.
- Successful therapy requires frequent and prolonged administration of medication. Hourly eyedrops may be necessary

for the first 2 to 7 days and then tapered over the course of several weeks.

- Topical steroids have been associated with the progression of keratomycosis.
- Intravitreal amphotericin B (5 to 10 μg) has been used for the treatment of *Aspergillus* endophthalmitis. A repeat injection may be necessary if persistence of organisms is suspected 2 to 7 days after initial injection.
- The use of intravitreal steroids is controversial. Intravitreal dexamethasone (400 μg) as an adjunct to intravitreal amphotericin B has been described.

Surgical

- Mechanical debridement of the fungal growth allows better penetration of antifungal medications.
- A penetrating keratoplasty may be required in cases of keratomycosis refractory to medical therapy. A lamellar keratoplasty is contraindicated.
- A vitrectomy may be necessary for treatment of intraocular *Aspergillus* infection.
- Orbital aspergillosis is a life-threatening condition. Prompt orbital debridement combined with systemic medical therapy is necessary.

REFERENCES

Bennett JE: *Aspergillus* species. In: Mandell GL, Bennett JE, Dolin R, eds: Mandell, Douglas, and Bennett's principles and practice of infectious diseases. 4th edn. New York, Churchill Livingstone, 1995, vol 2.

Foster CS: Fungal keratitis. Infect Dis Clin North Am 6:851–857, 1992.

Gassry GG, Hornblass A, Harrison W: Itraconazole in the treatment of orbital aspergillosis. Ophthalmology 103:1467–1470, 1996.

Hunt KE, Glasgow BJ: *Aspergillus* endophthalmitis: an unrecognized endemic disease in orthotopic liver transplantation. Ophthalmology 103:757–767, 1996.

Levin LA, Avery R, Shore JW, et al: The spectrum of orbital aspergillosis: a clinicopathological review. Surv Ophthalmol 41:142–154, 1996.

Rao NA, Hidayat AA: Endogenous mycotic endophthalmitis: variations in clinical and histopathologic changes in candidiasis compared with aspergillosis. Am J Ophthalmol 132:244–251, 2001.

Weishaar PD, Flynn HW, Murray TG, et al: Endogenous aspergillus endophthalmitis: clinical features and treatment outcomes. Ophthalmology 105:57–65, 1998.

6 BACILLUS SPECIES INFECTIONS 041.8

Franco M. Recchia, MD
Nashville, Tennessee
Sean P. Donahue, MD, PhD
Nashville, Tennessee
Denis M. O'Day, MD
Nashville, Tennessee

Bacillus is a genus of nearly ubiquitous, aerobic, gram-positive, spore-forming rods increasingly recognized as a cause of ocular infection. The species *B. cereus*, *B. anthracis*, *B. subtilis*, *B. lichenformis*, *B. thurigiensis* and *B. circulans* have all been reported to cause ocular infection, most importantly a rapidly progressive and devastating endophthalmitis. *Bacillus* is the most common cause of posttraumatic endophthalmitis occurring in the rural setting. It usually enters the eye as a result of penetrating trauma with a contaminated foreign body, although it can also occur following intraocular surgery or as a metastatic infection related to intravenous drug use. Most cases of *Bacillus* endophthalmitis result in extremely poor visual outcomes. Many patients require enucleation or evisceration. *Bacillus* species are usually resistant to penicillins and cephalosporins but are sensitive to vancomycin, clindamycin, and fourth-generation fluoroquinolones (e.g. levofloxacin and gatifloxacin).

Infection with *B. cereus* typically causes a rapid and fulminant endophthalmitis, which may progress to panophthalmitis, often accompanied by fever and leukocytosis. Characteristically, a ring abscess of the cornea develops in 24 to 48 hours after infection. At this point, however, the infection is usually well established and portends an extremely poor prognosis for the return of vision. The severe ocular damage caused by *B. cereus* seems to be due to endotoxins.

ETIOLOGY/INCIDENCE

- Penetrating ocular trauma, usually in a rural setting.
- Contamination of contact lenses or solutions.
- Low-grade chronic endophthalmitis following cataract surgery (*B. circulans*).
- Intravenous drug use or immune compromise.

COURSE/PROGNOSIS

- Fulminant panophthalmitis.
- Acute onset in 12 to 48 hours.
- Postoperative retinal detachments.
- Phthisis, no light perception vision, and enucleation are extremely common.

DIAGNOSIS

Clinical signs and symptoms

- Corneal ring infiltrate, diffuse sub-epithelial infiltrates.
- Hypopyon.
- Vitritis.
- Systemic infection (fever, leukocytosis).

Laboratory findings

- Gram-positive rod on Gram stain.

Differential diagnosis

- Endophthalmitis caused by other organisms. Other leading causes of postoperative and traumatic endophthalmitis include coagulase-negative staphylococcal and streptococcal species. Chronic, low-grade post-surgical endophthalmitis is commonly caused by *Propionobacterium acnes*.
- Ring abscess secondary to *Pseudomonas aeruginosa* or *Proteus* species.

PROPHYLAXIS

- The only prophylaxis is prevention of the injury; thus, the use of protective eyewear cannot be overemphasized.

TREATMENT

A high index of suspicion and prompt institution of appropriate treatment are crucial to any chance of salvaging vision in cases of *Bacillus* endophthalmitis. Treatment consists of antibiotics (intravitreal, topical, possibly systemic) and vitrectomy surgery. Due to the accelerated and aggressive course of *B. cereus* endophthalmitis, vitreous tap with antibiotic injection alone is not recommended.

- Local therapy: fortified topical antibiotics (vancomycin HCl 50 mg/mL alternating hourly with fortified gentamicin 13 mg/mL); consider topical or subconjunctival corticosteroids.
- Intravitreal: vancomycin (1.0 mg in 0.1 cc injection).
- Systemic: Vancomycin, 1 g/day IV every 12 hours; clindamycin 40 mg/kg/day IV in divided doses; gentamicin 3–5 mg/kg/day IV in divided doses. (The fourth-generation fluoroquinolones levofloxacin and gatifloxacin achieve vitreous concentrations above the minimum inhibitory concentration (MIC90) for *Bacillus cereus*. However, their use as monotherapy for intraocular infection is not recommended.)
- Surgical: pars plana vitrectomy with intravitreal injection of vancomycin.

COMPLICATIONS

Ocular complications consist of the typical devastating visual outcome. Of 83 eyes reported on before 1996 with posttraumatic *Bacillus* endophthalmitis, 62 (75%) became phthisical, were enucleated, or had no light perception vision. The vast majority of the remaining cases had light perception vision. Foster and colleagues recently reported on five patients with *Bacillus* endophthalmitis who maintained acuities ranging from 20/25 to 20/200. All presented within 32 hours of injury and had vitrectomy within 48 hours of injury; all except one received intravitreal vancomycin. Retinal detachment, caused either by the acute injury or by associated intraocular inflammation, is common.

COMMENTS

The best hope of salvaging eyes infected with *Bacillus* lies with early diagnosis and prompt treatment; thus, penetrating trauma with a metallic foreign body or that occurring in a rural setting should always suggest the possibility of infection by this organism. Intravenous drug abuse is also an important risk factor for metastatic endophthalmitis caused by this organism. Fever and leukocytosis occurring with a fulminant endophthalmitis are especially suggestive of *Bacillus* spp. because most other organisms causing endophthalmitis do not typically produce systemic signs. When *Bacillus* spp. are suspected, an immediate diagnostic and therapeutic vitrectomy is indicated, with antibiotic therapy being initiated before surgery if an undue delay is anticipated. Intravitreal, intravenous, and topical antibiotics are important if vision is to be salvaged. Although the prognosis is extremely poor, retention of useful vision is possible.

REFERENCES

Boldt HC, Pulido JS, Blodi CF, et al: Rural endophthalmitis. Ophthalmology 96:1722–1726, 1989.

Chen JC, Roy M: Epidemic *Bacillus* endophthalmitis after cataract surgery II: chronic and recurrent presentation and outcome. Ophthalmology 107(6):1038–1041, 2000.

Donzis PB, Mondino BJ, Weissman BA: *Bacillus* keratitis associated with contaminated contact lens care systems. Am J Ophthlmol 105(2):195–197, 1988.

Drobniewski FA: *Bacillus cereus* and related species. Clin Microbiol Rev 6:324–338, 1993.

Essex RW, Yi Q, Charles PG, Allen PJ: Post-traumatic endophthalmitis. Ophthalmology 111(11):2015–2022, 2004.

Foster RE, Martinez JA, Murray TG, et al: Useful visual outcomes after treatment of *Bacillus cereus* endophthalmitis. Ophthalmol 103:390–397, 1996.

Shamsuddin D, Tuazon CU, Levy C, Curtin J: *Bacillus cereus* panophthalmitis: source of the organism. Rev Infect Dis 4:97–103, 1982.

Vahey JB, Flynn Jr HW: Results in the management of *Bacillus* endophthalmitis. Ophthalmic Surgery 22(11):681–686, 1991.

7 BLASTOMYCOSIS 116.0

Jeffrey D. Horn, MD
Nashville, Tennessee

Blastomycosis is an acute or a chronic systemic, potentially life-threatening fungal disease characterized by granulomatous lesions that may involve any part of the body, with a predilection for the lungs, skin and bones. With the exception of eyelid involvement, ocular disease is exceedingly rare. There are reported cases, however, of keratitis, endophthalmitis, choroiditis and orbital disease.

ETIOLOGY/INCIDENCE

- The causative organism is *Blastomyces dermatitidis*, a thermally dimorphic fungus that exists in the mycelial phase at 25°C and in the yeast phase at 37°C.
- Most cases are endemic and occur in the Ohio and Mississippi River Valleys, where the organism has been found in soil.
- Annual incidence is about 4 per 100,000 population in endemic areas with a male predominance.
- Initial infection is usually from inhalation of spores resulting in pulmonary disease, although percutaneous inoculation has rarely been reported.

COURSE/PROGNOSIS

- Pulmonary disease ranges from asymptomatic (up to 50%) to severe pneumonia and may resolve spontaneously. Acute disease resembles influenza or pneumonia symptomatically. Most diagnosed with blastomycosis have chronic pneumonia.
- Extrapulmonary disease results from hematogenous dissemination. It may occur during or after the pulmonary phase.

- The skin is the most common extrapulmonary site affected (80%), followed by bone (25% to 50%), genitourinary system (about 10% in men), and central nervous system (5% to 10%).
- The eyelid has been reported to be affected in 25% of cases, although the recent literature suggests a much lower incidence.
- Ophthalmic manifestations:
  - Eyelid: granulomas, cicatricial ectropion;
  - Conjunctiva: rare granulomas either contiguous or non-contiguous with corneal involvement;
  - Cornea: ulcer, perforation;
  - Choroiditis;
  - Orbit: cellulites;
  - Endophthalmitis/panophthalmitis.

DIAGNOSIS

- Skin lesion is usually papular with a verrucous border and an atrophic center.
- Extravasation of erythrocytes between the dermis and epidermis gives rise to multiple black dots that are characteristic of the disease.
- Culture is the definitive method of diagnosis, but can take up to 30 days.
- Broad-based budding yeast forms (8 to 15 μm) with double-contoured walls are seen best with periodic acid-Schiff and Gomori methenamine silver stains. Chemiluminescent DNA probes are available.

Differential diagnosis

- Tuberculosis.
- Staphylococcal infection.
- Squamous cell carcinoma.
- Leprosy.
- Cryptococcosis, and other deep mycoses.

TREATMENT

Systemic

- Amphotericin B is the treatment of choice for life-threatening disease. The initial intravenous dose is 5 mg, increasing slowly to 50 mg three times per week until a total dose of 2 to 2.5 g is reached.
- Itraconazole, an oral triazole antifungal agent, has been shown to be as effective as amphotericin B for non-life-threatening disease, excluding CNS involvement, without the severe toxic reactions associated with amphotericin B. The dose is 200 to 400 mg/day for 6 months.
- Ketoconazole, an imidazole that also is administered orally, is slightly less efficacious and less well tolerated than itraconazole. It also is much less expensive. The dose is 200 to 800 mg/day for 6 months.
- Fluconazole, another oral triazole antifungal agent, appears to be as efficacious at 400 to 800 mg/day for 6 months as ketoconazole and may be an alternative for patients who are intolerant of itraconazole. More studies are necessary.

Topical

- Topical therapy may be indicated in conjunction with systemic therapy for corneal involvement.
- Topical amphotericin B can be prepared by diluting an intravenous solution to a concentration of 0.15%. Optimal dosing frequency is not known.
- Miconazole is tolerated by subconjunctival injection at a daily dose of 5 mg of the undiluted intravenous preparation. It may be administered topically as a 1% solution and given every hour.

Surgical

- Surgical drainage of lid or orbit abscesses may be needed in addition to antifungal treatment.
- Penetrating or lamellar keratoplasty is indicated in cases of corneal perforation or scarring.

COMPLICATIONS

- Systemic amphotericin B toxicity can cause fever, chills, hypokalemia, renal failure, and anemia.
- Itraconazole toxicity is relatively uncommon but can cause nausea, vomiting, impotence and elevated plasma aminotransferase levels. Itraconazole requires an acid pH for absorption; therefore, patients on antacids or H_2 receptor blockers may have reduced plasma levels.
- Ketoconazole toxicity can cause nausea, vomiting, and testicular and adrenal dysfunction; fatal hepatocellular damage is rare.

SUMMARY

Blastomycosis requires systemic therapy, but for less severe or non-life-threatening disease, newer, safer, more convenient, and equally effective treatment modalities are available. Ocular infection is so rare that the most appropriate therapy remains an unanswered question. Experience with infection in other tissues indicates that treatment should be given for a prolonged period. When there is corneal involvement, consideration should be given to the topical administration of miconazole in combination with systemic therapy.

REFERENCES

Barr CC, Gamel JW: Blastomycosis of the eyelid. Arch Ophthalmol 104:96–97, 1986.

Bartley GB: Blastomycosis of the eyelid. Ophthalmology 102:2020–2023, 1995.

Dismukes WE, Bradsher RW, Cloud GC, et al: Itraconazole therapy for blastomycosis and histoplasmosis. Am J Med 93:489–497, 1992.

Johns KJ, O'Day DM: Pharmacologic management of keratomycoses. Surv Ophthalmol 33:178–188, 1988.

Pappas PG, Bradsher RW, Kauffman CA, et al: Treatment of blastomycosis with higher doses of fluconazole. Clin Infect Dis 25:200–205, 1997.

Powers TP, Carlson AN, O'Day DM: Deep mycoses. In: Mannis MJ, Macsai MS, Huntley AC, eds: Eye and skin disease. Philadelphia, Lippincott-Raven, 1996:583–590.

Safneck JR, Hogg GR, Napier LB: Endophthalmitis due to *Blastomyces dermatitidis*: case report and review of the literature. Ophthalmology 97:212–216, 1990.

8 BRUCELLOSIS 01.8
(Mediterranean Fever, Malta Fever, Gibralter Fever, Undulant Fever, Rock Fever, Cyprus Fever)

John D. Sheppard, Jr., MD, MMSc
Norfolk, Virginia
Suzanne C. Johnston, MD
Norfolk, Virginia

Brucellosis is a zoonotic disease caused by intracellular bacteria in the genus *Brucella*. This gram negative, aerobic, nonmotile coccobacillus causes a chronic, granulomatous infection. The organism responsible for brucellosis was discovered by David Bruce in 1886. Six species of *Brucella* have since been identified, four of which are known to be transmitted to humans:

1. *B. abortus*, carried mainly by cattle but also by sheep, goats, camels, yaks, horses and dogs.
2. *B. melitensis*, most common and most virulent species, carried by sheep and goats and less commonly by cattle.
3. *B. suis*, carried by swine.
4. *B. canis*, carried by beagle dogs.

ETIOLOGY/INCIDENCE

Brucellosis is most commonly transmitted to humans by the consumption of infected meat or unpasteurized dairy products. Less commonly, it is spread through inhalation of infected aerosolized particles and contact with skin creams prepared from animal products. Brucellosis can enter through mucous membranes or broken skin.

Brucellosis is rare in developed countries, with an incidence of about 1 per 1 million; 100 cases are reported annually in the United States. However, it is a relatively common health problem in developing countries, with 850 cases per 1 million reported annually in the Arabian Gulf countries, for example. These estimates are most likely low since brucellosis remains largely underreported.

COURSE/PROGNOSIS

Brucellosis has a variable presentation and course in humans. Length of incubation varies from a few days to several months with an average of three weeks. Humans and animals may initially be asymptomatic or may present with mild flu-like symptoms. If not treated appropriately, the acute phase can become chronic or relapsing.

DIAGNOSIS

Clinical signs and symptoms

Systemic

Acute systemic infection is characterized by:

- Fever (classically intermittent with diurnal variation);
- Headache;
- Abdominal pain;
- Arthralgia;
- Chills, excessive sweating;
- Anorexia, weight loss;
- Splenomegaly, hepatomegaly;
- Diffuse lymphadenopathy;
- Nervousness, depression.

In a recent prospective study Gungor et al found that 26% of participants with systemic brucellosis had some form of ocular involvement.

Ocular

Brucellosis can affect any ocular structure, with the most common being:

- Optic nerve involvement:
  - optic nerve edema,
  - retrobulbar neuritis,
  - optic nerve atrophy.
- Papilledema;
- Chiasmal arachnoiditis;
- Uveitis (may be acute or chronic with recurrent attacks, inflammation may be severe with hypopyon);
- Iritis (granulomatous or nongranulomatous);
- Choroiditis (multifocal and nodular or geographic);
- Panuveitis;
- Eyelid edema;
- Dacryoadenitis;
- Conjunctivitis;
- Episcleritis, scleritis;
- Extraocular muscle palsies (most commonly IV, VI, and VII);
- Keratitis, with coin-shaped subepithelial infiltrates;
- Corneal ulcers;
- Endophthalmitis (rare, occurs during bacteremic stage);
- Retinal edema, hemorrhages, or detachment.

Laboratory findings

The diagnosis of systemic brucellosis depends on:

- Clinical manifestations;
- Blood and tissue cultures.

Ocular brucellosis may be diagnosed via:

- Culture of tears and other ocular fluids;
- Detection of ocular (and systemic) *Brucella* antibodies (Witmer's coefficient);
- Increasing serum antibody titers (presumptive diagnosis).

Isolation of the organism decreases with chronic brucellosis making serologic assays more important:

- Serum agglutination test: most reliable.

Titers greater than 1:160 diagnostic when associated with characteristic clinical presentation. Titers greater than 1:640 indicate chronic infection.

- Complement fixation test;
- Radioimmunoassay (RIA): IgM predominates in acute cases, IgG predominates in chronic disease;
- Enzyme-linked immunosorbent assay (ELISA): IgG and IgM titers (useful in neurobrucellosis);
- Polymerase chain reaction assay (PCR).

TREATMENT

Systemic

The treatment of brucellosis requires four to eight weeks of therapy. More than one therapeutic agent is generally required to prevent relapses. Effective medications are listed:

- Doxycycline 100 mg twice daily for six weeks;
- Cefixime 400 mg daily in one to two doses;
- Rifampin 600–1200 mg/day for six weeks;
- Trimethoprim-sulfamethoxazole 960 mg twice daily for six weeks;
- Streptomycin 15 mg/kg/day IM for 2–3 weeks;
- Netilmicin 150 mg twice daily IM or (1.5–2 mg/kg/dose);
- Ofloxacin 400 mg b.i.d. for six weeks;
- Ciprofloxacin 500 mg twice daily for six weeks;
- Gentamicin 5 mg/kg/day in three divided IV doses for 5–7 days.

Various combinations of these medications have been used. The World Heath Organization issued guidelines in 1986 recommending doxycycline for six weeks in combination with either streptomycin for 2–3 weeks or rifampin for 6 weeks. Doxycycline/streptomycin has been associated with lower recurrence rates and may be preferable in areas where tuberculosis is also endemic given concern for community resistance to rifampin. Protracted administration of triple regimens may be necessary for neurobrucellosis.

Treatment should continue for one or two months if infection is localized in the heart bone or eye. Doxycycline should be avoided in children and pregnant women.

Ocular

Topical medications used during attacks of uveitis associated with brucellosis infection:

- Atropine;
- Corticosteroids.

Topical and systemic steroids have been used to minimize damage to the eye during the ocular phase of the disease. Relapses are common after tapering corticosteroid therapy. Steroids should be used cautiously and for brief periods if possible for ocular inflammation.

COMPLICATIONS

Systemic

Complications associated with brucellosis infection:

- Pneumonia;
- Hepatitis;
- Splenic abscess;
- Epididymitis/orchitis;
- Prostatitis;
- Endocarditis;
- Arthritis;
- Osteomyelitis;
- Meningoencephalitis.

Ocular

Ocular complications:

- Glaucoma;
- Cataract;
- Ocular hypotony;
- Cystoid macular edema;
- Retinal detachment;
- Phthisis bulbi;
- Optic neuropathy.

REFERENCES

Al-Kaff AS: Brucellosis. In: Fraunfelder FT, Roy FH, eds: Current ocular therapy. 5th edn. Philadelphia, WB Saunders, 2000:15–16.

Al-Kaff AS: Ocular brucellosis. Int Ophthalmol Clin 35:139–145, 1995.

Elrazak MA: *Brucella* optic neuritis. Arch Intern Med 151:776–778, 1991.

Gungor K, Bekir NA, Namiduru M: Ocular complications associated with brucellosis in an endemic area. Eur J Ophthalmol 12(3):232–237, 2002.

Lyall M: Ocular brucellosis. Trans Ophthalmol Soc UK 93:689–697, 1973.

Pappas G, Akritidis N, Bosilkovski M, Tsianos E: Medical progress: brucellosis. N Engl J Med 352(22):2325–2336, 2005.

Rabinowitz et al: Bilateral mutifocal choroiditis with serous retinal detachment in a patient with *Brucella* infection: case report and review of literature. Arch Ophthalmol 123:116–118, 2005.

Walker J, Sharma OP, Rao NA: Brucellosis and uveitis. Am J Ophthalmol 114(3):374–375, 1992.

Woods AC: Nummular keratitis and ocular brucellosis. Arch Ophthalmol 35:490, 1946.

Young E: Human brucellosis. Rev Infect Dis 5(5):821–842, 1984.

9 CAT-SCRATCH DISEASE 078.3

(Bartonella henselae Infection)

Terry D. Wood, MD
Portland, Oregon
Eric B. Suhler, MD
Portland, Oregon

Cat-scratch disease (CSD) is usually a benign, self-limited illness characterized by regional lymphadenopathy lasting weeks to months after local inoculation with the gram-negative bacillus *Bartonella henselae*. The majority of cases (60–80%) occur in persons under 21 years old. A 'typical' CSD infection is manifest by the appearance of a localized skin papule at the inoculation site 3–10 days after exposure. This progresses to a pustule, which may or may not be recalled by the patient. Regional lymphadenopathy follows 1 to 7 weeks later and may be the only sign or symptom detected. The lymph node is tender 80% of the time and suppurates in 15%. 'Typical' CSD encompasses 89% of all cases. Of the remaining 11% 'atypical' CSD cases, approximately half involve the ocular structures. The most common of these is Parinaud's oculoglandular syndrome, which encompasses 6% of all cases and presents as a unilateral granulomatous conjunctivitis. One to two percent develop neurologic findings; encephalopathy is the most common manifestation in this sub-category, and focal findings may involve the cerebral cortex, thalamus, or the basal ganglia. Neuroretinitis, a clinical syndrome comprised of papillopathy and an exudative maculopathy typically manifesting as a 'macular star,' is a relatively common neurologic sequelae, although it is often initially misdiagnosed as optic neuritis. It is however, important to note that neuroretinitis is not associated with multiple sclerosis, making the appearance of a macular star a welcome finding in a young patient presenting with optic nerve edema. Less commonly reported intraocular manifestations of *B. henselae* infection include central retinal artery occlusion, central retinal vein occlusion, peripapillary angiomatosis and neovascular glaucoma.

ETIOLOGY/INCIDENCE

- Causative agent, *Bartonella* (formerly *Rochalimea*) *henselae*.
- Removed from *Rochalimea* sp./order *Rickettsiales* when it was discovered not to be an obligate intracellular parasite.
- Fastidious, pleiomorphic, gram-negative bacillus.
- Most infections are caused by a scratch from a young, flea-infested bacteremic kitten, although transmission may also occur from a cat bite or lick (role of fleas in the transmission of human disease is unclear, although *B. henselae* DNA has been isolated from the fleas of bacteremic cats).
- Fleas appear to serve as the vector of transmission between cats.
- Bacteremic cats are usually less than 1 year old, are asymptomatic, and do not require treatment.
- Inoculation has also been reported from other animals (monkey, rabbit, squirrel).
- Infections are more common in the autumn and early winter months (60%).
- Mean age of onset is 12 years; predominance of patients are 7–30 years of age.
- Incidence of disease 1/10,000.
- May occur in intrafamilial epidemics in families with kittens.
- No evidence to support person-to-person transmission.

PARINAUD'S OCULOGLANDULAR SYNDROME (POGS)

- Most common form of 'atypical' CSD: accounts for 6% all cases of CSD.
- Theorized alternative route of inoculum is from wiping eye after touching cat fur harboring cat saliva with organism (residual from cat self-cleaning).

Clinical presentation characterized by:

- Unilateral granulomatous conjunctivitis;
- Single or multiple soft granulomas, 0.5–2.0 mm (may enlarge and ulcerate);
- Redness, irritation, chemosis and watery discharge;
- No serious corneal complications reported;
- Ipsilateral preauricular/submandibular lymphadenopathy, occasionally cervical.

May be accompanied by fever, malaise, anorexia, weight loss.

DIAGNOSIS/LABORATORY FINDINGS

- Histopathologic (best diagnostic indicator):
  - Warthin–Starry silver impregnation stain of biopsied lymph node or other involved tissue reveals clumps of tiny pleiomorphic bacilli;
  - Lymph nodes usually show evidence of granulomatous inflammation and stellate microabscesses which may coalesce.
- Skin test (Hanger–Rose):
  - Former hallmark of diagnosis, now largely abandoned due to concerns regarding transmission of viral/prion infections.
- Serum immunofluorescent assay (IFA):
  - Routinely available;
  - Sensitivity of 84%, specificity of 96%; positive predictive value of 91%;
  - Significant positive titers found in 3% of healthy controls;
- PCR gaining increasing use in diagnosis when serology is equivocal or inconclusive:
  - Culture: difficult;
  - Slow growing organism; requires 1–4 weeks.

Differential diagnosis

- Tularemia.
- Sporotrichosis.
- Tuberculosis.
- Lymphoma.
- Syphilis.

Less common: sarcoid, coccidiomycosis, actinomycosis, blastomycosis, infectious mononucleosis, mumps, pasteurellosis, yersiniosis, glanders, chancroid, lymphogranuloma venereum, rickettsiosis, listerelliosis, ophthalmia nodosa.

- Work up:
  - History and physical exam directed toward likely differential diagnoses, CBC, CXR, PPD with controls, RPR, FTA-ABS, *B. henselae* IFA;
  - If clinically indicated conjunctival or lymph node biopsies, blood cultures.

TREATMENT

- Symptomatic: warm compresses, analgesics, antipyretics.
- Aspiration of the lymph node only if distention causes pain:
  - Needle drainage from site 1–2 cm away in unaffected skin.

Direct incision and drainage may lead to persistent sinus formation and is contraindicated.

- Consider antibiotics in moderate to severe cases or if the patient is systemically ill. Treatment, if effective, will usually improve clinical course within 48 hours:
  - Rifampin, 10–20 mg/kg/d, PO q 12 or 24 hourly: dosing (87% effective).

Often used as adjuvant to other antibiotics as listed below.

- Ciprofloxacin, 20–30 mg/kg/d given PO q 12 hourly: dosing (84% effective);
- Gentamicin sulfate, 5–7 mg/kg/d IV given q 8 hourly for 7 days: dosing (73% effective);
- Trimethoprim/sulfamethoxazole (Bactrim/Septra); 6–12 mg/kg/day TMP and 30–60 mg/kg/day SMX given PO, q 12 hourly: dosing (58% effective);
- Macrolide and tetracycline antibiotics also deemed effective in many case reports — course of treatment: 4–6 weeks. Should be afebrile by 1 week, decreasing lymphadenopathy, no constitutional symptoms by 5–10 days.

BACILLARY ANGIOMATOSIS (EPITHELIAL ANGIOMATOSIS)

Clinical features

- Single or multiple cutaneous, subcutaneous, mucosal, visceral, or retinal lesions.
- Reddish vascular papules, nodules, or tumors, rarely plaque-like.
- Often similar in appearance to Kaposi's sarcoma; range in size from small papules to large, ulcerating, exophytic growths which may erode underlying bone.
- Ophthalmic structures reported involved have included the conjunctiva and optic nerve head/peripapillary retina.
- Systemic manifestations may include fever, chills, malaise, anorexia, headache.
- Occurs more commonly and is more severe in AIDS/immunocompromised patients.

DIAGNOSIS

Based on histopathologic finding on Warthin–Starry and H & E staining.

Differential diagnosis

Kaposi's sarcoma (must be ruled out histologically in HIV patients), pyogenic granuloma, angiosarcoma, hemangioma.

TREATMENT

Resolves rapidly with antibiotic regimens listed above. Standard course of 3–4 weeks.

NEUORETINITIS (LEBER'S IDIOPATHIC STELLATE NEURORETINITIS)

- First hypothesized association with CSD in 1984.
- Generally reported to occur in 1–2% cases of CSD.
- Twenty-six percent of confirmed cases *B. henselae* infection in one series.
- CSD is implicated $^{2}/_{3}$ of patients with the clinical presentation of neuroretinitis.

Clinical features

- Optic disk edema, usually diffuse, varies in severity, may see disk hemorrhage. Resolves over 2 weeks to 2 months.
- Optic atrophy may follow uncommonly. 'Macular star' lipid exudates. Protein/lipid rich exudation from the nerve spreads to Henle's layer in parafoveal region. Resolves over 6–12 months.
- May see residual RPE deficits.

May also see:

- Peripapillary or macular serous retinal detachments;
- Focal or multifocal retinal infiltrates/retinitis;
- Vitritis and/or anterior uveitis;
- Retinal vasculitis;
- Often an afferent pupillary defect, unless affected bilaterally;
- Variety of visual field deficits; often central, cecocentral 'disk fields'; also arcuate, altitudinal, general constriction;
- Primary site of pathology appears to be the optic nerve;
- Fluoroscein angiography shows leakage and/or staining of the disc but no leakage from the perifoveal capillaries;
- More often unilateral, however both sides may be involved clinically and/or angiographically;
- May present with sudden loss of visual acuity and/or field, transient visual obscurations, floaters, dyschromatopsia, or be completely asymptomatic;
- Visual acuity at presentation may vary from 20/20 to light perception; usually between 20/40 and 20/200.

DIAGNOSIS

Primarily clinical

- Serologic: acute and convalescent titers useful.
- PCR useful in cases where serology is equivocal.

Differential diagnosis

- Syphilis, Lyme, TB should be ruled out if clinically indicated.
- Also tularemia, toxoplasmosis, HSV, HZV, EBV, psittacosis, parasitic disease/DUSN, salmonella, leptospira, histoplasmosis, toxocara.
- Influenza, mumps, coxsackie viruses, sarcoid.
- Hypertensive retinopathy/increased intracranial pressure especially with bilateral disease.

TREATMENT

Atypical CSD with neurologic manifestations (i.e. neuroretinitis, others as below) are usually treated with antibiotic regimens as listed above.

There is no consensus on the duration of treatment; most reports 4–8 weeks, and there is no documented proof of efficacy of treatment versus nontreatment; anecdotal reports describe hastened visual recovery. Systemic steroids are controversial; they have been used in some series, but have not been shown to be beneficial or harmful.

PROGNOSIS

Most patients (>90%) have very good recovery of Snellen acuity (20/40 or better); a small subset will have profound, persistent visual loss.

In patients with excellent Snellen acuity, subtle subjective disturbance often remain (i.e. metamorphopsia, dyschromatopsia).

Other posterior pole manifestations of CSD (uncommon)

- Optic neuritis.
- Branch retinal arterial occlusions.
- Serous retinal detachments.
- Peripapillary angiomatosis.
- Inflammatory mass of the optic nerve head.
- Panuveitis (has been reported to mimic VKH).

Other systemic manifestations

May occur in either immunocompetent or immunosuppressed hosts, although tend to be more severe in the immunocompromised.

Infectious

Fever/bacteremia, culture negative endocarditis, tonsillitis, osteomyelitis, brain abscess.

Neurologic

Seizures, coma, aseptic meningitis, encephalitis, cerebral arteritis, transverse myelitis, polyneuritis, radiculitis, peripheral neuropathy, Bell's palsy.

Pulmonary

Hilar adenopathy, pleural effusion.

GI

Bacillary peliosis hepatitis and/or splenitis.

Other

Hemolytic anemia, erythema nodosum or annulare, arthralgias, generalized lymphadenopathy.

REFERENCES

Anbu AT, Foulerton M, McMaster P, Bakalinova D: Basal ganglia involvement in a child with cat-scratch disease. Pediat Infect Disease J 10:931–932, 2003.

Bafna S, Lee AG: Bilateral optic disk edema and multifocal retinal lesions without loss of vision in cat scratch disease. Arch Ophthalmol 114: 1016–1017, 1996.

Cunningham ET, Koehler JE: Ocular bartonellosis. Am J Ophthalmol 130(3):340–349, 2000.

Dreyer RF, et al: Leber's idiopathic stellate neuroretinitis. Arch Ophthalmol 102(8):1140–1145, 1984.

Gray AV, Michels KS, Lauer AK, Samples JR: *Bartonella henselae* infection associated with neuroretinitis, central retinal artery and vein occlusion, neovascular glaucoma, and severe vision loss. Am J Ophthalmol 137(1):187–189, 2004.

Huang MC, Dreyer E: Parinaud's oculoglandular conjunctivitis and cat-scratch disease. Int Ophthalmol Clinics 36(3):29–36, 1996.

Khurana RN, Albini T, Green RL, et al: *Bartonella henselae* infection presenting as a unilateral panuveitis simulating Vogt-Koyanagi-Harada syndrome. Am J Ophthalmol 138(6):1063–1065, 2004.

Labalette P, Bermond D, Dedes V, Savage C: Cat-scratch disease neuroretinitis diagnosed by a polymerase chain reaction approach. Am J Ophthalmol 132(4):575–576, 2001.

Lee WR, Chawla JC, Reid R: Bacillary angiomatosis of the conjunctiva. Am J Ophthalmol 118(8):152–157, 1994.

Margileth AM: Antibiotic therapy for cat-scratch disease: clinical study of therapeutic outcome in 268 patients and a review of the literature. Pediatr Infect Dis J 11:474–478, 1992.

Newsom RW, Martin TJ, Wasilauskas B: Cat-scratch disease diagnosed serologically using an enzyme immunoassay in a patient with neuroretinitis. Arch Ophthalmol 114(4):493–494, 1996.

Reed JB, et al: *Bartonella henselae* neuroretinitis in cat-scratch disease: diagnosis, management and sequelae. Ophthalmol 105(3):459–466, 1998.

Starck T, Madsen BW: Positive polymerase chain reaction and histology with borderline serology in Parinaud's oculoglandular syndrome. Cornea 21(6):625–627, 2002.

Suhler EB, Lauer AK, Rosenbaum JT: Prevalence of serologic evidence of cat scratch disease in patients with neuroretinitis. Ophthalmol 107(5): 871–876, 2000.

Wong MT, et al: Neuroretinitis, aseptic meningitis, and lymphadenitis associated with *Bartonella (Rochalimea) henselae* infection in immunocompetent patients and patients infected with human immmunodeficiency virus type 1. Clin Infect Dis 21(2):352–360, 1995.

10 COCCIDIOIDOMYCOSIS 114.9
(Valley Fever, San Joaquin Fever)

John Mourani, MD
Tucson, Arizona
Stephen A. Klotz, MD
Tucson, Arizona

ETIOLOGY/INCIDENCE

Coccidioidomycosis is an infectious disease caused by *Coccidioides immitis* or *C. posadasii*. It is a dimorphic fungus endemic in southwestern United States, Mexico, and parts of Central and South America.

The life cycle of *Coccidioides* species has a saprophytic phase wherein the fungus grows as a mold in the soil giving rise to arthroconidia. Primary infection occurs following inhalation of airborne arthroconidia that transform into spherules, thus beginning the parasitic phase.

Patients with altered immune function, diabetes mellitus, acquired immune deficiency syndrome (AIDS), recipients of corticosteroids, pregnant patients, or transplant patients, are at particular risk for relapsing infection and/or extrapulmonary dissemination. African-American and Filipinos are at high risk for dissemination as well.

COURSE/PROGNOSIS

During primary infection approximately 40% of patients will have a symptomatic illness consisting of influenza-like symptoms with fever, cough, myalgia and arthralgia. Nearly 5% will be left with pulmonary nodules or cavitary lesions. Less than 1% of patients develop disseminated disease.

Symptomatic ocular involvement is rare and initial ocular symptoms are non-specific. Asymptomatic chorioretinal scars were seen in as many as 9% of patients seeking medical attention. The majority of lesions resolve spontaneously without therapy.

Ocular involvement can be categorized as external or internal disease.

External involvement

- Phlyctenular conjunctivitis, scleritis, or episcleritis during primary pulmonary infection are hypersensitivity responses to coccidioidal antigen and usually subside without treatment.
- Corneal manifestations include a spectrum from superficial infiltrate to necrotic inflammatory foci and perforation. Corneal opacities, staphyloma and perforation have been described. Granulomatous lesions of the eyebrow, lids, lacrimal gland, and palpebral conjunctiva may be a manifestation of disseminated disease or the only presentation. Direct inoculation has been reported.
- Orbital, optic nerve and extraocular muscle disturbance is due to direct granulomatous involvement or secondary to central nervous system disease.

Internal involvement

- Anterior uvea (iris and ciliary body), iridocyclitis. With anterior chamber involvement, a white fluffy exudate can

be observed adherent to the iris surface. Other anterior chamber findings may include mutton-fat precipitates, flare, cells, and hypopyon, along with anterior or posterior synechiae, or both.
- Posterior uvea (choroid), retinitis, choroiditis and chorioretinitis. Acute lesions vary from a large three disk diameter perimacular chorioretinal exudates to whitish-yellow, metallic, small (0.1–0.25 disc diameter) oval, depigmented slightly elevated, edematous appearing choroidal or chroioretinal patches scattered randomly throughout the fundus. Vascular sheathing and striate retinal hemorrhages occur. Retinal edema with detachment is associated with active choroiditis. The vitreous reaction can vary from a mild cyclitis to a dense turbid inflammatory exudate containing spherules.

With resolution of the acute inflammation chorioretinal lesions shrink and appear as sharply demarcated, punched-out, scars evolving with varying degrees of hyperpigmentation and depigmentation.

Diagnosis
A high index of suspicion on the part of physicians is important in establishing this diagnosis. A history of living in endemic areas, travel to or temporary residence in such areas should alert the physician to the possibility of coccidioidomycosis.

Laboratory findings
Direct examination of tissue from biopsy or cytologic specimens, and anterior chamber fluid, may demonstrate endosporulating spherules and/or granulomas.
- *Coccidioides* species grow in most routine culture media as early as 3 to 4 days.
- Laboratory personnel need to be notified about the possibility of isolation of this fungus due to potential for infection.

Serologic testing
Serologic testing can detect IgM antibody demonstrating acute infection and IgG antibody, demonstrating present or past infection.

Differential diagnosis
Includes other fungal infections, and granulomatous lesions.

TREATMENT

Serious ocular infections need to be treated with systemic antifungal medications. The value and safety of intraocular injection is unproven, but amphotericin B has been administered topically and by intraocular injection. For systemic treatment, consultation with an infectious disease specialist is strongly recommended. Oral azoles are the mainstay of current therapy with fluconazole having the greatest documented efficacy.

Local
- Conjuncitivitis, scleritis, episcleritis during acute primary infection: inflammation resolves with resolution of primary infection, topical corticosteroid might help.
- Granulomatous inflammation of conjunctiva and/or cornea: topical amphotericin B (AmB) or conjunctival/subconjunctival administration, which is painful with poor penetration.
- Topical steroids should be used judiciously and sparingly to control inflammation once diagnosis of intraocular infection is confirmed and appropriate antifungal therapy is initiated.

Systemic
- Fluconazole 400 to 800 mg/day has been used with success in patients with systemic infection even with meningeal involvement and is the most commonly used medication. The drug achieves good ocular levels.
- Amphotericin B, (AmB) IV indicated in severe systemic disease (0.3 mg/kg to 1.0 mg/kg/day in life-threatening illness).
- Amphotericin B lipid complex and liposomal amphotericin B are available for patients who do not tolerate AmB due to nephrotoxicity; efficacy in treatment of ocular coccidioidomycosis is unknown (5 mg/kg/day).
- Itraconazole has been used for non-meningeal involvement.

The newer azoles (voriconazole and posaconazole) and echinocandin (caspofungin) have *in vitro* activity but their efficacy in treatment of ocular disease is unknown.

COMPLICATIONS

Local destruction, extraocular muscle palsies, corneal scarring and/or perforation, scleral necrosis and staphyloma, anterior and posterior synechiae, panophthalmitis, optic atrophy, and blindness.

An excellent source of information for physicians and patients alike is the Valley Fever Center for Excellence: http://www.vfce.arizona.edu/.

REFERENCES

Deresinski SC, Mirels LF, Kemper CA: *Coccidioides immitis*. In: Gorbach SL, Bartlett JG, Blacklow NR, eds: Infectious diseases. 3rd edn. Philadelphia, Lippincott Williams & Wilkins, 2004:2227–2245.

Luttrull JK, Wan WL, Kubak BM, et al: Treatment of ocular fungal infections with oral fluconazole. Am J Ophthalmol 119(4):477–481, 1995.

Moorthy RS, Rao NA, Sidikaro Y, Foos RY: Coccidioiomycosis iridocyclitis. Ophthalomol 101(12):1923–1928, 1994.

Rodenbiker HT, Ganley JP, Galgiani JN, Axline SG: Prevalence of chorioretinal scars associated with coccidioidomycosis. Arch Ophthalmol 99(1):71–75, 1981.

Rodenbiker HT, Ganley JP: Ocular coccidioidomycosis. Surv Ophthalmol 24(5):263–290, 1980. Review.

11 DERMATOPHYTOSIS 110.9

Sanjay V. Patel, MD
Rochester, Minnesota
Alan Sugar, MD
Ann Arbor, Michigan

Dermatophytosis is an infection by any of the keratinophylic fungi known as the ringworm fungi, most commonly *Trichophyton, Epidermophyton* and *Microsporum* spp., involving superficial skin, hair and nails. Dermatophytes are ubiquitous and have very low infectivity. Clinically, they are classified according to the area of skin involved, such as tinea capitis (ringworm of the scalp), tinea faciei (face), tinea corporis (body), tinea pedis (athlete's foot) and onychomycosis (nails). Skin lesions are superficial and begin as red scaly papules that expand to become circular patches. As the lesion expands and the center clears, an annular pattern develops that is typical of ringworm. The lesions may be vesicular and single or multiple and often are intensely pruritic. Facial lesions may take a butterfly configuration. The rings may be multiple or biconcentric 'bull's eyes.'

ETIOLOGY

- *Trichophyton, Epidermophyton, Microsporum* spp.
- Specific species may be acquired from soil, farm animals, household pets, or by direct or indirect human contact.

DIAGNOSIS

Clinical signs and symptoms

- The enlarging lesion typically leaves a ringworm pattern with little inflammation.
- Occasionally, a severe inflammatory reaction called kerion occurs.
- Untreated lesions may become chronic.
- Allergic reactions to fungi, known as dermatophytid, or 'tid,' reactions, cause noninfected vesicles, usually on the hands, and, rarely, an allergic conjunctivitis.
- Clinical findings may be more severe and atypical in immunosuppressed and human immunodeficiency virus-infected patients.
- Animal-derived infections are more acute than human — or soil-derived infections.
- Ocular findings:
  - Eyelids: blepharitis, dermatitis, edema, madarosis, ulceration, preseptal cellulitis;
  - Eyebrows: folliculitis, madarosis, scaly rash;
  - Conjunctiva: infectious or allergic conjunctivitis;
  - Cornea: fungal corneal ulcer (rare).

Laboratory findings

- Keratinized tissue can be scraped from the lesion border.
- Septate hyphae branches on 20% potassium hydroxide stain.
- Culture on selective media requires 2 to 3 weeks to grow at room temperature.
- Rapid identification by polymerase chain reaction is possible.

TREATMENT

Local

Antifungal creams are useful for milder lesions. Creams should be applied twice daily to affected skin after cleansing; continue for 1 week after lesion clears. Available topical agents are:

- Butenafine 1%;
- Ciclopirox olamine 1%;
- Clotrimazole 1%;
- Econazole 1%;
- Haloprogin 1%;
- Miconazole 2%;
- Oxiconazole nitrate 1%;
- Sertaconazole nitrate 2%;
- Sulconazole 1%;
- Terbinafine 1%;
- Tolnaftate 1%.

Systemic

The trend is toward early systemic use, especially for extensive lesions and those unresponsive to topical agents. Tinea capitis requires systemic treatment. In the past, the standard for systemic use was oral griseofulvin 125 to 250 mg (for children) and 500 mg (for adults) of microsize crystalline form once daily for at least 4 to 6 weeks. Newer agents offer greater effectiveness with a shorter treatment course, usually 2 to 4 weeks; these include:

- Ketoconazole 200 mg/day;
- Fluconazole 100 mg/day;
- Itraconazole 100 mg/day;
- Terbinafine 250 mg/day.

The azole antifungals can cause hepatotoxicity, can increase the anticoagulant effect of coumadin and raise blood levels of several drugs, including cyclosporin A, digoxin, antiepileptic agents and oral hypoglycemic agents. Terbinafine and itraconazole have been shown to be safe and efficacious in children.

PRECAUTIONS

- Corticosteroids topically or systemically may mask the appearance of dermatophytoses and increase their severity and duration.
- Lesions may relapse if antifungal agents are discontinued prematurely.

COMMENTS

Ocular and periocular involvement by these fungi are rare. They usually result from extension from involved facial or scalp skin. Scalp ringworm occurs most frequently in children in hot, humid weather. Scalp ringworm is rare in adults and may be a sign of altered immunological status.

REFERENCES

Fedukowicz HB, Stenson S: External infections of the eye: bacterial, viral and mycotic. 3rd edn. East Norwalk, CT, Appleton-Century-Crofts, 1985:194–196.

Meis JF, Verweij PE: Current management of fungal infections. Drugs 61(Suppl 1):13–25, 2001.

Velazquez AJ, Goldstein MH, Driebe WT: Preseptal cellulitis caused by *Trichophyton* (ringworm). Cornea 21:312–314, 2002.

Warnock DW: Superficial fungal infections. In: Cohen J, Powderly WG, eds: Infectious diseases. 2nd edn. St Louis, Mosby, 2004:173–180.

Weitzman I, Summerbell RC: The dermatophytes. Clin Microbiol Rev 8:240–259, 1995.

Zaias N, Glick BP, Rebell G: Superficial mycoses. In: Mannis MJ, Macsai MS, Huntley AC, eds: Eye and skin disease. Philadelphia, Lippincott-Raven, 1996:573–582.

12 DIPHTHERIA 032.9

F. Hampton Roy, MD, FACS
Little Rock, Arkansas

Diphtheria is an acute infectious disease caused by the gram-positive bacillus *Corynebacterium diphtheriae*. It is characterized by a primary lesion, usually within the respiratory tract and more generalized symptoms caused by release and spread of bacterial exotoxins throughout the body. It most commonly affects children younger than 10 years.

Conjunctivitis diphtheria has the property of exciting profuse exudation in the tissue of the conjunctivae, which has great tendency to coagulate, leading to necrosis of the infiltrated tissue. Diphtheria can be life threatening because the exotoxins produced by the bacteria cause tissue necrosis and accumulation of the host's leukocytes and erythrocytes in respiratory exudates, which can occlude the trachea and other air passages. In addition, the toxins circulating in the patient's bloodstream can be deposited throughout the body; lesions may occur in the kidneys, heart and nerves, resulting in acute nephritis and serious cardiac debility.

ETIOLOGY/INCIDENCE

Diphtheria is an acute infectious disease caused by *C. diphtheriae*, a gram-positive, club-shaped organism. Only strains that are latently infected by a bacterial virus, diphtheria phage B, produce exotoxin and are capable of producing diphtheria. The toxin is responsible for the most common systemic complications of diphtheria, affecting the heart and nervous system; cranial nerve involvement can include the third, fourth and sixth nerves. *C. diphtheriae* is essentially a surface saprophyte, most commonly affecting the nasopharyngeal area; cutaneous diphtheria seems to be more frequently associated with external ocular involvement.

The incubation period is 2 to 5 days after exposure.

About 200 cases of nonocular diphtheria are reported annually in the United States, usually among individuals without adequate immunization histories. Widespread immunization of infants and children against diphtheria has limited the incidence recently to scattered outbreaks. However, a single inoculation does not confer lifetime immunity and booster injections of the protective toxoid are necessary every 3 to 5 years, particularly for children, who appear more susceptible to overt disease. Newborns usually are protected by transplacental globulin from the mother, although a few severe, nonocular infections in neonates have been reported. Healthy carriers of the *C. diphtheriae* organism, although not susceptible themselves, are a source of infection to others, but this means of transmission has become less important in populations with widespread immunization. The disease may occasionally be seen in fully immunized persons, but the infection is usually mild and rarely fatal; death is most frequent in the very young and the elderly. As a rule, the longer the delay in administration of antitoxin, the greater the incidence of complications and death.

DIAGNOSIS

Clinical signs and symptoms

The external ocular manifestations of diphtheria may include:

- Tender, red, swollen eyelids;
- Entropion;
- Meibomianitis;
- Trichiasis;
- Xerophthalmia, symblepharon;
- Ptosis;
- Accommodative spasm or paralysis of extraocular muscles;
- Convergence paralysis, divergence paralysis;
- Paralysis of third, fourth, or sixth nerve;
- Dacryoadenitis, dacryocystitis;
- Conjunctival hyperemia, petechiae;
- Catarrhal, membranous, pseudomembranous, or purulent conjunctivitis;
- Keratitis;
- Corneal ulcer, perforation.

Diphtheria also may result in serious intraocular complications, including:

- Cataract;
- Central retinal artery occlusion;
- Optic neuritis.

Laboratory findings

Because diphtheria is an acute, serious illness, suspect cases should be promptly treated, even before a positive diagnosis is confirmed. Swabs of the throat of a suspected case, plated onto slides and stained with methylene blue or toluidine blue (in addition to samples for Gram's stain), will demonstrate non-motile rods that are roughly club shaped but pleomorphic, with granular and uneven staining. The intracellular granules take on a reddish, refractive appearance and are characteristic of the bacterium. Specimens also may be inoculated onto Loeffler coagulated serum slant tubes, blood agar plates and tellurite plates for diagnostic confirmation.

TREATMENT

Systemic

A combination of antibiotics and antitoxin is necessary to effectively combat diphtheria; the patient should be treated promptly, if necessary even before a positive diagnosis is available, because the diphtheria toxins bind irreversibly to cells and the antitoxin then is ineffective except on circulating toxins. *The severity of the disease depends on the amount of exotoxin absorbed before treatment is initiated; once clinical manifestations of the toxins appear, they cannot be neutralized by antitoxin administration.*

Treatment is begun by administering a small test dose of antitoxin subcutaneously and observing the patient for 1 to 2 hours for a localized reaction to the antitoxin or the horse serum in which it is prepared, or both. After ruling out anaphylactic reactions, a therapeutic dose of:

- Diphtheria antitoxin 10,000 to 100,000 units in 100 or 200 mL of isotonic saline may be administered intravenously over 30 minutes.

Although antibiotics are thought to have little effect on the clinical course of the respiratory diphtheria infection, they may be of benefit in terminating toxin production. Antibiotic therapy is also of value because diphtheria infection typically is mixed with other bacteria, including staphylococci and pneumococci and many other organisms; in severe cases, streptococci are often present and there is evidence that tissue damage is due to the mixed infection rather than to the diphtheria toxin alone. Additional benefits of antibiotics are hastened clearance of the carrier state and prevention of spread of the organism to others:

- Penicillin is the drug of choice (procaine penicillin G 600,000 units IM twice daily for 7 to 16 days);
- Penicillin V PO may be substituted after the third day in patients with uncomplicated infections;
- Penicillin G (4 to 6 million units IV daily divided in four equal doses) may be used with IV solutions.

In patients allergic to penicillin:

- Erythromycin (25 to 50 mg/kg/day IV for 10 to 14 days) may be substituted. However, erythromycin resistance has occurred in some recent diphtheria outbreaks; *C. diphtheriae* also is frequently resistant to cephalexin, colistin, lincomycin and oxacillin. The organism is usually sensitive to ampicillin, clindamycin, tetracycline and rifampin. Regardless of the antibiotic, therapy should be continued for at least 7 days.

Steroids have been used to prevent or ameliorate myocarditis associated with diphtheria, but recent opinion holds that corticosteroids or corticotrophins are not of value in the treatment of diphtheria or any of its complications.

Ocular

Treatment of external ocular diphtheria has two goals: neutralization of toxin and eradication of live organisms. There are several regimens for the topical and systemic administration of antitoxin and the amount given is often based on empiric decision. In general, the more severe the disease or the more extensive the membrane formation, the greater the amount of antitoxin required.

After giving a test dose to rule out anaphylaxis:

- Diphtheria antitoxin 10,000 to 100,000 units is applied topically to the affected eye every 4 to 6 hours for 24 to 48 hours;
- A subconjunctival injection of diphtheria antitoxin also may be considered as an alternative to topical application.

Commercially available immune and hyperimmune globulin preparations have low diphtheria antitoxin titers and thus are not particularly useful; however:

- A high-titer γ-globulin preparation made from the blood of persons with high titers of antitoxin is available as an investigational preparation that may be useful in special circumstances, such as for a patient who is highly allergic to the horse serum used to prepare commercial antitoxin. Intended for use in prophylaxis, it is obtainable from the Communicable Disease Division, State Department of Public Health, Lansing, Michigan. The treatment dose has not been established; *this preparation should never be given intravenously.*

Antibiotics are not effective against diphtheria toxin but are indicated for the eradication of the bacilli and superinfections. Frequent instillations of penicillin G sodium ointment 1000 units/g or erythromycin (0.5%) ointment are administered in addition to systemic antibiotics.

If the infection involves the eyelid skin, cutaneous diphtheria responds well to local application of compresses soaked in penicillin solution 250 to 500 units/mL and diphtheria antitoxin 20,000 units IM.

A canthotomy *should not be done* in an effort to separate the lids because the incision invariably becomes infected and actually increases the area of toxin absorption.

Diphtheria membranes usually slough away spontaneously during convalescence; membranes should not be peeled off because this leaves a raw, suppurating surface and facilitates absorption of toxin. With this caveat, however, a glass rod or cotton-tipped applicator moistened with sterile saline may be used at intervals to break early symblepharon formation in the fornices.

Supportive

Patients with diphtheria should be isolated and hospitalized; bedrest is important for 3 weeks because of the frequency of myocardial involvement. Aspirin and codeine may be indicated for relief of pain.

Precautions

Before antitoxin administration, tests for hypersensitivity to horse serum are mandatory. If the patient is allergic to horse serum, antitoxin may be administered after desensitization, or, if available, human diphtheria immune globulin may be substituted. Rarely, a patient may exhibit such marked hypersensitivity that antiserum cannot be administered without the risk of death. The heart rate of all patients should be monitored carefully during the administration of diphtheria antitoxin because anaphylaxis may occur. In addition, all patients with diphtheria should receive careful cardiac monitoring for developing myocarditis. Drugs with depressant effects on the heart must be used with extreme caution in patients with diphtheria.

Patients with diphtheria should be quarantined until two successive cultures of the eye, skin, or other infected areas, taken at 24-hour intervals, are negative. If antibiotics have been given, cultures should not be taken until at least 24 hours after cessation of therapy.

REFERENCES

Burkhard C, Choi M, Wilhelm H: Optic neuritis as a complication in preventive tetanus-diphtheria-poliomyelitis vaccination: a case report. Klin Monatsbl Augenheilkd 218(1):51–54, 2001.

Chandler JW, Milam DF: Diphtheria corneal ulcers. Arch Ophthalmol 96:53–56, 1978.

Dittmann S, Wharton M, Vitek C, et al: Successful control of epidemic diphtheria in the states of the Former Union of Soviet Socialist Republics: lessons learned. J Infect Dis 181(Suppl 1):S10–S22, 2000.

Duke-Elder S, ed: System of ophthalmology. St Louis, CV Mosby, 1976: 46.

Eller JJ: Diphtheria. In: Conn HF, ed: Current therapy. 6th edn. Philadelphia, WB Saunders, 1982:15–19.

Harnisch JP: Diphtheria. In: Isselbacher KJ, et al, eds: Harrison's principles of internal medicine. 9th edn. New York, McGraw-Hill, 1980:671–675.

Rogell G: Infectious and inflammatory diseases. In: Duane TD, ed: Clinical ophthalmology. Hagerstown, MD, Harper & Row, 1982:33:9–10.

Top FH, Wehrle PF: Diphtheria. In: Wehrle PF, Top FH, Sr, eds: Communicable and infectious diseases. 9th edn. St Louis, CV Mosby, 1981: 197–210.

13 EPIDEMIC KERATOCONJUNCTIVITIS 077.1

Paul Jorge Botelho, MD
Baltimore, Maryland
John D. Gottsch, MD
Baltimore, Maryland

Epidemic keratoconjunctivitis (EKC) is an acute, highly contagious, follicular or papillary viral conjunctivitis associated with preauricular adenopathy, conjunctival pseudomembranes and diffuse superficial keratitis. Adenovirus, the causative agent in EKC, is a double-stranded DNA viruses classified according to serotype (1 to 49) and subgenus (A to F). Certain members of adenovirus subgroup D have been reported to cause significant outbreaks of EKC (primarily serotypes 8, 19 and 37). Others adenoviral serotypes associated with keratoconjunctivitis include 2–5,7–11,14,16,21–23 and 29. Adenoviruses have also been identified in cases of pharyngoconjunctival fever and hemorrhagic conjunctivitis.

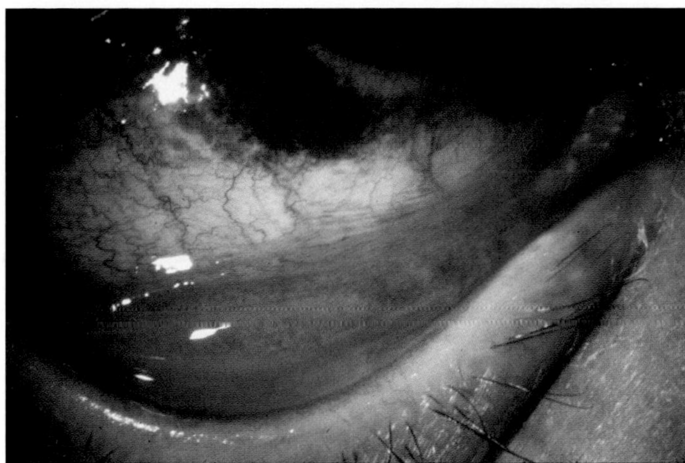

FIGURE 13.1 Epidemic keratoconjunctivitis with conjunctival hemorrhages.

DIAGNOSIS

Clinical signs and symptoms

Following a 5- to 14-day incubation period, EKC presents as acute unilateral and then bilateral (75% of cases bilateral) papillary, follicular or mixed conjunctivitis. Other signs include hyperemia, chemosis, serous discharge, subconjunctival hemorrhages and fibrin conjunctival pseudomembranes. Often patients present with foreign body sensation associated with diffuse, punctuate superficial keratitis during the first week. The lesions become raised and stain with fluorescein during the second week. After 14 days, subepithelial opacities may develop in up to 50% of patients. These opacities may be associated with pain, photophobia and decreased vision. The lesions usually spontaneously resolve over several months to years and are not associated with scarring or vascularization.

The conjunctivitis and viral shedding can persist for up to two weeks. The patient and the clinician must take precautions to avoid transmitting the pathogen.

Ocular and periocular manifestations

- Preauricular adenopathy, eyelid edema and serous discharge with lid matting.
- Diffuse papillary or follicular conjunctivitis with hyperemia, chemosis, subconjunctival hemorrhages and membrane or pseudomembrane formation (33% of cases) (Figure 13.1).
- Cornea diffuse superficial punctuate keratitis within the first week, followed by focal elevated punctuate epithelial lesions that stain with fluorescein during week two and in up to 50% of patients subepithelial opacities develop after 2 weeks associated with photophobia and blurred vision.

Laboratory findings

Laboratory testing for the presence of adenovirus serotypes linked to eye infections in suspected cases of EKC may assist the clinician in confirming the diagnosis and implementing measures to control nosocomial outbreaks. Cases of follicular conjunctivitis with superficial keratitis, especially when unilateral, may pose a diagnostic challenge. In the differential diagnosis are herpes simplex virus and adult inclusion conjunctivitis from *Chlamydia trachomatis* serotypes D–K.

- The gold standard for confirmatory diagnosis is viral isolation on cell culture from conjunctival scrapings. Viral isolation can take 1–2 weeks for completion. Recently, a shell-vial technique employing accelerated virus isolation and identification can reduce viral isolation time to three days. Because viable viral sample from conjunctival scrapings is needed, the sensitivity of this method is reduced compared to other techniques. It remains the definitive test of serotype identification in cases associated with epidemic outbreaks.
- Direct fluorescent anibody assay (DFA) is a rapid screening technique for adenoviral detection. Vigorous swabbing of the conjunctiva is performed to obtain an adequate sample size to avoid false negatives. Expertise is required to interpret the immunofluorescent results. Other methods of adenovirus antigen include enzyme immunoassay and immunochromatography.
- Polymerase chain reaction (PCR) assay for adenoviral detection is more sensitive than antigen detection and viral isolation methods. A comparison of PCR to a commercial immunoassay (adenoclone) found the PCR assay was positive in 46 of 58 adenoclone negative cases and positive in 11 of 11 adenoclone positive, culture positive swabs. It also maintains high specificity to common adenoviral pathogens. Newly designed primers in PCR assays have improved the sensitivity for adenoviral DNA recognition allowing for detection of most adenoviral subgroups associated with eye infections. Currently, PCR assays can be performed in several hours.
- Multiplex PCR assay can simultaneous screen for the presence of known viral and chlamydial pathogens associated with follicular keratoconjunctivitis. Using a series of primers in one reaction, the sensitivity of detecting adenovirus, herpes simplex virus and *Chlamydia trachomatis* using the multiplex PCR assay was equal to or greater than with conventional means for each pathogen individually. The test, which can be performed in seven hours, may reduce diagnostic confusion and allow the clinician to initiate the proper treatment plan and isolation precautions promptly.

TREATMENT

- Currently there are no effective topical or systemic antivirals agents in the management of EKC. No clinical trials have documented efficacy of antivirals with regards to duration of symptoms, severity of disease, reduction of viral shedding or decreased incidence of persistent subepithelial infiltrates.
- Supportive treatment including topical artificial tears four times daily, topical decongestants, topical antihistamines and cold packs can be offered.
- Patients with pain, photophobia and decreased vision associated with epithelial keratitis or subepithelial infiltrates may benefit from topical corticosteroids. In chronic cases of subepithelial infiltrates, judicious use of a mild topical corticosteroid such as fluorometholone 0.1% can improve comfort and vision.
- Phototherapeutic keratectomy (PTK) has been described as an alternative to topical corticosteroid use in the management of persistent nummular superficial subepithelial infiltrates following EKC. A reduced rate of recurrent nummuli following PTK was reported in several studies.
- Cidofovir [(S)-1-(3-hydroxy-2-phosphonylmethoxypropyl)ade nosine] or S-HPMPA, a broadspectrum, long-acting nucleoside analogue which inhibits viral DNA polymerase, was evaluated *in vivo* by Gordon et al. The authors found that pretreatment with topical 0.1% cidofovir reduced the peak viral titer when given 1 day before inoculation into New Zealand white rabbits infected with adenovirus type 5. The topical cidofovir was administered six times a day for five days. However, a rebound increase in viral titers were noted in 25% of cases. A subsequent *in vivo* study (same pathogen and animal model) using cidofovir 0.2% topically 6 times a day for 10 days demonstrated a decrease in viral titers and reduction in the number of days of viral shedding. Delayed onset nasolacrimal blockage was reported in this study. Clinical trials comparing topical cidofovir to placebo in cases of EKC have not been reported to date.

PREVENTION OF TRANSMISSION INCLUDING NOSOCOMIAL INFECTIONS

- Modes, duration and ease of transmission of adenovirus in acute cases of EKC are discussed with the patient in detail. Patients with acute EKC are excused from work or school for up to two weeks while convalescing.
- Of paramount importance when managing a suspected case of EKC is the implementation of a procedure policy to prevent transmission to other patients. Numerous reports of nosocomial EKC epidemics have been described, including transmission of EKC via an ophthalmologist's hands or instruments after managing an in-office case to a neonatal intensive care unit. Patients suspected to have acute conjunctivitis should be relatively isolated from other patients. Sources of transmission during an office visit include magazines, chair rests, slit lamp patient handles and multidose bottles of topical fluorescein. Following examination of any patient with communicable conjunctivitis, thorough cleaning of all examination equipment with chloramine-T should be performed immediately.
- Published guidelines regarding prevention and control of EKC at teaching eye institutes concluded that the following steps may decrease cases of rate of nosocomial infections; patient screening and isolation, handwashing, instrument disinfectants, furlough of infected employees, wearing disposable gloves for every patient, cleaning all therapeutic or diagnostic contact lenses for 30 minutes in chloramine-T, use of disposable occluders and soaking tonometers for 30 minutes in chloramine-T solution following each use.

COMMENTS

Outbreaks of EKC can present a significant health risk with ocular morbitity and loss of revenue. With the aid of several new PCR based adenoviral detection assays, prompt diagnosis and management of cases of EKC may limit the transmission of this highly contagious viral pathogen.

REFERENCES

Chaberny IE, Schnitzler P, Geiss HK, Wendt C: An outbreak of epidemic keratoconjunctivitis in a pediatric unit due to adenovirus type 8. Infect Control Hosp Epidemiol 24(7):514–519, 2003.

Cheung D, Bremner J, Chan JTK: Epidemic keratoconjunctivitis-do outbreaks have to be an epidemic? Eye 17:356–363, 2003.

Cooper RJ, Yeo AC, Bailey AS, Tullo AB: Adenovirus polymerase chain reaction assay for rapid diagnosis of conjunctivitis 40(1):90–95, 1999.

Elnifro EM, Cooper RJ, Klapper PE, et al: Diagnosis of viral and chlamydial keratoconjunctivitis: which laboratory test? Br J Ophthalmol 83:622–627, 1999.

Elnifro EM, Cooper RJ, Klapper PE, et al: Multiplex polymerase chain reaction for diagnosis of viral and chlamydial keratoconjunctivitis. Invest Ophthalmol Vis Sci 41(7):1818–1822, 2000.

Gordon YJ, Romanowski EG, Araullo-Cruz T: Topical HPMPC inhibits adenovirus type 5 in the New Zealand rabbit ocular replication model. Invest Ophthalmol Vis Sci 35(12):4135–4143, 1994.

Gottsch JD, Froggatt JW, III, Smith DM, et al: Prevention and control of epidemic keratoconjunctivitis in a teaching hospital. Ophthalmic Epidemiol 6(1):29–39, 1999.

Kaufman HE: Treatment of viral diseases of the cornea and external eye. Progress in Retinal and Eye Research 19(1):69–85, 2000.

Percivalle E, Sarasini A, Torsellini M, et al: A comparison of methods for detecting adenovirus type 8 keratoconjunctivitis during a nosocomial outbreak in a neonatal intensive care unit. J Clin Virol 28:257–264, 2003.

Quentin CD, Tondrow M, Vogel M: Phototherapeutic keratectomy (PTK) after epidemic keratoconjunctivitis 96(2):92–96, 1999.

14 ERYSIPELAS 035
(St. Anthony's Fire)

Richard L. Abbott, MD
San Francisco, California

Erysipelas is an acute, localized inflammation of the skin and subcutaneous tissue that is characterized by redness, edema and induration.

ETIOLOGY/INCIDENCE

The pathogenic organisms are usually group A β-hemolytic *streptococcus*, although occasional group B, C and G strains have been identified. It is a disease affecting primarily adults between 60 and 80 years old, but its incidence is increasing in younger age groups.

COURSE/PROGNOSIS

The site of infection is the extremities or face. The primary facial infection often is a nasopharyngitis, from which the organism is transferred to the skin through an abrasion or a minute wound.

Erysipelas may begin with an abrupt onset of fever, chills, malaise and nausea. A definite zone of redness soon appears, with edema, tenderness and a well-defined, advancing border. In more severe cases, vesicles may form on the surface. Typically, the infection involves the lymphatic spaces and is spread through these channels to neighboring areas. Constitutional symptoms include high temperature, headache, vomiting and localized pain. Without treatment, the disease is usually self-limited and runs its course within 4 days to several weeks. As the facial lesions spread, ocular involvement often occurs, consisting of marked edema and erythema of the lids. The edema is frequently extensive enough to prevent opening of the eyes. The disease may also progress to gangrene of the eyelids. Although less common, inflammation spreads from the lids to the conjunctiva, producing chemosis and external ophthalmoplegia. Other complications include dacryoadenitis, orbital thrombophlebitis, cellulitis, abscess and cavernous sinus thrombosis. A late result in chronic infections may be a solid edema or elephantiasis of the eyelids.

DIAGNOSIS

Clinical signs and symptoms

Ocular or periocular manifestations

- Conjunctiva: chemosis, exudative or membranous conjunctivitis.
- Cornea: superficial punctate keratitis secondary to bacterial toxins or exposure with lid ectropion (late), ulcerative keratitis.
- Eyelids: abscess, blepharitis, ectropion, elephantiasis, erythema, gangrene, madarosis, marked edema necrosis, trichiasis.
- Iris: iridocyclitis.
- Lacrimal system: dacryoadenitis, dacryocystitis.
- Orbit: abscess, cellulitis, thrombophlebitis.
- Vitreous or retina: chorioretinitis, metastatic vitreous abscess.

Laboratory findings

- Most often, it is difficult to definitively identify the inciting organism.
- The use of blood cultures, needle aspirates, or biopsy specimens has yielded fewer than 10% positive cultures.
- Detection of *Streptococcus* spp. in skin specimens with direct immunofluorescence is helpful.

Differential diagnosis

- Ophthalmic herpes zoster.
- Allergic contact dermatitis.
- Myosis of collagen disease.
- Trichinosis.
- Angioneurotic edema.

TREATMENT

Systemic

- Penicillin G is the drug of choice in treating erysipelas.
- Treatment should be instituted promptly and continued for 10 to 14 days to prevent the possibility of systemic spread.
- Intravenous penicillin G should be given in a minimum divided daily dosage of 6 million units.
- Once there is evidence of clinical improvement, the route of administration can be changed to oral medication.
- Penicillin V potassium should be given daily in four divided doses of 250 mg for the duration of the 10- to 14-day therapy period.
- In patients sensitive to penicillin, erythromycin may be substituted.
- Erythromycin may be given orally at an initial dosage of 500 mg four times daily for several days and then reduced to 250 mg four times daily for 10 days.
- In severely ill patients, erythromycin 500 mg IV should be given twice a day for the first 2 or 3 days before oral therapy is begun.

Ocular

- In severe cases resulting in tissue destruction and lid necrosis, meticulous cleaning and debridement of the wounds on a daily basis should be the mainstay of local therapy.
- The wounds are surgically debrided and cleansed with a 1:1 solution of hydrogen peroxide and sterile saline and repacked daily with iodoform gauze.
- The use of warm saline compresses and topical broad-spectrum antibiotic ointments helps accelerate the healing process and may prevent secondary bacterial contamination.
- The application of topical erythromycin ointment within the cul-de-sac helps prevent the occurrence of a secondary bacterial conjunctivitis.
- If there is a significant degree of lid contracture in the healing process, exposure keratitis may develop.
- This condition is best treated initially with tear substitute and lubricating ointments.
- Surgical repair of a cicatricial ectropion or other lid deformities may be required.
- It is prudent, however, to wait a minimum of 3 to 6 months before considering surgical intervention to allow the healing process to stabilize and reduce the likelihood of an undercorrection or overcorrection.

Supportive

- Attention should be given to the patient's physical, nutritional, emotional and recreational activity needs.
- Hospitalization is usually indicated, with the patient on bedrest.
- The patient should be isolated until the fever subsides and strict hygienic measures should be used by all hospital personnel who have contact with an infected patient.
- Alcohol and tepid sponge baths may be used to reduce high temperature.
- Vital signs should be monitored regularly.

PRECAUTIONS

- Because erysipelas usually begins abruptly and may progress rapidly, appropriate antimicrobial therapy must be instituted as soon as possible.
- The diagnosis may be made on the basis of the clinical presentation of the illness and intravenous penicillin G or its substitute should be started immediately.
- Regardless of which drug is used, it is essential that treatment in full doses be given over a period of at least 10 days because relapses are relatively common.
- Continuous antibiotic prophylaxis is indicated only in patients with a high recurrence rate.
- Cultures and sensitivities should be obtained for confirmation of the diagnosis only if there is exudate readily available for these studies.
- Needle aspiration from the lids or orbit is contraindicated in patients with erysipelas because of the possibility of spread of infection and injury to other structures.

COMMENTS

Although lower extremity involvement is most common, when affecting the face, the erysipelas exanthem most frequently appears in the region of the eye, with the sites of predilection being the eyelid and the inner canthus. The pathophysiology of lid necrosis seems to be related to the release of proteolytic enzymes by the streptococcal organisms, which dissolve connective tissue bridges and allow rapid spread of the bacteria. Because the skin of the lid is so thin, large amounts of fluid can accumulate, thereby raising the tissue pressure and shutting off capillary circulation. The combination of diffuse bacterial spread and diminished blood supply leads to destruction and necrosis of the lid tissue.

For treatment to be effective, one must make an early diagnosis and institute maximum parenteral antibiotic therapy combined with local debridement and topical antibiotic application. It is recommended that this therapy be continued for a minimum of 10 to 14 days until all evidence of the infection has resolved. Long-term therapy consists of lid plastic surgery after all healing processes have stabilized.

REFERENCES

Abbott RL, Shekter WB: Necrotizing erysipelas of eyelids. Ann Ophthalmol 11:381–384, 1979.

Bratton RL, Nesse RE: St Anthony's fire: diagnosis and management of erysipelas. Am Fam Phys 51:401–404, 1995.

Chartier C, Grosshans E: Erysipelas. Intl J Dermatol 35:779–781, 1996.

Feingold DS, Weinberg AN: Group A streptococcal infections: an old adversary reemerging with new tricks? Arch Dermatol 132:67–70, 1996.

McHugh D, Fison PN: Ocular erysipelas. Arch Ophthalmol 110:1315, 1992.

Ochs MW, Dolwick MF: Facial erysipelas: report of a case and review of the literature. J Oral Maxillofac Surg 49:1116–1120, 1991.

Ronnen M, Suster S, Satewach-Millet M, et al: Erysipelas. Changing faces. Intl J Dermatol 24:169, 1986.

Scott PM, Bloome MA: Lid necrosis secondary to streptococcal periorbital cellulitis. Ann Ophthalmol 13:461–465, 1981.

15 ESCHERICHIA COLI 008.0

Donny W. Suh, MD, FAAP

West Des Moines, Iowa

The genus Escherichia is named after Theodor Escherich who isolated the type species of the genus in 1885. *Escherichia coli* is a facultatively anaerobic gram-negative rod that is found as a normal commensal in the gastrointestinal tract, from which it may spread to infect contiguous structures when normal anatomic barriers are interrupted. This bacillus can also be found in association with other pathogenic organisms in perforated or inflamed conditions. *Escherichia coli* has both a fermentative and respiratory type of metabolism.

ETIOLOGY/INCIDENCE

Recent estimates suggest that more than 100,000 illnesses annually are attributable to shiga-toxin-producing *E. coli*, up to 50% of which are strains other than O157:H7. The urinary and gastrointestinal tracts are the usual portals of entry; however, once infection has occurred in a primary focus, further spread to distant organs may occur by means of the bloodstream. Septicemia is the most serious complication of *E. coli* infections. It occurs frequently in immunodeficient patients, in debilitated elderly patients with diabetes mellitus, in patients with urinary tract infection or biliary or intraperitoneal sepsis and after abortions or pelvic surgery. The most important are enterotoxigenic *E. coli* (ETEC), a cause of travelers' diarrhea; enteropathogenic *E. coli* (EPEC), a cause of childhood diarrhea; enteroinvasive *E. coli* (EICE), a cause of dysentery-like disease; and enterohemorrhagic *E. coli* (EHEC), a cause of hemorrhagic colitis and the hemolytic-uremic syndrome in children.

Ocular involvement is rare and may result in a mucopurulent conjunctivitis, most often in the elderly. Metastatic endophthalmitis may occur from *E. coli* septicemia and the usual portal of entry is the central retinal artery. The course of the endophthalmitis is acute; necrosis of the intraocular tissues and loss of vision can occur in less than 24 hours.

DIAGNOSIS

Clinical signs and symptoms

Ocular or periocular manifestations

- Anterior chamber: iritis, gas bubbles, hyphema, hypopyon.
- Conjunctiva: chemosis, hyperemia, pseudomembranous or purulent conjunctivitis, subconjunctival hemorrhage.
- Cornea: edema, keratitis, corneal ulcers, corneal infiltrates.
- Globe: panophthalmitis, purulent endophthalmitis.
- Other: increased intraocular pressure, ocular pain, anterior and/or posterior uveitis, chorioretinitis.

TREATMENT

Systemic

The choice of an appropriate antimicrobial agent in *E. coli* infections depends on the site and type of infection, as well as its severity. A number of antibiotics are effective against the bacillus, but no particular drug is uniformly active against all strains of *E. coli*, so sensitivity testing should guide the choice of antibiotics. Antimicrobial resistance occurs through plasmid-mediated determinants, several of which can be found in the same plasmid. These multiresistent plasmids can be transferred by conjugation.

For less severe *E. coli* infections, the initial treatment of choice may be ampicillin 2 to 4 g/day IM or IV. One may also consider other penicillins with β-lactamase inhibitor, cephalosporins, nitrofurantoin and trimethoprim-sulfamethoxazole. For more severe infections, the dose of ampicillin/sulbactam could be 3 g every 6 hours IV. One may also consider imipenem cilastatin, ciprofloxacin IV or cefotaxime.

Aminoglycoside antibiotics are most commonly used against coliform bacillary infections, including *E. coli*; they include kanamycin, gentamicin, amikacin and tobramycin.

Kanamycin is generally indicated for the initial treatment of serious *E. coli* infections. Severe urinary tract infections that seem to be resistant to other antimicrobial agents have responded to daily doses of kanamycin 15 mg/kg IM in divided doses every 6 to 8 hours.

Alternative treatment may be a total daily dose of parenteral gentamycin 3 to 5 mg/kg administered in divided doses every 8 hours. In severe infections that appear to be resistant to kanamycin and gentamicin, amikacin is indicated. Amikacin is given in daily doses of 15 mg/kg in two or three equally divided doses.

In severe cases of sepsis, a combination of antibiotics is given, which includes ampicillin and an aminoglycoside, the choice of which is based on knowledge of local susceptibility patterns. Ampicillin-sulbactam or cefatazime (a potent third-generation cephalosporin) is a suitable alternative, especially if an aminoglycoside-resistant nosocomial organism is suspected.

Neomycin appears to be most effective against *E. coli* gastroenteritis. An oral daily dose of 25 mg/kg is usually indicated for 1 or 2 days.

Ocular

In *E. coli* conjunctivitis, topical ciprofloxacin, ofloxacin, gatifloxacin, levofloxacin, moxifloxacin, or 0.3% tobramycin ophthalmic solutions are applied topically approximately six to eight times daily until the infection appears to be resolved. For a severe case, a more aggressive dose should be given during the first 24 to 48 hours in about 12 to 24 doses daily. For example, loads of three every 2 hours (drop at 8:00 a.m., 8:05 a.m. and 8:10 a.m.; then 10:00 a.m., 10:05 a.m. and 10:10 a.m.; and so on) for a total of 24 installations daily. Use of the concept of loading with well-tolerated topical antibiotics enhances compliance and optimizes effective microbial killing.

Early systemic and local antibiotic therapy is essential for *E. coli* endophthalmitis. Blanket local antibiotic therapy should consist of 20 mg of subconjunctival gentamicin or tobramycin. Also, for topical treatment 0.3% tobramycin ophthalmic solution or 3rd and 4th generation quinolones, such as gatifloxacin, levofloxacin and moxifloxacin, 12 to 24 doses daily, may be added. In most cases of *E. coli* endophthalmitis, intravitreal injection of gentamicin or tobramycin 100 to 300 μg can be used. Amikacin can also be used at 400 μg. Intravitreal injection consists of a total of 0.1 mL.

Systemic or local corticosteroids administered in combination with antibiotics may reduce the massive inflammatory response of the eye, which often is as destructive as the infection. Their use should be considered when highly effective antibiotics are being used at optimal dosing and there is a need to control the retinitis occurring.

Secondary involvement of the uveal tract may necessitate the use of a cycloplegic/mydriatic. Scopolamine 0.25% drops may be applied topically twice daily to aid in the relief of uveitis.

Supportive

Hospitalization is necessary for *E. coli* endophthalmitis infection.

PRECAUTIONS

The serum levels of aminoglycosides should be monitored to gauge therapeutic levels and to avoid toxicity because the ratio of therapeutic dose to toxic dose is very narrow. Ototoxicity and nephrotoxicity may occur even when serum levels have been appropriately monitored, so the risks should be weighed. The concurrent and/or sequential systemic use of potentially neurotoxic or nephrotoxic drugs should be avoided.

Isolation and antimicrobial therapy of contacts are essential to abort epidemic infantile diarrhea. Many *E. coli* infections are hospital acquired, so strict hygienic measures are essential.

COMMENTS

E. coli is rarely found in the normal flora of the conjunctiva. It is most commonly seen as a source of infection in ophthalmia neonatorum. *E. coli* endophthalmitis is a rare complication of *E. coli* septicemia. It has a poor prognosis and early diagnosis and treatment are essential if useful vision is to be retained.

REFERENCES

Aronson SB, Elliott JH: Ocular inflammations. St Louis, CV Mosby, 1972: 103–105, 112–114, 228–230.

Balestrazzi A, Blasi MA, Primitivo S, Balestrazzi: *Escherichia coli* endophthalmitis after trans-scleral resection of uveal melanoma. Eur J Ophthalmol 12(5):437–439, 2002.

Barnett BJ, Stephens DS: Urinary tract infection: an overview. Am J Med Sci 314(4):245–249, 1997.

Bonadio WA, Smith DS, Madagame E, et al: *Escherichia coli* bacteremia in children: A review of 91 cases in 10 years. Am J Dis Child 145:671–674, 1991.

D'Amico DJ, Caspers-Velu L, Libert J, et al: Comparative toxicity of intravitreal aminoglycoside antibiotics. Am J Ophthalmol 100:264, 1985.

Eisenstein BI: *Escherichia coli* infections. In: Isselbacher KJ, Braunwald E, Wilson JD, et al, eds: Harrison's principles of internal medicine. 13th edn. New York, McGraw-Hill, 1994:661–663.

Endophthalmitis Vitrectomy Study Group: Results of the endophthalmitis vitrectomy study: a randomized trial of immediate vitrectomy and of intravenous antibiotics for the treatment of postoperative bacterial endophthalmitis. Arch Ophthalmol 113:1479, 1995.

Glasser DB, Baum J: Antibacterial agents. In: Tabbara K, Hyndiuk RA, eds: Infections of the eye. Little, Brown, Boston, 1996:207–230.

Hyndiuk RA, Cokington CD: Bacterial keratitis. In: Tabbara K, Hyndiuk R, eds: Infections of the eye: diagnosis and management. Little, Brown, Boston, 1996:323–347.

Shammas HF: Endogenous *E. coli* endophthalmitis. Surv Ophthalmol 21:429–435, 1977.

Turck M, Schaberg D: Infections due to enterobacteriaceae. In: Isselbacher KJ, Adams RD, Braunwald E, eds: Harrison's principles of internal medicine. 9th edn. New York, McGraw-Hill, 1980:629–634.

16 GONOCOCCAL OCULAR DISEASE 098.4

Carlos M. Isada, MD
Cleveland, Ohio
David M. Meisler, MD, FACS
Cleveland, Ohio

Gonorrhea is one of the oldest described diseases of humans and it remains one of the most common sexually transmitted diseases, with an estimated 800,000 new cases occurring in the United States annually. It is an infection that primarily involves mucosal surfaces, particularly columnar or cuboidal epithelium. Gonorrhea presents most commonly with involvement of the genital tract (urethra, cervix), anorectal region and pharynx. Disseminated gonococcal infection can also occur in both the neonate and the adult; this condition is characterized by a petechial rash, arthralgias, fever, or septic arthritis. This is caused by bacteremia from strains of *Neisseria gonorrhoeae* that produce minimal or no genital inflammation.

Gonococcal ocular infection is a condition described since antiquity. It can affect newborns who are infected at the time of delivery, children and adolescents who are the victims of sexual abuse and sexually active adults who become infected through hand-eye inoculation. Gonococcal conjunctivitis is considered a medically urgent condition because of the potential of the organism to penetrate the intact cornea and progress rapidly to cause corneal ulceration and permanent vision loss.

ETIOLOGY/INCIDENCE

The causative organism is *N. gonorrhoeae*, an oxidase- and catalase-postive, gram-negative diplococcus. In clinical specimens containing purulent secretions, the organism may be seen as intracellular bean-shaped bacteria within polymorphonuclear leukocytes or closely associated with leukocytes. Several other organisms can appear identical to *N. gonorrhoeae* on Gram's stain, such as *N. meningitidis* and other nonpathogenic *Neisseria* spp. Structurally, the organism has an envelope (similar to other gram-negative bacteria) and pili, which mediate attachment to mucosal surfaces. Many strains carry plasmids that produce a β-lactamase enzyme that confers resistance to penicillin, termed a TEM-1 penicillinase. Tetracycline resistance is also plasmid mediated and these resistance-conferring plasmids are easily transferred to other gonococci. Antibiotic resistance can also occur via several chromosomal mutations, which tend to decrease the permeability of the outer membrane to β-lactam antibiotics and alter penicillin-binding proteins.

Humans are the only natural reservoir for *N. gonorrhoeae* and transmission occurs primarily via sexual contact with the reservoir in asymptomatically infected persons. The disease is most common in individuals 20 to 24 years old.

ADULT GONOCOCCAL CONJUNCTIVITIS

Although gonorrhea remains a common sexually transmitted disease, ocular involvement remains relatively infrequent. Nationwide statistics for the incidence of adult gonococcal conjunctivitis (AGC) are not kept specifically, but in some large series of patients with adult conjunctivitis, AGC occurs in fewer than 1% of cases. In the adult, gonococcal conjunctivitis is most commonly acquired after direct or manual contact with infected genital secretions or urine. The incubation period is usually less than one week from a potential exposure, but may be up to 3 weeks. Urethral symptoms (when present) usually precede ocular symptoms by 1 or more weeks, but notably, patients may never develop urethral symptoms. The prevalence of asymptomatic ocular colonization with *N. gonorrhoeae* in adults who have urogenital gonorrhea is unknown. Rare cases have been reported after the instillation of urine eyedrops as part of a folk remedy and after accidental laboratory inoculation. Because *N. gonorrhoeae* is capable of surviving outside the body for limited periods of time, the possibility of fomite transmission has been raised but likely is insignificant compared with hand-eye transmission.

PEDIATRIC AND ADOLESCENT GONOCOCCAL OCULAR DISEASE

Although uncommon, the finding of gonococcal conjunctivitis in children after the neonatal period is strongly associated with sexual abuse or assault. AGC may be due to either sexual abuse or early sexual activity, with the same considerations as for the adult. In the limited number of cases described, the clinical course in this age group appears to be similar to that of adults.

GONOCOCCAL OPHTHALMIA NEONATORUM

Gonococcal ophthalmia neonatorum (GON) has been described in the medical literature since antiquity. Neonatal conjunctivitis is the most common ocular disease of newborns, occurring in 1.6% to 12% of births.

The epidemiology of this syndrome has changed dramatically after the introduction of the use of a 2% silver nitrate solution for the prophylaxis of ophthalmia neonatorum. In later years, the widespread use of prenatal screening helped decrease the incidence of GON from 10% to less than 1% in industrial countries. This has led some countries, such as the United Kingdom, to discontinue prophylaxis for ophthalmia neonatorum. Sweden likewise discontinued prophylaxis but still requires its use in neonates born to mothers who do not receive comprehensive prenatal care.

In the United States, *C. trachomatis* is the most common cause of ophthalmia neonatorum, mirroring the increase in this organism as the leading sexually transmitted disease worldwide. The incidence of ophthalmia neonatorum in the United States secondary to *C. trachomatis* is about 8.2 in 1000 live births compared with 0.3 in 1000 live births secondary to *N. gonorrhoeae.* In other parts of the world, such as Africa, GON remains a serious concern due to the frequency of maternal gonococcal infection and the lack of systematic ocular prophylaxis. In some areas of Africa, the prevalence has been as high as 30 to 40 in 1000 live births.

GON is almost always acquired via direct inoculation of the eyes during passage through an infected birth canal. The incubation period in neonates is generally 1 to 3 days. Occasional cases of delayed GON have been reported up to 19 days after delivery.

COURSE/PROGNOSIS

In the largest reported series of AGC, 21 cases of culture-confirmed *N. gonorrhoeae* conjunctivitis were retrospectively analyzed. Most patients were between 20 and 26 years old, a distribution similar to that of other gonococcal infections. The median time between the onset of conjunctivitis and presentation to the physician was 4 days. The majority of patients denied exposure to *N. gonorrhoeae* from their partners or active genital infection themselves. However, 57% of patients were found to have concurrent urethritis on testing. Bilateral eye involvement was noted in 38%, with visual acuity of 20/40 in more than 50% at initial presentation. In nearly all patients, the degree of conjunctivitis on presentation was severe, with copious purulent drainage; only one patient presented with a mild conjunctivitis. Three patients also had superficial ulceration and two had perforating ulcerative keratitis on presentation. After antibiotic therapy, more than 90% of the involved eyes had a visual acuity of 20/50 or better. No patients progressed to ulcerative keratitis after therapy was initiated. The two individuals who presented with perforating ulcerative keratitis did poorly and remained with only light perception acuity after antibiotics and keratoplasty.

DIAGNOSIS

Clinical signs and symptoms

Adult gonococcal conjunctivitis

AGC is characterized by profuse purulent discharge, severe conjunctival injection and marked edema and hyperemia of the eyelids. Early in the course, AGC is limited to the mucosal surfaces. Rare cases of asymptomatic AGC have been described, but the prevalence of asymptomatic or minimally symptomatic gonococcal conjunctival infection is unknown. Some cases may be complicated by extension to the corneal epithelium, leading to varying degrees of chemosis and stromal or epithelial keratitis. The degree of corneal involvement varies considerably, but when it does occur findings commonly include subepithelial or stromal infiltrates and marginal corneal melt. *N. gonorrhoeae* is one of the few organisms that can penetrate intact corneal epithelium. If treatment is delayed, there may be rapid progression to ulcerative keratitis and perforation. This observation of a potentially fulminant course led the Centers for Disease Control and Prevention (CDC) in 1986 to recommend immediate hospitalization and intravenous antibiotics for 5 days. This approach has since been liberalized, but the potential for fulminant disease remains well recognized and is an important aspect of management.

Gonoccocal ophthalmia neonatorum

The clinical presentation of GON is similar to that of the AGC, as described, with copious purulent conjunctival discharge, hyperemia and edema. GON is considered a medical emergency because untreated cases commonly progress rapidly to corneal penetration and perforation of the globe, at times within 24 hours. Other localized manifestations of *N. gonorrhoeae* infection also may occur, including anorectal disease and rhinitis. Disseminated gonococcal infection can occur with neonatal infectious arthritis and meningitis. Neonates may acquire *N. gonorrhoeae* in utero if an infected mother develops premature rupture of membranes. This may result in a syndrome characterized by chorioamnionitis, meningitis, septicemia and pneumonia; *N. gonorrhoeae* can be recovered from orogastric aspirates of the neonate. Infants delivered by cesarean section also have been reported to have GON from in utero infection.

Differential diagnosis

The differential diagnosis of ophthalmia neonatorum is wide and includes chemical conjunctivitis, bacterial infection (*Moraxella catarrhalis*, *Staphylococcus aureus*, *Haemophilus* spp., *Streptococcus pneumoniae*, *Pseudomonas aeruginosa*, enterococci and *N. gonorrhoeae*), *Chlamydia trachomatis* and herpes simplex virus. In the late 1800s, *N. gonorrhoeae* was the major cause of ophthalmia neonatorum, occurring in 10% of children in Europe with GON.

Laboratory findings

The diagnosis of gonococcal ocular disease should be suspected in all newborns who present several days after delivery with conjunctivitis, particularly if any of the following risk factors are present:

- The mother lacked routine prenatal care.
- The mother has a history of sexually transmitted disease or substance abuse.
- The infant did not receive ophthalmia prophylaxis.

Definitive diagnosis of GON cannot be made on clinical grounds alone and requires laboratory confirmation. Evaluation for other causes of ophthalmia neonatorum is imperative, particularly detection of *C. trachomatis*. Chlamydia ophthalmia can be diagnosed by both specific tissue culture tests and non-culture tests such as immunoassays, nucleic acid amplification tests and direct fluorescent antibody tests. Gonococcal ocular disease in the adult is much more difficult to recognize because of its rare occurrence. The findings of copious purulent conjunctivitis with or without corneal involvement should suggest the diagnosis; a positive history of current urethral or urinary symptoms in the patient (or partner) is very helpful, but its absence does not exclude *N. gonorrhoeae* infection.

A Gram's stain smear is essential for the rapid diagnosis of *N. gonorrhoeae*. A 'positive' Gram's stain is defined by the finding of typical gram-negative diplococci within polymorphonuclear leukocytes in conjunctival exudates. Many clinicians consider a positive Gram's stain in the appropriate clinical setting to be compelling evidence for the presence of *N. gonorrhoeae*, even if a subsequent culture is negative. A Gram's stain is considered 'negative' if no organisms are seen on oil immersion field, even in the presence of many neutrophils. An 'equivocal' Gram's stain is characterized by (1) typical gram-negative diplococci that are found on the smear but are not cell associated or (2) atypical organisms that are neutrophil associated. The sensitivity of the Gram's stain for detecting *N. gonorrhoeae* varies depending on the anatomic site, with a sensitivity of 95% to 100% from the male urethra (symptomatic) to 40% to 50% from the rectum. Limited data are available concerning the sensitivity of the Gram's stain in gonococcal ocular disease, but it probably is high (more than 90% in one study). The specificity also is likely to be high, but occasionally *Neisseria* spp. other than *N. gonorrhoeae* can be detected. A positive or equivocal Gram's stain of conjunctival exudate from a newborn is sufficient laboratory evidence to begin appropriate therapy. Treatment may be initiated in the newborn with conjunctivitis and a negative Gram's stain if there is a high index of suspicion for gonococcal ocular disease based on the risk factors cited.

The definitive diagnosis of *N. gonorrhoeae* infection rests on laboratory confirmation of the organism. Isolation of the gonococcus in culture remains the gold standard and specimens should routinely be submitted for culture and antimicrobial susceptibility testing. Newer methods for the diagnosis of *N. gonorrhoeae* are increasingly popular and include nucleic acid probe technology and nucleic acid amplification techniques such as polymerase chain reaction (PCR). *N. gonorrhoeae* is a fastidious organism and requires specific culture techniques. Optimal isolation in culture requires a selective medium such as a chocolate agar, which contains antibiotics and incubation in 5% CO_2. Several such media are effective, including Thayer–Martin medium (chocolate agar with vancomycin, colistin and nystatin), modified Thayer–Martin medium (trimethoprim, vancomycin, colistin and nystatin) and Martin–Lewis medium. Ideally, specimens should be inoculated onto appropriate chocolate agar as soon as possible because the organisms do not survive drying. Plates can be held at room temperature in candle extinction jars for several hours before incubation in CO_2 at 35° to 37°C. With proper collection and handling, growth of the organism can be seen within 24 to 48 hours. Alternatively, several commercially available transport systems can be used in settings in which immediate inoculation of media is not feasible. These systems preserve the viability of most of the organisms for a short period of time before plating onto selective media; if such a system is used, the specimen should be transported promptly to the laboratory.

In some laboratories, nonculture techniques such as PCR, probes and enzyme immunoassays are being used routinely for the detection of *N. gonorrhoeae* from genital sites. The relative merits of these newer assays compared with traditional culture techniques are matters of some debate, particularly for nongenital specimens. These assays have not been formally studied (or approved) for the detection of *N. gonorrhoeae* from conjunctival exudates or scrapings and are not legally acceptable in suspected cases of child abuse. The optimal management of gonococcal eye infections requires isolation of the organism in traditional culture.

TREATMENT

The treatment of AGC has evolved due to the emergence of strains that are resistant to penicillin by plasmid-mediated β-lactamase production, along with strains resistant to tetracyclines and some cephalosporins. Penicillinase-producing and non-penicillinase-producing strains of *N. gonorrhoeae* can cause AGC. Ceftriaxone is a parenteral third-generation cephaloporin recommended for the first-line treatment of more common manifestations of gonococcal infection, such as genital infection, pharyngitis and anorectal infection. This agent has the longest half-life of all of the available cephalosporins and is chemically stable in the presence of the β-lactamases produced by *N. gonorrhoeae.* The prolonged half-life results in sustained bactericidal levels of drug in the conjunctival sac.

ADULT GONOCOCCAL CONJUNCTIVITIS

Only a limited number of studies have examined the efficacy of ceftriaxone in AGC. In the largest series reported, 12 adults with culture-proved gonococcal conjunctivitis were treated in an unblinded fashion with 1 g of ceftriaxone IM along with a single ocular saline lavage. The mean patient age was 26 years old. Symptoms consistent with urethritis were present in 69%. Corneal epithelial erosions were present on initial examination in 31%, but none had infiltration of the corneal stroma. All patients responded clinically with a significant decrease in the ocular discharge within 12 hours. There also was evidence of rapid microbiologic resolution, with all conjunctival scrapings taken at 6 hours negative in culture for *N. gonorrhoeae.*

Based on this and other studies, the CDC in 2002 recommended that uncomplicated AGC should be treated with 1 g ceftriaxone IM in a single dose, with a single lavage of the infected eye with a saline solution. There are no consensus recommendations for individuals with more serious corneal ulcerations; such patients should be hospitalized immediately and treated with extended courses of ceftriaxone on an individual basis.

Limited data are available regarding the use of fluoroquinolones in the treatment of AGC. In one study, oral norfloxacin was administered to 15 patients with culture-proved gonococcal conjunctivitis. Seven patients received 1200 mg norfloxacin PO for 3 days and eight patients received a single dose of 1200 mg. There was no progression of the corneal lesions during treatment and no significant toxicity was reported. Although quinolones are first-line agents for uncomplicated gonococcal infections of the urethra, cervix, rectum and pharynx, the CDC has not recommended the use of fluoroquinolones in AGC (as of 2005). In addition, there has been an increase of fluoroquinolones-resistant *N. gonorrhoeae* in Southeast Asia, areas in the Pacific, Hawaii, California; this has led the CDC in 2002 to advise against empiric quinolone use for the empiric treatment of genital *N. gonorrhoeae* in these areas. In 2004 a similar recommendation was made by the CDC to avoid the empiric treatment of genital gonorrhea infection with quinolones in men who have sex with men because of an increase in quinolone-resistant *N. gonorrhoeae* in this group in the US.

In 2003, the World Health Organization (WHO) recommended the following as first-line regimens for AGC:

- Ceftriaxone, 125 mg IM, as a single dose; or
- Spectinomycin, 2 g IM, as a single dose; or
- Ciprofloxacin, 500 mg PO, as a single dose.

In areas of the world where these antimicrobials are not available, an alternative regimen is kanamycin 2 g IM, as a single dose. The WHO also noted that these regimens were likely to be effective, although there was no specific published data to support their use in AGC.

Adults with gonococcal conjunctivitis require examination and testing for other sexually transmitted diseases, particularly *Chlamydia trachomatis*. Available studies suggest a significant coinfection rate with syphilis and a nontreponemal serologic test for syphilis should be considered, such as the rapid plasma reagin (RPR). Patients with AGC should also be told to refer their sex partner or partners for evaluation and treatment. There are no published series of gonococcal conjunctivitis in persons infected with human immunodeficiency virus (HIV). The CDC has recommended that HIV-infected persons with gonococcal infections of the cervix, urethra, rectum and pharynx be treated with the same regimens used for those who are negative for HIV. Individuals with AGC of unknown HIV status should be offered HIV testing.

PEDIATRIC AND ADOLESCENT GONOCOCCAL OCULAR DISEASE

There are no published studies regarding the optimal treatment regimen in this age group. Gonococcal infections in children involving more common sites such as the urethra, pharynx and rectum are treated with the same regimen recommended for adults (1 g ceftriaxone IM as a single dose) if the child weighs more than 45 kg or 125 mg ceftriaxone IM as a single dose if the child weighs less than 45 kg. This regimen should be adequate for uncomplicated ocular disease as well. Quinolones (ciprofloxacin, ofloxacin, levofloxacin and others) have previously been avoided in children based on toxicity data to articular damage in animal studies. In 2002, the CDC noted that there was no data showing this articular damage occurred in children; treatment of gonococcal infections in children <18 years of age could also include the flurorquinolones. Because of the implications of gonococcal infection in children, referral should be made to experts who have experience and training in the evaluation of sexual assault or abuse.

GONOCOCCAL OPHTHALMIA NEONATORUM

Optimal therapy for GON has similarly changed due to the increasing incidence of β-lactamase-producing gonococci. Previous recommendations by the CDC supported the use of aqueous crystalline penicillin G parenterally for non-β-lactamase-producing strains. However, penicillin has since been abandoned as first-line therapy for GON, given the prevalence of penicillinase-producing *N. gonorrhoeae* of more than 60% in some areas and the widespread development of chromosomally mediated resistance to penicillin in many strains of *N. gonorrhoeae* that do not produce β-lactamase. In a randomized clinical trial, 105 newborns in Kenya with GON were randomized to one of three regimens:

- A single dose of 125 mg ceftriaxone IM;
- A single dose of 75 mg kanamycin IM and 1% gentamicin ointment instilled in the eye q.i.d. for 7 days;
- A single dose of 75 mg kanamycin IM plus 1% tetracycline ointment in the eyes q.i.d. for 7 days.

All newborns who received ceftriaxone were clinically and microbiologically cured. One of 26 neonates receiving the kanamycin plus tetracycline ointment had persistent conjunctivitis and 2 of 24 neonates receiving kanamycin and gentamicin ointment were treatment failures. Ceftriaxone also was effective in eradicating extraocular *N. gonorrhoeae.*

In 2002, the CDC recommended GON treatment of 25 to 50 mg/kg ceftriaxone IV or IM in a single dose, not to exceed 125 mg. Topical therapy alone is not recommended and is considered unnecessary if systemic therapy is used. The World Health Organization also recommends ceftriaxone as the agent of choice; in areas of the world where ceftriaxone is not available alternatives include kanamycin 25 mg/kg IM as a single dose, to a maximum of 75 mg, or spectinomycin 25 mg/kgy IM as a single dose to a maximum of 75 mg. Ceftriaxone should be used with caution in infants with hyperbilirubinemia, especially those born prematurely, due to the liver metabolism of ceftriaxone. The CDC recommends hospitalization for infants with GON and careful observation for signs of disseminated infection such as meningitis and pneumonia. A single dose of ceftriaxone is likely curative for GON, although some clinicians prefer to continue daily dosing until cultures are negative at 2 to 3 days.

Treatment failures with ceftriaxone may be due to simultaneous infection with *C. trachomatis*, which is intrinsically resistant to cephalosporins. It is important to test initially for *C. trachomatis* at the same time as for *N. gonorrhoeae* because the former is more common and the clinical presentations may be indistinguishable. Both culture and nonculture tests are available for the diagnosis of *C. trachomatis*; nonculture tests include direct fluorescent antibodies, enzyme immunoassays and nucleic acid amplification tests. For testing of *C. trachomatis*, the specimen should contain conjunctival cells and not only exudates. Ophthalmia neonatorum caused by *C. trachomatis* should be treated with 50 mg/kg/day erythromycin base or ethylsuccinate orally divided into four doses daily for 14 days.

The mothers of infants with GON should be tested for other sexually transmitted diseases and treated with standard regimens for gonococcal infections in the adult; current recommendations for uncomplicated infections of the cervix, urethra and rectum include one of the following:

- Cefixime 400 mg PO in a single dose (limited availability);
- Ceftriaxone 125 mg IM in a single dose;
- Ciprofloxacin 500 mg PO in a single dose;
- Ofloxacin 400 mg PO in a single dose.

Each of the regimens should include simultaneous treatment for *C. trachomatis* such as 1 g azithromycin PO in a single dose or 100 mg doxycycline PO b.i.d. for 7 days. The sex partners of mothers of infants with GON should be referred for evaluation.

OPHTHALMIA NEONATORUM PROPHYLAXIS

The prevention of ophthalmia neonatorum is best accomplished by good prenatal care in pregnant women, with active screening for gonococcal and chlamydial infections. However, prenatal care may be insufficient or unavailable to some. The instillation of a prophylactic ointment or solution into the eyes of all newborns to prevent gonococcal ophthalmia is a law in most states in the United States. Historically, Credá, as reported in 1881, demonstrated that a 2% silver nitrate solution applied topically rapidly reduced the incidence of GON infection. Silver nitrate administration, however, is associated with chemical conjunctivitis and gives incomplete protection against *Chlamydia*. This has led to recommended prophylaxis to also include 0.5% erythromycin or 1% tetracycline ophthalmic ointment administered in a single application. In a prospective study, all three-topical silver nitrate solution and erythromycin and tetracycline ointments were found to be equivalent in preventing GON. Nevertheless, with increasing resistance to both tetracycline and erythromycin, alternative prophylaxis has been explored. Povidone-iodine is a potent antiseptic and in a 5% solution, a single drop applied is well tolerated by the external eye. Povidone-iodine in vitro has shown efficacy against *N. gonorrhoeae* as well as herpes simplex and *C. trachomatis.* In a controlled trial of prophylaxis against ophthalmia neonatorum, a 2.5% povidone-iodine solution was equally effective against gonococcal conjunctivitis as silver nitrate and erythromycin and more effective against *Chlamydia* than either of the two. However, the CDC does not recommend the routine use of povidone-iodine for ophthalmia prophylaxis until further information is available.

The regimens recommended in 2002 by the CDC are as follows:

- Silver nitrate 1% aqueous solution in a single application;
- Erythromycin 0.5% ophthalmic ointment in a single application;

- Tetracycline 1% ophthalmic ointment in a single application.

One of the three regimens should be instilled immediately after delivery, regardless of whether the delivery is vaginal or by cesarean section. Povidone-iodine is not recommended due to inadequate studies and bacitracin is not efficacious.

Similarly, infants born to mothers with untreated infection with *N. gonorrhoeae* should receive some form of prophylactic therapy, even in the absence of ocular or disseminated disease. Due to the high risk of postnatal infection, it is recommended that such newborns receive 25 to 50 mg/kg ceftriaxone IV or IM, not to exceed 125 mg, in a single dose.

REFERENCES

Centers for Disease Control and Prevention: 2002 Guidelines for treatment of sexually transmitted diseases. MMWR 51(RR-6):36–42, 2002.

Fruchtman Y, Greenberg D, Shany E, et al: Ophthalmia neonatorum caused by multidrug-resistant *Neisseria gonorrhoeae.* IMAJ 6:180–181, 2004.

Handsfield HH, Sparling PF: *Neisseria gonorrhoeae.* In: Mandell GL, Bennett JE, Dolin R, eds: Principles and practice of infectious diseases. 6th edn. New York, Churchill Livingstone, 2005:2514–2529.

Ingram DL: *Neisseria gonorrhoeae* in children. Pediatr Ann 23:341–345, 1994.

Isada CM: *Neisseria gonorrhoeae.* In: Isada CM, Kasten BL, Goldman MP, et al, eds: Infectious diseases handbook 1997–98. Cleveland, Lexii-Comp, 1998:201–203, 478–481.

Isenberg SJ, Apt L, Wood M: A controlled trial of povidone-iodine as prophylaxis against ophthalmia neonatorum. N Engl J Med 332:562–566, 1995.

Judson FN: Treatment of uncomplicated gonorrhea with ceftriaxone: a review. Sex Transm Dis 13:199–202, 1986.

Kestelyn P, Bogaerts J, Stevens AM, et al: Treatment of adult gonococcal keratoconjunctivitis with oral norfloxacin. Am J Ophthalmol 108:516–523, 1989.

Pareek SS: Conjunctivitis caused by beta-lactamase-producing *Neisseria gonorrhoeae.* Sex Transm Dis 12:159–160, 1985.

Podgore JK, Holmes KK: Ocular gonococcal infection with little or no inflammatory response. JAMA 3:246–242, 1981.

Ulman S, Roussel RJ, Forster RK: Gonococcal keratoconjunctivitis. Surv Ophthalmol 32:199–208, 1987.

Wan WL, Farkas GC, May WN, et al: The clinical characteristics and course of adult gonococcal conjunctivitis. Am J Ophthalmol 102:575–583, 1986.

World Health Organization: Guidelines for the management of sexually transmitted diseases, 2003. Online. Available at: http://www.who.int/reproductive-health/publications/rhr_01_10_mngt_stis/. Accessed June 2005.

Zajdowicz TR, Kerbs SB, Berg SW, et al: Laboratory-acquired gonococcal conjunctivitis: successful treatment with single-dose ceftriaxone. Sex Transm Dis 11:28–29, 1983.

17 HAEMOPHILUS INFLUENZAE 041.5

Chandak Ghosh, MD, MPH
New York, New York
Anouk Amzel, MD, MPH
New York, New York

Prior to the development and implementation of the *Haemophilus influenzae* type b (Hib) vaccine, *H. influenzae* was a significant and important cause of meningitis and other serious bacterial infections in childhood. Today, this genus of pathogens is still implicated in a number of different diseases. *H. influenzae* is a small, pleomorphic, gram-negative coccobacillus with 8 biotypes and 6 serotypes. The biotypes (1 through 8) are based on the presence or absence of indol, urease and ornithine decarboxylase. The serotypes (a through f) are based on the presence six types of polysaccharide capsules. Unencapsulated strains are called 'nontypeable.' The natural habitat of the *H. influenzae* bacteria is exclusively human upper respiratory tract. Transmission of the bacteria is by direct contact with respiratory secretions or inhalation of aerosolized respiratory droplets. Asymptomatic colonization is common.

Diseases *H. influenzae* can cause include:

- Ophthalmologic: conjunctivitis, orbital cellulitis, corneal ulcer, endophthalmitis;
- Non-ophthalmologic: otitis media, sinusitis, epiglottitis, pneumonia, empyema, septic arthritis, cellulitis, meningitis, occult bacteremia, purulent pericarditis, endocarditis, osteomyelitis, peritonitis, glossitis, uvulitis, septic thrombophlebitis.

ETIOLOGY/INCIDENCE

The terminology 'invasive' *H. influenzae* disease is used to describe the more life-threatening conditions predominantly found in children below the age of five (i.e. meningitis, bacteremia, epiglottitis, and pneumonia).

High risk factors for *H. influenzae* invasive disease are:

- Age less than 5 years;
- Male;
- African American, Alaska Native, Apache, Navajo (confounded by issues of socioeconomic status and household crowding);
- Childcare attendee, children living in crowded conditions, non-breastfed infants;
- Immunocompromised: HIV, certain congenital immunodeficiencies, asplenia, sickle cell, certain malignant neoplasms.

H. influenzae was previously a major cause of pediatric invasive infection, with over 95% caused by the b serotype. Since the initiation the Hib vaccine, pediatric invasive *Haemophilus* disease has become rare. Now, diseases secondary to *Haemophilus* bacteria are caused mainly by non-typeable strains (not covered by the Hib vaccine). These are predominantly non-invasive diseases. Disease secondary to *H. influenzae* usually occurs in winter. The risk of secondary cases in family members is over 500-fold.

DIAGNOSIS

Typically, diagnosis is based on clinical presentation of the specific diseases that *H. influenzae* bacteria cause. For example, when a patient presents with orbital cellulitis, the possibility of *H. influenzae* infection (along with other bacteria) is presumed. Health professionals should have increased suspicion in hosts with high risk factors. CT or MRI Scan is used when surgery is indicated for a non-improving orbital cellulitis.

Clinical signs and symptoms

- Clinicians should consider *H. influenzae* infection in patients with a past history of upper respiratory infection, sinusitis, trauma, and sinus or eye surgery.

- Different ocular disease states can have some or all of the following: pain, blurred or double vision, headache, injected conjunctiva (with or without chemosis), eyelid edema, restricted ocular motility (with or without pain), and proptosis.
- Specific to preseptal/periorbital cellulitis secondary to *H. influenzae* infection is a violaceous discoloration of eyelids with an associated conjunctivitis.

Laboratory findings

- *H. influenzae* infection can be confirmed by eye (conjunctival, corneal, vitreal), blood, or cerebro-spinal fluid (CSF) gram stain and culture, as indicated.
- Chocolate agar medium is used specifically for culturing *H. influenzae* bacteria.
- In cases of corneal ulcer, Giemsa stain can also be done.

TREATMENT

Treatment is started presumptively based on disease prior to laboratory confirmation.

Conjunctivitis and ulcers

- Topical fluoroquinolone eye drops four times per day to hourly, depending on the severity.

Endophthalmitis

- Broad-spectrum intravitreal antibiotics (e.g. vancomycin with either amikacin or ceftriaxone).
- Add topical *fortified* antibiotics eye drops.
- Vitrectomy indicated for vision of light-perception or worse.
- If endogenous endophthalmitis, intra-venous antibiotics are added to treat the underlying source of infection.

Preseptal/periorbital cellulitis

- Start a trial of oral antibiotics with amoxicillin. Up to 26% of *H. influenzae* isolates are β-lactamase resistant, therefore consider augmentin, second generation cephalosporins (e.g. cefuroxime), or macrolides (e.g. erythromycin) if drug resistance is a concern.
- If no improvement within one to two days, consider hospitalization and treatment with intravenous ceftriaxone and vancomycin.

Orbital cellulitis

- Hospitalization and treatment with intravenous ceftriaxone and vancomycin.
- Consider surgical drainage if non-responsive to antibiotics alone.

COMMENTS

Since the introduction of the Hib vaccine in 1987, rates of invasive *H. influenzae* type b infection have decreased by 99% in countries that use the vaccine. Today, patients rarely present with epiglottitis, meningitis, and bacteremia caused by *H. influenzae*. Thus, the vast majority of *H. influenzae* infections are of the non-invasive variety. Although there have been reports of decreased rates of orbital cellulitis after initiation of the Hib vaccine, as the majority of upper respiratory infections (the most significant precursor to orbital cellulitis) are caused by nontypable *H. influenzae*, it remains doubtful that the vaccine is the sole cause.

REFERENCES

Buznach N, Dagan R, Greenberg D: Clinical and bacterial characteristics of acute bacterial conjunctivitis in children in the antibiotic resistance era. Pediatr Infect Dis J 24(9):823–828, 2005.

Ghosh C: Periorbital and orbital cellulitis after *H. influenzae* B vaccination (Letter). Ophthalmology 108(9):1514–1515, 2001.

Gilsdorf JR, Marrs CF, Foxman B: *Haemophilus influenzae*: Genetic variability and natural selection to identify virulence factors. Infect Immun 72(5):2457–2461, 2004.

Iannini P: Prevention and management of antibacterial resistance for primary care patients with respiratory tract infections. South Med J 96(10):1008–1017, 2003.

Jacobs MR: Worldwide trends in antimicrobial resistance among common respiratory tract pathogens in children. Pediatr Infect Dis J 22(8 Suppl): S109–S119, 2003.

MMWR: Progress toward eliminating *Haemophilus influenza* type b disease among infants and children-United States, 1987–1997. Morb Mortal Wkly Rep 47:993; 1998.

Murphy TF: Respiratory infections caused by non-typeable *Haemophilus influenzae*. Curr Opin Infect Dis 16(2):129–134, 2003.

Starkey CR, Steele RW: Medical management of orbital cellulitis. Pediatr Infect Dis J 20(10):1002–1005, 2001.

Swingler G, Fransman D, Hussey G: Conjugate vaccines for preventing *Haemophilus influenzae* type b infections. Cochrane Database of Systematic Reviews (4):CD001729, 2003.

Yoder DM, Scott IU, Flynn HW, Jr, Miller D: Endophthalmitis caused by *Haemophilus influenzae*. Ophthalmol 111(11):2023–2026, 2004.

18 HERPES SIMPLEX 054.9

F. Hampton Roy, MD, FACS
Little Rock, Arkansas

Herpes simplex virus is a large, complex DNA virus that commonly infects the skin and mucous membranes in the regions of the mouth, genitalia, and eyes. The initial attack in adults is generally self-limited and often subclinical. However, herpetic disease is recurrent, and a wide range of clinical manifestations can result from an infection with this agent. Herpes simplex in the neonate is frequently accompanied by devastating complications of system wide infection, particularly in the central nervous system.

ETIOLOGY/INCIDENCE

Transmission is typically via sexual contact or hand-to-eye spread; the virus can infect a fetus in utero through the placenta, but more commonly the neonate is infected via the mother during passage through the birth canal.

DIAGNOSIS

Primary ocular herpes is often difficult to distinguish from acute follicular conjunctivitis due to adenovirus infection. The diagnosis usually is a clinical one, based on the presence of lid lesions, a characteristic dendrite, or both.

Clinical signs and symptoms

Ocular

Primary herpes infection of the eye is typically a unilateral blepharoconjunctivitis, characterized by:

- Vesicles on the skin of the eyelids;
- Follicular conjunctivitis, hyperemia;
- Preauricular adenopathy;
- Punctate keratitis (occasionally).

After primary infection, *recurrent disease* is usually in the form of a dendritic ulceration of the cornea.

However, epithelial ulceration can occasionally assume an amoebic or a geographic form. This more severe form of *epithelial herpetic keratitis* frequently appears in patients who are immunocompromised by the long-term use of topical corticosteroid preparations or by conditions such as infection with human immunodeficiency virus.

Between 10% and 20% of patients with herpetic corneal ulceration subsequently develop stromal inflammation, stromal scarring, or both.

The stromal involvement may be necrotizing, often associated with deep vascularization.

The stromal involvement may be non-necrotizing (most commonly disciform in configuration) due to severe endothelial disease and associated stromal edema.

The stromal patterns of involvement are associated with uveitis, iris atrophy and corneal hypesthesia.

Other manifestations and complications of ocular herpes simplex infection can include cataract, hypopyon, descemetocele, scleritis and occlusion of the nasolacrimal canaliculi.

Indolent (metaherpetic) ulceration occurs when healing of the epithelium is compromised by the underlying stromal inflammation, or it can be secondary to medication toxicity.

Laboratory findings

Laboratory diagnosis is made with viral cultures, immunohistochemistry, or polymerase chain reaction.

TREATMENT

Since most cases of HSV epithelial keratitis resolve spontaneously within 3 weeks, the rationale for treatment is to minimize stromal damage and scarring.

Local

Although *primary ocular herpes* is self-limited, treatment is recommended to limit corneal involvement. Treatment options include one of the following:

- Trifluridine 1.0% drops nine times daily for 10 days;
- Vidarabine 3.0% ointment five times daily for 10 days;
- Aciclovir 2 g/day PO for 10 days.

Oral aciclovir is the preferred treatment in patients who have good renal function and are unable to tolerate the topical medications. A cycloplegic agent may be added for relief from ciliary spasm.

Recurrent herpetic dendritic or *geographic epithelial keratitis* usually resolves spontaneously in 3 to 4 weeks if left untreated. However, treatment is recommended to reduce corneal damage from both the infection and the immune response to the infection.

Recommended treatment includes a combination of debridement and antiviral therapy with trifluridine, vidarabine, idoxuridine, or aciclovir.

Debridement is performed after the instillation of a topical anesthetic agent (4.0% cocaine or 0.5% proparacaine) into the conjunctival sac. The loose epithelium at the edges of the dendritic figure is wiped away with sterile cotton-tipped applicators or with the edge of a knife blade or platinum spatula.

Antiviral medications to be used after corneal debridement can be trifluorothymidine (trifluridine), idoxuridine, or vidarabine. Trifluridine, a pyrimidine analog, is the drug of choice in the United States for topical ophthalmic antiviral therapy. Although similar in structure to idoxuridine, it is twice as potent, and because of its biphasic solubility, it is 10-fold more soluble and so can achieve therapeutic intraocular concentrations. It is also considered more efficacious than vidarabine in the treatment of geographic ulcers. Of the three antiviral agents, trifluridine is the least vulnerable to resistant viral strains; there is no cross-allergenicity among trifluridine, idoxuridine, and vidarabine.

For recurrent herpetic episodes, the following are recommended doses:

- Trifluridine 1.0% drops nine times daily for 10 days and then tapered;
- Idoxuridine 1.0% drops once every waking hour and every 2 hours at night;
- Vidarabine 3.0% ointment five times daily.

Oral aciclovir is considered the treatment of choice for patients with recurrent disease in whom chronic suppression is desired or who are allergic to the available topical therapies. The recommended aciclovir dosage for active disease is 200 mg PO five times daily; for chronic suppression, as little as one 200-mg tablet every other day may be sufficient.

A study performed by the Herpetic Eye Disease Study Group showed no benefit by the addition of oral aciclovir to a regimen of topical trifluridine for the treatment of epithelial disease or for preventing the development of stromal disease or iridocyclitis.

Aciclovir is the most recent ophthalmic agent available for the treatment of herpes simplex; it is a prodrug that is activated through phosphorylation by a virus-specific thymidine kinase but only minimally activated by host cells. This gives aciclovir 3000 times greater effect against herpes simplex virus than against the host; its toxicity in the ointment form (not yet available in the United States) compares favorably with that of trifluridine, vidarabine, and idoxuridine. Aciclovir and trifluridine are equally effective in the treatment of epithelial disease.

Cidofovir (Vistide), a drug largely used against cytomegalovirus infections, may be effective in aciclovir-resistant cases.

Cimetidine has been studied recently in connection with augmentation or modification of the immunologic status of the patient with herpes as an adjunct to standard antiviral therapy. The efficacy of this combination modality has not been fully established.

In vitro studies using both fusion proteins (which block the interaction of T cells with antigen-presenting cells) and basic fibroblast growth factors have shown a beneficial effect of these as adjunctive treatments in decreasing the incidence of stromal keratitis and iridocyclitis.

Stomal herpetic keratitis occurs in 10% to 15% of patients with recurrent disease and carries the greatest visual morbidity risk. Stromal disease is believed to be a cell-mediated response to viral antigen; if the stromal involvement is accompanied by a concomitant epithelial defect, it is treated similarly to epithelial keratitis, with topical antiviral medication and a cycloplegic agent until the epithelium has healed. Both necrotizing and non-necrotizing stromal disease without associated epithelial defect are treated with topical corticosteroids and topical or oral antiviral agents.

These agents are recommended to prevent or limit epithelial disease during the course of treatment with corticosteroids.

The strategy for topical corticosteroid therapy is frequent initial administration (every 1 to 4 hours), followed by tapering the dose to the lowest effective amount; prophylactic trifluridine is initiated and tapered at the same rate as the steroid until corticosteroid therapy is tapered down to once daily, at which time the topical antiviral is discontinued.

Elevated intraocular pressure associated with steroid use should be treated with timolol and systemic acetazolamide as necessary.

Indolent stromal ulceration is managed with antiviral and corticosteroid therapy, along with a soft contact lens to prevent corneal drying. When there is herpetic melting of the cornea, care must be taken *not* to abruptly stop corticosteroid therapy because doing so may result in 'rebound' inflammation and increase the melting process, which may proceed to perforation.

The anticollagenolytic activity of tetracycline may help to retard corneal melting when applied as a topical ointment. There also is a risk of medication-induced corneal toxicity or an anesthetic cornea when faced with chronic nonhealing epithelial defect or defects.

Supportive

Epithelial herpetic disease usually runs a short course of several days, and an initial dose of a short-acting cycloplegic, such as homatropine 5.0% is usually sufficient for ciliary spasm and pain; for stromal herpetic keratitis, uveitis, or both, the longer-acting effect of atropine is preferred.

The presence of *bacterial infection* complicating herpetic keratitis is sufficiently uncommon to make the routine administration of antibiotics unnecessary. However, any abrupt change in the nature of the corneal lesion should arouse suspicion of a bacterial complication, and appropriate tests and treatment measures should be instituted promptly.

Surgical

If a descemetocele has formed and corneal perforation is imminent, penetrating keratoplasty must be considered; if the cornea perforates, the best management is keratoplasty, performed as expediently as possible. In such an emergency, it is possible to seal a perforated descemetocele using tissue adhesive and a bandage soft contact lens to allow reformation of the anterior chamber in preparation for definitive corneal transplantation.

Keratoplasty for corneal scarring secondary to stromal herpes simplex virus should be contemplated with caution; most corneal surgeons prefer to have the patient remain without recurrent disease for 6 to 12 months before considering the procedure.

PRECAUTIONS

A major problem related to therapy for recurrent herpetic keratitis is the difficulty in achieving a thorough and precise debridement that does not damage Bowman's layer. Some forms of debridement are particularly injurious; the use of sharp instruments, cryotherapy, or strong chemicals such as phenol or iodine should be avoided because they are unnecessarily damaging. Adequate debridement usually can be achieved by brushing the epithelial lesion or lesions with a cotton-tipped applicator, a technique that is both convenient and effective in that epithelial healing is rapid (usually within 24 hours) with an early resolution of the patient's pain and discomfort. Any tendency for recurrent lesions to form in the early period after healing can be overcome by using a topical antiviral agent for 7 to 10 days after debridement.

Topical corticosteroids are effective in suppressing the inflammatory response of herpetic keratitis; however, their inappropriate use may result in severe epithelial disease or stromal necrosis, an increased tendency toward recurrence, elevation of intraocular pressure, and the possibility of cataract formation. Patients requiring topical corticosteroids for suppression of the inflammatory response usually must use the drug for a period of months, and withdrawal often is complicated by recurrence of inflammation. The immunosuppressive complications of steroid administration can largely be avoided by the concurrent use of antiviral therapy. Patient cooperation is a prerequisite for the safe administration of corticosteroids in herpetic keratitis.

There also exists a fine balance between the beneficial anti-inflammatory action of steroids in the battle of host versus virus and the toxicity of the antiviral compounds. All topical antiviral medications available for clinical use in the United States are toxic to a degree; the signs of toxicity are similar for all such drugs. Punctate epithelial keratopathy, limbal follicles, a follicular conjunctival response, ptosis, punctal stenosis, and contact dermatitis may occur at any time after 10 to 14 days of antiviral therapy. In mild cases of antiviral toxicity, epithelial changes may be the only manifestation. Idoxuridine is the most toxic topical antiviral agent in clinical use, whereas vidarabine and trifluridine seem to be less toxic; topical aciclovir is not yet available in the United States. Oral aciclovir should be used with caution in patients who have renal disease.

COMMENTS

The major difficulties in treating herpetic keratitis are related to the tendency for recurrence and the management of stromal disease. Several mechanisms seem to be responsible for the recurrences. In its latent form, herpes simplex virus can be asymptomatically present in the cells of the cornea and in the central connections of the trigeminal nerve, particularly in the trigeminal ganglion. Disturbance of the nerve results in reactivation of the virus and its subsequent passage centrifugally along the nerve, with shedding from the nerve endings. Lesions tend to occur when the balance between latency and host defenses is disturbed, such as during febrile illness, during menses, or on exposure to sunlight.

The toxic potential of antiviral agents should always be considered in patients who heal poorly because these agents are inhibitors of cell division. Although continuous ocular drug delivery systems are currently under investigation, the limitations of such systems in preventing recurrences are related to the unacceptable toxicity from the chronic use of presently available topical medications.

REFERENCES

Chong EM, Wilhelmus KR, Matoba AY: Herpes simplex virus keratitis in children. Am J Ophthalmol 138(3):474–475, 2004.

Cohn J, Malet F, Chastel C: Acyclovir in herpetic anterior uveitis. Ann Ophthalmol 23:28–30, 1991.

Ekatomatis P: Herpes simplex dendritic keratitis after treatment with latanoprost for primary open angle glaucoma. Br J Ophthalmol 85(8):1008–1009, 2001.

Herbort CP, Buechi ER, Matter M: Blunt spatula debridement and trifluorothymidine in epithelial herpetic keratitis. Curr Eye Res 6:225–228, 1987.

Herpetic Eye Disease Study Group: A controlled trial of oral acyclovir for the prevention of stromal keratitis or iritis in patients with herpes simplex virus epithelial keratitis. Arch Ophthalmol 115:703–712, 1997.

Malouf DJ, Oates RK: Herpes simplex virus infections in the neonate. J Paediatr Child Health 31:332–335, 1995.

Ohashi Y, Nishida K, Yamamoto S, et al: Demonstration of herpes simplex virus DNA in idiopathic corneal endotheliopathy. Am J Ophthalmol 112:419–423, 1991.

Rong BL, Pavan-Langston D, Weng QP, et al: Detection of herpes simplex virus thymidine kinase and latency-associated transcript gene sequences in human herpetic corneas by polymerase chain reaction amplification. Invest Ophthalmol Vis Sci 32:1808–1815, 1991.

Wilhelmus KR, Dawson CR, Barron BA: Risk factors for herpes simplex virus epithelial keratitis recurring during treatment of stromal keratitis or iridocyclitis. Herpetic Eye Disease Study Group. Br J Ophthalmol 80:969–972, 1996.

19 INCLUSION CONJUNCTIVITIS 077.0 *(Paratrachoma, Chlamydial Conjunctivitis)*

F. Hampton Roy, MD, FACS
Little Rock, Arkansas

ETIOLOGY/INCIDENCE

The *Chlamydiae* are obligate intracellular organisms derived from bacteria and comprise four species: *Chlamydia trachomatis*, *C. psittaci*, *C. pneumoniae*, and *C. pecorum*. *C. trachomatis* is exclusively a human pathogen and includes the agents of classic trachoma (always associated with serotypes A, B, Ba, and C) and of inclusion conjunctivitis or paratrachoma (serotypes D, E, F, G, H, I, J, and K). These organisms infect transitional epithelium of mucous surfaces. *C. trachomatis* also includes the agents of lymphogranuloma venereum (serotypes L1, L2, and L3), which infect epithelial cells and macrophages and are more pathogenic in human and animal models.

Serotypes D through K are sexually transmitted, and secondary eye involvement in adults occurs in about 1 of 300 genital cases. Infection of the eyes occurs by the transfer of infected genital discharges from the patients or their sexual partners on the hands or by oral-genital sexual activities. Genitally transmitted chlamydial infections are the major cause of nongonococcal urethritis in males and of cervicitis and salpingitis in females.

Infants exposed to chlamydial infection from the mothers' cervix during birth develop chlamydial ophthalmia neonatorum at 5 to 12 days of age; of infants exposed during delivery, approximately 35% to 50% contract the disease. From 10% to 20% also develop chlamydial respiratory disease with pneumonia as late as 6 months postpartum; the infection also involves the gastrointestinal tract.

DIAGNOSIS

Clinical signs and symptoms

Patients with neonatal ophthalmia present with tearing, moderate discharge and swelling of the lids.

The eye is usually hyperemic, with infiltration and swelling of the conjunctiva and lids. If untreated, chlamydial conjunctivitis in newborns may resolve spontaneously in 5 to 9 months, but it has been known to persist for years with development of chronic follicular conjunctivitis, corneal neovascularization (vascular pannus) and conjunctival scarring.

Infants with chlamydial pneumonitis may present from 6 weeks to 6 months of age with rhinitis, cough, a pertussis-like inspiratory whoop, and eosinophilia.

In adults, ocular chlamydial infection produces chronic follicular conjunctivitis with keratitis. Because this adult disease is difficult to distinguish from the clinical findings in early trachoma, the term 'paratrachoma' has been used to describe the entire spectrum of eye disease with genitally transmitted chlamydial infection. Ocular chlamydial disease occurs most frequently in those 15 to 30 years old. The eye disease usually has an acute onset in one eye, with:

- Watering;
- Mucopurulent discharge and sticking of lids on waking;
- Foreign body sensation;
- Swelling of the lids;
- An ipsilateral swollen preauricular node;
- Follicular conjunctivitis with hyperemia;
- Diffuse infiltration;
- Superficial keratitis, including macropunctate epithelial erosions;
- Subepithelial infiltrates (like those of epidemic keratoconjunctivitis);
- Limbal infiltration; and
- Superficial neovascularization.

Rarely, *C. psittaci* strains produce follicular conjunctivitis in humans exposed to the appropriate animal hosts, specifically parrots and other psittacine birds (psittacosis agent) or young cats (feline pneumonitis agent). *C. pneumoniae* is an important cause of pneumonia in humans and can infect the eye. Both species cause a follicular conjunctivitis similar to that of *C. trachomatis*.

Laboratory findings

Laboratory procedures to identify *C. trachomatis* infections are necessary to confirm the diagnosis and include:

- Giemsa staining of smears;
- Isolation in cell culture (definitive method, although time intensive);
- Direct fluorescent monoclonal antibodies (DFAs) to stain smears;
- Enzyme immunoassays (EIAs);
- DNA probes;
- DNA amplification tests (including the polymerase chain reaction and ligase chain reaction); and
- Serum antibody tests (including the complement fixation and microimmunofluorescent tests but less useful than the demonstration of agent due to preexisting antibody titers).

Microscopic examination of Giemsa-stained conjunctival smears is most useful in detecting neonatal chlamydial infections because the inclusions are so numerous, but it is much less sensitive for adult inclusion conjunctivitis. The DFAs and EIAs are widely available and equally sensitive. The DNA amplification tests are highly sensitive and specific for identifying *C. trachomatis* infection in the conjunctiva and genital tracts of both adults and neonates. Cell culture is the definitive technique but is less available and is less sensitive than DNA amplification procedures.

The presence of serum IgM antibodies against *Chlamydiae* in newborns suggests a systemic infection, particularly pneumonia, but serologic tests have little use in diagnosing other *C. trachomatis* infections.

Most tests for *C. trachomatis* do not detect *C. psittaci* or *C. pneumonia*, but tests based on the detection of chlamydial genus-specific antigen detect *C. psittaci* and *C. pneumoniae* (e.g. DFA test [LPS, Ortho] that identifies all three species).

PROPHYLAXIS

The recommended prophylaxis for neonates to prevent both gonococcal neonatal ophthalmia and chlamydial ophthalmia is one application of tetracycline or erythromycin ointment within 1 hour after delivery. Credé prophylaxis with 1% silver nitrate is equally effective in preventing chlamydial eye infection of the newborn.

TREATMENT

Systemic

Because *C. trachomatis* infection is not limited to the eye in either neonatal infants or adults, it is necessary to use systemic antimicrobial treatment. Moreover, the sexual consorts of adults and the parents of infants must also receive a full course of therapy. Simultaneous treatment of all sexual partners is important to prevent reinfection. It also is prudent to examine all sexual partners for other venereal diseases, such as gonorrhea, syphilis, and HIV.

For infants, effective therapy is provided by erythromycin suspension 50 mg/kg/day PO in four equal doses for 2 weeks.

Children older than 4 months can be treated with azithromycin pediatric suspension 200 mg/5 ml in a single dose of 20 mg/kg body weight.

For adults with chlamydial eye infections one 1-g dose of oral azithromycin for genital *C. trachomatis* infections; a repeat dose at 1 week may be considered for those with eye infection.

Alternative treatment regimens for adults include one of the following:

- Doxycycline 100 mg b.i.d. for 2 weeks;
- Erythromycin base 500 mg PO four times a day for 7 days; or
- Ofloxacin 300 mg twice a day for 7 days (not for use in patients under 18 years or in pregnant or lactating women); or
- Amoxicillin 500 mg PO three times a day for 7 days.

C. psittaci and *C. pneumoniae* eye infections are treated with the same drugs and dosages for 4 to 6 weeks.

Ocular

Because chlamydial infections are systemic, local therapy alone should be discouraged; it has been shown that topical treatment alone is extremely slow and only partially effective in treating adult or neonatal inclusion conjunctivitis and that relapses are frequent. Local antimicrobial treatment with tetracycline or erythromycin ointment to the eye is not necessary for patients on full oral therapeutic doses of antibiotic. Topical sulfonamide alone is even less effective than topical tetracyclines or erythromycin; topical rifampin ointment has been used in the treatment of ocular chlamydial infections but, as with other topical antimicrobial agents, is of limited use.

For the occasional adult patient who develops an anterior iritis with inclusion conjunctivitis, the use of topical corticosteroids carries no more risk than to any other patient as long as the patient is under systemic treatment with antimicrobial agents or has received a full course of systemic antimicrobial treatment. When used without systemic antichlamydials, topical corticosteroids are definitely contraindicated for the treatment of chlamydial conjunctivitis or keratitis because the medications prolong the disease.

PRECAUTIONS

The use of erythromycin estolate or ethylsuccinate is known to carry a high risk of toxic hepatitis, and erythromycin is also generally less well tolerated than oral tetracyclines. Although sulfonamides have been given in the past, they carry a high risk of systemic toxicity, which precludes their use for chlamydial infection.

Nongranulomatous anterior uveitis may develop as a response to chlamydial infection in patients who are positive for HLA B27. The uveitis does not respond to antimicrobial treatment alone but can be suppressed with adequate doses of topical corticosteroids. Recurrent episodes of uveitis occur with this syndrome but are unrelated to further chlamydial infection.

REFERENCES

Bersudsky V, Rehany U, Tendler Y, et al: Diagnosis of chlamydial infection by direct enzyme-linked immunoassay and polymerase chain reaction in patients with acute follicular conjunctivitis. Graefes Arch Clin Exp Ophthalmol 237(8):617–620, 1999.

Carta F, Zanetti S, Pinna A, et al: The treatment and follow up of adult chlamydial ophthalmia. Br J Ophthalmol 78(3):206–208, 1994.

Dean D, Shama A, Schachter J, Dawson CR: Identification of an avian strain of *Chlamydia psittaci* causing severe keratoconjunctivitis in a bird fancier. Clin Infect Dis 20:1179–1185, 1995.

Grossman M, Schachter J, Sweet R, et al: Prospective studies in chlamydia in newborns. In: Mardh P-A, Holmes KK, Oriel JD, et al, eds: Chlamydial infections. Amsterdam, Elsevier Biomedical, 1982:213–216.

Lietman T, Dawson CR, Schachter J, Dean D: Chronic follicular conjunctivitis associated with *Chlamydia pneumoniae* and *Chlamydia psittaci*. Clin Infect Dis 26:1335–1340, 1998.

MMWR: 1998 guidelines for treatment of sexually transmitted diseases. MMWR 47:53–59, 1998.

20 INFECTIOUS MONONUCLEOSIS 075 *(Epstein–Barr Virus)*

Matilda Frances Chan, MD, PhD
Rochester, New York
Steven S. T. Ching, MD
Rochester, New York

Infectious mononucleosis (IM) is a clinical syndrome that is characterized by the triad of fever, tonsillar pharyngitis and lymphadenopathy. Epstein–Barr virus (EBV), the primary agent of infectious mononucleosis, is a widely disseminated herpesvirus that is spread by intimate contact between susceptible persons and asymptomatic EBV shedders. Contact of EBV with oropharyngeal epithelial cells followed by viral replication and infection of neighboring lymphoid B cells leads to dissemination of infection throughout the lymphoreticular system of which the lacrimal gland and conjunctiva are components. Other acute infections known to cause mononucleosis syndromes include cytomegalovirus, *Toxoplasma* spp., human immunodeficiency virus, human herpesvirus type 6, hepatitis virus and possibly human herpesvirus type 7.

ETIOLOGY/INCIDENCE

EBV infection occurs worldwide. Approximately 90 to 95% of adults are EBV-seropositive. The rate of EBV exposure and development of antibodies by the age of four is close to 100% in developing countries and between 25 to 50% in sociologically underprivileged communities in the United States. The majority of primary EBV infections throughout the world are subclinical and the risk of development of clinical symptoms depends on the age of exposure. In children younger than 6 years, EBV infection may be asymptomatic or present as an upper respiratory infection. EBV infection is the etiologic agent in 75% of children and adolescents manifesting the IM syndrome. The vast majority of adults are not susceptible to infection because of immunity due to prior exposure.

DIAGNOSIS

Clinical signs and symptoms

Systemic

The clinical course of the systemic illness is characterized by the following classic signs:

- Two to five days of prodrome of malaise, headache and low grade fever;
- Subsequent development of moderate to high fever, tonsillitis and/or pharyngitis and lymphadenopathy;
- Acute symptoms resolve in one to two weeks, but fatigue often persists for months.

Other systemic manifestations associated with infectious mononucleosis include the following:

- Severe fatigue;
- Splenomegaly (50 to 60%);
- Skin rash (associated with antibiotic use);
- Neurologic syndromes (Guillain–Barré syndrome, cranial nerve palsies, meningoencephalitis, aseptic meningitis, transverse myelitis, peripheral neuritis);
- Hematologic abnormalities.

Ocular

- Conjunctiva: follicular, granulomatous, or membranous conjunctivitis; subconjunctival hemorrhage, hyperemia.
- Cornea: punctuate epithelial keratitis, dendritic keratitis, stromal keratitis (subepithelial infiltrates, nummular opacities, ring-shaped granular opacities, multilevel stromal infiltrates), intrastromal neovascularization, keratoconjunctivitis sicca, linear endotheliitis.
- Lacrimal system: dacryoadenitis, dacryocystitis, Sjögren's syndrome, aqueous tear deficiency.
- Sclera: episcleritis, scleritis.
- Uvea: iritis, vitritis, multifocal choroiditis, retinitis (punctuate, hemorrhagic), intraocular posttransplant lymphoproliferative disorder.
- Neuro-ophthalmologic: accommodation paresis, convergence deficiency, hemianopsia, nystagmus, ophthalmoplegia, optic neuritis, papilledema.

Laboratory findings

Hematologic

Peripheral blood smear characterized by atypical lymphocytes (more than 10%) and lymphocytosis (60–70%).

Serologic

- Heterophile antibodies — Paul–Bunnell and Monospot tests are sensitive and specific for IM and antibodies appear within one week of clinical symptoms and remain positive for up to one year.
- Specific EBV antibodies — levels of IgM and IgG antibodies against viral capsid antigens (VCA) and nuclear antigen (EBNA) are used for heterophil-negative mononucleosis.

The current recommendation is that patients with clinical suspicion for IM should have a white blood cell count with differential and a heterophile test. If the heterophile test is negative but there is still a strong clinical suspicion, EBV antibody levels should be measured.

The direct detection of EBV genome fragments in ocular tissues can be achieved using polymerase chain reaction (PCR).

TREATMENT

Systemic

- Rest, fluids and acetaminophen are recommended. Aspirin should not be given to children or teenagers because of the risk for the development of Reye's syndrome.
- Avoid strenuous activity and contact sports to decrease the risk of splenic rupture.
- The use of systemic steroids is unproven, but they can be used for special circumstances such as airway restriction, hematologic or neurologic complications and uveitis.
- Aciclovir and immunomodulating drugs such as interleukin-2 and interferon alpha have not been proven to alter clinical course.

Ocular

- Topical steroids have been used to treat stromal keratitis and uveitis.
- The therapeutic benefits of topical aciclovir or topical trifluridine have not been well studied.

COMMENTS

Dendritic and stromal keratitis have only rarely been reported for this disease. However, the lesions may be indistinguishable from some manifestations of herpes simplex keratitis; therefore, caution is advised in the use of steroids.

As demonstrated by reports on stromal infiltration and neovascularization, this entity should be considered in the differential diagnosis of interstitial keratitis. A case report describing a patient with acute EBV infection and with corneal findings of stromal edema with a distinct line of endothelial keratic precipitates suggests that EBV infection should be considered in the differential diagnosis of linear endotheliitis (BJ Shin, SS Ching, ARVO abstract, 2002).

SUMMARY

IM is a disease of children and young adults caused by EBV infection. Fortunately, ocular involvement is usually mild and requires no intervention. However, because the virus can affect the ocular system in multiple areas, the possibility of this entity should be kept in mind when the practitioner encounters puzzling ocular inflammation.

REFERENCES

Al-Attar L, Berrocal A, Warman R, et al: Diagnosis by polymerase chain reaction of ocular posttransplant lymphoproliferative disorder after pediatric renal transplantation. Am J Ophthalmol 137:569–571, 2004.

Aronson MD: Infectious mononucleosis in adults and adolescents. Online. Available at: UptoDate online version 12.3. http://www.uptodate.com. Accessed December 13, 2004.

Chodosh J, Gan Y, Sixbey JW: Detection of Epstein–Barr virus genome in ocular tissues. Ophthalmology 103:687–690, 1996.

Kaye SB, Baker K, Bonshek R, et al: Human herpesviruses in the cornea. Br J Ophthalmol 84:563–571, 2000.

Matoba AY: Ocular disease associated with Epstein–Barr virus infection. Surv Ophthalmol 35:145–150, 1990.

Matoba AY, Wilhelmus KR, Jones DB: Epstein–Barr viral stromal keratitis. Ophthalmology 93:746–751, 1986.

Palay DA, Litoff D, Krachmer JH: Stromal keratitis associated with Epstein–Barr virus infection in a young child. Arch Ophthalmol 111:1323–1324, 1993.

Pflugfelder SC, Crouse CA, Atherton SS: Ophthalmic manifestations of Epstein–Barr virus infection. Int Ophthalmol Clin 33:95–101, 1993.

21 INFLUENZA 487.1

Daniel H. Spitzberg, MD, FACS
Indianapolis, Indiana

ETIOLOGY/INCIDENCE

Influenza is an acute respiratory infection of specific viral etiology. There are three distinct antigenic types of influenza virus, designated A, B, and C; although type C usually produces only a minor illness, antigenic types A and B can cause major epidemics. The disease often occurs sporadically or in localized outbreaks, particularly in schools or military camps, and usually in fall or winter.

DIAGNOSIS

Clinical signs and symptoms

Systemic

The characteristics of influenza include the sudden onset of:

- Headache;
- Fever, which gradually subsides over 2 to 3 days;
- Malaise;
- Muscular aching;
- Substernal soreness;
- Nasal stuffiness, coryza;
- Mild pharyngeal infection, sore throat;
- Nonproductive cough;
- Nausea.

Influenza may cause necrosis of the respiratory epithelium, predisposing the body to secondary bacterial infections. Contracted early in pregnancy, influenza has been implicated in multiple congenital deformities of the fetus, including anencephaly and congenital cataract.

Ocular

Complications of influenza in the eye include:

- Conjunctival redness, subconjunctival hemorrhages;
- Acute catarrhal conjunctivitis;
- Superficial punctate or interstitial keratitis;
- Dendritic ulcer due to opportunistic herpes simplex;
- Palpebral edema;
- Dacryoadenitis, dacryocystitis;
- Secondary bacterial infections of the cornea, conjunctiva, or both;
- Bilateral, self-limited nongranulomatous anterior uveitis;
- Retinal angiospasm, edema, exudates, hemorrhages, stellate retinopathy;
- Venous thrombosis;
- Extraocular muscle myalgias, paralysis of third or fourth cranial nerve, tendonitis;
- Accommodative spasm, episcleritis, mydriasis, myopia;
- Cellulitis, panophthalmitis;
- Cataract (congenital);
- Optic neuritis (associated with encephalitis);
- Bilateral simultaneous corneal graft rejection after influenza vaccination;
- Optic neuritis after influenza vaccination;
- Bilateral optic neuropathy associated with influenza vaccination.

Uveitis associated with influenza can become chronic, with exacerbations and remissions.

TREATMENT

Systemic

Prophylactically, amantadine protects 50% to 70% of recipients exposed to influenza A viruses and is indicated for patients older than 1 year during influenza A outbreaks, especially individuals for whom influenza would pose a grave risk, such as the elderly. It may be most effective in individuals who already have antibodies against influenza A virus strains; therefore, previous vaccination does not interfere with and may augment its effect. Amantadine also may have therapeutic value if given promptly after the first symptoms of infection appear. The administration of amantadine 100 mg twice daily should be continued for at least 10 days.

Ocular

In cases of mild uveitis homatropine 5% solution should be applied topically four times daily to control pain.

Influenzal uveitis can become chronic, with exacerbations and remissions; patients with this type of uveitis respond well to topical ocular corticosteroid therapy for short time periods.

Prednisolone topical 0.12% ophthalmic solution can be applied two or three times daily for 1 week to control low-grade uveitis.

Catarrhal marginal ulcers are an immunologic response to the viral infection and should be treated with 0.12% prednisolone solution four times daily.

Supportive

Bedrest and gradual return to full activity are advisable to reduce complications; the patient's cough reflex can be depressed with codeine (adult dose 15 to 60 mg PO).

Codeine is more effective than salicylates for the treatment of influenzal headache and myalgia; salicylates often increase discomfort by causing sweats and chills. Antibiotics should be reserved for treating bacterial complications.

PROPHYLAXIS

Routine yearly immunization with polyvalent influenza virus vaccine is strongly recommended for high-risk groups, including pregnant women and persons older than 65 years regardless of their health status. Persons of all ages who have chronic rheumatic heart disease, other cardiovascular disease, chronic bronchopulmonary disease, diabetes mellitus, or Addison's disease should be considered for prophylactic treatment.

PRECAUTIONS

If the fever persists for longer than 4 days, if the cough becomes productive, or if the white cell count rises above 12,000/mm^3, secondary bacterial infection should be ruled out or verified and treated.

Although the duration of uncomplicated influenza is 1 to 7 days and complete recovery is the rule, preexisting respiratory disease or secondary bacterial pneumonia can lead to a fatal outcome. Most fatalities are due to bacterial pneumonia; pneumococcal pneumonia is most common, but staphylococcal pneumonia is most serious.

In general, serious ocular complications of influenza are rare; however, secondary bacterial infections must be watched closely. The cornea is the usual site of most serious ocular complications; this area and the anterior chamber are in the areas in which the main follow-up examinations should be focused.

REFERENCES

Giraldi C, Paterni F, Cecchini S, et al: Paralysis of the parasympathetic ocular nerve after influenza syndrome. Rev Neurol 61:180–182, 1991.

Grossman M, Jawetz E: Infectious diseases: viral and rickettsial. In: Krupp MA, Chatton MJ, eds: Current medical diagnosis and treatment. Los Altos, CA, Lange, 1982:821–822.

Hull TP, et al: Optic neuritis after influenza vaccination. Am J Ophthalmol 124(5):703–704, 1997. PMID: 9372734; UI: 98040003.

Knight V: Influenza. In: Isselbacher KJ, Adams RD, Braunwald E, et al, eds: Harrison's principles of internal medicine. 9th edn. New York, McGraw-Hill, 1980:785–789.

Majde JA, Brown RK, Jones MW, et al: Detection of toxic viral-associated double-stranded RNA (ds RNA) in influenza-infected lung. Microb Pathol 10:105–115, 1991.

Rabon RJ, Louis GJ, Zegarra H, Gutman FA: Acute bilateral posterior angiopathy with influenza A viral infection. Am J Ophthalmol 103:289–293, 1987.

Ray CL, et al: Bilateral optic neuropathy associated with influenza vaccination. J Neuroophthalmol 16(3):182–184, 1996. PMID: 8865010; UI: 97018394.

Schlaegel TF, Jr: Uveitis associated with viral infections. In: Duane TD, ed: Clinical ophthalmology. Hagerstown, MD, Harper & Row, 1982: 4(46):1–13.

Solomon A, et al: Bilateral simultaneous corneal graft rejection after influenza vaccination. Am J Ophthalmol 121(6):708–709, 1996. PMID: 8644815; UI: 96243666.

22 KOCH–WEEKS BACILLUS 372.03

Alan Sugar, MD
Ann Arbor, Michigan
Roni Mintz, MD
Ann Arbor, Michigan

ETIOLOGY/INCIDENCE

Koch–Weeks bacillus is also known as *Hemophilus influenzae* biogroup *aegyptius*. It is a small, gram-negative, slender rod or coccobacillus. This organism was originally isolated as a cause of secondary infection in eyes with trachoma and as a cause of epidemic 'pink eye.' Despite some early confusion with classification, Koch–Weeks bacillus is considered to be a subspecies of *H. influenzae.*

Acute *H. aegyptius* conjunctivitis affects children during hot weather, especially in the tropical and subtropical climates of the Middle East and North Africa. Transmission is by flies and contact with ocular secretions. There is a 24-hour incubation period. Severe conjunctivitis develops rapidly with injection, chemosis, subconjunctival hemorrhage, and purulent discharge. Infection may follow or coincide with acute trachoma, although the relationship between these infections is not fully understood.

Although most patients do not develop systemic illness, a fulminant bacteremia may follow the resolution of conjunctivitis in patients infected with a distinct *H. aegyptius* strain known as the Brazilian purpuric fever (BPF) clone. This infection is associated with hemorrhagic skin lesions and often is rapidly fatal.

COURSE/PROGNOSIS

- There is rapid onset of injection, chemosis, and subconjunctival hemorrhage.
- Severe mucopurulent discharge occurs for about 3 days.
- Lid edema and preauricular node tenderness occur.
- Pseudomembrane may develop, especially in infants.
- Resolution usually occurs in 10 to 14 days without treatment.
- There may be relapse or chronic papillary conjunctivitis.
- Inferior limbal corneal ulcers may occur in the first few days.
- Phlyctenular conjunctivitis and conjunctival scarring may follow.
- Central corneal ulceration and perforation are rare.
- BPF follows resolution of conjunctivitis and is characterized by fever, vomiting, skin hemorrhage, hypotensive shock, and death if untreated.

DIAGNOSIS

Laboratory findings

- Thin, poorly staining gram-negative bacilli or coccobacilli on scrapings.
- Culture on chocolate agar or blood agar in high-CO_2 environment.
- Enhanced growth in presence of another organism.

TREATMENT

Local

- Hourly antibiotic eyedrops during the day and ointment at bedtime usually lead to resolution in 3 days.

Agents used include:

- Fluoroquinolones;
- Chloramphenicol;
- Sulfacetamide;
- Polymyxin B;
- Gentamicin;
- Tobramycin;
- Tetracycline;

Adequate treatment is helpful in preventing chronic conjunctivitis.

Systemic

Intravenous treatment for BPF with:

- Amoxicillin;
- Ampicillin;
- Azithromycin;
- Third-generation cephalosporins;
- Imipenem;
- Meropenem.

The use of oral rifampin in children with conjunctivitis in endemic areas for BPF may prevent onset of systemic illness.

COMPLICATIONS

- Chronic papillary conjunctivitis.
- Conjunctival scarring, especially when superimposed on trachoma.
- Periorbital or orbital cellulitis.
- BPF (as discussed).

REFERENCES

Brenner DJ, Mayer LW, Carlone GM, et al: Biochemical, genetic, and epidemiologic characterization of *Haemophilus influenzae* biogroup *aegyptius* (*Haemophilus aegyptius*) strains associated with Brazilian purpuric fever. J Clin Microbiol 26:1524–1534, 1988.

Dawson CF: Epidemic Koch–Weeks conjunctivitis and trachoma in the Coachilla Valley of California. Am J Ophthalmol 49:801–808, 1960.

Morrissey I, Burnett R, Viljoen L, et al: Surveillance of the susceptibility of ocular bacterial pathogens to the fluoroquinolone gatifloxacin and other antimicrobials in Europe during 2001/2002. J Infect 49:109–114, 2004.

Perkins BA, Tondella ML, Bortolotto IM, et al: Comparative efficacy of oral rifampin and topical chloramphenicol in eradicating conjunctival carriage of *Haemophilus influenzae biogroup aegyptius*: Brazilian Purpuric Fever Study Group. Pediatr Infect Dis J 11:717–721, 1992.

23 LEPROSY 023
(Hansen's Disease)

Timothy J. Ffytche, LVO, FRCS, FRCOphth
London, England

ETIOLOGY/INCIDENCE

Leprosy is a chronic granulomatous infection caused by the acid-fast bacillus *Mycobacterium leprae.* It is communicable and probably transmitted via droplets, although other methods of spread may occur.

The organisms have an affinity for neural tissue in parts of the body where the temperature is relatively low; thus, the skin, peripheral nerves, mucous membranes, testes and eyes are primarily involved. The disease leads to disfigurement and loss of mobility and in a significant number of patients, the deformities may be accompanied by visual impairment. In many countries, leprosy still carries a social stigma due to ignorance that has persisted for centuries.

DIAGNOSIS

Clinical signs and symptoms

The clinical picture of the disease is influenced by the immunity of the host, which is highest in the paucibacillary form (PB) and lowest in the multibacillary form (MB). Ocular involvement may occur through five main pathways:

- Directly in MB disease through invasion of the anterior part of the globe, which is susceptible because of its relatively low temperature;
- Indirectly in both types of leprosy through the effects of damage to the superficial branches of the fifth and seventh cranial nerves;
- During the two forms of acute inflammatory reaction that occur when there is a sudden alteration in the disease immunity; these are known as reversal reactions and erythema nodosum leprosum (ENL) and may develop spontaneously or as a result of changes in therapy, an intercurrent infection, or stress;
- Through damage to the adnexa;
- Through secondary infection.

Ocular and periocular

- Cornea: corneal hypesthesia, corneal ulcer, exposure keratopathy, leproma, pannus, superficial stromal keratitis, thickened corneal nerves.
- Episclera and sclera: episcleritis, scleritis, staphyloma.
- Eyebrows: madarosis; nodules, thickening of the skin.
- Eyelids: dermatochalasis, distichiasis, ectropion, entropion, lagophthalmos, madarosis, nodules, trichiasis.
- Iris: iridocyclitis (acute or chronic), iris atrophy, iris pearls, nodular leproma, synechiae (Figure 23.1).
- Lacrimal system: dacryocystitis, (acute or chronic), epiphora, nasolacrimal duct obstruction.
- Pupil: anisocoria, corectopia, diminished or absent response to light, miosis, occlusio pupillae, polycoria, seclusio pupillae.

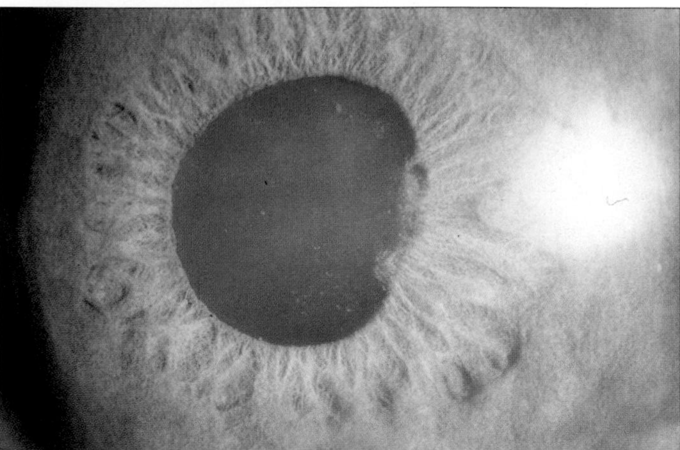

FIGURE 23.1 Anterior synechiae and adjacent iris nodule in patient with leprosy.

- Others: decreased intraocular pressure, paralysis of seventh nerve, phthisis bulbi, secondary cataract, secondary glaucoma.

TREATMENT

Systemic

The development of resistant organisms to standard antileprosy drugs, together with noncompliance, has led to a radical reappraisal of the therapy for the disease over the past two decades with the universal introduction of multidrug therapy (MDT).

Paucibacillary disease

The regimen recommended by the World Health Organization (WHO) consists of dapsone 100 mg/day as self-medication and rifampicin 600 mg once a month under surveillance, with treatment continued for at least 6 months.

Multibacillary disease

The WHO recommends dapsone 100 mg/day and clofazimine 50 mg/day as self-medication and once-monthly supervised doses of rifampicin 600 mg and clofazimine 300 mg. Treatment in MB cases should be continued for at least 1 year and preferably until negative skin smears are obtained. Doses are reduced proportionately for children. Patients who cannot take clofazamine can be treated with combinations of ofloxacin and minocycline.

Acute reactions

In leprosy, acute reactions require prompt and energetic therapy to avoid permanent neural and ocular damage; treatment includes the use of systemic corticosteroid preparations, doses starting at 40 mg of prednisone daily and analgesic agents. In addition, control of the reaction can be facilitated by the use of clofazimine and thalidomide (if available).

MDT has now become standard leprosy treatment everywhere, although a few of the more traditional therapies, such as chaulmoogra oil and herbal remedies, still persist in some parts of the world. Prophylactic vaccination with the bacillus Calmette–Guérin has been found to provide some protection in several areas where the disease is endemic.

Ocular

The ocular manifestations of leprosy are influenced by many factors and may vary according to ethnic groups. There are four main causes of blindness that can occur singly or in combination:

- Lagophthalmos, leading to exposure keratopathy;
- Corneal hypesthesia, predisposing to corneal ulceration;
- Acute or chronic iridocyclitis;
- Secondary cataract.

Medical and surgical treatments have an important role in preventing sight-threatening complications and in treating ocular and adnexal disease.

Medical

Exposure keratopathy may result from facial nerve involvement, especially if combined with corneal hypesthesia. It can occur after an acute neuritis in a reversal reaction or as part of chronic paralysis. To protect the cornea, it should be treated energetically with lubricating eyedrops and broad-spectrum antibiotic drops and ointment and the neuritis may respond to systemic steroid therapy. Lid surgery may be necessary in the later stages.

Acute iridocyclitis that occurs in ENL responds to conventional anti-inflammatory treatment with local mydriatic and steroid drops. During an attack, 1% atropine t.i.d. should be used with dexamethasone every hour; the dosage can be reduced as the inflammation subsides. In severe cases, subconjunctival injections of steroids and mydriatic agents may be necessary. If secondary glaucoma develops, oral hypotensive agents, such as acetazolamide 250 mg q.i.d., should be added to this regimen.

Chronic iridocyclitis occurs in MB disease, resulting in iris atrophy; a profound miosis may develop and cause considerable visual loss. This condition does not respond to local mydriatic or steroid therapy in the late stage, but attempts can be made to dilate the pupils with daily instillations of 5% phenylephrine or 1% atropine before the atrophy becomes too advanced.

Surgical

Lid surgery is designed to prevent corneal damage from exposure caused by facial nerve paralysis; procedures range from simple lateral tarsorrhaphy to more elaborate operations, such as temporalis transfer. Malpositions of the lids also require surgical correction to avoid secondary corneal disease and an infected lacrimal sac, which can provide a reservoir of infection, should be removed.

Intraocular surgery is tolerated reasonably well by the leprous eye as long as there is no active inflammation and such procedures as optical iridectomy, cataract surgery and corneal grafts may be performed safely. There is no contraindication to intraocular lens implantation in PB cases, but it should be avoided in MB disease when chronic iridocyclitis is present.

PRECAUTIONS

The institution of multidrug therapy has been the most significant factor in the control of eye complications and supervised administration in order to encourage compliance with treatment is very important for its success.

- Dapsone toxicity includes anorexia, nausea and vomiting, neuropathy, anemia and agranulocytosis and the drug should not be given to patients with glucose-6-phosphate dehydrogenase deficiency.

- Clofazimine can provoke diarrhea and causes red discoloration of the skin, conjunctiva and urine, which may be disturbing to the patient.
- Rifampicin may give rise to gastrointestinal and respiratory symptoms, acute renal failure, thrombocytopenic purpura, hepatic reactions and skin rashes.
- Steroids given either topically or systemically should be monitored carefully to avoid steroid-induced glaucoma and secondary cataract.

COMMENTS

Visual impairment in leprosy is caused mainly by damage to the cornea through paralysis of the facial and trigeminal nerves, by cataract and by the complications of acute and chronic iridocyclitis. Patients are often unaware of ocular involvement and therefore it may go undetected at a stage when preventive measures would be most effective. The education of leprosy workers to screen for eye disease and of patients on self-care and drug compliance therefore becomes fundamentally important.

The aim of therapy should be the prevention of ocular changes through attention to eye protection and hygiene and to the early diagnosis of intraocular disease. Once the eye is affected, continuous supervision should be the goal, even after the patient has completed multidrug therapy and is classified as 'cured.' Whenever late complications develop, attempts should be made to preserve useful vision by medical and surgical measures. This may often mean that long-standing prejudices and the stigma of the disease must be overcome to avoid blindness, which is especially tragic in these individuals who are already disabled and disadvantaged.

REFERENCES

Brand MB: The care of the eye in Hansen's disease. 3rd edn. Carville, LA, Gillis W. Long Hansen's Disease Centre, 1993.

Courtright P, Johnson GJ: Prevention of blindness in leprosy. Rev edn. London, International Centre for Eye Health, 1991.

ffytche TJ: The prevalence of disabling ocular complications of leprosy: a global study. Ind J Lepr 70:49–59, 1998.

Hogeweg M: Ocular leprosy. Int J Lepr 69:30–35, 2001.

Joffrion VC: Ocular leprosy. In: Hastings leprosy. 2nd edn. Edinburgh, Churchill Livingstone, 353–364, 1994.

WHO Expert Committee on Leprosy, Seventh Report. Geneva, World Health Organization, 1998 (Technical Report Series No. 874).

24 LEPTOSPIROSIS 100.9

S. R. Rathinam, MNAMS
Madurai, Tamal Nadu, India
Emmett T. Cunningham, Jr., MD, PhD, MPH
San Francisco, California

ETIOLOGY

Leptospirosis, borreliosis, and syphilis are three important spirocheatal diseases, each of which can manifest both as a primary systemic infection and/or following a latent period with associated secondary uveitis. *Leptospira interrogans*, the causative agent of leptospirosis, is a gram-negative, microaerophilic bacterium that belongs to the family *Spirochaetaceae*. *Leptospira* are very thin, spiral-shaped, motile, and best visualized by dark field microscopy. The antigenic specificity of the *Leptospira* allows classification into different serovars. Antigenically related serovars are grouped as serogroups whose members cross agglutinate with each other, but they do not cross agglutinate with members of other serogroups. There are nearly 270 serovars grouped into 23 serogroups. Rats are the most common reservoir. However, many other mammals have been identified as reservoirs, including cattle, dogs, pigs, raccoons, skunks and opossums. Urine of infected animals is the most common vehicle of transmission. Unlike *Trepanema*, *Leptospira* have the ability to survive outside the body in diverse environments and can live freely in alkaline soil and water for up to months. When the host is exposed to a contaminated source, the *Leptospira* enter the body through breaks in the skin and mucous membranes. After an average incubation period of 2 to 7 days, hematogenous dissemination and multiplication of *Leptospira* occur in various organs producing a diverse array of clinical manifestations.

DIAGNOSIS

Clinical findings

Systemic leptospirosis is a multi-system disorder, but the severity and disease course varies considerably, from mild to lethal. The clinical picture depends, to a large extent, on the organ systems involved. Anicteric systemic illness occurs in 85% to 90% of case. A minority develop icteric, septecemic leptospirosis, or Weil's syndrome. The most notable feature of severe leptospirosis is the progressive impairment of hepatic and renal function, and renal failure is the most common cause of death. Damage to the endothelial lining of the capillaries and subsequent interference with blood flow appear to be responsible for the lesions associated with leptospirosis. Common systemic clinical findings include any of the following:

- Abrupt onset of fever and rigor;
- Intense headache, myalgia and prostration;
- Muscle tenderness — particularly involving the calves and lumbar area;
- Scleral icteris with or without conjunctival injection;
- Meningeal irritation;
- Delirium/psychosis;
- Anuria or oliguria;
- Jaundice;
- Multi-organ hemorrhages;
- Cardiac arrhythmia or failure.

Physicians may easily miss the diagnosis, as symptoms are extremely variable, and can mimic other infectious diseases. The differential diagnoses of systemic leptospirosis includes:

- Dengue fever;
- Influenza;
- Hanta virus infection;
- Viral hepatitis;
- Hemorrhagic yellow fever;
- Malaria;
- Typhoid;
- Relapsing fever;
- Meningitis;

- Encephalitis;
- Rickettsial disease.

Systemic findings usually last for about a week, when development of immunoglobulins in the plasma coincides with rapid immune clearance of the organisms. However, even after clearance from the blood, *Leptospira* can remain in immunologically privileged sites, including the renal tubules, brain, and anterior chamber of the eye, for weeks to months. Uveitis is, therefore, an important late complication of leptospirosis. The precise incidence of uveitis in patients with systemic leptospirosis is not known, but has been estimated to be as low as 3% and as high as 92%. Intraocular inflammation may manifest as quickly as 2 days after infection, or may be delayed for up to 4 years. Most cases of leptospiral uveitis occur around six months following the onset of systemic disease. The onset and severity of leptospiral uveitis is quite variable and the severity does not appear to correlate with the severity of systemic disease. Uveitis may occur as single or recurrent episodes. The primary anatomical location of inflammation in patients with uveitis tends to be either anterior or diffuse. Anterior uveitis is usually insidious and mild in contrast to the severe, acute, and relapsing course characteristic of diffuse inflammation.

Ocular manifestation

The spectrum of ocular manifestation leptospirosis includes:

- Septecemic phase:
  - Conjunctival chemosis;
  - Scleral icteris.
- Immune phase:
  - Interstitial keratitis;
  - Iritis;
  - Hypopyon;
  - Vitreous cells;
  - Membranous vitreous opacities;
  - Papillitis;
  - Retinal vasculitis;
  - Cataract;
  - Cranial nerve palsies;
  - Neuroretinitis.

LEPTOSPIRAL UVEITIS

Leptospiral uveitis is one of the most common causes of hypopyon uveitis in leptospiral endemic areas. Early onset and a rapid progression of cataract, while relatively uncommon, is a unique feature in this entity. While dense vitreous inflammation with the formation of veil like membranous vitreous opacities are commonplace and may persist for several months, most patients regain excellent vision. Disc hyperemia and edema are more common than cranial nerve paresis, which can involve the third, fourth, sixth, and seventh cranial nerves. Retinal vasculitis with perivascular sheathing of the vein is frequently seen leptospiral uveitis, however occlusion and neovascularization are not common. Although leptospiral uveitis is one of the most frequent entities, it remains under diagnosed mainly because of its varying clinical manifestations.

Differential diagnoses of leptospiral uveitis includes

- HLA-B27-associated anterior uveitis.
- Behçets disease.
- Sarcoidosis.
- Syphilis.
- Tuberculosis.
- Lyme disease.
- Toxoplasmosis.
- Endogenous endophthalmitis.
- Acute retinal necrosis.

PROGNOSIS

Leptospiral uveitis carries a good prognosis. When the inflammation is transient, complete resolution with restoration of good vision is the rule. Cataract and occasionally corticosteroid induced ocular hypertension can complicate the course. Intraocular pressure lowering therapy and/or cataract extraction followed by intra-ocular lens implantation usually carry an excellent prognosis.

Laboratory work up

Routine laboratory findings in leptospirosis are often non-diagnostic.

CBC may reveal:

- Neutrophilia;
- Elevated ESR;
- Thrombocytopenia;
- Azotemia; and
- Anemia.

Urine examination may reveal:

- Microscopic hematuria;
- Proteinuria;
- Pyuria; and
- Granular casts.

In cases of systemic leptospirosis, isolation of the organisms from body fluids such as blood, urine, or cerebrospinal fluid can confirm the diagnosis. Isolation is possible within one week of infection, but is successful only in 50% of cases, even at this early stage. Unlike *Treponema pallidum*, *Leptospira* can be grown only in special media such as Ellinghausen McCullough Johnson Harris (EMJH) medium. Urine cultures become positive during the second week of illness and remain positive for up to 30 days. Beyond ten days of systemic infection, the Microscopic Agglutination Test (MAT) is the prefered assay. The MAT involves mixing motile bacteria in liquid medium with titrated amounts of patients serum. When the serum contains antibodies, agglutination is seen under dark field microscopy. Seroconversion or a fourfold or greater rise in paired serum samples or a titer above 1:400 dilution in the presence of a compatible clinical illness is considered diagnostic for systemic leptospirosis. In the chronic stage of leptospirosis, a titer of 1:100 dilutions is usually taken as significant. Other serological tests that are available, including ELISA, macroscopic agglutination, indirect hemagglutination, lepto dipstick, microcapsule agglutination tests, and lateral flow assays.

TREATMENT OF SYSTEMIC LEPTOSPIROSIS

There remains some controversy concerning the use of antimicrobial treatment of leptospirosis. However, several case series have reported a shortened duration of illness when antibiotic therapy was administered within 2–4 days. Leptospires are sensitive *in vitro* to most antimicrobial agents, including penicillin, amoxicillin, doxycycline and ceftriaxone. In practice, severe systemic leptospirosis is treated with intravenous penicillin G administered as 1.5 million units every 6 hours for one week. Ceftriaxone can also be used and has the benefit of reduced frequency of administration. For mild to moderate cases, doxycycline may be given in doses of 100 mg twice daily for one week.

In addition to antimicrobial agents, supportive therapy is mandatory in cases of severe infection. Depending upon the organ system involved, the following measures may need to be considered:

- Dialysis in patients with renal failure,
- Mechanical ventilation and airway protection in patients with respiratory compromise;
- Continuous cardiac monitoring;
- Management of electrolytes loss in patients with dehydration, hypotension and hemorrhage; and
- Administration of vitamin K in patients with hypoprothrombinemia.

Chemoprophylaxis may be impractical to administer in highly endemic areas, but is likely to be useful for travelers and military personnel who visit endemic areas, or following accidental laboratory infection. Doxycycline (200 mg/week) may have a significant protective effect in reducing morbidity and mortality.

TREATMENT OF LEPTOSPIRAL UVEITIS

Corticoteroids are the mainstay of treatment for leptospiral uveitis. The preferred mode of delivery depends upon the severity, laterality and anatomical location of the inflammation. Options include:

- Hourly topical application of a corticosteroid such as prednisolone acetate, 1%, together with a cycloplegic/mydriatic agent in severe anterior uveitis;
- A posterior sub-tenon depot-corticosteroids injection, such as triamcinolone acetonide, 40 mg, in diffuse uveitis; and
- Oral corticosteroids (0.5–1.5 mg/kg body weight/day) in bilateral diffuse uveitis.

It is not known whether the systemic antibiotic treatment during the systemic phase of illness has any protective role on long term complications such as uveitis.

PREVENTION

Leptospirosis is a re-emerging waterborne, zoonotic, spirochetal disease recognized throughout the world, especially in tropical — countries with heavy rainfall. The clinical presentation of leptospirosis varies and is not sufficiently characteristic, making the diagnosis of both systemic leptospirosis and leptospiral uveitis difficult. Currently recognized risk factor for contracting leptospirosis include:

- Occupational exposure — rice field workers, mining ranchers, abattoir workers, veterinarians, sewer workers and military personnel;
- Recreational activities — fresh water swimming, canoeing, kayaking, and trail biking;
- Household exposure — infestation by infected rodents and exposure to infected pet dogs and domesticated live stock.

Prevention is best accomplished by effective control and avoidance of known contaminated sources.

REFERENCES

Bharti AR, Nally JE, Ricaldi JN, et al: Leptospirosis: a zoonotic disease of global importance. Lancet Infect Dis 3:757–771, 2003. Review.

Duke-Elder S, ed: Diseases of the uveal tract system of ophthalmology. London, Hendry Kimpton, 1966:II:322–325.

Faine S, Alder B, Bolin C, et al: Leptospira and leptospirosis. 2nd edn. Melbourne, Australia, Medisci, 1999.

Heath CW, Alexander AD, Galton MM: Leptospirosis in the United States: 1949–1961. New Engl J Med 273:857–864, 915–922, 1965.

Levett PN: Leptospirosis. Clin Meicobiol Rev 14:296–326, 2001.

Martins MG, Matos KTF, da Silva MV, de Abreu MT: Ocular manifestations in the acute phase of leptospirosis. Ocular Immunol Inflam 6:75–79, 1998.

Panaphut T, Domrongkitchaiporn S, Vibhagool A, et al: Ceftriaxone compared with sodium penicillin g for treatment of severe leptospirosis. Clin Infect Dis 36:1507–1513, 2003.

Rathinam SR, Namperumalsamy P, Cunningham ET, Jr: Spontaneous cataract absorption in patients with leptospiral uveitis. Br J Ophthalmol 84:1135–1141, 2000.

Rathinam SR, Rathnam S, Selvaraj S, et al: Uveitis associated with an epidemic outbreak of leptospirosis. Am J Ophthalmol 124:71–79, 1997.

Sturman RM, Laval J, Weil VJ: Leptospiral uveitis. Arch Ophthalmol 61:633–639, 1959.

Woods AC, ed: Endogenous uveitis. Baltimore, Williams & Wilkins, 1960: 76–78.

25 LYME DISEASE 104.8

Gerald W. Zaidman, MD, FAAO, FACS
Valhalla, New York

Lyme disease is the most common arthropod-related disease in the United States, Europe and portions of Japan. Currently more than 15,000 cases occur each year.

ETIOLOGY/INCIDENCE

Lyme disease is transmitted by the bite of an *Ixodes* tick infected with *Borrelia burgdorferi*. Ehrlichiosis and babesiosis are also transmitted by the *Ixodes* tick. The disease is a multisystem spirochetal disorder that can mimic many other diseases. As in syphilis, another spirochetal illness, Lyme disease occurs in three stages.

The *Ixodes* tick life cycle consists of three stages – larval, nymphal and adult. Mice and deer are most commonly involved in this life cycle, but any mammal can serve as the tick's host. The nymphal stage is the most aggressive; ticks in this stage feed in mid to late spring. Because of their extremely small size, *Ixodes* ticks may not be noticed on the skin and their bite may not be remembered by the victim.

Seventy-five percent of cases occur during the summer months. There is a bimodal distribution of age groups with 2 peaks, one in children between 5 and 14, the other in adults between 30 and 59.

Clusters of Lyme disease occur in three geographic areas of the United States:

1. The northeast, especially southern Connecticut and Westchester County and Long Island in the state of New York.
2. The upper midwest in Minnesota and Wisconsin.
3. The northwest, in Washington, Oregon and northern California.

DIAGNOSIS

Clinical signs and symptoms

Systemic

The clinical manifestations of untreated Lyme disease occur in three stages.

Stage 1
- Localized bull's eye skin rash, or erythema chronicum migrans.
- Pathognomonic skin rash begins 3 to 30 days after tick bite (as many as 18% of patients can present without the skin rash).

Stage 2
- Follows weeks to months later.
- Neurologic (15% of patients), cardiac (5%), or arthritic manifestations (60%); neurologic signs can include.
  - Cranial neuropathy (especially Bell's palsy).
  - Meningitis.
  - Headache.
  - Neuritis.

Stage 3
- Follows weeks to months later.
- Chronic Lyme arthritis most common manifestation.
- Chronic neurologic syndromes include.
  - Neuropsychiatric disease.
  - Peripheral neuropathy.

Ocular

Ocular manifestations of Lyme disease may involve any portion of the eye and will vary depending on the stage of the disease.

Stage 1
- Conjunctivitis.
- Photophobia.

These symptoms are mild and transient and ophthalmologists are not usually consulted.

Stage 2

Significant ophthalmic complications first appear; the most common are various neuro-ophthalmologic signs. Typically, the patient may first present with a seventh cranial nerve palsy (Bell's palsy); some individuals may display the triad of Lyme neuroborreliosis:
- Cranial nerve palsy;
- Meningitis;
- Radiculopathy.

Blurred vision also can be noted during this stage, secondary to:
- Papilledema;
- Optic atrophy;
- Optic or retrobulbar neuritis;
- Pseudotumor cerebri.

Optic nerve disease may be unilateral, bilateral, solitary, or associated with other neurologic or neuro-ophthalmologic manifestations. There is some evidence that children are more predisposed to optic nerve disease than adults.

Late Stage 2 or Stage 3

Most of the severe ocular signs of the disease are seen, including:
- Episcleritis;
- Symblepharon;
- Keratitis;
- Iritis;
- Posterior or intermediate uveitis;
- Pars planitis;
- Vitreitis;
- Chorioretinitis;
- Exudative retinal detachment;
- Retinal pigment epithelial detachment;
- Cystoid macular edema;
- Branch retinal artery occlusion;
- Retinal vasculitis;
- Cranial nerve palsies.

Of this group, keratitis, vitreitis and pars planitis are the most common. The keratitis usually is a bilateral, patchy, nummular stromal keratitis. Posterior segment inflammatory disease generally presents as a bilateral pars planitis associated with granulomatous iritis and vitreitis. Many of these patients also will have granulomatous keratic precipitates and posterior synechiae.

PATHOGENESIS

The pathogenesis of the disease is not well understood but the symptoms are believed to be due to direct infection and a delayed hypersensitivity mechanism. A very controversial aspect of the disease is the form of the disease known as 'late' or 'chronic' Lyme disease. Some patients may develop chronic or relapsing inflammation (including uveitis). It is unknown if these patients truly have Lyme disease and if they represent treatment failures, persistence of organism, infection with another tick borne pathogen or an autoimmune phenomenon.

Laboratory findings

Because many patients with suspected Lyme disease do not recall the causative tick bite or the skin rash, laboratory tests are important in establishing the diagnosis; however, much confusion can occur in interpreting the tests used for Lyme disease. The organism and its DNA have been detected in CSF, urine and sera but only early in the disease. PCR is superior to cultures but it is not standardized and not widely available.

The two most frequently used tests are the immunofluorescent assay (IFA) and the enzyme-linked immunosorbent assay (ELISA); the principal limitation of these serologic tests has been the high frequency of both false-negative and false-positive results. False-negative results occur during the acute phase of Lyme disease, before patients have developed a sufficient antibody response to give a positive serologic test. False-positive readings are due to serologic cross-reactivity among Lyme disease, syphilis, Rocky Mountain spotted fever and other disorders.

To improve diagnostic accuracy, some laboratories use the immunoblot (Western blot) test; this test is more specific, sensitive and reliable than the ELISA. The National Conference on Lyme disease recommends a two-step protocol for disease testing. The first step is to use either Lyme IFA or ELISA and a Venereal Disease Research Laboratory and a fluorescent treponemal antibody absorption test should be done at the same time. Any positive or equivocal test mandates that IgG and IgM immunoblots be performed.

PROPHYLAXIS

Preventive measures for Lyme disease rely on personal protection; people in endemic areas should wear long pants and light-colored clothing and use insect repellent whenever venturing into the wooded areas preferred by *Ixodes*. The Food and Drug Administration has approved two preparations of a vaccine against Lyme disease that are being tested in the United States; limited trials of the vaccine have shown its safety and effectiveness in some animals and in adults. These vaccines are expected to be available in late 1998 or early 1999.

Lymerix, the vaccine for Lyme disease, was approved by the Food and Drug Administration in December 1998. Vaccination against Lyme disease requires three injections given over a 13-month period. The vaccine confers protection about 80% of the time. It protects people for a few years and booster shots are required to maintain protection. It is not available for children.

TREATMENT

Systemic

Stage 1

All patients with stage 1 Lyme disease should be treated with any one of the following oral antibiotics for 2 to 3 weeks:
- Tetracycline 500 mg q.i.d.;
- Doxycycline 100 mg b.i.d.;
- Phenoxymethyl penicillin 500 mg q.i.d.; or
- Amoxicillin 500 mg t.i.d. or q.i.d.

Children, pregnant women, patients who cannot tolerate tetracycline and patients who are allergic to penicillin may be given erythromycin 500 mg q.i.d.

Stages 2 and 3

Patients in the later stages of Lyme disease can be treated with oral antibiotics as well, but these patients usually require 30 days of therapy.

Patients with severe disease, such as meningitis, neuroborreliosis, or carditis, require parenteral therapy with β-lactam antibiotics, such as 14–21 days of one of the following:
- Penicillin G 3 to 4 million units IV every 4 hours;
- Ceftriaxone 2 g/day IV in divided doses;
- Parenteral penicillin and ceftriaxone in combination; or
- Roxithromycin and cotrimoxazole in combination.

Combination therapy may be worthwhile in patients who do not respond to monotherapy. Physicians should observe the patient closely for possible Jarisch–Herxheimer reactions after the institution of therapy; this allergic/inflammatory response may manifest in the skin, mucous membranes, viscera, or nervous system.

Ocular

Stage 1 Lyme conjunctivitis and photophobia require no therapy; stage 2 Bell's palsy is self-limited but requires supportive therapy to prevent the complications of exposure keratitis. Keratitis and episcleritis benefit from topical corticosteroids, usually a short course of either of the following:
- Prednisolone acetate 1.0%; or
- Fluorometholone 0.1%.

No treatment regimen for severe neuro-ophthalmic disease (involving the optic nerve) or posterior segment disease (e.g. pars planitis, vitreitis) has yet been established. Oral corticosteroids should not be used without concomitant antibiotics. The best approach for these patients might be a 'therapeutic antibiotic trial,' in which the patient can receive 2–3 weeks of intravenous penicillin or ceftriaxone; if the patient responds to treatment, the trial is successful, ocular Lyme disease is diagnosed and no further therapy is needed. Recurrences of Lyme uveitis, once adequate IV therapy has been given, can be treated with judicious corticosteroids

REFERENCES

Bergloff J, Basser R, Feigl B: Ophthalmic manifestations in Lyme borreliosis: a review. J Neuroophthalmol 14:14–20, 1994.

Johnson BTB, Robbins KE, Bailey RE, et al: Serodiagnosis of Lyme disease: accuracy of a two-step approach using a flagella-based ELISA and immunoblotting. J Infect Dis 174:346–353, 1996.

Karma A, Seppala I, Mikkala H, et al: Diagnosis and clinical characteristics of ocular Lyme borreliosis. Am J Ophthalmol 119:127–135, 1995.

Lesser RL: Ocular manifestations of Lyme disease. Am J Med 98:605–625, 1995.

Lesser RL, Kornmehl EW, Pachmer AR, et al: Neuroophthalmologic manifestations of Lyme disease. Ophthalmology 97:699–706, 1990.

Magnarelli LA: Current status of laboratory diagnosis for Lyme disease. Am J Med 98:105–125, 1995.

Mikkila HO, Seppala IJT, Viljanen MK, et al: The expanding clinical spectrum of ocular Lyme borreliosis. Ophthalmology 107:581–587, 2000.

Nadelman RB, Wormser GP: A clinical approach to Lyme disease. Mt Sinai J Med 57:144–156, 1990.

Rothermel H, Hedges TR, Steere AC: Optic neuropathy in children with Lyme disease. Pediatrics 108:477–481, 2001.

Steere AC: Medical progress-Lyme disease. N Engl J Med 345:115–125, 2001.

Steere AC, Sikand VK: The presenting manifestations of Lyme disease and the outcomes of treatment. N Engl J Med 348:2472–2474, 2003.

Winward KE, Lawton Smith J, Culbertson WW, Paris-Hamelin A: Ocular Lyme borreliosis. Am J Ophthalmol 108:651–657, 1989.

Wormser GP: Prospects for a vaccine to prevent Lyme disease in humans. Clin Infect Dis 5:1267–1274, 1995.

26 MICROSPORIDIAL INFECTION 104.8

Penny J. McAllum, MBChB
Toronto, Ontario

ETIOLOGY/INCIDENCE

Microsporidia are obligate intracellular, spore-forming, mitochondria-lacking, eukaryotic protozoan parasites. The rate of occurrence of ocular microsporidiosis is not known, although it is thought to be rare. Ocular infection typically presents as a chronic, bilateral keratoconjunctivitis in immunocompromised patients, particularly patients with acquired immunodeficiency syndrome (AIDS) and a significantly reduced CD4⁺ T lymphocyte count. There are also recent reports of unilateral and bilateral microsporidial keratoconjunctivitis in well patients, mostly with a history of topical steroid use. Much less commonly, ocular microsporidiosis presents as a unilateral stromal ulcerative keratitis in immunocompetent individuals. There is one reported case of microsporidial sclerouveitis.

Four genera and five species have been the reported agents in ocular microsporidiosis: *Encephalitozoon hellem*, *E. cuniculi* and *Septata intestinalis* are the causes of keratoconjunctivitis, and *Vittaforma (Nosema) corneae* and *Trachipleistophora hominis* are the causes of ulcerative keratitis. The source and method of transmission remain unclear. Some cases have been associated with exposure to household pets or contaminated water. Ocular inoculation may occur by horizontal transmission from nasopharyngeal, gastrointestinal or urinary tract colonization in immunocompromised individuals or from trauma or contact lenses.

COURSE/PROGNOSIS

Keratoconjunctivitis

If untreated, chronic infection of the conjunctival and corneal epithelium persists. In the absence of retinal complications associated with AIDS and with effective treatment, the visual prognosis is excellent.

Ulcerative keratitis

Keratitis presents as a slowly progressive, indolent corneal ulcer. It may involve the visual axis, lead to perforation of the cornea, or both, resulting in a guarded visual prognosis.

DIAGNOSIS

Keratoconjunctivitis

Clinical signs and symptoms

- Intense foreign body sensation.
- Marked photophobia.
- Blepharospasm.
- Nonspecific or papillary conjunctival hyperemia.
- Diffuse, coarse, punctate, intraepithelial corneal opacities with focal epithelial surface erosions. Occasionally mild anterior stromal infiltrates. May mimic adenoviral keratoconjunctivitis.
- No intraocular inflammation.

Laboratory findings

- Immune status: significant decrease in CD4⁺ T lymphocytes and human immunodeficiency virus (HIV) seropositivity in many cases.
- Gram's stain smear of conjunctival or corneal scrapings: numerous gram-positive, ovoid spores in the cytoplasm of epithelial cells.
- Electron microscopy of centrifuged conjunctival or corneal scrapings: characteristic wide ovoid, 2–5 μm spores and species-specific features.
- *In vivo* confocal microscopy: may be useful for rapid, noninvasive identification of corneal intraepithelial spores.
- Other techniques: fluorescent microscopy using species-specific antisera; periodic acid-Schiff, Grocott-methenamine silver and modified trichrome stains may be positive.
- Culture of conjunctival or corneal scrapings negative for bacteria, viruses and fungi and viral PCR negative.

Ulcerative keratitis

Clinical signs and symptoms

- Foreign body sensation.
- Photophobia.
- Decreased vision.
- Slowly progressive, often central, corneal ulcer with variable clinical appearance; from disciform stromal infiltrate which may mimic herpes simplex stromal keratitis, to suppurative ulceration with epithelial breakdown, to severe corneal thinning and perforation.
- Anterior chamber reaction and conjunctival injection.
- Refractory to topical antibiotic and anti-inflammatory therapy.

Laboratory findings

- Immune status: normal.
- Gram's stain of corneal biopsy: spores may be seen within stromal keratocytes.
- Electron microscopy of corneal biopsy or penetrating keratoplasty recipient button required to make the diagnosis and characterize the species involved in all reported cases.

PROPHYLAXIS

Handwashing may help prevent transmission of *Encephalitozoon* spp. in immunocompromised patients, particularly if there is a genitourinary tract microsporidial infection.

TREATMENT

Keratoconjunctivitis

Local

- Topical fumagillin 70 μg/mL can be prepared from fumagillin bicyclohexylammonium salt (Fumadil B). Sixty milligrams is dissolved in 20 mL of sterile Dacriose. The solution is passed through a 0.22-μm filter into three opaque, sterile dropper bottles (10 mL). Keep refrigerated. Remains stable for 1 to 3 weeks. Use hourly while awake as initial therapy, decreasing to three or four times daily for maintenance treatment.

Systemic

- Albendazole, an orally administered broad-spectrum antihelminthic agent, has been reported to be useful in combination with topical fumagillin in treating ocular microsporidial infection, particularly in the presence of multiorgan microsporidiosis. There is one report of successful treatment with debridement and oral itraconazole.

Ulcerative keratitis

- There are no reported cases of microsporidial ulcerative keratitis cured with topical fumagillin. Penetrating corneal transplantation appears to be the only treatment that has proven successful.

COMPLICATIONS

Microsporidial keratoconjunctivitis may persist as chronic infection, but remains confined to epithelial cell layers. Ulcerative keratitis, however, tends to progress and may lead to corneal perforation. Recurrence of keratitis following penetrating keratoplasty has not been reported.

COMMENTS

Topical antibiotics, anti-inflammatories, propamidine and metronidazole have all proved to be ineffective in the treatment of microsporidial keratoconjunctivitis.

REFERENCES

Cali A, Meisler D, Lowder CY, et al: Corneal microsporidiosis: characterization and identification. J Protozool 38:S215–S217, 1991.

Chan CML, Theng JTS, Li L, et al: Microsporidial keratoconjunctivitis in healthy individuals. Ophthalmol 110:1420–1425, 2003.

Font RL, Samaha AN, Keener MJ, et al: Corneal microsporidiosis: report of case, including electron microscopic observations. Ophthalmol 107:1769–1775, 2000.

Font RL, Su GW, Matoba AY: Microsporidial stromal keratitis. Arch Ophthalmol 121:1045–1047, 2003.

Gritz DC, Holsclow DS, Neger RE, et al: Ocular and sinus microsporidial infection cured with systemic albendazole. Am J Ophthalmol 124:241–243, 1997.

Lewis NL, Francis IC, Hawkins GS, et al: Bilateral microsporidial keratoconjunctivitis in an immunocompetent non-contact lens wearer. Cornea 22:374–376, 2003.

Lowder CY, McMahon JT, Meisler DM, et al: Microsporidial keratoconjunctivitis caused by *Septata intestinalis* in a patient with acquired immunodeficiency syndrome. Am J Ophthalmol 121:715–717, 1996.

Rauz S, Tuft S, Dart JK, et al: Ultrastructural examination of two cases of stromal microsporidial keratitis. J Med Microbiol 53:775–781, 2004.

Rosberger DF, Serdarevic ON, Erlandson RA, et al: Successful treatment of microsporidial keratoconjunctivitis with topical fumagillin. Cornea 12:261–265, 1993.

Sridhar MS, Sharma S: Microsporidial keratoconjunctivitis in a HIV-seronegative patient treated with debridement and oral itraconazole. Am J Ophthalmol 136:745–746, 2003.

27 MOLLUSCUM CONTAGIOSUM 078.0

Alan B. Leahey, MD
Allentown, Pennsylvania
Frank G. Baloh, MD
Allentown, Pennsylvania

ETIOLOGY/INCIDENCE

Molluscum contagiosum is a large, enveloped, double-stranded DNA virus of the Poxviridae family that can produce small, pearly pink and white umbilicated lesions on the skin and, less commonly, on mucous membranes. The periocular skin, eyelid and ocular surface can be infected, as can be the face, abdomen and groin. This poxvirus replicates in the cytoplasm of epidermal cells inducing cell lysis. It is a mildly contagious skin disease that is usually self-limited and the lesions can be asymptomatic or inflamed, depending on the location and stage of the lesion. The average incubation period is 2 to 3 months but may range between 1 week to 6 months.

Molluscum contagiosum has a bimodal incidence in otherwise healthy individuals. Children and adolescents are often infected by direct contact, whereas young adults may acquire the virus through sexual contact. When the mode of transmission is sexual, lesions usually are also present on the inner thighs and lower abdomen. Overall, the greatest incidence is between the ages of 15 and 35 years of age. Most of the lesions are 2 to 3 mm long and have a central umbilication with a caseous material. Usually, there are fewer than 10 lesions and often only two or three lesions around the lids.

The incidence, size and number of lesions can be much greater in immunocompromised individuals; there may be more than 20 lesions on an upper and a lower eyelid and they can range in size from 1 to 6 mm. These atypical lesions may coalesce; atypical presentation may be a sign of an immunocompromised host, such as a patient with acquired immune deficiency syndrome, who has undergone chemotherapy, who receives corticosteroids, who has atopic dermatitis, who has undergone splenectomy and who has Wiskott–Aldrich syndrome.

COURSE/PROGNOSIS

The virus can be spread through direct contact or fomites. It is contagious in moist, close-contact conditions such as in swimming pools and saunas and during wrestling or sex. No exclusion from school, work or swimming pools is necessary. Direct hand-to-eye contact and infected cosmetics can be modes of transmission. There is no evidence of acquired immunity. The virus replicates in the epithelial cells; cellular destruction occurs, causing the central umbilication. The virus particles go from lid lesions to tear film, thus affecting all ocular surfaces and often causing a toxic keratoconjunctivitis. The lesions may resolve spontaneously in 2 to 12 months, but there may be recurrences for as long as 8 years. Surgical treatment is usually required, but immunocompromised individuals may still have recurrences in 6 to 8 weeks.

DIAGNOSIS

Clinical signs and symptoms

The lesions of molluscum contagiosum can affect the eye and the lid by infecting the periocular skin surface and the lid margin, causing a toxic follicular keratoconjunctivitis. The limbus, bulbar conjunctiva and cornea can also be involved. The typical umbilicated lesions can occur on any of these ocular surfaces and cause further inflammation, such as conjunctival scarring, punctate epithelial keratopathy, pannus, pseudodendrite, subepithelial infiltrates, corneal ulceration, corneal perforation and punctal occlusion. The follicular conjunctivitis can cause pseudotrachoma with superior epithelial keratitis and corneal scars; thus, if left untreated when the ocular surface is involved, significant visual loss can result.

The umbilicated, dome-shaped, pearly pink and white papules are 2 to 3 mm and usually smooth and elevated. Cheesy-type material is present in the central craters. Usually, several lesions are seen in the periocular area.

Laboratory findings

The craters in acanthotic epidermis are filled with epithelial cells with large eosinophilic intracytoplasmic inclusion bodies (molluscum or Henderson–Patterson bodies) as viewed with light microscopy when virus particles are deep in the epidermis. As virus particles migrate to the granular layer of the epidermis, the inclusion bodies become basophilic.

Immunocompromised individuals have a dense mononuclear infiltrate at the base of the lesions.

Differential diagnosis

- Warts.
- Verrucae vulgaris.
- Papillomas.
- Milia.
- Sebaceous cysts.
- Herpes simplex virus.
- Lichen planus.
- Keratoacanthoma.
- Sebaceous cell carcinoma.
- Chlamydial infection.

TREATMENT

Local

- Spontaneous resolution.
- Excision.
- Curettage.
- Chemical cauterization (trichloroacetic acid, phenol, iodine, triretinoin).
- Cryotherapy.
- Liquid nitrogen.
- Cidofovir cream 3% (nucleotide analog of deoxycytidine) in patients positive for human immunodeficiency virus (HIV).
- Cantharidin 0.9% (blistering agent).
- Imiquimod cream 5% (immune response modifier).

Systemic

- Intravenous cidofovir in patients positive for HIV.

Many of these lesions will resolve in 2 to 12 months, but many require a surgical or medical option described above. Curettage of the central lesion will speed resolution by bleeding into the central cavity. Often, a combination of treatments such as excision or curettage and double freeze-thaw cryotherapy is required to remove lid lesions that cause ocular complications. Immunocompromised individuals are more difficult to treat because there may be recurrence in 6 to 8 weeks.

COMPLICATIONS

Loss of vision secondary to corneal vascularization, corneal perforation and scarring from a toxic keratoconjunctivitis or primary corneal lesions must be prevented. The overzealous treatment of lid lesions could lead to entropion or ectropion with resultant exposure keratitis.

COMMENTS

Atypical numerous, confluent molluscum contagiosum lesions may be an indicator of systemic immunocompromise and HIV status should be determined because of the association of a venereal disease in adult transmission. Prevalence of molluscum contagiosum in HIV patients may be as high as 5–18%. These individuals should also undergo a dilated retinal examination to rule out another opportunistic infection that could affect the eye, such as cytomegalovirus.

SUMMARY

Molluscum contagiosum of the periocular skin and lid margin is best diagnosed on the basis of clinical appearance and confirmed through excisional biopsy. Numerous local surgical therapies have been described, but excision or curettage combined with cryotherapy seems to be the most effective in non-immunocompromised individuals. In immunocompromised individuals, recurrence rates are much higher regardless of the treatment. Atypical molluscum lesions require that the HIV status of the infected individual be determined.

REFERENCES

Charles NC, Friedberg DN: Epibulbar molluscum contagiosum in acquired immune deficiency syndrome: case report and review of the literature. Ophthalmology 99:1123–1126, 1992.

Charteris DG, Bonshek RE, Tullo AB: Ophthalmic molluscum contagiosum: clinical and immunopathological features. Br J Ophthalmol 79:476–481, 1995.

Goodman DS, Teplitz ED, Wishner A, et al: Prevalence of cutaneous disease in patients with acquired immunodeficiency sysndrome (AIDS) or AIDS-related complex. J Am Acad Dermatol 17(2 Pt 1):210–220, 1987.

Hoeprich PD, Jordan MC, Ronald AR, eds: Infectious diseases: a treatise of infectious processes. 5th edn. Philadelphia, JB Lippincott, 1994.

Krachmer JH, Mannis MJ, Holland EJ: Cornea: fundamentals of cornea and external disease. St Louis, Mosby, 1997.

Lucius RW, Santander S: Opportunistic infections of the anterior segment in the HIV population. Ophthalmol Clin North Am 10:85–96, 1997.

Meadows KP, Tyring SK, Pavin AT, et al: Resolution of recalcitrant molluscum contagiosum virus in lesions in human immunodeficiency virus-infected patients with cidofovir. Arch Dermatol 133:1039–1041, 1997.

Robinson MR, Udell IJ, Garber PF, et al: Molluscum contagiosum of the eyelids in patients with acquired immune deficiency syndrome. Ophthalmology 99:1745–1747, 1992.

Seitz B: Chronische einseitige Keratokonjunktivitis bei Molluscum contagiosum der Oberlidkante. Klin Monatsbl Augenheilkd 204:142–143, 1992.

Theos AU, Cummins R, Silverberg NB, Paller AS: Effectiveness of imiquimod cream 5% for treating childhood contagiosum in a double-blind, randomized pilot trial. Cutis 74(2):134–138, 141–142, 2004.

28 MORAXELLA 372.02

Audina M. Berrocal, MD
Miami, Florida
Jaime R. Gaitan, MD
Miami, Florida

ETIOLOGY/INCIDENCE

Moraxella organisms are aerobic, oxidase positive, gram-negative diplococci or coccobacilli morphologically indistinguishable from *Neisseria*. It has been isolated from patients with external ocular diseases such as angular blepharoconjunctivitis and corneal ulcers but it has also been the culprit in cases of intraocular infections. In all cases of endophthalmitis they have been bleb-associated.

Moraxella species (formerly known as *Branhamella*) are associated with otititis media and sinusitis in children, endocarditis, laryngitis, bronchitis, pneumonia, meningitis, osteomyelitis, septic arthritis, stomatitis, vaginitis and bacteremia. These have been *M. lacunata*, *M. osloensis*, *M. phenylperuvica*, *M. liquefasciens*, *M. nonliquefasciens*, and *M. catarrhalis*.

DIAGNOSIS

Clinical signs and symptoms

- Blepharoconjunctivitis.
- Follicles.
- Mucopurulent discharge.
- Erythematous, eczematoid, or macerated appearance of skin at lateral canthus.
- Chronic blepharitis.
- Severe corneal ulcers (superficial or deep, central or peripheral).
- Hypopyon.

TREATMENT

Ocular

Moraxella spp. tend to be sensitive to:

- Fluoroquinolones;
- Penicillin;
- Aminoglycosides;
- Amoxycillin/clavulanate;
- Macrolides;
- Cephalosporins;
- Clindamycin.

The treatment of the blepharoconjunctivitis is relatively simple. Proteases produced by the organism cause the maceration of the skin at the canthus.

- Zinc sulfate 0.25% or 0.5% eyedrops or ointment counteracts the effects of these proteases.

After cultures have been obtained and drug sensitivity tests have been performed, both a topical antibiotic (selected on the basis of sensitivities) and zinc sulfate should be administered three or four times daily until the blepharoconjunctivitis disease process has resolved.

The treatment of a *Moraxella* spp. corneal ulcer should conform to the initial treatment of any suspected corneal ulcer. The treatment for *Moraxella* spp. endophthalmitis should conform to the initial treatment of any suspected endophthalmitis.

COMMENTS

Moraxella spp. ocular infections tend to occur most frequently in a derelict, malnourished, alcoholic population, in whom compliance with treatment is often a problem. *Moraxella* intraocular infections have been associated to delayed-onset bleb-associated endophthalmitis or trauma.

Patients with *Moraxella* endophthalmitis present with 1–2 day history or redness, pain and decreased vision. In the cases where there has been a bleb there is either a leak on the bleb or an inferiorly placed bleb with exposure. Resistance to antibiotics tend to be against vancomycin, ampicillin and trimethoprim/sulfa. Visual outcomes in these patients are generally favorable unless there are coexistent ocular comorbidities.

REFERENCES

Bergren RL, Tasman WS, Wallace RT, Katz LJ: *Branhamella (Moraxella) catarrhalis* endophthalmitis. Arch Ophthalmol 111:1169–1170, 1993.

Berrocal AM, Scott IU, Miller D, et al: Endophthalmitis caused by *Moraxella osloensis*. Graefe's Arch Clin Exp Ophthalmol 240:329–330, 2002.

Berrocal AM, Scott IU, Miller D, et al: Endophthalmitis caused by *Moraxella* species. Am J Ophthalmol 132:788–790, 2001.

Garg P, Mathur U, Athmanathan S, et al: Treatment outcome of *Moraxella* keratitis: our experience with 18 cases-a retrospective review. Cornea 18:176–181, 1999.

Jacobs MR, Dagan R: Antimicrobial resistance among pediatric respiratory tract infections: clinical challenges. Semin Pediatr Infect Dis 15:5–20, 2004.

Laukeland H, Bergh K, Bevanger L: Posttrabeculectomy endophthalmitis caused by *Moraxella nonliquefaciens*. J Clin Microbiol 40:2668–2770, 2002.

Lipman RM, Deutsch TA: Late-onset *Moraxella* catarrhalis endophthalmitis after filtering surgery. Can J Ophthalmol 27:249–250, 1992.

Orden Martinez B, Martinez Ruiz R, Millan Perez R: Bacterial conjunctivitis: most prevalent pathogens and their antibiotic sensitivity. An Pediatr (Barc) 61:32–36, 2004.

Sherman MD, York M, Irvine AR, et al: Endophthalmitis caused by beta-lactamase-positive *Moraxella nonliquefaciens*. Am J Ophthalmol 15(115):674–676, 1993.

Verduin CM, Hol C, Fleer A, et al: *Moraxella catarrhalis*: from emerging to established pathogen. Clin Microbiol Reviews 15:125–144, 2002.

29 MUCORMYCOSIS 117.7
(Phycomycosis)

Damon B. Chandler, MD
Philadelphia, Pennsylvania
Mark L. Moster, MD
Philadelphia, Pennsylvania

ETIOLOGY/INCIDENCE

Mucormycosis is a severe, acute infection caused by fungi of the order Mucorales and the class Phycomycetes. The most common genera causing orbital infection are *Mucor* and *Rhizopus*, with *Absidia* less likely. Infection begins in the nasal mucosa with contiguous spread from the paranasal sinuses to the orbit and CNS. This infection pattern is known as rhino-orbital-cerebral mucormycosis. Incidence is difficult to determine given the paucity of reported cases.

Phycomycetes are saprophytic fungi found throughout the environment. Intact immune defenses, particularly phagocytosis, normally prevent infection despite ubiquitous airborne Phycomycetes spores. Opportunistic infection occurs with suppressed immune function and rarely in immunocompetent hosts. The most common associated conditions include:

- Diabetes mellitus (especially with ketoacidosis);
- Corticosteroid use;
- Hematologic malignancy (leukemia, lymphoma, myeloma);
- Acquired immune deficiency syndrome;
- Chronic immunosuppressive drugs.

Mucorales fungi have a propensity for angioinvasion resulting in vascular occlusion and tissue necrosis. Tissue infarction is responsible for the classically described 'black eschar,' a late clinical finding associated with poor prognosis. Mucormycosis may enter the CNS via the orbital apex or cribiform plate. This can lead to thrombosis of retinal, internal carotid, and middle cerebral arteries, as well as the cavernous sinus. Obtundation, stroke, and death may follow CNS infiltration.

COURSE/PROGNOSIS

- Almost a universally fatal disease in the first half of the 20th century, mortality rates for mucormycosis have dropped substantially over the last 30 years. Recent series indicate mortality rates of 15% to 35%.
- Early recognition of the condition and its particular clinical presentation may increase patient survival.

DIAGNOSIS

Clinical signs and symptoms

- Early symptoms include fever, headache, localized pain, sinusitis, pharyngitis, or nasal discharge.
- Ophthalmic complaints include orbital pain (unilateral or bilateral), visual loss, diplopia, and facial numbness.
- The nasal discharge is foul smelling and seropurulent.
- Early orbital signs include eyelid edema and mild conjunctival chemosis.
- Patients usually have pyrexia and leukocytosis and coexisting bacterial infection.
- Central retinal artery occlusion may occur, causing acute vision loss.
- Disease progression may lead to an orbital apex syndrome with vision loss, afferent pupillary defect, ophthalmoplegia, and proptosis.

Late findings of intracranial extension including severe headache, altered mental status, obtundation, or stroke.

- A high level of suspicion aids the clinician in the early stages of presentation, particularly in a diabetic patient with new facial or orbital pain and/or obtundation.

Laboratory findings

- Tissue biopsy and culture of paranasal sinuses demonstrate the presence of the fungi, which appear as broad, irregular, nonseptate, branching hyphae on H&E staining. The large fungi are often visible even without special fungal stains.
- Vascular invasion and tissue necrosis is often seen.
- Blood cultures and lumbar puncture are usually negative for fungus.

Imaging

- Computed tomography (CT) scanning of the head and orbits defines the extent of sinus disease, and helps guide surgical planning.
- CT may demonstrate sinus disease affecting the maxillary, ethmoid, frontal, and sphenoid sinuses (affected in decreasing order). Sinus disease manifests as nodular mucosal thickening, opacification with hyperdense material, and infrequent air/fluid levels. Bone erosion, orbital extension and intracranial extension are late findings.
- Magnetic resonance imaging (MRI) reveals particular features of infected sinuses, including T2 hyperintensity, which may be due to iron and manganese in fungal infected tissue. MRI may demonstrate intracranial extension seen as regions of cerebral infarction or inflammation.
- Flow sensitive gradient-echo MR sequences or magnetic resonance angiography (MRA) aid in determining vascular thrombosis.

Differential diagnosis

- Orbital cellulitis (bacterial).
- Aspergillosis.
- Less common fungal organism (*Rhizopus, Absidia*).
- Idiopathic orbital inflammatory syndrome.
- Necrotizing fasciitis.

TREATMENT

- Early diagnosis and improved treatment protocols have resulted in a major reduction in mortality rates.
- Due to the rarity of the condition, treatment protocols have not undergone clinical trials. However, appropriate treatment consists of local antifungal therapy, surgical debridement, and systemic antifungal agents.

Local

- Local therapy can be performed by bathing orbital tissues with an amphotericin B solution.
- The orbit may be packed with antifungal soaked gauze or an orbital irrigation catheter can be placed at the time of surgical debridement to irrigate infected tissues 3–4 times daily.
- Local treatment allows amphotericin B access to poorly perfused tissues.
- One series showed an orbital irrigation catheter to be an excellent adjunct to limited debridement surgery when combined with systemic treatment.

Systemic

- Amphotericin B is the mainstay of treatment and its use necessitates familiarity with the drug's systemic toxicity and extensive side-effect profile.
- Liposomal formulations of amphotericin B are available which allow for a greater therapeutic index with decreased systemic and renal toxicity.
- If possible, systemic immune suppression should be reversed.
- Metabolic disturbances such as diabetic ketoacidosis must be corrected.
- Hyperbaric oxygen may offer some benefit, but this is not well established.

Surgical

- Surgical therapy is directed at the removal of necrotic and nonviable tissue and multiple surgical debridements may be required.
- Surgical debridement can result in significant morbidity and cosmetic deformity and the extent of surgical resection

must be weighed carefully against the threat to the patient's life and sight.

- An orbital irrigation catheter may be placed at the time of surgery for postoperative irrigation of orbital tissues with antifungal agents.
- Disease progression may require aggressive removal of devitalized tissue, including orbital exenteration, sinus surgery, and possible adjunctive craniotomy.

COMPLICATIONS

- Blindness.
- Loss of eye.
- Death.
- Severe neurologic disability.
- Cosmetic disfigurement.

COMMENTS

Mucormycosis is a vision and life threatening condition. The only hope for preserving life and vision is early recognition and aggressive medical and surgical treatment.

REFERENCES

Fairley C, Sullivan TJ, Bartley P, et al: Survival after rhino-orbital-cerebral mucormycosis in an immunocompetent patient. Ophthalmology 107:555–558, 2000.

Ferry AP, Abedi S: Diagnosis and management of rhino-orbitocerebral mucormycosis (phycomycosis): a report of 16 personally observed cases. Ophthalmology 90:1096–1104, 1983.

Newman RM, Kline LB: Evolution of fundus changes in mucormycosis. J Neuro-ophthalmol 17:51–52, 1997.

Peterson KL, Wang M, Canalis RF, Abemayor E: Rhinocerebral mucormycosis: evolution of the disease and treatment options. Laryngoscope 107:855–862, 1997.

Radner AB, Witt MD, Edwards JE, Jr: Acute invasive rhinocerebral zygomycosis in an otherwise healthy patient: case report and review. Clin Infect Dis 20:163–166, 1995.

Seiff SR, Choo PH, Carter SR: Role of local amphotericin B therapy for sino-orbital fungal infections. Ophthalmic Plast Reconstr Surg 15:28–31, 1999.

Strasser MD, Kennedy RJ, Adam RD: Rhinocerebral mucormycosis: therapy with amphotericin B lipid complex. Arch Int Med 156:337–339, 1996.

Thomas PA: Current perspectives on ophthalmic mycoses. Clin Microbiol Rev 16:730–797, 2003.

Yohai RA, Bullock JD, Aziz AA, Markert RJ: Survival factors in rhino-orbital-cerebral mucormycosis. Surv Ophthalmol 39:3–22, 1994.

30 MUMPS 072.9

Ian H. Kaden, MD
Randolph, New Jersey
Roger F. Meyer, MD
Ann Arbor, Michigan

ETIOLOGY/INCIDENCE

Mumps is an acute contagious disease caused by the mumps virus. It is usually spread by aerosolized saliva, secondary to coughing, sneezing, or even speech of infected individuals. The incubation period averages 18 days and can range from 12 to 25 days. A generalized viremia carries the virus to susceptible tissues. The parotid and other salivary glands are usually affected, and their enlargement characterizes the illness. Mumps can also affect the brain, resulting in meningitis or encephalitis. In males it may cause inflammation in the testicles and in females in the ovaries. Infection can cause pancreatitis and hearing loss in some individuals. Mumps is commonly considered a disease of childhood, but can cause serious illness in adults. It may induce birth defects in pregnant women. Before 1967, when a vaccine was introduced in the United States, more than 200,000 cases were reported per year. Now, fewer than 1000 cases are reported per year and epidemics are rare.

COURSE/PROGNOSIS

Children usually recover from mumps in about 10 to 12 days. About 1 child in every 10 who gets mumps develops symptoms of meningitis and symptoms of encephalitis are seen much less often. About 1 out of every 4 teenage or adult men who contract mumps develops orchitis. In rare cases of mumps, temporary or permanent hearing loss develops in one or both ears. Abdominal pain associated with pancreatitis or inflammation of the ovaries is observed infrequently. Ocular disease generally does not present until 10 days to three weeks after the onset of the acute illness. Ocular disease may be prolonged, however, lasting weeks or months.

DIAGNOSIS

Clinical signs and symptoms

Mumps presents with fever of up to 103°F (39.4°C), headache and loss of appetite. Swelling of the cheeks and jaw become quickly apparent. Other symptoms may include hearing loss, abdominal pain, or scrotal pain and swelling in males. Nervous system involvement may result in complaints of stiff neck, severe headache, nausea and vomiting, drowsiness, and convulsions.

Ocular symptoms may present from 10 days to 3 weeks after the onset of the acute systemic mumps infection. These ocular complications, in approximate decreasing order of frequency, can include dacryoadenitis, optic neuritis, conjunctivitis, scleritis, keratitis, uveitis, retinitis, oculomotor palsies, opsoclonus, and transient elevation of intraocular pressure.

Laboratory findings

The diagnosis of mumps should be suspected from the history and physical examination during the acute phase and can be confirmed by acute and convalescent serologic studies. The mumps virus has been shown to be present in the saliva as long as 7 days before and 9 days after the appearance of parotid swelling.

Differential diagnosis

Early symptoms of fever and headache in mumps may be confused with other viral illness, including the common cold. The subsequent development of parotid swelling makes the diagnosis of mumps infection, more likely. Abdominal pain associated with cases of orchitis and pancreatitis has been confused with acute appendicitis. Ocular complications seen in cases of mumps resemble problems seen after numerous other systemic viral infections. The temporal sequence of acute mumps infection and the subsequent onset of ocular disease, generally leads to appropriate ophthalmologic diagnosis.

PROPHYLAXIS

A live, attenuated mumps virus vaccine was licensed in the United States in 1967. It is safe and highly effective. The current vaccine results in protective immunity in over 90% of vaccinated persons. Adverse reactions are unusual, and consist primarily of reports of low grade fever and swollen glands. Rare cases of neurologic problems have been reported. The vaccine is provided in combination with measles and rubella vaccines and is recommended for routine immunization of children older than 1 year. In the United States, laws requiring school children to be immunized against mumps exist in 43 of the 50 states. States without school requirements have been shown to have a higher incidence of disease.

A recent resurgence of mumps infection has been observed among young adults, many of whom belong to what is thought to be a relatively underimmunized cohort of children born between 1967 and 1977. Seronegativity may be as high as 15% in these individuals. Serologic screening and revaccination is recommended for these patients.

TREATMENT

Systemic

Because there is no specific antiviral treatment for mumps infection, therapy should be directed toward the relief of symptoms and the prevention of complications. Temperature should be regularly monitored and recorded. Non-aspirin medications such as acetaminophen or ibuprofen can be given to reduce fever. Warm or cold packs can be helpful to soothe swollen parotid glands. Patients should be served a soft, bland diet that does not require a lot of chewing and should be encouraged to drink fluids. Testicular swelling may also benefit from cool packs and may require a narcotic pain reliever.

Vaccination after exposure to an infected individual, is not necessarily protective, but is not harmful and may avert later disease. Mumps immune globulin is not effective at preventing illness after a person has been exposed. Because of the potential hazard of corticosteroid therapy, its use in mild cases is not recommended. Antimicrobial drugs are of no value, except when secondary bacterial infections are present.

Ocular

Symptomatic relief for the ocular complications of mumps infection can include the following:

- Cool, moist compresses can ease periocular swelling;
- Atropine 1.0% 1 or 2 drops in each eye may be used to put the ciliary body at rest if iritis is present (cycloplegia begins within 25 minutes and persists for 3 to 5 days);
- Topical corticosteroids (1% prednisolone 1 or 2 drops b.i.d. to q.i.d.) can shorten the course of mumps-associated scleritis, keratitis, or uveitis;
- Elevated intraocular pressure has been responsive to topical prednisolone and oral acetazolamide;
- Oral or intravenous steroids may be indicated for more severe uveitis and for optic neuritis or neuroretinitis.

COMPLICATIONS

Aspirin should generally be avoided in the treatment of children with mumps because of the potential for development of Reye's syndrome, which can lead to liver failure and death. Before there was a mumps vaccine, many children had hearing loss caused by mumps. Other complications involve organs such as the heart, pancreas and ovaries. Lasting visual system disease is rare, but corneal scarring and optic nerve injury may cause vision loss.

REFERENCES

Centers for Disease Control: Mumps-United States, 1985–1988. MMWR 3:101–105, 1989.

Darin N, Hanner P, Thiringer K: Changes in prevalence, aetiology, age at detection and associated disabilities in children with hearing impairment born in Goteborg. Dev Med Child Neurol 39:797–802, 1997.

Foster RE, Lowdee CY, Meislee DM, et al: Mumps neuroretinitis in an adolescent. Am J Ophthalmol 110:91–93, 1990.

Hayden GF, Preblud SR, Orenstein WA, et al: Current status of mumps and mumps vaccine in the United States. Pediatrics 62:965–969, 1978.

Kelly PW, et al: The susceptibility of young adult Americans to vaccine-preventable infections. JAMA 266:2724–2729, 1991.

Krishna N, Lyda W: Acute suppurative dacryoadenitis as a sequel to mumps. Arch Ophthalmol 59:350–351, 1958.

Meyer RF, Sullivan JH, Oh JO: Mumps conjunctivitis. Am J Ophthalmol 78:1022–1024, 1974.

Nussinovitch M, Volovitz B, Varsano I: Complications of mumps requiring hospitalization in children. Eur J Pediatr 154:732–734, 1995.

Polland W, Thorburn W: Transient glaucoma as a manifestation of mumps: a case report. Acta Ophthalmol 54:779–782, 1976.

Riffenburgh RS: Ocular manifestations of mumps. Arch Ophthalmol 66:739–743, 1961.

Saijo M, Fujita K: Central nervous system infection caused by the mumps virus. Nippon Rinsho 55:870–875, 1997.

31 NEWCASTLE DISEASE 077.8

Laurent Lamer, MD, FRCS(c)
Montreal, Quebec

ETIOLOGY/INCIDENCE

Newcastle disease is caused by a paramyxovirus and is primarily a serious epizootic pneumoencephalitic infection of fowls that occurs throughout the world. In humans, the disease usually is transmitted by contact with infected poultry, primarily to poultry-farm workers and laboratory personnel. Although human-to-human transmission has not been documented, it seems likely that it may occur.

DIAGNOSIS

Clinical signs and symptoms

Systemic

- Fatigue.
- Slight elevation of temperature.
- Headaches.
- Mild arthralgia.
- Preauricular lymphadenopathy.

Ocular

The first indications of Newcastle disease infection usually appear in the eye with the sudden onset of:

- Burning;
- Foreign body sensation;
- Pain;
- Chemosis;
- Lacrimation; and
- Photophobia.

The infection progresses to an acute follicular conjunctivitis, with the following:

- Serous or mucopurulent discharge;
- Subconjunctival hemorrhages, exudates, or both.

The eyelids usually are affected, becoming edematous and developing follicles; the cornea can occasionally become involved, with:

- Fine keratic precipitates;
- Round subepithelial opacities.

Other ocular symptoms include:

- Decreased visual acuity;
- Decreased accommodation.

TREATMENT

Ocular

There is no specific treatment for Newcastle disease; it is a benign, self-limited condition that normally runs its course in 7 to 10 days. Therapy should be directed toward preventing complications such as secondary bacterial infection and toward relieving symptoms. The use of topical ocular broad-spectrum antibiotics, such as neosporin (neomycin, polymyxin B, and bacitracin) may be of some value, although this has not been definitively demonstrated. The application of hot compresses gives some symptomatic relief.

Systemic

Bedrest may be indicated in more severe cases; the patient should be instructed to avoid eyestrain or any activity that might increase the severity of the ocular symptoms.

PRECAUTIONS

Although Newcastle disease usually runs its course in 7 to 10 days, in rare instances some blurring of vision or difficulty of accommodation may persist longer.

There is some concern that the Newcastle disease virus may develop into a more severe human pathogen. The virus, a parainfluenza type, has demonstrated its genetic plasticity by assuming four pathologic forms.

Recent efforts to develop effective poultry vaccines have resulted in unexpected adverse effects of some vaccines on immune system functions, further suggesting the possibility of viral mutation and subversion of the host's immune response.

REFERENCES

Charan S, Mahajan VM, Rai A, Balaya S: Ocular pathogenesis of Newcastle disease virus in rabbits and monkeys. J Comp Pathol 94:159–163, 1984.

Duke-Elder S, ed: System of ophthalmology. St Louis, CV Mosby, 1965: VIII:369–372; 1976:XV:110.

Hanson RP: Paramyxovirus infections. In: Hubbert WT, McCulloch WF, Schnurrenberger PR, eds: Diseases transmitted from animals to man. 16th edn. Springfield, Charles C Thomas, 1975:851–858.

Lamer L: Sur un cas de conjonctivite de la maladie de Newcastle. Can J Ophthalmol 4:390–393, 1969.

Montgomery RD, Maslin WR, Boyle CR: Effects of Newcastle disease vaccines and Newcastle disease/infectious bronchitis combination vaccines on the head-associated lymphoid tissues of the chicken. Avian Dis 41:399–406, 1997.

Schemera B, Toro H, Herbst W, et al: Conjunctivitis and disorders of general health status in humans caused by infection with Newcastle disease virus. DTW 94:383–384, 1987.

Zehetbauer G, Kunz C, Thaler A: Cases of pseudo fowl plague (Newcastle disease) in man in lower Austria. Wien Klin Wochenschr 83:878–880, 1971.

32 NOCARDIOSIS 039

John D. Bullock, MD, MPH, MSc
Dayton, Ohio
Ronald E. Warwar, MD
Dayton, Ohio

ETIOLOGY/INCIDENCE

Nocardiosis is typically caused by *Nocardia asteroides*, which is named for the star-like appearance of the colonies on agar plate. Once thought to be a fungus, it is classified in the bacterial family Nocardiaceae, which includes the aerobic *Actinomycetes*. The organism reproduces through fragmentation of its hyphae into bacillary and coccoid elements. It is distinguished by a propensity for filamentary growth with true branching. It is a ubiquitous natural soil saprophyte often found in decaying organic matter. *N. asteroides* is a facultative, intracellular parasite that can persist and grow within macrophages. The basis of nocardial pathogenicity is its cell wall composed of complex lipids, peptides and polysaccharides, making it resistant to macrophage phagolysosomal fusion.

Nocardiosis typically affects debilitated, immunosuppressed patients, but 20% to 50% of patients may be otherwise healthy.

Systemic nocardiosis

- Typically respiratory tract entry.

Ocular nocardiosis

- Exogenous.
- Extraocular or intraocular infection most often associated with trauma, also associated with previous ocular surgery (including refractive surgery/LASIK), contact lens use and corticosteroid use.
- Endogenous.
- Via hematogenous spread to the eye.
- Mean patient age is 46 years; male-to-female ratio of 4:1.
- Bilateral in 30%.
- Occurs in 3% of systemic cases.

DIAGNOSIS

Clinical signs and symptoms

Systemic nocardiosis

- Bronchitis or pneumonia.
- Often presents with cough and low-grade fever.
- Malaise, weight loss and night sweats possible.
- On chest radiograph, typically shows rapidly developing lobar or segmental infiltrate.
- Sites of dissemination: central nervous system (25% to 40%), skin and subcutaneous tissues, kidney, liver and lymph nodes.
- Mycetoma (maduromycosis or Madura foot).
- Chronic, deep subcutaneous tissue and bone infection; usually involves lower extremities.

Ocular nocardiosis

- Keratitis.
- Symptoms of pain, photophobia, blepharospasm and lid swelling.
- Classically appears as patchy anterior stromal infiltrates with scalloped margins arranged in a ring-like or wreath pattern surrounding or underlying an epithelial defect.
- May appear as nonspecific punctate epitheliopathy.
- Iritis with or without hypopyon may be present.
- Deep corneal infiltration and vascularization may be seen with prolonged infection.
- Chorioretinitis, subretinal abscess, scleritis, endophthalmitis, dacryocystitis, periorbital and orbital cellulites.
- Poor prognosis with frequent loss of vision.

Mortality rates

- Otherwise healthy patients: 15%.
- Nonimmunosuppressed patients with underlying disease: 20%.
- Patients receiving immunosuppressive agents: 80% to 100%.

Laboratory findings

- Blood culture, sputum culture, or culture of material directly aspirated.
- Gram's stain.
- Gram-positive filamentous structures with an intermittent or a beaded staining pattern; weakly acid-fast.
- Grocott–Gomori methenamine-silver nitrate and periodic acid-Schiff stains.
- Culture.
- Slow growing; may take 2 to 4 weeks to appear, but its isolation is significant as it rarely represents a contaminant.
- Will grow on virtually any medium without antibiotics; yield may be increased by the use of selective media such as Thayer–Martin agar with antibiotics or paraffin agar.
- Antibiotic susceptibility tests are often unreliable.
- Histopathologic features of nocardial endophthalmitis: suppurative and necrotizing inflammatory response in the choroid and retina.

TREATMENT

Systemic nocardiosis

- Sulfadiazine or sulfisoxazole 6 to 10 g/day, or amikacin 15 mg/kg/day; if immunocompetent, treat for 6 weeks; if immunosuppressed, treat for 1 year.

Ocular nocardiosis

- Keratitis/scleritis.
- Topical: sulfacetamide 15% to 30% or amikacin 2.5% to 5% with or without topical trimethoprim 16 mg/mL-sulfamethoxazole 80 mg/mL every 15 to 30 minutes until clinical improvement.
- Systemic: oral trimethoprim 1.6 g-sulfamethoxazole 320 mg b.i.d. or intravenous amikacin 15 mg/kg/day.
- Consider subconjunctival injection: trimethoprim-sulfamethoxazole.
- Endophthalmitis.
- Vitrectomy and/or intravitreal amikacin with or without cefazolin.

REFERENCES

Brooks JG, Mills RAD, Coster DJ: Nocardial scleritis. Am J Ophthalmol 114:371–372, 1992.

Bullock JD: Endogenous ocular nocardiosis: a clinical and experimental study. Trans Am Ophthalmol Soc 81:451–531, 1983.

Chen CJ: *Nocardia asteroides* endophthalmitis. Ophthalmic Surg 14:502–505, 1983.

Climenhaga DB, Tokarewicz AC, Willis NR: *Nocardia* keratitis. Can J Ophthalmol 9:284–286, 1984.

Donnenfeld ED, Cohen EJ, Barza M, Baum J: Treatment of *Nocardia* keratitis with topical trimethoprim-sulfamethoxazole. Am J Ophthalmol 99:601–602, 1985.

Ferry AP, Font R, Weinberg RS, et al: Nocardial endophthalmitis: report of two cases studied histopathologically. Br J Ophthalmol 72:55–61, 1988.

Gregor RJ, Chong CA, Augsburger JJ, et al: Endogenous *Nocardia asteroides* subretinal abscess diagnosed by transvitreal fine-needle aspiration biopsy. Retina 9:118–121, 1989.

Katten HM, Pflugfelder SC: *Nocardia* scleritis. Am J Ophthalmol 110:446–447, 1990.

King LP, Furlong WB, Gilbert WS, Levy C: *Nocardia asteroides* infection following scleral buckling. Ophthalmic Surg 22:150–152, 1991.

Sridhar MS, Gopinathan U, Garg P, et al: Ocular *Nocardia* infections with special emphasis on the cornea. Surv Ophthalmol 45:361–378, 2001.

Zimmerman PL, Mamalis N, Alder JB, et al: Chronic *Nocardia asteroides* endophthalmitis after extracapsular cataract extraction. Arch Ophthalmol 111:837–840, 1993.

33 OCULAR CANDIDIASIS 112.89

Srilakshmi Maguluri, MD
Nashville, TN
Franco M. Recchia, MD
Nashville, TN
Sean P. Donahue, MD, PhD
Nashville, TN
Denis M. O'Day, MD, FACS
Nashville, TN

ETIOLOGY/INCIDENCE

Candida species usually are part of the normal flora on the mucocutaneous surfaces of the human gastrointestinal, genitourinary and respiratory systems. These yeasts can be isolated from the oropharynx and gastrointestinal tract of up to 50% of healthy asymptomatic individuals. *Candida* can also be recovered from soil, food and other areas in the environment. Although *Candida albicans* is by far the most common species isolated, followed by *C. parapsilosis*. Ocular infection has also been reported from other species of *Candida* such as: *C. tropicalis, C. glabrata, C. quilliermondi and C. krusei*.

RISK FACTORS

Ocular involvement with *Candida* species may be secondary to local inoculation or from endogenous colonization. Altered host resistance locally or systemically is critical to development of ocular disease. Risk factors include intravenous drug abuse, prolonged antibiotic therapy, systemic corticosteroids, immunosuppressive treatment, immunodeficiency syndromes, diabetes mellitus, non-ocular malignancy, post keratoplasty, intraocular surgery, corneal anesthetic abuse, contact lens wear and laser in situ keratomileusis (LASIK). Infection has also been reported following induced abortion and tattooing in an asplenic patient. When ocular *Candida* infections occur in children the risk factors appear to be prematurity and underlying candidemia. Gago et al described a case of bilateral *Candida* endogenous endophthalmitis in an extremely premature infant with stage 3 ROP. Drohan et al reported the development of a lens abscess in a 28 week gestational age infant. In both cases underlying candidemia was likely the inciting cause.

Generalized candidiasis is uncommon, but it can occur in two settings: systemic immunosuppression as described above and chronic mucocutaneous candidiasis (CMCC). CMCC is a distinct clinical entity involving immune or immunoregulatory dysfunctions, or both. Four types of CMCC have been described: early, late-onset, familial and juvenile familial polyendocrinopathy with candidiasis.

COURSE AND PROGNOSIS

A delay in the diagnosis and treatment of candidal keratomycosis may lead to stromal ulceration and scarring with neovascularization. Corneal perforation is uncommon because the infection is usually not deeply invasive. During the past two decades, the increased awareness and recognition of the clinical signs of fungal keratitis and more effective treatment have led to earlier diagnosis, improved management and better clinical outcome.

Management of candidal endophthalmitis, on the contrary, has until recently been less effective. Delays in diagnosis, poor intravitreal penetration of amphotericin B, (the agent of choice until recently for yeast infections) and a compromised host defense mechanism have all contributed to this poorer prognosis. However, with the advent of the triazoles, fluconazole and itraconazole and most recently voriconazole, the prognosis for saving the eye and preserving vision is considerably improved. However, chorioretinitis can still occur despite early intervention. Empiric treatment may be reasonable when suspicious lesions are noted in a patient with risk factors or with known candidemia.

DIAGNOSIS

Clinical signs and symptoms

Anterior segment

Eyelid involvement is uncommon but may include: calcareous cast, dacryocystitis, epiphora, occlusion of lacrimal canaliculi, blepharitis, cheesy material expressed from the meibomian glands, eczema, granuloma, pustules and ulceration at the base of an eyelash.

Rarely, *conjunctival* involvement may present as a purulent conjunctivitis with patchy white lesions on the palpebral conjunctiva. Pseudomembranes, cicatrisation and phlyctenulosis have also been reported.

The *cornea* is the most common site for *Candida* infection in the anterior segment. The appearance is typically in the form of a dry, gray, slightly elevated stromal infiltrate with feathery edges or a shallow ulcer. Deeper corneal involvement is unusual except following penetrating keratoplasty, *Lasik* and crystalline keratopathy.

Posterior segment

In the posterior segment, there is a spectrum of involvement ranging from: positive blood cultures without any posterior segment abnormailities, chorioretinitits without vitritis, mild vitritis and dense vitritis with vitreous opacifications. The latter two are classified as endophthalmitis. Infection usually extends from the choroid anteriorly into the vitreous.

In the *choroid/retina Candida* infection typically manifests as a creamy-white, round or oval, circumscribed chorioretinal lesion with overlying vitreous cells and debris (Figure 33.1). Other findings include: focal perivascular inflammatory deposits, intraretinal hemorrhages, exudative retinal detachment, white centered hemorrhages, focal retinal atrophy and choroidal neovascularization. *Vitreous* involvement may manifest as vitreoretinal membrane formation, free-floating snowball-like vitreous opacities.

Rarely the *optic nerve* may demonstrate a granuloma, papillitis, or perivasculitis.

Laboratory findings

The diagnosis of candidal chorioretinitis or endophthalmitis is made in the context of known risk factors coupled with the clinical appearance of the lesion. Since the clinical features are not pathognomonic for *Candida* infection, isolate recovery

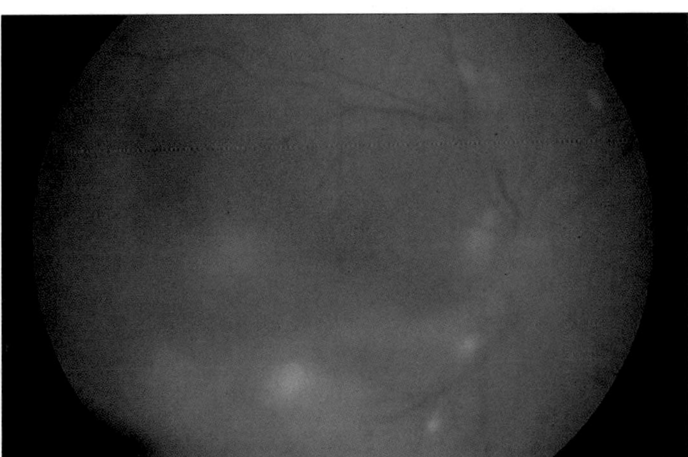

FIGURE 33.1 Chorioretinal lesions with vitritis in eye with ocular candidiasis.

directly from the eye should be attempted to confirm the presence of the organism.

Isolate recovery and identification

Most *Candida* species are readily isolated on blood agar and Sabourauds dextrose agar. A pasty, white colony appears 24 to 48 hours after inoculation. A number of rapid species identification diagnostic kits are available, as well as polymerase chain reaction (PCR) for organism identification from tissue and fluid samples. *Candida* species are easily visualized on smear with Gram stain as well as with special fungal stains such as Gomori methenamine silver stain and KOH.

Isolate recovery from cornea

In the case of a keratitis or corneal ulceration, corneal scrapings should be obtained for culture and smear. If the site of the suspected infection is deeper in the corneal stroma, corneal biopsy or elevation of a LASIK flap may be necessary to obtain an adequate specimen.

Periocular infections

Periocular infections caused by *Candida* species can be diagnosed by culturing conjunctival and eyelid scrapings and any reflux material obtained after irrigation of the lacrimal sac.

Specimen recovery from posterior segment

Vitreous biopsy is performed in the case of chorioretinits, vitritis, or endophthalmitis. In addition, a complete diagnostic microbiologic workup should be performed if a fungal etiology is suspected and not already documented. Serial blood cultures are necessary as part of the complete workup if the patient does not already have culture-positive candidemia.

TREATMENT

Topical medical treatment for anterior segment involvement

Most infections respond rapidly to a loading dose of 0.15% amphotericin B every 5 minutes for 1 hour and then hourly for the first 48 hours. Topical natamycin 5% suspension is less effective. The penetration of both drugs into deeper stroma is poor. Removal of corneal epithelium dramatically enhances the penetration and efficacy of these agents. Triazoles are also useful as topical agents. Fluconazole can be applied topically as a 0.2% solution in a balanced salt solution with adequate corneal and aqueous levels attainable. A new triazole, voriconazole, also shows promise when administered as a 1% solution topically.

Clotrimazole, an older imidazole, applied as a cream 8 to 12 times per day has also been successfully used. Subconjunctival injections are unnecessary and are of unproven efficacy. In those rare situations where systemic therapy is indicated fluconazole or voriconazole are likely to be the most efficacious.

Medical management of posterior segment involvement

Systemic

Systemic treatment is indicated for suspected candidal chorioretinitis or endophthalmitis. Intravenously administered amphotericin B can be used in this context. Efforts should be made to reach a dosage of 0.7 to 1.0 mg/kg/day as quickly as possible. Treatment may be also given on alternate days to increase drug tolerance. The drug is infused slowly over 4 to 6 hours in 500 mL of 5% dextrose in water. In treating early cases of *Candida* chorioretinitis, in which the lesions are confined to the retina and choroid, a minimal cumulative dose of 200 to 500 mg may be adequate to control the infection. If there is significant vitreous involvement, i.e. endophthalmitis, therapy should be continued until the total cumulative dose of amphotericin B is between 1000 and 1500 mg. Due to potential life-threatening complications with amphotericin B treatment, ophthalmologists should manage antifungal therapy with the aid of an internist who is skilled in infectious diseases.

Fluconazole and voriconazole are emerging as better systemic agents than amphotericin B in terms of coverage and toxicity profiles. *In vitro* investigation of voriconazole treatment for *Candida* endophthalmitis shows 100% susceptibility of *Candida* species. These newer agents can be a good alternative to amphotericin B for treatment of refractory cases, or those with significant systemic toxicity to amphotericin B. Further prospective studies are needed to corroborate their efficacy and lack of toxicity in the management of candidal endophthalmitis.

Local delivery of intravitreal therapy for endophthalmitis

Intravitreal injections of amphotericin B have been used in patients with chorioretinitis without vitritis and mild vitritis. Both 5- and 10-microgram doses of intravitreal amphotericin B have been shown to have no retinal toxicity. Su et al report the use of 5 to 10 microgram per 0.1 cc of fluconazole intravitreally to successfully treat candidal endophthalmitis in 8 patients. However, further large scale prospective randomized clinical trials need to corroborate the efficacy and document lack of retinal toxicity before these newer agents become standard intravitreal treatment.

Surgical treatment for anterior and posterior segment

In the absence of descemetocele formation, perforation or visually significant scarring, *penetrating keratoplasty* is rarely required for candidal corneal infections.

Therapeutic vitrectomy combined with intravitreal amphotericin B is indicated for eyes with prominent vitreous involvement. Vitrectomy removes inflammatory debris and fungal elements as well as scaffolding for vitreoretinal traction bands and epiretinal membranes that contribute later to the development of macular pucker and retinal detachment. It also allows intravitreal delivery of amphotericin B. Because of the frequent association of endogenous candidal endophthalmitis with systemic candidiasis, intravitreal amphotericin B should be an adjunct to intravenous therapy rather than a substitute.

Sub macular surgery and membrane removal may be beneficial in the setting of choroidal neovascular membrane without underlying fibrosis.

COMMENTS

The use of systemic steroids, topical corticosteroids, or both, in the management of patients with keratitis or endophthalmitis caused by *Candida* species, is controversial. Corticosteroids can inhibit the severe inflammatory host response that is sometimes highly destructive to the eye. Some clinicians believe that it is possible and desirable to halt such destruction without simultaneously depressing the host immune response. The use of steroid therapy adjunctively in a patient with fungal keratitis is complex and may be unwise.

REFERENCES

Alexandriou A, Reginald AY, Stavrou P, et al: *Candida* endophthalmitis after tattooing in an asplenic patient. Arch Ophthalmol 120:518–519, 2002.

Abbasoglu OE, Hosal BM, Sener B, et al: Penetration of topical fluconazole into human aqueous humor. Exp Eye Res 72:147–151, 2001.

Borne MJ, Elliott JH, O'Day DM: Ocular fluconazole treatment of *Candida parapsilosis* endophthalmitis after failed intravitreal amphotericin B. Arch Ophthalmol 111:1326–1327, 1993.

Breit SM, Hariprasad SM, Mieler WF, et al: Management of endogenous fungal endophthalmitis with Voriconazole and Capsofungin. Am J of Ophthalmol 139:135–140, 2005.

Brod RD, Flynn HW, Jr, Clarkson JG, et al: Endogenous *Candida* endophthalmitis. Ophthalmol 97:666–674, 1990.

Chen SJ, Chung YM, Liu JH: Endogenous *Candida* endophthalmitis after induced abortion. Am J Ophthalmol 125:873–875, 1998.

Chern KC, Meisler DM, Wilhelmus KR, et al: Corneal anesthetic abuse and *Candida* keratitis. Ophthalmol 103:37–40, 1996.

Donahue SP, Greven CM, Zuravleff JJ, et al: Intraocular candidiasis in patients with candidemia: clinical implications derived from a prospective multicenter study. Ophthalmol 101:1302–1309, 1994.

Drohan L, Colby CE, Brindle Me, et al: *Candida* (amphotericin-sensitive) lens abscess associated with decreasing arterial blood flow in a very low birth weight preterm infant. Pediatrics 110:e65, 2002.

Gago LC, Capone A, Jr, Trese MT: Bilateral presumed endogenous candida endophthalmitis and stage 3 retinopathy of prematurity. Am J Ophthalmol 134:611–613, 2002.

Hariprasad SM, Mieler WF, Holz ER, et al: Determination of vitreous, aqueous and plasma concentrations of orally administered Voriconazole in humans. Arch Ophthalmol 122:42–47, 2004.

Hidalgo JA, Alangaden GJ, Eliott D, et al: Fungal endophthalmitis diagnosis by detection of *Candida albicans* DNA in intraocular fluid by use of a species-specific polymerase chain reaction assay. J Infect Dis 181:1198–1201, 2000.

Jampol LM, Sung J, Walker JD, et al: Choroidal neovascularization secondary to *Candida albicans* chorioretinitis. Am J Ophthalmol 121:643–649, 1996.

Kostic DA, Foster RE, Lowder CY, et al: Endogenous endophthalmitis caused by *Candida albicans* in a healthy woman. Am J Ophthalmol 113:593–595, 1992.

Luttrull JK, Wan WL, Kubak BM, et al: Treatment of ocular fungal infections with oral fluconazole. Am J Ophthalmol 119:477–481, 1995.

Marangon FB, Miller D, Giaconi JA, et al: In vitro investigation of Voriconazole susceptibility for keratitis and endophthalmitis fungal pathogens. Am J Ophthalmol 137:820–825, 2004.

Merchant A, Zacks CM, Wilhelmus K, et al: Candidal endophthalmitis after keratoplasty. Cornea 20:226–229, 2001.

Recchia FM, Shah GK, Eagle RC, et al: Visual and anatomical outcome following sub macular surgery for choroidal neovascularization secondary to *Candida* endophthalmitis. Retina 22:323–329, 2002.

Schmid S, Martenet AC, Oelz O: Candidal endophthalmitis: clinical presentation, treatment and outcome in 23 patients. Infection 19:21–24, 1991.

Solomon R, Biser SA, Donnenfeld ED, et al: *Candida parapsilosis* keratitis following treatment of epithelial ingrowth after laser in situ keratomileusis. Eye Contact Lens 30:85–86, 2004.

Stern JH, Calvano C, Simon JW: Recurrent endogenous candidal endophthalmitis in a premature infant. J AAPOS 5:50–51, 2001.

Todd Johnston W, Cogen MS: Systemic candidiasis with cataract formation in a premature infant. J AAPOS 4:386–388, 2000.

34 OCULAR HISTOPLASMOSIS 115.12

Diana V. Do, MD
Baltimore, Maryland
Barbara S. Hawkins, PhD
Baltimore, Maryland

Originally described in 1951, the classic triad of the ocular histoplasmosis syndrome (presumed ocular histoplasmosis syndrome) consists of peripapillary chorioretinal scarring, punched-out 'inactive' chorioretinal scars, and hemorrhagic or neurosensory macular lesions or disciform macular scars. (See Figures 34.1 and 34.2.)

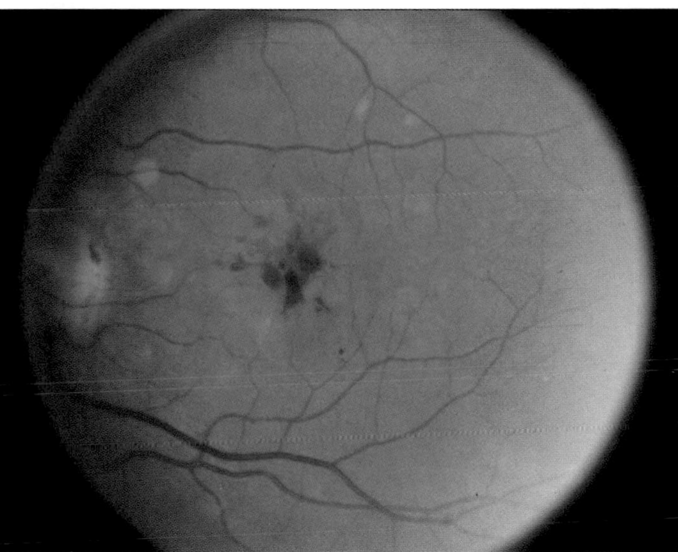

FIGURE 34.1 Fundus photograph of an eye with characteristic findings seen in ocular histoplasmosis syndrome: peripapillary atrophy, histo spots, and subretinal fluid and hemorrhage in the macula suggestive of choroidal neovascularization.

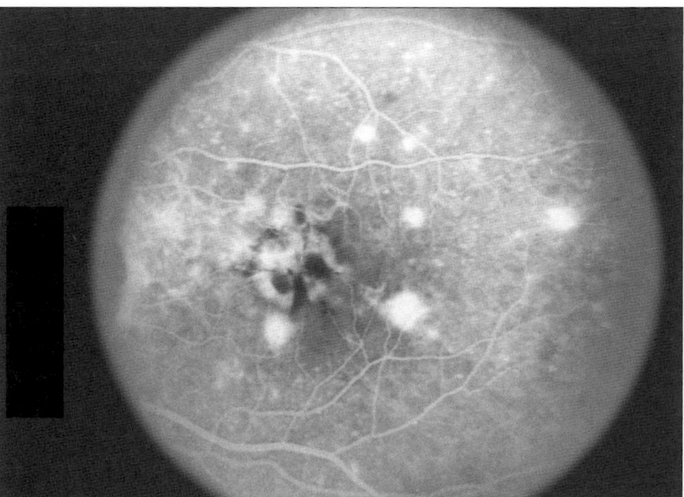

FIGURE 34.2 Fluorescein angiogram shows abnormal hyperfluorescence and leakage in the fovea consistent with CNV along with areas of blocked fluorescence due to subretinal blood.

ETIOLOGY/INCIDENCE

Ocular histoplasmosis is prevalent in North America, especially within the Mississippi and Ohio River valleys in which exposure to *Histoplasma capsulatum*, a bimorphic fungus with spores in the soil, is endemic. It has been estimated that ocular findings are present in approximately 2 million individuals, among whom 100,000 are at risk of losing vision in 1 or both eyes due to choroidal neovascularization (CNV). CNV associated with the ocular histoplasmosis syndrome is a vision-threatening complication that primarily affects working-age adults.

The etiology of ocular histoplasmosis is believed to begin with systemic infection with *H. capsulatum* via the respiratory tract, resulting in a mild upper respiratory-type infection. Although no serologic confirmation of *H. capsulatum* infection in patients with ocular histoplasmosis has been reported, it is generally believed that asymptomatic focal infection of the choroid occurs at the time of the initial benign systemic infection. This focal infection may resolve as an atrophic scar that disrupts Bruch's membrane. However, the infection may affect the retinal pigment epithelium and choriocapillaris and can result in serous and hemorrhagic retinal detachments associated with CNV. The initiator for CNV development is unknown and likely multi-factorial as genetic predisposition, immune system function, and initial inoculum of the fungus each may play a role.

DIAGNOSIS

Clinical signs and symptoms

The diagnosis of ocular histoplasmosis can be made on a clinical basis when findings of the classic triad of peripapillary chorioretinal scarring, punched-out 'inactive' chorioretinal scars, and hemorrhagic or neurosensory macular lesions or disciform macular scars are noted. In addition, there is a complete absence of vitreous inflammation.

Because chorioretinal scars are usually asymptomatic, it is usually not until CNV compromises the fovea that individuals seek ophthalmologic attention. The presenting symptoms in most patients are blurred central vision, metamorphopsia, micropsia, and central scotomas.

Laboratory findings

In a large portion of the Ohio and Mississippi River valleys, 60% or more of the adult population reacts positively to histoplasmin skin testing; thus a positive skin test is not proof of ocular histoplasmosis. Additional ancillary studies, such as serologic testing, are also not helpful, and the diagnosis is primarily made clinically when the patient presents with visual symptoms and ocular findings that are consistent with ocular histoplasmosis. Fluorescein angiography is used to assess for CNV and guide the physician with clinical treatment.

TREATMENT

Systemic

Although *H. capsulatum* is postulated but not proven to play a direct role in the development of ocular histoplasmosis, attempts at treating the disease with antimycotics failed and were abandoned. Although systemic corticosteroids were widely used at one time, oral steroids have not shown to be beneficial in treating CNV associated with ocular histoplasmosis and this type of treatment is not routinely used.

Ocular

Laser photocoagulation

In randomized clinical trials, the Macular Photocoagulation Study demonstrated that argon and krypton laser photocoagulation is effective in treating extrafoveal and juxtafoveal CNV lesions secondary to ocular histoplasmosis. From 1 year through 5 years of follow-up, 10% of eyes treated with laser photocoagulation versus approximately 40% of observed eyes had visual acuity that was six or more lines worse than at baseline. Thermal laser photocoagulation is not recommended for subfoveal CNV lesions given the immediate visual loss that results from a foveal scotoma.

Photodynamic therapy with verteporfin

Photodynamic therapy with verteporfin (Visudyne©; Norvartis Ophthalmics, Basel, Switzerland), termed verteporfin therapy, was developed as an alternative to thermal photocoagulation for the treatment of subfoveal CNV. A large randomized clinical trial confirmed the benefit of verteporfin therapy for CNV in age-related macular degeneration. Unlike laser photocoagulation, verteporfin therapy has been shown to selectively occlude vessels of experimentally induced CNV in animal models with minimal effects on the overlying retina and underlying choroid. Two-year results from an uncontrolled clinical study of 26 patients with ocular histoplasmosis revealed improvement of visual acuity from baseline as well as an absence of serious adverse events.

Surgery

The Submacular Surgery Trials (SST) Group H Trial was a randomized trial to compare surgical removal vs observation of subfoveal CNV lesions due to ocular histoplasmosis or idiopathic causes. Although the findings from the SST Group H do not support submacular surgery in similar patients with an initial visual acuity of 20/100 or better, surgery should be considered when presenting visual acuity is worse than 20/100. Quality-of-life findings were consistent with a beneficial affect of surgery.

SUMMARY

The diagnosis of presumed ocular histoplasmosis is made primarily by finding the typical clinical findings of peripapillary scarring, chorioretinal scars, and a serous or hemorrhagic detachment of the macula. Loss of central vision is caused by the development of CNV. Laser photocoagulation has proved to be effective in the treatment of extrafoveal and juxtafoveal CNV lesions, and verteporfin therapy has been effective and safe in a small case series of subfoveal CNV patients.

Although the risk of CNV in the second eye is less than 2% per year, there is no evidence that the risk diminishes over time. Patients who have CNV in one eye should be counseled regarding the lifetime risk of CNV developing in the second eye and the need to consult the ophthalmologist if any visual symptoms are noted in the fellow eye.

REFERENCES

Edwards LB, Acquaviva FA, Livesay VT, et al: An atlas of sensitivity to tuberculin, PPD-B, and histoplasmin in the United States. Am Rev Resp Dis 99:1–132, 1969.

Gass JDM: Stereoscopic atlas of macular diseases. Diagnosis and treatment. St Louis, Mosby, 1987:I.

Godfrey WA, Sabates R, Cross DE: Association of presumed ocular histoplasmosis with HLA-B7. Am J Ophthalmol 85:854–858, 1978.

Gunby P: Ocular histoplasmosis. JAMA 243:626–627, 1980.

Hawkins BS, Alexander J, Schachat AP: Ocular histoplasmosis. In: Ryan SJ, Schachat AP, eds: Retina. 3rd edn. St Louis, Mosby, 2001:1687–1701.

Kaplan HJ, Waldrep JC: Immunological basis of presumed ocular histoplasmosis. Int Ophthalmol Clin 23:19–31, 1983.

Krause AC, Hopkins WG: Ocular manifestation of histoplasmosis. Am J Ophthalmol 34:564–566, 1951.

Macular Photocoagulation Study Group: Argon laser photocoagulation for ocular histoplasmosis: results of a randomized clinical trial. Arch Ophthalmol 101:1347–1357, 1983.

Macular Photocoagulation Study Group: Argon laser photocoagulation for neovascular maculopathy: three year results from randomized clinical trials. Arch Ophthalmol 104:694–701, 1986.

Makley TA, Long JW, Suie T, Stephan JD: Presumed histoplasmic chorioretinitis with special emphasis on the present modes of therapy. Trans Am Acad Ophthalmol Otolaryngol 69:443–457, 1965.

Miller J, AW W, Kramer M: Photodynamic therapy of experimental choroidal neovascularization using lipoprotein-delivered benzopophyrin. Arch Ophthalmol 113:810–818, 1995.

Rosenfeld PJ, Saperstein DA, Bressler NM, et al: Photodynamic therapy with verteporfin in ocular histoplasmosis: uncontrolled, open-label 2-year study. Ophthalmology 111(9):1725–1733, 2004.

Smith RE: Natural history and reactivation studies of experimental ocular histoplasmosis in a primate model. Trans Am Ophthalmol Soc 80:695–757, 1982.

Submacular Surgery Trials research Group. Surgical removal vs. observation for subfoveal choroidal neovascularization, either associated with ocular histoplasmosis syndrome or idiopathic: I. Ophthalmic findings from a randomized clinical trial: submacular surgery trials (SST) group H trail: SST Report No.9. Arch Ophthalmol 122:1597–1611, 2004.

Submacular Surgery Trials Research Group: Surgical removal vs. observation for subfoveal choroidal neovascularization, either associated with ocular histoplasmosis syndrome or idiopathic: II. Quality-of-life findings from a randomized clinical trial: SST group H trial: SST Report No.10. Arch Ophthalmol 122:1616–1628, 2004.

35 PHARYNGOCONJUNCTIVAL FEVER 372.02

Aaron D. Smalley, MD
Hershey, Pennsylvania
Ingrid U. Scott, MD, MPH
Hershey, Pennsylvania

ETIOLOGY

Pharyngoconjunctival fever (PCF) is one of several presentations of adenoviral ocular infection, caused most often by serotypes 3, 4 and 7. Other serotypes have been implicated, namely 1, 5, 6, and 14 because of their isolation from culture of conjunctiva, nasopharynx and feces. Transmission of the virus is usually via droplet contact with ocular or respiratory tract secretions or water contamination with feces. Contact may occur directly through respiratory droplets or indirectly from a contaminated finger, instrument or medicine dropper coming in contact with the ocular surface. Symptoms appear after an incubation period of 5–12 days. Because of the high communicability of adenoviruses, PCF occurs more frequently in children or institutionalized persons with epidemics during warm weather, among families, schools or military organizations and inadequately chlorinated swimming pools.

DIAGNOSIS

Clinical signs and symptoms

Patients with PCF present most commonly with an acute follicular conjunctivitis, pharyngitis and fever. Upper respiratory infection and fever may precede the conjunctivitis by a few days and may mimic influenza. Conjunctivitis tends to present after an incubation period of 5 to 12 days with unilateral involvement, worse on the lower eyelid with progression to similar but less severe findings in the other eye. Other helpful diagnostic clues include development of tender preauricular lymphadenopathy, chemosis, conjunctival hemorrhages, non-purulent watery discharge, photophobia, and mild periorbital pain or edema. Epithelial keratitis and subepithelial infiltrates occur much less often than other adenoviral ocular diseases like epidemic keratoconjunctivitis (EKC) (5% versus 50%). Clinical symptoms usually resolve within 15 days after their onset.

Laboratory findings

Testing is usually not necessary because of spontaneous resolution of symptoms in most patients.

Cell culture of virus from conjunctival or nasopharyngeal swab is considered conclusive evidence for adenoviral infection and allows for more precise identification of serotype. Adenoviral antibody titer, while also useful for diagnosis, has the disadvantage of being delayed and is dependent upon the patient's immune system responding appropriately with a fourfold or greater increase in humoral antibody to adenovirus. The time to obtain culture and serology results is often too long for such tests to be useful for clinical decision-making. Because of implications for possible systemic treatment decisions, cell culture isolates are the preferred method of testing in immune-compromised patients.

Recent development of commercially available rapid antigen testing may provide faster results, but are not sufficiently sensitive to rule out adenoviral infection. Automated nucleic acid amplification techniques such as polymerase chain reaction (PCR) have been shown to be more sensitive and rapid, but may be limited by availability of proper equipment, technicians and quality control methods.

TREATMENT

Systemic

In most cases, no systemic antiviral treatment is recommended for PCF. Research is ongoing regarding systemic treatment for disseminated adenoviral infections in immune-compromised patients in whom systemic organ involvement may be life-threatening.

Topical

Topical treatments are generally not recommended, but may alleviate patient discomfort and prevent secondary bacterial infections. Medications that have been used, depending on patient symptoms, include:

- Artificial tears;
- Antihistamine drops as needed for severe itching;
- Antibiotics if mucopurulent discharge or uncertain diagnosis;
- Non-steroidal anti-inflammatory drops (diclofenac, ketorolac);
- Cidofovir (shown effective in early studies, but with concerning lacrimal stenosis toxicity, thus development was abandoned in the US and not FDA approved).

Supportive

This is the usual treatment of choice in most cases. It generally consists of:

- Patient education regarding the expected time course until resolution of symptoms and the rare occurrence of serious complications;
- Cold compresses to the eyelids as needed;
- Antipyretics as needed;
- Hand washing before and after contact with the eye or other respiratory secretions;
- Cleaning or disposal of pillow cases, towels, tissues or other surfaces that contact the eye.

PRECAUTIONS

Human adenoviral infections are highly contagious and have been implicated in several epidemic outbreaks.

Concern for chronic infections and delayed transmission of viral pathogens are supported by isolation of different serotypes of adenovirus in feces or tear secretions of patients months to years after onset of symptoms. These patients tended to have a more severe presentation and were more likely to have been prescribed topical steroids early on in their disease course.

Topical ophthalmic medication bottles may provide an additional mechanism for viral spread, especially to patient family members. This may be a reason to limit the use of topical medication according to the patient's symptoms and to counsel patients regarding the high transmissibility of virus. In addition, patients should be counseled to consider a leave of absence for at least 2 weeks, especially those with close contact with coworkers (schools, nursing homes, military housing or summer camps) or those providing healthcare to immune-compromised patients.

SUMMARY

Pharyngoconjunctival fever (PCF) is one of several disease presentations of ocular adenoviral infection that tends to be self-limited and typically responds well to supportive treatment alone. Consistent hand washing and other hygiene methods seem to be the most effective ways to reduce the incidence and spread of PCF to close contacts.

REFERENCES

Elnifro EM, Cooper RJ, Klapper PE, et al: Diagnosis of viral and chlamydial keratoconjunctivitis: which laboratory test? Br J Ophthalmol 83:622–627, 1999.

Kaye SB, Lloyd M, Williams H, et al: Evidence for persistence of adenovirus in the tear film a decade following conjunctivitis. J Med Virol 77:227–231, 2005.

Kinchington PR, Romanowski EG, Gordon YJ: Prospects for adenovirus antivirals. J Antimicrobial Chemotherapy 55:424–429, 2005.

Koidl C, Bozic M, Mossböck G, et al: Rapid diagnosis of adenoviral keratoconjunctivitis by a fully automated molecular assay. Ophthalmology 112:1521–1527, 2005.

Kojaoghlanian T, Flomenberg P, Horwitz MS: The impact of adenovirus infection of the immunocompromised host. Rev Med Virol 13:155–171, 2003.

Hillenkamp J, Reinhard T, Ross RS, et al: The effects of cidofovir 1% with and without cyclosporin A 1% as a topical treatment of acute adenoviral keratoconjunctivitis: a controlled clinical pilot study. Ophthalmology 109:845–850, 2002.

Pavan-Langston D: Viral diseases of the cornea and external eye. In: Albert DM, Jakobiec FA, eds. Principles and practices of ophthalmology. 2nd edn. Philadelphia, WB Saunders, 2000:878–879.

Shenk T: *Adenoviridae.* In: Knipe DM, Howley PM, eds: Fields virology. Philadelphia, Lippincott-Williams & Wilkins, 2001:2265–2228.

Uchio E, Ishiko H, Aoki K, Ohno S: Adenovirus detected by polymerase chain reaction in multidose eyedrop bottles used by patients with adenoviral keratoconjunctivitis. Am J Ophthalmol 134:618–619, 2002.

Vastine DW, Wilner BI: *Adenoviridae.* In: Darrell RW, ed: Viral diseases of the eye. Philadelphia, Lea & Febiger, 1985:131–146.

36 PNEUMOCOCCUS 041.2
(Streptococcus pneumoniae)

F. Hampton Roy, MD, FACS
Little Rock, Arkansas

ETIOLOGY/INCIDENCE

Commonly known as pneumococcus, *Streptococcus pneumoniae* is a gram-positive, lancet-shaped coccus characteristically appearing as diplococcus but occasionally appearing singly or as short chains. The normal habitat of the pneumococcus is the upper respiratory tract of humans; it is also present in the eyes of a small percentage of healthy individuals.

Pneumococcus is the primary etiologic agent in all types of pneumonia and the most frequent cause of otitis media in children; the organism also has been implicated in meningitis and septicemia. Pneumococcal infection is spread through aerosol dispersal of droplets released by infected persons.

DIAGNOSIS

Clinical signs and symptoms

Pneumococcal pneumonia is often preceded by an upper respiratory infection.

Systemic

- Sudden onset.
- Shaking chills.
- Fever.
- Sharp pain in the involved hemithorax.
- Cough with early sputum production.
- Headache.
- Gastrointestinal symptoms.

Ocular

Ocular disease occurs through direct invasion by the organism via aerosol or hand-to-eye contact; ocular pneumococcus infection may present as:

- Acryocystitis;
- Ophthalmia neonatorum in newborns;
- Orbital cellulites;
- Acute catarrhal conjunctivitis;
- Membranous, pseudomembranous, purulent, or ulcerative conjunctivitis;
- Hypopyon;
- Exudative anterior uveitis.

S. pneumoniae is also a true corneal pathogen and can lead to:

- Anterior staphyloma;
- Epithelial keratitis;
- Leukoma;
- Serpiginous ulcers;
- Perforation.

Secondary glaucoma can occur as a complication of such infections; endophthalmitis or panophthalmitis also can ensue.

Laboratory findings

A Gram's stain can be of great value in identifying *S. pneumoniae* in corneal scrapings. With this stain, the organisms are seen as gram-positive cocci in pairs, with the unattached end of each coccus slightly pointed outward, giving the organism its lancet shape. A capsule surrounding each pair of cocci often can be seen as well.

TREATMENT

Systemic

With few exceptions, *S. pneumoniae* is susceptible to penicillin, bacitracin, the cephalosporins, chloramphenicol, clindamycin, erythromycin, trimethoprim, and vancomycin. The quinolone ciprofloxacin is somewhat less active than the β-lactam agents against *S. pneumoniae.*

The treatment of choice is 300,000 to 600,000 units procaine penicillin at 12-hour intervals for pneumococcal pneumonia. It is inadvisable to rely on oral therapy for acutely ill patients; however, patients with a mild infection who are otherwise healthy can be treated safely with an initial intramuscular injection of 300,000 to 600,000 units procaine penicillin, followed by 250 mg penicillin V PO every 6 hours for 10 days. For patients with overwhelming disease and the potential for cardiovascular collapse, 40,000 to 50,000 units/kg aqueous potassium penicillin G can be divided in four equal portions and given every 6 hours.

Alternative drugs that may be used for the patient allergic to penicillin include 250 mg erythromycin every 6 hours and 500 mg vancomycin every 12 hours. Cefazolin 1 g every 8 hours and other cephalosporins are effective; however, clinical cross-sensitivity reactions to penicillin occur in about 8% to 15% of patients.

In the United States, 5% to 10% of *S. pneumoniae* strains are resistant to penicillin. Bacteremia and meningitis caused by highly resistant strains and meningitis due to intermediately resistant strains should be treated with agents other than penicillin. Therapy for these infections may include chloramphenicol (depending on susceptibility), cefotaxime, ceftriaxone, or vancomycin, possibly with the addition of rifampin, depending on the patient's response and such factors as the serum bactericidal activity. Pneumonias caused by intermediately resistant strains may be treated in most cases with high-dose penicillin alone.

Ocular

Topical ophthalmic antibiotics normally suffice for the treatment of conjunctivitis due to pneumococcus. Becitracin 10,000 units/mL should be given every hour during the first day and then four times daily for 1 week. Erythromycin ophthalmic ointment 0.5% may be substituted for the bacitracin.

For suppurative keratitis, central corneal ulcers due to *S. pneumoniae,* 100,000 units/mL topical fortified aqueous penicillin G should be administered every 30 minutes during the day and every hour during the night. Bacitracin 10,000 units/mL or cefazolin 50 mg/mL topically may be substituted for the penicillin. Subconjunctival cefazolin 50 to 100 mg or penicillin 0.5 to 1.0 million units also should be given every 12 to 24 hours for the first few days. If perforation seems imminent, systemic antibiotics as outlined under the information on endophthalmitis should be started.

For endophthalmitis caused by pneumococcus, 2.25 mg intravitreal cefazolin should be administered immediately after the aspiration of vitreous or vitrectomy. A daily dose of 20 to 40 million units aqueous penicillin G, divided into four equal portions, should be administered intravenously. In patients with a history of hypersensitivity to penicillin, 15 mg/kg/day cefazolin divided into three equal doses, 15 to 20 mg/kg/day erythromycin divided into four equal doses, or 600 mg lincomycin t.i.d. may be given intravenously in place of the penicillin. Subconjunctival injections, as outlined for the treatment of corneal ulcers, also should be given.

Cycloplegic agents are indicated to reduce pain and prevent posterior synechiae in patients with suppurative keratitis or endophthalmitis. One or two drops of 1% atropine or 1% cyclopentolate qd to t.i.d. may be instilled.

Orbital cellulitis caused by pneumococcal infection should be treated with aqueous penicillin G intravenously as outlined previously. An otolaryngologist should evaluate and treat the paranasal sinuses, if indicated.

Acute dacryocystitis caused by pneumococcus requires prompt and adequate drainage of the lacrimal sac. When the dacryocystitis is no longer acute, the patency of the nasolacrimal system should be reestablished. If periodacryocystitis has occurred, either 250 mg penicillin V PO every 6 hours or 600,000 units/day aqueous procaine penicillin G IM may be used. In addition, drainage of the nasolacrimal sac should be reestablished. In instances of hypersensitivity to penicillin, 250 to 500 mg erythromycin PO q.i.d. may be substituted.

Secondary glaucoma, which can occur in central corneal ulcers or endophthalmitis, may require the use of a systemic carbonic anhydrase inhibitor or a topical beta blocker. The usual oral adult dosage is 250 mg acetazolamide q.i.d.

Supportive

A new pneumococcal capsular polysaccharide vaccine is recommended for the prevention of pneumococcal infection in high-risk patients, including the elderly, patients with underlying disease that compromises pulmonary function, and immunosuppressed individuals. The vaccine is not indicated for more widespread use at this time but may be indicated in the future if penicillin-resistant pneumococci become more common.

PRECAUTIONS

Systemic therapy for ocular pneumococcal infection, except for endophthalmitis and orbital cellulitis, offers little or no advantage over topical and subconjunctival therapy. In addition to the risk of toxicity, systemic therapy yields relatively low levels of the appropriate drug in the affected ocular tissues. The organism usually is resistant to neomycin, gentamicin, and polymyxin B; thus, Neosporin®, of which the principal constituents are neomycin, polymyxin B, and bacitracin, is a poor choice for the treatment of pneumococcal infections. The same may be said for all of the fluoroquinolones, which have an extremely variable effect.

Strict guidelines for the use of corticosteroids in the treatment of pneumococcal infections are not presently available and there should be caution in the use of these agents.

REFERENCES

Applebaum PC: World-wide development of antibiotic resistance in pneumococci. Eur J Clin Microbiol 6:367–373, 1987.

Conte JE, Barriere SL: Manual of antibiotics and infectious diseases. 5th edn. Philadelphia, Lea & Febiger, 1984:25–26.

Hoeprich PD: Bacterial pneumonias. In: Hoeprich PD, ed: Infectious diseases. 3rd edn. Hagerstown, Harper & Row, 1983:347–360.

Klugman KP: Pneumococcal resistance to antibiotics. Clin Microbiol Rev 3:171–196, 1989.

Lentnek A, LeFrock JL, Molavi A: *Streptococcus pneumoniae.* In: Levison ME, ed: The pneumonias: clinical approaches to infectious diseases of the lower respiratory tract. Littleton, John Wright, 1984:261–271.

Mandell GL, Sande MA: Antimicrobial agents: penicillins and cephalosporins. In: Gilman AG, Goodman LS, Gilman A, eds: The pharmacological basis of therapeutics. 7th edn. New York, Macmillan, 1985:1115–1145.

Wilkins J, Whitcher JP, Margolis TP: Penicillin-resistant *Streptococcus pneumoniae* keratitis. Cornea 15:99–100, 1996.

37 PROPIONIBACTERIUM ACNES 040

James K. Leong, MD
Sydney, Australia
Peter J. McCluskey, MD, FRACO
Sydney, Australia

ETIOLOGY/INCIDENCE

Propionibacterium acnes is a gram-positive, pleomorphic, nonspore forming bacillus that is considered part of the normal eyelid and conjunctival anaerobic flora. This low-virulence fastidious organism has the predilection to cause persistent mild inflammation. It has been implicated in a number of periocular and ocular infections including conjunctivitis, chronic blepharitis, corneal ulcers, periorbital cellulitis and endophthalmitis following trauma and surgery.

P. acnes is an opportunistic pathogen that gained prominence as it became increasingly recognized in the pathogenesis of chronic endophthalmitis following cataract surgery. It is suggested that it may adhere to the intraocular lens at the time of surgery. Once introduced it resists host defenses by inhibiting suppressor T-cell lymphocytes and the nature of its cell wall structure protects against degradation by neutrophils and macrophages allowing the organism to remain viable within the eye and cause a chronic inflammatory response. Additionally sequestration of viable organisms within capsule remnants or between an intraocular lens and posterior capsule further protects the organism from host defenses and is thought to act as a nidus for recurrent infections.

P. acnes endophthalmitis may become clinically obvious following neodymium-yttrium aluminum garnet laser posterior capsulotomy and also may develop following glaucoma drainage device surgery.

COURSE/PROGNOSIS

- *P. acnes* may cause either acute or indolent chronic keratitis; usually in the context of compromised corneas.
- *P. acnes* is generally associated with delayed endophthalmitis that typically presents several months to two years postoperatively.
- Endophthalmitis due to *P. acnes* characteristically presents as an indolent low-grade anterior uveitis. There is frequently a transient response to topical corticosteroids and such cases may be initially misdiagnosed as sterile postoperative inflammation.
- Recurrence of *P. acnes* endophthalmitis is relatively common, particularly after more conservative initial management.
- *P. acnes* endophthalmitis is associated with relatively good final visual outcomes. The average final visual acuity in the two largest series documented was 20/40 or better.
- Rarely, poor visual outcomes have been reported secondary to diffuse intraretinal hemorrhages complicating the infection.

DIAGNOSIS

Clinical signs and symptoms of *P. acnes* endophthalmitis:

- Patients may present with decreased vision and occasionally pain;
- The hallmark sign of *P. acnes* endophthalmitis is a white intracapsular plaque that represents collections of organisms (40–100% of cases);
- Vitritis (100%);
- Conjunctival injection (100%);
- Granulomatous keratic precipitates (31–81%);
- Anterior chamber cells (80%);
- Hypopyon (31–63%);
- Beaded fibrin strands in the anterior chamber (33%).

Laboratory findings

- Aerobic and anaerobic cultures for *P. acnes* must be incubated for 14 days due to its fastidious nature and slow growth rates.
- A high index of suspicion for *P. acnes* endophthalmitis is essential in patients with chronic postoperative uveitis and aqueous and vitreous aspirates for microscopy and culture are required. Poor sensitivity results in a high false-negative rate. Polymerase chain reaction techniques may improve detection rates.
- Capsular biopsy may reveal sequestered intracellular and extracellular bacilli and may also be used for diagnostic culture.

TREATMENT

- In general *P. acnes* is sensitive to tetracycline, clindamycin, chloramphenicol and a wide variety of penicillins, cephalosporins and quinolones.
- Vancomycin however is usually the antibiotic of choice; topical (50 mg/mL), intravitreal (1 mg/0.1 mL) or systemic (initiate with 1 g IV every 12 hours and titrate according to renal function and drug levels).

Treatment options for postoperative *P. acnes* endophthalmitis include:

- Intravitreal antibiotics (recurrence rate 50–100%);
- Pars plana vitrectomy with intravitreal antibiotics (recurrence rate 50%);
- Pars plana vitrectomy with partial capsulectomy and intravitreal antibiotics (recurrence rate 14–44%);
- Pars plana vitrectomy with total capsulectomy, intravitreal antibiotics and intraocular lens removal or exchange (definitive curative procedure usually indicated for recurrent cases).

Despite potential recurrences, the initial therapy selected for *P. acnes* endophthalmitis does not appear to significantly influence the final visual outcome.

The risk of recurrence versus the risks associated with the various therapeutic interventions should be considered when selecting an appropriate initial therapy.

Long-term follow-up is essential to detect late recurrences.

SUMMARY

P. acnes is a low virulence organism and postoperative endophthalmitis in particular presents with a characteristic indolent low-grade uveitis. This fastidious organism is often difficult to culture and often presents a diagnostic dilemma. Molecular techniques hold great promise to improve detection. A number of effective therapeutic options are available with pars plana vitrectomy, total capsulotomy and intraocular lens removal being the definitive procedure. A significant number of patients may be successfully managed with more conservative treatment. Final visual outcomes are relatively good despite frequent recurrences of infection.

REFERENCES

Aldave AJ, Stein JD, Deramo VA, et al: Treatment strategies for postoperative *Propionibacterium acnes* endophthalmitis. Ophthalmology 106:2395–2401, 1999.

Clark WL, Kaiser PK, Flynn HW, et al: Treatment strategies and visual acuity outcomes in chronic postoperative *Propionibacterium acnes* endophthalmitis. Ophthalmology 106:1665–1670, 1999.

Deramo VA, Ting T: Treatment of *Propionibacterium acnes* endophthalmitis. Curr Opin Ophthalmol 12:225–229, 2001.

Hall GS, Pratt-Rippin K, Meisler DM, et al: Minimum bactericidal concentrations of *Propionibacterium acnes* isolates from cases of chronic endophthalmitis. Diagn Microbiol Infect Dis 21:187–190, 1995.

Lohmann CP, Linde H, Reischl U: Improved detection of microorganisms by Polymerase Chain Reaction in delayed endophthalmitis after cataract surgery. Ophthalmology 107:1047–1052, 2000.

Underdahl JP, Florakis GJ, Braunstein RE, et al: *Propionibacterium acnes* as a cause of visually significant corneal ulcers. Cornea 19:451–454, 2000.

38 PROTEUS 041.9

Howard M. Leibowitz, MD
Boston, Massachusetts

ETIOLOGY/INCIDENCE

Proteus spp. (*P. mirabilis, P. vulgaris* and *P. penneri)* are gram-negative bacilli found as free-living saprophytes in water and soil and in dead or decaying organic substances. These organisms are enterobacteria, a component of the normal intestinal flora, but in a weakened host they may cause opportunistic infection at many sites, including the eye. Ocular *Proteus* infections include scleritis, keratitis, necrotic inflammation of the eyelid, dacryocystitis, endophthalmitis and panophthalmitis. Such infections are uncommon, generally are encountered after trauma or intraocular surgery and often are severe with a relatively poor prognosis.

DIAGNOSIS

Clinical signs and symptoms

- Conjunctiva: conjunctival inflammation, edema, exudates.
- Cornea: epithelial loss, stromal infiltration and/or ulceration, edema, folds in Descemet's membrane, descemetocele, perforation.
- Eyelids: edema, infiltration, gangrene, necrosis.
- Globe: intraocular inflammation (endophthalmitis; panophthalmitis).
- Sclera: scleral inflammation and necrosis (scleritis).
- Other: anterior chamber cells and flare, hypopyon, dacryocystitis, paralysis of seventh nerve.

Laboratory findings

- Gram-stained smear.
- Culture and antibiotic sensitivities.

Differential diagnosis

- Ocular infection by other gram-negative bacilli.

PROPHYLAXIS

- Adequate gram-negative antibiotic coverage prior to surgery and following ocular trauma.

TREATMENT

Ocular antibiotics

- A fortified aminoglycoside, (gentamicin or tobramycin ophthalmic drops — 14 mg/mL) initially is administered hourly (or more often) for infections of the external eye.
- Third (ceftazidine) and fourth (cefepime) generation cephalosporins are effective and may be administered concurrently with an aminoglycoside for severe *Proteus* infections. (Ophthalmic products are not commercially available; the drug must be formulated for this purpose.)

- Fluoroquinolones (ciprofloxacin 0.3%; ofloxacin 0.3%; moxifloxacin 0.5%; gatifloxacin 0.3%) ophthalmic solutions are effective alternatives.

Systemic antibiotics

- Intraocular infections and infection of the sclera or eyelids require systemic antibiotic therapy with the same drugs recommended for topical administration. The virulence of *Proteus* infection mandates parenteral administration.

Surgical

- Endophthalmitis generally requires pars plana vitrectomy and injection of antibiotic into the vitreous cavity (ceftazidine 2.25 mg/0.1 mL).

PRECAUTIONS

Aminoglycosides are potentially nephrotoxic and can cause vestibular and auditory dysfunction. Cephalosporins and fluoroquinolones also have well-documented toxicity. Patients on systemic antibiotics must be carefully monitored.

COMPLICATIONS

Complications include eyelid and scleral necrosis, corneal scarring and perforation, retinal necrosis and loss of vision.

COMMENTS

The rarity of cases precludes specific recommendations of an optimal antibiotic regimen; the initial regimen is administered empirically while awaiting the results of *in vitro* antibiotic sensitivities.

REFERENCES

Aras C, Ozdamar A, Ozturk R, Karacoriu M, Ozkan S: Intravitreal penetration of cefepime after systemic administration to humans. Ophthalmologica 216:261–264, 2002.

Eifrig CWG, Scott IU, Flynn HW, et al: Endophthalmitis after pars plana vitrectomy: incidence, causative organisms and visual acuity outcomes. Amer J Ophthalmol 138:799–802, 2004.

Hariprasad SM, Mieler WF, Holz ER: Vitreous and aqueous penetration of orally administered gatifloxacin in humans. Arch Ophthalmol 121:1408–1409, 2003.

Kunimoto DY, Tasman W, Rapuano C, et al: Endophthalmitis after penetrating keratoplasty: microbiologic spectrum and susceptibility of isolates. Amer J Ophthalmol 137:343–345, 2004.

Leibowitz HM: Antibacterial effectiveness of ciprofloxacin 0.3% ophthalmic solution in the treatment of bacterial keratitis. Am J Ophthalmol 112:34S–47S, 1991.

McKeag D, Kamal Z, McNab AA, Sheorey H: Combined coliform and anaerobic infection of the lacrimal sac. Clin and Exp Ophthalmol 30:52–54, 2002.

O'Brien TP, Maguire MG, Fink NE: Efficacy of ofloxacin vs. cefazolin and tobramycin in the therapy for bacterial keratitis. Arch Ophthalmol 113:1257–1265, 1995.

Parunovic A: *Proteus mirabilis* causing necrotic inflammation of the eyelid. Am J Ophthalmol 76:543–544, 1973.

Solberg R, Meberg A, Schoyen R: Neonatal conjunctivitis in a nursery and a neonatal unit. Tidsskr Nor Laegeforen 111:1230–1232, 1991.

39 PSEUDOMONAS AERUGINOSA
041.7

Mehdi Ghajarnia, MD
Pittsburgh, Pennsylvania
Regis P. Kowalski, MS, [M]ASCP
Pittsburgh, Pennsylvania
Deepinder K. Dhaliwal, MD
Pittsburgh, Pennsylvania

ETIOLOGY/INCIDENCE

Pseudomonas aeruginosa is a Gram-negative rod that is ubiquitous in water, soil and plants. It is commonly found in the hospital environment and is an important nosocomial pathogen. Often affecting immunocompromised hosts or patients with specific susceptibility factors (i.e. cystic fibrosis), it nevertheless has important virulence factors that render it a formidable pathogen. Its most common ocular manifestation is infectious keratitis and less commonly endophthalmitis.

Pseudomonal keratitis can be one of the most serious and sight threatening infections of the cornea. Virulence factors such as alkaline protease (AP), elastase (LasB) and a novel virulence factor, protease IV, may contribute to the rapid course by which the bacillus can cause liquifactive stromal necrosis and perforation. In addition, secreted exotoxin, ExoU and ExoT contribute to the pathogen's ability to cause cytotoxicity and inhibit phagocytosis by epithelial cells.

Prior to the introduction of sterile fluorescein strips, fluorescein sodium solutions were an important source of epidemic pseudomonal keratitis. More recently, *P. aerugenosa* has become a common source of corneal infection secondary to the increasing use of soft contact lens wear, which has been clearly identified as a risk factor in the development of pseudomonal ulcerative keratitis. While most studies reveal Gram-positive organisms as the predominant pathogen in bacterial keratitis, *P. aerugenosa* is typically the most common Gram-negative isolate and the most common pathogen in contact lens wearers.

Evidence suggests that pseudomonal keratitis can only develop in a cornea which has had its epithelial barrier broken down. In the outpatient setting, contact lens wearers are at increased risk secondary to corneal microtrauma from the insertion/removal of lenses as well as from frequent epithelial breakdown from toxic injury secondary to hypoxia, lens solutions, or lens deposits. Hydrophilic lenses are particularly prone to colonization with *P. aeruginosa* as the regular deposition of mucin and protein onto the soft lens polymers facilitate the adherence of the bacteria; this is believed to readily serve as the source by which transfer from contact lens to injured epithelium and subsequent corneal infection takes place. Several *P. aeruginosa* surface molecules including pili, flagella, outer membrane proteins and lipopolysaccharide (LPS) can modulate adherence to the cornea. Although poor lens hygiene and overnight wear significantly raise the risk of acquiring pseudomonal keratitis, even proper lens care and disposable contact lenses have caused corneal ulcers. Corneal infections secondary to mascara injury and contaminated ocular cosmetics have also been a frequent observation in the outpatient setting.

Inpatient pseudomonal ulcers are frequently seen in patients with concurrent non-ophthalmic infections, in particular burn patients and patients receiving respiratory assistance.

Endophthalmitis caused by *P. aeruginosa* is a less frequent occurrence. In the Endophthalmitis Vitrectomy Study, only 4 out of 420 cases had confirmed infection with pseudomonal species. However, cases of *P. aeruginosa* endophthalmitis have been documented in cases of postoperative cataract extraction, corneal transplantation, glaucoma valve surgery, trabeculectomy, pars plana vitrectomy, as well with corneal ulcers. Moreover, epidemics related to contaminated irrigation solutions have been documented. In general, endophthalmitis caused by *P. aeruginosa* is associated with very poor visual outcome despite rapid treatment with appropriate antibiotics.

DIAGNOSIS

Clinical signs and symptoms

Patients typically present with sudden onset of symptoms that initially include foreign body sensation with progressively worsening pain, conjunctival injection and photophobia. A mucopurulent discharge and blurry vision related to the location of the ulcer are associated symptoms. Corneal ulceration (epithelial defect with stromal infiltrate) is usually central or paracentral though peripheral infections near the limbus may occur and can extend to the sclera by means of a satellite subconjunctival abscess; the prognosis in cases of scleral involvement is typically very poor. Anterior chamber reaction and hypopyon formation can also occur (Figure 39.1). Corneal melting with progressive thinning to subsequent perforation occurs in a small percentage of cases. Careful evaluation for signs and symptoms of possible pseudomonal endophthalmitis is important given the different treatment strategies.

Laboratory findings

Any vision threatening or aggressive ulcerative keratitis should be cultured for identification of pathogen and antibiotic susceptibility testing, preferably before the initiation of antibiotics if it does not cause significant delay in treatment. Corneal scrapings should be collected for Gram's staining and Giemsa stain. The eye should be anesthetized with topical proparacaine (5%) rather than tetracaine as the latter is more likely to interfere with recovery of organisms. In addition, culturing contact lenses and lens solutions can provide valuable susceptibility information when corneal cultures remain negative. Antibiotic susceptibility testing should be done on any other bacterial isolate that grows from a mixed infection. Lastly, in cases of suspected endophthalmitis, intravitreous and/or aqueous samples for culture should be drawn prior to any administration of intravitreal antibiotics.

P. aeruginosa appears as slender Gram-negative rods that are aerobic and grow easily on routine isolation media (trypticase soy agar supplemented with 5% sheep blood) as grayish or greenish, metallic appearing to very gelatinous colonies. The colonies exude a sweet, grape like odor and exhibit a characteristic blue-green pigment called pyocyanin when grown on uncolored media such as Muller–Hinton media. However, not all strains of *P. aeruginosa* produce pyocyanin and others may produce other pigments that can mask pyocyanin. Colonies can grow rather rapidly at a rate of 3 to 5 mm in diameter within 48 hours under incubation at 35–37°C.

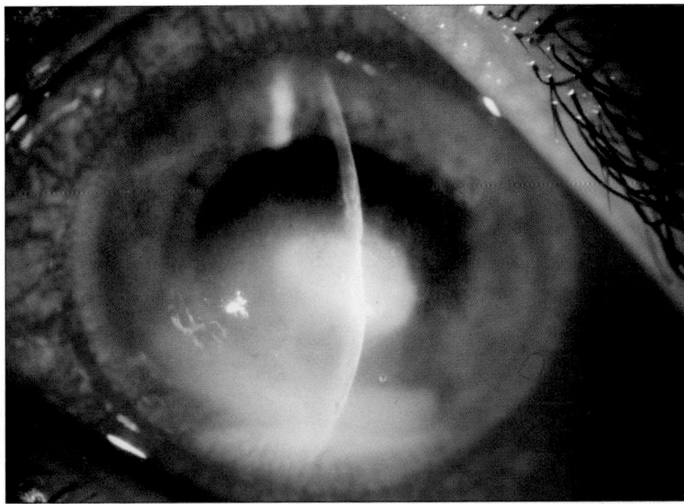

FIGURE 39.1 Pseudomonal keratitis in a soft contact lens wearer. Note the presence of hypopyon and corneal thinning.

TREATMENT

Topical therapy

Topical therapy with broad-spectrum antibiotics has been the mainstay initial treatment of bacterial keratitis since the causative organism is not known. Treatment consisting of gram-positive coverage with a first-generation cephalosporin and an aminoglycoside active against most Gram-negative organisms has been generally employed. The following combination has often been used:

- Fortified tobramycin 14 mg/mL;
- Fortified cefazolin 50 mg/mL.

Due to excellent coverage of Gram-negative organisms by fluoroquinolones (Table 39.1), we substitute a topical fluoroquinolone (such as ciprofoxacin) for fortified tobramycin to minimize ocular toxicity seen with frequent dosing. Dosing is generally every 15 minutes for the first 6 hours, then every 30 minutes until bedtime. Hourly treatment is then continued around the clock for the first 24–48 hours. Once the culture results and susceptibilities are known, therapy is adjusted. Also, the frequency of antibiotic administration is tapered based on clinical evidence of improvement: decreased density of the stromal infiltrate, improved demarcation of infiltrate borders, decreased anterior chamber inflammation, re-epithelialization of the epithelial defect and decreased pain.

Cycloplegia is recommended to reduce photophobia and prevent synechiae. Due to the rapid rate of keratolysis with pseudomonal infections, use of a systemic anticollagenolytic agent (e.g. doxycycline) is recommended.

Systemic

Systemic therapy is usually not necessary for bacterial keratitis, including that caused by *P. aeruginosa*, unless the infection involves the limbus and sclera, or when endophthalmitis is suspected. Systemic therapy may also be indicated in cases when compliance with frequent topical therapy is not possible (i.e. pediatric patient). In the past, gentamicin offered adequate coverage, but with the emergence of gentamicin-resistant *P. aeruginosa*, tobramycin has become an alternative initial choice. Currently, either of the following intravenous regimens may be used:

- Tobramycin 4 mg/kg qd;
- Ciprofloxacin 500 mg b.i.d.

TABLE 39.1 – *In vitro* susceptibility of keratitis isolates of *Pseudomonas aeruginosa* to common ophthalmic antibiotics from 1993–2004

Antibiotic	Isolates	% Susceptible	% Intermediate	% Resistant
bacitracin	145	0	0	100 (145)
chloramphenicol	120	0	5.8 (7)	94.2 (113)
vancomycin	144	0	0	100 (144)
gentamycin	145	93.8 (136)	1.4 (2)	7 (4.8)
ciprofloxacin	143	95.1 (136)	0	4.9 (7)
ofloxacin	143	90.9 (130)	1.4 (2)	7.7 (11)
trimethoprim	80	0	0	100 (80)
polymixin B	145	0	0	100 (145)
cefazolin	144	0	0	100 (144)
tobramycin	145	97.2 (141)	0.7 (1)	2.1 (3)
sulfacetamide	145	1.4 (2)	6.2 (9)	92.4 (134)
gatifloxacin	25	88 (22)	0	12 (3)
moxifloxacin	25	88 (22)	0	12 (3)

(Source: The Charles T. Campbell Ophthalmic Microbiology Laboratory, University of Pittsburgh Medical Center.)

Concurrent coverage for Gram-positive pathogens may be necessary in suspected or proven cases of mixed infections when using tobramycin. Other antibiotics to which *P. aeruginosa* has shown a high degree of sensitivity include arbekacin, ceftazidime, imipenem, ofloxacin and piperacillin. Given the potential renal toxicity associated with aminoglycocides such as tobramycin, systemic therapy required peak and trough serum levels 30 minutes before and 30 minutes after infusion of the antibiotic and monitoring of renal function. There is one study that reports the successful treatment of serious *P. aeruginosa* scleritis with a combination of intravenous ceftazidime plus an aminoglycoside and topical antibiotics.

Surgical

In cases of *P. aeruginosa* endophthalmitis immediate injection of antibiotics is warranted if there is any hope of salvaging vision in these patients. Addition of intravitreal corticosteroids have not demonstrated proven benefit or harm and this remains at the discretion of the treating ophthalmologist. Immediate vitrectomy plus antibiotic injection may be required in more severe presenting cases. In cases of severe infection with pain and no visual potential, evisceration or enucleation may be necessary.

PRECAUTIONS

The addition of corticosteroids in treatment of bacterial keratitis remains controversial especially if the etiologic agent is *P. aeruginosa*. The goals of concomitant topical steroid use are: to reduce corneal inflammation, to facilitate epithelial and stromal healing and to minimize corneal opacification, neovascularization and destruction. However, potential risks of steroid use include enhanced microbial replication and recrudescence and accelerated stromal loss with increased risk of perforation. To minimize these risks in cases of pseudomonal keratitis, steroids should not be used in the early stages of infection. After there is definite clinical response, topical steroids may be added to concomitant bactericidal antibiotic therapy with close monitoring.

COMPLICATIONS

The feared complication of pseudomonal keratitis is perforation, which can occur within 24 hours after the onset of corneal ulceration. Therefore, patients with pseudomonal keratitis should be treated aggressively and followed closely.

COMMENT

P. aeruginosa is a virulent organism that is a common cause of contact lens-related infectious keratitis. Adherence of the bacteria to the mucin coating on soft contact lenses greatly facilitates subsequent corneal invasion after epithelial microtrauma. Due to several virulence factors, *P. aeruginosa* can cause rapid liquifactive necrosis and even perforation. Topical fluoroquinolones or fortified tobramycin are the agents of choice in treating pseudomonal keratitis.

REFERENCES

Asbell P, Stenson S: Ulcerative keratitis: survey of 30 years' laboratory experience. Arch Ophthalmol 100:77–80, 1982.

DiGaetano M, Stern GA, Zam AS: The pathogenesis of contact lens-associated *Pseudomonas aeruginosa* corneal ulceration, II: an animal model. Cornea 5:155–158, 1986.

Eifrig CWG, Scott IU, Flynn HW, Jr, Miller D: Endophthalmitis caused by *Pseudomonas aeruginosa*. Ophthalmology 110:1714–1717, 2003.

Fleiszig SMJ, Evans DJ: The pathogenesis of bacterial keratitis: studies with *Pseudomonas aeruginosa*. Clin Exp Optom 85:271–278, 2002.

Hehm CJ, Holland GN, Webster RG, Jr, et al: combination of intravenous ceftazidime and aminoglycosides in the treatment of pseudomonal scleritis. Ophthalmology 104:838–843, 1997.

Mela EK, Giannelou IP, Koliopoulos JX, et al: Ulcerative keratitis in contact lens wearers. Eye and Contact Lens: Science & Clinical Practice 29: 207–209, 2003.

O'Brien T, Mauire MG, Fink NE, et al: Report from the Bacterial Keratitis Study Research Group: efficacy of ofloxacin vs cefazolin and tobramycin in the therapy for bacterial keratitis. Arch Ophthalmol 113:1257–1256, 1995.

Ooishi M, Miyao M: Antibiotic sensitivity of recent clinical isolates from patients with ocular infections. Ophthalmologica 211(Suppl 1):15–24, 1997.

Stern GA: *Pseudomonas* keratitis and contact lens wear: the lens/eye is at fault. Cornea 9(Suppl 1):S36–S38, 1990.

Wilhelmus KR: Indecision about corticosteroids for bacterial keratitis. An evidence-base Update. Ophthalmology 109:835–844, 2002.

40 **Q FEVER** 083.0

Richard B. Hornick, MD, MACP
Orlando, Florida

Q fever is the name given to the infection initiated by *Coxiella burnetii.* The name originated from the frustration that Derrick encountered when he was unable to isolate a bacterial pathogen from workers in an Australian abattoir who were part of an outbreak of a febrile illness; thus, he called the infection Q (for *query*) fever.

ETIOLOGY/INCIDENCE

C. burnetii is a small gram-negative rod that is classified with the other Rickettsiae. Like the other organisms in this group, it grows inside eukaryotic cells. Chronic infection occurs when phagosomes in monocytes fail to mature and defective killing of the organisms results. It is a highly infectious pathogen; because infection by only one organism may cause disease in humans, diagnosis is made with serologic tests rather than isolation of the organism. Most persons who acquire the organism develop an asymptomatic infection that can be detected only through the use of serologic surveys. These surveys have demonstrated antibodies to *C. burnetii* in 10% to 20% of populations exposed to sheep, goats, cats and cattle. However, using reverse-transcription-polymerase chain reaction, over 90% of milk samples demonstrate *C. burnetii.*

COURSE/PROGNOSIS

The majority of patients who develop this disease have a fever, a headache that often is severe and a flu-like syndrome. This illness may abate spontaneously. About half of these patients will have pneumonitis as demonstrated through radiographic procedures. Ten percent of the patients develop hepatitis, but as many as 85% of patients may have abnormal liver function tests. Rarely, chronic infection of the heart valves occurs; this is a difficult condition to treat with antibiotics, but 2 to 3 years of therapy may result in a cure. A rash may be present in a small percentage of patients; it presents with maculopapular or purpuric lesions.

DIAGNOSIS

Clinical signs and symptoms

This organism infects both endothelial cells and hepatocytes, so vasculitis, the hallmark of all rickettsial infections, ensues in various organ systems throughout the host. The inflammatory reaction to the infected liver cells can lead to granulomas, sometimes doughnut shaped. Similar granulomas are in patients infected with *Mycobacterium tuberculosis.* In addition, autoantibodies such as smooth muscle and phospholipid can be demonstrated.

Ocular involvement is unusual and ocular manifestations as the only evidence of the disease are very rare.

Ocular lesions

- In conjunctival infection, there is no exudate and lesions clear as the infection abates.
- Uveitis is a rare occurrence and there is no evidence that *C. burnetii* is the cause of uveitis as primary disease.
- Retinal hemorrhage is unusual but can occur as a manifestation of vasculitis.
- Episcleritis is remote and secondary to an autoimmune reaction.
- There is one case report of Miller–Fisher variant of Guillain–Barré syndrome, in which the symptoms of bilateral ptosis, bilateral sixth nerve paralysis and upgaze paralysis persisted for 7 months.
- Q fever meningoencephalitis is characterized by low-grade fever, cerebrospinal fluid pleocytosis, abducens nerve paralysis and optic neuritis.
- Partial third nerve palsy.

Laboratory findings

In most clinical laboratories, serologic diagnosis is recommended. Attempts at isolating organisms require appropriate safety equipment to prevent disease in laboratory workers.

- The serologic test complement fixation is specific but lacks sensitivity and indirect immunofluorescence is both highly specific and sensitive.
- A positive antibody titer for phase II antigen of *C. burnetii* indicates recent infection. The presence of antibodies to phase I antigen are compatible with chronic infection, such as endocarditis.
- Laboratory results include normal leukocyte count in 90% of patients, thrombocytopenia in 25%, increased transaminase levels in 75%, smooth muscle antibodies in 65% and phospholipid antibodies in 50%.

Differential diagnosis

An acute illness with nonspecific, severe retro-orbital headache and fever plus an association with parturient or newborn animal provides strong diagnostic aid. Other rickettsial diseases may cause similar diseases, but the antibiotic will cover both.

PROPHYLAXIS

- Antibiotic prophylaxis after contact with infected placenta from sheep, goats and cats is not effective; it will prolong the incubation period.
- Prevention includes the avoidance of aerosols generated by infected animals. Placentas can be heavily contaminated.

Laboratory animals, such as sheep, must be proved to be free of *C. burnetii.* Abattoir workers are at risk.

- A vaccine is used in Australia, but it is not available in the United States.

TREATMENT

Systemic

- Doxycycline can be given at 200 mg/day for 14 to 21 days.
- Ciprofloxacin (and other quinolones) have been effective.
- The use of alkalinizing agents to increase pH in lysosome enhances doxycycline activity. The experimental use of chloroquine and doxycycline in selected patients appears to be effective.
- Tetracycline and chloramphenicol 0.5 g every 6 hours have been successful in the treatment of patients with pneumonitis.
- The duration of treatment for patients with optic neuritis is unknown.

Ocular

Local therapy includes steroid drops for episcleritis plus a systemic antibiotic.

COMPLICATIONS

- Rare patients have persistent blindness after the evolution of optic neuritis.
- Diminished vision has been described in patients recovering from meningoencephalitis.

SUMMARY

C. burnetii is an organism that is well suited for aerosol dissemination. It is found in the feces, placentas, urine and milk of infected but asymptomatic animals. These hardy organisms survive for long periods in the inanimate environment and can be readily dispersed by wind and thereby infect persons remote from the animal sources. Infections are probably more common than realized and not diagnosed because of the self-limited nature of the infectious process. Because so few cases of acute Q fever occur in the United States, the diagnosis may be missed. This may lead to the development of chronic disease or serious complications. A careful history of potential contact with animals is the key to making the right diagnosis and initiating appropriate and prompt antibiotic therapy.

REFERENCES

Derrick EH: 'Q' fever, a new fever entity: clinical features, diagnosis and a laboratory investigation. Med J Aust 11:281–299, 1937.

Ferrante MA, Dolan MJ: Q fever meningoencephalitis in a soldier returning from the Persian Gulf War. Clin Infect Dis 16:489–496, 1993.

Ghigo E, Honstettre A, Capo C, et al: Link between impaired maturation of phagosomes and defective *Coxiella burnetii* killing in patients with chronic Q fever. J Infect Dis 190:1767–1772, 2004.

Ortuno AD, Maeztu C, Munoz JA, et al: Miller Fisher syndrome associated with Q fever. J Neurol Neurosurg Psych 53:615–616, 1990.

Peres-Flores E, Delas MA, et al: Partial third nerve palsy caused with chronic Q fever. European J of Neurology 6:619–620, 1999.

Raoult D, Marrie T: Q fever: state-of-the-art clinical article. Clin Infect Dis 20:489–496, 1995.

Tselentis Y, Gikas A, Kofteridis D, et al: Q fever in the Greek island of Crete: epidemiologic, clinical and therapeutic data from 98 cases. Clin Infect Dis 20:1311–1316, 1995.

41 RABIES 071

Edsel Ing MD, FRCSC
Toronto, Ontario
Amal Al-Sayyed, MD
Toronto, Ontario

Rabies is a potentially fatal, acute progressive encephalitis caused by single-stranded RNA neurotropic viruses (genus Lyssavirus, family Rhabdoviridae). This viral zoonotic disease is transmitted from the saliva or neuronal tissue of infected animals. Any mammal can potentially become infected with rabies. In North America, wild animals such as raccoons, skunks, bats, foxes, woodchucks and beavers are the major reservoirs of infection, since domesticated animals have been vaccinated. Bat bites in particular may go unrecognized due to the small bite marks and because patients may be bitten when they are sleeping. Inhalation of rabies can also occur in bat caves. Domestic animals that can get rabies include dogs, cats, cattle, guinea pigs and rabbits. Developing countries such as Africa and Asia more commonly have dog rabies since preventive treatment for rabies may be hard to maintain.

ETIOLOGY/INCIDENCE

Rabies has an almost world wide distribution practically and causes approximately 30,000 deaths per year worldwide. However in the United States, fewer than 3 deaths are reported per year. Between 1993 and 2002, the number of human and canine rabies cases in the Americas' region fell by approximately 80%; there were 39 human cases in 2002, 63% of them transmitted by dogs. This sharp reduction is attributable mainly to the control measures implemented in the Americas, such as the mass vaccination of dogs and prophylactic treatment for people who have been exposed. Human to human spread of rabies via corneal transplant has been well documented by the Centers for Disease Control and other references since 1979.

COURSE/PROGNOSIS

Infectious material can enter percutaneously or through the mucous membranes (e.g. eye, nose, mouth or wound.) The virus is excreted abundantly in saliva. After inoculation, the virus can incubate in host cells (usually muscle cells) from 9–90 days. After a sufficient concentration of infectious units is reached, the virus crosses the myoneural junction to enter the peripheral nerves to the central nervous system. The long incubation period usually affords adequate time for postexposure prophylaxis treatment. If the virus crosses the nerve axons, infection cannot be prevented by immunization.

DIAGNOSIS

Clinical signs and symptoms

Local symptoms include pain or itching around the wound site. Early systemic symptoms are non-specific and include headache, fever, vomiting and loss of appetite. Patients may then become anxious and agitated in the excitatory phase of the disease. At this stage they may develop extreme difficulty with drinking. During attempts to swallow fluids painful expulsion may occur from spasmodic contraction of the muscles of deglutition and respiration, such that even the sight, sound or smell of liquids can provoke fear (hydrophobia). Seizures are common. Some patients may develop paralysis or intense muscle spasm.

Ocular

Ophthalmic findings in rabies include photophobia, retinal hemorrhages, disc edema, pupillary irregularities, loss of the corneal reflexes and paralysis or the extraocular muscles. Antirabies vaccination has been associated with cases of optic neuritis and neuroretinitis.

Laboratory findings

Multiple tests are required to diagnose rabies ante-mortem in humans; no single test is adequate. Testing can be performed on saliva, serum, spinal fluid, skin and cornea. Saliva can be tested by virus isolation or reverse transcription followed by polymerase chain reaction. Serum and spinal fluid are tested for antibodies to rabies virus. Rabies neutralizing antibodies may be detected in the serum 6–13 days post exposure. Skin biopsy specimens are examined for rabies antigen in the cutaneous nerves at the base of hair follicles. Immunofluorescent antibody staining of the epithelial cells on corneal impression test has also been suggested as part of the antemortem work-up in patients with suspected rabies.

Whenever possible the suspected infectious animal should be captured, assessed by a veterinarian and quarantined for 10 days. If the animal is suspected to be infected, it should be euthanized and the brain tissue analyzed for rabies virus or Negri bodies (cytoplasmic inclusion bodies). Direct fluorescent antibody test and immunhistochemistry stains are frequently used to diagnose rabies and are more sensitive and specific than the finding of Negri bodies.

TREATMENT/PROPHYLAXIS

Ocular adnexal injury due to bite of a rabid animal is a life-threatening condition for which patients should be administered prompt rabies prophylaxis.

Animal bites should be flushed vigorously for ten minutes with a soapy solution followed by 1% povidone-iodine. Antibiotics and tetanus prophylaxis should be administered.

Rabies can be prevented if rabies postexposure prophylaxis (PEP) is administered before the onset of clinical signs. PEP consists of one dose of immune globulin and five doses of rabies vaccine over a 28 day period. The immune globulin and first rabies vaccine is given as soon as possible following exposure. Subsequent doses of rabies vaccine are given on days 3, 7, 14 and 28 after the first vaccination. Current vaccines are relatively painless. Rabies is almost always fatal once symptoms begin. There is a recent case report of a 15-year-old surviving from rabies after medical induction of coma while a native immune response matured.

Differential diagnosis

The differential diagnosis of rabies includes any acute encephalitis. Silent or radiculomyelitic rabies can present with ascending paralysis like Guillian–Barré syndrome, especially after postexposure prophylaxis.

COMMENTS

Rabies virus-mediated eye disease provides a new model for studying mechanisms regulating immune privilege during viral infection. In mouse models, following brain infection, the Challenge Virus Standard strain of rabies virus infects the retina. Rabies virus ocular infection induces the infiltration of neutrophils and predominantly T cells into the eye. Rabies virus is also used as a retrograde transneuronal tracer in the experimental mapping the oculomotor system and investigation of the cerebral cortical control of orbicularis oculi motoneurons.

REFERENCES

Belotto A, Leanes LF, Schneider MC, et al: Overview of rabies in the Americas. Virus Res 111(1):5–12, 2005.

Gode GR, Bhide NK: Two rabies deaths after corneal grafts from one donor. Lancet 2(8614):791, 1988.

Gupta V, Bandyopadhyay S, Bapuraj JR, Gupta A: Bilateral optic neuritis complicating rabies vaccination. Retina 24(1):179, 2004.

Houff SA, Burton RC, Wilson RW, et al: Human-to-human transmission of rabies virus by corneal transplant. N Engl J Med 300(11):603–604, 1979.

Javadi MA, Fayaz A, Mirdehghan SA, Ainollahi B: Transmission of rabies by corneal graft. Cornea 15(4):431–433, 1996.

Rupprecht CE, Gibbons RV: Prophylaxis against rabies. N Engl J Med 351:2626–2635, 2004.

Tabbara KF, al-Omar O: Eyelid laceration sustained in an attack by a rabid desert fox. Am J Ophthalmol 119:651–652, 1995.

Willoughby RE, Jr, Tieves KS, Hoffman GM, et al: Survival after treatment of rabies with induction of coma. N Engl J Med 352(24):2508–2514, 2005.

Zaidman GW, Billingsley A: Corneal impression test for the diagnosis of acute rabies encephalitis. Ophthalmology 105:249–251, 1998.

42 RHINOSPORIDIOSIS 117.0

James J. Reidy, MD, FACS
Buffalo, New York

Rhinosporidiosis is a rare fungal infection, primarily affecting the mucous membranes of the nose and eye, caused by *Rhinosporidium seeberi*. Infection with this organism results in a chronic, granulomatous tissue response characterized by the formation of a highly vascular, polypoid mass that may be single or multiple, sessile or pedunculated. The nasal mucosa is the most frequently affected site, followed by the bulbar conjunctiva. Other sites of infection that have been reported less frequently include: the respiratory mucosa, vaginal mucosa, skin and metastatic-like involvement of the internal organs.

The geographic distribution of *Rhinosporidium seeberi* is extremely wide, with the majority of the cases of disease reported in the Indian subcontinent. Cases of rhinosporidiosis have also been reported in North America, South America, Africa, the Middle East, Asia and Europe.

The mode and means of *R. seeberi* infection are not well understood. It has been proposed that the infection is spread by means of direct exposure to contaminated water (ponds, lakes, rivers) or field dust. Infected livestock or waterfowl may contaminate the water either via spore containing nasal discharge or by way of contaminated feces. Dust containing spores from fields contaminated with feces from infected animals could be inhaled, thereby accounting for the predilection for infection of the nasal mucosa. Alternatively, runoff from contaminated fields into nearby lakes, streams and ponds could secondarily contaminate the water. The conjunctiva could be exposed to either contaminated dust or water. None of the cases reported in the literature suggest that rhinosporidiosis is transmitted from person to person.

Rhinosporidium seeberi has been classified as a Phycomycete, a lower order non-septate, spore-forming fungus. Once the spores have infected the epithelium, they incite a reaction in the surrounding tissue resulting in a highly vascular polypoid or sessile growth. These masses contain fibromyxomatous connective tissue that contains trophocytes and sporangia in all stages of development and degeneration, surrounded by a mononuclear inflammatory infiltrate.

Disease of the eye accounts for about 15% of rhinosporidiosis infections. Most cases of ocular disease have been reported in warmer climatic regions. The typical conjunctival lesion is a freely mobile, granular, pink or red, sessile or pedunculated lesion that is usually attached at the upper or lower conjunctival fornix, or tarsal conjunctiva. Involvement of the limbus, caruncle and canthi have been reported. Lesions are initially small and flat, painless and often go unnoticed by the patient. As the lesion(s) gradually enlarge, patients may note: tearing, injection, photophobia, deformation of the eyelid and occasionally, secondary conjunctival infection. Typically, ocular lesions are solitary and unilateral.

Complete surgical excision remains the most effective treatment of this disease. Application of cautery or cryopexy to the base of the excised lesion may be an effective adjunct to prevent recurrence. Use of systemic dapsone, when used as an adjunct to surgical excision, has also met with some success in preventing recurrences.

REFERENCES

Jimenez JF, Young DE, Hough AJ, Jr: Rhinosporidiosis: a report of two cases from Arkansas. Am J Clin Path 62:611–615, 1984.

Nair KN: Clinical trial of diaminodiphenylsulfone (DDS) in nasal and nasopharyngeal Rhinosporidiosis. Laryngoscope 89:291–295, 1975.

Reidy JJ, Sudesh S, Olivier C: Rhinosporidiosis of the conjunctiva: a case report from Western New York. Surv Ophthalmol 41:409–413, 1997.

Rippon JW: Medical mycology: the pathogenic fungi and the pathogenic actinomycetes. 3rd edn. Philadelphia, WB Saunders, 1988.

Savino DF, Margo CE: Conjunctival rhinosporidiosis: light and electron microscopic studies. Ophthalmolgy 90:1482–1489, 1983.

43 ROCKY MOUNTAIN SPOTTED FEVER 082.0

Byron L. Lam, MD
Miami, Florida

ETIOLOGY/INCIDENCE

Rocky Mountain spotted fever is the most common rickettsial disease in the United States and occurs throughout the Western hemisphere. It is caused by *Rickettsia rickettsii*, an obligate, intracellular gram-negative coccobacilli that contains both DNA and RNA. Ticks that serve as vectors and reservoirs for Rocky Mountain spotted fever are *Dermacentor andersoni*, the wood tick, in the Rocky Mountain states; *Dermacentor variabilis*, the dog tick, in the eastern and southern states; and *Amblyomma americanum*, in Texas. The disease is transmitted to humans through tick bites, which often occur unnoticed.

The organism invades the endothelial and smooth muscle cells of the blood vessels, producing a systemic vasculitis with increased vascular permeability. Loss of serum proteins, decreased blood volume, and thrombi over damaged endothelial cells result in hypoperfusion and circulatory failure. A recent survey in children with immunofluorescence antibody assay suggests infections with *R. rickettsii* or related spotted-fever group rickettsiae may be subclinical and occur more commonly than previous thought.

Most cases occur during the spring and summer, with sporadic cases occurring throughout the year. Risk factors include exposure to wooded areas and to dogs. Infection should also be considered in family members and contacts who have febrile illness and share environmental exposures with the patient.

COURSE/PROGNOSIS

The incubation period is 2 to 14 days. Ninety percent of symptomatic patients develop a maculopapular rash between days 3 and 5 of the illness. The rash gradually becomes petechial and progresses to ecchymoses. Necrosis and gangrene occur rarely.

Untreated symptomatic cases usually result in death within 15 days of the onset of symptoms. The mortality rate is 6.5% if treatment is begun within 5 days of the onset of disease; the rate increases dramatically if treatment is delayed.

DIAGNOSIS

Clinical signs and symptoms

The rash may have a variable distribution, although classically it first involves the distal extremities, including the palms and soles, and subsequently spreads toward the trunk.

A high fever (more than 102°F) and headaches occur in at least 90% of patients. Other symptoms include lethargy, myalgia, abdominal pain, diarrhea, and nausea and vomiting. Dehydration and edema often follow.

Systemic

- Splenomegaly.
- Hepatomegaly.

- Interstitial pneumonitis.
- Myocarditis.
- Encephalitis.

Ocular

- Petechial conjunctivitis.
- Anterior uveitis.
- Retinal hemorrhages.
- Cotton-wool spots.
- Retinal vascular engorgement and tortuosity.
- Branch retinal arteriolar occlusion.
- Optic disk edema due to ischemia and inflammation.
- Neuroretinitis.
- Orbital edema due to increased extravascular volume.

Laboratory findings

Early diagnosis is based on clinical and epidemiologic grounds. When available, polymerase chain reaction has high sensitivity and specificity. The immunofluorescence test on skin biopsy is specific but not highly sensitive. Serologic tests do not become reliably positive for 7 to 10 days after the onset of symptoms because serum antibodies to the organism are detectable only during convalescence.

TREATMENT

In most cases, systemic intravenous tetracycline and chloramphenicol should be started as soon as possible. Oral doxycycline, tetracycline, and chloramphenicol may be considered but only in patients who are not acutely ill. Therapy is continued for 7 to 10 days or until the patient is afebrile for 2 to 3 days. The antibiotics are rickettsiostatic, and final elimination of the organism is achieved by host immune mechanisms.

Intravenous fluids and electrolyte management are crucial to overcome dehydration and to support blood pressure. Anticonvulsant, analgesic and antipyretic agents; oxygen; mechanical ventilation; and other methods may be necessary depending on the involvement of different organ systems.

Moderate to severe uveitis may be treated with topical cycloplegic agents and corticosteroids, although no reliable information on efficacy is available.

COMMENTS

Rocky Mountain spotted fever is a potentially fatal disease and early treatment with appropriate antibiotics is the key prognostic factor. Therapy should be instituted as soon as the disease is suspected clinically. Ophthalmologists rarely participate in the management of patients with Rocky Mountain spotted fever when fulminant systemic symptoms overwhelm mild ocular manifestations. The ocular changes are probably underestimated and usually resolve within 3 weeks of therapy.

REFERENCES

Cherubini TD, Spaeth GL: Anterior nongranulomatous uveitis associated with Rocky Mountain spotted fever. Arch Ophthalmol 81:363–365, 1969.

Duffey RJ, Hammer E: The ocular manifestations of Rocky Mountain spotted fever. Ann Ophthalmol 19:301–306, 1987.

Eremeeva ME, Dasch GA, Silverman DJ: Evaluation of a PCR assay for quantitation of Rickettsia rickettsii and closely related spotted fever group rickettsiae. J Clin Microbiol 41:5466–5472, 2003.

Kamper C: Treatment of Rocky Mountain spotted fever. J Pediatr Health Care 5:216–222, 1991.

Kirk JL, Fine DP, Sexton DJ, Muchmore HG: Rocky Mountain spotted fever: a clinical review based on 48 confirmed cases, 1943–1986. Medicine 69:35–45, 1990.

Kirkland KB, Wilkinson WE, Secton DJ: Therapeutic delay and mortality in cases of Rocky Mountain spotted fever. Clin Infect Des 20:1118–1121, 1995.

Marshall GS, Stout GG, Jacobs RF, et al: Tick-Borne Infections in Children Study Group. Antibodies reactive to *Rickettsia rickettsii* among children living in the southeast and south central regions of the United States. Arch Pediatr Adolesc Med 157:443–448, 2003.

Presley GD: Fundus changes in Rocky Mountain spotted fever. Am J Ophthalmol 67:263–267, 1969.

Smith TW, Burton TC: The retinal manifestations of Rocky Mountain spotted fever. Am J Ophthalmol 84:259–262, 1977.

Sprach DH, Liles WC, Campbell GL, et al: Tick-borne diseases in the United States. N Engl J Med 329:936–947, 1993.

Weber DJ. Walker DH: Rocky Mountain spotted fever. Infect Dis Clin North Am 5:19–35, 1991.

44 RUBELLA 056.9
(German Measles)

Vivien Boniuk, MD, FRCS(C)
New York, New York

ETIOLOGY/INCIDENCE

Rubella has been known as a clinical entity for almost 200 years. It is caused by a member of the togavirus group with one antigenic type. In 1941, Gregg observed that a peculiar type of congenital cataract was associated with the occurrence of a rubella epidemic 9 to 10 months earlier. This observation led to the description of the congenital rubella syndrome (CRS), which is a well-defined and well-described group of ocular, cardiac, and other organ system abnormalities resulting from exposure to the rubella virus during embryonic life. The rubella epidemic of 1964/1965 afforded an opportunity for a multidisciplinary study of the effects of the rubella virus and led to the development of a vaccine, resulting in a 98% to 99% reduction in the incidence of rubella and CRS since 1969. In countries where there is no national rubella vaccination program, the yearly incidence of new cases ranges from 8.1–12.7 cases per 100,000 live births. There are still more than 100,000 infants born with CRS every year, world-wide.

In the United States, in spite of the goal of eliminating rubella and CRS by 2000, there are still approximately 300 cases of rubella annually with less than a handful of CRS (4–5 cases) reported annually, and mostly in Hispanic foreign workers.

Because rubella infrequently causes significant ocular and systemic complications during the postnatal period, attention here is directed only to CRS. Although several cases of acute rubella retinal pigment epitheliitis have been reported in adults, they have not led to serious sequelae. The effects in utero are explained by the observation that chronic infection with the rubella virus causes cells to have a prolonged doubling time and shortened survival time; therefore, organ systems infected with virus during their active growing period will be underdeveloped and abnormal.

DIAGNOSIS

Depending on the stage of gestation during which rubella is acquired, there is a wide spectrum of systemic features, ranging from stillbirth to the most minimally detectable damage to the retinal pigment epithelium and the pigmented epithelium in the organ of Corti of the inner ear. Other systemic abnormalities are prematurity by weight and mental and physical developmental retardation that persists into childhood. Other signs are thrombocytopenic purpura, pancytopenia, large skull with bulging anterior fontanelle, encephalitis, various neurologic anomalies, hepatosplenomegaly, radiologically observable bone changes, pancreatic insufficiency, esophageal atresia and cleft palate. Various types of cardiac anomalies may be present and are frequently associated with other defects.

Clinical signs and symptoms

Ocular

The most common ocular findings in CRS are:

- Retinopathy (Figure 44.1);
- Peculiar central, often eccentric, dense nuclear cataract;
- Microphthalmos.

Less frequent findings include:

- Iris hypoplasia with pigment epithelial defect;
- Nystagmus and strabismus;
- Congenital glaucoma;
- Corneal haze due to transient keratitis, which may leave a permanent scar.

The pigmentary changes of the retina may show progression in early childhood, and there have been 10 reported cases of subretinal neovascularization and disciform macular detachment as late complications. CRS must be considered in the differential diagnosis of subretinal neovascular membranes in the pediatric age group.

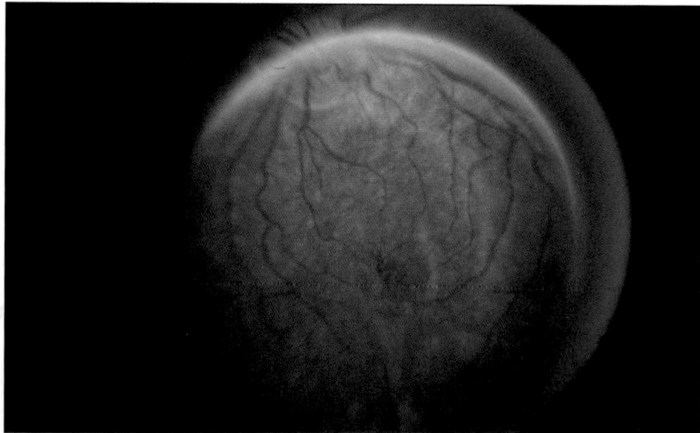

FIGURE 44.1 Rubella retinopathy.

TREATMENT

Surgical

- As soon as the child's condition permits, the congenital rubella cataract should be completely aspirated.
- Postoperative treatment with mydriatic agents should be intensive and continued for at least 3 months.
- Parents should be cautioned about the importance of punctal occlusion after eyedrop administration.
- Early optical correction of aphakia is essential.

The glaucoma secondary to the CRS behaves as a phenotypic congenital glaucoma. Other ocular abnormalities, such as strabismus, are treated in a manner consistent with basic therapeutic principles.

PRECAUTIONS

A multidisciplinary approach to the treatment of these children is essential because of the presence of multiple abnormalities associated with physical and mental developmental delay. It is essential that children affected with CRS be followed in centers familiar with coordination of therapy to maximize their development.

COMMENTS

The incidence of rubella in pregnancy is directly related to the pool of susceptible women in the childbearing age group and their exposure to those recently infected with rubella virus. Epidemiologic data indicate that most reported cases now occur in young adults (older than 15 years), a group that includes women of childbearing age who are at high risk. (Previously, prevalence predominated in those younger than 14 years.) Therefore, congenital rubella syndrome may still occur.

In the United States, laws require vaccination against rubella for school entry. Special attention (state mandated) is paid to the rubella immunization status of healthcare workers. The risk of severe congenital malformation after rubella vaccination is low, even if it is administered to pregnant women; however, to avoid this risk, women known to be pregnant should not be vaccinated and conception should be avoided for 3 months after vaccination. CRS has been reported in the offspring of previously vaccinated women. Rubella immunity should be tested before each pregnancy. It is not surprising to find severe ocular congenital anomaly concomitant with high rubella titers in a neonate.

REFERENCES

Bloom S, et al: Congenital rubella syndrome burden in Morocco: a rapid retrospective assessment. Lancet 365:135–141, 2005.

Bonuk V: Rubella. Int Ophthalmol Clin 15:229–241, 1975.

Collis WJ, Cohen DN: Rubella retinopathy: a progressive disorder. Arch Ophthalmol 84:33, 1970.

Condon R, Bower C: Congenital rubella after previous maternal vaccination (Letter). Med J Aust 156:882, 1992.

Deutman AF, Grizzard WS: Rubella retinopathy and subretinal neovascularization. Am J Ophthalmology 85:22, 1978.

Gerber SL, Helveston EM: Subretinal neovascularization in a 10-year-old child. J Pediatr Ophthalmol Strabismus 29:250–251, 1992.

Gerstle C, Zinn KM: Rubella-associated retinitis in an adult: report of a case. Mt Sinai J Med NY 43:303–308, 1976.

Greaves WL, Orenstein WA, Stetler HC, et al: Prevention of rubella transmission in medical facilities. JAMA 248:861–964, 1982.

Hayashi M, Yoshimura N, Knodo T: Acute rubella retinal pigment epitheliitis in an adult. Am J Ophthalmol 93:285–288, 1982.

Porges Y: Congenital conjunctiva: limbo-corneal choristoma associated with marginal keratopathy. Cent Afr J Med 42:49–50, 1996.

Preblud SR, Stetler HC, Frank JA, Jr, et al: Fetal risk associated with rubella vaccine. JAMA 246:1413–1418, 1981.

Reef SE, et al: The changing epidemiology of rubella in the 1990s. JAMA 287:464–472, 2002.

World Health Organization: Guidelines for surveillance of congenital rubella syndrome and rubella field testing version. Geneva, WHO, 1999.

45 RUBEOLA 045
(Measles, Morbilli)

Nick W. H. M. Dekkers, MD, PhD
Tilburg, The Netherlands

ETIOLOGY/INCIDENCE

Rubeola, caused by paramyxovirus, is an acute, extremely communicable disease that primarily affected school-aged children. In the developed world, measles is now a rarity due to the high rate of immunization. In developing countries, depending on the immunization rate, crowding and poverty, primarily the very young (6 months to 2 years) are affected.

DIAGNOSIS

Clinical signs and symptoms

The prodromal phase consists of a catarrhal inflammation of the respiratory tract, with fever, cough, rhinitis, and a subepithelial conjunctivitis.

In the exanthematous stage, a characteristic maculopapular rash develops, beginning on the head. Late in the prodromal phase and continuing into the exanthematous stage, the great majority of patients develop a strictly epithelial conjunctivitis, in the exposed parts of the conjunctiva. This conjunctivitis is followed by an epithelial keratitis consisting of coarse punctate lesions, with a characteristic form, stainable by vital stains (fluorescein, rose bengal, lissamin green). The keratitis starts at the limbus and progresses toward the central cornea. Separate lesions can coalesce into large corneal erosions. The main symptom of this self-limiting keratitis is photophobia.

PROPHYLAXIS

Vaccination with live, attenuated measles virus is very effective. Adult patients can develop measles when their vaccine-induced immunity wanes or when they get immune-compromised (HIV, chemotherapy).

Measles and nutritional status

Protein-energy malnutrition

- Higher infection rates with a high morbidity and mortality due to pulmonary infections and gastroenteritis characterize measles in malnourished children. In severe protein-energy malnutrition, the patient is immune-compromised, and the measles runs its course without the characteristic rash; the diagnosis of measles is easily missed.
- Measles is an important cause of acute progression of marginal malnutrition (stunting, marasmus) into a full-blown kwashiorkor.
- Kwashiorkor destabilizes the collagen in the skin and cornea, which enhances corneal ulceration and necrosis.

Vitamin A

- Vitamin A protects against infections; in children with (marginal) vitamin A deficiency, infections are more common.
- Vitamin A deficiency causes night blindness, xerosis and colliquative necrosis of the cornea. In measles, this can occur very rapidly, within the course of days.
- Measles depletes the liver stores of vitamin A and can considerably lower the serum retinol level.

TREATMENT

Ocular

- Eye ointment (tetracycline/chloramphenicol/simplex), three or four times a day, can be used to protect the cornea against secondary bacterial infection and exposure. Specific antiviral treatment for the self-limited measles keratitis is not available or needed.

Systemic

- Mild antipyretic and analgesic (nonsteroidal anti-inflammatory drugs) agents are used.
- Systemic antibiotics are needed only for secondary bacterial infection.
- Supplementation with vitamin A 200,000 IU on two consecutive days may be indicated.

Supportive

- Low-level illumination is used.

COMPLICATIONS

- Measles keratitis is self-limited, without sequelae.
- Exposure ulcers can occur in severely debilitated children.
- Anterior segment blindness occurs in developing countries in as many as 1% of the patients. Corneal ulcers (usually at the 6 o'clock position) perforations, and endophthalmitis can occur due to any combination of measles keratitis, exposure ulcers, protein-energy malnutrition, vitamin A deficiency, secondary infections, and the application of harmful substances to the eye. The use of traditional eye medicines is an important cause of severe corneal damage, especially in developing countries.

COMMENTS

In affluent societies, the number of cases of measles is low due to a high level of immunization, and when measles is contracted, it runs a mild course. When the level of immunization is low, classic epidemics of measles are possible; even then, however, measles is essentially a benign disease, with a low mortality rate. When malnourished children contract measles, complications are common. It is customary to ascribe these complications primarily to vitamin A deficiency, but this underestimates the role of measles, protein energy malnutrition, exposure and traditional eye medicines. Prevention of post-measles blindness involves all causative factors.

REFERENCES

Dekkers NWHM, Treskes M: Measles keratitis. Ophthalmol Clin North Am 7:567–576, 1994.

Kayikcioglu O, Kir E, Soyler M, et al: Ocular findings in a measles epidemic among young adults. Ocul Immunol Inflamm 8:59–62, 2000.

Perry RT, Halsey NA: The clinical significance of measles: a review. JID 189(Suppl 1):4–15, 2004.

Whitcher JP, Srinivasan M, Upadhyay MP: Corneal blindness: a global perspective. Bulletin of the World Health Organization 79:214–221, 2001.

World Health Organization (WHO): The child, measles and the eye (booklet and slides for education and training). Geneva, WHO, 2004.

46 SPOROTRICHOSIS 117.1

Ramin Tayani, MD, MPH
San Clemente, California
Robert A. Hyndiuk, MD
Milwaukee, Wisconsin
Ayat Kazerouni, BS, BA
San Clemente, California

ETIOLOGY/INCIDENCE

Sporotrichosis is a widespread but relatively uncommon chronic infectious disease. The disease occurs worldwide and affects all ages but is most common in adult farmers, gardeners, laborers and certain types of miners. It is a mycosis caused by the filamentous branching fungus *Sporothrix schenckii*, also known as *Sporothrichum schenckii*, or *Sporotrichum beurmani* and *Sporotrichum asteroides*. It is classified as a subcutaneous mycosis of an exogenous origin; soil, wood and decaying vegetation carry the spores that enter lesions after trauma. For this reason, the infection primarily occurs in the upper and lower extremities.

The eye has been implicated in many reports, with the lids, conjunctiva, lacrimal sac, eyebrow, orbit, cornea, limbus, uveal tract and lacrimal canal involved. Not all reports of the disease include a traumatic history. Alvarez and Lopez-Villegas reported a case involving the conjunctiva in which there was no history of trauma. Another conjunctival involvement was described by Hampton, Adesina and Chodosh. Retinal involvement was described by Font and Jakobiec. Curi and Felix reported retinal granuloma caused *Sporothrixs schenckii*. Scleritis was reported by Brunette and Stulting. Endophthalmitis has been reported with and without systemic infection. Chin and Hyndiuk reported that sporotrichosis is a common cause of Parinaud's oculoglandular syndrome, which is an entity in which there is a unilateral granulomatous conjunctivitis (with or without ulceration, follicles, or both), often in association with a large preauricular or submandibular lymph node on the affected side. Fever and other systemic signs may or may not be present.

DIAGNOSIS

Clinical signs and symptoms

The sporotrichum causes a chronic noncontagious infection. The disease is manifested in various ways, with the most common being a localized lymphangitic form in which a nodule is formed that breaks down to form a chronic ulcer; within a few weeks, new subcutaneous nodules arise consecutively along the course of the regional lymphatics in a more or less linear fashion. The other forms are disseminated subcutaneous, epidermal, mucosal, osseous and muscular.

Laboratory findings

- The diagnosis is readily made in the ulcerous and cutaneous forms, but the lesion must be differentiated from lesions of syphilis, tuberculosis, or mycoses of other origin.
- The organism is cultured on Sabouraud dextrose agar; cream-colored to black, folded, leathery colonies develop within 3 to 5 days and consist of thin, septate, branching hyphae that cause clusters of pear-shaped conidia at the end of lateral branches.
- Histologic examination reveals no specific lesions.
- Granulation tissue with giant cells and epithelioid cells is seen.
- Gridley's stain is also helpful in detecting the fungus in chronic cases.

Ocular

The fungus may infect all parts of the globe and its adnexa but has its greatest affinity for the conjunctiva and eyelids.

- Eyelids: primary infection of the eyelids may occur on upper or lower eyelid. Palpebral sporotrichosis usually begins like a chalazion and develops like a tuberculous gumma. Features of ulcerative and suppurative, localized folliculitis with edema and regional hyperemia can occur in eyelid sporotrichosis.
- Lacrimal system: sporotrichotic dacryocystitis develops like tuberculosis of the lacrimal sac. Fistula formation is common. The preauricular and submaxillary glands are often swollen.
- Orbit: the orbit is rarely involved. Orbital osteitis and periostitis with abscess and erosion of the bony wall occur. Fistula formation also occurs.
- Conjunctiva: the palpebral conjunctiva is mainly involved. Small, yellowish nodules, sometimes ulcerated, occur with granulomatous or purulent conjunctivitis.
- Cornea: there is yellowish infiltration of the cornea with keratitis, ulceration and perforation.
- Sclera: the sclera is generally resistant to sporotrichotic invasion. It is one of the last preserved structures in eyes

otherwise extensively destroyed by necrotizing endophthalmitis caused by *Sporothrix schenkii.* It may show a yellowish paralimbal scleral nodule leading to scleritis and abscess formation.

- Intraocular infection/endophthalmitis: exogenously or endogenously, this infection will usually lead to loss of the eye.
- Retina: this infection may begin as retinitis and lead to retinochoroiditis. Endophthalmitis is relatively common if the retina is implicated.

TREATMENT

- Potassium iodide: this mechanism of action is unknown. The typical dosage is 15 drops t.i.d. of a saturated solution of potassium iodide (usually 50 mg/drop), with gradual increases to 30 to 40 drops t.i.d. This should be continued for at least 1 month after clinical recovery.
- Amphotericin B: this is reserved for more severe forms of infection, in visceral and intraocular or orbital involvement. Depending on the severity of the disease, amphotericin B (1.5 mg/mL in 5% dextrose in water) eyedrops may be sufficient to treat sporotrichosis involving the conjunctiva.
- Sulfa drugs and other antibiotics: these drugs are useless, including other antifungal agents, such as nystatin, miconazole, flucytosine, ketoconazole and griseofulvin.
- Local irrigation and warm compresses: these have been helpful in cases in which the disease also involves the canaliculi or the sac.

REFERENCES

Alvarez RG, Lopez-Villegas A: Primary ocular sporotrichosis. Am J Ophthalmol 62:150–151, 1966.

Brunette I, Stulting RD: *Sporothrix schenckii* scleritis (Letter). Am J Ophthalmol 114:370–371, 1992.

Cartwright MJ, Promersberger M, Stevens GA: *Sporothrix schenckii* endophthalmitis presenting as granulomatous uveitis. Br J Ophthalmol 77:61–62, 1993.

Cassady JR, Forester HC: *Sporotrichum schenckii* endophthalmitis. Arch Ophthalmol 85:71–74, 1971.

Chin G: Parinaud oculoglandular conjunctivitis. In: Tasman W, ed: Duane's clinical ophthalmology. External diseases. Diseases of the uvea, Revised edn. Philadelphia, Lippincott Williams & Wilkins, 1998: IV:1–6.

Curi AL, Felix S, Azevedo KM, Estrela R, et al: Retinal granuloma caused by *Sporothrix schenckii*. Am J Ophthalmol 136(1):2005–2007, 2003.

Font RL, Jakobiec RA: Granulomatous necrotizing retinochoroiditis caused by *Sporotrichum schenckii*: report of a case including immunofluorescence and electron microscopical studies. Arch Ophthalmol 94:1513–1519, 1976.

Gordon DM: Ocular sporotrichosis. Arch Ophthalmol 37:56, 1947.

Hampton DE, Adesina A, Chodosh J: Conjunctival sporotrichosis in the absence of antecedent trauma. Cornea 21(8):831–833, 2002.

Kurosawa A, Pollock SC, Collins MP, et al: *Sporothrix schenckii* endophthalmitis in a patient with human immunodeficiency virus infection. Arch Ophthalmol 106:376–380, 1988.

Streeten BW, Rabuzzi DD: Sporotrichosis of the orbital margin. Am J Ophthalmol 77:750–755, 1974.

Witherspoon CD, Kuhn F, Owens D, et al: Endophthalmitis due to *Sporothrix schenckii* after penetrating ocular injury. Ann Ophthalmol 22:385–388, 1990.

47 STAPHYLOCOCCUS 041.1

Thomas L. Steinemann, MD
Cleveland, Ohio
Sangeeta Khanna, MD
Cleveland, Ohio

ETIOLOGY/INCIDENCE

Staphylococci are gram-positive bacteria of the family Micrococcaceae. They are aerobic (facultatively anaerobic) and nonmotile and tend to grow in grape-like clusters. The Micrococcaceae family can be further divided into two groups based on coagulase production. Coagulase, an enzyme that causes plasma to coagulate, has been regarded as a marker for virulence. Although most severe staphylococcal infections are caused by coagulase-positive organisms and many researchers believe that coagulase production indicates the likelihood that a strain is potentially pathogenic, there is no evidence that coagulase itself is directly responsible for disease signs and symptoms.

Coagulase-positive organisms compose one species (*Staphylococcus aureus*), but coagulase-negative staphylococci are divided into 28 species. In the past, most coagulase-negative staphylococci were collectively referred to as *S. albus* because of the white colony growth pattern on agar plates; in contrast, *S. aureus* elaborates a golden pigment. More recently, *S. albus* has been referred to as *S. epidermidis.* The term *S. epidermidis* is still used by some to include all coagulase-negative staphylococci in a generic sense, strictly speaking, however, coagulase-negative staphylococci have been further speciated by biotyping, a scheme based on specific biochemical properties.

Components of the cell wall of *S. aureus* include peptidoglycan, protein A, and teichoic acid polymers, all of which may contribute to pathogenicity. *S. aureus* also produces several enzymes and toxins that have been implicated as important pathogenic factors. These secreted extracellular enzymes include hyaluronidase and lipase, which may help the organism survive in tissues. Many strains also produce toxins, which damage membranes and exert a cytotoxic effect on a variety of cells, including leukocytes, fibroblasts, and epithelial cells of the cornea and conjunctiva. Most of the staphylococci isolated from skin infections are *S. aureus. S. aureus* organisms gain access to underlying tissues, often after surgery or trauma, creating a characteristic local abscess lesion. Colonization of the nose, skin and scalp may begin early in childhood and continue throughout life. These sites probably serve as a source of ocular infection.

Coagulase-negative staphylococci have historically been regarded as contaminants when recovered in culture media, probably because they are the predominant normal skin flora and often are present on mucous membranes. Rarely do they cause skin infections; however, they are clearly recognized as opportunistic pathogens of increasing importance, especially in hospital-acquired infections. Multiresistant coagulase-negative staphylococci commonly colonize the skin and mucous membranes, serving as a reservoir for antibiotic-resistant genes (*mecA, blaZ*), which can be transferred among staphylococcal organisms. They are most commonly associated with infections involving prosthetic devices, such as intraocular lenses and intravenous lines. It has been shown that many strains produce an exopolysaccharide ('slime': or 'biofilm' substance) that facilitates bacterial adherence to prosthetic surfaces and may be a factor in resistance to host defenses and antimicrobial therapy.

DIAGNOSIS

Clinical signs and symptoms

Staphylococci may infect any portion of the eye or orbital structure. Lid infections are common and may be chronic. They often reflect lowered host resistance; the infection can be directly spread from the conjunctiva or nasolacrimal system. Atopy is a common predisposing condition. Staphylococci remain a common cause of acute and chronic conjunctivitis, suppurative keratitis, marginal corneal (catarrhal) infiltrates, phlyctenulosis and hordeola. Orbital infections can occur, either from staphylococcal septicemia or via direct spread from contiguous structure, such as lid abscess, periosteal orbital abscesses, or infected teeth. Staphylococci are the most common cause of acute or delayed endophthalmitis in postoperative cataract patients. In the Endophthalmitis Vitrectomy Study, 70% of 323 isolates were coagulase-negative staphylococci, and 9.9% were *S. aureus*. Coagulase-negative staphylococcal endophthalmitis can present as delayed-onset, chronic, painless inflammation. Familiarity with the clinical presentation is essential because prompt treatment is often associated with a good visual recovery.

Ocular or periocular

- Anterior chamber: cells and flare, hypopyon.
- Conjunctiva: hyperemia, papillary response, purulent conjunctivitis, chemosis, phlyctenulosis, post-trabeculectomy 'blebitis'.
- Cornea: punctate epithelial keratopathy, suppurative keratitis, perforation, marginal (catarrhal) infiltrates, phlyctenulosis, crystalline keratopathy.
- Eyelids: collarettes, lid margin vascularization, tylosis, meibomianitis, lash follicle folliculitis, lid margin ulceration, eczematoid dermatitis, angular blepharitis, trichiasis, madarosis, poliosis, hordeolum, chalazion, ectropion, entropion, edema, abscess, cellulitis, pseudoptosis.
- Globe: endophthalmitis, panophthalmitis, intraocular lens contamination, scleral ulceration.
- Iris: nongranulomatous anterior uveitis, posterior synechiae.
- Orbit: cellulitis, osteomyelitis, periosteitis.
- Other: dacryocystitis, increased intraocular pressure, dacryoadenitis, cavernous sinus thrombosis.

TREATMENT

Systemic

Specific antimicrobial therapy is chosen based on the site and severity of the infection and the antimicrobial sensitivities of the organism involved. The increasing prevalence of staphylococcal infections reflects the frequency with which the organism has developed antimicrobial resistance; in fact, fewer than 30% of community strains of staphylococcal species are still sensitive to penicillin G. However, many community-acquired staphylococcal infections are still sensitive to synthetic penicillinase-resistant penicillins. For these, methicillin, nafcillin and dicloxacillin are effective. Amongst nososcomial staph species (*S. aureus* and *S. epidermidis*), 80% are resistant to methicillin.

> **BOX 47.1 – Systemic treatment**
>
> **Community-acquired staphylococcal infections**
>
> **Parenteral**
>
> - Methicillin/nafcillin 150 to 200 mg/kg IV every 4–6 hours (1–2 g)
>
> **Oral**
>
> - Dicloxacillin 500 mg PO q.i.d.
> - Cephalexin 250 to 500 mg PO every 6 hours
>
> **Hospital-acquired (nosocomial), methicillin-resistant staphylococcal infections or history of penicillin-related anaphylaxis**
>
> **Parenteral**
>
> - Vancomycin 500 mg IV every 6 hours
>
> **Oral (do not use a single agent with methicillin–resistant staphylococci)**
>
> - Ciprofloxacin 200 to 400 mg PO every 12 hours
> - Rifampin 330 to 600 mg PO every 12 hours

Cephalosporins are an acceptable alternative to semisynthetic penicillinase-resistant penicillin in patients who have had prior reactions to penicillin. Cefazolin can be given intramuscularly or intravenously in a maximum dosage of 1 g every 6 hours. Oral preparations, such as cephalexin, can be given for less serious infections; the usual oral dosage is 250 to 500 mg every 6 hours. However, methicillin resistant staphylococci are all resistant to cephalosporins since they produce β-lactamases.

For infections caused by methicillin-resistant staphylococci, vancomycin remains the drug of choice for parenteral treatment. Doses of 500 mg are given over a 1 hour period every 6 hours. Vancomycin levels of more than 30 μg/mL should be avoided because of potential renal damage and ototoxicity. Oral rifampin may be particularly useful as an adjunctive treatment to either parenteral or local therapy. The emergence of resistance, however, is rapid, and this drug should never be used as a single antistaphylococcal agent. Oral doses of 300 to 600 mg are usually given every 12 hours. Rifampin may also be useful in combination with other antimicrobial agents for the elimination of the staphylococcal carrier state.

Fourth generation fluoroquinolones such as gatifloxacin and moxifloxacin are newer agents that show great promise in treatment of resistant staph infections. Fourth generation fluoroquinolones require two mutations to establish resistance: one in the topoisonmerase IV and a second one in the DNA gyrase gene. Therefore, these provide better coverage against gram-positive bacteria that were already resistant to previous generation fluoroquinolones that only require a single mutation to establish resistance. Fourth generation agents have activity against methicillin sensitive and methicillin resistant staphylococci. Also, studies have shown good penetration of oral gatifloxacin into the vitreous cavity in non-inflamed eyes after oral administration. However, resistance has been increasingly documented in both methicillin resistant species and methicillin sensitive, so fluoroquinolones should not be used as a single

BOX 47.2 – Local treatment

Blepharitis

- Bacitracin ointment 5000 units/g
- Sulfacetamide 10% ointment
- Erythromycin 0.5% ointment

Conjunctivitis

- Topical fluoroquinolone, one drop every 6 hours
- Sulfacetamide 10% 1 drop every 6 hours
- Trimethoprim sulfate 0.1% and polytrim B sulfate 10,000 units/mL

Conjunctivitis (methicillin-resistent staphylococci)

- Vancomycin hydrochloride in phosphate-buffered artificial tears 25 to 50 mg/mL

Keratitis

- Fluoroquinolones
- (4th generation: gatifloxicin or moxifloxacin) combined with fortified aminoglycoside 14 mg/mL drops
- Fortified cefazolin 50 mg/mL drops

Keratitis (methicillin-resistent staphylococci)

- Vancomycin hydrochloride in phosphate-buffered artificial tears 50 mg/mL drops

Endophthalmitis

- Vancomycin 1.0 mg in 0.1 mL intravitreal injection in conjunction with vitrectomy if indicated, and vancomycin 50 mg/mL drops

agent in the treatment of methicillin resistant staphylococcal infections.

Ocular

Staphylococcal infections of the lid may be treated with a variety of antimicrobial ointments, including sulfacetamide (10%), erythromycin (0.5%), or bacitracin (5000 units/g). There is a definite trend of increased resistance of coagulase-negative staphylococci to erythromycin. Frequency and duration of treatment should be based on the severity of the infection and the clinical response. Less severe forms of conjunctivitis also usually respond to 10% sulfacetamide ophthalmic drops every 6 hours. Polytrim combines trimethoprim sulfate (0.1%) and polymyxin B sulfate (10,000 units/mL). Trimethoprim is effective against many aerobic gram-positive bacteria, including many strains of staphylococci.

Chronic staphylococcal blepharitis and meibomian keratoconjunctivitis can be treated effectively with oral tetracycline. Treatment is initiated at 1 to 2 g/day until the signs and symptoms are controlled. After control is attained, low-dose (250 mg/day) maintenance therapy is continued for months or years to prevent recurrences. The mechanism of action seems to be mediated by reducing staphylococcal lipase production, not by eliminating the bacteria.

Conjunctivitis caused by methicillin-resistant staphylococci has been increasingly recognized, especially in patients in long-term care facilities. In these cases, topical vancomycin is effective and can be prepared by dissolving injectable vancomycin hydrochloride in phosphate-buffered artificial tears at a concentration of 25 to 40 mg/mL.

Keratitis is typically treated with topical antibiotic drops as primary therapy based on corneal scrapings obtained for culture and sensitivity. The empiric use of fortified antibiotic concentrations to obtain higher corneal drug levels is widely accepted. Fortified amnioglycosides (14 mg/mL gentamicin) and cephalosporins (50 mg/mL cefazolin) are usually effective in treating staphylococcal keratitis. Methicillin-resistant staphylococcal keratitis has, however, recently been reported. For these infections, vancomycin (50 mg/mL) every 30 minutes and alternating with fourth generation quinolone every 30 minutes should be started.

Other common corneal diseases caused by staphylococci include marginal (catarrhal) infiltrates and phlyctenulosis. Both are caused by chronic staphylococcal colonization of the external ocular surface and lids and are thought to represent an immune reaction to staphylococcal exotoxins deposited in the cornea or conjunctiva. Treatment is directed at eliminating the antigen load through the use of frequent lid scrubs, mild shampoo, and antibiotic drops or ointment. This therapy is sometimes used in conjunction with topical steroids to diminish immunologically medicated inflammation.

Staphylococcal endophthalmitis is typically treated with intravitreal injection of vancomycin 1.0 mg in 0.1 mL augmented by vitrectomy if vision is less than or equal to light perception. A complete discussion of the management of endophthalmitis is beyond the scope of this chapter. Please see Section 23, Bacterial endophthalmitis and Fungal endophthalmitis, for details.

Supportive

Inspissated secretions glandular structures of the lid may occur both externally (glands of Zeis) or internally (meibomian glands). These secretions often contribute to chronic staphylococcal surface disease, such as blepharitis or hordeolum, and may be treated by applying moist, warm compresses to the lid. Excessive oil secretion may also be treated by gently expressing the material with fingertip pressure or with cotton-tipped applicators. Daily lid hygiene to remove oil, lid debris, and scaling is accomplished with a mild baby shampoo or commercially available lid hygiene packs. Localized abscesses that do not spontaneously drain with moist heat may require incision and draining.

PRECAUTIONS

The emergence of methicillin-resistant *S. aureus* and penicillin and methicillin-resistant *S. epidermidis* is a concern in nosocomial infections. Every attempt should be made to isolate the organism and perform sensitivity tests to a wide range of antimicrobial agents. Sensitivity patterns may differ from hospital to hospital.

Fluoroquinolones have an increased trend of resistance because these are concentrated dependent antibiotics so when bacteria are exposed to sublethal concentrations they can induce resistance. Alternating different classes of antibiotics has been recommended in protracted therapy to minimize resistance.

COMMENTS

Staphylococci are common worldwide causes of blepharitis, conjunctivitis and keratitis. In the past, *S. aureus* was implicated as the most responsible organism for endophthalmitis. Recent reports indicate that *S. epidermidis* that the most commonly cultured intraocular pathogen, accounting for 70% of postoperative endophthalmitis. This is consistent with the finding of *S. epidermidis* as the most common isolate from conjunctival cultures. Also, molecular techniques have established that in most cases of postoperative endophthalmitis, the coagulase-negative staphylococci arise from the patient's eyelid flora. In a recent study regarding antibiotic susceptibility of bacterial isolates from endophthalmitis, about 63% of isolated coagulase-negative staph were methicillin sensitive and 75% of the isolated *S. aureus* were methicillin sensitive. Both staph isolates were 100% sensitive to vancomycin. Because these organisms can be resistant to penicillinase-resistant penicillins, treatment should be guided by culture and sensitivity results.

REFERENCES

Archer GL: *Staphylococcus epidermidis* and other coagulase-negative staphylococci. In: Mandell GL, Bennett JE, Dolin R, eds: Principles and practice of infectious diseases. 5th edn. New York, Churchill Livingstone, 2000:2092–2100.

Bannerman TL, Rhoden DL, McAllisster SK, et al: The source of coagulase-negative staphylococci in the Endophthalmitis Vitrectomy Study. Arch Ophthalmo 115:357–361, 1997.

Ha DP, Wisniewski SR, Wilson LA, et al: Spectrum and susceptibilities of microbiological isolates in the Endophthalmitis Vitrectomy Study. Am J Ophthalmol 122:1–17, 1996.

Kowalski RP, Karenchak LM, Romanowski EG: Infectious disease: changing antibiotic susceptibility. Ophthalmology Clinics of North America 16(1):1–11, 2003.

Mather R, Karenchak LM, Romanowski EG, Kowalski RP: Fourth generation fluoroquinolones: new weapons in the arsenal of ophthalmic antibiotics. Am J Ophthalmol 133(4):L463–L466, 2002.

Sotonzo C, Inagaki K, Fujita A, et al: Methicillin-resistant *Staphylococcus aureus* and methicillin-resistant *Staphylococcus epidermidis* infections in the cornea. Cornea 21(7 suppl):S94–S101, 2002.

Tungsiripat T, Sarayba MA, Kaufman MB, et al: Fluoroquinolone therapy in multi-drug resistant staphylococcal keratitis after lamellar keratectomy in a rabbit model. Am J Ophthalmol 136(1):76–81, 2003.

Waldvogel FA: *Staphylococcus aureus* (including toxic shock syndrome). In: Mandell GL, Bennett JE, Dolin R, eds: Principles and practice of infectious diseases. 5th edn. New York, Churchill Livingston, 2000:2069–2092.

48 STREPTOCOCCUS 041.0

Rookaya Mather, MD, MBBCh, FRCS(C), DABO
London, Ontario

ETIOLOGY/INCIDENCE

Streptococci are gram-positive cocci that grow in pairs or chains. Most pathogenic streptococci are facultative anaerobes. Many species of streptococci constitute the normal flora of the respiratory, gastrointestinal, and genitourinary tracts. These organisms cause disease either directly by invasion of tissues or indirectly through the elaboration of toxins.

Streptococci may be classified based on the antigenic composition of cell wall carbohydrates. To date, Lancefield serogroups A to H and K to V have been identified.

Another useful classification scheme is based on the ability of the organism to produce zones of hemolysis around the colony when cultured on blood agar. α-Hemolysis is characterized by a zone of partial hemolysis, which often appears as a greenish hue on the agar. A clear zone of complete hemolysis characterizes β-hemolysis. γ-Hemolysis indicates the absence of hemolysis.

The most important pathogen in the a-hemolytic group is *Streptococcus pneumoniae*, commonly referred to as pneumococcus. It is a common cause of pneumonia, meningitis, endocarditis, and otitis media. The *S. viridans* group consists of several a-hemolytic species (*S. mitis*, *S. sanguis*, *S. salivarius*, *S. mutans*, and *S. anginosus*). These bacteria can cause acute and subacute endocarditis and dental and brain abscess.

Among the streptococci, the β-hemolytic groups are the most common pathogens. *S. pyogenes* (group A) can give rise to pharyngitis, impetigo, necrotizing fasciitis, cellulitis, toxic streptococcal syndrome, and scarlet fever. In addition, this organism is known to trigger the postinfectious syndromes of acute rheumatic fever and poststreptococcal glomerulonephritis. *S. agalactiae* (group B) is a frequent cause of neonatal sepsis and meningitis. *S. equi* (group C) has been identified as a cause of cellulitis and endocarditis.

Enterococci, formerly designated as group D streptococci, exhibit variable hemolysis. These bacteria cause urinary tract infections, wound infections, peritonitis, and endocarditis.

Streptococcal infections of the eye and its adnexa are relatively common. The orbit, eyelids, lacrimal sac, conjunctiva, cornea, uvea, and globe may be involved.

COURSE/PROGNOSIS

- *S. pyogenes* causes membranous or pseudomembranous conjunctivitis, which can lead to corneal infiltration, ulceration, and eventual perforation.
- *S. pneumoniae* conjunctivitis is usually self-limited. Topical antibiotics are typically prescribed to shorten the duration of the infection, reduce the risk of developing complications and possibly reduce epidemic spread of the pathogen.
- Endophthalmitis caused by streptococci has a poor prognosis for vision. *S. pyogenes* and *S. pneumoniae* infections tend to have the worst outcomes, whereas *S. viridans* have the best. *Streptococcus* species account for the majority of post-penetrating keratoplasty endophthalmitis.
- *S. pneumoniae* and *S. viridans* can cause keratitis following refractive surgery. Management of these infections may require LASIK flap amputation and/or subsequent penetrating keratoplasty.

DIAGNOSIS

Clinical signs and symptoms

- *S. pyogenes* can cause preseptal and orbital cellulitis, conjunctivitis, suppurative keratitis, postinfectious uveitis, and endophthalmitis.
- Preseptal cellulitis usually occurs in children in the form of erysipelas, impetigo, or nonsuppurative cellulitis.
- Severe and at times life-threatening group A streptococcal infections occur, including toxic shock-like syndrome and necrotizing fasciitis.

- *S. pneumoniae* can cause preseptal and orbital cellulitis, dacryocystitis, conjunctivitis, suppurative keratitis, crystalline keratopathy and endophthalmitis.
- Group B streptococci causes conjunctivitis in neonates, keratitis, and endophthalmitis.
- They are a common cause of bleb-associated endophthalmitis.
- They are a major cause of sepsis and meningitis in neonates.
- *S. viridans* can cause keratitis, crystalline keratopathy and endophthalmitis.
- Enterococci can cause conjunctivitis in neonates, keratitis, crystalline keratopathy and endophthalmitis.
- Group C streptococci can cause conjunctivitis and endophthalmitis.

Laboratory findings

Infected tissues should be examined microbiologically with culture and serologic typing. Most streptococci are fastidious organisms. Sheep blood agar is especially useful, and growth is enhanced at reduced oxygen levels.

PROPHYLAXIS

- Group B streptococcus: Identification and treatment of high-risk carrier mothers may have a role in preventing group B streptococcal infections. GBS has shown continued sensitivity to ampicillin and penicillin but increased resistance to erythromycin and clindamycin. Intravenous antibiotics should be administered during labor and until delivery for at least 4 hours. Vancomycin is reserved for GBS resistant to clindamycin and erythromycin
- *Streptococcus pneumoniae* is a major cause of morbidity and mortality in infants, children and the elderly. Although, the 23-valent polysaccharide vaccine is protective in most adults and children over 5 years of age, it fails to protect children under 2 years of age. Conjugate vaccines are efficacious in preventing invasive diseases in this risk group. Unfortunately, protection is confined to a limited number of pneumococcal serotypes.
- *Streptococcus pneumoniae* has gradually become resistant to penicillins, macrolides and older generation fluoroquinolones. The selection of antibacterials used for treatment and prophylaxis should be based upon local resistance patterns. Penicillin resistance has risen to 80% of isolates in some parts of Asia. In the US, intermediate-level resistance of pneumococcus to penicillin was found to be 27.8% and high-level resistance was 16%. There is considerable regional variability. In addition, high-level penicillin resistance predicts resistance to other (β)-lactams, macrolides and cotrimoxazole. Telithromycin and linezolid may prove to be potent new drugs for treating pneumococcal disease.
- *S. pyogenes:* penicillin has been the drug of choice. Alternative drugs include 2nd generation cephalosporins, tetracyclines, chloramphenicol, erythromycin, clindamycin, vancomycin and bacitracin. Erythromycin is the preferred agent in patients who are hypersensitive to penicillin.
- *S. viridans:* penicillin is the drug of choice. Alternative drugs include cephalosporins, tetracyclines, chloramphenicol, erythromycin, clindamycin, vancomycin and bacitracin. Erythromycin is the preferred agent in patients who are hypersensitive to penicillin. Although, high-level penicillin resistance is rare in the United States, viridans streptococci resistance to antibiotics is increasing. Possible resistance to penicillin should be considered when selecting empiric therapy. Vancomycin is the drug-of-choice for serious viridans streptococcal infection until susceptibility data are available. Imipenem has been shown to be highly active against viridans streptococci *in vitro*.
- Enterococci: penicillin alone is usually ineffective. Penicillin or vancomycin, in combination with an aminoglycoside, is the treatment of choice. Enterococci are resistant to cephalosporins. Emergence of high-level resistance to vancomycin in the US and some other parts of the world during the 1990s has severely constrained therapeutic options for management of serious infection because enterococci already possess intrinsic and acquired resistance to most other antimicrobials.
- Group C streptococci: penicillin is the drug of choice. Aminoglycosides may be synergistic in some infections. The majority of GCS and GGS strains demonstrate *in vitro* susceptibility to penicillins, vancomycin, erythromycin and cephalosporins.

Ocular

- Impetigo: oral penicillin or cephalexin for 10 days with topical antibiotic ointment, hot compresses and gentle debridement of skin crusts are recommended. There is no standard therapy and treatment guidelines differ widely. There is good evidence that the topical antibiotics mupirocin and fusidic acid are equal to or possibly more effective than oral treatment. Based on the available evidence, there is no clear preference for β-lactamase resistant narrow-spectrum penicillins such as cloxacillin, dicloxacillin and flucloxacillin, versus broad spectrum penicillins such ampicillin and amoxicillin plus clavulanic acid, cephalosporins and macrolides. Although, there is no evidence to support oral antibiotics over topical for serious and extensive forms of impetigo, oral antibiotics may be an easier option for people with very extensive impetigo.
- Preseptal cellulitis: Streptococci are now the most common organisms causing bacteremia in patients with periorbital cellulitis. In young children, *S. pneumoniae* is the most common organism; in older children, group A streptococcus is more likely. Adults and older children can be managed conservatively with oral antibiotics, such as penicillin or moxifloxacin for a total of 7 to 10 days. Children younger than 5 years should receive parenteral therapy regardless of the severity of infection. If the orbit or optic nerve are involved orbital imaging and aggressive intervention are required. Patients who have had recent surgery are at risk for developing endophthalmitis. Complaints of pain or a red eye indicate intraocular infection until ruled out.
- Orbital cellulitis: management requires a multispecialty team including infectious diseases, otolaryngology and ophthalmology. Patients should be examined at least daily by an ophthalmologist to assess vision and extraocular muscle function. Repeat CT scan should be obtained in 24 to 48 hours if there has been no clinical improvement. Parenteral treatment with penicillin is recommended. Patients with a large, well-defined abscess, complete ophthalmoplegia and/or significant visual impairment should undergo surgical drainage of the abscess and sinus(es). Antimicrobial therapy for empiric treatment should to cover *S. pneumoniae*, *Staphylococcus aureus* and other *Streptococcus* spp. Orbital cellulitis caused by *H. influenzae* type b is now rare.

- Dacryocystitis: oral penicillin (or alternative) and topical antibiotics are recommended for 7 to 10 days. Dacryocystorhinostomy may be necessary to prevent recurrence.
- Conjunctivitis: treatment of bacterial conjunctivitis is often empirical and initiated before bacteriological culture. Empiric antibiotic therapy should have broad spectrum of antimicrobial activity. Topical fluoroquinolone antibiotics are widely used for the treatment of acute bacterial conjunctivitis. The newer 4th generation fluoroquinolones (moxifloxacin and gatifloxacin) exhibit improved bactericidal activity by inhibiting two essential bacterial topoisomerase enzymes, DNA gyrase (topoisomerase II) and topoisomerase IV. Topical polymyxin-trimethoprim, or neomycin-polymixin drops are alternatives. If *S. pyogenes* is the cause of conjunctivitis, 250 mg penicillin VK q.i.d. PO for 10 days should be considered for prophylaxis against poststreptococcal sequelae.
- Keratitis: streptococcal corneal ulceration must be treated aggressively to maintain corneal integrity. Topical cefazolin 50 mg/mL, or vancomycin 50 mg/mL should be administered at least hourly for the first 24 or 48 hours and then tapered to four times daily, based on the therapeutic response. Topical erythromycin, ciprofloxacin or bacitracin ointments may be applied nightly as the fortified antibiotic is tapered. Supplementation with subconjunctival antibiotic injections may be considered in some cases. Moxifloxacin and gatifloxacin have shown improved potency against previously fluoroquinolone-resistant strep isolates. These agents provide improved penetration into ocular tissues. Systemic therapy in keratitis is generally unnecessary unless the threat of intraocular spread, scleritis or sepsis is present. Corneal perforation or scarring may require penetrating keratoplasty.
- Post-laser refractive surgery keratitis: laser refractive surgery procedures involve breakdown of the epithelial barrier of the cornea with an inherent risk of infectious complication. Since laser in situ keratomileusis (LASIK) has become widely available, numerous cases of LASIK-associated infectious keratitis have been reported. In such cases, the corneal flap must sometimes be lifted and stromal bed cultured, irrigated or amputated in addition to aggressive topical antibiotic therapy.
- Uveitis: streptococcus-associated uveitis should be treated with topical corticosteroids and cycloplegics. Corticosteroids may be used hourly, depending on the degree of inflammation. Poststreptococcal reactive arthritis (PSRA) can occur concomitantly with uveitis.
- Endophthalmitis: streptococci are currently the second most frequent group of bacteria recovered from patients with post-cataract endophthalmitis. Streptococcal endophthalmitis is a visually devastating infection that requires prompt and aggressive therapy with topical, intravitreal, and sometimes systemic antibiotics and pars plana vitrectomy, depending on severity. At the time of vitreous tap or vitrectomy, a broad-spectrum cocktail consisting of 1 mg of vancomycin and 2.25 mg of ceftazadime is injected into the vitreous cavity. Additionally, dexamethasone may be injected. Once an organism is identified, the choice of antibiotic must be tailored to the in vitro susceptibility results. Topical cefazolin 50 mg/mL, vancomycin 50 mg/mL, or penicillin 100,000 units/mL may be applied. Systemic antibiotics such as the 4th generation fluoroquinolones, cefazolin, penicillin G and vancomycin have been used. Filtering blebs infected with streptococci usually require revision or excision.

COMMENTS

Streptococci are common causes of bacterial infection of the eye and its adnexa. Most streptococci are sensitive to the β-lactam family of antibiotics. Emerging strains of penicillin-resistant organisms pose a threat to the treatment of streptococcal infections on an empiric basis. A specimen for culture and in vitro antimicrobial susceptibility testing should be obtained whenever possible. Because resistance patterns of streptococci causing ocular infections change over time, outcomes of studies dating back more than 10 years, may not be applicable to the current prevalence of infecting agents. Also, resistance between regions and countries may vary considerably. Up-to-date, local characteristics and resistance patterns of the causative bacteria should always be taken into account when choosing antibiotic treatment. Local health authorities and other relevant bodies may advise against prescribing certain antibiotics in order to restrict the development of bacterial resistance and reserve these drugs for more serious infections.

REFERENCES

Bisno AL: Group A streptococcal infections and acute rheumatic fever. N Engl J Med 325:783–793, 1991.

Bogaert D, Hermans PWM, Adrian PV, et al: Pneumococcal vaccines: an update on current strategies. Vaccine 22(17–18):2209–2220, 2004.

Givner LB: Periorbital versus orbital cellulitis. Pediatric Infect Disease J 21(12):1157–1158, 2002.

Koning S, Verhagen AP, van Suijlekom-Smit LW, et al: Interventions for impetigo. Cochrane Database of Systematic Reviews. (2):CD003261, 2004.

Kunimoto DY, Tasman W, Rapuano C, et al: Endophthalmitis after penetrating keratoplasty: microbiologic spectrum and susceptibility of isolates. Am J Ophthalmol 137(2):343–345, 2004.

Meisler DM, Langston RH, Naab TJ, et al: Infectious crystalline keratopathy. Am J Ophthalmol 97:337–343, 1984.

Neralla S, Meyer KC: Drug treatment of pneumococcal pneumonia in the elderly. Drugs & Aging 21(13):851–864, 2004.

Platt JS, O'Brien WF: Group B streptococcus: prevention of early-onset neonatal sepsis. Obstetrical & Gynecological Survey 58(3):191–196, 2003.

Schaefer F, Bruttin O, Zografos L, et al: Bacterial keratitis: a prospective clinical and microbiological study. Br J Ophthalmol 85(7):842–847, 2001.

49 TETANUS 037
(Lockjaw)

Terry D. Wood, MD
Portland, Oregon
Eric B. Suhler, MD
Portland, Oregon
Robert A. Egan, MD
Portland, Oregon

ETIOLOGY/INCIDENCE

Tetanus is an ancient malady. It was described by Hippocrates as early as the fifth century BCE. Its effects were perhaps most graphically depicted in a sketch by Charles Bell showing a 19th century British soldier locked in agonizing opisthotonus. The causative organism is *Clostridium tetani*, a gram positive, spore-forming bacterium found in many environments, including soil and the gastrointestinal tracts of humans and many animals. *C. tetani* is an obligate anaerobe; as a result, it is most commonly found in places where oxygen tensions are low. This also accounts for its propensity to flourish in deep puncture wounds, especially if devitalized tissue is present. Contrary to popular belief, however, tetanus can develop in the setting of very superficial wounds, including insect bites. Parenteral drug abuse can also represent a portal of entry *C. tetani*.

Spore formation occurs in the presence of conditions unfavorable for vegetative growth. The spore is quite resistant to standard methods of disinfection. Spores may remain viable after treatment with chemical microbicides and can withstand boiling in water for up to an hour. This very hardy organism is able to produce infection after surviving for years in the spore form.

The clinical disease of tetanus occurs via elaboration of tetanospasmin by *Clostridia tetani* in the active, vegetative state. This very potent neurotoxin acts primarily at the pre-synaptic terminal of alpha motor neurons. It prevents release of the inhibitory neurotransmitters glycine and gamma aminobutyric acid (GABA). The result is sustained, uncontrolled muscular contraction. In addition to derangement of somatic muscle control, autonomic dysfunction frequently occurs due to loss of feedback inhibition at the adrenal gland. Excessive catecholamine secretion results in a hypersympathetic state that is the proximal cause of death in affected patients.

Clinical tetanus has become a rare entity in the developed world, due in large part to vaccination efforts. In the United States, the year 2002 saw only 25 reported cases. In less developed regions, however, tetanus remains a significant cause of morbidity and mortality. Worldwide, approximately one million new cases are estimated to occur each year, with upwards of 270,000 attributable deaths annually.

COURSE/PROGNOSIS

- The incubation period for *C. tetani* ranges from 3 to 21 days. The time of onset for symptoms is directly related to the distance from the original wound to the central nervous system.
- Tetanospasmin is elaborated within the wound and travels in retrograde fashion along neurons.
- Tetanospasmin passes across synaptic clefts to invade connecting neurons.
- Although spinal inhibitory neurons are most affected, acetylcholine release may also be inhibited, causing muscle paralysis rather than spasm.
- Trismus is the classic early finding.
- Increased tone in masseter muscle group causes 'lockjaw.'
- Facial muscle spasm progresses, leading to *risus sardonicus* or 'fixed grin.'
- Dysphagia and laryngospasm occur commonly.
- Tetanus is classically divided into one of three forms, depending upon predominant clinical presentation.
  1. Generalized tetanus, occurring most commonly, represents a descending pattern. Trismus is followed by nuchal rigidity, dysphagia, then rigidity of the abdominal muscles. Hyperthermia (two to four degrees Celsius above normal), hypertension, tachycardia, and diaphoresis are commonly observed.
  2. Cephalic tetanus, a rare variant, typically originates from head wounds or otitis, and is limited to cranial nerve involvement, often presenting as cranial nerve palsies. It may progress to the generalized form.
  3. Local tetanus is anatomically limited to the region of the inciting wound. It may remain self-limited or progress to generalized tetanus.
- Neonatal tetanus is a significant cause of infant mortality in developing countries. It most commonly arises in the setting of inadequate care of the umbilical stump following delivery.
- Ophthalmic manifestations of tetanus.
- Blepharospasm is the most common eye finding in generalized and cephalic tetanus. It is usually bilateral. Tonic spasm may mimic ptosis.
- True ptosis may occur in the setting of a cranial nerve III palsy.
- Alignment and motility disturbances are frequently observed. These findings typically have nuclear or infranuclear origins.
- Supranuclear gaze palsies have been described.
- Downbeat nystagmus has been observed in the setting of bilateral cranial nerve IV palsy.
- Internal ophthalmoplegia may occur, usually in association with cranial nerve III dysfunction.
- Isolated accommodative paresis has been described.

DIAGNOSIS

Clinical signs and symptoms

History and clinical signs are fundamental to the diagnosis of tetanus. Diagnosis of tetanus in an individual with current vaccination status should be viewed with skepticism, as protection rates in appropriately vaccinated patients approaches 100%.

Laboratory findings

Laboratory studies are of little value in the diagnosis, as clostridia can often be found in non-disease states, and conversely, culturing *C. tetani* in known cases of clinical tetanus is often impossible. Cerebrospinal fluid is typically normal in tetanus.

Differential diagnosis

A broad and etiologically diverse differential diagnosis should be considered when evaluating potential tetanus.

- Strychnine poisoning.
- Black widow spider bite.
- Alcohol or narcotic withdrawl.
- Dystonic phenothiazine reaction.
- Rabies.
- Meningitis.
- Subarachnoid hemorrhage.
- Seizures.
- Hypocalcemic tetani.

PREVENTION

Appropriate vaccination is the cornerstone of prophylaxis. This is accomplished via subcutaneous injection of tetanus toxoid (inactivated tetanospasmin). Current recommendations call for a series of four injections as part of a childhood vaccination regimen. Tetanus toxoid is usually co-administered with diphtheria and acellular pertussis vaccine. Boosters are recommended at 10 year intervals. It should be noted that a prior episode of tetanus does not confer immunity. This is because the very potent nature of tetanospasmin (lethal dose: 2.5 ng/kg of body weight) typically means that levels are too small to produce an adequate immune response.

Nearly any wound can potentially lead to tetanus. Wounds that are deeper than one centimeter, involve environmental contamination, or have extensively de-vitalized tissue are particularly at risk. Wounds that have not been cleaned within six hours of injury represent additional risk.

Ocular wounds that involve corneal or scleral penetration or perforation are considered to be tetanus-prone. Signs of endophthalmitis should prompt consideration of tetanus. Eyelid and periorbital injuries should be treated as having a tetanus risk equivalent to similar non-ocular injuries. Simple corneal abrasions are not associated with increased risk of tetanus.

TREATMENT

Treatment begins with proper wound management. Wounds should be cleaned in a fashion appropriate to type and location. Devitalized tissue should be debrided. Wounds should be examined carefully for foreign bodies; if present, they should be removed. Depending on immune status, administration of tetanus toxoid vaccine following injury may be part of the treatment algorithm. This does not, however, provide protection against the development of tetanus in the setting of acute injury, as development of vaccine mediated immunity is far slower than the development of disease.

In the setting of clinical tetanus, the mainstay of therapy is Tetanus Immune Globulin (TIG). TIG is given intramuscularly, but should not be administered at the same site as a recent tetanus toxoid injection. TIG is very effective at neutralizing free tetanospasmin, can only neutralize toxin that has not yet entered the nervous system. Unlike tetanospasmin, it is unable to cross the blood–brain barrier and cannot enter a neuron. There does not appear to be any advantage to administering TIG at the wound site. Intrathecal administration is advocated by some clinicians, but its superiority over the intramuscular route is debated.

Antibiotic control of infection is, however, an important part of treatment of tetanus. Penicillin has historically been considered the first line agent against *C. tetani*, but metronidazole shows similar efficacy.

Long term supportive measures are frequently required for the tetanus patient. Depending on area and degree of involvement, ventilatory support may be needed. Medical treatment of associated conditions, especially autonomic dysfunction, is complex and often requires admission to an intensive care unit. Benzodiazepines can increase release of GABA and reduce muscle spasm. Neuromuscular blockade can be achieved with several agents, such as pancuronium bromide. Beta blockers and alpha-2 agonists may be used to address the hyper-sympathetic state and autonomic instability that is a frequent cause of death in tetanus patients.

REFERENCES

Abrahamian FM: Management of tetanus: a review. current treatment options in infectious disease. 3:209–216, 2001.

Biglan AW, Ellis FD, Wade TA: Supranuclear oculomotor palsy and exotropia after tetanus. Am J Ophthalmol 86(5):666–668, 1978.

De Barros Miranda-Filho D, Arraes de Alencar Ximenes R, Barone AA, et al: Randomized controlled trial of tetanus treatment with antitetanus immunoglobulin by the intrathecal or intramuscular route. BMJ 328(7440):615. 2004.

Meienberg O, Burgunder JM: Sacchadic eye movement disorder in cephalic tetanus. Europ Neurol 24(3):182–190, 1985.

Orwitz JI, Galetta SL, Teener JW: Bilateral trochlear nerve palsy and downbeat nystagmus in a patient with cephalic tetanus. Neurology 49(3):894–895, 1997.

Purvin VA: Bacterial diseases. Bacterial diseases. In: Walsh and Hoyt's clinical neuro-ophthalmology. 5th edn. Baltimore, Williams and Wilkins, 1998:IV:4109–4117.

50 TRACHOMA 076

Anthony W. Solomon, MBBS, PhD
London, England
David C. W. Mabey, DM, FRCP
London, England
Allen Foster, OBE, FRCS
London, England

ETIOLOGY/PREVALENCE

Trachoma is caused by serovars A, B, Ba and C of the obligate intracellular bacterium *Chlamydia trachomatis*. These serovars have a predilection for conjunctival and nasopharyngeal epithelium. Infection is passed from person to person by eye-seeking flies, by direct contact with infected secretions on fingers and fomites (such as bed sheets and shared cloths), and possibly by droplet spread.

Trachoma is endemic in 55 countries in Africa, Asia, the Middle East, Latin America, and Australia. An estimated 84 million people worldwide have active trachoma, and some 1.3 million are blind from the disease, making it the leading cause of infectious blindness. Trachoma is found in communities where access to water, sanitation and medical care are inadequate and personal and environmental hygiene are poor. Such communities are generally located in hot, dry, remote areas.

Conjunctival *C. trachomatis* infection and the associated clinical signs of active trachoma are most common in preschool children. In adults, the prevalence of infection and active disease is usually higher in women than in men, perhaps because women usually take primary responsibility for child care and are therefore more frequently exposed to infection. The complications of trachoma leading to visual loss and blindness are seen more commonly with advancing age, with several times increased risk for women.

COURSE/PROGNOSIS

The clinical course is not strictly linear. Manifestations can be classified as being either acute (*active*) or late-stage (*cicatricial*), but multiple episodes of active trachoma are required for later development of cicatricial disease, and active and cicatricial signs can occur at the same time in the same individual.

After an incubation period of 5–10 days, conjunctival *C. trachomatis* infection may be marked by injection of conjunctival vessels and production of scant mucopurulent exudate. After several weeks, the more specific signs of *active trachoma* may appear. Though these are signs of acute disease, they represent a chronic inflammatory process:

- Development of subepithelial follicles subjacent to the conjunctiva of the tarsal plates (Figure 50.1b), the fornices, and the limbus;
- Papillary hypertrophy (Figure 50.1c); and
- Thickening of the conjunctiva (Figure 50.1c).

Pannus (in-growing vessels) on the superior cornea can be associated with active disease, but rarely progresses to impair vision. A superficial punctate keratitis may also be noted. Repeated or prolonged episodes of severe active trachoma over many months constitute a risk factor for later development of cicatricial disease.

Inflammation results in deposition of conjunctival scar. With repeated infection over many years, accumulated scar may become visible in the everted conjunctivae (Figure 50.1d). In some individuals, contraction of scar eventually causes individual lashes or the whole upper eyelid to turn inwards, producing trichiasis (Figure 50.1e) and/or entropion. Corneal abrasion and opacification (Figure 50.1f) may ensue. Direct corneal damage from misdirected lashes is compounded by secondary bacterial and fungal infections of the cornea, and corneal drying due to trachomatous scarring of lacrimal and Meibomian glands.

DIAGNOSIS

Clinical signs and symptoms

Active trachoma is generally asymptomatic or mildly irritating. Trichiasis may be symptomatic, with the degree of discomfort dependant on the number of lashes touching the globe, the position of those lashes, and the presence or absence of blepharospasm and the other complications described above.

Examination requires use of binocular magnifying loupes (×2.5) and sunlight or strong torchlight. The eyelashes and cornea should be carefully inspected, and the upper lid everted to allow inspection of the tarsal conjunctivae, one eye at a time. Signs of interest are described above.

Laboratory findings

In most endemic areas, because laboratory tests are expensive and often unavailable, diagnosis relies on the clinical appearance. Laboratory confirmation of *C. trachomatis* conjunctival infection is possible using a commercial polymerase chain reaction (PCR)-based assay, which has high sensitivity and specificity. Various other assays are available, but all are less sensitive than PCR.

Differential diagnosis

The differential diagnosis of active trachoma includes:

- Bacterial conjunctivitis;
- Adult inclusion conjunctivitis (caused by infection by genital serovars of *C. trachomatis*);
- Viral conjunctivitis;
- Allergic conjunctivitis; and
- Toxic follicular conjunctivitis secondary to topical medications or cosmetics.

In areas where trachoma is endemic, pannus, conjunctival scarring, and trichiasis are nearly always attributable to trachoma. Corneal opacity, however, has many possible aetiologies.

Grading

The WHO simplified trachoma grading system is widely used for research and programme monitoring purposes. The system includes five signs (Figure 50.1):

- Trachomatous inflammation — follicular (TF): the presence of five or more follicles at least 0.5 mm in diameter in the central part of the upper tarsal conjunctiva;
- Trachomatous inflammation — intense (TI): pronounced inflammatory thickening of the upper tarsal conjunctiva obscuring more than half the normal deep tarsal vessels;
- Trachomatous scarring (TS): the presence of easily visible scars in the tarsal conjunctiva;
- Trachomatous trichiasis (TT): at least one eyelash rubs on the eyeball, or evidence of recent removal of in-turned eyelashes;
- Corneal opacity (CO): easily visible corneal opacity over the pupil, so dense that at least part of the pupil margin is blurred when viewed through the opacity.

The presence or absence of each sign should be independently determined for each person examined. In the WHO system, the presence of TF and/or TI in one eye is necessary and sufficient to confer a diagnosis of active trachoma.

PREVENTION AND CONTROL

Because corneal grafting is difficult in (and generally unavailable to) patients with trachomatous corneal opacity, blindness from trachoma is difficult to cure. It is, however, possible to prevent:

- Primary prevention occurs through provision of adequate water and hygiene facilities combined with education to promote facial cleanliness and the use of hygiene facilities;
- Secondary prevention occurs through antibiotic treatment to clear ocular *C. trachomatis* infection;
- Tertiary prevention occurs through trichiasis surgery for individuals with trichiasis.

These activities are represented by the acronym SAFE: *s*urgery for trichiasis, *a*ntibiotics to clear infection, and *f*ace washing and *e*nvironmental improvement to reduce transmission. The SAFE strategy is endorsed by WHO, and involves much more than treatment of symptomatic individuals presenting to medical facilities: it is a comprehensive package of interventions delivered at the community level, requiring the coordination and cooperation of organizations from multiple sectors. Using this strategy, WHO and its partners aim to eliminate trachoma as a cause of blindness by the year 2020.

Surgery

Individuals with trichiasis/entropion need corrective surgery. The recommended procedure is bilamellar tarsal rotation. This involves full-thickness division of the upper lid and external rotation of the margin using three sutures. It can be performed by trained eye nurses or other paramedical staff. Correction of trichiasis halts progression of visual loss; it may also marginally improve existing vision by reducing corneal oedema. Case identification is labor-intensive. Having identified people who need it, surgery should be offered within the village or at a nearby health facility, at low or no cost to the patient. After surgery, patients remain at risk for recurrence and require long-term intermittent follow-up.

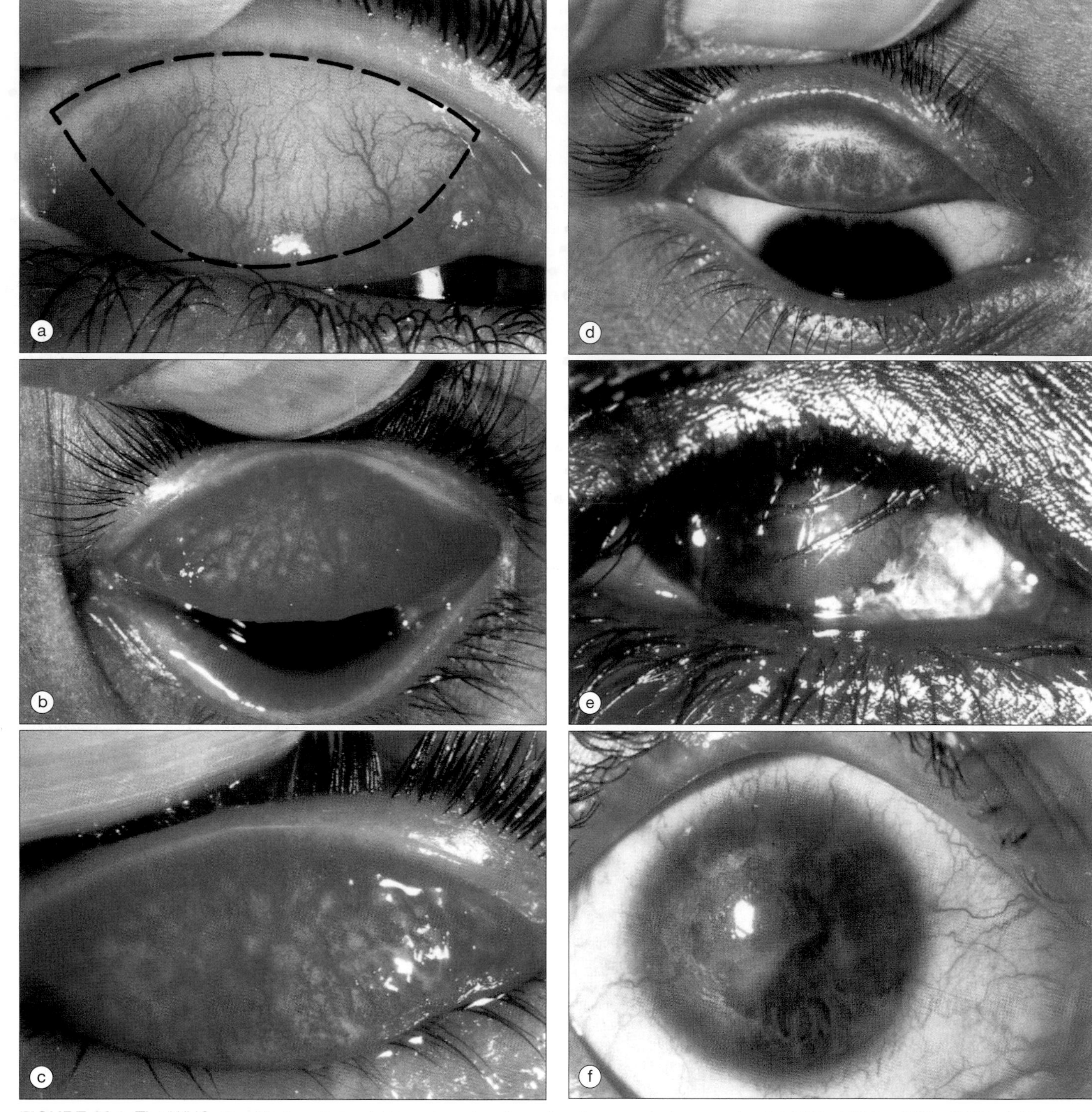

FIGURE 50.1. The WHO simplified system. a) Normal conjunctiva, showing area to be examined. b) TF. c) TI (and TF). d) TS. e) TT. f) CO. (© World Health Organization. Reproduced with permission.)

Antibiotics

Two antibiotic regimens are recommended for trachoma: 6 weeks of twice-daily 1% tetracycline eye ointment, or a single oral dose of azithromycin 20 mg/kg body weight, to a maximum of 1 g. Azithromycin is expensive if not donated, but is easy to administer, well tolerated and allows monitoring of compliance by direct observation of treatment. Tetracycline ointment is inexpensive, but stings on application and requires a prolonged course: compliance in the community is thought to be poor. In areas where the prevalence of TF in 1–9-year-old children is 10% or more, WHO currently recommends annual mass antibiotic treatment of the entire community. Where the prevalence of TF in 1–9-year-old children is 5% or more but <10%, family treatment (identification and treatment of families in which there are one or more members with TF or TI) should be considered. Where the prevalence of TF in 1–9-year-old children is <5%, community-based antibiotic treatment is not recommended.

Facial cleanliness

Facial cleanliness in children should reduce active trachoma prevalence, probably by reducing transmission of *C. trachomatis* by eye-seeking flies. However, changing personal hygiene habits is difficult, particularly in water-insecure communities.

Environmental improvement

Once highly endemic in Europe and North America, trachoma disappeared from those continents in the early twentieth century, as living standards improved. Socioeconomic development takes decades; in the interim, specific interventions to reduce transmission of ocular *C. trachomatis* have been suggested, including improving access to water, and control of flies (specifically *Musca sorbens*) through provision of latrines or spraying of residual insecticide. Proof of the effectiveness of sustainable environment-improving interventions is still awaited.

REFERENCES

Emerson PM, Lindsay SW, Alexander N, et al: Role of flies and provision of latrines in trachoma control: cluster-randomised controlled trial. Lancet 363:1093–1098, 2004.

Emerson PM, Lindsay SW, Walraven GE, et al: Effect of fly control on trachoma and diarrhoea. Lancet 353:1401–1403, 1999.

Mabey DC, Solomon AW, Foster A: Trachoma. Lancet 362:223–229, 2003.

Reacher M, Foster A, Huber J, Bauer B: Trichiasis surgery for trachoma: the bilamellar tarsal rotation procedure (WHO/PBL/93.29). Geneva, World Health Organization, 1993.

Schachter J, West SK, Mabey D, et al: Azithromycin in control of trachoma. Lancet 354:630–635, 1999.

Solomon AW, Holland MJ, Alexander ND, et al: Mass treatment with single-dose azithromycin for trachoma. N Engl J Med 351:1962–1971, 2004.

Solomon AW, Holland MJ, Burton MJ, et al: Strategies for control of trachoma: observational study with quantitative PCR. Lancet 362:198–204, 2003.

Solomon AW, Peeling RW, Foster A, Mabey DC: Diagnosis and assessment of trachoma. Clin Microbiol Rev 17:982–1011, 2004.

Thylefors B, Dawson CR, Jones BR, et al: A simple system for the assessment of trachoma and its complications. Bull World Health Organ 65:477–483, 1987.

West SK, Munoz B, Lynch M, et al: Impact of face-washing on trachoma in Kongwa, Tanzania. Lancet 345:155–158, 1995.

51 TUBERCULOSIS 010.0

Dieudonne Kaimbo Wa Kaimbo, MD, PhD

Kinshasa, Democratic Republic of Congo

Tuberculosis is an acute or chronic communicable disease caused by the acid-fast bacterium *Mycobacterium tuberculosis*, which most commonly involves the lungs but may affect virtually any organ or tissue in the body. Tuberculosis is a leading cause of mortality and morbidity worldwide. Ocular tuberculosis can show a variety of different clinical presentations ranging from an amelanotic choroidal mass to panophthalmitis. It can simulate ocular neoplasms. A high degree of clinical suspicion is important in suspecting and managing this condition. Late diagnosis and delay in management can result in loss of the eye and can even be life-threatening.

ETIOLOGY/INCIDENCE

The tubercle bacilli can gain entrance to the body by several routes. The only one of practical importance is the respiratory tract. Tuberculosis is transmitted by airborne particles that are 1 to 5 μm in diameter, the *Mycobacterium tuberculosis* spreads by droplet infection from coughing or sneezing; the organisms spread from the lungs to regional lymph nodes, producing lymphadenitis. Subsequently, lymphatic drainage delivers the tubercle bacilli to the systemic circulation, whence it has the potential to spread to all organs of the body. During this primary phase of tuberculosis the infection is usually subclinical; the likehood that the disease is radiographically or clinically apparent is approximately 5%.

The most common outcome for the initial infection with *Mycobacterium tuberculosis* is healing with granuloma formation; this occurs over a period of months and is for most people accompanied by the development of tuberculin skin test reactivity. Generally, the granulomas remain stable, and frequently they calcify. In a minority of cases (5 to 15%), occasionally, the granulomas break down; tubercle bacilli multiply and disperse, producing systemic disease. Active tuberculosis is defined as tissue invasion by *Mycobacterium tuberculosis* bacilli that may progress to produce signs and symptoms. Approximately 5% of infected patients may develop a progressive primary disease and an additional 5% may reactivate in future years. Although the majority of cases of active tuberculosis are thought to arise from a reactivation of latent infection, exogenous reinfection with a second strain of *Mycobacteriim* can occur, particularly in profoundly immunocompromised persons and in those heavily exposed to new bacilli.

According to the World Health Organization, it is estimated that one-third of the world's population is infected with *Mycobacterium tuberculosis*, with an annual incidence approaching 8.7 million. There are remarkable geographic variations in the distribution of tuberculosis and 22 countries, including India, China, Indonesia, Bangladesh, Pakistan, Nigeria, Philippines and South Africa, have been identified as contributing 80% of the world's total burden of tuberculosis. In the United States, the prevalence of tuberculosis has been rising after decades of decline.

Although the lung is the primary site of disease in 80 to 84% of cases of tuberculosis, extrapulmonary tuberculosis has become more common with the extent of HIV infection, and the risk of tuberculosis increases as immunosuppression progresses. The most commonly reported extrapulmonoray sites of disease are the lymph nodes, pleura and bones or joints. Other sites include the genitourinary system, the central nervous system, the abdomen and pericardium, and in rare cases, virtually any other organ. The incidence of ophthalmic manifestations is approximately 1 to 2%. Ocular and periocular involvement may occur as a consequence of active infection from hematogenous or contiguous spread of viable bacilli or as a local manifestation of an allergic or hypersensitivity reaction to circulating tuberculoproteins.

DIAGNOSIS

Clinical signs and symptoms

Ocular

- Tuberculosis of the eyelids may present as a localized nodule or an abscess simulating chalazion. Lupus vulgaris, a progressive form of cutaneous tuberculosis, can involve the lids, the lacrimal sac area, and the conjunctiva. Association with systemic tuberculosis occurs in 9 to 19% of patients, and biopsy should be performed to confirm the diagnosis. Tuberculous dacryocystitis is a rare secondary cause of nasolacrimal duct obstruction. Conjunctival involvement may be bilateral and may present as a swelling or painless infiltration responsible for a red eye. Phlyctenulosis, a rare and uncommon presentation, is a localized hypersensitivity reaction to antigens of *Mycobacterium tuberculosis*. A nodule is formed at the limbus and occurs more frequently in children with malnutrition. Phlyctenules may occur on the conjunctiva, but are more frequently observed at the limbus. Phlyctenulosis may be associated with lymph node enlargement of the neck and responds promptly to topical application of steroids. Primary tuberculosis of nasolacrimal mucosa may occur without any symptoms. Therefore, pathologic examination and PCR have been used to confirm the presence of *Mycobacterium tuberculosis*. The cornea may be involved during tuberculosis or nontuberculous mycobacterial infections. Interstitial keratitis is rare but usually unilateral and painless. It may occur as isolated finding or in association with scleritis. Nontuberculous mycobacteria are the most frequently reported agents causing keratitis (*M. kansasii, M. fortuitum*, and *M. chelonei*). Interstitial keratitis secondary to tuberculosis may be associated with uveitis. Tuberculosis is a rare, but classic, cause of scleritis, which is usually anterior and necrotizing, associated with scleral ulceration. Scleral perforation may occur if patients are not treated. Lacrimal gland involvement by the *Mycobacterium tuberculosis* leads to localized granuloma.

- Orbital infection is uncommon; it represents as a lid abscess or a soft tissue mass causing proptosis and resulting from tuberculous periostitis or/and preseptal cellulitis, often with fever, lymphadenopathy, ophthalmoplegia, cutaneous fistula. It may result from either hematogenous spread or from adjacent structures such as the paranasal sinuses or lacrimal gland. The clinical presentation can include panophthalmitis.

Intraocular

- Uveitis is usually granulomatous, with mutton-fat keratic precipitates, iris granulomas, and posterior synechiae. Vitritis can be associated with vasculitis, retinal vein occlusion with subsequent retinal ischemia, and macular edema. Anterior uveitis secondary to tuberculosis is characterized by mutton-fat keratic precipitates. The iris shows both Koeppe and Busacca nodules. Posterior synechiae occur in patients with chronic uveitis and may cause posterior adhesions to the anterior lens capsule, which may cause papillary block angle closure glaucoma. The lens may become cataractous, and the anterior vitreous shows evidence of vitritis secondary to involvement of the ciliary body.
- Ciliary body masses respond very slowly to treatment and may cause secondary angle-closure glaucoma. This can mimic a tumor but can be differentiated on B-scan, which will show variable internal reflectivity consistent with an inflammatory process.
- Solitary or multiple iris nodules can occur.
- Multifocal choroiditis with one to five lesions varying in size from 0.3 to 4.0 mm appear mainly in the posterior pole. The choroidal tubercles are yellow to gray-white. Retinal tuberculosis is rare, but a periphlebitis due to direct infection, a hypersensitivity reaction, or both may occur. However, it is more common for the retinal blood vessels to be normal. On fluorescein angiography, the choroidal tubercles are initially hypofluorescent and then show a late hyperfluorescence that increases in size. After treatment, a chorioretinal scar will remain and may occur with or without a subretinal neovascular membrane. The scars are hyperfluorescent and have sharp margins.
- Solitary choroidal tuberculoma as solitary elevated masslike lesion (4 to 14 mm in size) may be present. The lesion results from a progressive, liquefied caseation necrosis with rapid multiplication of tubercular bacilli and tissue destruction.
- Endophtalmitis may be present as acute onset endogenous endphthalmitis due to rapidly progressive disease, which does not respond to antitubercular therapy. In young children, clinically the endophthalmitis may simulate retinoblastoma.
- Tubercular neuroretinitis is usually seen as a retrobulbar optic neuritis complicating meningitis.

Systemic

- Central nervous system involvement can encompass meningoencephalitis, spinal column disease, and intracranial tuberculomas. Isolated brain stem tuberculomas can be present in association with ocular involvement.

Laboratory findings

- Cultures of sputum, urine, or feces are most commonly done, but any sterile body fluid, including aqueous and vitreous fluids, can be cultured if thought to be infected. Sputum collection exhibits a higher yield of positive cultures than bronchoalveolar lavage or biopsy. Microscopic examination and smear of any fluid for acid-fast bacilli can be done but are much less sensitive than culture. Cultures should be done on both liquid albumin and solid media (Lowenstein–Jenson/egg and Middlebrook/agar base) and kept for a minimum of 8 weeks. A DNA fingerprint pattern of the suspicious isolate can be compared with other laboratory isolates and, if they are identical, the isolate is readily identified as a false-positive result.
- Fine needle aspirate or biopsy with culture is most frequently done on lymph nodes, bone marrow, or liver, (i.e. extrapulmonary tuberculosis).
- Polymerase chain reaction is sensitive for pulmonary infection (89%) but is somewhat less sensitive (42%) for nonpulmonary infections. Clinical trials for an automated Q-beta replicase amplification assay for mycobacteria are being carried out, and so far they have been positive in 69% of smear-negative, culture-positive samples; the specificity is 97%.
- Blood-soluble antigen fluorescent antibody and enzyme-linked immunosorbent assay can be used to detect systemic mycobacterial antigens (even with ocular involvement) as well as antibodies in the aqueous and vitreous fluids.
- The degree of tuberculin test reactivity can correlate to the likelihood of infection in immunocompetent patients, but even 5 mm of reactivity is significant in immunocompromised patients. The bacille Calmette–Guérin (BCG) vaccination can also serve as a test; reactivity within 3 days of vaccination is considered evidence of prior infection.

Differential diagnosis

Establishing the diagnosis of ocular tuberculosis can be challenging because presentations can be varied and similar to other conditions that are often difficult to confirm except with tissue or culture. Tuberculous uveitis must be differentiated from other granulomatous infections such as sarcoidosis, brucellosis, leprosy, cat-scratch disease, syphilis, toxoplasmosis, and fungal infection. Choroidal tubercles can resemble metastatic foci from breast, lung, prostate, and other primary sites.

Acute posterior multifocal placoid pigment epitheliopathy (APMPPE) has been associated with several agents, including pulmonary tuberculosis. The typical lesions of APMPPE were multiple flat, gray-white lesions of the retinal pigment epithelium occurring posterior to the equator. A granulomatous anterior uveitis with mutton-fat precipitates and Koeppe's nodules has also been associated with APMPPE.

PROPHYLAXIS

An efficacious and safe vaccine is not available. BCG vaccination causes tuberculin skin test conversion, but the duration of hypersensitivity varies, and the size of induration fades with time. The BCG vaccine is also more effective at preventing disseminated disease in children than in preventing pulmonary disease in adults. BCG causes disseminated infection in patients with symptomatic human immunodeficiency virus infection or AIDS; BCG also is not recommended for health care workers exposed to multiple-drug-resistant tuberculosis.

TREATMENT

Topical

Topical isoniazid and streptomycin can be used to enhance the systemic treatment of external and anterior segment lesions. Topical corticosteroids and mydriatric agents can also be useful in tuberculous uveitis and should be used while systemic antimycobacterial treatment is under way. Nontuberculous mycobacterial keratitis, especially *M. fortuitum*, is responsive to topical ciprofloxacin; amikacin is less effective.

Systemic

Treatment of tuberculosis has changed over the past decades. For the patient with documented systemic tuberculosis, medical therapy should be administered by an internist or specialist in infectious diseases. A course of 4-drug combination chemotherapy (isoniazid, rifampin, pyrazinamide and ethambutol or streptomycin) for a period of 6 months has been advocated for systemic tuberculosis. Similar therapy is recommended for active ocular tuberculosis. Resolution of the ocular condition depends on treatment of the underlying disease. The initial phase of treatment lasts for 2 months and is followed, depending upon the circumstances, by a 4–7 month continuation phase to complete therapy. Ethambutol is usually discontinued 2 months after the initiation of therapy, and the remaining 3 drugs can be continued for 4 months. This drug regimen has been found to be as effective as standard 9-month course. In adults, the dosage for isoniazid is 300 mg orally per day (10 to 15 mg/kg/d, maximum dose of 300 mg/kg/d), rifampin 600 mg orally per day (10 to 20 mg/kg/d, maximum dose of 600 mg/kg/d), pyrazinamide 2 g orally per day (15 to 30 mg/kg, maximum dose of 2 g/d in children), and ethambutol 800 mg orally per day (15 to 25 mg/kg/d, maximum dose of 2.5 g); pyridoxine 50 mg orally per day (15 to 30 mg/kg/day in children) should be given to prevent isoniazid neurotoxicity. Alternative drugs for adults include amikacin, ciprofloxacin, clofazimin, cycloserin A, ethionamide, ofloxacin, and rifabutin. The Centers for Disease Control recommends that all tuberculosis patients be observed taking their medication by healthcare providers (direct observed therapy, DOT).

The treatment period for immunocompromised patients is extended to 6 months after negative cultures first appear.

Surgical

A tissue biopsy can be considered if diagnosis cannot be established any other way. Procedures for secondary glaucoma may be necessary for patients with ciliary body tuberculosis because the masses respond slowly to medical therapy. Cataract surgery can be performed in patients with complicated cataract and quiet eyes.

COMPLICATIONS

General considerations

The incidence of adverse hepatic reactions is greater when rifampin is combined with isoniazid, but it is not statistically significant; the therapeutic response rate is much better with combination treatment. The threat of optic neuritis and optic atrophy resulting from the use of isoniazid, rifampin, and ethambutol mandates color vision monitoring while these agents are being used. Pattern-reversal visual evoked potentials may detect an early prolongation of the P100 wave secondary to these agents before clinical signs appear.

Specific drug considerations

Isoniazid

A hypersensitivity reaction can occur. Hepatotoxicity, peripheral neuropathy and CNS effects also are possible. Overdose may be fatal. Drug interactions include coumadin, benzodiazepines, theophylline, phenytoin, alcohol, disulfiram and aluminum-containing antacids.

Rifampin

Causes orange-pink discoloration of body fluids, secretions (urines, sweat, tears, etc.) and contact lenses. Antacids may reduce the absorption of rifampicin. Hypersensitivity reactions can occur, as well as hematologic abnormalities such as anemia, thrombocytopenia, leucopenia, hepatotoxicity and influenza-like syndrome. Drug inhibits effects of warfarin, corticosteroids, oral contraceptives, theophylline, dapsone, ketoconazole, protease inhibitors and nonnucleoside reverse-transcriptase inhibitors, digoxin diazepam, quinidine, methadone and oral hypoglycemic agents.

Pyrazinamide

Reactions include hepatitis, hyperuricemia, nausea, vomiting and drug fever. It can cause thrombocytopenia and sideroblastic anemia; mild arthralgias.

Ethambutol

An optic neuritis and retinal ganglion cell toxicity are the most common and serious side effects, but skin rash and hyperuricemia can also occur. It decreases red-green discrimination and visual acuity.

Streptomycin

Ototoxicity (vestibular and auditory) is the most common and serious side effect. Neuromuscular blockage can occur. Renal toxicity and hypersensitivity with skin rash and fever are uncommon. The drug potentiates the action of neuromuscular blocking agents.

Rifabutin

The most common side effect is hepatotoxicity; other complications include hypopyon iritis, fever, flushing pruritus, intestinal nephritis, rash, orange-colored body fluids, neutropenia and rarely thrombocytopenia. This orange staining in the tear film can permanently color soft contact lenses.

Miscellaneous

Drug resistance should be considered if there are any of the following:

- Treatment failure;
- Poorly compliant patient;
- Contact with known resistant strains of tuberculosis;
- Large inoculum;
- Positive cultures after 3 months of therapy.

REFERENCES

Biswas J, Shome D: Choroidal tubercles in disseminated tuberculosis diagnosed by the polymerase chain reaction of aqueous humor. Ocul Immunol Inflamm 10:293–298, 2002.

Bodaghi B, LeHoang P: Ocular tuberculosis. Curr Opin Ophthalmol 11:443–448, 2000.

Demirci H, Shields CL, Shields JA, Eagle RC: Ocular tuberculosis masquerading as ocular tumors. Surv Ophthalmol 49:78–89, 2004.

Gupta A, Gupta V: Tubercular posterior uveitis. Int Ophthalmol Clin 45:71–88, 2005.

Myers JP: New recommendations for the treatment of tuberculosis. Curr Opin Infect Dis 18:133–140, 2005.

Small PM, Fujiwara PI: Management of tuberculosis in the United States. N Engl J Med 345:189–200, 2001.

Tabbara KF: Ocular tuberculosis: anterior segment. Int Ophthalmol Clin 45:57–69, 2005.

Torres RM, Calonge M: Macular edema as the only ocular finding of tuberculosis. Am J Ophthalmol 138:1048–1049, 2004.

52 TYPHOID FEVER 002.0
(Enteric Fever)

Theodore H. Curtis, MD
Portland, Oregon
David T. Wheeler, MD
Portland, Oregon

ETIOLOGY/INCIDENCE

Typhoid fever is an acute febrile illness caused by the ingestion of and intestinal invasion by *Salmonella enterica* serotype *typhi*, a gram-negative bacillus found only in humans. Prevalent in those regions of the world lacking in sanitary water and sewage systems, its transmission can occur through ingestion of contaminated food or water, contact with an acute case of typhoid fever, or contact with an asymptomatic carrier. Adults and children of all ages and both genders appear equally susceptible to infection. Transmission through direct fecal-oral contact is more common among children.

Sustained fever, abdominal pain or other manifestations of gastroenteritis, and non-specific symptoms such as headache, chills, diaphoresis, anorexia, cough, sore throat, dizziness and myalgias characterize typhoid fever. The onset is usually gradual and, without antibiotics, the illness achieves maximum severity during the second or third week with marked weakness, abdominal discomfort and distension, skin rash (rose spots), cervical adenopathy, hepatosplenomegaly, and occasional neuropsychiatric manifestations such as delirium or seizures. Recovery, characterized by declining fever, begins by the end of the third or fourth week. The most prominent major complications are intestinal hemorrhage and perforation, which can occur during the third week and is often heralded by a sudden drop in temperature and increased pulse.

Ocular manifestations of typhoid fever are rare and may include lid edema or abscess, dacryoadenitis, conjunctival petechiae or chemosis, corneal ulceration, uveitis, vitreous hemorrhage, retinal hemorrhage and detachment, stellate maculopathy, pigmentary retinopathy, optic neuritis, internal or external ophthalmoplegia, and orbital hemorrhage or abscess. These complications are probably a result of direct invasion by the organism into ocular tissues, but some may be hypersensitivity phenomena, such as vitreous hemorrhage reported after first generation typhoid vaccination.

COURSE/PROGNOSIS

Following penetration of intestinal mucosa, *S. enterica typhi* replicate in mononuclear phagocytes of ileal Peyer's patches and mesenteric lymph nodes. After incubation of 1 to 3 weeks, hematogenous spread occurs to spleen, liver and bone marrow where further replication takes place. Bacteremia and humoral mediators are responsible for fever and other non-specific symptoms of illness. A relative bradycardia (given the degree of fever) occurs in up to 50% of patients. Rose spots can occur on the trunk, consisting of erythematous maculopapules 1 to 5 mm in diameter, which initially blanch with pressure but may become hemorrhagic. Altered mental status out of proportion to systemic illness may occur; seizures are more common in children. Intestinal manifestations are caused by hyperplasia of Peyer's patches with ulceration of overlying mucosa resulting in pain, diarrhea, bleeding or perforation. Without antibiotic therapy, fever and most symptoms resolve by the fourth week of infection in approximately 90% of individuals who survive.

Typhoid fever carried a case fatality rate of 15% in the pre-antibiotic era. Mortality was reduced to 2% after chloramphenicol became available. Case fatality rates >10% continue to be reported in developing countries despite availability of antibiotics, whereas developed countries show case fatality rates <1%. With antibiotic treatment, most patients become afebrile within 4 to 7 days. There is a 10% relapse rate.

Around 3% of patients develop a chronic carrier state after recovery; this rate is higher in women and older men and is associated with biliary abnormalities. Most carriers are asymptomatic and up to 25% have no history of typhoid, making identification difficult.

DIAGNOSIS

Laboratory findings

- Isolation of *S. enterica typhi* from blood culture is most likely in the first two weeks of illness but is positive in only 50% to 70% of cases.
- Stool cultures are positive less frequently but may increase the diagnostic yield; other sources include urine, rose spots and gastric or intestinal secretions.
- Bone marrow culture is the most sensitive (positive in nearly 90% of cases) and can be used when diagnosis is crucial or following antibiotic treatment.
- The time honored Widal test for agglutinating antibodies to H or O antigen is of limited value; recent agglutination tests to Vi antigen are more sensitive and specific. PCR to this antigen has been developed but is not commercially available.
- Anemia, thrombocytopenia, and relative neutropenia of variable severity may be present.
- Liver function tests may show elevated aminotransferases and bilirubin.
- Renal failure is an infrequent complication.

Differential diagnosis

- In travelers returning from developing countries, infections such as hepatitis, malaria, typhus, amoebiasis, shigellosis, visceral leishmaniasis, Dengue fever, or leptospirosis should be considered.
- In non-travelers, infections associated with prolonged fever such as the rickettsioses, brucellosis, tularemia, miliary tuberculosis, bacterial endocarditis, infectious mononucleosis, cytomegalovirus infections, influenza, or meningococcemia must be ruled out.
- Non-infectious causes of fever (such as lymphoma or connective tissue disease) should be considered.
- Ocular manifestations are rare and will generally only be seen in the setting of systemic illness.

PROPHYLAXIS

Improvement of environmental sanitation, including water supplies and sewage disposal, sharply reduces the incidence of typhoid fever. Travelers to developing countries should avoid consuming untreated water, drinks served with ice, peeled fruits, and other food not served hot as the organism is resistant to drying and cooling. American international travelers face an overall risk of developing typhoid fever of <1 case in 10,000 trips but this increases to 4 in 10,000 with travel to high-risk countries. Immunization is at best an adjunct to typhoid avoidance because of limited vaccine efficacy.

The traditional heat-killed, phenol-extracted whole typhoid vaccine is no longer recommended because of its limited efficacy, short duration of protection, and the high frequency of local reactions and fever. Children over 6 years of age and adults can receive three doses of a first-generation live oral vaccine (Ty21a) that is invasive but metabolically defective, so dies after a few cycles of replication. This vaccine is safe, provides as much protection as the killed vaccine (42% to 67%), and continues to be protective for at least several years. One parenteral dose of purified Vi polysaccharide vaccine has proved as effective (55% to 77%) and long-lasting as multiple doses of Ty21a and may be used in children over 2 years of age and in at-risk HIV-infected patients. Genetically engineered live typhoid vaccine strains are being developed. No ocular complications have been reported with use of any modern typhoid vaccines.

TREATMENT

Systemic

- Since 1989, numerous reports have surfaced regarding multi-drug resistant strains of *S. typhi* on the Indian subcontinent and throughout Southeast Asia, Africa and the Middle East. This has influenced the medical treatment of typhoid fever.

Ocular

- Ocular infection should be treated with ophthalmic chloramphenicol (0.5% solution or 1% ointment) or ciprofloxacin (0.3% solution), frequency correlated with severity of infection (from BID for conjunctivitis to hourly for corneal ulceration). Although newer generation fluoroquinolones (gatifloxacin, levofloxacin, moxifloxacin) are likely effective, there are no clinical trials on their efficacy. Smears for culture and sensitivity should be obtained prior to initiating chemotherapy.
- Lid or orbital abscesses require surgical drainage and debridement, copious irrigation and appropriate cultures. The only ophthalmic ointment with activity against *S. enterica typhi* is 1% chloramphenicol.
- Uveitis (iritis, iridocyclitis or choroiditis) should be treated with appropriate topical, periocular or systemic corticosteroids or non-steroidal anti-inflammatory agents based on the clinical presentation. Patients with anterior uveitis should also receive topical mydriatic-cycloplegic medication and severe intraocular inflammation (e.g. endophthalmitis or panophthalmitis) may require systemic analgesics.
- Retinal detachment is rare. Reported cases have been due to serous detachment from presumed choroiditis. Medical management with systemic corticosteroids may hasten resolution and improve visual outcome. Choroiditis is also blamed for stellate maculopathy and pigmentary retinopathy.
- The specific etiology of dacryoadenitis, optic neuritis and ophthalmoplegia is unknown and treatment is therefore directed at the underlying systemic infection and inflammatory response as outlined above.

Medical

- Oral chloramphenicol, introduced in 1948, is no longer the drug of choice due to widespread resistance, high rates of relapse and chronic carriage, and the risk of bone marrow toxicity.
- Alternative antibiotics include trimethoprim-sulfamethoxazole, ampicillin, amoxicillin, and third generation cephalosporins and can be used if the risk of multi-drug resistance is thought to be low or if sensitivities are available.
- The current drug of choice for adults is oral ciprofloxacin (500 mg b.i.d. for 10–14 days). Although there have been increasing reports of organisms resistant to quinolone therapy, especially in Asia, this drug is the most effective and has the additional advantage of excellent penetration into macrophages and the biliary system which may reduce the incidence of relapse and carrier states.

- The current drug of choice for children or pregnant women is parenteral ceftriaxone (50–80 mg/kg qd for 5–7 days). Quinolone use has been shown experimentally to damage cartilage in young animals and should probably be avoided in these patients.
- Third generation cephalosporins and azithromycin are useful for drug-resistant strains.
- Patients in shock or with altered mental status may benefit from corticosteroid administration, usually parenteral dexamethasone (3 mg/kg followed by 1 mg/kg every 6 hours for 48 hours).
- Supportive care, consisting of intravenous fluids and occasionally transfusion, is often required. The use of aspirin is relatively contraindicated due to reported hypothermia, hypotension and gastrointestinal mucosal irritation.
- Treatment of patients who relapse is generally identical to the initial infection, although the choice of antibiotic should ideally be guided by sensitivity. It may be reasonable to use ciprofloxacin or ceftriaxone if not used initially.
- Treatment of the chronic carrier state is difficult as anatomical abnormalities are often present (e.g. biliary or renal stones). Most clinical experience has involved amoxicillin or trimethoprim-sulfamethoxazole; eradication rates of >80% are reported following 6 weeks of therapy. Due to their excellent penetration, quinolones have a theoretical advantage and several small studies have shown efficacy with these drugs over a 4-week course. Chronic carrier state is rare in children, but amoxicillin would be the drug of choice.

Surgical

- Prompt surgical intervention for severe intestinal bleeding or bowel perforation has been shown to reduce mortality substantially.
- There may be a role for cholecystectomy in management of the chronic carrier state if there is underlying biliary disease.

COMPLICATIONS

In about 10% of patients, intestinal bleeding or perforation occurs, usually after the second week of illness. Bleeding occurs from ileal ulcers and may present as melena or bright red blood in stools. Perforation most often occurs unexpectedly after a few days of treatment when a patient has started to improve. Other unusual complications of typhoid fever include pneumonia, myocarditis, acute cholecystitis, hepatitis, nephritis, parotitis, orchitis, osteomyelitis and acute meningitis.

COMMENTS

Approximately 500 reported cases of typhoid fever occur each year in the United States. The percentage of these cases contracted abroad has increased to >70%, most of whom are children, adolescents or young adults. Most domestically acquired cases occur in outbreaks or among at-risk patients with underlying medical disease; the rate among patients with HIV is sixty times greater than the general population. Typhoid fever is a reportable disease in the United States.

REFERENCES

Bajpai PC, Dikshit SK: Bilateral optic neuritis and encephalitis complicating typhoid fever. J Indian Med Assoc 30:54–57, 1958.

Dhir SP, Jain IS, Kumar P, et al: *Salmonella* lid abscess. Indian J Ophthalmol 24:27–28, 1977.

Duke-Elder S: Typhoid fever. In: Duke-Elder S, ed: System of ophthalmology, (summary of systemic ophthalmology). St Louis, CV Mosby, 1976: XV:163–164.

Fusco R, Magli A, Guacci P: Stellate maculopathy due to *Salmonella typhi*: a case report. Ophthalmologica, Basel 192:154–158, 1986.

Keusch G: Salmonellosis. In: Fauci AS, et al, eds: Harrison's principles of internal medicine. 14th edn. New York, McGraw-Hill, 1998:950–956.

Lewis PJ, Jones BL: Vitreous haemorrhage after typhoid cholera inoculation. Med J Aust 2:914, 1974.

Mathur JS, Nema HV, Char JN, et al: Post typhoid retinal detachment. J All-India Ophthalmol Soc 18:135–137, 1970.

Miller SI, Hohmann EL, Pegues DA: *Salmonella* (including *Salmonella typhi*). In: Mandell GL, Bennett JE, Dolin R, eds: Principles and practice of infectious diseases. 4th edn. New York, Churchill Livingstone, 1995:2013–2033.

Parry CM, Hein TT, Dougan G, et al: Typhoid fever. N Engl J Med 347:1770–1782, 2002.

Rowe B, Ward LR, Threlfall EJ: Multidrug-resistant *Salmonella typhi*: a worldwide epidemic. Clinical Infectious Diseases 24(Suppl 1):S106–S109, 1997.

van Basten JP, Stockenbrugger R: Typhoid perforation: a review of the literature since 1960. Tropical and Geographical Medicine 46:336–339, 1994.

53 VARICELLA AND HERPES ZOSTER 052.9

Thomas J. Liesegang, MD
Jacksonville, Florida

Varicella

ETIOLOGY/INCIDENCE

Varicella-zoster virus causes two distinct syndromes. Primary infection presents as varicella (or chickenpox), a contagious and usually benign childhood illness that occurs in epidemics among susceptible children. The reactivation of the virus, usually associated with decline in cell-mediated immunity, occurs as herpes zoster (shingles). Varicella is spread through droplet infection with an initial viremia, and then viral spread to the skin and the eye. It is easily disseminated to susceptible individuals. Ninety-five percent of the population has serological evidence of prior VZV infection with or without symptomatic varicella. The incidence of varicella has diminished 70% after implementation of the varicella vaccine in 1995.

DIAGNOSIS

Varicella is an acute infectious exanthem characterized by fever, myalgias, anorexia, headache, sore throat, and vesicular eruptions on the skin. The disease is more severe in neonates, adults, and the immunosuppressed in whom complications such as pneumonitis and encephalitis may occur. Serological tests can confirm prior varicella infection.

TREATMENT

Systemic

This common, self-limiting disease requires minimal supportive therapy. Varicella in immunocompromised individuals may require aciclovir, famvir, or valaciclovir. These antivirals shorten the duration of illness; however, it is unclear whether the medication cost justifies use in otherwise healthy children. Zoster immune globulin can induce passive immunity within 96 hours of exposure in susceptible individuals at risk for severe infection. Systemic steroids are usually not indicated or are frequently contraindicated.

OCULAR COMPLICATIONS AND TREATMENT

Varicella may be accompanied by a temporary conjunctivitis and episcleritis, which require no specific treatment. Rarely, microdendritic keratitis, nummular keratitis, disciform keratitis, mucous plaque keratitis, sclerokeratitis, and iritis may occur which require topical steroid treatment.

Herpes zoster

ETIOLOGY/INCIDENCE

The second clinical entity of VZV, herpes zoster disease, occurs from reactivation of VZV after initial establishment of latency within cells of the dorsal root ganglia throughout the body. Herpes zoster occurs in about 500,000 individuals annually in the US. Declining virus-specific cell-mediated immune responses, which occur naturally as a result of aging or are induced by immunosuppression, increase the frequency and severity of shingles. In patients with AIDS the incidence is 15 times greater than a non-AIDS population. In Africa HZ is especially common and severe.

DIAGNOSIS

Herpes zoster is an acute painful, vesicular eruption within a dermatomal distribution. Herpes zoster ophthalmicus (HZO), which defines the involvement of the ophthalmic division of the fifth cranial nerve, comprises about 20% of cases, and the eye is involved in 50% of these cases. The prodromal period before skin eruptions may feature fever, malaise, headache, and pain in the eye. The rash is initially erythematous, and then macules, papules, vesicles, pustules, and crusts develop. If the rash involves the nasociliary nerve distribution, there is a high rate of ocular complications.

COMPLICATIONS OF HZO

The ocular complications may vary markedly in severity and are complicated by contributing factors associated with the infection, with the inflammatory and immune changes (especially to blood vessels), with the neural damage, and with the subsequent tissue scarring.

With herpes zoster ophthalmicus the following complications may occur:

Eyelid

Rash, edema, ptosis, and late scarring with the development of entropion, ectropion, notch defects, or full-thickness lid loss.

Episclera/sclera

Affected during the acute stages of HZO or months later. Scleritis and episcleritis may persist for months. Scleritis has a tendency to progress toward limbal vasculitis and a sclerokeratitis. Posterior scleritis may result from an infiltrative perivasculitis and perineuritis.

Conjunctiva

Changes may include a papillary or follicular reaction, chronic hyperemia, and/or pseudomembrane formation with resultant conjunctival scarring.

Cornea

There is a wide range of complications:

- Pseudo dendrites and punctate epithelial keratitis: transient and rarely give rise to chronic keratitis;
- Nummular anterior stromal keratitis: resolves within the first month. Rarely becomes chronic and gives rise to lipid keratopathy and facet formation;
- Keratouveitis/endotheliitis with localized stromal edema: may represent direct viral infection of the endothelium or an immune reaction. Associated with uveitis, glaucoma, and iris atrophy;
- Disciform keratitis with deep disc-shaped area of stromal edema: may represent a VZV infection of the endothelium to an immune reaction. Resolves within a few months or may become chronic with a lipid keratopathy;
- Corneal mucous plaques: occur several months after HZO in a quiescent eye. They are variable in size, migratory in nature, and transitory around the cornea. May be immune related or represent chronic viral infection;
- Interstitial keratitis/lipid keratopathy: long-term corneal inflammation usually results in extensive corneal vascularization;
- Neurotrophic keratopathy: diminution of corneal sensation with subsequent a loss of epithelial integrity. May occur abruptly months following HZO with diffuse epitheliopathy, and chronic surface problems with calcareous plaque formation. It may progress to perforation or severe scarring;
- Corneal edema: temporary or permanent even in the absence of scarring and vascularization and is probably related to endothelial destruction by VZV;
- Exposure keratopathy: associated with a cicatricial eyelid changes leading to corneal desiccation.

Eye muscles

External ocular motor palsies with transient diplopia and involvement of the third, fourth, or sixth nerve may develop in 20%.

Retina and optic nerve

Rare complications include retinal perivasculitis, acute retinal necrosis, progressive outer retinal necrosis or ischemic optic neuritis.

Neurological

Acute neuralgia, post herpetic neuralgia (PHN), contralateral hemiplegia, encephalitis, or myelitis. The incidence and the duration of post herpetic neuralgia are correlated with age (about 7% of patients).

TREATMENT

Systemic

A course of systemic antiviral agents (aciclovir, valaciclovir, or famvir) is advised for all patients with defects of cell-mediated immunity. Controversy lingers regarding the use of antivirals for localized zoster in the normal host although they are recommended for all patients with HZO. Although any of the 3 systemic antivirals may lessen the complications of ocular zoster, there does not appear to be convincing or consistent evidence of the benefit of the systemic antivirals in preventing or treating the most severe complications of HZO. The drugs should be administered within 72 hours of the onset of the rash. Patients receiving combined corticosteroids and antivirals have an acceleration in cutaneous healing rates and a better quality of life, decreased use of analgesics, a decrease in the time to uninterrupted sleep, and a decrease in time to resumption of normal activities of daily living compared to those with antiviral alone. Steroids should not be used in those with depressed cell-mediated immunity. Aciclovir-resistant VZV have been reported in patients with advanced AIDS, requiring therapy with alternative drugs (e.g. foscarnet). There is no role for topical antiviral drugs in the management of herpes zoster.

Most treatment plans for PHN have anecdotal reports rather than controlled trials, so effectiveness is both complex and difficult to evaluate. Early antiviral appears to modify later PHN only marginally. For persistent cases, management in conjunction with a pain expert and a multifaceted approach is recommended. A variety of pharmacologic therapies exist for those who are not helped by mild analgesia. Clinical trials have shown that opioids, tricyclic antidepressants, and gabapentin reduce the severity or duration of post herpetic neuralgia, either as single agents or in combination.

Ocular

Topical steroids are recommended for chronic episcleritis and keratitis and for all cases of iritis. Careful monitoring of the use of topical steroids with very slow reduction and withdrawal prevents rebound effects and detects steroid responders.

Complications from severe neurotrophic keratopathy or exposure keratitis can require surgical intervention such as a partial tarsorrhaphy. Occasionally corneal surgery may be required in cases of perforation from neurotrophic corneas. Following a penetrating keratoplasty, HZO patients require close monitoring and therapy with lubrication and possibly lateral tarsorrhaphies. Cataract and glaucoma operations are generally uncomplicated, but topical steroids must be used postoperatively. Systemic steroids are indicated for markedly hemorrhagic rashes, proptosis with external ophthalmoplegia, optic neuritis and contralateral hemiplegia.

PROPHYLAXIS

The varicella vaccine has created a decline in varicella disease but there are concerns about the long-term efficacy of vaccination and whether the vaccine will lead to an increase in adult varicella as well as an increase in the incidence of herpes zoster. About 3% of childhood and 30% of adult vaccinees will have a breakthrough infection, but is usually much less severe than primary varicella. Epidemiologists predict that the more effective vaccination is at preventing varicella, the larger the future increase in zoster incidence. A vaccine trial is currently underway to assess whether varicella immunization of children affects the incidence of herpes zoster later in life. A separate trial is investigating whether periodic vaccination can prevent herpes zoster in the elderly.

REFERENCES

Liesegang TJ: Varicella-zoster virus eye disease. Cornea 18:511–531, 1999.

Severson EA, Baratz KH, Hodge DO, Burke JP: Herpes zoster ophthalmicus in Olmsted County, Minnesota: have systemic antivirals made a difference? Arch Ophthalmol 121:386–390, 2003.

Starr CE, Pavan-Langston D: Varicella-zoster disease: mechanisms of pathogenesis and corneal disease. Ophthalmol Clin N Amer 15:7–15, 2002.

Vafai A, Berger M: Zoster in patients infected with HIV: a review. Am J Med Sci 321:372–380, 2001.

Vazquez M: Varicella zoster virus infections in children after the introduction of live attenuated varicella vaccine. Curr Opin Pediatr 16:80–84, 2004.

Vrabec TR: Posterior segment manifestations of HIV/AIDS. Surv Ophthalmol 49:131–157, 2004.

54 YERSINIOSIS 020.9

K. Matti Saari, MD, MedScD, FEBO
Turku, Finland

ETIOLOGY/INCIDENCE

Yersiniosis is caused by infection with one of the invasive rod-shaped *Yersinia* bacteria; these organisms are small, nonmotile, gram-negative coccobacilli. The two species that cause disease in humans are *Y. enterocolitica* and *Y. pseudotuberculosis*; they are closely related to the bubonic plague bacillus *Y. pestis*.

Y. enterocolitica serotypes 3, 4, 5, 8, and 9 and *Y. pseudotuberculosis* are the principal causes of yersiniosis; the yersinioses are distributed worldwide. The bacilli have been isolated from a wide variety of domestic and wild animals, and although the mode of transmission of *Yersinia* spp. is not fully certain, the primary mode appears to be through the ingestion of fecally contaminated water or food. Transmission to humans through contact with infected animals, especially swine, and from person to person can occur in rare instances.

The incubation period is 4 to 10 days.

DIAGNOSIS

Clinical signs and symptoms

Systemic

Yersiniosis may show a wide range of clinical manifestations, varying according to the age and condition of the patient.

- In infants, gastroenteritis with high fever is common.
- Older children often experience acute abdominal symptoms, such as acute terminal ileitis or mesenteric adenitis.
- Adults may present with enteritis, including diarrhea, nonspecific abdominal pain, nausea, vomiting and fever.
- In young and middle-aged adults with HLA-B27 antigen, nonpurulent reactive arthritis, often with myalgia and sacroiliitis, is more common.
- In women of later middle age, erythema nodosum is a frequent symptom.

Less common symptoms of yersiniosis include the following:
- Carditis;
- Septicemia;
- Glomerulonephritis;
- Hepatitis;
- Hemolytic anemia.

Although septicemia with serious complications may occur in debilitated and elderly patients, the prognosis for *Yersinia* infections is generally good, especially if diagnosed early and treated promptly.

In children, the diarrhea associated with *Y. enterocolitica* often is self-limited, and the role of antibiotic therapy is unclear; subacute localizing forms of infection sometimes occur with *Y. pseudotuberculosis*, particularly in patients with concurrent underlying disease.

Ocular

Pyogenic intraocular involvement (microbial invasion of the eye) is very rare in patients with yersiniosis, but the following have been reported:
- Parinaud's oculoglandular syndrome with:
  - Corneal perforation; and
  - Panophthalmitis;
  - Leading to visual loss.

Reactive ocular inflammation is occasionally associated with patients with HLA-B27 antigen; the causative agent cannot be isolated from the eye. Symptoms in these patients include:
- Acute anterior uveitis;
- Conjunctivitis;
- Reiter's syndrome.

Reactive acute anterior uveitis may follow from 5 days to 1 month after the onset of *Yersinia* infection, with the following consistent signs:
- Conjunctival redness;
- Photophobia;
- Ocular pain;
- Decreased vision;
- Increased lacrimation;
- Pericorneal ciliary injection;
- Aqueous cells and flare;
- Fine keratic precipitates.

Other signs and symptoms of *Yersinia* can include the following:
- Vasodilation of iris vessels;
- Fibrinous exudation in the aqueous humor;
- Cells in the vitreous humor;
- Macular edema.

In most cases, the uveitis is unilateral, and its duration may vary from 3 weeks to 3 months; the inflammatory signs usually resolve completely, but in 30% to 50% of cases, the uveitis may recur after a lapse of 1 month to 3 years.

Reactive conjunctivitis may occur in one or both eyes from 4 to 17 days after the onset of *Yersinia* infection; conjunctival symptoms are mostly mild, although the patient may complain of ocular redness and a burning sensation. More rarely, slight ocular pain, palpebral edema, and purulent exudate may be found.

Reactive conjunctivitis resolves spontaneously in 7 days.

Laboratory findings

Because yersiniosis may present with such a wide spectrum of symptoms, diagnosis may easily be missed. This infection should always be considered in patients with fever and abdominal symptoms of unknown origin after appendicitis has been ruled out.

When a diagnosis of yersiniosis is suspected, cultures should be made of:
- Stool samples;
- Conjunctival discharges.

A presumptive diagnosis can be made from serologic test results on the demonstration of:
- Enzyme-linked immunosorbent assay for detection of IgA and IgM antibodies to *Yersinia* spp. showing elevated antibody levels, indicating a recent infection;
- An elevated erythrocyte sedimentation rate, characteristic for yersiniosis in patients of all ages.

Patients with reactive ocular inflammation after *Yersinia* infection are HLA-B27 positive.

TREATMENT

Systemic

Most *Y. enterocolitica* strains are sensitive to:
- Ceftazidime;
- Chloramphenicol;
- Ciprofloxacin;
- Gentamicin;
- Tetracycline;
- Tobramycin;
- Trimethoprim-sulfamethoxazole.

However, success with these drugs is not uniform, and *Yersinia* spp. have been found to be resistant to amoxicillin, ampicillin, carbenicillin, cephalosporin, and penicillin.

Drug therapy must be started promptly when *Yersinia* infection is suspected; the usual drugs of choice are:
- Tetracycline 250 to 500 mg PO every 6 hours for 10 days;
- Chloramphenicol 250 to 500 mg PO every 6 hours or 500 mg IV every 6 hours.

Alternatives are:
- Sulfamethoxazole 800 mg and trimethoprim 160 mg PO b.i.d. or t.i.d.;
- Gentamicin 0.8 mg/kg IM initially followed by 0.4 mg/kg IM every 6 hours.

Therapy should be continued for at least 24 to 48 hours after the fever and other symptoms have subsided.

Ocular

For pyogenic conjunctival *Yersinia* infections:

- Fortified gentamicin 14 mg/mL eyedrops should be administered *hourly* for 8 days and then tapered to 1 drop every 6 hours until the infection is resolved.

With corneal involvement:

- Gentamicin 20 to 40 mg/day by sub-Tenon's injection for 4 to 5 days should be given; this series may be followed by two additional injections on alternate days;
- Topical atropine solution 1% 1 drop every 6 hours may be used for uveitis;
- Scopolamine 0.25% 1 drop every 6 hours may be substituted for patients sensitive to atropine.

Reactive conjunctivitis associated with *Yersinia* infection usually resolves in 1 week without treatment.

Reactive iritis should be treated with topical corticosteroids such as:

- Dexamethasone 0.1%;
- Prednisolone 0.5% or 1%.

Either of these drugs should be administered as eyedrops every hour while awake and in an equivalent concentration in ointment form at night, plus:

- Scopolamine 0.25% drops t.i.d.

In patients with reactive ocular inflammation associated with yersiniosis, antibiotic therapy should be administered only in cases in which high levels of IgM antibodies indicate recent infection, when *Yersinia* organisms can be cultured from stool samples, or when diarrhea, abdominal pain, or both are still present or closely connected with the illness.

In cases with fulminant onset of reactive ocular inflammation, systemic corticosteroids such as:

- Prednisolone 40 to 60 mg/day PO may be used; the dose should be tapered as soon as the inflammation has subsided.

The management of *Y. enterocolitica* endophthalmitis or panophthalmitis is extremely difficult, and usually eyesight is lost at this stage of the disease.

Surgical

In cases of *Yersinia* endophthalmitis or infectious keratitis, surgery may become necessary in an effort to salvage the eyes. If corneal perforation occurs:

- A corneal patch graft may be indicated to seal the perforation;
- Emergency pars plana vitrectomy may be indicated.

Vitrectomy is performed to remove infectious organisms, to confirm their identity and antibiotic sensitivity by vitreous culture, and to enable the:

- Intravitreal injection of ceftazidime 2.25 mg in 0.1 mL of isotonic saline.

The postoperative therapeutic regimen should include systemic antibiotics, daily sub-Tenon's injections of 20 to 40 mg of either gentamicin or tobramycin, or of 100 mg of ceftazidime, and the topical instillation of 14 mg/mL fortified gentamicin or 11 mg/mL fortified tobramycin every 30 minutes for the first few days, which can then be tapered as indicated.

PRECAUTIONS

Adverse effects caused by tetracyclines include nausea, enterocolitis, superinfections, and photosensitivity. Patients taking tetracyclines should not sunbathe. Products containing aluminum, magnesium, or calcium ions (antacids, milk, and milk products) decrease the absorption of tetracyclines and should not be taken during the hour before or 2 hours after an oral dose of tetracycline. Tetracyclines should be avoided during pregnancy and in children younger than 8 years because of irreversible deposition of the substance in growing bones and teeth.

Gentamicin must be used with caution in patients who have renal impairment; both nephrotoxicity and neurotoxicity with involvement of the eighth cranial nerve have been reported with the use of gentamicin.

Chloramphenicol may have severe side effects, although they are rather uncommon. Adverse effects reported with this drug include skin rashes, fever, gastrointestinal disturbance, bone marrow depression, and the gray-baby syndrome.

COMMENTS

Pyogenic ocular involvement in patients with *Yersinia* infection is very uncommon but may cause Parinaud's oculoglandular syndrome with hyperemia, edema, necrosis, and ulcer of the conjunctiva; clouding, ulcer, and perforation of the cornea; hypopyon and cataract; vascular constriction and hemorrhages of the retina; and endophthalmitis or panophthalmitis and visual loss. Pyogenic ocular manifestations in patients with yersiniosis should be treated aggressively with systemic and local antibiotics and with emergency pars plana vitrectomy if necessary.

Reactive ocular inflammation after *Yersinia* infection provides the best example of an association among acute anterior uveitis or reactive conjunctivitis, HLA-B27, and an identified infectious agent. Acute anterior uveitis is typically unilateral and resolves during corticosteroid therapy, on average during the first 6 weeks. Reactive conjunctivitis is generally mild and resolves in 1 week without any treatment. Reactive ocular inflammation associated with *Yersinia* infection often occurs with reactive arthritis, myalgia, and sacroiliitis.

REFERENCES

Cancino-Diaz JC, Vargas-Rodriguez L, Grinberg-Zylberbaum N, et al: High levels of IgG class antibodies to recombinant HSP60 kDa of *Yersinia enterocolitica* in sera of patients with uveitis. Br J Ophthalmol 88:247–250, 2004.

Chin GN, Noble RC: Ocular involvement in *Yersinia enterocolitica* infection presenting as Parinaud's oculoglandular syndrome. Am J Ophthalmol 83:19–23, 1977.

Mattila L, Granfors K, Toivanen A: Acute anterior uveitis after yersinia infection. Br J Ophthalmol 66:209–212, 1982.

Saari KM: The eye and reactive arthritis. In: Toivanen A, Toivanen P, eds: Reactive arthritis. Boca Raton, CRC, 1988:113–124.

Saari KM, Laitinen O, Lierisalo M, et al: Ocular inflammation associated with *Yersinia* infection. Am J Ophthalmol 89:84–95, 1980.

Saari KM, Maki M, Paivonsalo T, et al: Acute anterior uveitis and conjunctivitis following yersinia infection in children. Int Ophthalmol 9:237–241, 1986.

SECTION

2 Parasitic Diseases

55 ACANTHAMEBIASIS 136.9 (Acanthamoeba *Keratitis*)

John Everett Sutphin, MD
Kansas City, Kansas

ETIOLOGY/INCIDENCE

Four genera of the free-living amoebae are known to cause human disease: *Acanthamoba* spp., *Balamuthia mandrillaris, Naegleria fowleri* and *Sappinia diploidea. Naegleria* spp. were first associated with fatal meningoencephalitis in 1965. Most subsequent rapidly fatal cases have been associated with *Naegleria fowleri,* which enters through the mucous membranes and causes death within 5 to 7 days.

The more chronic form of granulomatous encephalitis has been attributed to several species of *Acanthamoeba.* In 1973, the first case of iridocyclitis attributed to *Acanthamoeba* was described, and in 1974, *Acanthamoeba* keratitis was recognized. *Acanthamoeba* spp. have been implicated in other infections, including disseminated granuloma of the skin, pneumonitis, external otitis and osteomyelitis. Keratitis is reported with eight species of *Acanthamoeba* (*A. castellani, A. polyphaga, A. hatchetti, A. culbertsoni, A. lugdunensis, A. quina, A. rhysodes* and *A. griffini*). All are in the cyst morphologic Group II except *A. culbertsoni* in Group III. These species are found predominantly in genotype group T4, but also in T3, T6, and T11.

Acanthamoeba keratitis (Figure 55.1a,b) has been reported from North and South America, Europe, Asia, Africa and Australia. The genus *Acanthamoeba* is found ubiquitously in nature, commonly in fresh water and soil, but it has also been isolated from dust, hot tubs, air filters, cooling towers, sewage, salt water and, most ominously, contact lens cases. The annual instance among contact lens wearers may be as high as 1 in 30,000.

The organism exists in the free-living form (trophozoite) and in the encysted form. Encystation is induced by changes in the environmental osmolarity or other noxious stimuli. Cysts are highly resistant to freezing, desiccation, and disinfection, including standard chlorination of the water supply.

Acanthamoeba organisms can be found as part of the normal flora of the human mouth and pharynx, and serologic evidence of immunity is present in over 80% of the population. The peak of the epidemic of keratitis in the United States was in the mid-1980s, but the infection continues to occur at a steady or an increasing rate despite improved methods of disinfection and recognition of the risk factor of the use of tap water or nonsterile saline in caring for contact lenses. *Acanthamoeba* spp. may harbor waterborne bacterial endosymbiants such as *Legionella pneumophila* and *Mycobacterium avium* among others.

COURSE/PROGNOSIS

Clinical keratitis can range from very mild, which may mimic epidemic keratoconjunctivitis or have the distinctive sign of perineuritis, to severe, with ring infiltration, descemetocele formation and perforation. The keratitis is commonly confused in its early phases with herpes simplex keratitis and may even coexist with herpes simplex. The clinician must maintain a high index of suspicion for this condition.

Keratitis typically follows exposure of an epithelially compromised cornea to a contaminated water source. Epithelial compromise includes any form of contact lens wear (daily disposable soft lenses, extended-wear soft lenses, gas-permeable, or hard polymethylmethacrylate), epithelial disease such as dry eye, herpes simplex keratitis and ocular injuries, such as abrasions or foreign bodies. Exposure to a contaminated water source can result from contact lens cases or solutions, municipal water supply, brackish water, pond or lake water, hot-tub water, or water that has been contaminated by animals. Trophozoites feed on gram-negative bacteria and cyanobacteria. Organisms prefer an environment of 25° to 35°C. The most common species are *A. culbertsoni, A. polyphaga,* and *A. castellani.*

DIAGNOSIS

Early infection begins as epitheliopathy, which progresses to subepithelial changes, followed by inflammation along the nerves; finally, as the organism progresses deeper, a double ring is seen.

- Initial stage: redness, irritation, foreign body sensation, photophobia, localized punctate staining or microcysts, pseudodendrite or corneal epithelial lines, radial perineuritis, limbitis, and mild iritis.
- Transient stage: stromal infiltrates progress to form a ring or double ring (almost pathognomonic).
- Final stage: corneal abscess, central stromal edema similar to disciform keratitis, delayed-onset subepithelial infiltrates, neurotrophic keratitis, descemetocele, severe iritis and hypopyon.

There is severe pain in any of the three stages. Steroid therapy delays diagnosis, and prognosis worsens with diagnosis that

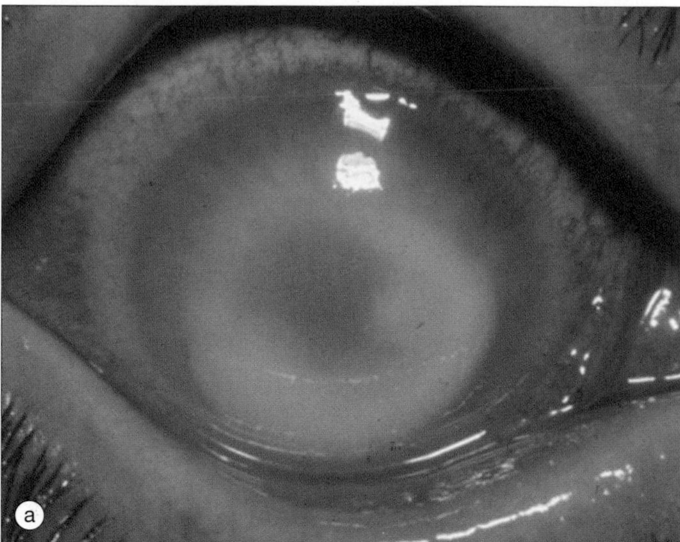

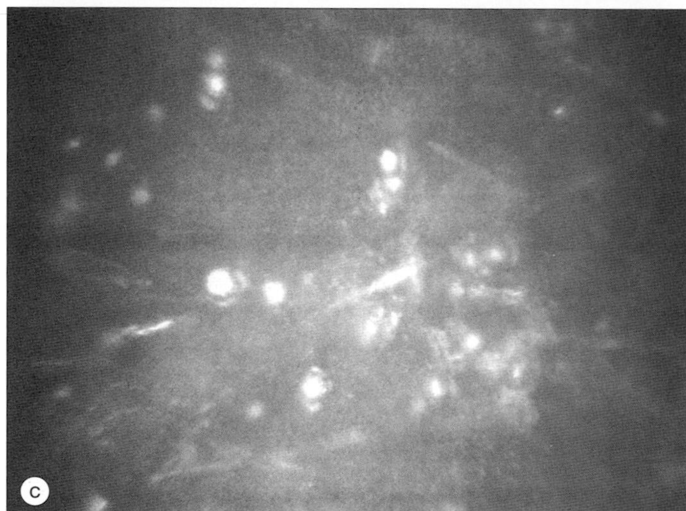

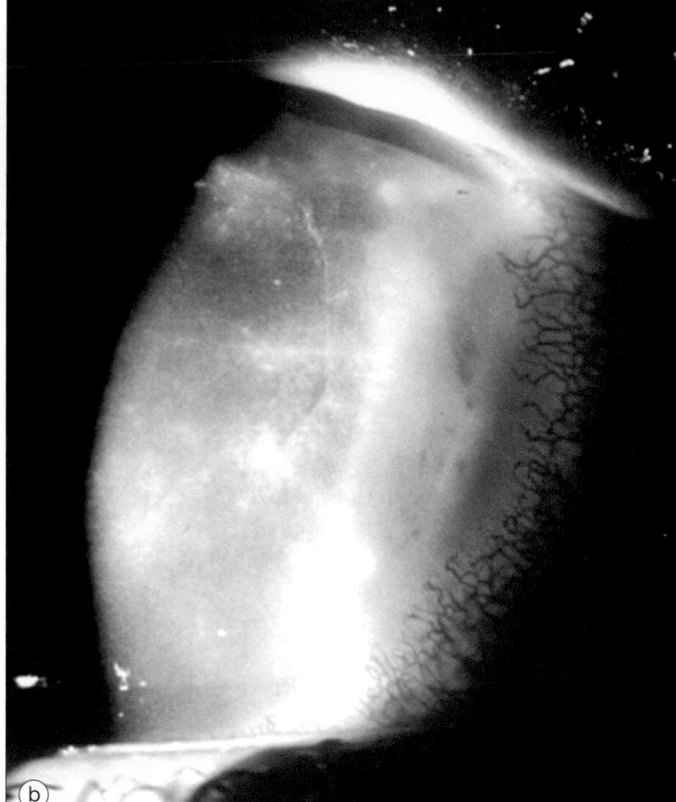

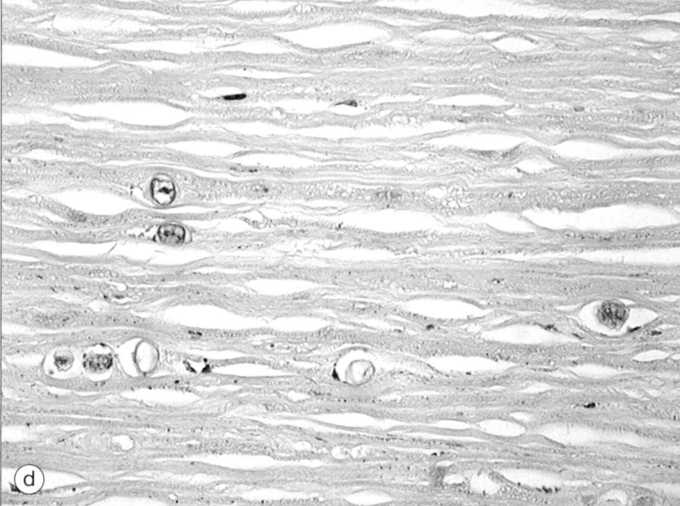

FIGURE 55.1. a) Clinical picture of advanced acanthamoeba keratitis ring infiltrate. b) Clinical picture of early acanthamoeba keratitis with perineuritis. c) Confocal microscopy showing double walled cysts of acanthamoeba. d) Histopathology of corneal button showing cysts and trophozoites in the deep cornea. (H and E)

occurs more than 4 weeks from the onset. Clinicians must have a high index of suspicion, particularly when a patient with keratitis fails to respond to the usual antibacterial, antiviral, or antifungal therapies. In a contact lens wearer with severe pain, the diagnosis must be considered early.

Laboratory findings

- Corneal scrapings under bright-field or phase-contrast microscopy or stained with hematoxylin and eosin, Gram's, Giemsa, or cellufluor white.
- Typical polygonal, double-walled cysts.
- Trophozoites show spiky appearance on electron microscopy or sharp borders with prominent karyosome and foamy cytoplasm under light microscopy.
- Cultures plated on blood agar, chocolate agar, or nonnutrient agar overlaid with killed *Escherichia coli* or *Klebsiella* spp.
- Observe plates with microscope for typical tracks of the trophozoite.
- Immunofluorescent staining of cultured amoeba or original scraping.
- Polymerase chain reaction (PCR) of amoebic RNA or DNA (mitochondrial or genomic).
- Confocal microscopy (Figure 55.1c); recognition of refractile spots of appropriate size (20 to 40 μm) representing trophozoites and cysts in the epithelium and anterior stroma.
- Advanced cases, corneal biopsy or therapeutic keratoplasty specimen for histopathology or culture (Figure 55.1d).

Differential diagnosis

- Early: herpes simplex, dendritic keratitis, epidemic keratoconjunctivitis, Thygeson's superficial punctate keratitis.
- Late: herpes simplex disciform keratitis, bacterial or fungal suppurative keratitis, other interstitial keratitis.

PROPHYLAXIS

- Contact lens care system with amoebecidal disinfection (e.g. chlorhexidine, PHMB or hydrogen peroxide).
- Avoidance of contaminated water.

TREATMENT

Diagnosis and initiation of treatment earlier than 4 weeks after onset results in a much-improved prognosis. Treatment requires intense therapy for 72 to 96 hours followed by continuing treatment for at least 6 to 12 months. Confocal can be used to determine if persisting inflammation is from residual infection or toxicity of the medications (Figure 55.2).

Ocular

- Debridement of affected epithelium (may have to be repeated).
- Combination therapy.
- A biguanide:
  - Polymeric-polyhexamethyl biguanide (PHMB) 0.02% (Baquacil) or bisbiguanide-chlorhexidine 0.02%;
  - Used every hour in the affected eye for 72 to 96 hours, then every 2 hours for 2 to 4 weeks and gradual reduction to 4 times a day for 6 to 12 months; and
- A diamidine:
  - Hexamidine 0.1% (Desmomodine, available in France) or propaminidine 0.1% (Brolene, available in the United Kingdom);
  - Used every hour for 24 to 48 hours, followed by 4 times a day for 2 to 4 months or as tolerated.
- Additional topical treatment: neomycin, paromycin (Humatin), ketoconazole, or clotrimazole.

Combination of PHMB and chlorhexidine for difficult cases. Rarely chlorhexidine 0.04% or 0.10% has been used.

Systemic

- Imidazoles or triazoles including voriconazole itraconazole, ketoconazole, and fluconazole for deeper lesions and scleritis.
- Pentamidine isethionate (4 mg/kg Q 24 hours) intravenously for recalcitrant keratitis, scleritis or endophthalmitis.

Surgical

- Repeat debridement of epithelium with persisting stromal disease despite adequate topical treatment to remove organisms and improve drug penetration.
- Penetrating keratoplasty best after medical control, which may take 12 months.
- Deep anterior lamellar keratectomy, particularly if the infection threatens the sclera.
- Gunderson or total conjunctival flaps do not work to resolve the infection.
- Adjunctive cryotherapy not helpful.

Other

- Choice of biguanide (PHMB or chlorhexidine) may depend on availability and purity of base chemical.
- Effectiveness depends on lipid permeability (hexamidine greater than propamidine).
- Topical and systemic steroid use controversial; steroid therapy not associated with worse prognosis other than from delay in diagnosis; systemic steroid needed for scleritis; steroid use requires adequate amebicidal therapy concurrently.
- Direct antiamoebic sensitivity testing of clinical isolate needed for recalcitrant cases.
- PHMB and chlorhexidine may be synergistic.
- Some authorities use PHMB or chlorhexidine as single agent.

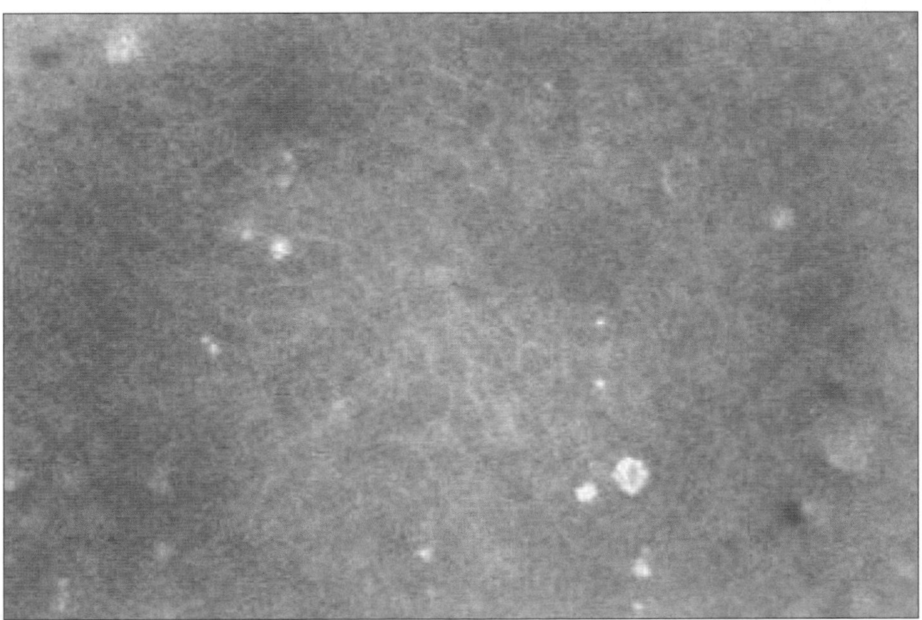

FIGURE 55.2. Confocal microscopy in the resolving phase of acanthamoeba keratitis showing persistent organisms.

- Epithelial toxicity may be confused with ongoing infection; repeat diagnostic testing such as epithelial scraping or confocal microscopy may guide therapeutic decisions.

COMPLICATIONS

- Indolent course requiring long-term treatment or adjunctive therapy with bandage contact lens.
- Progression to stromal necrosis or endophthalmitis.
- Descemetocele.
- Corneal perforation.
- Intractable pain.
- Inflammatory glaucoma.
- Keratoplasty.
- Enucleation.
- Drug toxicity; pain and burning; conjunctival ulceration; keratopathy.

SUMMARY

Acanthamoeba keratitis may mimic mild corneal disease in its early stages but can progress to severe intractable pain associated with the typical perineuritis followed by a ring infiltrate. Although commonly associated with contact lens wear and improper sterilization, it is also seen following other forms of ocular injury in which there is a history of contamination by soil or brackish or inadequately treated water. Early diagnosis is key to effect medical cure, and the prognosis of surgical therapy improves following adequate medical treatment with a biguanide, minimally, but preferably in association with a diamidine. Systemic imidazole or triazole (antifungal) therapy may be helpful in the deeper forms of keratitis or scleritis.

REFERENCES

Graham MD, Dart JKG, Morlet N, et al: Outcome of *Acanthamoeba* keratitis treated with polyhexamethyl biguanide and propamidine. Ophthalmology 104:1587–1592, 1997.

Johns KJ, Head WS, O'Day DM: Corneal toxicity of propamidine. Arch Ophthalmol 106:68–69, 1988.

Kahn NA: Pathogenesis of *Acanthamoeba* infections. Microbial Pathogenesis 34:277–285, 2003.

Kirkness CM, Hay J, Seal DV, et al: *Acanthamoeba* keratitis. Ophthalmol Clin North Am 7:605–616, 1994.

Mathers WD, Goldberg MA, Sutphin JE, et al: Coexistent *Acanthamoeba* keratitis and herpetic keratitis. Arch Ophthalmol 115:714–718, 1997.

McClellan K, Howard K, Niederkorn JY, Alizabeh H: Effects of steroids on *Acanthamoeba* cysts and trophozoites. IOVS 42(12):2885–2893, 2001.

Nwachuku N, Gerba CP: Health effects of *Acanthamoeba* spp. and its potential for waterborne transmission: Rev Environ Contam Toxicol 180:93–131, 2004.

Schuster FL, Visvesvara GS: Opportunistic amoebae: challenges in prophylaxis and treatment. Drug Resistance Updates 7:41–51, 2004. Review.

Seal D: *Acanthamoeba* keratitis update — incidence, molecular epidemiology and new drugs for treatment. Eye 17:893–905, 2003.

Seal D, Hay J, Kirkness C, et al: Successful medical therapy of *Acanthamoeba* keratitis with topical chlorhexidine and propamidine. Eye 10(pt. 4):413–421, 1996.

Zanetti S, Fiori PL, Pinna A, et al: Susceptibility of *Acanthamoeba castellanii* to contact lens disinfecting solutions. Antimicrob Agents Chemother 39:1596–1598, 1995.

56 BAYLISASCARIS 363.05

(A Type of Diffuse Unilateral Subacute Neuroretinitis, Ocular Larva Migrans)

Lawrence A. Raymond, MD
Cincinnati, Ohio

The size and morphology and the serologic and epidemiologic findings provide evidence that the common raccoon roundworm, *Baylisascaris procyonis*, is a cause of the large-nematode variant of diffuse unilateral subacute neuroretinitis (DUSN). DUSN represents a type of ocular larva migrans (OLM) in which loss of vision is due to parasite-induced inflammation of the retina, retinal vessels, and optic disk. A motile nematode in the patient's retina confirms the diagnosis of DUSN. OLM or DUSN develops from the chance migration of a nematode larva to the eye by ingestion of a single infective egg. Laser treatment destroys the migrating worm in the retina of patients.

ETIOLOGY/INCIDENCE

- *Baylisascaris procyonis, Toxocara canis* (from puppy or young dog), and *Ancylostoma caninum* have been linked as potential causes of DUSN and OLM.
- Clinical and pathologic lesions in the eyes of experimental animals infected orally with *B. procyonis* correlate well with suspected human cases of DUSN and OLM.
- The length of the motile larva in the retina of *B. procyonis* ranges between 400 and 2000 microns, although the usual length is between 1000 and 2000 microns. The retinal larva of *T. canis* is smaller, ranging between 350 and 445 microns. It is a possible cause of the small-nematode variant of DUSN and OLM.
- *B. procyonis* is a widespread and important cause of visceral larva migrans and brain disease in lower animals in North America. Raccoons are commonly infected with *B. procyonis*, with prevalence rates as high as 68%–82%.

COURSE/PROGNOSIS

- Typical of the clinical course is the first report of a motile retinal nematode, matching the size of *B. procyonis* and causing DUSN in a 13-year-old healthy girl in 1976. She had acquired a pet raccoon 6 weeks prior to her monocular symptoms of a moving shadow, night blindness, a constricted visual field, and blurred central vision.
- In an otherwise healthy patient, the prognosis for stabilization of vision and visual field is excellent if the motile nematode larva in the retina is treated promptly with laser photocoagulation, avoiding the fovea. The motile worm will sometimes disappear from view in the retina and then reappear, so prompt laser treatment is needed.
- Two deaths were reported in 1984 and 1985 in children as a result of eosinophilic meningoencephalitis. *B. procyonis* was confirmed as the parasite during examination of the brain tissue.

DIAGNOSIS

Clinical signs and symptoms

- Retina: retinal or subretinal tracks with or without motile worm, recurrent evanescent gray-white lesions of retinitis, absent or a few small hemorrhages, focal or diffuse hypopigmented tracks in the pigment layer, pigment migration, sheathed or narrowed vessels or both, subretinal mass (granuloma).
- Choroid: sometimes small infiltrates or scars.
- Optic disk: edema, pallor.
- Vitreous: vitreitis.
- Ciliary body: snowbanking in pars plana.
- Iris: iritis.
- Transient unilateral blackouts in vision lasting a few seconds may indicate optic disk edema.

Laboratory findings

The motile nematode in the retina is diagnostic of DUSN or OLM. The subretinal tracks, created by the larger-nematode larva such as *B. procyonis*, are commonly visible nearby. The Goldmann fundus contact lens or the 78D or 90D funduscopic lenses are useful to find the motile larva.

- Serum can be examined for antibodies to *B. procyonis* by indirect immunofluorescence and *T. canis* by enzyme-linked immunosorbent assay (ELISA) and Western blot analysis. *Toxocara* ELISA is available from the Centers for Disease Control and Prevention (Atlanta, GA).
- Unless peripheral eosinophilia or neurologic disease (neural larva migrans) is present, no further investigation is necessary.

Differential diagnosis

- Pigment mottling in the retina caused by the tracks of a motile worm (pseudoretinitis pigmentosa) resembles retinitis pigmentosa.

PROPHYLAXIS

- Risk of transmission of *B. procyonis* to humans exists through ingestion of eggs from feces of raccoons. These eggs remain viable and infective in the soil for months to years.
- Risk of transmission is increased because raccoons commonly live in residential and recreational areas.
- Children are especially at risk through accidental hand-to-mouth transfer of infective *B. procyonis* eggs.
- Raccoons defecate on downed logs, on hearths or decks of homes and in barns.
- Places where raccoons have nested or have been caged should be avoided.
- Handwashing should be done immediately after contact with soil or waste material contaminated by raccoons.

TREATMENT

Systemic

- The anthelmintic oral agent, thiabendazole, appears to have varying success for small-nematode larva such as *T. canis* in DUSN.

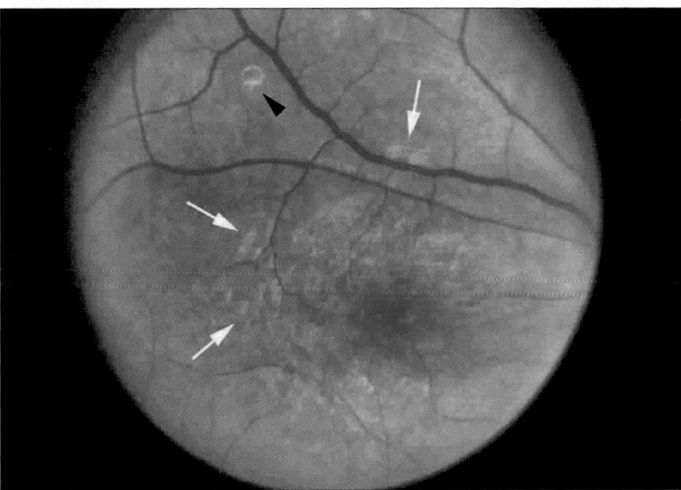

FIGURE 56.1. A 2000 micron long motile larva (arrowhead) is superotemporal to the right macula, with hypopigmented subretinal tracks (arrows) in a 13-year-old girl, who had a pet raccoon. Prompt photocoagulation destroyed the larva.

Laser surgery

- Prompt laser photocoagulation of the motile worm in the retina is preferred as the most effective treatment of DUSN. The fovea is avoided during laser treatment (Figure 56.1).

Surgery

- Difficulty in identifying the worm has been reported with surgical excision of the motile nematode larva.

REFERENCES

Fox AS, Kazacos KR, Gould NS, et al: Fatal eosinophilic meningoencephalitis and visceral larva migrans caused by the raccoon ascarid, *Baylisascaris procyonis.* N Engl J Med 312:1619–1623, 1985.

Gass JDM, Callanan DG, Bowman CB: Oral therapy in diffuse unilateral subacute neuroretinitis. Arch Ophthalmol 110:675–680, 1992.

Gass JDM, Gilbert WR, Jr, Guerry RK, Scelfo R: Diffuse unilateral subacute neuroretinitis. Ophthalmology 85:521–545, 1977.

Goldberg MA, Kazacos KR, Boyce WM, Ai E, Katz B: Diffuse unilateral subacute neuroretinitis: morphometric, serologic, and epidemiologic support for *Baylisascaris* as a causative agent. Ophthalmology 100:1695–1701, 1993.

Huff DS, Neafie RC, Binder MJ, et al: The first fatal *Baylisascaris* infection in humans: an infant with eosinophilic meningoencephalitis. Pediatr Pathol 2:345–352, 1984.

Kazacos KR, Raymond LA, Kazacos EA, Vestre WA: The raccoon ascarid: a probable cause of human ocular larva migrans. Ophthalmology 92:1735–1744, 1985.

Kazacos KR, Vestre WA, Kazacos EA, Raymond LA: Diffuse unilateral subacute neuroretinitis syndrome: probable cause. Arch Ophthalmol 102:967–968, 1984.

Mets MB, Noble AG, Basti S, et al: Eye findings of diffuse unilateral subacute neuroretinitis and multiple choroidal infiltrates associated with neural larva migrans due to *Baylisascaris procyonis.* Am J Ophthalmol 135:888–890, 2003.

Pork SY, Glaser C, Murray WJ, et al: Raccoon roundworm (*Baylisascaris procyonis*) encephalitis: case report and field investigation. Pediatrics 106:56–60, 2000.

Raymond LA, Gutierrez Y, Strong LE, et al: Living retinal nematode (filarial-like) destroyed with photocoagulation. Ophthalmology 85:944–949, 1978.

57 COENUROSIS 123.8

Lihteh Wu, MD
San José, Costa Rica
J. Fernando Arévalo, MD
Caracas, Venezuela
Teodoro Evans, MD
San José, Costa Rica
Saylin Iturriaga, MD
San José, Costa Rica

ETIOLOGY/INCIDENCE

When an intermediate host becomes infected with the cystic larval stage of any of the four species of dog tapeworm: *Taenia multiceps*, *Taenia serialis*, *Taenia glomerata* and *Taenia brauni*, the ensuing disease is known as coenurosis. A coenurus is a fluid filled thin-walled cyst containing many scoleces that are attached in rows on its internal membrane. It measures from a few millimeters to several centimeters in diameter. The absence of daughter cysts differentiates it from the hydatids. The multiple scoleces distinguish it from the cysticercus that has a single scolex.

Adult tapeworms develop in dogs or other canids that ingest coenuri in the tissues of various intermediate hosts. These hosts include sheep, goats, hares, rabbits, rodents, gerbils and other herbivores. Each scolex within a coenurus can mature into an adult tapeworm after ingestion by a canid host. Adult worms produce eggs, which are passed in the feces. Human coenurosis results when humans accidentally ingest mature eggs, usually in contaminated fruits or vegetables, becoming incidental intermediate hosts. The coenuri are carried by the bloodstream into the central nervous system (CNS), eye, orbit, subcutaneous or intramuscular tissues. In a very rare case, subperitoneal spread ocurred pressing on bile ducts and causing obstructive jaundice. Larvae may be inoculated directly into a child's conjunctiva and skin as the child plays on contaminated ground.

Approximately 100 cases of coenurosis have been reported, primarily in Africa, with the remainder in Europe, North and South America. Only a handful of cases of ocular coenurosis have been reported in the literature.

DIAGNOSIS

Clinical signs and symptoms

Symptoms are the result of toxic and allergenic metabolites and pressure effects. Interestingly, the cases in central Africa rarely involved the CNS, whereas more than 75% of the cases elsewhere had CNS involvement. Coenuri cysts in the brain may cause ventricular obstruction, giving rise to raised intracranial pressure. Patients with coenurosis present with headache and papilledema. Other neurological findings include jacksonian epilepsy, hemiplegia, monoplegia, cerebellar ataxia and spastic paraplegia.

The initial ocular manifestations are rather nonspecific. Slight pain, redness may be present. If the cyst bursts severe glaucoma and uveitis ensues. Visual loss depends on the size and site of the cyst and vitreous haze. Several cases have been documented in the subretinal space and in the periocular tissues.

Laboratory findings

If the cyst is located sunconjuntivally, in the anterior segment or the vitreous it is easily identified by direct examination. There are no specific diagnostic tests. On CT scans viable cysts appear as lucent lesions surrounded by a contrast-enhanced peripheral rim. Multiple echo MRI sequences reveal that the intensity of the cyst contents is similar to that of CSF. False positive Casoni and hydatid complement fixation tests do occur. Eosinophilia may be present in 3% of cases.

TREATMENT

Medical

There is no specific pharmacologic therapy for coenurosis. Since 50 mg/kg/day of praziquantel in divided doses for 14 days has been successful in the treatment of cysticercosis, it has been recommended in coenurosis. If a response is not seen within a week, surgical evacuation should be attempted. Specific ocular manifestations such as glaucoma and uveitis should be treated accordingly with hypotensive agents, cycloplegics and steroids.

Surgical

The natural history of an intraocular coenurus is very poor, often requiring enucleation. Therefore surgical extraction should always be attempted. The surgical approach will depend on the exact location of the coenurus. Wide angle viewing coupled to modern vitreoretinal techniques including subretinal surgery, should permit access to the cyst in most cases.

REFERENCES

Boase AJ: *Coenurus* cyst in eye. Br J Ophthalmol 40:183–185, 1956.

Epstein E, Proctor NSE, Heinz J: Intraocular coenurosis infestation. S Afr Med J 33:602–604, 1959.

Ibechukwu BI, Onwukene KE: Intraocular *Coenurus*. Br J Ophthalmol 75:430–431, 1991.

Ing MB, Schantz PM, Turner JA: Human coenurosis in North America: case reports and review. Clinical Infectious Diseases 27:519–523, 1998.

Manschot WA: *Coenurus* infestation of eye and orbit. Arch Ophthalmol 94(6):961–964, 1976.

Williams PH, Templeton AC: Infection of the eye by tapeworm *Coenurus*. Br J Ophthalmol 55:766–769, 1971.

58 CYSTICERCOSIS 123.1

Shishir Agrawal, MS, DNB, FRCS, MRCOphth, FRF
Meerut, Uttar Pradesh, India
Jaya Agrawal, MS, DNB, MNAMS, FRCS
Meerut, Uttar Pradesh, India
Trilok P. Agrawal, MS
Meerut, Uttar Pradesh, India

ETIOLOGY/INCIDENCE/PATHOGENESIS

The two commoner tapeworms/flatworms (cestodes) are *Taenia saginata* and *Taenia solium*; these cause taeniasis. Cysticercosis is the infestation of humans by *Cysticercus cellulosae*, the larval form of *Taenia solium* or the pork tapeworm. It is the most common ocular tapeworm infestation occurring in endemic regions such as Africa, South-East Asia (Indian subcontinent), Mexico, South America and Eastern Europe. Cysticercosis continues to be a public health problem even in the developed nations due to easy air travel.

Man is the definitive host. The adult worm, consisting of a head or scolex with its double row of hooks and four suckers, neck and segments or proglottids, inhabits the human small intestine. The terminal gravid segments are passed into the feces and eaten by pig, the usual intermediate host. On reaching its alimentary canal, these hatch, penetrate the gut wall to gain entrance into the systemic circulation and the naked oncospheres are ultimately filtered out into the striated muscles and various tissues, where they undergo development, encyst and expand into fluid-filled bladders to form cysticerci. These are ellipsoid bodies with an opalescent transparency measuring 0.1 to 2 cm with a dense milky white spot at the side where the scolex remains invaginated. Man can also act as an intermediate host and harbor the cyst, which is termed as cysticercosis. In humans, ingestion of ova via improperly cooked pork, or food (vegetables)/water contaminated with eggs, or by autoinfection (either from contaminated hands or by reverse peristaltic movements) leads to cysticercosis. It is to be noted that infection can occur even in those who don't eat pork via food prepared by an infected individual from an endemic region.

DIAGNOSIS

Clinical signs and symptoms

Systemic

Taeniasis causes only minor clinical problems in the form of gastrointestinal disturbances and pruritis ani. Cysticerci can be found in subcutaneous tissue, skeletal muscles, central nervous system, viscerae and eyes. Although only a mild tissue reaction occurs with a few viable cysticerci, heavy infestation can cause more marked generalized symptoms. Symptoms in cysticercosis occur mainly from invasion of the central nervous system (parenchymal, meningeal, ventricular and spinal). There could be mild neurological manifestations to severe epileptiform attacks, when the patient may fall and be injured. In neurocysticercosis, acute meningoencephalitic symptoms may ensue. Other symptoms include headache, lethargy, weakness, etc. Intracranial hypertension and hydrocephalous, and death may occur from blockage of the circulatory pathway of cerebrospinal fluid. Both living and calcified dead cysts cause neurological disturbances. Cysticerci can remain alive for 3 to 5 years. Subcutaneous nodules may be palpable.

Ocular

In and around the eye, the cyst can invade almost any ocular, orbital or adnexal tissue:

- Retina (subretinal or intraretinal);
- Vitreous;
- Orbit (extraocular muscle or retro-orbital space);
- Conjunctiva (subconjunctival);
- Eyelid;
- Optic nerve;
- Anterior chamber;
- Lens;
- Iris;
- Cornea; or
- Lacrimal gland.

Intraocular posterior segment cysticercosis, i.e. vitreal and subretinal, is a common occurrence. Cysticerci reach the subretinal space through posterior ciliary arteries, from where they migrate into the vitreous through a pre-existing retinal break or by perforating the retina, which usually seals with inflammatory reaction forming a chorioretinal scar. The parasite has a predilection for the macular region, presumably because of vascularity of the region (Figure 58.1a). The patient presents with a painless diminution of vision. The subretinal cyst may initially present as an acute retinitis with exudates and hemorrhages; peripheral cysticercus may be asymptomatic, or the patient presenting with floaters. The clinical picture of a translucent cyst in the vitreous with a scolex, which may be invaginated or evaginated, is unmistakable. Contractions and undulating movements of the cyst are often observed, more so on throwing ophthalmoscopic indirect light, when the scolex will invaginate (Figure 58.1b). As a reaction to the cyst, serous

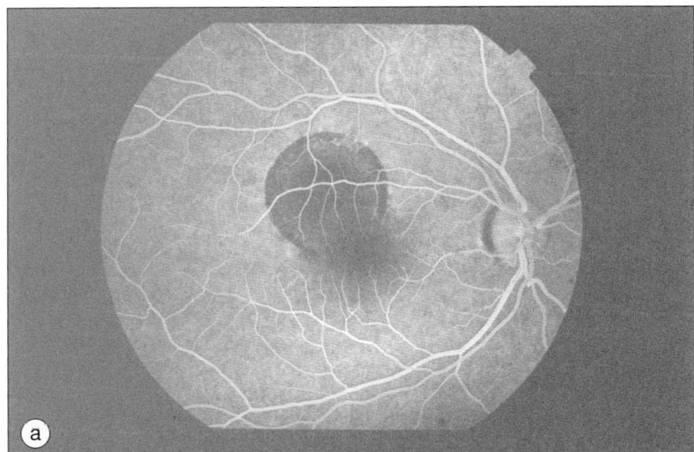

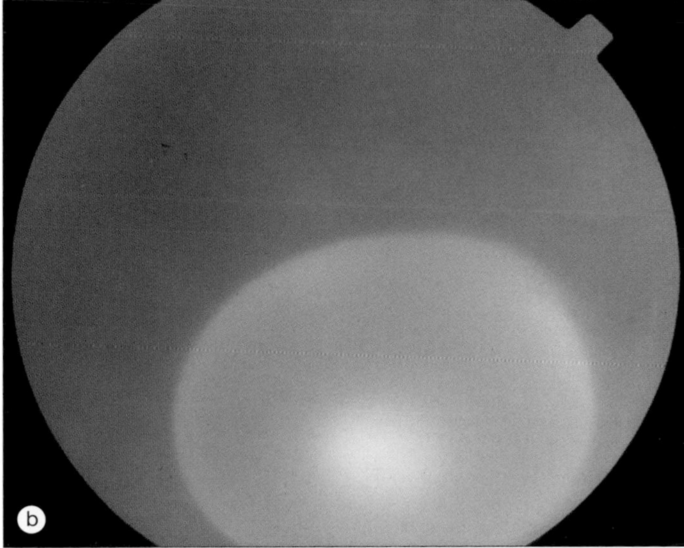

FIGURE 58.1. Intraocular and orbital/adnexal cysticercosis. a) Subretinal cysticercus, seen as a black shadow (from masking of the background fluorescence) on this fluorescein angiogram. The macula is the preferred site because of vascularity of the area. There is an absence of inflammatory reaction at this early stage. The patient presents with a painless diminished vision initially (in this case of 4 days). b) Intravitreal cysticercosis having a dense white spot suggestive of the scolex.

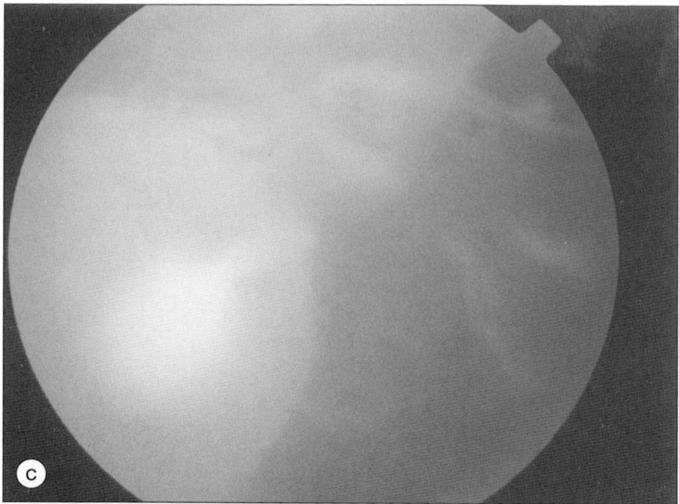

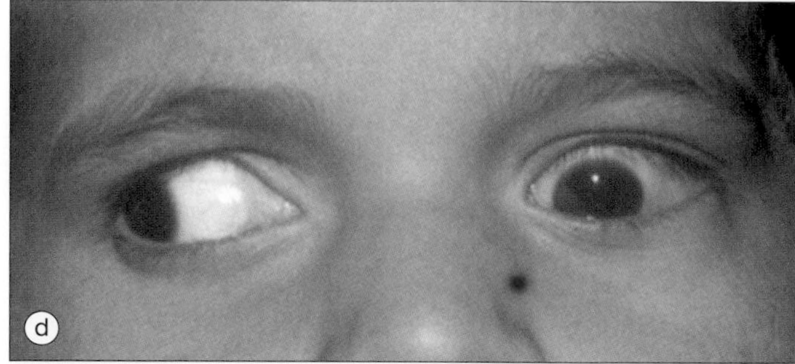

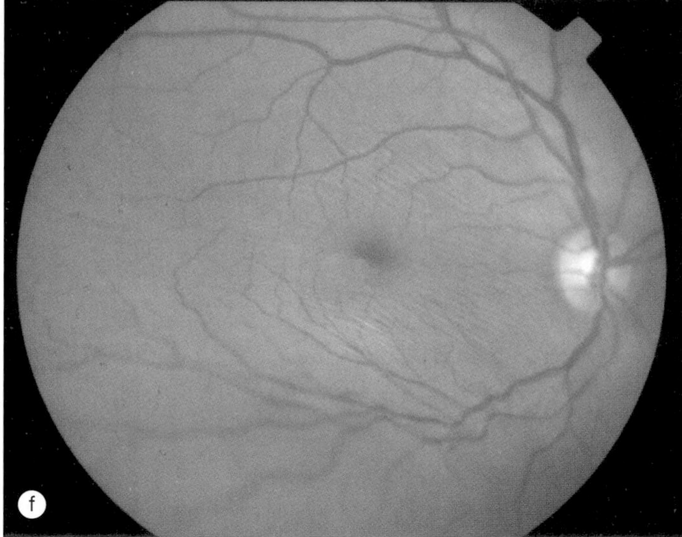

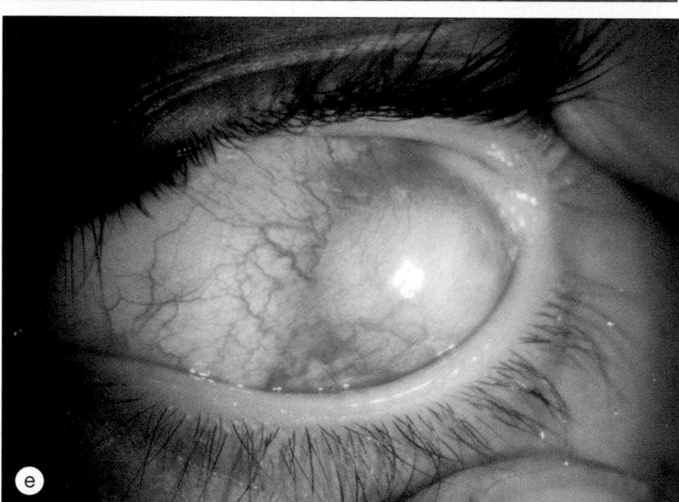

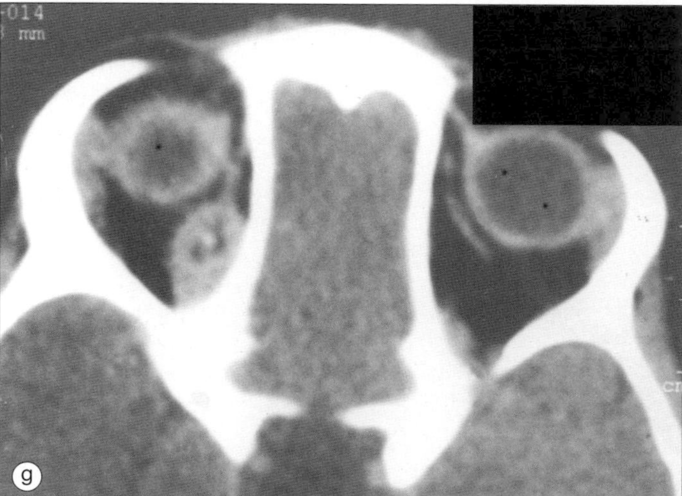

FIGURE 58.1., cont'd c) Subretinal cysticercosis presents with a loss of vision; there is severe intraocular inflammation with an exudative retinal detachment. d) Orbital myocysticercosis. A child typically presents with proptosis, restricted ocular motility and redness. He is a vegetarian; the infection is commonly acquired through contaminated food in endemic regions such as India. On dextroversion, there is a restricted left eye movement. The cyst is present along the left lateral rectus, which was confirmed on CT scanning. This clinical picture is pathognomonic. e) A subconjunctival cysticercus, which will extrude out any time. It commonly extrudes spontaneously, the patient sometimes coming with the cyst in his hand. At times, this might have to be removed by giving a small cut on the conjunctiva and tenon's capsule, when the cysticercus comes out along with a pus bead. f) Pseudo-retinal detachment. A solid-looking retinal elevation with striae caused by an orbital cysticercus, pushing the eyeball and indenting it. The patient presented with diminished vision in the presence of symptoms and signs of orbital inflammation. g) CT scan showing the cysticercus along the medial rectus, with an eccentric shadow of the scolex.

or exudative retinal detachment occurs (Figure 58.1c). Chorioretinitis, vitritis and severe anterior uveitis will often ensue; pain and redness from uveitis follows. Inflammation can cause tractional or combined tractional-rhegmatogenous retinal detachment; fibrous proliferations occur. Retinal detachment and proliferative vitreoretinopathy may form. Once the cyst dies its contents are spilled; the panuveitis secondary to release of toxins can lead to destruction of the globe and phthisis bulbi. Bilateral multiple cysticerci may be found.

Extraocular muscle and subconjunctival tissue are the two commonest sites of presentation of extraocular/adnexal cysticercosis; involvement occurring probably through anterior ciliary arteries. These have been more common in reports from India. Extraocular muscle cysticercosis, the commonest form of orbital cysticercosis, typically presents with signs of orbital inflammation — a red eye, restricted ocular motility and/or proptosis. A painful inflammatory proptosis with restricted ocular motility when present in an individual with a history of exposure to an endemic area is diagnostic of myocysticercosis. Though it occurs at any age, the majority of patients are usually children and young adults in their first two or three decades. The lesion excites a recurrent severe inflammatory reaction resulting in considerable pain accompanied by edema and chemosis. There is a decreased ocular motility in the direction of action of the involved muscle and a restriction of the opposite movement (diplopia) (Figure 58.1d). The presentation is characteristic and pathognomonic. A localized redness and nodule formation is present (Figure 58.1e). Although mentioned as two different primary sites, in our experience, subconjunctival cysts appear to be secondary to extrusion from extraocular muscles, which is the actual primary site. We have seen it in a large number of orbital cysticerci cases (49 patients) that myocysticerci are precursors of subconjunctival cysticerci, which finally extrude out spontaneously (Agrawal S, unpublished work, 2003). Involvement of levator palpebrae superioris results in ptosis. Superior oblique muscle cysticercosis may present as Brown syndrome. Myocysticerci cases usually have a single cyst with no systemic involvement. Bilateral/multiple cysts are rarely found.

At times, fundus appearance of a solid-looking retinal detachment caused by orbital cysticercosis mechanically indenting the eyeball can be seen, all the three coats of the eyeball pushed in from outside (very well supported by ultrasonography (USG) and computed tomography (CT) scan). The term pseudo-retinal detachment has been coined for it because it is not a true retinal detachment, there being no subretinal fluid. Retinal striae support the mechanical nature of the lesion (Figure 58.1f). Such patients present with diminished vision and associated signs of orbital inflammation — localized recurrent inflammation with conjunctival congestion, restriction of ocular movements and/or proptosis.

Other forms are less common. Cysticercus may present with cranial nerve palsies, papilledema or optic neuritis. Rarely it can pass the vitreous and lens, and enter the anterior chamber, where it causes a severe anterior uveitis. The leucocytes in the anterior chamber are mostly eosinophils.

Investigations

The segments/eggs can be found in the fecal sample; perianal swabbing is important in diagnosis of taeniasis. An adult patient presenting with epilepsy for the first time should be suspected of having neurocysticercosis, especially with history of exposure to a hyperendemic area. These patients may have subcutaneous nodules (in 50%). Radiologic examination of the limbs and skull may show calcified cysts. Contrast-enhanced CT scan and magnetic resonance imaging (MRI) are required for brain and other lesions. USG may also be required for different visceral pathologies. Skin/subcutaneous nodule biopsy is diagnostic. Eosinophilia may be found in blood. Serological tests like indirect hemagglutination (IHA) (positive in 85% of patients and titers of 1 : 64 considered diagnostic) and complement fixation may be used; however, these cross-react with hydatid antigen, etc., and also give false positives in patients who only have adult worm infestation. A cerebrospinal fluid complement fixation test is more specific. ELISA (enzyme-linked immunosorbent assay) for anticysticercus IgG is more sensitive but again cross-reacts with *Taenia saginata/Echinococcus/Coenurus*. Enzyme-linked immunoelectro transfer blot (EITB) assay is highly sensitive and specific (98%).

When clinical presentation suggests ocular cysticercosis but doubts arise (e.g. due to hazy media), diagnostic aids such as USG, CT scan or MRI are useful. Orbital/adnexal cysticercosis is conclusively diagnosed by these methods (Figure 58.1g) — USG being most economical. Finding a cyst with an eccentric shadow of the scolex is pathognomonic. Fluorescein angiography may delineate a subretinal cyst. Aqueous humor tap can be screened for circulating antibody and antigen.

Differential diagnosis

Epilepsy, brain tumors, and other types of neurologic and psychiatric disorders may be simulated in neurocysticercosis. Diagnosis of ocular cases may be difficult in the presence of media haze from inflammation; in children different causes of leukocoria have to be ruled out. Orbital cases may present as cellulitis, pseudotumor or subconjunctival abscess.

PROPHYLAXIS

Infection is prevented by eating thoroughly cooked pork (56°C for 5 minutes), properly washed and boiled vegetables, drinking clean water and by maintaining personal hygiene.

TREATMENT — MEDICAL AND SURGICAL

Systemic

Praziquantel (50 mg/kg/day) had been the drug of choice for taeniasis and cysticercosis. Albendazole (15 mg/kg/day) has been found to be more effective (penetrates better and achieves larvicidal concentrations) and cheap, and is fast replacing other drugs. Stools should be rechecked in 3 months. For cysticercosis, systemic removal of the cyst is recommended whenever possible. Destruction of the cysts in cerebral cysticercosis by anticysticercals may induce severe side effects from an inflammatory response. Corticosteroids (1.5 mg/kg/day) are used in these cases. Niclosamide (2 g) is another drug used. Old dead cysts are left as such. Asymptomatic subcutaneous nodules do not require treatment.

Ocular

The best course in cases of intraocular cysticercosis is the removal of the cyst by surgery, lest it causes irreversible damage. There has been concern of an exaggerated inflammatory response from release of toxins leading to destruction of the globe and phthisis bulbi following death of the parasite; hence antihelminthics are avoided. As a result of reaction to the cyst and its content, inflammation/exudative retinal detachment is often present. Corticosteroids are used to control the intraocular inflammation when present, and surgery should be performed under cover of steroids. Pars plana vitrectomy and removal of the intravitreal cyst should be undertaken at the earliest opportunity. The cyst can be aspirated into the port of the cutter — this requires care to be taken as it tends to shy away from the endoilluminator light. If the cyst is damaged, a thorough lavage of the vitreous cavity with fluid is in order to reduce the resulting severe inflammatory response. Subretinal cysts can be easily evacuated transvitreally by the vitrectomy procedure via retinotomy, or transclerally by giving a nick on the sclera over the base of the cyst (after it has been accurately localized), treatment of the scleral bed with diathermy and incision of the choroid, ensuring that the cyst has not moved during preparation of the site, with or without scleral buckling. Postoperatively, corticosteroids will have to be continued for a few weeks to suppress inflammation.

As with intraocular cysticercosis, it is better that the orbital cysts be extruded rather than killed inside. However, surgery for orbital myocysticercosis is fraught with complications as it may damage important orbital structures (because the cyst is adherent to the surrounding structures) or cause inflammatory reactions, and is best avoided. Corticosteroids and anti-inflammatory drugs are given to suppress the inflammation. Recently, cysticidal drugs such as albendazole (200–400 mg twice daily for one month) and praziquantel have been given to kill the parasite with good results, confirmed by USG. We have noticed that the cysticerci of the extraocular muscles travel forward, come to lie in a subconjunctival location and then extrude spontaneously. We have adopted a policy to wait and watch in these cases. We avoid giving steroids and antihelminthics as these suppress inflammation and delay the movement of the cyst outward, and hence, its extrusion. A subconjunctival cyst will usually extrude spontaneously; however, sometimes it requires to be removed by making a nick on the conjunctiva and tenons, allowing it to squeeze out along with any pus.

Cysts occurring in other places are best removed whenever possible.

REFERENCES

Agrawal S, Agrawal J, Agrawal TP: Orbital cysticercosis-associated scleral indentation presenting with pseudo-retinal detachment. Am J Ophthalmol 137(6):1153–1155, 2004.

Agrawal S, Agrawal J, Agrawal TP: Traveling cysticercosis — from orbital (extraocular muscle) to subconjunctival location and the final extrusion/ surgical removal. Video presented at: American Academy of Ophthalmology annual meeting, New Orleans, Louisiana, USA, October 23–26, 2004.

Cano MR: Ocular cysticercosis. In: Ryan SJ, ed: Retina. 3rd edn. St Louis, Mosby, 2001:1553–1557.

Pushker N, Bajaj MS, Chandra M, et al: Ocular and orbital cysticercosis. Acta Ophthalmol Scand 79(4):408–413, 2001.

Ryan ET, Maguire JH: Cysticercosis. In: Albert DM, Jakobiec FA, eds: Principles and practice of ophthalmology. 2nd edn. Philadelphia, Saunders, 2000:4930–4931.

Sekhar GC, Lemke BN: Orbital cysticercosis. Ophthalmology 104(10):1599–1604, 1997.

Sharma T, Sinha S, Shah N, et al: Intraocular cysticercosis: clinical characteristics and visual outcome after vitreoretinal surgery. Ophthalmology 110(5):996–1004, 2003.

Sihota R, Honavar SG: Oral albendazole in the management of extraocular cysticercosis. Br J Ophthalmol 78(8):621–623, 1994.

59 DEMODICOSIS 133.8

William D. Mathers
Portland, Oregon

ETIOLOGY/INCIDENCE

Demodectic infestation of humans is characterized by the presence of two congenic species on the same host: *Demodex folliculorum*, which is found in the hair and eyelash follicles, and *Demodex brevis*, which infests the meibomian and sebaceous glands and the gland component of the pilosebaceous unit. Recently, on routine sectioning of eyelids, this shorter acarid was also noted in a follicle, as the section included its egg. These metazoans are ubiquitous in the adult population with the highest infestations found in the facial area — the eyelids, eyebrows, forehead, and nasal region. They are also found in the oral, mammary, axillary, and pubic regions. All phases of their development can be seen, including the immature and mature stages.

D. folliculorum lies in the hair follicle with its head downward and feet facing the epithelial surface. The sharp chelicerae puncture epithelial cells, allowing evacuation of cytoplasm by the parasite. Later, its trifid claws shred these damaged cells as they move upward, contributing to the diagnostic cuffs seen in infestation. *D. brevis* consumes glandular cells in its particular locus and in heavy infestation may affect the lipid layer of the tear film.

Demodex infestation may cause blepharitis although symptoms of infestation are relatively non-specific and indistinguishable from other forms of blepharitis. The presence of mites does not necessarily constitute disease. Patients may complain of itching and burning eyelids, with crusting and loss of lashes. The pruritus is often episodic and may parallel oviposition activity. Normally, the parasite's existence is a torpid one; however, in egg-laying there is increased activity lasting several hours. The acarid can cause granulomas of the skin that are characterized by pain and swelling of tissue.

Many crumpled, dead parasites are observed, often unwittingly, by the ophthalmologist in the daily office routine, as they are located in lid margin debris and sometimes straddle cilia. In short, the observer is scanning a graveyard of mites. Parasites are best viewed after the lid has been scrubbed with a moist cotton-tipped applicator that is then placed in a droplet of saline on a slide and examined with a microscope. The organisms are 0.3mm in length and are nearly transparent.

Demodectic mites undergo two molting periods in development, and the cast exoskeletons of immature specimens are also seen with high magnification. The observer is sometimes rewarded with an exquisite view of the empty exoskeleton.

D. brevis can migrate from its epithelial niche into dermal tissue and produce a granuloma of the eyelid which may also be found in other skin. Mites may be found in chalazia and in basal cell carcinomas. Proof that this is more than an incidental finding remains illusive. Infestation of the lid is very common in the elderly — more than 80% can be affected-but it is uncommon in babies and children.

The relationship between rosacea and *Demodex* infestation is illustrative of the difficulty in attributing causation of disease to this organism. Patients with rosacea do not have a higher incidence of *Demodex* although they demonstrate higher concentrations of organisms. The reason for this is unclear but may be related to an altered immunologic response.

Immunosuppression may be relevant and may worsen the condition but the majority of patients with demodicoses have an intact immune response.

DIAGNOSIS

Clinical signs and symptoms

- Infestation may result in follicular distention, hyperplasia, hyperemia, hyperkeratinization and madarosis.
- Deposition of exoskeletons of adult mites, acarid exuviae, and broken, evacuated eggshells of mites are found on the lid margin; these objects are composed of chitin and may be responsible for the condition referred to in the vernacular as 'sleep.'

- When heavy infestation occurs, cuffing and formation of mite nests occur on the eyelashes.

Laboratory findings

Diagnosis of demodicosis is confirmed by the presence of parasites on epilated eyelashes. They can be identified when cilia are deposited in a droplet of saline on a slide and subjected to microscopy.

PROPHYLAXIS

- It is not known if the acarid is transmitted by personal contact.
- *D. canis*, which is taxonomically similar to *D. brevis*, produces mange in dogs and in earlier times was thought to be transferrable to humans.

TREATMENT

Ocular

Treatment consists primarily of lid scrubs using mild soap. Ether is not recommended. Topical antibiotics may be useful to alter lid flora and further reduce lid inflammation. Skin infestations may also be treated with topical acaricidal medications after facial washing on well-dried skin (crotamiton 10% in the morning and crotamiton 10% plus benzyl benzoate 12% in the evening). Simply washing the skin daily probably helps reduce the level of infestion considerably.

Systemic

Systemic therapy is used in demodectic management in canines with good effect. It is not recommended for humans.

COMMENTS

Demodicosis is associated with specific pathology of the eyelids. *Demodex* infestation is more common than is generally appreciated by the ophthalmic community. The degree to which it causes or contributes to ocular symptoms is still controversial and often difficult to determine unless the infestation is rather heavy. Demodectic mites have been recorded carrying *Mycobacterium leprae* bacilli and fungi, and this feature causes concern. Since treatment includes basic measures for treating blepharitis such as lid scrubs, the presence of mites in a symptomatic patient warrants treatment.

REFERENCES

Baima B, Sticherling M: Deomodicidosis revisited: Acta dermato-Venereolog 82(1):3–6, 2002.

Bonnar E, Eustace P, Powell FC: The *Demodex* mite population in rosacea. J Am Acad Dermatol 28:443–448, 1993.

English FP, Cohn D, Groeneveld ER: Demodectic mites and chalazion. Am J Ophthalmol 100:482–483, 1985.

English FP, Zhang GW, McManus DP, Campbell P: Electron microscopic evidence of acarine infestation of the eyelid margin. Am J Ophthalmol 109:239–240, 1990.

Erbagci Z, Erbagci I, Erkilic S: High incidence of dermodicosis in eyelid basal cell carcinomas. Int J of Dermatol 42(7):567–571, 2003.

Forton F, Germaux MA, Brasseur T, et al: Demodicosis and rosacea: epidemiology and significance in daily dermatologic practice. J Am Acad Dermatol 52(10):74–87, 2005.

Karincaoglu Y, Bayram N, Aycan O, Esrefoglu M: The clinical importance of *Demodex folliculorum* presenting with nonspecific facial signs and symptoms. J Dermatol 31(8):618–626, 2004.

Kemal M, Summer Z, Toker MI, et al: The prevelance of *Demodex folliculorum* in blepharitis patients and the normal population. Ophthalmic Epidemiology 12(4):287–290, 2005.

Smith S, MaCullough C: *Demodex folliculorum palpebrarum*. Can J Ophthalmol 4:3–15, 1969.

Wolf R, Ophir J, Avigad J, Lengy J, Krakowski A: The hair follicle mites (*Demodex* sp.). Acta Dermatol Venereol (Stockholm) 68:535–536, 1988.

60 ECHINOCOCCOSIS 122.9

F. Hampton Roy, MD, FACS
Little Rock, Arkansas

ETIOLOGY/INCIDENCE

Echinococcosis is an infection caused by the larval forms of the genus *Echinococcus*. *E. granulosus* is the most common of the species, which also includes *E. multilocularis*, *E. oligoarthus* and *E. vogeli*. The worms of all species live in the intestines of the host, which is usually a dog. The human acts as an intermediate host, becoming infected by ingestion of the eggs of the organism through contaminated food or water. Eggs hatch in the intestines, and the embryos penetrate the intestinal wall to gain the portal to circulation. The parasite forms a vesicle containing fluid in the internal organs, which is called a hydatid cyst; the disease is called hydatid disease. Usually only one slowly growing cyst develops, but it may persist for many years.

The hydatid cyst has an outer acellular laminated membrane and an inner germinative layer. The outer (or cuticular) layer is surrounded by an adventitial layer that is a granulamatous reaction produced by the host. Secondary cysts (brood capsules) bud from the germinative layer, in which protoscoleces are produced. Accidental rupture of the cyst may give rise to anaphylactic reactions.

DIAGNOSIS

Clinical signs and symptoms

Clinical manifestations are determined by the locations of the cysts. The liver is the most common site for hydatid disease, accounting for 60% to 70% of cases. The pulmonary form is found in about 30% of cases. Less frequently, the spleen, kidney, central nervous system, or heart may be involved.

Only 1% of cases of echinococcosis may have an ophthalmologic location, which is usually situated in the orbit. Few cases of anterior chamber, vitreous, or subretinal cysts have been reported. Orbital hydatid cysts are more commonly found in young adults. Patients present with progressive, unilateral, nonpulsating exophthalmos with a duration of approximately 1 month to 2 years. The cysts tend to be located superiorly and may erode the orbital roof, invading the cranial cavity. Pain may be present, as well as ocular motion restriction, papilledema, and retinal striae. Advanced cases may present conjunctival chemosis, lid edema, and exposure keratitis.

Laboratory findings

Hydatid cyst should be included in the differential diagnosis of unilateral proptosis in patients from countries where echinococcosis is endemic.

- Plain orbital radiographs may show enlarged orbital diameters and increased soft-tissue density.
- Ultrasonography demonstrates a cystic lesion without internal reflectivity.
- Computed tomography discloses a well-defined cystic mass.
- Magnetic resonance imaging reveals a low-intensity signal on T1-weighted images and a high-intensity signal on T2-weighted images.
- Because of the integrity of the cyst, serologic tests (like the detection of arc-5 antigen) may be negative in orbital hydatid disease.

TREATMENT

Medical

Medical treatment of echinococcosis is usually carried out in patients for whom surgery cannot be performed or in cases in which the cyst has ruptured. Mebendazole or albendazole is used in these cases.

Surgical

The treatment of choice for orbital hydatidosis is surgical. Various surgical approaches can be used, although lateral osteoplastic orbitotomy (the Krönlein–Berke procedure) is the most common. Once the cyst is observed, puncture and aspiration of its liquid content is performed. The content of the cyst is replaced with 1% formaldehyde in saline, hypertonic solution, or 70% alcohol and is left in place for 5 minutes, followed by surgical excision of the parasitic membrane and its contents.

COMMENTS

Although echinococcosis may occur throughout the world, it constitutes a major health problem in particular areas. *E. granulosus* has a worldwide distribution, with high incidence in North Africa, the Middle East, Australia, South America, and certain rural areas of central Utah, California, New Mexico and Arizona in the United States. *E. multilocularis* is more frequent in Central Europe, whereas *E. oligarthrus* and *E. vogeli* are found in Central and South America. Preventive measures should include education of the public in order to eliminate the feeding of infected waste materials to dogs. Contact with infected dogs should be avoided, and treatment of these animals should be instituted.

REFERENCES

De Silva N, Guyatt H, Bundy D: Antihelmintics: a comparative review of their clinical pharmacology. Drugs 53:769–788, 1997.

Ergun R, Okten AI, Yuksel M, et al: Orbital hydatic cysts: report of four cases. Neurosurg Rev 20:33–37, 1997.

Fry G: Anti-helminthic therapy. Curr Opin Infect Dis 10:461–465, 1997.

Gomez Morales A, Croxatto JO, Crovetto L, et al: Hydatic cyst of the orbit: a review of 35 cases. Ophthalmology 95:1027–1032, 1988.

Jones TC: Cestodes. In: Mandell GL, et al, eds: Principles and practice of infectious diseases. Edinburgh, Churchill Livingstone, 1990:2155–2156.

Lerner SF, Gomez Morales A, Croxatto JO: Hydatic cyst of the orbit. Arch Ophthalmol 109:285, 1991.

Mandell GL: Echinococcosis (hydatid and alveolar cyst disease). In: Mandell, Douglas, eds: Bennett's principles and practice of infectious diseases. 5th edn. Philadelphia, Churchill Livingstone, 2000: 2962–2963.

Schmidt GD, Roberts LS: Foundations of parasitology. 6th edn. New York, McGraw-Hill, 2000:338–342.

Sinav S, et al: A primary intraocular hydatic cyst. Acta Ophthalmologica 69:802–804, 1991.

61 OCULAR TOXOCARIASIS 128.0

Carlos Walter Arzabe, MD
Santa Cruz, Bolivia

ETIOLOGY/INCIDENCE

Two nematode larvae can cause toxocariasis. Both are round worms found in the intestine of dogs (*T. canis*) and cats (*T. cati*). Eggs eliminated in the feces of these animals are not infective and require an incubation period in the soil to embryonate, in which they can remain latent and infectious for many years. Puppies usually contract the *T. canis* from the mother before birth or from her milk. When the puppies are 3–4 weeks old, produces large number of eggs that contaminates the environment through their feces. Warm, humid climates help survival of eggs in the soil. Patients can become infected after accidentally swallowing infective *Toxocara* eggs from contaminated soil or feces.

Toxocariasis is one of the most commonly reported zoonotic helminth infections in the world. It may develop at any age, although the initial infection typically occurs in childhood, because young children's are more likely to ingest the eggs of the worm from contaminated soil or by their permanent contact with infected puppies that have not been dewormed. Consequently, toxocariasis is found more commonly in individuals who have contact with soil, e.g. children and farmers.

T. canis L3 larvae deposit excretory-secretory (ES) antigens in the eye. The ES antigen activates complement, attracts eosinophils, and stimulates T cells and other immune cells. Acute inflammation develops around the parasite or deposited ES antigen. The inflammatory response can lead to retinal detachment with visual loss.

DIAGNOSIS

Clinical signs and symptoms

There are three main clinical forms of the disease:

1. Symptomatic visceral larva migrans is caused by the host response to parasite-excreted surface antigen dropped by the larvae during their migration through the body. It is characterized by fever, irritability, pallor, anorexia, malaise, eosinophilia, hepatomegaly, coughing, asthma or pneumonia. Is a disease of young children (6 months–4 years of age). Fortunately, most systemic infections are mild and produce no serious morbidity.
2. Covert toxocariasis is a syndrome characterized by abdominal pain, anemia and eosinophilia.

3. Ocular toxocariasis is the least common presentation of toxocariasis. Eye involvement is usually unilateral, with bilateral lesions occurring in only 1%.

Laboratory findings

Eosinophilia is usually present in patients with visceral diseases but often absent in patients with ocular infection.

ELISA test is the test of choice to document systemic or ocular infection with *T. canis*. It is particularly useful for the diagnosis of visceral disease, in which antibody titers tend to be high. In contrast, in ocular disease, antibody levels are significantly lower according to the Centers for Disease Control, and a serum titer of 1 : 8 is sufficient to support the diagnosis if the patient has signs and symptoms compatibles with ocular toxocariasis.

ELISA testing of intraocular fluids (vitreous and aqueous humor) is of great value in the diagnosis.

Standardized echography can be of help in the diagnosis of this ocular disease.

In the ocular form, one or more larvae become trapped in the eye, causing a granuloma in the retina. This nematode may be located beneath or within the retina, or may extend into the choroid and vitreous.

- Posterior pole 'granuloma' (usually, patients with 6–14 years old).
- Peripheral granuloma (with a quiet eye, range in age from 6–40 years old).
- Children with diffuse chronic endophthalmitis (usually, patients with 2–9 years old).
- Uveitis.
- Unilateral pars planitis.
- Macular scarring.
- RPE changes.
- Retinal detachment.

The nematode it may remain viable for several years in the eye.

In many instances, the child does not present for medical attention until permanent ocular damage has taken place. (See Figure 61.1.)

The nematode may enter the eye via central retinal artery (peripheral granuloma), or via the short posterior ciliary arteries (optic disc, macula or posterior pole).

Differential diagnosis

- Retinoblastoma.
- Retrolental fibroplasia.
- Familial exudative vitreoretinopathy.
- Coats' disease.
- Persistent hyperplastic primary vitreous.
- Pars planitis and other uveitis.

PROPHYLAXIS

Education is important. Wash hands often, especially after playing with a pet.

Dogs and cats should be dewormed regularly, starting before they are 4 weeks old.

Dogs release *T. Canis* in their stool. A single dog feces can contain approximately 1 million eggs. The eggs are resistant and can survive for over 10 years. Freshly deposited feces are not infectious and can safely removed. *Toxacara* eggs become infectious when they embryonate, this is usually 2–3 weeks after they have been deposited by the dog.

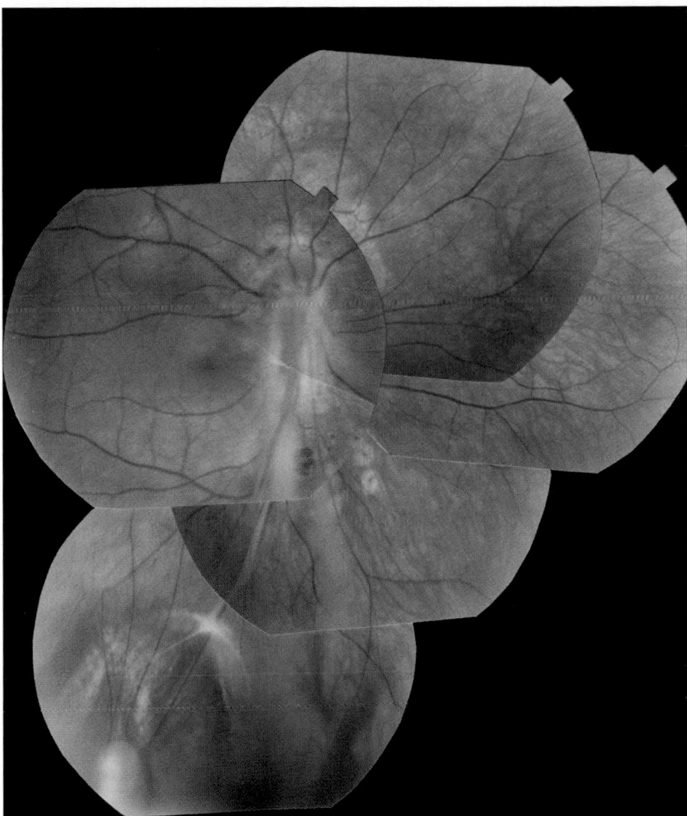

FIGURE 61.1. A 15-year-old boy with a localized, white, elevated peripheral 'granuloma' caused by *Toxocara canis*, and typical fibrocellular stalk running to the optic nerve, as well as the macular area in which a macular ectopia and dragging of the macular vessels has developed due to the transvitreal traction bands.

TREATMENT

The natural history of toxocariasis is to resolve spontaneously over a period of weeks to months, so visceral larva migrans often is treated conservatively. If treatment is necessary, 5 mg/kg albendazole b.i.d. can be used. Diethylcarbamazine has been recommended by some.

Treatment of the inflammatory stage of the ocular disease is with antinflamatory/cycloplegic eye drops, and periocular depomethylprednisolone (40–60 mg), repeated every 7–14 days until the process resolves itself.

If antihelminthic therapy is used, it should always be coupled with steroids because *T. canis*, is not a self-replicating organism. A common combination is Thiabendazole, 500 mg PO q.i.d. or 20 mg/kg/day in divided doses for 5 days; plus 40 mg of prednisone PO qd for 10 days tapered as warranted by the rate of resolving intraocular inflammation.

Surgery may be indicated to manage the complications of ocular toxocariasis, including repair of retinal detachment. Detachment is usually caused by vitreous bands that can be removed only by vitrectomy. Vitrectomy may also be indicated to remove the opaque vitreous secondary to inflammation.

Cryocoagulation and photocoagulation also kill the larvae effectively but should not be used within the foveal area.

COMPLICATIONS

The main complications are endophthalmitis, macular scarring, anterior uveitis and retinal detachment.

COMMENTS

It is reasonable to assume that all puppies are born with *Toxocara canis*, and they will produce larger numbers of eggs than adult dogs. This is why it is very important for dog owners to worm their dogs regularly, to rid their animals of infestation, and for them to remain free, as the dogs will themselves become re-infested when they come into contact with the eggs.

REFERENCES

Magnaval JF, Glickman PD, Morassin B: Highlights of human toxocariasis. Korean J Parasitology 39(1):1–11, 2001.

Ryan SJ, Schachat AP, Murphy RB: Retina. 2nd edn. St Louis, Mosby, 1994.

Gillespie SH, Dinning WJ, Voller A, Crowcroft NS: The spectrum of ocular toxocariasis. Eye 7:415–418, 1993.

Glickman LT: The epidemiology of human toxocariasis. In: Lewis JW, Maizels RM, eds: *Toxocara* and toxocariasis: clinical, epidemiological and molecular perspectives. London, Institute of Biology, 1993.

Holland CV, O'Lorcain P, Taylor MR, Kelly A: Sero-epidemiology of toxocariasis in school children. Parasitology 110:535–545, 1995.

Van Knapen F, Buijs J: Diagnosis of *Toxocara* infection. In: Lewis JW, Maizels RH, eds: *Toxacara* and toxocariasis: clinical, epidemiological and molecular perspectives. London, Institute of Biology, 1993.

Sowka JW, Gurwood AS, Kabat AG: Handbook of ocular disease management. Online. Available at: www.revoptom.com/handbook/oct02_sec5_4.htm., 2006.

62 PEDICULOSIS AND PHTHIRIASIS 132.9

William D. Mathers, MD
Portland, Oregon

ETIOLOGY/INCIDENCE

Pediculosis refers to infestation by *Pediculus humanus corporis* and *Pediculus humanus capitis*, body and head lice, respectively. These two variants are similar to each other in appearance, and they interbreed freely. *Pediculus* lice are 2 to 4 mm long and have long slender legs that allow them to move about freely. They are typically passed from person to person by close contact with an infested person or by contact with contaminated items. Pediculosis of the ocular region is extremely rare and is generally an extension of heavy scalp infestation.

Infestation by *Phthirus pubis*, the pubic or crab louse, is called phthiriasis. It is by far the most common type of louse infestation of the ocular region and typically involves the lashes. It can be considered a sexually transmitted disease. At 2 mm, the louse is smaller than *Pediculus* spp. and has a broad, shield-like body. It also has serrated tarsal claws that allow traction over flat, hairless areas and thus it can navigate the entire skin surface. It usually prefers sites where the distance between adjacent hairs is similar to its grasping span, preferring particularly pubic hair but also axillary, chest, and beard hair, as well as the eyelashes. *Phthirus* sp. also causes 1% of all lice infestations of scalp hair.

Both types of lice lay eggs on the hair shafts; the eggs, or nits, are firmly adherent, and resist both mechanical and chemical removal. Although lice infestation is popularly considered a sign of poor hygiene, this may not be accurate. Lice can survive in soap and water for protracted periods. Lice infestation affects all socioeconomic groups, and the incidence appears to be increasing. This is attributable to several factors including insecticide resistance, reliance on physical methods of removal which are not very effective, and increased sexual activity in the adolescent population.[3,5,9]

Lice are spread by close contact with an affected person or with objects the person has very recently contacted, such as bedding, stuffed animals, combs and brushes. Lice do not survive unless they have ready access to human blood.

DIAGNOSIS

Clinical signs and symptoms

- Eyelids: lice and nits on lashes, reddish-brown louse feces, maculae ceruleae (blue spots on the skin caused by louse bites), pruritus, blepharitis, secondary infection (preauricular lymphadenopathy).
- Cornea: marginal keratitis (rare).
- Conjunctiva: follicular conjunctivitis (rare).

TREATMENT

Local

Physical removal in cooperative children and adults can be done using a slit lamp. Periodic re-examination for 10 to 14 days is necessary to remove new nits. Removal from the scalp requires combing with a metal comb that has narrowly spaced teeth, after shampooing with a pediculocidal agent. Efficacy of physical removal has been questioned.

Topical white petrolatum, a smothering agent, for 10 days b.i.d.; the ointments for dry eyes are petrolatum-based.

Dimeticone lotion has no conventional insecticide activity. It has recently been demonstrated to be effective against head lice. Application to lashes has not been investigated.

Lindane (* benzene hexachloride) 1% shampoo is toxic and may not be as effective as other agents. It can cause nausea, vomiting, eye irritation and pain. Because of these side effects, the drug has recently undergone increase regulation in the United States.

Permethrin shampoo, and Malathion which is not available in the United States, are now less effective for lice with the development of resistance.

Oral Ivermectin, an insecticide, has recently been shown to be effective in the treatment of phthiriasis in children. This is a promising development.

Cholinesterase inhibitors such as physostigmine ointment help to immobilize and kill the adult lice but not the nits.

Argon laser therapy and cryotherapy to lashes have also been reported.

Miscellaneous

Wash clothing, bedding, hairbrushes, and combs in hot water (50°C) or dry clean, as appropriate. Sprays can be used on nonwashable items that the affected person has recently come into contact with. Cosmetics should be discarded.

Because it is harder to remove or kill the nits, reexamine in 7 to 10 days for signs of recurrence, and re-treat as indicated.

Infestation may be acquired through sexual contact. Increased sexual activity in adolescents may have contributed to the recent rise in prevalence.

REFERENCES

Awan K: Argon laser phototherapy of phthiriasis palpebrum. Ophthalmic Surgery 17:813–814, 1986.

Awan K: Cryotherapy in phthiriasis palpebrarum. Am J Ophth 83:906, 1997.

Burgess I, Brown C, Lee P: Treatment of head louse infestation with 4% dimeticone lotion: randomised controlled equivalence trial. BMJ doi:10.1136, 1–4, 2005.

Burkhart CN, Burkhart CG: Oral ivermectin therapy for phthiriasis palpebrum. Arch Ophthalmol 118:134–135, 2000.

Burns D: The treatment of *Pthirus pubis* infestation of the eyelashes. Br J Ophthalmol 117:741–743, 1987.

Couch J, Green W, Hirst L, De La Cruz Z: Diagnosing and treating Phthirus pubis palpebrum. Survey Ophthalmol 26:219–225, 1982.

Forrester M, Sievert J, Stanley S: Epidemiology of Lindane exposures for pediculosis reported to poison control centers in Texas. J Toxicol 42:55–60, 2004.

Mutavdzic A: Head lice and their treatment. S Afr Med J 66:923–924, 1984.

Plastow L, Luthra M, Powell R, et al: Head lice infestation: bug-busting vs traditional treatment. J Clin Nurs 10:775–783, 2001.

Rundle P, Hughes D: *Phthirus pubis* infestation of the eyelids. Br J Oophthalmol 77:815–816, 1993.

63 TOXOPLASMOSIS 130.9

Jean D. Vaudaux, MD
Lausanne, Switzerland
Gary N. Holland, MD
UCLA, Los Angeles

CAUSE/INCIDENCE

Toxoplasma gondii, an obligate intracellular protozoan parasite, is found extensively in human populations worldwide. The prevalence of serum anti-*T. gondii* IgG antibodies depends on geographic location and socio-economic status. Overall age-adjusted seroprevalence has been estimated to be 22.5% in the United States, but is much higher in many other parts of the world. The cat is the only definitive host. Other animals acquire infection through ingestion of tissue cysts (from infected food animals) or oocysts (from vegetables or water contaminated with cat feces), with subsequent asexual reproduction of the parasite. Infection may also be congenital.

COURSE/PROGNOSIS

Following infection, host immunity controls replication, which causes the organism to become encysted within cells (tissue cysts), establishing latent infections that may reactivate later in life. The stimulus for reactivation is unknown. In immunocompetent individuals, the most common site of clinically apparent reactivation is the retina, where localized replication of *T. gondii* produces retinochoroiditis. The traditional concept that toxoplasmic retinochoroiditis primarily results from reactivation of congenitally-acquired infection has been questioned; postnatally acquired infection is probably responsible for a higher proportion of cases than previously thought.

DIAGNOSIS

Diagnosis is clinical, based on the typical appearance of a yellow-white focus of active retinochoroiditis, often adjacent to a preexisting retinochoroidal scar. Intraocular inflammation is generally present, albeit in variable amounts.

Clinical signs and symptoms

Anterior segment

- Keratic precipitates (variable).
- Anterior chamber cells and flare (usually mild; associated with redness and photophobia).

Posterior segment

- Vitreous humor cells and haze (can be severe).
- Retinochoroiditis (may or may not be associated with preexisting scars) (Figure 63.1).
- Neuroretinitis (uncommon as sole finding).
- Papillitis (uncommon as sole finding).
- Retinal vasculitis (usually associated with retinochoroiditis).

Laboratory findings

Serologic tests for anti-*T. gondii* antibodies will support a clinical diagnosis by confirming exposure to the organism; because antibodies are common in the general population, a positive test does not confirm the diagnosis, however.

Differential diagnosis

Clinical features may vary in certain hosts. Immunosuppressed individuals or the elderly may have extensive areas of retinitis, sometimes mimicking necrotizing herpetic retinopathies. Newborns with lymphocytic choriomeningitis virus retinitis can have lesions resembling toxoplasmic retinochoroiditis.

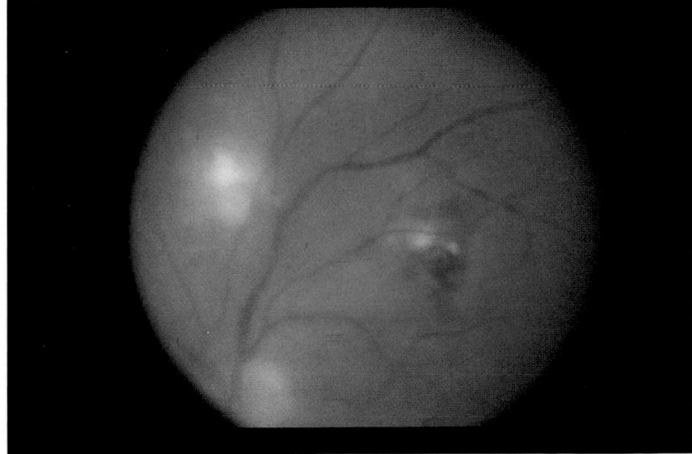

FIGURE 63.1. Toxoplasmosis with vein occlusion.

PROPHYLAXIS

Drug treatment is not used to prevent primary infection; prevention of infection is based on public health measures. (See Treatment section below for discussion of secondary prophylaxis.)

TREATMENT

Active retinochoroiditis in an immunosuppressed host, elderly patient, or newborn should always be treated. Toxoplasmic retinochoroiditis in immunocompetent individuals is a self-limited infection, suggesting that not every patient requires treatment. A decision to treat will depend on the clinician's judgment and experience, and on potential contraindications to treatment, such as drug intolerance. The goal of treatment is to shorten the time to resolution and to reduce symptoms associated to inflammation. Indications for drug therapy in immunocompetent children and adults include the following: decrease in visual acuity; active retinochoroiditis located in the posterior pole (involving macula, optic disc, papillomacular bundle, or major vascular arcades, and threatening central vision); vitreous inflammation that is associated with substantial vision loss or obscuration of the fundus; and lesion size.

An evidence-based review of published, randomized clinical trials failed, however, to demonstrate any benefit of short-term anti-*T. gondii* treatment in terms of duration of inflammation or visual prognosis. There have been few such studies, however, and based on animal studies and clinical experience, most uveitis specialists believe that treatment is beneficial, in at least some cases. There is no consensus regarding the superiority of one drug versus another, however. Consequently, there is no 'standard' treatment.

Systemic drug therapy

Ocular toxoplasmosis in the immunocompetent host

In general, multiple drugs are used simultaneously to treat ocular toxoplasmosis. The most commonly used combination, sometimes referred to as 'classic therapy,' consists of pyrimethamine, sulfadiazine, and prednisone. Therapy is usually maintained for 4 to 6 weeks. Pyrimethamine is a potent dihydrofolate reductase inhibitor. A loading dose of 50 to 200 mg is followed by 25 to 50 mg PO daily in one or two divided doses. If side effects occur, the dosage can be reduced to 25 mg daily. Systemic side effects include nausea and bone marrow suppression through inhibition of folate metabolism; the latter is generally prevented by adding 5 mg leucovorin (folinic acid) two to three times a week to the drug regimen. Serial blood counts should be obtained to rule out hematopoietic toxicity. Sulfadiazine is used at a dose of 1 g PO q.i.d. Systemic side effects include allergic reactions, ranging from benign cutaneous manifestations to the more severe Stevens–Johnson syndrome. Prednisone is used only in combination with at least one antimicrobial agent; oral corticosteroids alone have been associated with severe exacerbation of infection. The primary goal of oral corticosteroid therapy is to decrease intraocular inflammation, thus contributing to faster visual recovery. A dosage of 1 mg/kg PO qd is typically initiated 24 hours after antimicrobial therapy is started.

Other commercially available combinations of dihydrofolate reductase inhibitors and sulfonamides, such as trimethoprim-sulfamethoxazole (160 mg/800 mg PO b.i.d.) have become popular as alternatives to classic therapy because of lower rates of adverse effects.

Other drugs may be effective in the treatment of ocular toxoplasmosis, and are used in particular cases, such as in patients who are intolerant of dihydrofolate reductase inhibitors or sulfonamides. They include clindamycin, the macrolides, and atovaquone. Clindamycin is usually administered at a dose of 300 mg PO q.i.d. Diarrhea is a common side effect; a more severe complication is pseudomembranous colitis, warranting immediate discontinuation of therapy.

Ocular toxoplasmosis in the immunosuppressed host

To prevent further suppression of host defenses, oral corticosteroid therapy is generally eliminated from the therapeutic regimen. Some clinicians advocate the use of alternative agents such as atovaquone or clindamycin in people with AIDS because of a higher occurrence of sulfonamide-associated adverse effects in this population. In addition, continued use of at least one drug as 'maintenance therapy' is generally administered as long as immunosuppression persists. In HIV-infected individuals, discontinuation of maintenance therapy may be contemplated if immune reconstitution is achieved by use of potent antiretroviral drugs.

Ocular therapy

Topical corticosteroids are commonly used to treat the associated anterior chamber reaction, but the need for such therapy has never been confirmed. Vitrectomy is occasionally performed to obtain samples for diagnostic testing using polymerase chain reaction techniques, and may be necessary to manage complications, such as retinal detachment or persistent vitreous opacities. Cryotherapy or laser photocoagulation of active retinochoroiditis have been described, but their efficacy remains uncertain.

Secondary prophylaxis

Prevention of recurrences through long-term intermittent therapy has been subject to limited study; one prospective, randomized trial demonstrated a reduced rate of recurrences with intermittent trimethoprim-sulfamethoxazole therapy in a high-risk population. The benefit of such treatment for patients in general has not been determined.

COMMENTS

Ocular toxoplasmosis remains the most common cause of posterior uveitis in immunocompetent individuals. Currently available drugs may shorten the time to resolution of active retinochoroiditis and produce symptomatic improvement, but none of these agents kills *T. gondii* cysts, making recurrence an issue. Therapeutic decisions should be based upon clinical factors, including visual acuity, location of lesions, and the host's immune status, as well as risks associated with medical therapy.

REFERENCES

Holland GN, Lewis KG: An update on current practices in the management of ocular toxoplasmosis. Am J Ophthalmol 134:102–114, 2002.

Holland GN: Ocular toxoplasmosis: a global reassessment. Am J Ophthalmol 136:973–988, 2003 (Part I); 137:1–17 (Part II), 2004.

Jones JL, Kruszon-Moran D, Wilson M: *Toxoplasma gondii* infection in the United States: seroprevalence and risk factors. Am J Epidemiol 154:357–365, 2001.

Silveira C, Belfort R, Jr, Muccioli C, et al: The effect of long-term intermittent trimethoprim/sulfamethoxazole treatment on recurrences of toxoplasmic retinochoroiditis. Am J Ophthalmol 134:41–46, 2002.

Stanford MR, See SE, Jones LV, Gilbert RE: Antibiotics for toxoplasmic retinochoroiditis — an evidence-based systematic review. Ophthalmology 110:926–932, 2003.

64 TRICHINOSIS 124

Khalid F. Tabbara, MD, ABO, FRCOphth
Riyadh, Saudi Arabia

ETIOLOGY/INCIDENCE

Trichinosis, also known as trichinellosis or trichiniasis, is an infection caused by the nematode larva *Trichinella spiralis.* The disease is acquired by the ingestion of undercooked pork or ground beef contaminated by pork in the grinder. *Trichinella* larvae tend to invade skeletal muscle where they encyst and cause localized inflammation and edema in the orbicularis and extraocular muscles. The disease may be asymptomatic or may lead to manifestations varying from mild edema of the eyelid to generalized systemic symptoms of fever, myalgia and eosinophilia.

Trichinosis has a worldwide distribution except some Pacific islands and Australia. The disease occurs in Asia, Europe, North America and Central and South America. The prevalence of wild trichinosis and human trichinosis has decreased over the past three decades primarily because of tighter regulations of the swine industry, including restrictions on feeding of raw garbage to animals. Major reservoirs of trichinosis occur among hogs in Europe and North America, among bear, fox and walrus in Alaska, Canada, and other northern regions of the world, and among bush pigs in East Africa and Senegal.

In Europe, there are four species of the genus Trichenella that have been identified:

1. *T. spiralis*;
2. *T. britovi*;
3. *T. native*; and
4. *T. pseudospiralis.*

T. spiralis and T. britovi parasites are present in wild and domestic animals in Poland. In the period of 1997–2001, there were 72 cases reported to the CDC in Atlanta. Thirty one (43%) cases were associated with eating wild game including bear meat in 29, cougar meat in one, and boar meat in one, and only 12 (17%) were associated with eating commercial pork products. Nine (15%) of the cases were associated with eating noncommercial pork from home-raised or directly from swine farm where United States industry standards and regulations do not apply.

COURSE

Humans can acquire the infection by eating raw or uncooked pork, horse meat, boar meat, bear meat, cougar meat or any raw or undercooked meat containing the larvae. Adult intestinal worms usually disappear within 2 to 3 months after infecting and feeding. The adult female trichina measures 2 to 4 mm in length and 60 μm in width. The adult male worm measures 1.5 mm in length. The average life span is 4 months.

Following the ingestion of encysted larvae in contaminated meat, the cyst wall is digested by the gastric enzymes, releasing the larvae. The larvae burrow and attach to the duodenal and jejunal mucosae, where they molt to produce sexually mature worms. The adult worms mate and produce larvae that reach the bloodstream and are distributed throughout the body. Depending on the number of larvae reaching striated muscles, patients with trichinosis may have asymptomatic illness or may have symptoms varying from mild edema of the eyelid to death secondary to myocarditis or encephalitis. Larvae that encyst mature, and may remain viable and infective for many years in calcified cysts. The released larvae gain access to the bloodstream and are carried to all parts of the body, reaching the striated muscles, extraocular muscles, orbicularis, diaphragm, tongue and throat. It may rarely cause carcinoma of the larynx. The larvae grow rapidly to about 10 times their birth size in 3 weeks, and they coil up between muscle fibers and become encapsulated. The encysted larvae may remain infective for many years.

DIAGNOSIS

Clinical signs and symptoms

Humans may harbor both adult worms and larvae of *T. spiralis.*

Clinical findings consist of the following:

- Malaise;
- Fever;
- Generalized muscular tenderness and pain;
- Headache;
- Burning sensation in the eyes;
- Arthralgias;
- Respiratory manifestations.

Trichinosis is the only helminthic infection that causes consistent fever during its course.

The ophthalmologic manifestations of trichinosis result from the invasion of the larvae into extraocular and orbicularis muscles. Patients may present with:

- Periorbital edema;
- Swelling of the eyelids;
- Conjunctivitis;
- Conjunctival chemosis;
- Subconjunctival hemorrhages.

Some patients may present with bilateral edema of the eyelids with or without chemosis of the conjunctiva, but with no other systemic or ocular manifestations. The swelling of the eyelids occurs 1 week after acquiring the infection and may remain for 2 to 3 weeks. Patients with trichinosis may also complain of pain on moving the eye because of myositis of the extraocular muscles. Retinal hemorrhages and papilledema may occur. Patients with trichinosis may develop optic neuritis and neuroretinitis.

Myocarditis, bronchopneumonia, encephalitis and nephritis may cause death. In rare cases, exophthalmos, strabismus, photophobia, or nystagmus may be observed. The four cardinal signs of trichinosis are:

1. Fever;
2. Bilateral edema of the eyelid and periorbital edema;
3. Myalgia;
4. Eosinophilia.

The ophthalmologist may be the first to make the diagnosis of trichinosis.

IMMUNOLOGY

Following infection with *T. spiralis*, the gastrointestinal mucosa attempts to expel the nematode with a pronounced mast cells infiltration mediated by a Th2 type response involving IL-4, IL-10, and IL-13. It appears that rIL-12 can result in significant suppression of intestinal mast cell responses and delayed worm expulsion with increased muscle larvae burden. IL-10 can also protect the liver from necrosis during the murine infection with *T. spiralis*. IL-10 is most evident in the first 20 days following muscle infection. Between 20 and 50 post infection days, the inflammatory response is noted to diminish in both the wild-type and IL-10 deficient mice. It appears that IL-10 can limit local and regional inflammation during the early stages of muscle infection and that chronic inflammation is controlled by an IL-10 independent mechanism that is co-incident with a Th2 response.

Laboratory findings

Patients with trichinosis develop leukocytosis and eosinophilia. There is also specific elevation of the serum levels of muscle enzymes such as lactate dehydrogenase, aldolase, and creatine phosphokinase in 50% of cases. Adult worms and larvae can be detected in stools during the acute phase of the infection, but this is not a helpful test in making the diagnosis because of the transient residence of the adult worms in the intestine. Serologic tests are available, and the standard test is bentonite flocculation. Complement fixation, indirect hemagglutination and immunofluorescence tests are also available. Serologic tests become positive 3 to 4 weeks after the infection. The enzyme-linked immunosorbent assay (ELISA) for *T. spiralis* is more sensitive than the other serologic tests. The definitive diagnosis of trichinosis is confirmed by histopathologic examination of a biopsy specimen of a muscle such as the deltoid muscle. A skin test for trichinosis is also available. The random amplified polymorphic DNA (RAPD) technique was successfully used to produce genetic fingerprints of *T. spiralis*. The RAPD technique requires no prior knowledge of the molecular biology of the organism and therefore appears to be a promising tool in parasitology.

Molecular identification of *T. spiralis* and *T. britovi* can be performed by diagnostic multiprimer large mitochondrial rRNA amplification.

Differential diagnosis

All conditions that lead to bilateral eyelid swelling and periorbital edema should be considered in the differential diagnosis. They include:

- Angioneurotic edema;
- Erysipelas;
- Mumps;
- Chronic renal disease;
- Insect bites.

PREVENTION

The disease may be prevented by proper control of the swine-raising industry, including restrictions on the feeding of raw garbage to animals. The larvae of *T. spiralis* in infected pork are killed by freezing at −15°C for at least 20 days. The practice of storing meat in a freezer before consumption may kill the larvae. In addition, larvae in meat may be killed by cooking in a microwave oven and maintaining temperatures above 77°C.

TREATMENT

Systemic

Systemic treatment in mild cases consists of supportive therapy of nonsteroidal anti-inflammatory drugs such as ibuprofen along with hydration. When the diagnosis of trichinosis is made early, patients may be given mebendazole 200 to 400 mg orally three times daily for 3 days, then 400 mg three times daily for a period of 10 days. This therapy helps to reduce the number of larvae released from the intestines. Thiabendazole may be given at a dosage level of 25 mg orally twice daily for 7 days to eliminate the gut-swelling adult trichinosis and larvae. Thiabendazole was used in the past but mebendazole has replaced it and is better tolerated. Both thiabendazole and mebendazole are contraindicated in pregnancy and do not cross the blood-brain barrier.

In severe cases, patients must be given systemic corticosteroid in the form of prednisone 0.5 to 1 mg/kg/day in conjunction with the antihelminthic agent mebendazole. In life-threatening conditions and myocarditis, one may have to consider the administration of pulse therapy with intravenous methylprednisolone 500 mg to be given daily with the antihelminthic therapy.

Topical

Topical therapy is aimed at the relief of ocular pain, swelling, and chemosis of the conjunctiva. Patients may be given prednisolone acetate 1% eyedrops q.i.d. and dexamethasone 0.1% ophthalmic ointment once at bedtime. In patients with extraocular muscle involvement, subconjunctival or posterior subtenon injection of triamcinolone acetonide 40 mg may be given through the inferior fornix.

Hospitalization

Hospitalization is recommended for patients with severe trichinosis and evidence of myocarditis or encephalitis.

REFERENCES

Astudillo LM, Arlet PM: Images in clinical medicine. The chemosis of trichinosis. N Engl J Med 351(5):487, 2004.

Bandi C, LaRosa G, Comincini S, et al: Random amplified polymorphic DNA technique for the identification of *Trichinella* species. Parasitology 107:419–424, 1993.

Beiting DP, Bliss SK, Schlafer DH, et al: Interleukin-10 limits local and body cavity inflammation during infection with muscle-stage *Trichinella spiralis*. Infect Immun 72(6):3129–3137, 2004.

Bliss SK, Alcaraz A, Appleton JA: IL-10 prevents liver necrosis during murine infection with *Trichinella spiralis*. J Immunol 171(6):3142–3147, 2003.

Borsuk P, Moskwa B, Pastusiak K, Cabaj W: Molecular identification of *Trichinella spiralis* and *Trichinella britovi* by diagnostic multiprimer large mitochondrial rRNA amplification. Parasitol Res 91(5):374–377, 2003.

Cabie A, Bouchaud O, Houze S, et al: Albendazole versus thiabendazole as therapy for trichinosis: a retrospective study. Clin Infect Dis 22:1033–1035, 1996.

Centers for Disease Control and Prevention (CDC): Trichinellosis associated with bear meat — New York and Tennessee, 2003. MMWR Morb Mortal Wkly Rep 53(27):606–610, 2004.

Cvorovic L, Milutinovic Z, Kiurski M: *Trichinella spiralis* and laryngeal carcinoma: a case report. Eur Arch Otorhinolaryngol 262(6):456–458, 2005.

Dworkin MS, Gamble HR, Zarlenga DS, Tennican PO: Outbreak of trichinellosis associated with eating cougar jerky. J Infect Dis 174:663–666, 1996.

Dzik JM, Golos B, Jagielska E, et al: A non-classical type of alveolar macrophage response to *Trichinella spiralis* infection. Parasitc Immunol 26(4):197–205, 2004.

Gurish MF, Bryce PJ, Tao H, et al: IgE enhances parasite clearance and regulates mast cell responses in mice infected with *Trichinella spiralis*. J Immunol 172(2):1139–1145, 2004.

Helmby H, Grencis RK: IFN-gamma-independent effects of IL-12 during intestinal nematode infection. J Immunol 171(7):3691–3696, 2003.

Laurichesse H, Cambon M, Perre D, et al: Outbreak of trichinosis in France associated with eating horse meat. Commun Dis Rep CDR Rev 7:69–73, 1997.

Roy SL, Lopez AS, Schantz PM: Trichinellosis surveillance — United States, 1997–2001. MMWR Surveill Summ 52(6):1–8, 2003.

Siriyasatien P, Yingyourd P, Nuchprayoon S: Efficacy of albendazole against early and late stage of *Trichinella spiralis* infection in mice. J Med Assoc Thai 86(Suppl 2):S257–S262, 2003.

Wakelin D: *Trichinella spiralis*: Immunity, ecology, and evolution. J Parasitol 79:488–494, 1993.

SECTION

3 Nutritional Disorders

65 INFLAMMATORY BOWEL DISEASE 555.9 (Crohn's Granulomatous Enterocolitis, Regional Enteritis, Ulcerative Colitis)

F. Hampton Roy, MD, FACS
Little Rock, Arkansas

ETIOLOGY/INCIDENCE

Neither Crohn's disease nor ulcerative colitis has a clearly defined etiology that explains all cases. Multifactoral influences are being defined.

Genetic factors are clear to those who have seen enough patients and heard from patients about other family members with the same disorder. Parents and children, cousins, aunts, uncles and grandparents have had the same syndrome.

Several familial subgroups of Crohn's disease have similar clinical presentations, symptoms, signs, and courses. The first subgroup involves oral and gastroduodenal-jejunal disorders. The second focuses around the ileocecal junction, with focal inflammation and obstructions. The third clustering affects the rectum and tends to produce fistulas.

Genetic anticipation occurs; the second generation is likely to be affected earlier than was the first generation. The children of a father with Crohn's disease are more likely to be affected than are those whose mother has Crohn's disease.

Allergic mechanisms in some patients explain exacerbations provoked by the ingestion of foods such as cow's milk and milk products or of drugs. Smoking more than 10 cigarettes per day is associated with more severe Crohn's disease.

Stress, either recent or chronic, is often associated with initial presentation or with exacerbations.

COURSE/PROGNOSIS

Chronicity, remission, and recurrence are common to the clinical courses of both these disorders. Prognosis varies, in part related to genetic factors, which are currently being recognized and clarified. Some patients respond to medical regimens and experience long-lasting subsidence of symptoms and signs. Others respond and then, as drug dosages are reduced, find that symptoms and signs return. A small number of patients do not respond, and surgery is required to remove affected segments of the small or large bowel. In some cases of ulcerative colitis, total colectomy is advised to remove intractable bowel or stop progression of liver disease.

Fistulas caused by Crohn's disease usually require surgical removal, particularly when they have formed connections with the vagina, bladder, or urethra.

Both Crohn's disease and ulcerative colitis are associated with increased risk of developing cancer, so patients require regular monitoring by means of office visits, interval histories, physical examinations, and radiocontrast and endoscopic examinations.

DIAGNOSIS

These disorders are characterized by both gastrointestinal and systemic symptoms and signs. Generalized malaise, fevers, arthralgia, anemia, erythema nodosum, pyoderma gangrenosum, large oral ulcers, weight loss, and growth delay are the systemic symptoms and signs. Elevated white blood cell (WBC) count and erythrocyte sedimentation rate are often present. Crampy abdominal pain, diarrhea with or without blood, excess mucus, and obstructions are the intestinal presentations.

Crohn's disease, usually insidiously but occasionally acutely, produces focal inflammation at any point from mouth to anus, most commonly in the terminal ileum. Fistulas may form from bowel to bowel or bowel to vagina, skin, or bladder. Radiography can demonstrate the 'string sign' of narrowed lumen in the terminal ileum. Biopsies of ulcers reveal granulomatous inflammation with giant cells in 30% of cases.

Ulcerative colitis can have a chronic, indolent onset or a fulminant presentation with explosive diarrhea, fever, and systemic toxicity. Endoscopy reveals eroded, often hemorrhagic colonic mucosa. Biopsy and histopathology demonstrate acute inflammatory cells. Arthralgias and skin lesions are seen. Persistence of active disease can produce liver dysfunction, damage, and sclerotic cirrhosis. In patients with liver disease, colectomy stops progression of the hepatopathy.

TREATMENT

Treatment is difficult, primarily because etiologic mechanisms have not been defined. Family physicians, internists, gastroenterologists, and general surgeons, all with slightly different educations, experiences and psychologic natures, are the primary and secondary managers of these patients. In their desperation, patients often seek care from many different physicians. *Ophthalmologists should not try to manage these patients alone* but should work closely with other experienced practitioners.

- Systemic corticosteroids are the most commonly used agents. They are familiar, available, standardized and effective. Initial high dosages rapidly reduce abdominal pain, nausea, fever and diarrhea. Gradual tapering over weeks to months often brings stability to patients.
- Sulfa-containing drugs such as sulfasalazine are used for chronic maintenance therapy.
- Metronidazole is another useful agent.
- Severe refractiveness to these therapies forces the use of cytotoxic agents such as azathioprine.
- General supportive measures such as liquid or low-residue diets, pain medication and antispasmodic drugs give relief.
- Oral multivitamin use is important.

Surgical intervention is indicated as mentioned above. In some instances, removal of affected bowel is followed by a general systemic improvement, implying that something toxic in the gut has had a systemic effect.

COMPLICATIONS

Ocular complications occur in about 10% of patients with Crohn's disease and less frequently in patients with ulcerative colitis. Ocular problems may present before a gastrointestinal diagnosis is made. Crohn's disease begins with episcleritis, the most common symptom, and a peculiar subepithelial keratopathy, the most specific. Limbal corneal infiltrates, iritis, iridocyclitis, macular edema, retinal vasculitis, papillitis, choroiditis, and orbital myositis are primary complications. Ulcerative colitis seems to have iritis or iridocyclitis as its major ocular complication.

Ocular complications can be divided into three groups:

Primary

Primary complications associated with the activity of Crohn's disease occur frequently and respond to systemic therapy, such as systemic corticosteroids or surgical excision. The primary complications of Crohn's disease include specific epithelial and anterior stromal keratopathy, limbal corneal infiltrates, subconjunctival hemorrhage, episcleritis, scleritis, acute iritis, chronic iridocyclitis, macular edema, retinal vasculitis, and papillitis. Orbital inflammation can produce proptosis, pain, and limited movement caused by myositis or general inflammation. Optic neuritis or chiasmal involvement can cause the loss of vision in one or both eyes. Episcleritis has been, in the author's experience, the most common ocular complication of Crohn's disease; thus, it is a diagnostic point in the differentiation of Crohn's from ulcerative colitis and an indicator of the activity of the basic disease.

Secondary

Secondary complications of Crohn's disease include night blindness and dry eyes caused by vitamin A deficiency induced by patients' reduced intake of vegetables, which irritate the gut, and by an absent or a diseased ileum that prevents the normal absorption of vitamins. Refraction changes occur when patients start or stop taking systemic corticosteroids. Cataracts occur after the prolonged use of corticosteroids or because of chronic iridocyclitis. Exudative retinal detachment has been seen in two patients. Only after drainage of a psoas abscess did one patient improve. The other patient had posterior scleritis that improved with systemic corticosteroids. Optic disk edema occurred in two patients, presumably from posterior scleritis. Scleromalacia caused by scleritis occurred in one patient, and *Candida* endophthalmitis caused by intravenous nutrition occurred in another.

Coincidental

Coincidental complications occur so frequently that they are considered not related. They can include conjunctivitis, recurrent corneal erosion, glaucoma, and generalized retinal artery narrowing. Ulcerative colitis is complicated in the eyes by iritis and iridocyclitis.

MANAGEMENT

Treatment of ocular complications begins with identification of the type of complication. *Primary complications* require attention to the intestinal disease and clarification of its status. More aggressive treatment, either medically or surgically, may be indicated.

- Acute iritis requires topical corticosteroids, cycloplegics, and, at times, systemic corticosteroids.
- Limbal corneal infiltrates and episcleritis commonly respond to topical steroids.
- Chronic iridocyclitis is closely associated with active gut disease and has responded to excision of involved intestinal tissue. Systemic corticosteroids given for both conditions help but are not curative.
- The characteristic keratopathy of Crohn's disease does not impair vision and is not painful, so it requires no therapy.
- Macular edema syndromes usually respond to systemic corticosteroids.

Secondary complications require first the recognition that an intervening process exists and then that it be identified and treated.

- Dry eyes and night blindness are managed by giving the patient vitamin A, either parenterally or in a liquid preparation for oral ingestion and easy absorption.
- Exudative retinal detachment requires clarification of whether it is secondary to scleritis or from a remote abscess.
- Cataract is managed according to its nature. Early posterior subcapsular opacities have, in the author's experience, stopped progressing when systemic corticosteroids were stopped. However, the activity of the intestinal disease may require continuation of corticosteroids. In young people, visually disabling cataract is well managed by extracapsular, irrigation-aspiration techniques through a small limbal incision.
- Papillitis from posterior scleritis usually responds to systemic corticosteroids.
- Endophthalmitis caused by bacteria or fungi can be aggressively managed by diagnostic and therapeutic vitrectomy, which provides an organism for culture and removes the mass of infected vitreous. Appropriate antimicrobial therapy depends on identification and sensitivity studies.

Coincidental ocular disease requires only that the ophthalmologist recognize that it is not related to the intestinal disorder. Management is the same as would be given to any patient.

Management of a patient with an ocular complication of Crohn's disease or ulcerative colitis is difficult and time-consuming. Efforts must be expended to clarify the status of the intestinal disease and to communicate with the other physicians involved.

REFERENCES

Baldassano VF, Jr: Ocular manifestations of rheumatic diseases. Curr Opin Ophthalmol 9(6):85–88, 1998.

Bayless TM, Tokyer AZ, Polito JM, II, et al: Crohn's disease: concordance for site and clinical type in affected family members-potential hereditary influences. Gastroenterology 111:573–579, 1996.

Blase WP, Knox DL, Green WR. Granulomatous conjunctivitis in 2 patients with Crohn's disease. Br J Ophthalmol 68:901–903, 1984.

Bredvik BK, Trocme SD: Ocular manifestations of immunological and rheumatological inflammatory disorders. Curr Opin Ophthalmol 6(6):92–96, 1995.

Carty E, Rampton DS: Evaluation of new therapies for inflammatory bowel disease. Br J Clin Pharmacol 56(4):351–361, 2003.

Cheung O, Regueiro MD: Inflammatory bowel disease emergencies. Gastroenterol Clin North Am 32(4):1269–1288, 2003.

Hopkins DJ, Horan E, Burton IL, et al: Ocular disorders in a series of 332 patients with Crohn's disease. Br J Ophthalmol 58:732–737, 1974.

Lindberg E, Janerot G, Huitfeldt B: Smoking in Crohn's disease: effect on localization and clinical course. Gut 33:779–782, 1992.

Polito JM, II, Childs B, Mellits ED, et al: Crohn's disease: Influence of age at diagnosis on site and clinical type of disease. Gastroenterology 111:580–586, 1996.

Polito JM II, Rees RC, Childs B, et al: Preliminary evidence for genetic anticipation in Crohn's disease. Lancet 347:798–800, 1996.

Rudy AJ, Jampol LM: Crohn's disease and retinal vascular disease. Am J Ophthalmol 110:349–353, 1990.

Salmon JF, Wright JP, Bowen RM, Murray AD: Granulomatous uveitis in Crohn's disease: A clinicopathologic case report. Arch Ophthalmol 107:718–719, 1989.

66 HYPOVITAMINOSIS 066
(Xerophthalmia, Keratomalacia, Nutritional Blindness)

Ejaz A. Ansari, BSc(Hons), MBBCh, FRCOphth, MD
Maidstone, England

ETIOLOGY/INCIDENCE

Several different vitamins and minerals are required for eye health, although vitamin A has a pivotal role. The need for adequate vitamin A to prevent xerophthalmia and night blindness, especially in developing countries, is well described. Xerophthalmia impairs the vision of 5–10 million children annually, causing irreversible blindness in 500,000 of these. Children and women in developing countries, and even immigrants who follow their traditional dietary patterns, become deficient because of poor dietary consumption of preformed vitamin A (egg yolk, liver, dairy products) or provitamin A carotenoid-containing foods (green leafy vegetables, carrots, mango). Poor diets are exacerbated by diarrhea, gastroenteritis, and parasitic infections that reduce absorption of vitamin A and by frequent respiratory and other infectious diseases that increase vitamin A excretion or demand.

In developed nations, vitamin A deficiency and xerophthalmia are most commonly a consequence of poor absorption (regional enteritis, cystic fibrosis), liver disease (cirrhosis, hepatitis), poor diet (alcoholism, certain vegetarian diets) or self-imposed bizarre diets.

Vitamin A (retinol) is a necessary component of rhodopsin; deficiency results in impaired adaptation to darkness. As retinoic acid, vitamin A is essential for normal differentiation of mucus-secreting epithelia in the eye and many other epithelial-lined organs such as the respiratory and genitourinary tracts. Retinoic acid regulates the expression of more than 300 genes, affecting the immune response and therefore the risk of severe infectious disease.

Vitamin-B deficiency may also cause visual loss. Nutritional amblyopia, manifesting as scotomas, can result from hypovitaminosis B_1. Keratitis (hypovitaminosis B_2), corneal neovascularisation (hypovitaminosis B_6) and optic neuropathy (hypovitaminosis B_{12}) can also occur, and can be improved with adequate vitamin supplementation. Ocular hemorrhage is associated with vitamin C deficiency, or scurvy.

COURSE/PROGNOSIS

Simple, gradual depletion of vitamin A results in the appearance of xerophthalmia of sequentially increasing severity (XN, X1, X2, X3). Acute decompensation leads to the sudden occurrence of corneal ulcers, keratomalacia, or both. The milder forms (XN through X2, XF) respond rapidly within 1 to 7 days to vitamin A therapy, without leaving sequelae. Localized corneal ulcers also heal rapidly, usually within 1 to 2 weeks, leaving a localized scar of varying density. Localized keratomalacia heals more slowly, leaving a dense leucoma adherens. Limbus-to-limbus keratomalacia is gradually replaced by an opaque fibrovascular scar. The anterior chamber is invariably lost, with resulting staphyloma or phthisis. Treatment can still save the other eye, if involvement is less severe, as well as increase the likelihood of survival.

DIAGNOSIS

Vitamin A deficiency results in systemic and ocular manifestations. The systemic consequences are protean and often overlooked: increased severity of infectious disease, increased mortality, growth retardation and anemia. The ocular manifestations are almost pathognomonic and are summarized in the classification by ten Doeschate (see Table 66.1).

Salient characteristics that point to hypovitaminosis are:

- Corneal ulcers (sometimes secondarily infected) but otherwise lacking a ragged, inflamed appearance.
- History of preexisting night blindness in cases of gradually occurring deficiency.
- Presence of underlying causal factors for vitamin A deficiency (e.g. cystic fibrosis).
- Impaired dark adaptation.
- Depressed serum retinol.

Differential diagnosis

- Hereditary causes of night blindness.
- Traumatic or infectious ulcer or both.
- Superficial measles keratitis.

PROPHYLAXIS

The most important preventive measure is a well-balanced diet. In the developing world, prevention is achieved by periodic

TABLE 66.1 – Vitamin A deficiency ocular manifestations (Adapted from Tasman T, Jaeger EA, Duane's Ophthalmology 2006 Edition. Lippincott Williams and Wikins, Philadelphia US, Oct. 2005)	
Classification	**Signs**
XIA	Conjunctival xerosis (thickened, corrugated skin-like changes — keratinizing metaplasia)
X1B	Bitot's spots (foamy/cheesy perilimbal accretions — subepithelial inflammatory infiltration)
X2	Corneal xerosis (dry, hazy, irregular corneal surface)
X3A	Corneal ulceration with xerosis (initially small, peripheral and anterior chamber maintained)
X3B	Keratomalacia (full thickness corneal necrosis with loss of anterior chamber)
XN	Night blindness (early sign)
XF	Xerophthalmic fundus (spotty retinal depigmentation, reversible field defects)
XS	Corneal scars

NOTES: Xerophthalmia includes all ocular changes, from night blindness to corneal necrosis.

Keratomalacia represents only full-thickness necrosis.

The disease does not necessarily evolve through a series of clinical stages, but may manifest any stage alone.

supplementation with high-dose oral vitamin A (200,000 IU every 4 months, half this dose for children 6 to 11 months). Women of childbearing age are particularly susceptible to deficiency during the third trimester of pregnancy. Because of the risk of teratogenicity from high doses, pregnant women should receive not more than 10,000 IU daily.

In developed countries, alcoholics and others with poor diets should improve their diets or receive daily RDA supplements. People with chronic malabsorption, particularly those with cystic fibrosis, need larger oral doses. Adequacy should be periodically assessed by serum retinol determination. Unusually refractory cases of cystic fibrosis may require periodic intramuscular injection of water-miscible vitamin A (oil-miscible preparations should never be injected, as they are poorly absorbed from the injection site).

TREATMENT

The presence of vitamin A deficiency, particularly advanced deficiency with ocular involvement (xerophthalmia), is a medical emergency and a threat to sight and life.

Local

- Corneal ulceration or keratomalacia should be protected from secondary infections (or existing infections treated) with appropriate antibiotics.
- The globe should be protected from undue pressure, particularly in children.

Systemic

- Vitamin A 200,000 IU, water-miscible, PO immediately and again the next day.

Surgical

- There is rarely, if ever, a need for surgical intervention (e.g. tectonic grafts), as peripheral ulcers usually are plugged by iris and heal rapidly; limbus-to-limbus keratomalacia presents with the anterior chamber already lost.

COMMENTS

Vitamin A deficiency is a systemic disease that ophthalmologists are often in the position to detect first. Adequate attention must be paid to potential systemic effects and the need for supportive therapy.

REFERENCES

Ansari EA, Sahni K, Etherington C, et al: Ocular signs and symptoms and vitamin A status in patients with cystic fibrosis treated with daily vitamin A supplements. Br J Ophthalmol 83(6):688–691, 1999.

Mares JA, La Rowe TL, Blodi BA: Doctor, what vitamins should I take for my eyes? Arch Ophthalmol 122:628–635, 2004.

Sommer A, Green WR, Kenyon KR: Clinicohistopathologic correlations in xerophthalmic ulceration and necrosis. Arch Ophthalmol 100:953–963, 1982.

Sommer A, Hussaini G, Muhilal H, et al: History of nightblindness: a simple tool for xerophthalmia screening. Am J Clin Nutr 33:887–891, 1980.

Sommer A, West KP, Jr: Vitamin A deficiency: health, survival and vision. New York, Oxford University Press, 1996.

Underwood BA, Arthur P: The contribution of vitamin A to public health. FASEB J 10:1040–1048, 1996.

SECTION

4 Diorders of Protein Metabolism

67 OCULOCEREBRORENAL SYNDROME 270.8
(Lowe Syndrome)

Deborah M. Alcorn, MD
Stanford, California

Oculocerebrorenal syndrome of Lowe (OCRL), or Lowe's syndrome, is an X-linked recessive multisystem metabolic disorder involving the eyes, nervous system and kidneys. It is characterized by congenital cataracts, glaucoma, motor retardation, intellectual impairment, muscular hypotonia, seizures, renal tubular dysfunction (Fanconi's syndrome), metabolic acidosis, proteinuria, and aminoaciduria. These patients often exhibit a characteristic facial appearance of frontal bossing, enophthalmos, and full cheeks. Female carriers demonstrate characteristic lenticular opacities, though they have normal renal and neurologic functions.

OCRL has been mapped to Xq25–26. The OCRL 1 gene has been cloned. The gene encodes a phosphatidylinositol-4,5-biphosphate 5-phosphatase in the trans-Golgi complex.

ETIOLOGY/INCIDENCE

- Caused by reduction of phosphatidyliositol-4,5-biphosphate 5-phosphatase and accumulation of phosphatidylinositol-4,5-biphosphate (PIP2) with a disequilibrium of the phosphoinositides.
    - PIP 2 is known to be involved with cellular signallng, protein trafficking and actin polymerization, but the exact mechanism responsible for the disease remains uncertain.
- Rare disease: 1 in 200,000 to 500,000 live births.
- The vast majority of patients are male. A few cases are reported in females, often with X autosome translocation involving the OCRL1 locus.

COURSE/PROGNOSIS

Congenital bilateral cataracts are the hallmark of this disease. Lens abnormalities have been described in 20- and 24-week fetuses. Bilateral leukokoria is evident at birth, often with miosis, shallow chamber, and microphthalmos. These cataracterous lenses are small and discoid and histopathology shows an absence of demarcation between nucleus and cortex, indicating a retarded maturation. The posterior capsule is irregular, with warty excrescenses indicating abnormal function of posterior lens epithelium. If untreated, they may develop nystagmus and dense amblyopia. Best corrected visual acuity is infrequently better than 20/70 despite optimal management. Glaucoma is usually detected within the first year of life and develops in 50% to 70% of patients, usually by age 6. It is usually bilateral and of a primary nature. Corneal keloids may develop in up to 25% of patients, usually after age 5. They extend through the entire thickness of the cornea.

The initial neurologic manifestation of the disease is infantile hypotonia. After 1 year of age, deep tendon reflexes are absent. Up to 50% of patients have seizures, but there is no characteristic seizure type. There is a poorer prognosis for intellectual development with early-onset seizures and inadequately controlled seizures. The diagnosis of OCRL is compatible with normal intelligence with approximately 25% of patients having IQs in the 'normal' range (≥70). Their intelligence appears to be stable over their lifetime, excluding decline to intercedent illness. There is a high incidence of behavioral abnormalities, including tantrums and aggressive and self-injurious behavior.

The last of the clinical triad is renal dysfunction. Renal function and histology are normal in utero but may not always be normal at birth. There is subsequent development of proximal renal tubular acidosis, phosphaturia, aminoaciduria, and proteinuria. Acidosis leads to failure to thrive and metabolic collapse, if untreated. By the second to third decade there is gradual loss of creatinine clearance, with progressive renal failure.

Additional manifestations include arthropathy, joint swelling, and tenosynovitis. Half of the patients over 20 years old have diffuse swellings of both small and large joints and nodules of fingers and feet, which may represent excessive growth of fibroblasts. Fractures are common, particularly in the early childhood years.

At birth, these patients are within the normal growth curve, but fall in length, height, and weight especially by their early 20s. Up to 40% have cryptorchidism.

Patients with appropriate therapy may live to be 30 to 40 years old, generally dying from renal failure, respiratory distress, infection, or status epilepticus in the 2nd to 4th decade of life.

DIAGNOSIS

- Clinical.
- Biochemical.
    - Enzyme deficiency analysis, >99% sensitivity.

- DNA analysis:
  - Detection of mutations in OCRL1, about 90% sensitivity for affected males;
  - Detection of carrier females with a definite family history of Lowe's syndrome (known mutation).
- Prenatal diagnosis.
  - Families with identified mutation in the OCRL1 gene.
  - Enzymatic testing on males fetuses if no known mutation.

Clinical signs and symptoms

Clinical triad

- Congenital cataracts.
- Neonatal or infantile hypotonia with cognitive impairment and areflexia.
- Renal tubular dysfunction.

Confirming features

- Positive family history.
- Glaucoma.
- Characteristic facies: frontal bossing, enophthalmos, full cheeks.
- Positive laboratory testing.

Carrier status: lenticular changes

Detected in 94% by slit lamp examination

- Multiple (15 to >100) punctate gray-white cortical opacities.
- Located outside the nucleus.
- Wedge-shaped aggregates.
- Seen in increasing numbers with increasing age.
- Also seen in the general population, but with less numerous opacities.

Subcapsular cataract, usually posterior

- Increases in size and density with age.

Laboratory findings

Urinalysis

- Aminoaciduria, proteinuria, calciuria and phosphaturia.
- Urine ph is usually between 6.0 and 7.5 with bicarbonate loss evident in the urine with proximal renal tubular acidosis.
- Low urine osmolality and elevated 24 hour volumes.
- Elevated retinal binding protein (RBP) and n-acetyl-glucosaminidase (NAG) (both are sensitive markers of proximal tubular integrity).

Serum

- Elevated acid phosphatase.
- Elevation of aspartate aminotransferase (AST), lactate dehydrogenase (LDH), creatine phosphokinase (CPK) and glutamic oxaloacetic transaminase (SGOT).
- Elevated total cholesterol (increased HDL) with normal serum triglycerides.
- Elevated a-2 band on serum protein electrophoresis.

Imaging studies

- Brain MRI: Mild ventriculomegaly is evident in about one third of cases. White matter changes in the periventricular region. The increased signal intense areas may correspond to cysts with as yet no known clinical significance.
- Ocular ultrasound.
- If no view posteriorly, secondary to cataract, need to assess status of posterior segment R/O mass or RD.

Differential diagnosis

Many, diverse systemic diseases are associated with bilateral cataracts, such as:

- Bilateral cataracts and glaucoma:
  - Rubella;
  - Anterior segment dysgenesis.
- Bilateral cataracts and hypotonia:
  - Congenital myotonic dystrophy;
  - Congenital myopathies;
  - Congenital infections;
  - Peroxisomal disorders.
- Bilateral cataracts and neurologic features:
  - Syphilis;
- Bilateral cataracts and renal disease.
  - Alport's syndrome.

PROPHYLAXIS

- Prenatal diagnosis and carrier detection.

TREATMENT

Systemic

Ocular

- Cataract extraction if indicated and as early as possible.
- Appropriate aphakic prescription (glasses, contact lenses or intraocular lenses).
- Monitor and appropriate treatment of glaucoma as indicated, medical or surgical.
- Appropriate amblyopia treatment.
- Monitor for potential strabismus.
- Minimize corneal epithelial trauma.

Renal

- Consistent periodic monitoring for renal complications.
- Alkalizing agents to manage metabolic acidosis.
- Citrates (sodium and/or potassium citrate).
- Oral phosphate and vitamin D (for rickets).
- Replacement of fluids, if polyuria.
- Calcium supplementation, as indicated.
- Carnitine may be indicated if abnormally low blood levels.

General

- Anticonvulsants in patients with seizures.
- Speech or physical therapy or both, as indicated by developmental delay.
- Behavioral modification as needed, especially for maladaptive behaviors.
- Feeding therapy, particularly with severe hypotonia.

Genetic counseling

- Thirty percent of affected males have *de novo* mutations.

X-linked recessive.

COMMENTS

Appropriate and prompt diagnosis is imperative in conjunction with the initiation of proper treatment. OCRL heterozygotes must be identified. Lenticular changes may be identified by means of dilatation and slit-lamp examination.

Support group

Lowe Syndrome Association
222 Lincoln Street
West Lafayette, IN 47906
(317) 743–3634

REFERENCES

Kruger SJ, Wilson ME, Jr, Hutchinson AK, et al: Cataracts and glaucoma in patients with oculocerebrorenal syndrome. Arch Ophthalmol 121(9):1234–1237, 2003.

Lavin CW, McKeown CA: The oculocerebrorenal syndrome of Lowe. Int Ophthalmol Clin 33:179–191, 1993.

Lin T, Lewis RA, Nussbaum RL: Molecular confirmation of carriers for Lowe Syndrome. Ophthalmol 106(1):119–122, 1999.

Lowe CU, Terrey M, MacLachan EA: Organic aciduria, decreased renal ammonia production, hydrophthalmos, and mental retardation: a clinical entity. Am J Dis Child 83:164–184, 1952.

Lowe M: Structure and function of the Lowe syndrome protein OCRL1. Traffic 6:711–719, 2005.

Nussbaum RL, Orrison BM, Janne PA, et al: Physical mapping and genomic structure of the Lowe syndrome gene OCRL 1. Hum Genet 99:145–150, 1997.

Tripathi RC, Cibis GW, Tripathi BJ: Pathogenesis of cataracts in patients with Lowe's syndrome. Ophthalmol 93:1046–1051, 1986.

Walton DS, Katsavounidou G, Lowe CU: Glaucoma with the oculocerebrorenal syndrome of Lowe J Glaucoma 14(3):181–185, 2005.

68 TYROSINEMIA II 270.2
(Pseudodendritic Keratitis, Recessive Keratosis Palmoplantaris, Richner–Hanhart Syndrome)

Stephen P. Christiansen, MD
Minneapolis, Minnesota

ETIOLOGY/INCIDENCE

Tyrosinemia II is a rare autosomal recessive metabolic disorder characterized by herpetiform corneal ulcers and painful keratoses of the hands and feet. It is caused by deficiency of hepatic cytoplasmic tyrosine aminotransferase (cTAT). The gene for this enzyme has been mapped to chromosome 16q 22.1–q22.3. Hepatic mitochondrial TAT levels are normal. Cytoplasmic TAT catalyzes the conversion of tyrosine to p-hydroxyphenylpyruvic acid. Deficiency of c-TAT results in elevated plasma tyrosine concentration, tyrosinuria, and tyrosyluria.

COURSE/PROGNOSIS

Tyrosine crystallizes within cells, initiating an inflammatory cascade. Ocular involvement is usually heralded by pain, photophobia, tearing and conjunctival injection. The keratitis has been described as stellate or branching and is initially restricted to the epithelium. Most patients develop bilateral pseudodendritic keratitis early within the first year of life. Onset is variable, however, and ranges from 2 weeks of age to late in the second decade. Some patients never develop ocular findings. As the disease progresses, corneal ulceration, subepithelial and stromal scarring and corneal neovascularization may occur with resultant visual loss. Cataracts and glaucoma have also been described in untreated patients. Nystagmus and exotropia have been noted in some patients with tyrosinemia II; these may be a consequence of visual loss rather than a primary effect of the disease.

Cutaneous lesions typically occur with or after the eye lesions. They begin as blisters or erosions on the palms and soles, particularly on the tips of the digits and the thenar and hypothenar eminences. The blisters crust and eventually become hyperkeratotic. The lesions are painful but not pruritic and often present in a linear distribution. The severity of cutaneous involvement may wax and wane independently of systemic or topical therapy. Some authors have described symptomatic improvement in ocular and cutaneous symptoms during the summer months. Mental retardation, learning disability, behavioral anomalies, microcephaly, growth retardation, and seizures have been noted in some patients with tyrosinemia II, but are, at best, inconsistent findings.

DIAGNOSIS

Laboratory findings

Serum

- Tyrosinemia is diagnostic. Plasma tyrosine ranges from 16 to 62 mg/dL (normal, 0.6 to 2.1 mg/dL).

Urine

- Tyrosinuria and tyrosyluria.
- Elevated tyrosine metabolites.
- No other amino acids elevated.

Liver biopsy

- Decreased cTAT activity.

Differential diagnosis

- Herpes simplex keratitis: bilateral presentation, minimal staining with fluorescein or rose bengal, negative viral studies, normal corneal sensation and lack of response to topical antiviral therapy allow one to rule out a herpetic etiology.

TREATMENT

Systemic

- Dietary restriction of tyrosine and phenylalanine intake. This diet may be initiated with a prepared formula, such as the Mead Johnson 3200 AB diet. As plasma tyrosine levels decrease, the diet may be liberalized, with the goal of therapy being to maintain plasma tyrosine in the range of 10 mg/dL. Reduction of plasma tyrosine results in fairly rapid resolution of both ocular and cutaneous lesions, both of which will recur if an unrestricted diet is resumed. The effect of dietary control on the occurrence of mental retardation in tyrosinemia II is unknown.

Ocular

- Symptomatic: the early ocular manifestations of tyrosinemia II respond rapidly to dietary therapy. Therefore, initial ocular therapy is usually symptomatic. Topical cortisteroid, antiviral, and antibiotic therapy have all been shown to be ineffective.

Medical

- Oral retinoids have been used to control cutaneous lesions even when dietary compliance is poor. No other systemic or topical treatments have proven effective to date, including steroids.

Surgical

- Lamellar or penetrating keratoplasty may be necessary if corneal scarring or neovascularization has affected the visual axis. However, failure to address the underlying metabolic defect will promote recurrence of keratitis in the graft.
- Excimer laser photokeratectomy may be useful in this disorder if corneal scarring and neovascularization are superficial.

COMMENTS

Patients with tyrosinemia II may first present with ocular symptoms and signs. Thus, it is imperative that the ophthalmologist consider this metabolic cause of keratitis during this initial evaluation. Clinical suspicion of this disorder can be easily confirmed with amino acid studies. Early diagnosis and dietary intervention may ultimately prevent visual loss.

Tyrosinemia II is distinct from tyrosinemia I, another recessive disorder caused by a deficiency of fumarylacetoacetate hydrolase. Patients with tyrosinemia I also have elevated levels of tyrosine and its metabolites. However, these patients do not have the cutaneous or ocular findings of patients with tyrosinemia II. Rather, they characteristically have hepatic and renal dysfunction and failure.

SUPPORT GROUPS

National Coalition for PKU & Allied Disorders, P.O. Box 1244, Mansfield, MA 02048

www.pku-allieddisorders.org

Contact Person: Trish Mullaley, Phone: (877) 996-2723, E-mail: coalition4pkuad@aol.com

REFERENCES

Scott CR: The genetic tyrosinemias. Am J Med Genet, Part C, Semin Med Genet 142C:121–126, 2006.

Heidemann DG, Dunn SP, Bawle EV, et al: Early diagnosis of tyrosinemia type II. Am J Ophthalmol 107:559–560, 1989.

Macsai MS, Schwartz TL, Hinkle D, et al: Tyrosinemia type II: nine cases of ocular signs and symptoms. Am J Ophthalmol 132:522–527, 2001.

Natt E, Kida K, Odievre M, et al: Point mutations in the tyrosine aminotransferase gene in tyrosinemia type II. Proc Nat Acad Sci 89:9297–9301, 1992.

Shear CS, Nyhan WL: Tyrosinemia II, Oregon type. In: Buyse ML, ed: Birth defects encyclopedia. Dover, MA, Center for Birth Defects Information Services, 1990.

SECTION

5 Disorders of Carbohydrate Metabolism

69 DIABETES MELLITUS 250.0

F. Hampton Roy, MD, FACS
Little Rock, Arkansas

ETIOLOGY/INCIDENCE

Diabetes mellitus is a complex disorder of carbohydrate, lipid, and protein metabolism characterized clinically by hyperglycemia and a relative or total lack of insulin. It is a common disorder that is prevalent worldwide. The development of diabetes is influenced by multiple factors, both genetic and environmental. The disease may develop in the first or second decade of life (type I) or in middle or late life (type II); more than half of diabetic individuals older than 40 years are overweight. A family history of diabetes is positive in 25% of patients. The disease is generally transmitted as a recessive trait without sex linkage.

The increased life span of diabetics due to the use of insulin and other hypoglycemic agents has also resulted in a longer duration of the disease. This is associated with an increased incidence of accelerated atherosclerosis and a triad of retinopathy, nephropathy and neuropathy. The degree of hyperglycemia is also thought to influence the incidence and severity of complications.

Diabetic retinopathy is the most serious ocular manifestation of diabetes mellitus and it causes more blindness among working-age Americans than any other disease. More than 20 million people worldwide are estimated to be blind due to complications from diabetes. Having diabetes increases the risk of blindness by 25%. The etiology is multifactorial and is still not fully understood, but there is evidence to suggest strong relationships between retinopathy and the duration of diabetic disease and high levels of blood glucose.

There is an increasing incidence of diabetes in the United States; an estimated 6% of the population is affected. Of the estimated 16 million diabetics in the United States, about half have retinopathy. Type II diabetes and its complications affect minority populations more than the white population. Native Americans, blacks, and Hispanics have twofold to sixfold higher incidence rates. The rate of clinically detectable retinopathy is less than 25% in patients with a known diabetes of less than 5 years, about 50% with a history of 5 to 15 years, and more than 75% with a history of more than 15 years.

The exact cause of diabetic microvascular disease is not known; possibly, prolonged exposure to hyperglycemia results in glycosylation of tissue proteins with ultimate endothelial damage. Specific changes that have been noted are the loss of intramural pericytes and basement membrane thickening, which results in obstruction of the capillary lumen and a breakdown of the blood-retina barrier.

Ocular or periocular

- Ciliary body: glycogen deposits in pigment epithelium, thickening of basement membrane.
- Cornea: endothelial pigment deposits, hypesthesia, poor epithelial healing.
- Extraocular muscles: paralysis of third or sixth cranial nerve.
- Iris: ectropion uveae, glycogen deposits in pigment epithelium, pupillary abnormality, rubeosis iridis.
- Lens: cataracts, pigment deposits on epithelium, premature presbyopia.
- Macula: edema, ischemia, exudates, hemorrhage.
- Optic nerve: atrophy, papillopathy.
- Retina: microaneurysms, hard exudates, hemorrhages, cotton-wool spots, venous abnormalities, intraretinal microvascular abnormalities (IRMAs), neovascularization, detachment, arteriolar sclerosis.
- Vitreous: asteroid hyalosis, detachment, hemorrhage.

Diabetic retinopathy

Diabetic retinopathy is the most common and one of the most serious ocular manifestations of diabetes mellitus. Visual loss, often severe, can result through one or more of the following mechanisms: macular edema due to breakdown of the blood–retina barrier, macular ischemia due to occluded perifoveal capillaries, fibrovascular proliferation with associated complications of vitreous hemorrhage, traction detachment of macula, and neovascular glaucoma.

Classification and clinical features of diabetic retinopathy

Two stages are recognized: the early, or nonproliferative (NPDR), stage and the more advanced, or proliferative (PDR), stage. Macular edema can develop during either stage.

NPDR is further described as mild, moderate, severe and very severe. Mild NPDR is characterized by the presence of microaneurysms; retinal edema, or 'thickening'; and hard exudates. The Early Treatment Diabetic Retinopathy Study (ETDRS) coined the term *clinically significant macular edema* (CSME) to indicate situations in which edema or hard exudates involved or threatened to involve the center of the fovea. Moderate NPDR additionally presents with cotton-wool spots, IRMAs and venous beading. Severe NPDR is characterized by the presence of four quadrants of significant retinal hemorrhages, two quadrants of significant venous beading, or one quadrant of significant IRMA. This is known as the ETDRS *4, 2, 1 rule.* Very severe NPDR is defined as the presence of two or more of these criteria. Severe NPDR can progress to high-risk PDR in 15%, and very severe NPDR can progress to PDR in 45% of patients within 1 year. Venous beading, IRMAs, and extensive capillary nonperfusion on fluorescein angiography are important indicators of significant retinal ischemia.

PDR is further described as early, high risk, or advanced. It is said to occur with the formation of new vessels on the disk (NVD) or elsewhere on the retina (NVE) and with associated proliferation of fibrous tissue. High-risk PDR, as defined by the Diabetic Retinopathy Study (DRS), presents with three or more of the following high-risk characteristics:

- Vitreous or preretinal hemorrhage.
- New vessels.
- New vessels at or within one disk area of the disk.
- Moderate to severe new vessels (NVD equal to or more than one third of the disk area or NVE equal to or more than one half of the disk area).

Advanced PDR is associated with recurrent vitreous hemorrhage, retinal detachment, and neovascular glaucoma. Vision is seriously compromised, and a serious threat of blindness exists.

Fluorescein angiography is of value in the early detection of microangiopathy and in the assessment of macular edema and retinal ischemia. It also aids in photocoagulation.

PROPHYLAXIS

The best way to prevent the major complications of diabetes is probably to keep blood glucose levels as close to normal as possible. The Diabetes Control and Complications Trial (DCCT) has demonstrated that tight blood glucose control through intensive insulin therapy can delay the onset and slow the progression of retinopathy, nephropathy, and neuropathy in type I diabetics. Tightening of blood glucose control is seen to cause a deterioration in retinopathy in some patients with mild or moderate NPDR. This generally stabilizes with time.

TREATMENT

The use of desperate measures such as pituitary ablation has been abandoned because of the associated morbidity and mortality rates. Various pharmacologic agents have been used to treat diabetic retinopathy; the past use of drugs like clofibrate, calcium dobesilate, aspirin, and aldose reductase inhibitors largely reflected the prevalent thinking regarding the possible causes of retinopathy. The ETDRS evaluated the role of aspirin in dosages of 650 mg/day for a possible role in treatment because of its antiplatelet aggregation and fibrinolytic actions. The Sorbinil Retinopathy Trial likewise evaluated the role of an aldose reductase inhibitor (sorbinil) aimed at blocking the effect of the enzyme aldose reductase and thus preventing the formation of toxic levels of sorbitol through the polyol metabolic pathway. None of these drugs have been found to be of value.

Contemporary management of diabetic retinopathy consists of good medical control of diabetes, retinal photocoagulation, and additional vitreous surgery when needed.

Medical

The DCCT has clearly established the value of tight control of blood glucose levels in type I diabetics. Good metabolic control not only helps to prevent retinopathy but also helps to slow down its progression. Type II diabetes in persons whose diabetes cannot be controlled by diet alone or those who are unwilling or unable to adhere to a restrictive diet can be controlled with oral hypoglycemic agents, insulin, or both. Most type I diabetics require insulin.

Photocoagulation

Retinal photocoagulation is the most successful tool in the treatment of diabetic retinopathy; the landmark studies of DRS and ETDRS have clearly established its value. The DRS proved the value of panretinal photocoagulation (PRP) in high-risk PDR and severe NPDR. The ETDRS, on the other hand, demonstrated the usefulness of macular photocoagulation (grid or focal) in CSME.

Photocoagulation is commonly performed with lasers emitting in the green wave band such as argon or frequency-doubled YAG lasers. Lasers emitting in the red or yellow ranges are useful when there is blood in the vitreous or when treatment is needed very close to the fovea. The treatment technique used for PDR is called 'panretinal' or 'scatter.' It consists of the application of several hundred 500-μm-diameter burns to the midperipheral and peripheral portions of the retina. Treatment extends posteriorly to two disk diameters from the center of the macula in the temporal quadrants and to one-half disk diameter nasal to the optic disk. In addition, focal treatment using moderate-intensity confluent burns may be applied to new vessels on the surface of the retina. The total number of burns is usually 1200 to 1600, depending on the severity of the retinopathy. Each burn is of a duration of 0.1 to 0.2 second. Power is adjusted to achieve a moderately white burn. The treatment is applied on an outpatient basis with the patient under topical or retrobulbar anesthesia. Focal treatment to new vessels on the optic disk is not necessary.

The regression of neovascularization is usually apparent soon (weeks to months) after treatment, but it is not always complete or permanent. When substantial regression of neovascularization is not obtained or not maintained, one or more additional scatter treatments over previously untreated retina are often followed by satisfactory regression.

The ETDRS recommended treatment of CSME and formulated guidelines that consist of the identification and treatment of all leaking microvascular abnormalities located in an area 500 to 3000 μm from the center of the fovea. The treatment would be focal or in the form of a grid pattern, depending on the nature of the leakage. The burns used to treat the macula are smaller and mild.

The complications of photocoagulation are generally mild and often transient; they include a decrease in light sensitivity, contraction of peripheral visual field, loss of accommodation, and nyctalopia. Intense treatments in a single session have been associated with more serious complications of detachment or hemorrhage of the choroid, macular pucker and subretinal neovascularization.

Surgical

The aims of pars plana vitreous surgery are to remove vitreous hemorrhage, to relieve all traction threatening the macula, and to remove the scaffolding on which fibrovascular proliferation grows. It is required in eyes with severe retinopathy in which there is either nonresolving or recurrent vitreous hemorrhage that prevents vision or the delivery of photocoagulation, increasing vitreoretinal traction posing a threat to the macula from traction detachment, combined traction and rhegmatogenous detachment, and progressive proliferation uncontrolled with photocoagulation, or, in some cases, with preretinal membrane. The Diabetic Retinopathy Vitrectomy Study emphasized the value of vitrectomy in severe proliferative disease and the usefulness of early vitrectomy (1 to 6 months) in eyes with vitreous hemorrhage in type I diabetics.

COMMENTS

Diabetic retinopathy poses a major threat of blindness to patients with diabetes mellitus. This blindness is preventable in most cases. Early detection and proper diabetic control through diet, exercise, medication, or a combination probably are still the best tools for controlling the disease. Equally important are regular examinations that include ophthalmoscopic examinations through dilated pupils. Should retinopathy be seen, progression should be monitored by an ophthalmologist who can seek specialized care, such as photocoagulation or vitrectomy, at the appropriate time. It must be recognized that pregnancy and concurrent cardiovascular disease are higher-risk situations that require greater care.

Photocoagulation with or without vitrectomy is largely an effective tool to retard the progression of retinopathy; however, it is an invasive procedure that involves some destruction of the retina. Some patients will complain of a decrease in visual acuity or a constriction of the visual fields after the procedure. Current emphasis therefore is on prevention and on the development of new drugs that are safe and have the potential of preventing or arresting the progress of retinopathy. Retinal ischemia is believed to result in the formation of a vascular endothelial growth factor, a molecule suspected to stimulate endothelial cells to multiply and cause neovascularization. Drugs that inhibit the formation of this molecule or block its vasoproliferative effect could play an important role in the management of PDR. Certain protein kinases could block the chemical trigger for angiogenesis. Antihistamines could be of value in preventing breakdown of the blood-retina barrier due to the liberation of bradykinin or serotonin. These agents are being investigated for their therapeutic potential.

REFERENCES

Aiello LP, Avery RL, Arrigg PG, et al: Vascular endothelial growth factor in ocular fluid of patients with diabetic retinopathy and other retinal disorders. New Engl J Med 331:1480–1487, 1994.

American Diabetes Association: Diabetes 1996: vital statistics. Alexandria, American Diabetes Association, 1996:32–33, 51–59.

Carter JS, Monterrosa A, Pugh JA: Non-insulin-dependent diabetes mellitus in minorities in the United States. Ann Intern Med 125:221–232, 1996.

Deb-Joardar N, Germain N, Thuret G, Manoli P, et al: Screening for diabetic retinopathy by ophthalmologists and endocrinologists with pupillary dilation and a nonmydriatic digital camera. Am J Ophthalmol 140(5):814–821, 2005.

Early Treatment Diabetic Retinopathy Study Research Group: Focal photocoagulation treatment of diabetic macular edema. ETDRS Report 19. Arch Ophthalmol 113:1144–1155, 1995.

El-Bradey M, Plummer DJ, Uwe-Bartsch D, Freeman WR: Scanning laser entoptic perimetry for the detection of visual defects associated with diabetic retinopathy. Br J Ophthalmol 90(1):17–19, 2006.

70 GALACTOSEMIAS 271.1
(Galactose-1-Phosphate Uridyl Transferase Deficiency, Galactokinase Deficiency, Galactose-6-Phosphate Epimerase Deficiency)

Deborah M. Alcorn, MD
Stanford, California

ETIOLOGY/INCIDENCE

Galactosemias are autosomal recessive disorders resulting from an error of galactose metabolism caused by a deficiency of any one of three enzymes: transferase, galactokinase, or epimerase. These enzymes catalyze the reactions in the Leloir pathway by which galactose is converted to glucose-1-phosphate. The main dietary source of galactose is mammalian milk, in which it is found in the form of disaccharide lactose. Lactose is then hydrolyzed with the release of the monosaccharides glucose and galactose.

Worldwide estimates of incidence vary from 1 in 18,000 to 1 in 187,000 persons. In the United States, the incidence is approximately 1 in 50,000; it is rare in Asia; and it is more frequent in Europe, with an incidence of 1 in 40,000 persons.

Classic galactosemia, which is the most common and the most severe form, is caused by the impairment of galactose-1-phosphate-uridyl-transferase (GALT). The gene has been mapped to chromosome 9p13 and cloned. Within days of consuming milk, these infants develop a toxicity syndrome characterized by vomiting, diarrhea, failure to thrive, lethargy, jaundice and hepatomegaly. If left untreated, sepsis (usually *E. Coli*) and shock are likely. Approximately 30% develop cataracts.

Galactokinase deficiency catalyzes the first step in galactose metabolism (phosphorylation of galactose). The deficiency results from mutation in the *GALK1* gene on 17q24. Toxicity in galactokinase deficiency is milder, resulting primarily only in cataracts, usually occurring in the first year of life. The exact prevalence of GALK deficiency is unknown, but felt to be <1/100,000.

The third and rarest type is deficiency of uridine diphosphate (UDP) galactose-4-epimerase, GALE deficiency. UDP galactose-4-epimerase catalyzes the third step of galactose metabolism. Two types of epimerase deficiency have been described; one involves only red and white blood cells without metabolic derangement in other tissues and is clinically benign. The other, generalized epimerase deficiency has clinical manifestations similar to those of transferase deficiency and responds to dietary restrictions. GALE deficiency should be considered in patients with liver disease, failure to thrive, increased red blood cell galactose-1-phosphate but with normal GALT enzyme activity.

In infants, the clinical manifestations are toxicity syndromes resulting from exposure to galactose. All three enzyme deficiencies can cause lenticular opacities.

Pathophysiology

Classic galactosemia results in the accumulation of galactose-1-phosphate and galactose in varying organs with resultant toxicity. In addition, galactitol and galactonate are present in significant amounts. Cataract formation is secondary to galactose-1-phosphate accumulation in the lens with its reduction to galactitol with resultant osmotic swelling. This causes loss of plasma membrane redox potential and subsequent cell death.

Proposed theories for the long-term sequelae include *in utero* damage, chronic self-intoxication by endogenous galactose formation, or depletion of key metabolites.

COURSE/PROGNOSIS

Galactokinase deficiency is the mildest form, manifesting primarily in cataracts. Some patients present with pseudotumor cerebri. These children do not present with the additional systemic manifestations that occur in patients with transferase and epimerase deficiency. Cataracts may develop in heterozygotes.

In transferase and generalized epimerase deficiency, neonatal illness presents soon after the initiation of milk feedings, manifesting with vomiting, failure to thrive, jaundice, hepatomegaly, *Escherichia coli* sepsis, and cataracts. Most patients present with jaundice in the first few weeks of life distinguishable from physiologic hyperbilirubinemia of the newborn by the degree of elevation in serum total bilirubin or time of onset. Untreated, patients will eventually manifest hepatomegaly, abnormal liver function tests, ascites and renal failure. The mortality rate is high if there is no treatment.

Infant classic galactosemics develop 'oil droplet' cataracts in the central lens as well as in the nuclear fibers secondary to galactitol formation in the lens. If left untreated, they may progress to lamellar and, eventually, total cataracts. There may be some reversibility of the lenticular changes if galactose exclusion is initiated early (secondary to resolution of the nuclear edema). Vitreous hemorrhage has been reported, albeit rare.

Despite rapid treatment with strict lactose-galactose restriction, which alleviates the acute toxicity, dietary treatment alone is not sufficient to prevent long-term complications, particularly in transferase-deficient patients. Long-term sequelae consist of speech abnormalities, ovarian failure, ataxia, developmental delay and mental deficiency. Speech and language deficits, associated with a characteristic verbal dyspraxia, are the most recognizable sign of central nervous system dysfunction. Tremors, ataxia, and incoordination become evident during late childhood and adolescence in about one fourth of these patients. Despite dietary restriction, there is poor growth and physical development. There is a high incidence of ovarian failure and pregnancy is rare because of the high incidence of hypergonadotropic hypogonadism with ovarian atrophy. Overall, long term results are disappointing, which may be related to delayed diagnosis and poor dietary compliance.

DIAGNOSIS

Laboratory findings

- Newborn screening: utilizes blood to assay GALT enzyme activity and quantify total red blood cell galactose-1-phosphate concentration and galactose.
- Any infant with suspicious symptoms, positive newborn screening test, or a positive clinitest reaction and a negative glucostix reaction, deserves measurement of GALT activity.
- Urine for reducing substances: tube test, not dipstick (may be falsely negative if the infant is not feeding well or ingesting non-milk formula).
- Galactosemia: determined by quantitative measurement of erythrocyte galactose-1-phosphate uridyltransferase (GALT) activity and its isoforms by isoelectric focusing of GALT.
  - In classic (G/G) galactosemia, affected have GALT enzyme activity <5% of controls.
  - In Duarte Variant (D/G) galactosemia, affected have GALT enzyme activity between 5% and 20% of controls.
- Molecular testing:
  - Mutation analysis;
  - Sequence analysis.
- Prenatal testing available:
  - Using both GALT enzyme activity and known family mutations.
- GALE Deficiency: detection of reduced UDP-galactose-4-epimerase activity is diagnostic.
- Slit-lamp examination for any lenticular opacities (faint opacities may be overlooked on indirect ophthalmoscopy).

Additional findings

- Abnormal liver function tests.
- Albuminuria.
- Hyperchloremic metabolic acidosis.
- Hyperaminoaciduria.

Differential diagnosis

- Bilateral cataracts and metabolic disease:
  - Hypocalcemia;
  - Hypoglycemia;
  - Hyperferritinemia;
  - Hypoparathyroidism.
- Neonatal hepatotoxicity:
  - Alagille syndrome;
  - Wilson disease;
  - Niemann–Pick disease.
- Sepsis.

TREATMENT

Systemic

- Immediate dietary restriction of all lactose-containing foods and medicines (those that contain lactulose) for transferase and kinase patients:
  - Complete absence of galactose prevents formation of complex carbohydrates and galactolipids necessary for metabolic processes;
  - Includes not only milk but also some fruits and vegetables (especially watermelon and tomatoes);
  - Lifelong dietary commitment, though debated how stringent it should be after early childhood;
  - Generally, lactose restriction helps prevent severe liver disease, death from *Escherichia coli* sepsis, or significant cataracts but no significant effect on central nervous dysfunction or ovarian dysfunction.
- Calcium supplements.
- Speech therapy.
- Developmental evaluation.
- Metabolic geneticist.
- Endocrinologist (evaluation of ovarian status).

Ocular

- If lens opacifies and becomes visually significant or there are total cataracts, lens extraction indicated:
  - Maximize visual potential.
- For vitreous hemorrhage, possible surgical intervention.

SUPPORT GROUP

Parents of Galactosemic Children Inc.
2871 Stagecoach Drive
Valley Springs, CA 95252
(209) 772-2449
E-mail: www.galactosemie.org

REFERENCES

Beigi B, O'Keefe MO, Bowell R, et al: Ophthalmic findings in classical galactosaemia: prospective study. Br J Ophthalmol 77:162–164, 1993.

Burke JP, O'Keefe M, Bowell R, Naughten ER: Ophthalmic findings in classical galactosemia: a screened population. J Pediatr Ophthalmol Strabismus 26:165–168, 1989.

Gitzelmann R: Hereditary galactokinase deficiency, a newly recognized cause of juvenile cataracts. Pediatr Res 1:14, 1967.

Levy HL, Brown AE, Williams SE, de Juan E: Vitreous hemorrhage as an ophthalmic complication of galactosemia. J Pediatr 129:922–925, 1996.

Mason HH, Turner ME: Chronic galactosemia. Am J Dis Child 50:359, 1935.

Ridel KR, Leslie ND, Gilbert DL: An updated review of the long-term neurological effects of galactosemia. Pediatr Neurol 33(3):153–161, 2005.

Schweitzer-Krantz S: Early diagnosis of inherited metabolic disorders towards improving outcome: the controversial issue of galactosaemia. Eur J Pediatr 162 Suppl 1:S50–S53, 2003.

Stambolian D: Galactose and cataract. Surv Ophthalmol 32:333–349, 1988.

Walter JH, Collins JE, Leonard JV: Recommendations for the management of galactosaemia. UK Galactosaemia Steering Group. Arch Dis Child 80(1):93–96, 1999.

71 MUCOPOLYSACCHARIDOSIS IH 277.5 *(Dysostosis Multiplex, Hurler Syndrome, MPS IH, Pfaundler–Hurler Syndrome)*

Fernando H. Murillo-Lopez, MD
La Paz, Bolivia

ETIOLOGY/INCIDENCE

Mucopolysaccharidosis type I (MPS I), the most common of the mucopolysaccharidoses, is an autosomal recessive disease caused by mutations in the α-L-iduronidase (IDUA) gene (localized to the distal short arm of chromosome 4 at 4p16) α-L-iduronidase is the enzyme responsible for the breakdown of dermatan sulfate and heparan sulfate. As a result of this mutation, abnormal intracellular accumulations of glycosaminoglycans and interference with normal cell function take place. Corneal clouding results from abnormal accumulation of proteoglycans in abnormal vacuolated stromal cells and nearby stroma. To date, more than 46 mutations of the IDUA gene have been defined for MPS I. Since the cloning of this gene, mutation analysis has also provided some molecular explanations for the range of MPS I phenotypes. The overall frequency is 1 per 100,000 live births worldwide. Severe Hurler syndrome and mild Scheie's disease are extremes of the clinical spectrum caused by different IDUA mutations. Children affected by Hurler syndrome may develop normally for the first few months, but typical Hurler manifestations begin to appear in the first or second year of life. The primary manifestations include skeletal abnormalities, umbilical and inguinal hernias, enlargement of the spleen and liver, and mental retardation. Clouding of the cornea is present in all patients with this disease. Prenatal diagnosis is possible by measuring the iduronidase activity in cultured amniotic cells and in chorionic villi.

COURSE/PROGNOSIS

- Slowly progressive, if untreated it usually leads to death before the age of 14 years.
- Death commonly occurs from cardiac failure and chronic respiratory infection, although early death during infancy has occurred after endocardial fibroelastosis.
- There is a wide range of clinical phenotypes in MPS I, which makes the prediction of disease severity and genetic counseling difficult.

DIAGNOSIS

Early diagnosis is essential to achieve an acceptable outcome after bone marrow transplantation (BMT). The diagnosis is suggested by certain clinical and radiologic findings, as well as by a urine screening test, and it should be confirmed with enzyme assays of cultured fibroblasts or leukocytes. By the end of the first year of life, the clinical diagnosis becomes evident. The following are the most common clinical and radiologic findings associated with MPS I.

Clinical signs and symptoms

Systemic

Within 3 months of age

- Recurrent rhinitis.
- Recurrent inguinal hernias.

Within 6 months of age

- Skeletal abnormalities.
- Gibbus formation.
- Asymmetric chest.
- Prominent sternum.
- Bulging forehead.

After 9 months

- Decreased hearing secondary to recurrent ear infections.
- Coarse facial appearance.
- Hepatomegaly.

All age groups

- Nasal obstruction, sinus polyps, multiple ear, nose, and throat operations.
- Recurrent upper respiratory and sinus infections.

- Macrocephaly (secondary to calvarial thickening and hydrocephalus), microcephaly, hydrocephalus, craniosynostosis, kyphosis, scoliosis.
- Dysostosis multiplex, a group of skeletal abnormalities consisting of a large skull with a deep elongated, J-shaped sella; thickened, oar-shaped ribs; deformed, hook-shaped lower thoracic and upper lumbar vertebrae; pelvic dysplasia; shortened tubular bones with expanded diaphyses and dysplastic epiphyses.

Ocular

- Ocular manifestations include peripheral/central corneal clouding, megalocornea, buphthalmos, coarse eyelashes, lid edema, ptosis, retinal pigmentary degeneration, optic nerve atrophy, hypertelorism, chronic open-angle glaucoma, acute and chronic angle-closure glaucoma, goniodysgenesis, anisocoria and abnormal electroretinogram.

Laboratory findings

- Blood smears: abnormal cytoplasmic inclusions in lymphocytes.
- Urine: increased excretion of dermatan sulfate and heparan sulfate.
- Cultured cells: elevated iduronidase activity in leukocytes, cultured fibroblasts, cultured amniotic cells, or chorionic villus cells.
- Predicting disease severity in mucopolysaccharidosis I patients may be possible using a biochemical analysis of cultured skin fibroblasts.

TREATMENT

- Laronidase enzyme replacement therapy with aldurazyme (Genzyme), a polymorphic variant of the human enzyme α-L-iduronidase has shown significant improvement in walking capacity and pulmonary function in clinical trials.
- Allogeneic bone marrow transplantation has been an effective treatment for MPS I.
- Most patients who survive at least 5 years after BMT show an arrest or slowing down of psychomotor regression, although dysostosis multiplex continues to progress.
- Early diagnosis is essential in achieving an acceptable outcome after BMT.
- Since cloning of the IDUA gene, mutation analysis has provided more information that facilitates the selection and evaluation of patients undergoing experimental treatment protocols, including BMT.
- Due to a lack of matched related donors and unacceptable morbidity rates for matched unrelated transplantation, BMT is not available to all patients with Hurler syndrome.
- Transfer and expression of the normal gene in autologous bone marrow using techniques such as retroviral gene transfer into human bone marrow may offer the prospect for gene therapy in the near future.
- Surgical supportive treatment includes the repair of hernias and hydroceles, orthopedic surgery for skeletal deformities, and adenoidectomy to provide relief from persistent upper airway obstruction.
- Ocular treatment includes penetrating keratoplasty and trabeculectomy for corneal opacification and glaucoma, respectively.

COMPLICATIONS

- The administration of general anesthesia is complicated by excessive pharyngeal secretions, laryngospasm, cardiac abnormalities, increased frequency of cardiac arrest, hypoxia, and hypotension.
- Postoperative obstruction or infection may occur in the respiratory tract and requires tracheotomy.

COMMENTS

Understanding of the genotype/phenotype correlation in the mucopolysaccharidoses has increased significantly in the past 10 years. A complex picture of molecular heterogeneity has emerged and has provided some important clues into the structure and function of the IDUA gene. In the future, this knowledge will contribute to the development of successful gene therapy for these disorders. Until then, patients with Hurler syndrome still have a dismal prognosis, and their only hope lies in enzyme replacement therapy and/or early BMT. For this reason, making a timely clinical diagnosis is very important in this disorder, and a urine test for glycosaminoglycan excretion should be performed if there is any clinical suspicion, even in the presence of normal developmental progress.

REFERENCES

Cleary MA, Wraith JE: The presenting features of mucopolysaccharidosis type IH (Hurler syndrome). Acta Paediatr 84:337–339, 1995.

Fairbairn LJ, Lashford LS, Spooncer E, et al: Long-term in vitro correction of alpha-L-iduronidase deficiency (Hurler syndrome) in bone marrow. Proc Natl Acad Sci USA 93:2025–2030, 1996.

Francois J: Ocular manifestations of the mucopolysaccharidoses. Ophthalmologica 169:345–361, 1974.

Fuller M, Brooks DA, Evangelista M, et al: Prediction of neuropathology in mucopolysaccharidosis I patients. Mol Genet Metab. 84(1):18–24, 2005.

Grewal SS, Wynn R, Abdenur JE, et al: Safety and efficacy of enzyme replacement therapy in combination with hematopoietic stem cell transplantation in Hurler syndrome. Genet Med 7(2):143–146, 2005.

Huang Y, Bron AJ, Meek KM, et al: Ultrastructural study of the cornea in a bone marrow-transplanted Hurler syndrome patient. Exp Eye Res 62:377–387, 1996.

Scott HS, Bunge S, Gal A, et al: Molecular genetics of mucopolysaccharidosis type I: Diagnostic, clinical, and biological implications. Hum Mutat 6:288–302, 1995.

Stephen JM, Stevens JL, Wenstrup RJ, et al: Mucopolysaccharidosis I presenting with endocardial fibroelastosis of infancy. Am J Dis Child 143:782–784, 1989.

Vellodi A, Young EP, Cooper A, et al: Bone marrow transplantation for mucopolysaccharidosis type I: experience of two British centres. Arch Dis Child 76:92–99, 1997.

Wraith JE: The first 5 years of clinical experience with laronidase enzyme replacement therapy for mucopolysaccharidosis I. Expert Opin Pharmacother 6(3):489–506, 2005.

72 MUCOPOLYSACCHARIDOSIS IH/S 277.5 (Hurler–Scheie Syndrome, MPS IH/S)

Fernando H. Murillo-Lopez, MD
La Paz, Bolivia

ETIOLOGY/INCIDENCE

Mucopolysaccharidosis type I (MPS I) is an autosomal recessive disease caused by mutations in the α-L-iduronidase (*IDUA*) gene (localized to the distal short arm of chromosome 4) that result in abnormal intracellular accumulations of glycosaminoglycans and interference with normal cell function. Corneal clouding results from abnormal accumulation of proteoglycans in abnormal vacuolated stromal cells and nearby stroma. To date, more than 46 mutations of the *IDUA* gene have been defined for MPS I. Since the cloning of this gene, mutation analysis has also provided some molecular explanations for the range of MPS I phenotypes. Severe Hurler syndrome and mild Scheie's disease are extremes of the clinical spectrum caused by different *IDUA* mutations. Novel mutations are still being reported for Hurler–Scheie syndrome including single base changes. Patients with MPS IH/S have a phenotype intermediate between those of IH and IS that is caused by homozygous mutations or double heterozygosity of different *IDUA* gene mutations. The primary manifestations of MPS IH/S include skeletal abnormalities, enlargement of the spleen and liver, umbilical and inguinal hernias, and corneal opacities. Micrognathia and severe acne are features peculiar to this form of mucopolysaccharidosis; clouding of the cornea is also present in all patients with this disease. Prenatal diagnosis is possible by measuring the iduronidase activity in cultured amniotic cells and chorionic villi.

COURSE/PROGNOSIS

- Slowly progressive; if untreated the life expectancy of these patients is usually into the 20s.
- Mental deficiency and dwarfism are less severe than in Hurler syndrome, although the patterns of radiographic changes are similar.
- Death commonly occurs after protracted cardiac failure.
- There is a wide range of clinical phenotypes in MPS I (including MPS IH/S), which makes the prediction of disease severity and genetic counseling difficult.

DIAGNOSIS

Early diagnosis is essential to achieve an acceptable outcome after bone marrow transplantation (BMT). The diagnosis is suggested by certain clinical and radiologic findings, as well as by a urine screening test, and it should be confirmed with enzyme assays of cultured fibroblasts or leukocytes. The following are the most common clinical and radiologic findings associated with MPS I.

Clinical signs and symptoms

Systemic

- Mild to severe mental retardation.
- Recurrent rhinitis, nasal obstruction, sinus polyposis, multiple ear, nose, and throat operations.
- Recurrent inguinal hernias, hepatomegaly.
- Skeletal abnormalities, gibbus formation, asymmetric chest, prominent sternum, kyphosis, scoliosis, bulging forehead.
- Decreased hearing secondary to recurrent ear infections.
- Coarse facial appearance, coarse and bushy eyebrows.
- Recurrent upper respiratory and sinus infections.
- Macrocephaly (secondary to calvarial thickening and hydrocephalus), microcephaly, hydrocephalus, craniosynostosis.
- Grouped papules on the extensor surfaces on the upper portions of the arms and legs, progressive flexion contractures.
- Dysostosis multiplex, a group of skeletal abnormalities consisting of a large skull with a deep elongated, J-shaped sella; thickened, oar-shaped ribs; deformed, hook-shaped lower thoracic and upper lumbar vertebrae; pelvic dysplasia; and shortened tubular bones with expanded diaphyses and dysplastic epiphyses.

Ocular

- Ocular manifestations include peripheral/central corneal clouding, megalocornea, buphthalmos, coarse eyelashes, lid edema, ptosis, retinal pigmentary degeneration, optic nerve atrophy, hypertelorism, chronic open-angle glaucoma, acute and chronic angle-closure glaucoma, goniodysgenesis, anisocoria and abnormal electroretinogram.

Laboratory findings

- Blood smears: abnormal cytoplasmic inclusions in lymphocytes.
- Urine: increased excretion of dermatan sulfate and heparan sulfate.
- Cultured cells: elevated iduronidase activity in leukocytes, cultured fibroblasts, cultured amniotic cells, or chorionic villus cells.

TREATMENT

- To date, allogeneic BMT has been the only form of effective treatment for MPS I.
- BMT must be done at an early stage of the disease to achieve an acceptable outcome.
- Since cloning of the *IDUA* gene, mutation analysis has provided more information that facilitates the selection and evaluation of patients undergoing experimental treatment protocols, including BMT.
- Transfer and expression of the normal gene in autologous bone marrow using new techniques such as retroviral gene transfer into human bone marrow may offer the prospect for gene therapy in the near future.
- Treatment with recombinant human α L-iduronidase (laronidase) in patients with mucopolysaccharoridosis I is being reported as successful and well tolerated, particularly in the more severely affected patients.
- Surgical supportive treatment includes the repair of hernias and hydroceles, orthopedic surgery for skeletal deformities, and adenoidectomy to provide relief from persistent upper airway obstruction.

- Ocular treatment includes penetrating keratoplasty and trabeculectomy for corneal opacification and glaucoma, respectively.

COMPLICATIONS

- The administration of general anesthesia is complicated by excessive pharyngeal secretions, laryngospasm, cardiac abnormalities, increased frequency of cardiac arrest, hypoxia and hypotension.
- Postoperative obstruction or infection may occur in the respiratory tract and requires tracheotomy.

COMMENTS

Hurler syndrome and Scheie syndrome share a common metabolic defect; in both, the enzymatic deficiency is α-L-iduronidase. The mutation in both is presumed to be allelic, and thus it is thought that the inheritance of a Hurler gene and a Scheie gene results in a genetic compound with a phenotype intermediate in severity between those of the Hurler and Scheie syndromes: the Hurler–Scheie syndrome, or MPS IH/S. During the past decade, understanding of the genotype/phenotype correlation in the mucopolysaccharidoses has increased significantly, and a complex picture of molecular heterogeneity has emerged. Mutation analysis continues to provide some important clues into the structure and function of the *IDUA* gene, and in the near future, this knowledge will lead to the development of definitive gene therapy for these disorders.

REFERENCES

Francois J: Ocular manifestations of the mucopolysaccharidoses. Ophthalmologica 169:345–361, 1974.

Girard B, Hoang-Xuan T, D'Hermies F, et al: Mucopolysaccharidose de type I, phenotype Hurler-Scheie avec atteinte oculaire: Etude clinique et ultrastructurale. Journal Francais d' Ophthalmologie 17:286–295, 1994.

Hein LK, Bawden M, Muller VJ, et al: Alpha-L-iduronidase premature stop codons and potential read-through in mucopolysaccharidosis type I patients. J Mol Biol 338(3):453–462, 2004.

MacArthur CJ, Gliclich R, McGill TJ, et al: Sinus complications in mucopolysaccharidosis IH/S (Hurler-Scheie syndrome). Int J Pediatr Otorhinolaryngol 26:79–87, 1993.

Mullaney P, Awad AH, Millar L: Glaucoma in mucopolysaccharidosis 1-H/S. J Pediatr Ophthalmol Strabismus 33:127–131, 1996.

Rimoin DL, Connor JM, Pyeritz RE, eds: Emery and Rimoin's principles and practice of medical genetics. 3rd edn. New York, Churchill Livingstone, 1996:2071–2079.

Schiro JA, Mallory SB, Demmer L, et al: Grouped papules in Hurler-Scheie syndrome. J Am Acad Dermatol 35(5 pt 2):868–870, 1996.

Scott HS, Ashton LJ, Egre JH, et al: Chromosomal localization of the human alpha-L-iduronidase gene (IDUA) to 4p16.3. Am J Hum Genet 47:802–807, 1990.

Scott HS, Litjens T, Nelson PV, et al: Identification of mutations in the alpha-L-iduronidase gene (IDUA) that cause Hurler and Scheie syndromes. Am J Hum Genet 53:973–986, 1993.

Tieu PT, Bach G, Matynia A, et al: Four novel mutations underlying mild or intermediate forms of alpha-L-iduronidase deficiency (MPS IS and MPS IH/S). Hum Mutat 6(1):55–59, 1995.

Vellodi A, Young EP, Cooper A, et al: Bone marrow transplantation for mucopolysaccharidosis type I: Experience of two British centres. Arch Dis Child 76:92–99, 1997.

Wraith JE, Clarke LA, Beck M, et al: Enzyme replacement therapy for mucopolysaccharidosis I: a randomized, double-blinded, placebo-controlled, multinational study of recombinant human alpha-L-iduronidase (laronidase) J Pediatr 144(5):561–562, 2004.

73 MUCOPOLYSACCHARIDOSIS II 277.5 *(Hunter Syndrome, MPS II)*

Sangeeta Khanna, MD
Cleveland, Ohio
Elias I. Traboulsi, MD
Cleveland, Ohio

Mucopolysaccharidosis II is the only known X-linked disorder of mucopolysaccharide metabolism. All others are inherited in an autosomal recessive fashion. Hunter syndrome is caused by mutations in the iduronate-2-sulfatase (*IDS*) gene. *IDS* deficiency causes accumulation of undegraded dermatan and heparan sulfate in various tissues and organs. The disease is categorized as severe (type A) with substantial neurological dysfunction, and mild (type B) in which neurological impairment is not prominent. In the severe form (MPS IIA), mental retardation and neurologic changes are almost indistinguishable from those of mucopolysaccharidosis I-H or Hurler syndrome; they include gargoyle-like facies, dwarfism, hepatosplenomegaly, deafness, and death by age 15 years. In the mild type (MPS IIB), intelligence is not impaired, patients survive into adulthood and even procreate. Patients with MPS II have characteristic pebbly, ivory colored skin lesions over the back, neck, scapula, and thighs.

Corneal clouding is usually absent early in type B, although deposits of acid mucopolysaccharides are found histologically, even in clinically clear corneas. All patients have a pigmentary retinopathy with a severely reduced electroretinogram. This leads to visual impairment of varying degrees in all patients. About 20% of patients with Hunter syndrome may have elevated and blurred optic disc margins in the absence of elevated intracranial pressure. This is thought to result from compression of optic nerve fibers at the lamina cribrosa by a sclera that is thickened with mucopolysaccharides. This chronic papilledema leads to optic atrophy in some patients. Other rarely reported ocular findings include epiretinal membranes and uveal effusion syndrome secondary to scleral thickening.

ETIOLOGY

- The incidence of MPS II is 1 : 132,000 male newborns in the United Kingdom, and 1 : 34,000 in Israel.
- The two types of Hunter syndrome are allelic and are caused by mutations at the X-linked locus for the enzyme iduronate sulfate sulfatase. The gene is located on Xq28, distal to the fragile X site. Gene mutation analysis is possible.

COURSE/PROGNOSIS

- In MPS IIA, death usually occurs prior to the age of 15 years.
- In the milder type B, survival may extend past the age of 45. One patient has lived to age 87.

DIAGNOSIS

Laboratory findings

- Dermatan and heparan sulfate are present in the urine. Serum assay of *IDS* activity can also be used.
- A definitive diagnosis is made by assaying for the activity of sulfoiduronate sulfatase in fibroblasts or by demonstrating mutations in the gene.

Differential diagnosis

- Hurler syndrome in type IIA, other storage diseases.

PROPHYLAXIS

- Mucopolysaccharidosis II is an X-linked disorder. Hence, the disease is only transmissible from mother to son. Parents at risk should be informed that there is a 50% chance that a son will be affected and a 50% chance that a daughter will be a carrier. Carrier females do not manifest any signs of the disease. Carrier detection can be done by using direct dye primer sequencing of PCR products.
- Prenatal diagnosis is possible and is at the present time the most effective way to deal with MPS II. Amniocentesis or chorionic villus biopsy is performed in pregnancies where the mother has previously given birth to an affected son. Amniotic cells are cultured and examined for a deficiency of iduronate sulfatase or for mutations in the gene. If such is found, the pregnancy can be interrupted early. It is also possible to measure the levels of iduronate sulfatase in the mother's serum; these levels rise between the 6th and 12th week if the fetus is normal, but do not increase if the fetus is affected.

TREATMENT

- The physician should offer the parents sympathetic guidance in dealing with the deformities and resultant complications that characterize both forms of Hunter syndrome.
- Genetic counseling and prenatal diagnosis are offered to families with an affected child.
- Surgical treatment is supportive; repair of hernias or orthopedic surgery for skeletal deformities may be necessary. Patients with hydrocephalus and papilledema may require shunting if intracranial pressure is elevated.
- Allogeneic bone marrow transplantation has been tried in several patients with improvement in clinical findings. But it still remains controversial since it often fails to reverse CNS impairment and carries substantial mortality and morbidity.
- Enzyme and gene replacement therapies are under development.

ANESTHESIA CONSIDERATIONS

Administration of a general anesthetic may be complicated by excessive pharyngeal secretions, laryngospasm, cardiac abnormalities, and increased frequency of cardiac arrest, hypoxia or hypotension. Postoperative obstruction or infection may occur in the respiratory tract and may require tracheotomy. Many of these complications may be avoided if large doses of atropine are given in the preinduction period and if postoperative narcotics are withheld as much as possible.

SUPPORT GROUPS

The Canadian Society for Mucopolysaccharide & Related Disease, Inc.
P.O. Box 64714
Unionville, ON L3R 0M9
Phone/Fax (905) 479-8701
National MPS Society, Inc.
17 Kraemer Street
Hicksville, NY 11801
(516) 432-1797
Fax: (410) 538-4964

REFERENCES

Beck M, Cole G: Disc oedema in association with Hunter's syndrome. Ocular histopathological findings. Br J Ophthalmol 68:590–594, 1984.

Braun S, Aronovich E, Anderson R, et al: Metabolic correction and cross-correction of mucopolysaccharidosis type II (Hunter syndrome) by retroviral-mediated gene transfer and expression of human iduronate-2-sulfatase. Proc Natl Acad Sci USA 90:11830, 1993.

Caruso R, Kaiser-Kupfer M, Muenzer J, et al: Electroretinographic findings in the mucopolysaccharidoses. Ophthalmology 93:1612, 1986.

Collins MLZ, Traboulsi EI, Maumenee IH: Optic nerve head swelling and optic atrophy in the systemic mucopolysaccharidoses. Ophthalmology 97:1445–1449, 1990.

Hopwood JJ, Bunge S, Morris CP, et al: Molecular basis of mucopolysaccharidosis type II: mutations in the iduronate-2-sulphatase gene. Hum Mutat 2:435–442, 1993.

Legum CP, Schorr S, Berman ER: The genetic mucopolysaccharidosis, type II A (Hunter syndrome, severe). Ophthalmology 92:1772–1779, 1985.

Narita AS, Russell-Eggitt I: Bilateral epiretinal memebranes: a new finding in Hunter syndrome. Ophthalmic Genetics 17(2):75–78, 1996.

Neufeld EF, Muenzer J: The mucopolysaccharidoses. In: Scriver CR, Beudet AL, Sly WS, Valle D, eds: The metabolic and molecular bases of inherited disease. New York, McGraw-Hill, 1995:2465–2494.

Pan D, Jonsson JJ, Braun SE, et al: Supercharged cells for delivery of recombinant human iduronate-2-sulfatase. Mol Genet Metab 70(3):170–178, 2000.

Peters C, Krivit W: Hematopoietic cell transplantation for mucopolysaccharidosis IIB (Hunter's syndrome). Bone Marrow Transplantation 25(10):1097–1099, 2000.

Vellodi A, Young E, Cooper A, et al: Long-term follow-up following bone marrow transplantation for Hunter disease. J Inherit Metab Dis 22(5):638–648, 1999.

Vine AK: Uveal effusion in Hunter's syndrome. Evidence that abnormal sclera is responsible for the uveal effusion syndrome. Retina 6(1):57–60, 1986.

74 MUCOPOLYSACCHARIDOSIS III 277.5 *(MPS III, Sanfilippo Syndrome)*

Sangeeta Khanna, MD
Cleveland, Ohio
Elias I. Traboulsi, MD
Cleveland, Ohio

The Sanfilippo syndrome, or mucopolysaccharidosis III, is a lysosomal storage disease due to impaired degradation of heparan sulfate. Patients with Sanfilippo syndrome have severe central nervous system but only mild somatic disease. Clinical signs become apparent between two and six years of age. The mild somatic features often lead to a significant delay in diagnosis because a storage disease is not suspected. There may be moderate dwarfism, minimal skeletal dysostosis, and moderate hepatosplenomegaly. Some patients present with marked hyperactivity, or with destructive tendencies and behavioral problems. Four non-allelic subtypes, designated A, B, C, and D, may be difficult to distinguish clinically. Type A, however, is most severe, with an earlier onset, more rapid progression of symptoms and earlier death than types B, C or D.

The corneas of patients with MPS III remain clear, but retinal pigmentary degeneration is common. Collins and co-workers found papilledema in 5% of patients and optic atrophy in 14%.

ETIOLOGY/INCIDENCE

The four types of Sanfilippo syndrome can be differentiated by enzymatic assays. N-sulfated glucosamine residues are removed during the degradation of heparan sulfate through the sequential action of four enzymes which are defective in the Sanfilippo syndromes.

- In MPS IIIA, there is a deficiency of heparan N-sulfatase or sulfamidase that maps to chromosome 17q25.3.
- In MPS IIIB, α-N-acetyl-glucosaminidase (NAG) is lacking and maps to chromosome 17q21.
- In MPS IIIC, there is deficiency of acetyl CoA: α-glucosaminidase located on chromosome 14.
- In MPS IIID the defect is in N-acetyl glucosamine 6-sulfatase located on chromosome 12q14.

COURSE/PROGNOSIS

Mental and neurologic defects progress to extreme degrees within a few years and death usually occurs by 10 to 15 years of age.

DIAGNOSIS/LABORATORY FINDINGS

- Excessive heparan sulfate, but not dermatan sulfate, is excreted in the urine. The MPS urine spot test is positive.
- A precise diagnosis can be obtained by assaying for the specific enzymes in cultured fibroblasts.

Differential diagnosis

As the physical features of mucopolysaccharidosis III are usually minimal, this disorder may not be included in the differential diagnosis of a child with progressive central nervous system disorder, leading to a significant delay in diagnosis. The urine of patients suspected of having this disorder should be tested for excess mucopolysaccharides, and skin fibroblasts should be cultured and examined for the enzymatic defect.

PROPHYLAXIS

Prenatal diagnosis is possible. Amniocentesis or chorionic villus biopsy is performed in pregnancies where the mother has previously given birth to an affected child. Assays are performed on amniotic cells or chorionic villi for all of the enzymes involved in MPS III. If one of the enzymes is found to be deficient, pregnancy can be interrupted early.

TREATMENT

- Genetic counseling is indicated for parents who already have an affected child. They should be informed of the 25% statistical probability of having affected children in future pregnancies.
- Bone marrow transplantation (BMT) has been tried in some patients with some improvement in clinical findings. Successful BMT has been shown to improve systemic health, but not long term retinal function. It should only be used in selected cases with extensive pre-transplantation counseling and clinical assessment and with systematic long-term monitoring.
- Enzyme and gene replacement therapies are under development.

SUPPORT GROUPS

The Canadian Society for Mucopolysaccharide & Related Disease, Inc.
P.O. Box 64714
Unionville, ON L3R 0M9
Phone/Fax (905) 479-8701

National MPS Society, Inc.
17 Kraemer Street
Hicksville, NY 11801
(516) 432-1797
Fax: (410) 538-4964

REFERENCES

Caruso R, Kaiser-Kupfer M, Muenzer J, et al: Electroretinographic findings in the mucopolysaccharidoses. Ophthalmology 93:1612, 1986.

Collins MLZ, Traboulsi EI, Maumenee IH: Optic nerve head swelling and optic atrophy in the systemic mucopolysaccharidoses. Ophthalmology 97:1445–1449, 1990.

Del Monte MA, Maumenee IH, Green WR, Kenyon KR: Histopathlogy of Sanfilippo's syndrome. Arch Ophthalmol 101:1255–1262, 1983.

Gliddon BL, Hopwood JJ: Enzyme-replacement therapy from birth delays the development of behavior and learning problems in mucopolysaccharidosis type IIIA mice. Pediatr Res 56(1):65–72, 2004.

Gullingsrud EO, Krivit W, Summers CG: Ocular abnormalities in the mucopolysaccharidoses after bone marrow transplantation. Longer follow-up. Ophthalmology 105(6):1099–1105, 1998.

Lavery MA, Green WR, Jabs EW, et al: Ocular histopathology and ultrastructure of Sanfilippo's syndrome, type III-B. Arch Ophthalmol 101:1255–1262, 1983.

Neufeld EF, Muenzer J: The mucopolysaccharidoses. In: Scriver CR, Beudet AL, Sly WS, Valle D, eds: The metabolic and molecular bases of inherited disease. New York, McGraw-Hill, 1995:2465–2494.

Van de Kamp J, Niermeiyer M, Von Figura K, Giesberts M: Genetic heterogeneity and clinical variability in the Sanfillippo syndrome (Types A, B, C). Clin Genet 20:152, 1981.

Yogalingam G, Hopwood JJ: Molecular genetics of mucopolysaccharidosis type IIIA and IIIB: diagnostic, clinical, and biological implications. Hum Mutat 18(4):264–281, 2001.

75 MUCOPOLYSACCHARIDOSIS IV
277.5
(Chondro-Osteodystrophy, Keratosulfaturia, Morquio–Brailsford Syndrome, Morquio Syndrome, MPS IV)

F. Hampton Roy, MD, FACS
Little Rock, Arkansas

ETIOLOGY/INCIDENCE

Mucopolysaccharidosis IV (MPS IV) is a progressive autosomal recessive disorder characterized by dwarfism, spondyloepiphyseal and dental anomalies, corneal opacification, and normal intelligence. Although primarily a disease of the anterior segment, posterior pole involvement has recently been described. MPS IV is an enzyme deficiency of *N*-acetyl-galactosamine-6-sulfate sulfatase (type A) or of β-galactosidase (type B). It results in an abnormal accumulation of keratin sulfate in tissues with excretion in urine.

- Cornea: increase in stromal collagen fibril diameter and bulk density; corneal clouding most likely due to abnormal keratocytes and collagen-free areas.
- Lens: cataracts.
- Anterior chamber, trabecular meshwork: glaucoma.
- Retinal pigment epithelium: arteriolar narrowing, increased photopic b wave implicit time, decreased scotopic b wave amplitude, abnormal electro-oculogram.
- Optic nerve: optic atrophy.
- Brain low-density white-matter lesions, dilated ventricle, basal cisterns, subarachnoid space.

COURSE/PROGNOSIS

- Although the classic clinical and radiographic features of Morquio syndrome are present at birth, they become distinctive by 2 years of age.
- Joint laxity and shortness of stature require prompt medical attention.
- Advancing age brings exaggeration of the multiple skeletal abnormalities, with deficient linear growth beyond age 5.
- Cardiac manifestations occur secondary to respiratory failure caused by kyphoscoliosis and restricted chest movements.
- Aortic regurgitation may occur primarily.
- Teeth are severely affected and have thin enamel (type A).
- Subtle corneal changes may appear at an early age but are not usually appreciated until age 4.
- Glaucoma, cataracts, and retinal pigment epithelium changes have been reported.
- Note: retinal findings have been reported only in patients of an advanced age, suggesting that retinal involvement in the disease is mild but progressive and therefore cannot be seen in younger patients but becomes apparent in older patients.
- Despite normal intelligence, patients with Morquio syndrome who reach advanced age show characteristic computed tomography scan findings suggesting mucopolysaccharide deposition in cortical matter.
- Patients with MPS IV usually die in their third or fourth decade of life from cor pulmonale caused by the severe abnormalities of the chest and spine.
- Variations in the clinical manifestations are common; mild cases have been encountered.
- Patients with mild forms may survive into their 60s.

DIAGNOSIS

Diagnosis is made by radiographic confirmation by the demonstration of flat vertebrae (platyspondyly universalis) and odontoid hypoplasia, the presence of Reilly's granules in leukocytes, thin-layer chromatography of abnormal oligosaccharide excretion in urine, and the demonstration of profound deficiency of β-galactosidase activity in cultured fibroblasts. New synthetic fluorimetric substrate has provided a highly effective and sensitive method for the postnatal, prenatal, and retrospective diagnosis of Morquio syndrome type A.

TREATMENT

Systemic

- Methods to regulate the synthesis or to enhance the metabolism or excretion of mucopolysaccharides are not available.
- Direct gene replacement is futuristic.
- Small clinical trials involving enzyme replacement have been carried out.
- To date, the infusion of plasma and purified enzymes and the implantation of cultured fibroblasts and amnion cells (HLA negative) have failed to produce quantitative clinical effects.

Supportive

- The intelligence of patients with MPS IV is usually normal; with sympathetic guidance, these individuals can achieve age-appropriate levels of education.
- A hearing aid may be of some value in patients with hearing loss from recurrent otitis media.
- Parents of affected children have a 25% risk of having another affected child.
- Prenatal diagnosis can be made by enzyme assay from cultured amniotic fluid cells or by analysis of amniotic fluid MPS derived from fetal tissue.

Surgical

- Prophylactic posterior spinal fusion of the upper cervical spine can be performed to prevent atlantoaxial subluxation or translocation with resultant spinal cord compression and cervical myelopathy.
- Myringotomy can be performed for recurrent otitis media.
- Penetrating keratoplasty is generally not necessary.

PRECAUTIONS

There is no specific treatment for MPS IV. The risk of complications associated with anesthesia and postoperative respiratory obstruction must be appreciated before even simple procedures are undertaken. Hyperextension should be *avoided.*

SUMMARY

Morquio syndrome is a multisystem disorder whose hallmark is severe skeletal deformity. The ocular involvement is usually mild and confined to the anterior segment, with corneal clouding being the most common presenting ocular complaint. Management is inevitably multidisciplinary, with the primary care physician playing the primary role in the coordination of services. The major treatment issue centers on the prevention of cervical myelopathy. Prophylactic surgical intervention is recommended by many, but the timing and selection of patients are unclear. Parents of affected children need considerable support, and The Society for Mucopolysaccharide Diseases has afforded parents and affected individuals a much needed outlet for emotional and financial support.

SUPPORT GROUP

The Society for Mucopolysaccharide Diseases
55 Hill Avenue
Amersham, Bucks, UK HP6 5BX

REFERENCES

Cahane M, Treister G, Abraham FA, Melamed S: Glaucoma in siblings with Morquio syndrome. Br J Ophthalmol 74:382–383, 1990.

Dangel ME, Tsou BH: Retinal involvement in Morquio syndrome. Ann Ophthalmol 17:349–354, 1985.

Iwamoto M, Nawa Y, Maumenee IH, et al: Ocular histopathology and ultrastructure of Morquio syndrome. Graefes Arch Clin Exp Ophthalmol 228:342–349, 1990.

Leslie T, Lois N, Christopoulou D, et al: Photodynamic therapy for inflammatory choroidal neovascularisation unresponsive to immunosuppression. Br J Ophthalmol 89(2):147–150, 2005.

Leslie T, Siddiqui MA, Aitken DA, et al: Morquio syndrome electron microscopic findings. Br J Ophthalmol 89(7):925–926, 2005.

Northover H, Cowie RA, Wraith JE: Mucopolysaccharidosis type IV A (Morquio syndrome): Clinical review. J Inher Metab Dis 19:357–365, 1996.

Rawe IM, Leonard DW, Meek KM, Zabel RW: X-ray diffraction and transmission electron microscopy of Morquio syndrome type A cornea: Structural analysis. Cornea 16:369–376, 1997.

Rekhi GS: Morquio syndrome (MPS IV): a case report. Indian J Ophthalmol 39:78–81, 1991.

Zhao H, Van Diggelen OP, Kleijer WJ, Li P: Enzymatic diagnosis of Morquio A syndrome with a new fluorimetric substrate. Chin Med Sci J 6:9–13, 1991.

76 MUCOPOLYSACCHARIDOSIS VI 277.5 (MPS VI, Maroteaux–Lamy Syndrome)

La-ongsri Atchaneeyasakul, MD
Bangkok, Thailand
Richard G. Weleber, MD
Portland, Oregon

ETIOLOGY/INCIDENCE

Mucopolysaccharidosis VI (MPS VI) is a rare autosomal recessive disorder characterized by the intralysosomal storage and excessive urinary excretion of the glycosaminoglycan dermatan sulfate or chondroitin sulfate B. The syndrome is caused by a deficiency of the lysosomal enzyme sulfogalactosamine sulfatase (*N*-acetyl-galactosamine-4-sulfatase or arylsulfatase B, ASB). Clinical phenotypes have been described as mild, intermediate, or severe based on the age at onset, the organ of involvement, and the rate of disease progression. After the description of the arylsulfatase B gene, several mutant alleles have been identified suggesting a wide genetic heterogeneity of the syndrome.

COURSE/PROGNOSIS

Recent studies demonstrated some genotype/phenotype correlations that may contribute to the prediction of disease progression and the evaluation of various therapeutic approaches. The physical findings of MPS VI resemble those of MPS IH with respect to growth retardation, skeletal deformities, and coarse facial features; however, intellectual development is normal. A prominent forehead and sternal protrusion are frequently noted soon after birth. Restriction of joint motion may begin by the first year. Growth retardation is first noted at the age of 2 or 3 years, and skeletal growth may cease entirely after 8 years resulting in dwarfism. By the sixth year, all patients have hepatomegaly, and about half have enlarged spleens. Deafness and inguinal hernias are common. Most patients have corneal clouding, which can interfere with vision and adversely affect psychomotor development. Cardiac involvement (aortic and mitral valvular stenosis) is frequent and, with respiratory complications, is the most serious threat to patients. Generally, the life span is longer than that for patients with MPS IH, although with the severe phenotype, survival past the mid-20s is rare.

DIAGNOSIS

Clinical signs and symptoms

The significant ocular manifestations of MPS VI are corneal clouding, which is moderate in degree and develops early; glaucoma; and optic atrophy. Significant visual loss from corneal clouding usually develops during the first decade of life. The mechanism of glaucoma may be secondary angle closure due to thickening of the cornea or secondary open angle due to the obstruction of the trabecular meshwork by mucopolysaccharides. Papilledema has been reported and is thought to be associated with hydrocephalus.

Ocular or periocular

- Choroid: thinning.
- Ciliary body: acid mucopolysaccharide deposits.
- Cornea: acid mucopolysaccharide deposits in the epithelium, lamellar clefts in the anterior stroma, cytoplasm of keratocytes and endothelial cells, clouding, opacity, thickening.
- Eyebrows: bushy, coarse.
- Optic nerve: atrophy, cupping, papilledema, thickening of the optic nerve sheaths.
- Retina: detachment, macular edema, vascular tortuosity.
- Sclera: acid mucopolysaccharide deposits, thickening.
- Other: coarse eyelashes, decreased visual acuity, glaucoma.

TREATMENT

Systemic

Bone marrow transplantation

Bone marrow transplantation (BMT) in newborn rats with MPS VI may prevent many pathologic and clinical findings but still has unpredictable effects on the skeletal abnormalities. BMT has been tried in patients with several forms of mucopolysaccharidoses, including MPS VI, with subsequent normalization of ASB activity in white blood cells and glycosaminoglycans excretion. The treatment also improved cardiac and respiratory functions and the ultrastructural appearance of the liver and resulted in a decrease in hepatosplenomegaly and an increase in joint mobility. There is no change in bone pathology, facial appearance, and short stature. Clearing of corneal cloudiness, which has occurred with BMT in other forms of MPS, has not been observed in MPS VI. However, a follow-up of the corneal transplants after BMT demonstrated clear corneal grafts 13 years postoperatively. Considering the risks, high expense, and questionable outcome, BMT should be considered experimental and restricted to carefully selected and monitored patients.

Enzyme replacement therapy

An ongoing Phase I/II study of recombinant human *N*-acetylgalactosamine-4-sulfatase in MPS VI patients has recently reported that this treatment was well-tolerated and reduced lysosomal storage as evidenced by a dose-dependent reduction in urinary glycosaminoglycan. Functional status also improved as shown by an increase in distance walked, stair-climbing ability, shoulder range of motion, and decrease in pain and arthritis severity scores.

Gene therapy

Another experimental approach is the use of hematopoietic stem cell gene therapy through the construction of a retroviral vector containing the full-length human ASB cDNA and the use of this vector to transduce bone marrow cells in vitro from patients with MPS VI. Recent study in MPS VI cats showed that AAV-mediated subretinal delivery of the feline 4-sulfatase cDNA reduced lysosomal accumulation in the retinal pigment epithelial cells.

Supportive

The physician should offer sympathetic guidance in helping the parents deal with the skeletal deformities that develop in these patients. Parents should be informed of available inpatient clinic care facilities. Genetic counseling should be provided to parents and other potential carriers, as well as to patients who reach childbearing age. Both parents of an affected child are carriers of the deficient gene; however, because the gene defect is detectable in amniotic cell cultures, prenatal diagnosis is possible.

Surgical

Surgical treatment is supportive, with repair of hernias and hydroceles, orthopedic surgery for skeletal deformities, or adenoidectomy to provide relief from the persistent nasal discharge, as indicated. Penetrating keratoplasty or lamellar corneal grafting has been performed for significant corneal clouding. Although mucopolysaccharide can reaccumulate in corneal grafts within 1 year after transplantation, there are some patients with clear grafts and good visual outcomes after 5 years of follow-up. Hydrocephalus and associated papilledema may be relieved through the shunting of cerebrospinal fluid.

PRECAUTIONS

Atlantoaxial subluxation can occur as a result of hypoplasia of the odontoid process. In addition, neurologic deterioration from myelopathy due to thickening of the dura of the cervical spinal cord and consequent cord compression has been reported. Somatosensory evoked potential testing is useful to detect subclinical impairment of the cervical cord. Early surgical decompression seems to be beneficial.

COMMENTS

One of the most outstanding features of MPS VI is the normal intellectual capacity of the patients. They usually attend regular schools and pass their examinations without difficulties, although visual and physical handicaps eventually impede their psychomotor performance.

REFERENCES

Boor R, Miebach E, Bruhl K, Beck M: Abnormal somatosensory evoked potentials indicate compressive cervical myelopathy in mucopolysaccharidoses. Neuropediatrics 31:122–127, 2000.

Fillat C, Simonaro CM, Veyati PL, et al: Arylsulfatase B activities and glycosaminoglycan levels in retrovirally transduced mucopolysaccharidosis type VI cells. J Clin Invest 98:497–502, 1996.

Harmatz P, Whitley CB, Waber L, et al: Enzyme replacement therapy in mucopolysaccharidosis VI (Maroteaux-Lamy syndrome). J Pediatr 144:574–580, 2004.

Ho TT, Maguire AM, Aguirre GD, et al: Phenotypic rescue after adeno-associated virus-mediated delivery of 4-sulfatase to the retinal pigment epithelium of feline mucopolysaccharidosis VI. J Gene Med 4:613–621, 2002.

Jin WD, Jackson CE, Desnick RJ, Schuchman EH: Mucopolysaccharidosis type VI: Identification of three mutations in the arylsulfatase B gene of patients with the severe and mild phenotypes provides molecular evidence for genetic heterogeneity. Am J Hum Genet 50:795–800, 1992.

Litjens T, Brooks DA, Peters C, et al: Identification, expression, and biochemical characterization of N-acetylgalactosamine-4-sulfatase mutations and relationship with clinical phenotype in MPS-VI patients. Am J Hum Genet 58:1127–1134, 1996.

Neufeld EF, Muenzer J: The mucopolysaccharidoses. In: Scriver CR, Beaudet AL, Sly WS, Valle D, eds: The metabolic and molecular bases of inherited disease. 7th edn. New York, McGraw-Hill, 1995: II:2465–2494.

Simonaro CM, Haskins ME, Kunieda T, et al: Bone marrow transplantation in newborn rats with mucopolysaccharidosis type VI. Transplantation 63:1386–1393, 1997.

Ucakhan OO, Brodie SE, Desnick R, et al: Long-term follow-up of corneal graft survival following bone marrow transplantation in the Maroteaux-Lamy syndrome. CLAO J 27:234–237, 2001.

Van Dyke DL, Fluharty AL, Schafer IA, et al: Prenatal diagnosis of Maroteaux-Lamy syndrome. Am J Med Genet 8:235–242, 1981.

77 MUCOPOLYSACCHARIDOSIS VII
277.5
(β-Glucuronidase Deficiency, GUSB Deficiency, MPS VII, Sly Disease)

Chantal F. Morel, MD, FRCP(C)
Toronto, Ontario, Canada
Alex V. Levin, MD, MHSc, FAAP, FAAO, FRCSC
Toronto, Ontario, Canada

ETIOLOGY/INCIDENCE

β-Glucuronidase (GUSB) is a lysosomal enzyme that catalyzes the hydrolysis of β-glucuronide residues as part of the sequential degradation of the glycosaminoglycans chondroitin sulfate, dermatan sulfate and heparan sulfate. This enzyme is a homotetramer of four 651 amino acid chains. The autosomal recessive disorder known as mucopolysaccharidosis type VII (MPS VII, OMIM 253220) is due to deficiency of this enzyme which in turn leads to the accumulation of incompletely degraded glycosaminoglycans in secondary lysosomes in many tissues. The first patient was described by Sly in 1973. The incidence of the severe neonatal form is estimated at approximately 1 in 300,000 live births. Over 50 cases have been reported. The clinical manifestations are chronic and progressive, ranging from nonimmune hydrops fetalis to mild disease variants presenting in adults. Milder forms are less common. A pseudodeficiency is also known in which enzyme levels are reduced (>3%), the phenotype is normal, and there is no abnormal urinary excretion.

The *GUSB* gene has been cloned and found to contain 12 exons. It is located at chromosome 7q21.11. More than 50 mutations have been identified, including missense, nonsense, frame shifts, small deletions, and splice-site changes. Both homozygotes and compound heterozygotes have been reported. Most mutations are novel. Clinical heterogeneity is well recognized.

COURSE/PROGNOSIS

- Wide phenotypic variability categorized by some as mild, moderate, or severe and by others as juvenile, infantile, or neonatal/fetal, respectively.
- May present as *in utero* death and non-immune hydrops fetalis. Increased nuchal translucency in the first trimester of pregnancy has been observed.

Features of moderate to severe disease include:
- Characteristic coarse facies with epicanthus, midfacial hypoplasia, and telecanthus.
- Hepatosplenomegaly.
- Bone and joint abnormalities (dysostosis multiplex, kyphoscoliosis with vertebral deformities, sternum deformity), difficulties in ambulation.
- Recurrent respiratory disease.
- Cardiac abnormalities (myocardial thickening, valvular disease).
- Umbilical and/or inguinal hernia.
- Short stature.
- Mild to severe mental retardation, usually nonprogressive.
- Reduced life span, often with neonatal or infant death.

Ocular involvement may include:
- Progressive corneal clouding: usually mild and not noted until the end of the first decade but may be observed in some infants.
- Retinal dystrophy.
- Optic atrophy: late manifestation in survivors beyond the neonatal period.
- Papilledema.
- Abnormal storage of glycosaminoglycans in retinal pigmented epithelium, ciliary body epithelium, and corneal endothelium observed in animal models.

- Mild form that presents after the age of 4 years with variable severity of skeletal involvement, normal intelligence, normal facies, and clear corneas.

DIAGNOSIS

- High urinary excretion of glycosaminoglycans and large oligosaccharides.
- Vacuoles may be seen in peripheral lymphocytes and fibroblasts.
- Metachromatic granular inclusions (Alder bodies) in leukocytes; abnormalities also in some cells of obligate carriers or pseudodeficiency.
- Light and electron microscopy of neurons, muscle fibers, renal cells, hepatic cells or corneal stromal keratocytes show cytoplasmic inclusions representing partially degraded glycosaminoglycans in secondary lysosomes.
- Low leukocyte or fibroblast GUSB enzyme activity (0–2%).
- Gene mutation analysis.
- Prenatal diagnosis: measuring glycosaminoglycans in amniotic fluid, GUSB enzyme activity in cultured fetal cells, or molecular analysis of *GUSB* gene if proband's disease-causing mutations known.

TREATMENT

Systemic

- Direct enzyme replacement therapy (ERT) unsuccessful.
- Varying success with bone marrow transplantation: animal models show improved response following pre-treatment with ERT.

Ocular

- Penetrating keratoplasty or lamellar keratoplasty for significant corneal clouding, may result in visual gain although improvement may be moderated by retinal and/or optic nerve disease. Without systemic therapy, disease may recur in grafted cornea.
- Intraocular gene therapy in affected mice results in nearly normal levels of *GUSB* and decreased lysosomal storage within the retinal pigmented epithelium (RPE) and improved retinal function.
- Intravitreal gene therapy results in increased *GUSB* activity and reduced lysosomal storage in the certain areas of the CNS, suggesting diffusion and trans-synaptic transfer.
- BMT in mice with MPS VII decreases RPE lysosomal storage and improves retinal function.
- Systemic injection of recombinant adenovirus expressing *GUSB* in first 24 hours of life in affected mice may prevent

progression of corneal clouding, retinal degeneration and other systemic manifestations.

COMPLICATIONS

- Visual loss due to corneal, retinal or optic nerve involvement.
- Craniovertebral instability (potential risk at intubation for anaesthesia).
- Spinal cord compression.
- Hearing loss.
- Cardiac ischemia due to narrowing of coronary arteries.
- Obstructive airway disease.
- Joint stiffness, carpel tunnel syndrome.

COMMENTS

Corneal clouding is the most common ocular manifestation. Involvement of the retina and optic nerve occur less frequently. There are very few references in the medical literature describing the non corneal ocular phenotypes. The availability of animal models presents the opportunity for therapeutic trials, which may ultimately lead to a viable treatment in the realm of gene therapies.

SUPPORT GROUPS

National MPS (Mucopolysaccharidoses/Mucolipidoses) Society, Inc.
17 Kraemer Street
Hicksville, NY 11801
(516) 931-6338
Fax: (516) 822-2041
E-mail: Soc@aol.com
Home page: http://members.aol.com/mpssociety

Vaincre Les Maladies Lysosomales [French]
9 Place du 19 Mars 1962
Evry Cedex 91035, France
(331) 609-1750
E-mail: VML@provnet.fr
Home page: http://www.provnet.fr/VML/

Society of Mucopolysaccharidosis (MPS) Disease, United Kingdom
7 Chessfield Park
Buckinghamshire HP6 6RU, UK

Canadian Society for Mucopolysaccharidosis and Related Diseases, Inc.
Postal Box 64714
Unionville, Ontario, Canada L3R OM9
(905) 479-8701
Home page: http://neuro-www2mgh.harvard.edu/MPS/mpsmain.html

Lysosomal Storage Diseases: A Family Sourcebook Reference Chart
Home page: http://mcrcr2.med.nyu.edu/murphp01/lysosome/lysosome. htm

REFERENCES

Bergwerk KE, Falk RE, Glasgow BJ, Rabinowitz YS: Corneal transplantation in a patient with mucopolysaccharidosis type VII (Sly disease). Ophthalmic Genet 21:17–20, 2000.

Geipel A, Berg C, Germer U, et al: Mucopolysaccharidosis VII (Sly disease) as a cause of increased nuchal translucency and non-immune fetal hydrops: study of a family and technical approach to prenatal diagnosis in early and late pregnancy. Prenat Diagn 22:487–500, 2002.

Hennig AK, Levy B, Ogilvie JM, et al: Intravitreal gene therapy reduces lysosomal storage in specific areas of the CNS in mucopolysaccharidosis VII mice. J Neurosci 23:3302–3307, 2003.

Hennig AK, Ogilvie JM, Ohlemiller KK, et al: AAV-mediated intravitreal gene therapy reduces lysosomal storage in the retinal pigmented epithelium and improves retinal function in adult MPS VII mice. Mol Ther 10:106–116, 2004.

Kamata Y, Okuyama T, Kosuga M, et al: Adenovirus-mediated gene therapy for corneal clouding in mice with mucopolysaccharidosis type VII. Mol Ther 4:307–312, 2001.

Kamata Y, Tanabe A, Kanaji A, et al: Long-term normalization in the central nervous system, ocular manifestations, and skeletal deformities by a single systemic adenovirus injection into neonatal mice with mucopolysaccharidosis VII. Gene Ther 10:406–414, 2003.

Neufeld EF, Muenzer J: The mucopolysaccharidoses. In: Scriver CR, Beaudet AL, Sly WS, Vale D, eds: The metabolic and molecular basis of inherited disease. 8th edn. Toronto, McGraw-Hill, 2001:3421–3452.

Ohlemiller KK, Vogler CA, Roberts M, et al: Retinal function is improved in a murine model of lysosomal storage disease following bone marrow transplantation. Exp Eye Res 71:469–481, 2000.

Storch S, Wittenstein B, Islam R, et al: Mutational analysis in the longest known survivor of mucopolysaccharidosis type VII. Hum Genet 112:190–194, 2003.

SECTION

Disorders of Lipid Metabolism

78 FABRY DISEASE 272.7
(Angiokeratoma Corporis Diffusum Universale, Anderson–Fabry Disease, Glycolipid Lipidosis)

Koji Hirano, MD, PhD
Aichi, Japan

ETIOLOGY/INCIDENCE

Fabry disease is an X-linked inborn error of glycosphingolipid metabolism caused by a deficiency of the lysosomal hydrolase α-galactosidase A (α-Gal A). Typically, in affected males who have little if any residual α-Gal A activity, the first clinical manifestations occur in childhood when episodes of severe pain in the extremities (i.e. acroparesthesias), hypohidrosis, corneal and lenticular changes, and characteristic skin lesions (i.e. angiokeratomas) are noted. With advancing age, progressive kidney, cardiovascular, and cerebrovascular disease develop and are the major causes of mortality.

The complete clinical manifestations of Fabry disease occur only in males (hemizygotes); in heterozygous female carriers, Fabry disease is usually limited to the eyes, and life expectancy is near normal because renal and cerebrovascular involvement is uncommon.

COURSE/PROGNOSIS

Systemic

Fabry disease is not a symptomatic disease of early childhood but may be diagnosed before 10 years of age. Children may complain of:

- Pain in the extremities;
- Anhidrosis;
- Which can give rise to fevers.

With progression, there are complaints of:

- Easy fatigability, due to glycosphingolipids accumulating in skeletal muscle;
- Psychologic disturbances, due to decreased blood flow from thrombus formation in the brain;
- Multiple wine-red angiokeratomas involve the trunk, fingers, penis, lips and tongue; these lesions may be distributed in the swim-trunk region in hemizygous adults;
- Female carriers (heterozygotes) are involved to a lesser extent and usually develop symptoms at a later age; in hemizygous males, death usually occurs before the fourth or fifth decade due to renal or cardiac failure or cerebrovascular disease.

DIAGNOSIS

Clinical signs and symptoms

Ocular

Ocular findings in Fabry disease are often subtle but can result in compromised vision in several ways; the abnormal accumulation of intracytoplasmic lipid occurs throughout endothelial, perithelial, and smooth muscle cells of the eye. The epithelium of the conjunctiva, cornea, and lens can be affected, as well as the vasculature of the retina. Characteristic ocular symptoms include:

- Cornea verticillata: fine, whorl-like superficial corneal opacities that affect both males and females; on slit-lamp examination, golden-brown pigmentation is visible in the corneal epithelium.

Once thought to be a separate entity and termed the *familial corneal dystrophy of Fleischer–Gruber*, this vortex pattern is known to be a sign of Fabry disease and resembles the corneal changes found after the chronic ingestion of chloroquine, amiodarone, and other agents that cause a drug-induced lipidosis.

- Dilated, sausage-shaped conjunctival blood vessels (telangiectasia).
- Two specific types of cataracts occur in patients with Fabry disease.
- Granular anterior subcapsular deposits.
- An unusual spoke-like posterior subcapsular opacity that is best seen through retroillumination (termed *Fabry cataract*).
- Internuclear ophthalmoplegia can affect the extraocular muscles.
- Edema in the area of the optic disk, periorbitally, or both is possible.
- Tortuous retinal vessels common.
- Decreased visual acuity results primarily from occlusive retinal vascular disease or complications of hypertensive retinopathy.
- Profound vision loss from central retinal artery occlusion is sometimes the initial presenting symptom.

Laboratory findings

Affected males have the following:

- A reduced a-galactosidase A level in plasma, serum, leukocytes, tears, and skin fibroblasts;

- Elevated trihexosyl ceramide level in urine, plasma and skin fibroblasts;
- Abnormal intracytoplasmic and intracellular lipid deposits.

Ultrastructural examination of these inclusions in epithelial cells of the cornea, conjunctiva, and lens reveals that they consist of a single membrane surrounding concentrically arranged membranous lamellae; however; the myelin-like structures are not pathognomonic of Fabry disease.

The histopathologic basis for the whorl-like corneal pattern has been the subject of debate; increasing evidence indicates that the pattern is due to a combination of:

- Lysosomal granules in the epithelium (which have been detected even in fetal eyes);
- Duplication of the basal lamina of the corneal epithelium.

TREATMENT

Systemic

The intravenous administration of purified placental a-galactosidase has been investigated but offers little promise. Phlebotomy does not alter plasma or urinary levels of ceramide trihexoside, and plasmapheresis is ineffective in treating the acroparesthesia of Fabry disease.

Treatment of the pain associated with the disease is symptomatic and has been used with varying levels of success.

- Diphenylhydantoin 20 mg/24 hour; or
- Carbamazepine 200 mg/hour.

Surgical

No satisfactory treatment is available. Renal transplantation has been performed for amelioration of chronic uremia, and cardiac transplantation has been performed for the cardiovascular aspects of the disease; however, recurrence of the storage disease is common in the allografts.

The disproportionately high incidence of sepsis in some patients may be due to the deficient immunologic function of lipid-laden leukocytes.

Hemodialysis remains an alternative mode of therapy for uremia but does not alter the accompanying cerebrovascular or cardiovascular impairment and simply postpones renal failure.

Recently, attention has been given to modeling the disease in animals to permit exploration of various therapies; gene manipulation (especially at the carboxyl terminus) has begun to show some promise for the future.

PRECAUTIONS

Genetic counseling and recognition of female carriers are important. The pattern of inheritance is like that of all X-linked recessive disorders: there is no father-to-son transmission, but all daughters of an affected male will be carriers (heterozygotes), and half of the sons of affected daughters will also have Fabry disease. Identification of all female carriers has been difficult because 25% to 40% of suspected heterozygotes may have normal levels of a-galactosidase. Recent studies, however, have shown that carriers can be identified in more than 90% of cases through the use of multiple biochemical tests.

COMMENTS

The diagnosis of Fabry disease is easily missed, especially in female carriers. The ophthalmologist is in an excellent position to make the diagnosis because the ocular changes (corneal verticillata and spoke-like cataracts) are among the earliest and most consistent signs. Corneal changes occur in about 90% of affected male patients and may be the only ocular sign in female carriers. The posterior spoke-like cataracts may be pathognomonic of Fabry disease, and the whorl-like corneal opacities are highly indicative of the disease, especially if there has been no previous history of consumption of drugs such as chloroquine.

REFERENCES

Cantor WJ, Daly P, Iwanochko M, et al: Cardiac transplantation for Fabry disease. Can J Cardiol 14:81–84, 1998.

Dantas MA, Fonseca RA, Kaga T, et al: Retinal and choroidal vascular changes in heterozygous Fabry disease. Retina 21:87–90, 2001.

Hirano K, Murata K, Miyagawa A, et al: Histopathologic findings of cornea verticillata in woman heterozygous for Fabry's disease. Cornea 20:233–236, 2001.

Kleijer WJ, Hussaarts-Odijk LM, Sachs ES, et al: Prenatal diagnosis of Fabry's disease by direct analysis of chorionic villi. Prenat Diagn 7:283–287, 1987.

Mastropasqua L, Nubile M, Lanzini M, et al: Corneal and conjunctival manifestations in Fabry disease: in vivo confocal microscopy study. Am J Ophthalmol 14:709–718, 2006.

Miyamura N, Araki E, Matsuda K, et al: A carboxy-terminal truncation of human alpha-galactosidase A in a heterozygous female with Fabry disease and modification of the enzymatic activity by the carboxy-terminal domain: Increased, reduced, or absent enzyme activity depending on number of amino acid residues deleted. J Clin Invest 98:1809–1817, 1996.

Ohshima T, Murray GJ, Swaim WD, et al: Alpha-galactosidase A deficient mice: a model of Fabry disease. Proc Natl Acad Sci USA 94:2540–2544, 1997.

Rodriguez FH, Hoffmann EO, Ordinario AT: Fabry's disease in a heterozygous woman. Arch Pathol Lab Med 109:89–91, 1985.

Sakuraba H, Igarashi T, Shibata T, et al: Effects of vitamin E and ticlopidine on platelet aggregation in Fabry's disease. Clin Genet 31:349–354, 1987.

Sugimoto Y, Aksentijevich I, Murray GJ, et al: Retroviral coexpression of a multidrug resistance gene (MDR1) and human alpha-galactosidase A for gene therapy of Fabry disease. Hum Gene Ther 6:905–915, 1995.

Tsutsumi A, Uchida Y, Kanai T, et al: Corneal findings in a foetus with Fabry's disease. Acta Ophthalmol 62:923–931, 1984.

79 HYPERLIPOPROTEINEMIA 272.4

Ahmad M. Mansour, MD
Beirut, Lebanon
Mays El-Dairi, MD
Beirut, Lebanon

ETIOLOGY

Hyperlipoproteinemia is a metabolic disorder characterized by abnormally elevated plasma total cholesterol, low density lipoprotein-cholesterol, triglyceride, or apolipoprotein-B, or abnormally low high density lipoprotein (HDL)-cholesterol or apolipoprotein-A1.

DIAGNOSIS

Clinical signs and symptoms

Clinical manifestations are caused by deposition of lipids at various tendons, the vascular system, and the eye.

Ocular

Eye manifestations include corneal arcus, lipemia retinalis and xanthelasma.

- Corneal arcus is accumulation of lipid in peripheral cornea as part of ageing. Juvenile arcus is associated with familial hypercholesterolemia. Presenile corneal arcus is associated with types II-V hyperlipidemia. Unilateral arcus may be a sign of carotid artery disease or ocular hypotony.
- Xanthomas are localized infiltrates of lipid containing histiocytic foam cells. There are five types. Tendinous xanthoma (xanthoma IA) is associated with xanthelasma and beta-lipoprotein disturbance. Cerebrotendinous xanthomatosis (xanthoma IB) is associated with bilateral juvenile cataracts, xanthelasma, and elevated cholestanol level. Planar xanthoma (xanthoma II) is associated xanthelasma and hyperlipoproteinemia. Tuberous xanthoma (xanthoma III) is associated with broad beta disease. Eruptive xanthoma (xanthoma IV) is associated with lipemia retinalis and hypertriglyceridemia. Disseminated xanthoma (xanthoma V) is associated with corneal and scleral xanthoma with normal lipid profile.
- Lipemia retinalis is caused by elevation of serum triglyceride level above 2500 mg/dL. This occurs in types I and V hyperlipoproteinemia and more often is associated with diabetes mellitus, alcoholism, hypothyroidism, nephrotic syndrome, and biliary obstruction. In mild lipemia retinalis (triglyceride 2500–3500 mg/dL), only peripheral vessels have a creamy tint. In moderate lipemia retinalis (triglyceride 3500–5000 mg/dL), there is posterior extension of the creamy color. In severe lipemia retinalis (triglyceride >5000 mg/dL), there is whitening of all retinal vessels with inability to differentiate arteries from veins. Conjunctival and iris vessels might be creamy providing an easy slit-lamp follow-up for triglyceride level. Complications associated with lipemia retinalis include eruptive xanthoma, hepatosplenomegaly, acute pancreatitis, and atheroma.

Laboratory findings

A standard serum lipid profile consists of total cholesterol, triglycerides, and HDL-cholesterol. Lipoprotein analysis should be performed after 12 hours of fasting to minimize postprandial hyperlipidemia. Lipoprotein electrophoresis is expensive and is unnecessary for the diagnosis of most lipid disorders.

TREATMENT

Systemic

Weight reduction and diet low in saturated fat and cholesterol are advocated. Extreme fat and cholesterol restriction has been achieved with vegetarian diets. Alcohol and estrogen should be avoided in certain types of hyperlipoproteinemias. Aerobic exercise improves insulin sensitivity, HDL-C concentrations and reduces coronary artery disease risk. Lipid lowering drugs include fibric acid derivatives (clofibrate, gemfibrozil, fenofibrate), niacin, omega-3 fatty acids, and statins (atorvastatin, simvastatin, rosuvastatin, cerivastatin, pravastatin, lovastatin, fluvastatin).

Surgical

Ileal bypass or plasmapheresis are performed in selected cases of familial hypercholesterolemia. Liver transplanstation is rarely done in familial hypercholesterolemia.

COMMENTS

Patients with lipid disorder have a higher risk for occlusive vascular disease which is decreased by healthy diet, desirable weight, and regular exercise.

REFERENCES

Barchiesi BJ, Eckel RH, Ellis PP: The cornea and disorders of lipid metabolism. Surv Ophthalmol 36:1–22, 1991.

Crispin S: Ocular lipid deposition and hyperlipoproteinaemia. Prog Retin Eye Res 21:169–224, 2002.

Mansour AM, Raimer SS: Cerebrotendinous xanthomatosis and other xanthomas. In: Gold D, Weingeist TA, eds: The eye in systemic disease. Philadelphia: Lippincott, 1990:337–340.

Uwaydat S, Mansour AM: Infantile lipemia retinalis et conjunctivalis. J Ped Ophthalmol Strab 7:47–49, 2000.

SECTION

7 Hematologic and Cardiovascular Disorders

80 CAROTID CAVERNOUS FISTULA
853.0
(Dural Shunt Syndrome, Carotid Artery-Cavernous Sinus Fistula, Arteriovenous Communication or Arteriovenous Fistula)

M. Tariq Bhatti, MD
Durham, North Carolina
Keith Robertson Peters, MD, ABR, CAQ VIR, CAQ NR
Gainesville, Florida

INTRODUCTION

Carotid cavernous fistulas represent an abnormal arteriovenous communication between the cavernous sinus (a venous structure) and the carotid arterial system (internal and/or external carotid arteries). Carotid cavernous fistulas can be classified as: high flow vs. low flow, direct vs. indirect (dural) or traumatic vs. spontaneous. The Barrow classification categorizes the fistulas depending on the angiographic pattern of the arterial flow. Depending on the type of carotid cavernous fistula and the pattern of venous drainage (anterior or posterior) the clinical manifestations can be variable and diverse.

ETIOLOGY/INCIDENCE

Most carotid cavernous fistulas are of the direct type and caused by head trauma (70%–90%). Dural carotid cavernous fistulas are thought to be congenital in etiology and are more commonly seen in middle-aged or elderly women often associated with systemic arterial hypertension, atherosclerotic vascular disease and connective tissue disorders.

COURSE/PROGNOSIS

Direct carotid cavernous fistulas can be life threatening due to severe epistaxis or intracranial (intracerebral or subarachnoid) hemorrhage therefore nearly all require intervention. In comparison, if left untreated dural carotid cavernous fistulas rarely result in neurological sequela but can be associated with significant ocular morbidity. Up to 50% of dural carotid cavernous fistula will close without treatment. Acute worsening of the ocular manifestations may occur from increased blood flow through the fistula or spontaneous thrombosis of the superior ophthalmic vein.

DIAGNOSIS

Clinical signs and symptoms

(Figure 80.1)

- Red eye due to episcleral venous congestion (corkscrew episcleral vessels).
- Conjunctival chemosis.
- Eyelid or facial edema.
- Elevated intraocular pressure (asymmetric ocular pulse).
- Pulsating exophthalmos.
- Diplopia due to ocular motor cranial neuropathy or extraocular muscle congestion.
- Orbital (ocular) pain or headache.
- Orbital bruit (approximately 50% of dural fistulas).
- Retinal vascular congestion and hemorrhages.
- Visual loss due severe corneal exposure, glaucoma, retinopathy or optic neuropathy.

Laboratory findings

- Orbital ultrasonography: dilated superior ophthalmic vein and enlarged extraocular muscles.
- Computed tomography: dilated superior ophthalmic veins, dilated cerebral veins, and enlarged extraocular muscles.
- Magnetic resonance imaging: abnormal flow voids, dilated superior ophthalmic vein, enlarged extraocular muscles, and orbital congestion.
- Magnetic resonance angiography (maximum intensity projection and source images): flow signal abnormalities.
- Six-vessel cranial digital subtraction angiography (diagnostic procedure of choice): characterization of the arterial supply and venous drainage of fistula.

Differential diagnosis

- Chronic conjunctivitis.
- Orbital cellulites.
- Thyroid eye disease.
- Orbital arteriovenous malformation.

TREATMENT

Ocular

- Topical lubrication.
- Intraocular pressure lowering agents.

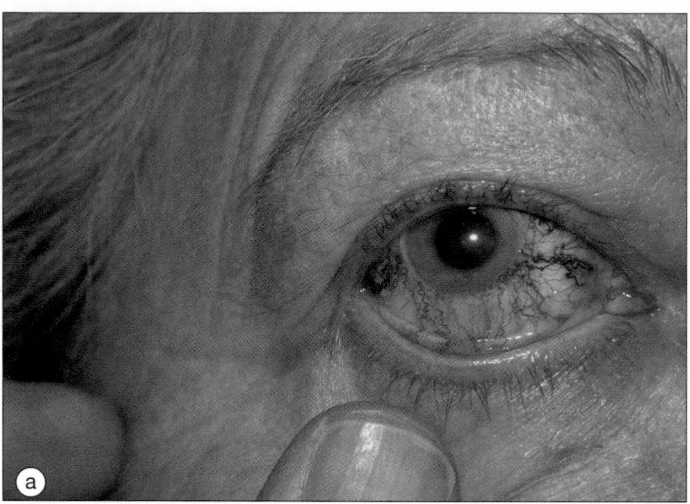

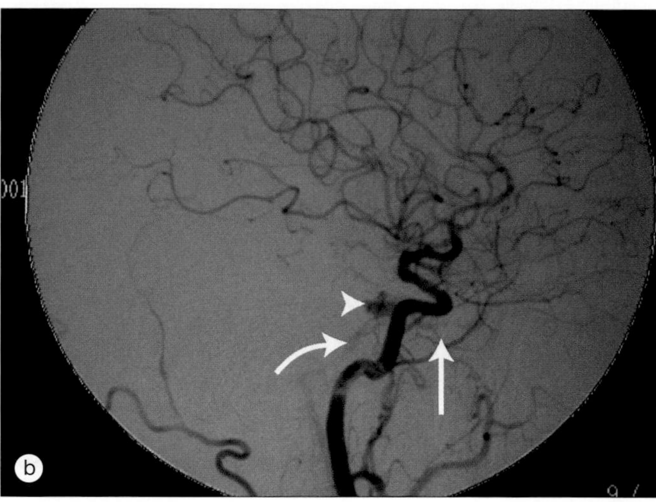

FIGURE 80.1. External photograph demonstrating arterialization (corkscrew appearance) of conjunctival vessels. The lateral digital subtraction angiogram of the right common carotid artery in early arterial phase demonstrates immediate dense contrast filling of the cavernous sinus (arrowhead) with drainage anteriorly through the superior ophthalmic vein (straight arrow) and posteriorly through the inferior petrosal sinus (curved arrow).

Medical

- Intermittent self-manual carotid artery compression.

Stereotactic radiosurgery
Direct cavernous sinus surgery
Endovascular embolization (recommended therapy of choice)

- Transarterial route.
- Transvenous route.
- Superior ophthalmic vein route.

Complications of endovascular embolization therapy

- Carotid artery occlusion resulting in ipsilateral cerebral hemisphere ischemia.
- Transient worsening of ocular and orbital manifestations.
- Partial closure of fistula with persistent posterior venous drainage and cortical venous arterialization.

COMMENTS

The clinical manifestations of direct and dural carotid cavernous fistulas may overlap with the signs and symptoms being more dramatic in direct fistulas. All direct carotid cavernous sinus fistulas should be treated. In contrast dural fistulas can often be observed expectantly and in many cases may close spontaneously or after a diagnostic angiogram.

REFERENCES

Barrow DL, Spector RH, Braun IF, et al: Classification and treatment of spontaneous carotid-cavernous sinus fistulas. J Neurosurg 62(2):248–256, 1985.

Goldberg RA, Goldey SH, Duckwiler G, Vinuela F: Management of cavernous sinus-dural fistulas. Indications and techniques for primary embolization via the superior ophthalmic vein. Arch Ophthalmol 114(6):707–714, 1996.

Grove AS, Jr: The dural shunt syndrome. Pathophysiology and clinical course. Ophthalmology 91(1):31–44, 1984.

Miller NR: Carotid-cavernous sinus fistulas. In: Miller NR, Newman NJ, Biousse V, Kerrison JB, eds: Walsh and Hoyt's clinical neuro-ophthalmology. 6th edn. Baltimore, Williams & Wilkins, 2005:2263–2296.

Sergott RC, Grossman RI, Savino PJ, et al: The syndrome of paradoxical worsening of dural-cavernous sinus arteriovenous malformations. Ophthalmology 94(3):205–212, 1987.

Tsai Y-F, Chen L-K, Su C-T, et al: Utility of source images of three dimensional time-of-flight magnetic resonance angiograpy in the diagnosis of indirect carotid-cavernous sinus fistulas. J Neuro-Ophthalmol 24:285–289, 2004.

81 SICKLE CELL RETINOPATHY 282.60

Hon-Vu Q. Duong, MD

Las Vegas, Nevada

ETIOLOGY/INCIDENCE

Sickle cell hemoglobinopathy encompasses a group of inherited genetic disorders, which cause erythrocytes to become sickled and affect multiple organ systems. The rigid sickled erythrocytes lead to vascular occlusion, which results in retinal hypoxia, ischemia, infarction, detachment, and neovascularization.

In sickle cell anemia (SS disease), the amino acid substitution valine for glutamate occurs on the β-chain at the sixth position. This substitution, combined with conditions that may promote sickling triggers the deoxygenated Hb S to polymerize, making the erythrocyte rigid. This rigidity is partially responsible for the vasoocclusion. Vasoocclusion is also in part due to the interaction between sickled cells and the vascular endothelium with the end result of vascular stasis, hemolysis, and vasoocclusion.

In the United States, sickle cell anemia primarily occurs in the black population, with approximately 0.2% of African-

American children afflicted by this disease. The prevalence in adults is lower because of the decrease in life expectancy. Sickle cell anemia is a homozygous-recessive disorder.

Sickle cell C disease is the second most common form, resulting from amino acid substitution of lysine for glutamic acid, and commonly seen in West African populations. Sickle cell thalassemia is the third most common form of sickle cell disease.

COURSE/PROGNOSIS

Systemic disease associated with sickle cell anemia is more common and more severe than ocular disease. Sickle cell C disease and sickle cell thalassemia tend to have mild systemic manifestations however, ocular manifestations can be severe.

Prognosis is fair to good if consistent follow-up care is maintained with both an internist/hematologist and an ophthalmologist.

DIAGNOSIS

Clinical signs and symptoms

Patients with a history of sickle cell anemia should undergo a dilated fundus exam based on retinal findings. Changes in the posterior segment are divided into 4 major categories: optic disc changes, macular changes, nonproliferative retinal changes, and proliferative retinal changes.

Optic disc

Intravascular occlusions primarily affect the small vessels on the surface of the optic disc and appear as dark red spots or clumps. They are often called the disc sign of sickling. They are self-limiting and do not produce any appreciable visual symptoms.

Macula

Vascular occlusion can lead to complete loss of vision or can lead to central or paracentral scotoma. A macular depression may be seen. Proliferative findings in the macular include macula hole, macula traction, enlarged segments of terminal arterioles, hairpin-shaped vascular loops, and abnormal foveal avascular zone.

Nonproliferative sickle cell retinopathy

While abnormal, nonproliferative changes are generally asymptomatic and do not require treatment. The nonproliferative changes include:

- *venous tortuosity* — common but not pathognomonic for sickle cell disease,
- *salmon patch hemorrhage* — intraretinal hematoma, found in the periphery, and confined to the neural retina,
- *black sunburst* — a pigmented chorioretinal scar, usually found in the periphery. These scars appear round or ovoid with stellate or speculate borders and often associated with iridescent spots,
- *angiod streaks* — breaks in Bruch membrane and appeared as pigmented striae that lie under the retinal vessels.

Proliferative retinopathy

Stage I — Peripheral arteriolar occlusion: areas of retinal ischemia secondary to nonperfusion become an abnormal grayish brown color.

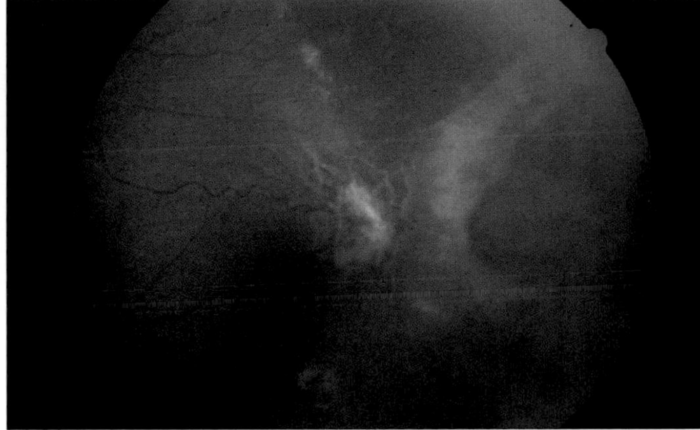

FIGURE 81.1. Sickle cell retinopathy.

Stage II — Arterioilar-venular anastomoses: shunting of blood from the occluded arterioles to the nearest venules. Often difficult to view by ophthalmoscopy an FA can demonstrate arteriovenous anastomoses that do not leak dye.

Stage III — Neovascular proliferation: classic finding for stage IIII is the 'sea fan –neovascularization' lesion. On FA, sea fan lesions leak profusely (Figure 81.1).

Stage IV — Vitreous hemorrhage: it may be spontaneous secondary to vitreous collapse and/or traction of the adherent neovascular tissue.

Stage V — Retinal Detachment: detachments may be rhegmatogenous and/or tractional.

Differential diagnosis

- BRVO CRVO.
- Eales disease.
- Hypertension.
- Retinopathy of prematurity.
- Proliferative diabetic retinopathy.
- Sarcoidosis.

TREATMENT

Medical

This condition is treated by an internist or hematologist.

Surgical/Ocular

The primary goal in treating proliferative sickle cell retinopathy is to minimize or eliminate neovascularization. Although treatments are not indicated for stages I and II, most advocate treatment with stage III.

Laser photocoagulation

It is relatively safe and one of the more commonly used therapeutic modality. Different techniques have been advocated and include scatter or feeder vessel photocoagulation.

Retinal cryotherapy

Cryotherapy often is limited to cases with cloudy ocular media. Single freeze-thaw and triple freeze-thaw have been advocated in treating PSR.

Vitrectomy

Vitrectomy is indicated in cases of nonresolving vitreous hemorrhage and retinal detachment.

COMPLICATIONS

Anterior segment ischemia

- The following measures can decrease complications.
- Preoperative partial exchange transfusion.
- Administer local anesthesia, stellate ganglion block.
- Cycloplegic (parasympathomimetics).
- Decrease IOP and should be kept less than 25 mmHg, preoperatively, intraoperatively, and postoperatively.
- Supplemental oxygen.

Recurrent retinal detachment

Hyphema

Neovascular glaucoma

COMMENTS

Early detection and treatment may help decrease the retinal complications. Special concern should include repeated blood transfusion, hyphema, and scleral buckling. Ophthalmic care is determined by the proliferative stage. Patients should be well informed of their current and potential long-term complications. These patients are strongly encouraged to enroll at a local or regional sickle cell clinic along with providing these patients with local support group. Patients with diagnosed sickle cell disease should seek genetic counseling prior to starting a family.

REFERENCES

Andreoli TE, et al: Disorder of red cells. In: Cecil's essentials of medicine. 4th edn. 1997:383–387.

Asdourian GK: Sickle cell retinopathy. In: Albert DM, Jakobiec FA, eds. Principles and practice of ophthalmology. 1994:II:1006–1018.

Beutler E: Disorders of hemoglobin. In: Fauci AS, et al, eds: Harrison's principle of internal medicine. 14th edn. 1998:645–652.

Bunn HF: Pathogenesis and treatment of sickle cell disease. New Engl J Med 337(11):762–769, 1997.

Fekrat S, Lutty G, Goldberg M: Hemoglobinopathies. In: Guyer D, et al: Retina-vitreous macula. 1999:I:438–458.

Ho AC: Hemoglobinopathies. In: Yanoff, M, Duker, JS, eds. Ophthalmology. 2nd edn. Mosby, 2004:Ch119:891–895.

Yanoff M, Fine BS: Sickle cell disease. In: Ocular pathology. 4th edn. 1996:377–378.

82 THE THALASSEMIAS 282.4

Stephen S. Feman, MD, FACS
St. Louis, Missouri
Levent Akduman, MD
St. Louis, Missouri
Ozgur Yalcinbayir, MD
St. Louis, Missouri

The thalassemias are a group of hereditary disorders characterized by decreased rates of hemoglobin polypeptide chain synthesis. They represent the clinical features of a series of pathologic alleles on chromosome 11 and 16. As a group, the thalassemias are the most common single-gene problem in humans. The chromosomal abnormalities can result in total gene deletion, rearrangements of genetic loci, mutations that impair transcription, defects in the processing of genetic information, and errors in the translation of RNA. In the past, these disorders had a variety of historic names (Cooley's anemia, thalassemia major, thalassemia minor, etc.). In an attempt to include all the manifestations of this disorder, a nomenclature related to the involved polypeptide chain has become popular (alpha-thalassemia for alpha polypeptide chain abnormalities, beta-thalassemia for beta polypeptide chain abnormalities, etc.).

The clinical manifestations of this disorder are the results of inadequate globin production and the accumulation of blood products. The clinical features are diverse and can range from asymptomatic states to death from anemia. The most common clinical characteristic of the thalassemias is the development of a hypochromic microcystic anemia. However, in some patients, the pathologic changes represent such a small fraction of total globin synthesis that this abnormality is difficult to measure.

In general, when a patient has one thalassemia gene and one normal gene, the disorder is called thalassemia trait (thalassemia minor in the older literature) and a relatively mild anemia is present. When two similar genes are present, there is a more severe impairment of hemoglobin synthesis and a more severe anemia (thalassemia major in the older literature). In addition, it is possible to describe the thalassemias in regard to the rate of hemoglobin polypeptide chain synthesis. Some recent publications use this to specify the relative amount of hemoglobin synthesis impairment and imply this information (i.e. severe, mild and silent form of thalassemia) is of greater clinical value than the other nomenclatures.

The most common variety of thalassemia was described by Cooley and Lee in 1925. It is caused by a defect in the rate of synthesis of the beta-polypeptide chain of hemoglobin A. This abnormality results in a relative increase in the levels of hemoglobin A2 and hemoglobin F, along with the development of a microcystic hypochromic anemia. As the years progress, splenomegaly, hepatomegaly and discoloration of the skin and sclera occur. At one time, this particular disorder was thought to have a specific geographic distribution that extended from the Mediterranean through the Middle East, India and Southeast Asia. Although there is a relatively high gene frequency in those areas (it can range from 2.5% to 15% in those regions), it has been found that the thalassemias have a worldwide distribution.

COURSE/PROGNOSIS

Infants are born free of anemia because of prenatal hemoglobin F production. In most patients, the clinical manifestations are first identified at about the 6th month of life. Without treatment, 80% of the patients with the classic form of this disorder will die within 5 years. In these young infants, the most common associated clinical features consist of pallor, irritability, growth retardation, abdominal swelling and jaundice. Transfusions to prevent the associated anemias have become a treatment standard.

Ocular or periocular manifestations

Conjunctiva

Focal regions of dilated and turtuous vessels.

Retina

Vascular tortuosity; pigmented chorioretinal scars (black sunburst pattern); iridescent intraretinal deposits; focal arterial occlusions; central retinal vein occlusion; neovascularizations; hemorrhages; angioid streaks which may be associated with subretinal neovascularization; macular pucker; and macular ischemia.

Vitreous

Hemorrhages.

THERAPY

Systemic

Transfusions to prevent the symptoms of anemia have been the standard of treatment for many years. In time, such therapy will result in an iron overload and hemosiderosis; this complication had been a common cause of death for these patients. However, with the use of iron chelators, such as deferoxamine and desferrioxamine, this danger is lessened. Nevertheless, splenomegaly can be a major problem for such patients and may need to be resolved with a splenectomy.

Ocular

The most serious threats to vision occur in patients with thalassemia and sickle cell trait. Such patients develop multifocal areas of peripheral retinal neovascularization that result in vitreous hemorrhages. The vessels feeding and draining the neovascular growth can be identified by fluorescein angiography, and photocoagulation to occlude these vessels can prevent such hemorrhages. Then, the surrounding area of ischemic retina can be treated with a scatter photocoagulation pattern to reduce the stimulus for recurrent neovascularization and to prevent future problems in that retinal region.

Precautions

Ocular complications indicate, in most cases, that the patient has a combination of thalassemia and some other hemoglobin abnormality. The treatment of the ocular manifestations associated with the other hemoglobin abnormality offers the greatest visual benefit to most patients. In addition, patients requiring frequent blood transfusions may show signs of retinal toxicity from the iron accumulation or from the desferrioxamine use. The clinical features of this type of retinal toxicity include night blindness, visual field defects and ERG changes.

COMMENTS

Whenever an intraocular hemorrhage, visual field defect, or retinal neovascular change is identified, one must search for an additional hemoglobin abnormality. If found, the treatment should be directed to the ocular and systemic manifestations of the other co-existing hemoglobinopathy to prevent additional visual loss.

Regular, or yearly, ophthalmic examinations are recommended for patients with the thalassemias in order to detect and treat possible ocular complications and to monitor the potential iron toxicity.

REFERENCES

Aessopos A, Farmakis D, Karagiorga M, et al: Pseudoxanthoma elasticum lesions and cardiac complications as contributing factors for strokes in beta-thalassemia patients. Stroke 28(12):2421–2424, 1997.

Aessopos A, Voskaridou E, Kavouklis E, et al: Angioid streaks in sickle-thalassemia. Am J Ophthalmol 117(5):589–592, 1994.

Al-Hazzaa S, Bird AC, Kulozik A, et al: Ocular findings in Saudi Arabian patients with sickle cell disease. Br J Ophthalmol 79(5):457–461, 1995.

Carney MD, Jampol LM: Epiretinal membranes in sickle cell retinopathy. Arch Ophthalmol 105(2):214–217, 1987.

Comings DE: Thalassemia. In: Williams WJ, Beutler E, Lichtman MA, et al, eds: Hematology. New York, Mc Graw-Hill, 328–345, 1972.

Condon PI, Serjeant GR: Ocular findings in sickle cell thalassemia in Jamaica. Am J Ophthalmol 74:1105–1109, 1972.

Cooley TB, Lee P: A series of cases of splenomegaly in children with anemia and peculiar bone changes. Trans Am Pediatr Soc 37:29–35, 1925.

Davies SC, Marcus RE, Hungerford JL, et al: Ocular toxicity of high-dose intravenous desferrioxamine. Lancet 2(8343):181–184, 1983.

Dennerlein JA, Lang GE, Stahnke K, et al: Ocular findings in Desferal therapy. Ophthalmologe 92(1):38–42, 1995.

Feman SS, Westrich DJ: Macular arteriolar occlusions in sickle cell beta-thalassemia. Am J Ophthalmol 101:739–740, 1986.

Goldberg MF, Charache S, Acacio I: Ophthalmologic manifestations of sickle cell thalassemia. Arch Intern Med 128:33–39, 1971.

Gupta A, Agarwal A, Bansal RK, et al: Ischaemic central retinal vein occlusion in the young. Eye 7(Pt 1):138–142, 1993.

Kinsella FP, Mooney DJ: Angioid streaks in beta thalassaemia minor. Br J Ophthalmol 72(4):303–304, 1988.

Magli A, Fusco R, Mettivier V, Pisapia R: Ocular manifestations in thalassemia minor. Ophthalmologica 184:139–146, 1982.

Theodossiadis G, Ladas I, Koutsandrea C, et al: Thalassemia and macular subretinal neovascularization. J Fr Ophtalmol 7(2):115–118, 1984.

SECTION

8 Dermatologic Disorders

83 ATOPIC DERMATITIS 691.8
(Atopic Eczema, Disseminated Neurodermatitis)

Carsten Heinz, MD
Muenster, Germany
Arnd Heiligenhaus, MD
Muenster, Germany

INCIDENCE/ETIOLOGY

Atopic dermatitis (AD) is a chronic disease with a prevalence of 10–20% in children and 1–3% in adults. In acute AD a Th2 dominated immune process with production of cytokines as IL-4, IL-5 and IL-13 is found, while in chronic AD the mircomilieu comprises of both Th1 and Th2 cytokines. AD may also be complicated by rhinitis or asthma. The etiology seems to be multivariant. Familial disease increases the risk 2 to 3 fold. The hygiene hypothesis proposes that an in utero and postnatal immune stimulation with infectious agents with a subsequent predominantly Th1 immune response results in a lower risk of atopic manifestation. Food allergens, aeroallergens, bacteria and also emotional stress have been implicated to stimulate AD. Serum IgE is often elevated in patients with AD and sensitization against a variety of environmental allergens is frequent. However, manifestation or exacerbation of AD also occurs in the absence of exposure to environmental allergens. The high level of IgE autoantibodies against a broad variety of human proteins often correlates with disease severity and may contribute to pathogenesis.

DIAGNOSIS

Atopic dermatitis is a chronic relapsing, inflammatory skin disease that is characterized by pruritic eczematous skin lesion. Predominant localization varies with the patient's age, with predilection on the extensor surfaces in young children and on the flexor surfaces in adults. Ocular involvement is reported in about 32%.

OCULAR

Eyelid

- Erythema, exudates, crusting, scaling, blepharitis, secondary infection.

Conjunctiva

- Conjunctival injection, chemosis, mucus discharge, papillary reaction, Trantas dots, squamous cell carcinoma.

Cornea

- Superficial punctate keratopathy (SPK), shield ulcer, scars, keratoconus, vascularization.

Lens

- Cataract formation.

Retina

- Detachment due to rubbing of the eyelids or traumatic slapping.

TREATMENT

Systemic

- Avoidance of identified allergens.
- Oral corticosteroids.
- Systemic tetracycline as blepharitis treatment.
- Immunosuppression in severe cases, e.g. with cyclosporin A.

Topical

Skin

Lid hygiene, topical corticosteroids, calcineurin inhibitors (e.g. tacrolimus or pimecrolimus), antibiotics.

Ocular

Unpreserved lubricants, mast cell stabilisators, antihistamines, cyclosporin A, topical corticosteroid, antibiotics, therapeutic contact lenses

Surgical

- Tarsorhaphie or punctual occlusion in SPK.
- Amniotic membrane transplantation in corneal epithelial defects or shield ulcers.
- Cataract extraction with IOL implantation.
- Keratoplasty for keratoconus.
- Retinal detachment surgery.

COMMENTS

Atopic dermatitis is a chronic skin disease that also affects the eyelid leading to severe discomfort. Treatment of the skin disease is often satisfactory and should be managed cooperatively with dermatologists. The severity of eye affections varies extremely and may lead to visual loss. Treatment strategies include lubricants, topical mast cell stabilizers antihistamines or topical ciclosporin, and systemic immunosuppression or surgical interventions may be required to preserve vision.

REFERENCES

Heinz C, Fanihagh F, Steuhl KP: Squamous cell carcinoma of the conjunctiva in patients with atopic eczema. Cornea 22(2):135–137, 2003.

Hida T, Tano Y, Okinami S, et al: Multicenter retrospective study of retinal detachment associated with atopic dermatitis. Jpn J Ophthalmol 44(4):407–418, 2000.

Hingorani M, Moodaley L, Calder VL, et al: A randomized, placebo-controlled trial of topical cyclosporin A in steroid-dependent atopic keratoconjunctivitis. Ophthalmology 105(9):1715–1720, 1998.

Leung DY, Bieber T: Atopic dermatitis. Lancet 361(9352):151–160, 2003.

Leung DY, Jain N, Leo HL: New concepts in the pathogenesis of atopic dermatitis. Curr Opin Immunol 15(6):634–638, 2003.

Novak N, Bieber T, Leung DY: Immune mechanisms leading to atopic dermatitis. J Allergy Clin Immunol 112(6 Suppl):S128–S139, 2003.

Schultz Larsen F, Diepgen T, Svensson A: The occurrence of atopic dermatitis in north Europe: an international questionnaire study. J Am Acad Dermatol 34(5 Pt 1):760–764, 1996.

Sturgill S, Bernard LA: Atopic dermatitis update. Curr Opin Pediatr 16(4):396–401, 2004.

Uchio E, Miyakawa K, Ikezawa Z, et al: Systemic and local immunological features of atopic dermatitis patients with ocular complications. Br J Ophthalmol 82(1):82–87, 1998.

84 CONTACT DERMATITIS 692.9
(Contact Allergy, Dermatitis Venenata)

Srini V. Goverdhan, MD, FRCSOphth
Southampton, England

ETIOLOGY/INCIDENCE

Contact dermatitis is a common immunologic skin condition which often presents to ophthalmologists as an eyelid or periorbital dermatitis. It results from exposure of the skin to a wide variety of substances with primary irritant properties commonly found in the environment, including drugs, dyes, plant resins, preservatives, cosmetics, resins, rubber derivatives and metals. Small incomplete hapten molecules bind to dermal protein, forming complete antigens. Initial exposure to haptens results in sensitization of $CD8^+$ T lymphocytes, a second application triggers release of cytokines, which amplify the inflammatory response in the skin. There are three varieties of contact dermatitis:

1. Allergic, which is the common form;
2. Atopic; and
3. Irritant.

Allergic contact dermatitis (ACD), unlike the irritant variety, occurs only in sensitized individuals and involves the mechanism of cell-mediated immunity. In ACD, an individual becomes sensitized to a given chemical or other sensitizing substance, and with re-exposure to the same chemical, an erythematous delayed hypersensitivity skin reaction is elicited. In Glaucoma, ACD has been seen with use of brimonidine or beta- blockers (timolol, befunolol, and carteolol) where cross-reactivity may occur as this is caused by a common aldehyde metabolite.

Atopic dermatitis (AD) is a common cause of chronic recurring eyelid dermatitis often developing as an atopic itchy red eye in childhood, but can also present in adulthood. Cell mediated immune defects within the skin and abnormal IgE levels have been described as possible mechanisms.

Irritant contact dermatitis (ICD) is caused by excessive moisture or by acids, alkalis, resins, or chemicals capable of injuring any person's skin if persistent contact is allowed. Allergy or hypersensitivity plays no role in irritant contact dermatitis.

DIAGNOSIS

History is essential in making the diagnosis of contact dermatitis; a personal and family history of hay fever, asthma, eczema or childhood atopy supports the diagnosis of ACD. History may be positive for exposure to irritative or sensitizing substances including topical ocular medications like neomycin, atropine derivatives, preservatives (benzalkonium chloride, benzyl alcohol, thimerosal, etc.) and anti-glaucoma medications (beta-blockers). Patch testing is often required for an adequate diagnosis of ACD or ICD. Withdrawal of the offending substance often alleviates signs and symptoms.

Clinical signs and symptoms

Signs and symptoms include erythematous, edematous, exudative, and pruritic skin lesions; scaling, ulceration, and edema of the eyelids; conjunctivitis and keratitis, especially inferiorly; and punctate corneal staining or infiltrates, especially inferiorly; itching of the skin and of the eye itself. With chronicity, the periorbital skin, particularly the upper eyelid becomes eczematous and lichenified.

TREATMENT

Systemic

- Poison ivy or poison oak dermatitis may require a course of oral corticosteroids. Desensitization may also be helpful. Antihistamines and mast-cell stabilizers can help control atopic symptoms in AD. Local reactions rarely require systemic therapy.

Local

- The allergen or irritant (determined by patch testing) should be removed from the patient's environment.
- Topical corticosteroids may lead to the rapid relief of symptoms.
- Saline compresses and steroid lotions are helpful for skin lesions.

SUMMARY

Contact sensitivity is a common ophthalmologic problem because of exposure to chemicals in eye drops. The best form of treatment is discontinuation or avoiding the offending substance. Steroid therapy can reduce symptoms, but it is not recommended on a long-term basis. Patch testing can be very helpful in determining the cause of contact dermatitis and in selecting alternative drugs to which the patient is not sensitive.

REFERENCES

Friedlaender MH: Allergy and immunology of the eye. New York, Raven, 1993:79–82.

Guin JD: Eyelid dermatitis: a report of 215 patients. Contact Dermatitis 50:87–90, 2004.

Holdiness MR: Contact dermatitis to topical drugs for glaucoma. Am J Contact Dermatitis 12:217–219, 2001.

Manni G, Centofanti M, Sacchetti M, et al: Demographic and clinical factors associated with development of brimonidine tartrate 0.2%-induced ocular allergy. J Glaucoma 13:163–167, 2004.

Zug KA, Palay DA, Rock B, et al: Dermatologic diagnosis and treatment of itchy red eyelids. Surv Ophthalmol 40:293–306, 996.

85 ERYTHEMA MULTIFORME MAJOR

695.1

(Erythema Multiforme Exudativum, Stevens–Johnson Syndrome, Toxic Epidermal Necrolysis)

Sharon S. Lehman, MD

Wilmington, Delaware

ETIOLOGY/INCIDENCE

Erythema multiforme, Stevens–Johnson (SJS) and toxic epidermal necrolysis (TEN) represent a spectrum of disease characterized by an acute mucocutaneous reaction caused by hypersensitivity reaction to infection or drugs with activated T-lymphocytes acting destructively at the dermo-epidermal junction.

Erythema multiforme is a disease ranging in severity from mild (erythema multiforme minor), which is a benign condition without mucosal involvement, to severe (erythema multiforme major), which is characterized by bullous-erosive mucocutaneous reactions.

SJS, a form of erythema multiforme major, has limited full thickness epidermal necrosis, marked constitutional symptoms and low mortality rate. TEN is characterized by epidermal necrosis involving greater than 30% of the body surface with marked long term complications and mortality.

COURSE/PROGNOSIS

- The prodromal period before skin lesion usually includes fever, malaise, sore throat and arthralgias.
- Erythematous macules, papules, and the characteristic bull's eye target skin lesions occur on the skin and ocular involvement includes:
  - Eyelid: edema, erythema, and crusting occur initially with later entropion, scarring and trichiasis;
  - Conjunctiva: initial chemosis and inflammatory pseudomembrane occur with later keratinization, scarring, symblepharon, ankyloblepharon, and a dry eye;
  - Cornea: epithelial defects, limbal stem cell deficiency, corneal ulcers, vascularization, scarring and perforation occur.

DIAGNOSIS

Clinical signs and symptoms

The target, or bull's eye, lesions of erythema multiforme are diagnostic and are recognized by the central, dark-purple area or a blister surrounded by a pale, edematous, circular zone, which in turn is surrounded by a peripheral rim of erythema. The characteristic involvement of the oral and conjunctival mucosa can also aid in the diagnosis of Stevens–Johnson syndrome.

TREATMENT

Systemic

- Multispecialty care, often in an ICU or burn unit, is required.
- Use of steroids is controversial.
- Use of antibiotics is based on clinical course and cultures.
- Immunosuppresive agents continue to be studied.

Ocular

- Gentle eyelid hygiene should be performed as necessary.
- Preservative free artificial tear ointment should be frequently and liberally applied.
- Use of antibiotics is based on clinical course and cultures.
- Use of steroids is controversial.
- Use of topical anesthetics should be limited because of ocular surface toxicity.
- Daily examination and disruption of symblepharon is required.
- Chronic dry eye requires continued use of preservative free artificial tear products and consideration may be given to the use of topical cyclosporin A.

Surgical

- Consider symblepharon ring for prevention of adhesions if tolerated by patient.
- Consider amniotic membrane transplantation (AMT) in acute phase in order to promote healing and inhibit inflammation, vascularization and scar.
- Treatment for chronic dry eye may require punctual occlusion and tarsarrhaphy.
- Treatment for trichiasis and entropion may require epilation, cryoablation, electolysis and eyelid reconstruction.
- Treatment of severely affected eyes requires consideration of AMT, limbal stem cell transplantation and corneal transplantation with possible immunosuppression.

COMMENTS

The treatment of erythema multiforme major, SJS and TEN remains challenging. New treatments such as immunomodulatory therapy offer new hope but require further testing for proof of therapeutic efficacy.

REFERENCES

Foulks GN: The evolving treatment of dry eye. Ophthalmol Clin N Am 16:29–35, 2003.

John T, Foulks GN, John ME, et al: Amniotic membrane in the surgical management of acute toxic epidermal necrolysis. Ophthalmology 109:351–360, 2002.

Lehman SL: Long-term ocular complication of Stevens-Johnson syndrome. Clin Pediatr 38:425–427, 1999.

McKenna JK, Leiferman KM: Dermatologic drug reactions. Immunol Allergy Clin North Am 24:399–423, 2004.

Metry DW, Jung P, Levy ML: Use of intravenous immunoglobulin in children with Stevens-Johnson syndrome and toxic epidermal necrolysis: seven cases and review of the literature. Pediatrics 112:1430–1436, 2003.

Samson CM, Nduaguba C, Baltatzis S, et al: Limbal stem cell transplantation in chronic inflammatory eye disease. Ophthalmology 109:862–868, 2002.

86 OCULAR ROSACEA 695.3

Vinicius Coral Ghanem, MD
Joinville, Santa Catarina, Brazil
Mark J. Mannis, MD, FACS
Sacramento, California

ETIOLOGY/INCIDENCE

Acne rosacea is a chronic cutaneous disease of unknown etiology. It affects up to 10% of the population, most notably fair-skinned women from 30 to 60 years of age. Theories of its pathogenesis have included gastrointestinal, psychological, infectious, climatic, pharmacological and immunological causes.

COURSE/PROGNOSIS

Rosacea is most commonly seen in adults although it has been reported in young children. The course may be characterized by recurrent inflammatory attacks of decreasing severity and frequency, or more commonly by chronic disease that lasts for more than 10 years, presenting chronic complications such as persistent facial edema, keratitis and rhinophyma. The prognosis of ocular rosacea is generally good. Nevertheless, corneal involvement may be as high as 30% in cutaneous rosacea and up to 85% in frank ocular rosacea.

DIAGNOSIS

Clinical signs and symptoms

Primary features include flushing (transient erythema), non-transient (persistent) erythema, papules, pustules and telangiectasias. The presence of one or more of these features with a central facial distribution is suggestive of rosacea. Secondary features include burning or stinging, plaques, dry appearance, edema, phymatous changes and involvement of more peripheral locations (neck, chest, scalp, ears and back). Persistent erythema and telangiectasia between acute episodes of inflammation are typical signs.

Ocular involvement, commonly referred to as ocular rosacea, occurs in more than 50% of patients, usually affecting both eyes simultaneously. Clinical findings may be confined to the eyes and may include:

- Eyelid: telangiectasias and erythema of the lid margin, meibomian gland dysfunction, anterior blepharitis, recurrent chalazion/hordeolum, madarosis, trichiasis;
- Conjunctiva: interpalpebral or diffuse hyperemia, papillary and/or follicular reaction, pinguecula, scarring;
- Cornea: punctate erosions, pannus, neovascularization, lipid deposition, spade-shaped infiltrates, scarring, thinning, ulceration, perforation, phlyctenule;
- Sclera: episcleritis, scleritis.

The prevalence of ocular complaints in patients with acne rosacea is estimated at between 45% and 85%. The primary symptoms include burning, itching, tearing, foreign body sensation, redness and pain; however, the symptoms may be out of proportion to the clinical signs of the disease.

Laboratory findings

None.

Differential diagnosis

- Blepharitis, meibomitis, recurrent chalazion, sebaceous gland carcinoma.
- Staphylococcal and seborrheic blepharokeratoconjunctivitis.
- Dry eye syndrome.
- Medication toxicity.
- Interstitial keratitis.
- Skin disease:
  - Acne vulgaris;
  - Seborrheic dermatitis;
  - Chronic topical corticosteroid therapy;
  - Alcohol abuse;
  - Phototherapy;
  - Lupus erythematosus, perioral dermatitis, essential telangiectasia, tuberculosis, syphilis, dermatomyositis, etc.

TREATMENT

Systemic

The use of systemic antibiotics is the mainstay of treatment in most cases. We would stress that the treatment goal is to reduce the signs and symptoms rather than effecting a cure. Tetracycline is the most common initial regimen, 250 mg orally every 6 hours for a time period of 3 to 4 weeks, tapering to a maintenance dosage with improvement of the clinical condition. Alternatively, one can use 100 mg of doxycycline taken orally two times daily for 3–4 weeks with a subsequent taper. Symptomatic improvement commonly occurs before the clinical signs ameliorate and generally occurs 2 to 4 weeks after initiation of treatment. Patients who have recurrent disease or potentially sight-threatening complications may require a maintenance dose of up to 250 mg of tetracycline or 50 mg of doxycycline daily or every other day indefinitely. Abrupt withdrawal of treatment may cause an exacerbation of the disease. Recently, a sub-antimicrobial-dose doxycycline (doxycycline hyclate, 20mg twice daily) has demonstrated results comparable to conventional doses of tetracyclines, but with significant fewer side effects. The effectiveness of this therapy has yet to be evaluated for ocular rosacea. Supplements rich in Omega 3 (flaxseed oil — 500 to 1000 mg 3 times per day) may also be helpful in reducing ocular symptoms.

For dermatologic disease, oral metronidazole or erythromycin can also be employed. These treatment methods are less effective for cases of persistent lymphedema and rhinophyma, while oral isotretinoin has been used successfully in resistant cases and in rhinophyma.

Ocular

Proper lid hygiene is fundamental in the successful treatment of ocular rosacea. Warm compresses, lid margin massage (meibomian gland expression), and careful cleaning of the cilia and lid margin with dilute baby shampoo or commercially available lid scrubs are very helpful. The frequency of lid hygiene depends on the severity of the disease and is generally performed 2–4 times per day.

Approximately 40% of rosacea patients have signs of keratoconjunctivitis sicca. For this reason, artificial tears, preferentially without preservatives, should be used frequently. Punctal plugs may be helpful. Systemic antibiotics, lid hygiene and artificial tears in combination, may aid in restoration of the ocular surface by reduction of *Staphylococcus aureus* toxins and toxic free fatty acids present on the tear film.

In cases of severe lid margin disease, topical antibiotic and corticosteroid ointment may be used cautiously for short periods of time to control the acute exacerbations. Corticosteroid eye drops may be used, but with caution and preferably only for severe ocular inflammatory signs and symptoms.

Topical

Topical medications are usually combined with systemic treatment for successful control of symptoms and signs, especially in the case of ocular disease. The use of metronidazole 0.75% or 1% gel, sodium sulfacetamide 10%/sulfa 5% as a topical formulation or azelaic acid have shown good results. Topical corticosteroids must be used cautiously and for short periods, since their chronic usage can cause worsening of vasodilatation and telangiectasias.

Surgical

Surgical treatment is reserved for the most severe cases of ocular rosacea that develop significant corneal thinning or impending or actual perforation. Surgical options may include: conjunctival flap, cyanoacrylate adhesive application, or lamellar or penetrating keratoplasty. Before considering a transplant for optical purposes, it is essential that any inflammatory signs be controlled. Even so, these corneas are usually vascularized and transplant surgery is high-risk. Maintenance of systemic and ocular treatment is vital.

Dermatological surgical treatment is reserved for selected cases of telangiectasias and rhinophyma.

COMPLICATIONS

The absorption of tetracycline may be hindered by food intake. Therefore, tetracycline should not be taken during meals or along with dairy products, antacids, or iron preparations. Doxycycline absorption, on the other hand, is not affected by food intake. Neither tetracycline nor doxycycline should be used in children under 12 years of age or in pregnant or nursing women. Patients using these drugs should be advised of gastrointestinal side-effects and photosensitivity.

COMMENTS

Rosacea is a relatively common and frequently under-diagnosed disease by ophthalmologists, who may not carefully examine the patient's face. Considering that there are no objective diagnostic tests currently available, both the ophthalmologist as well as the dermatologist must rely on clinical findings, which may be subtle. A careful facial examination with adequate illumination is essential. In 20% of the cases, ocular symptoms appear before skin disease, and since the ocular signs may be non-specific, the clinical diagnosis may be difficult. Nevertheless, if the ocular signs are diagnostic, empirical treatment should be initiated. Patient follow-up and management must be multidisciplinary, including not only the dermatologist but also the ophthalmologist.

REFERENCES

Akpek EK, Merchant A, Pinar V, et al: Ocular rosacea: patient characteristics and follow-up. Ophthalmology 104:1863–1867, 1997.

Alvarenga LS, Mannis MJ: Ocular rosacea. Ocul Surf 3(1):41–58, 2005.

Brown SI, Shahinian J, Jr: Diagnosis and treatment of ocular rosacea. Ophthalmology 85:779–786, 1978.

Browning DJ, Proia AD: Ocular rosacea. Surv Ophthalmol 31:145–158, 1986.

Frucht-Pery J, Chayet AS, Feldman ST, et al: The effect of doxycycline on ocular rosacea. Am J Ophthalmol 107:434–436, 1989.

Frucht-Pery J, Sagi E, Hemo I, et al: Efficacy of doxycycline and tetracycline in ocular rosacea. Am J Ophthalmol 116:88–92, 1993.

Ghanem VC, Mehra N, Wong S, et al: The prevalence of ocular signs in acne rosacea: comparing patients from ophthalmology and dermatology clinics. Cornea 22(3):230–233, 2003.

Macsai MS, Mannis MJ, Huntley AC: Acne rosacea. In: Mannis MJ, Macsai MS, Huntley AC, eds. Eye and skin disease. Philadelphia, Lippincott-Raven, 1996:335–341.

Quaterman MJ, Johnson DW, Abele DC, et al: Ocular rosacea: signs, symptoms, and tear studies before and after treatment with doxycyline. Arch Dermatol 133:49–54, 1997.

Sneddon IB: A clinical trial of tetracycline in acne rosacea. Br J Dermatol 78:649–652, 1966.

Wilkin J, Dahl M, Detmar M, et al: Standard grading system for rosacea: report of the national rosacea society expert committee on the classification and staging of rosacea. J Am Acad Dermatol 50(6):907–912, 2004.

87 PSORIASIS 696.1

Rubén Queiro, MD
Oviedo-Asturias, Spain
Juan J Barbón, MD
Avilés-Asturias, Spain
Daniel de la Mano, MD
Avilés-Asturias, Spain

ETIOLOGY/INCIDENCE

Psoriasis is a chronic skin disorder characterized by excessive proliferation of the epidermis. Epidermal cells in psoriatic patches have lost regulatory control and exhibit accelerated growth. It can begin at any age but most commonly arises in the third decade. It is more common in white people and its prevalence is similar in both sexes. Psoriasis affects 1% to 2% of general population, and 7% to 40% of these patients develop arthritis as the main systemic complication. Most patients have minimal disease, but 15% have severe generalized disease. Psoriasis typically lasts for life, and infections, psychological distress, trauma, and some therapies are common causes of exacerbation. The etiology is unknown, but genetical and immunological factors are relevant in the etiopathogenesis.

DIAGNOSIS

Clinical signs and symptoms

Systemic

- Characterized by sharply demarcated , geographically shaped, erythematous patches of skin covered with coarse, dry, silvery scales.
- When hyperkeratotic scales are removed, small blood droplets develop within seconds (Auspitz's sign).
- Scalp, nails, elbows, knees, extensor surfaces of the extremities, and sacral region most commonly affected.

Ocular

- Affects about 10% of patients with psoriasis.
- Lids:
  - May develop plaques.
  - Lid margins can be affected by scaling, with trichiasis and madarosis in severe cases.
  - An obstructive type of meibomian gland dysfunction has been described in psoriatic patients.
- Conjunctiva:
  - Nonspecific conjunctivitis.
  - Yellow plaque-like lesions.
  - Limbal phlyctenule-like lesions.
- Cornea:
  - Superficial and deep opacities.
  - Vascularization, infiltration, and melting can occur, especially peripherally.
  - Usually corneal involvement when there is active lid disease.
- Uveitis:
- The risk of uveitis is about 7% to 18%, especially in those affected by advanced spondylitis.
- Uveal inflammation may be anterior, posterior, and sometimes bilateral.

TREATMENT

Systemic

Systemic treatment is undertaken in coordination with a dermatologist, and in cases of psoriatic arthritis with a rheumatologist.

Local

Topical treatment

- Corticosteroids (most commonly fluorinated preparations such as halcinonide, fluocinonide, betamethasone, and triamcinolone) twice daily.
- Coal tar (2% to 5%) or tar derivate, with subsequent exposure to ultraviolet (UV) B light (Goeckerman regimen).
- Anthralin derivates (0.1% to 0.8%) with salicylic acid in a paste or ointment form and used in combination with tar and UV therapy (Ingram regimen).
- Waterproof adhesive dressings left in place for at least 1 week.
- Phototherapy through presensitization with psoralens and exposure to UVA light (320 to 400 nm).
- Intralesional injections of corticosteroids, such as 5 mg/mL triamcinolone.
- In severe cases, methotrexate 7.5 to 25 mg/week or cyclosporin A (CsA) 2.5 to 5 mg/kg/day.
- Oral retinoids, particularly in association with UV therapy.

Ocular

- Topical corticosteroids for lid lesions, conjunctivitis, and uveitis.
- Adhesive dressings and detergent scrubs may be also used for skin lesions.
- Topical tar, anthralin derivates, and UV therapy probably not appropriate for lid lesions.
- Corneal melting: lubrication, bandage contact lenses, tarsorrhaphy, and treatment of systemic disease; high doses of oral corticosteroids (1 to 2 mg/kg of prednisone or equivalent) and oral CsA appear to provide systemic relief most rapidly, but corticosteroids are not recommended because of the high doses necessary and the severe exacerbations that often occur after esteroids are stopped. Corneal involvement can be slow to respond and can result in vascularization and scarring.
- Severe cases of uveitis may need systemic corticosteroids and immunosupresants such as CsA, azathioprine, alfa-interferon or anti-TNF therapies.

COMPLICATIONS

Retinoids have been reported to cause dry eyes, blepharitis, corneal opacities, cataracts, and decreased night vision.

Conjunctival hyperemia, decreased lacrimation, and cataract have been described with psoralens and UVA, but the relationship is unclear. The use of adequate UV-blocking sunglasses after treatment is recommended.

Methotrexate-treated patients may show reduced full-field electroretinogram and decreased vision.

REFERENCES

Catsarou-Catsari A, Katambus A, Tkheodorpoulos P, et al: Ophthalmological manifestations in patients with psoriasis. Acta Derm Venereol (Stock) 64:557–559, 1984.

Cram DL: Corneal melting in psoriasis. J Am Acad Dermatol 5:617, 1981.

Eustace P, Pierse D: Ocular psoriasis. Br J Ophthalmol 54:810–813, 1970.

McClure SL, Valentine J, Gordon KB: Comparative tolerability of systemic treatments for plaque-type psoriasis. Drug Saf 25:913–927, 2002.

Ponjavic V, Granse L, Stigmar EB, et al: Reduced full-field electroretinogram (ERG) in a patient treated with methotrexate. Acta Ophthalmol Scand 82:96–99, 2004.

Queiro R, Torre JC, Belzunegui J, et al: Clinical features and predictive factors in psoriatic arthritis-related uveitis. Semin Arthritis Rheum 31:264–270, 2002.

See JA, Weller P: Ocular complications of PUVA therapy. Aust J Dermatol 34:1–4, 1993.

Zengin N, Tol H, Balevi S, et al: Tear film and meibomian gland functions in psoriasis. Acta Ophthalmol Scand 74:358–360, 1996.

88 URTICARIA AND HEREDITARY ANGIOEDEMA 708.9
(Angioneurotic Edema, Giant Edema, Giant Urticaria, Hives, Nettle Rash, Quincke's Disease)

Mitchell H. Friedlaender, MD
La Jolla, California

ETIOLOGY/INCIDENCE

Urticaria is a cutaneous eruption with multiple pathogenic mechanisms that may be immunologic or nonimmunologic. Its prevalence in the general population is estimated to be between 10% and 25%. No specific cause can be found in 50% of patients with chronic urticaria; in others, psychogenic, allergic and physical factors may play a role. The pathogenesis of urticaria is poorly understood. It is associated with uncontrolled mast cell degranulation and the release of mediators. Hereditary angioedema is an inherited deficiency of C1-esterase inhibitor.

Hereditary angioedema (HAE) is an autosomal dominant disease, and characterized by repeated attacks of epithelial edema involving the skin, respiratory tract, and gastrointestinal tract. Repeated episodes of angioedema involving the skin and respiratory tract may lead to death from pharyngeal edema and asphyxiation.

DIAGNOSIS

Clinical signs and symptoms

Erythematous, elevated, multiple, pruritic skin lesions may be localized or widespread. Hereditary angioedema is characterized by repeated attacks of epithelial edema involving the skin, respiratory tract and gastrointestinal tract. Pharyngeal edema may be life threatening. Abdominal attacks may mimic intra-abdominal crises.

TREATMENT

Systemic

- Antihistamines for urticaria or angioedema.
- β-Adrenergic drugs.
- Systemic corticosteroids.
- Cyclosporin A.
- Antifibrinolytic agents for hereditary angioedema (aminocaproic acid or tranexamic acid).
- Anabolic steroids and impeded androgens and fresh frozen plasma.
- C1 esterase inhibitor concentrate (for HAE).

Local

Subcutaneous injection or application of cotton pads soaked in 1 : 1000 epinephrine may be useful to treat severe conjunctival edema.

Surgical

If orbital edema develops to such an extent that the globe or optic nerve is threatened, relief from pressure should be provided. This may involve decompression of the lateral orbital wall. Surgery is rarely necessary.

SUMMARY

Urticaria has numerous causes, and its pathogenesis is poorly understood. Basically, it is associated with uncontrolled mast cell degranulation and release of mediators. Therapy is designed to prevent mast cell release or inhibit the mediators of inflammation.

Hereditary angioedema is an inherited deficiency of C1-esterase inhibitor and represents a chronic condition that is life threatening. Patients must be counseled intensively and emergency therapy must be available to them.

REFERENCES

Bielory L, Noble KG, Frohman LP: Urticarial vasculitis and visual loss. J Allergy Clin Immunol 88:819–821, 1991.

Bowen T, Cicardi M: Canadian 2003 international consensus algorithm for the diagnosis, therapy, and management of hereditary angioedema. J Allergy Clin Immunol 114:629–637, 2004.

Fay A, Abinun M: Current management of hereditary antio-oedema (C'1 esterase inhibitor deficiency). J Clin Pathol 55:266–270, 2002.

Friedlaender MH: Allergy and immunology of the eye. New York, Raven, 1993:85–86.

Kaplan AP: Chronic urticaria and angioedema. N Engl J Med 346:175–179, 2002.

Kaplan AP: Chronic urticaria: pathogenesis and treatment. J Allergy Clin Immunol 114:465–474, 2004.

Kozel MMA, Bossuyt PMM, Mekkes JR, Bos JD: Laboratory tests and identified diagnoses in patients with physical and chronic urticaria and angioedema: a systematic review. J Am Acad Dermatol 48:409–416, 2003.

Mathews KP: Urticaria and allergic conjunctivitis. Curr Opin Immunol 2:535–541, 1990.

Nzeako UC, Frigas E, Tremaine WJ: Hereditary angioedema: a broad review for clinicians. Arch Intern Med 161:2417–2429, 2001.

SECTION

9 Connective Tissue Disorders

89 AMYLOIDOSIS 277.3

Steven P. Dunn, MD
Southfield, Michigan
Jay H. Krachmer, MD
Minneapolis, Minnesota

ETIOLOGY/INCIDENCE

Amyloidosis is a disease complex that results in the accumulation of an amorphous, insoluble, fibrillar protein or aberrantly folded and assembled protein fragments in a variety of tissues. It is readily identified pathologically with polarizing light microscopy by it's characteristic apple-green birefringence after Congo red staining.

In recent years, the study of amyloid fibrils has led to the classification of amyloid on the basis of the biochemical composition of its subunit proteins. More than 25 fibrillar proteins have now been identified as precursor proteins in amyloidosis. The Nomenclature Committee of Amyloidosis has revised the classification scheme such that all forms are designated by 'A' + a suffix that denotes the precursor protein.

Most forms of amyloidosis can be categorized as localized or systemic forms. The two major types of systemic amyloidosis are AL (primary amyloidosis or myeloma-associated amyloidosis) and AA (secondary or reactive amyloid). AL results from deposition of terminal fragments of immunoglobulin kappa or lambda light chains: AA is associated with the acute phase reactant serum amyloid A (SAA) as the precursor protein.

The reported incidence of systemic AL amyloidosis is 1/100,000 persons in Western countries. AA amyloidosis, related to familial Mediterranean fever has a definite ethnic predilection among Sephardic Jews, Armenians, Turks and Arabs having a higher incidence. An increased incidence is seen in patients with tuberculosis, leprosy, anklylosing spondylitis, rheumatoid arthritis and Crohn's disease. Senile amyloidosis is thought to occur in almost all individuals over the age of 85.

Six types of primary familial amyloidosis have now been described, and they appear to be related most frequently to an abnormality in transthyretin (prealbumin); however, mutations of apolipoprotein A-I, gelsolin, fibrinogen A and lysozyme are also seen. Amyloid deposits resulting from these conditions are usually associated with an autosomal dominant form of inheritance. These forms of amyloidosis are seen in greater frequency among patients originating from Portugal, northern Sweden, Japan, Iceland and Finland.

DIAGNOSIS

Clinical signs and symptoms

Multisystem involvement is characteristic of primary systemic amyloidosis. Progressive peripheral polyneuropathy, cardiomyopathy, and gastrointestinal and skin involvement are seen most frequently. The eye may be involved in a number of ways; linear and veil-like vitreous opacities associated with slowly progressive visual loss, however, are virtually diagnostic of this disease. Discrete, bilateral, yellow-white, xanthoma-like subconjunctival nodules, occasionally with petechiae and hemorrhage, may be the initial findings. Involvement of the lacrimal and parotid glands may produce dryness of the eyes and mouth. Proptosis and external ophthalmoplegia have been attributed to amyloid deposits in the extraocular muscles. Pupillary abnormalities are thought to be due to amyloid neuropathy, or possibly secondary to deposits in the iris sphincter and dilator muscles. Neurotrophic keratitis and glaucoma may also be seen.

Localized, primary amyloidosis may also affect the eye in the form of small pink-red nodules in the lids or conjunctiva. This form of the disease is usually bilateral and affects young adults in their 20s and 30s. A number of forms of primary corneal amyloidosis exist. The most commonly recognized is lattice corneal dystrophy, which has now been broken down into three subtypes based on inheritance pattern and clinical findings.

Type I lattice corneal dystrophy is the classic form; it is autosomal dominant and presents with central, anterior, and midstromal lattice lines and dots and stromal haze. It is not associated with any systemic disorders and typically presents in patients between the ages of 10 and 40. A variant, Avellino dystrophy, has clinical and histologic features of both lattice and granular dystrophies. A mutation in the transforming growth factor beta-induced (*TGFBI*) gene on chromosome 5q31 is responsible for these conditions.

Type II lattice corneal dystrophy, also known as Meretoja syndrome, is also autosomal dominant. It is actually a manifestation of a form of primary systemic amyloidosis known as Finnish hereditary amyloidosis. It is generally associated with blepharochalasis, bilateral facial nerve palsies, and peripheral neuropathy. Clinically, both peripheral and central lattice lines are found in the anterior stroma. Occasionally, conjunctival and adnexal deposits of amyloid may be seen. Recently, molecular genetics research has isolated a point mutation on the gelsolin gene in patients with clinical findings quite similar to those seen in Finnish hereditary amyloidosis.

Type III lattice corneal dystrophy typically presents in an older age group and is thought to be a recessive disorder characterized by markedly thickened lattice-like lines involving the anterior stroma centrally and paracentrally. On occasion, lattice lines may extend out to the periphery. This condition is not associated with any systemic abnormality.

Primary gelatinous drop-like keratopathy (GDLD) is a rare amyloid disorder seen most commonly in individuals of Japanese ancestry. The inheritance pattern is thought to be autosomal recessive with a low degree of penetrance. Clinical findings consist primarily of numerous small to moderate-sized subepithelial gelatinous excrescences that give the corneal surface a 'mulberry' or 'toad skin' appearance. Patients with this disorder tend to present before the age of 20 with symptoms of photophobia, lacrimation, redness, and foreign body sensation. No systemic disorders are associated with this condition. As yet, the precise type of amyloid in gelatinous drop-like keratopathy has not been elucidated. The altered gene responsible for GDLD is *M1S1* which is located on the short arm of chromosome 1.

A variety of chronic systemic disorders may be accompanied by secondary systemic amyloidosis. Deposits are found chiefly in the spleen, kidney, and liver. Occasionally, the eyelid may be involved.

Localized secondary amyloidosis may present as clinically detectable deposits in the lids, conjunctiva, and cornea. Clinically unrecognizable microdeposits of amyloid have been found in association with such conditions as basal cell carcinoma of the lid margin, conjunctival intraepithelial neoplasia, and conjunctival sarcoidosis. Microdeposits within the cornea have been seen with retinopathy of prematurity, phlyctenular keratoconjunctivitis, trachoma, trichiasis, keratoconus, and penetrating ocular trauma. Polymorphic amyloid degeneration, a condition typically seen in older patients without a history of ocular disease, is probably a form of primary localized amyloidosis.

Laboratory findings

Corneal lesions have a characteristic clinical appearance, but most other lesions require pathologic evaluation for a definitive diagnosis. Histopathologic features crucial to the diagnosis of amyloidosis include:

- Distinctive fibrillar ultrastructure;
- Staining of pathologic specimens with Congo red;
- Apple-green birefringence under polarized light.

Differential diagnosis

- Orbital tumors.
- Conjunctival sarcoidosis.
- Epibulbar rheumatoid nodulosis.
- Foreign body granuloma.
- Conjunctival lymphoid infiltrates (lymphomas, MALTomas).
- Multiple myeloma and cryoglobulin corneal deposits.

TREATMENT

Systemic

- All patients in this group require a thorough evaluation that includes the search for an underlying cause of the amyloidosis (i.e. inflammatory or neoplastic).
- Because some amyloid fibrils have an immunologic origin, therapeutic trials using melphalon, prednisone, colchicines or a combination of these have been tried.
- Chemotherapy with the iodinated anthracycline 4′-iodo-4′ deoxydoxorubicin has also demonstrated some clinical benefit in patients with immunocyte-derived (AL) amyloidosis.
- The observation that transthyretin is synthesized predominantly by the liver has led to liver transplantation or combined liver-kidney transplantation as therapy for this disease (familial amyloid polyneuropathy).

Local

- Localized disease is usually managed surgically; excision is performed for diagnostic as well as therapeutic reasons.
- The disease, however, has a strong tendency to recur.
- Reduced vision commonly leads to penetrating keratoplasty by the fourth or fifth decade in patients with lattice dystrophy.
- Keratoplasty may also be helpful in patients with gelatinous drop-like dystrophy and diffuse familial amyloidosis.
- Polymorphic amyloid degeneration does not usually require therapy.
- Total vitrectomy appears to be the treatment of choice for amyloid patients with dense vitreous opacities that interfere with vision.

PRECAUTIONS

There is a high incidence of recurrent amyloid deposition following surgery. This is particularly important when cosmetic surgery is planned. Regrafting or repeat vitrectomy is an option available to the patient with recurrent corneal and vitreal amyloidosis and visual deterioration.

COMMENTS

Localized amyloid deposits are by far the most common form of ocular amyloidosis. In some cases, amyloid deposits involving the eye may actually be an early localized manifestation of a generalized amyloidosis. This is particularly true with eyelid and vitreal amyloid deposits. The possibility that these deposits may be associated with an underlying disease process or immunologic abnormalities must always be considered.

REFERENCES

Brunt EM, Tiniakos DG: Metabolic storage diseases: amyloidosis. Clin Liver Disease 8:915–930, 2004.

Doughman DJ: Ocular amyloidosis. Surv Ophthalmol 13:133–142, 1969.

Falk RH, Comenzo RL, Skinner M, et al: The systemic amyloidoses. N Engl J Med 337:898, 1997.

Gorevic PD, Muroz PE, Gorgone G, et al: Amyloidosis due to a mutation of the gelsolin gene in an American family with lattice corneal dystrophy, type II. N Engl J Med 325:1780–1785, 1991.

Henderson JW: Orbital tumors. Philadelphia, WB Saunders, 1973: 602–608.

Hitchings RA, Tripathi RC: Vitreous opacities in primary amyloid disease: a clinical, histochemical, and ultrastructural report. Br J Ophthalmol 60:41–54, 1976.

Knowles DM II: Amyloidosis of the orbit and adnexae. Surv Ophthalmol 19:367–384, 1975.

Mannis MJ, Krachmer JH, Rodrigues MM, et al: Polymorphic amyloid degeneration of the cornea: A clinical and histopathologic study. Arch Ophthalmol 99:1217–1223, 1981.

Meretoja J: Familial systemic paramyloidosis with lattice dystrophy of the cornea, progressive cranial neuropathy, skin changes and various internal systems: a progressive, unrecognized, heritable syndrome. Ann Clin Res 1:310–312A, 1969.

90 BEHÇET DISEASE 136.1

Ilknur Tugal-Tutkun, MD
Istanbul, Turkey

ETIOLOGY/INCIDENCE

Behçet disease is a multisystem inflammatory disorder of unknown etiology. Although it has a worldwide distribution, it is more prevalent in the Mediterranean area, the Middle East and the Far East. Behçet disease is closely associated with HLA-B51 in endemic areas. Microbial antigens have long been proposed as the triggering factors. An antigen-driven specific inflammatory response superimposed on enhanced innate immune functions is implicated in the pathogenesis of vascular endothelial dysfunction and occlusive vasculitis.

COURSE/PROGNOSIS

Age of onset is usually around the end of the third decade. The frequency of ocular involvement is 50–70%. The disease has a relapsing remitting course. Male patients have a younger age of onset, more severe disease and a higher risk of visual loss compared to female patients. The risk of visual loss at 10 years has been estimated to be 30% in males and 17% in females. However, visual prognosis has improved in the last decade due to an earlier and more aggressive use of immunosuppressive therapy. Furthermore, a trend to milder disease and better visual outcomes has been reported from Japan. Mortality is associated with severe neurological, intestinal and cardiovascular involvement.

DIAGNOSIS

Clinical signs and symptoms

The diagnosis of Behçet disease is clinical. Systemic manifestations include recurrent oral and genital ulcers, skin lesions, arthritis, thrombophlebitis, arterial aneurysms, intestinal ulcers and neuropsychiatric symptoms. The typical form of ocular involvement is bilateral nongranuomatous panuveitis and retinal vasculitis. Explosive uveitis attacks and spontaneous remissions mark the disease course. Ocular findings include cells and flare in the anterior chamber, hypopyon, diffuse vitritis, retinal vasculitis, retinitis, retinal hemorrhages, retinal vein occlusions, macular edema, papilledema, papillitis, and rarely conjunctival ulcers, episcleritis, scleritis and keratitis.

Laboratory findings

There are no laboratory findings specific for Behçet disease. HLA-B51 positivity may help to support a clinical diagnosis. Patients may have skin hyperreactivity, i.e. a positive pathergy test, defined as >2 mm erythema occurring 48 hours after a skin prick by a sterile needle. Patients may have leukocytosis, high erythrocyte sedimentation rates and high C-reactive protein levels during active disease.

Differential diagnosis

HLA-B27-associated uveitis, sarcoidosis, syphilis, viral retinitis and endophthalmitis.

TREATMENT

Ocular

In patients with only anterior uveitis topical corticosteroids and mydriatic agents are used.

Local corticosteroid injections, including intravitreal injection of triamcinolone acetonide may be required for the treatment of severe panuveitis attacks and/or cystoid macular edema.

Systemic

Corticosteroids are used for the treatment of uveitis attacks. Long-term immunosuppressive therapy is required in order to prevent recurrences in patients with posterior segment involvement. Colchicine does not have a proven effect on eye disease. Azathioprine (2 mg/kg/day) and cyclosporin A (5 mg/kg/day) have been found to be effective in controlled trials. Combination of cyclosporin A with antimetabolites is more effective than monotherapy. Ciclosporine is best avoided in patients with neuro-Behçet due to its potential neurotoxicity. Tacrolimus (FK506) (0.10–0.15 mg/kg/day) has an immunologic activity and side-effect profile similar to cyclosporin A. Alkylating agents (cyclophosphamide and chlorambucil) have been reserved for cases refractory to initial treatment with cyclosporin A and antimetabolites. Encouraging results have been recently reported on the use of new biologic agents, including interferon alfa and anti-TNF alfa monoclonal antibody, infliximab, in patients with uveitis resistant to conventional agents. Interferon alfa-2α is administered as monotherapy at an initial dose of 6 million units per day subcutaneously. The response rate has been reported to be 94%. Infliximab infusions (5 mg/kg) are usually given at 8-week intervals following a loading dose. In open trials, it has been shown to have a rapid antiinflammatory effect and reduce the frequency of uveitis attacks.

COMPLICATIONS

Cataract, posterior synechiae, secondary glaucoma, maculopathy, optic atrophy, retinal atrophy and scarring, disc or retinal neovascularizations, retinal detachment and phthisis.

COMMENTS

The etiopathogenesis of Behçet disease has not been elucidated yet. There are individual variations in disease course and severity. There is no single therapeutic regimen uniformly effective in all patients with Behçet disease.

REFERENCES

Kötter I, Gunaydin I, Zierhut M, et al: The use of interferon alfa in Behçet disease: review of the literature. Semin Arthritis Rheum 33:320–335, 2004.

Ohno S, Nakamura S, Hori S, et al: Efficacy, safety, and pharmacokinetics of multiple administration of infliximab in Behçet's disease with refractory uveoretinitis. J Rheumatol 31:1362–1368, 2004.

Okada AA: Drug therapy in Behçet's disease. Ocul Immunol Inflamm 8:85–91, 2000.

Sfikakis PP, Kaklamanis PH, Elezoglou A, et al: Infliximab for recurrent, sight-threatening ocular inflammation in Adamantiades-Behçet disease. Ann Intern Med 140:404–406, 2004.

Tugal-Tutkun I, Onal S, Altan-Yaycioglu R, et al: Uveitis in Behçet disease: an analysis of 880 patients. Am J Ophthalmol 138:373–380, 2004.

Verity DH, Wallace GR, Vaughan RW, et al: Behçet's disease: from Hippocrates to the third millennium. Br J Ophthalmol 87:1175–1183, 2003.

Yoshida A, Kawashima H, Motoyama Y, et al: Comparison of patients with Behçet's disease in the 1980s and 1990s. Ophthalmology 111:810–815, 2004.

91 COGAN SYNDROME 370.52

Rex M. McCallum, MD
Durham, North Carolina

ETIOLOGY/INCIDENCE

Cogan syndrome is a rare clinical entity of unknown etiology and unknown incidence first described by David Cogan, MD, in 1945. It occurs primarily in young adults and has an average age of onset of 28.6 in 47 patients evaluated at the National Institutes of Health and Duke University Medical Center.

COURSE/PROGNOSIS

The primary ocular manifestation, interstitial keratitis, is either acute and recurrent or chronic. It may vary in intensity from day to day and from eye to eye. In the acute stages, conjunctival hyperemia and patchy white infiltrates of the subepithelium are noted more often than deep or midcorneal stroma. Corneal infiltrates are more prominent at the periphery. Epithelial defects can be seen. In the later stages, corneal vascularization and opacity may be noted, typically at the corneal periphery. Posterior uveitis and other forms of ocular inflammation are rarely found.

Ocular outcome is excellent, with only 6% of patients having a visual acuity greater than 20/30 in either or both eyes. Auditory outcome, however, is less good; permanent loss of hearing occurs commonly, depending on use of oral corticosteroids. In patients *not* treated with oral corticosteroids, 17% had an auditory threshold of <60 db, whereas 81% of patients who were treated with oral corticosteroids had an auditory threshold of <60db. The primary systemic complication is the development of aortitis or large-vessel (Takayasu-like) vasculitis or both in 10% to 12% of patients.

DIAGNOSIS

Clinical signs and symptoms

The syndrome is characterized by inflammatory eye disease, typically nonsyphilitic interstitial keratitis, and vestibuloauditory dysfunction, typically Ménière-like disease. Presenting ocular complaints are ocular discomfort (90%), redness (79%) and photophobia (68%). Ocular examination reveals interstitial keratitis in 72%, conjunctivitis in 34%, iritis in 32%, and episcleritis/scleritis in 28%. The presenting vestibuloauditory symptoms are vertigo (85%), sudden hearing loss (79%), sudden nausea and vomiting (70%), tinnitus (53%), ataxia (45%) and gradual decrease in hearing (17%). Vestibuloauditory features include Ménière-like symptoms with hearing loss in 92%, nystagmus in 32%, oscillopsia in 15%, Ménière -like symptoms without hearing loss in 4%, and hearing loss in only 4%. Ocular symptoms and signs develop first in 50% of patients, vestibuloauditory complaints develop first in 25% of patients and both occur within 1 month of each other in 25% of patients. In 50% of patients, an antecedent upper respiratory illness has occurred.

Laboratory findings

- Leukocytosis in 75%:
  - Neutrophilia in 50%;
  - Mild eosinophilia in 17%.
- Relative lymphopenia in 25%.
- Anemia in 33%.
- Thrombocytosis in 30%.
- Erythrocyte sedimentation rate (ESR) of >20 in 75%.
- Rheumatoid factor ≤1 : 80 in 10%.
- Elevated cerebrospinal fluid protein or white blood cell count or both in 25% of patients studied.
- Audiogram almost always abnormal:
  - Most pronounced at the extreme frequencies;
  - Relative sparing of the midrange frequencies.
- Short-increment sensitivity index testing and brain stem auditory evoked potential studies suggest cochlear disease.
- Caloric testing is abnormal to absent in 96% of patients.

Differential diagnosis

- Infections:
  - Syphilis, congenital or acquired;
  - Lyme disease;
  - *Chlamydia*;
  - Virus.
- Vasculitis:
  - Polyarteritis nodosa;
  - Wegener granulomatosis;
  - Temporal arteritis;
  - Takayasu arteritis.
- Rheumatic diseases:
  - Rheumatoid arthritis;
  - Relapsing polychondritis;
  - Behçet disease.
- Toxins:
  - 3-Methyl-1-pentyn-3-yl acid phthalate (Whipcide);
  - Cobalt;
  - Desferioxamine.
- Others:
  - Sarcoidosis;
  - Vogt–Koyanagi–Harada syndrome;
  - Ménière disease with eye inflammation.

TREATMENT

Systemic

- Systemic corticosteroids are rarely necessary to control the symptoms and signs of acute interstitial keratitis, but they may be appropriate for the rare patient with posterior ocular inflammation associated with Cogan syndrome.
- Systemic corticosteroids are immediately indicated in the treatment of hearing loss associated with Cogan syndrome. Hearing loss may respond by showing significant improvement.
- An initial trial of daily oral corticosteroid at a dose of 1 to 2 mg/kg/day of prednisone-equivalent therapy is instituted.

This can be started in divided doses for 3 to 5 days in severely symptomatic patients, with subsequent consolidation to a single daily morning dose.

- If hearing improves, then the patient should undergo a taper to a qd regimen over 4 to 6 days followed by a tapering of corticosteroids over the subsequent 6 to 8 weeks, while clinical status is being monitored.
- Clinical parameters such as auditory symptoms, ESR, ocular inflammatory disease and audiogram establish the efficacy of therapy.
- If no response is noted in 2 to 3 weeks, the patient should be rapidly tapered off corticosteroids and a trial of other immunosuppressive therapy, such as methotrexate, azathioprine, cyclosporin A, or cyclophosphamide, should be considered. The effectiveness of immunosuppressive treatment has never been established.
- Immunosuppressive therapy is effective for 'steroid sparing' in some patients whose hearing loss responds to corticosteroid therapy but who cannot be tapered to an acceptably low dosage or who suffer unacceptable side effects from steroids.
- Salt restriction, diuretic therapy, or both may be effective in the treatment of hearing fluctuation secondary to cochlear hydrops. Diuretics commonly used are hydrochlorothiazide and chlorthalidone.

Ocular

- Topical 1% mydriatic solution or ointment is appropriate for the management of acute anterior uveitis.
- Topical corticosteroids, such as 1% prednisolone applied every 1 to 2 hours during the acute stages of inflammation and then tapered after appropriate response, are indicated for the control of corneal and ocular inflammation.
- Between flares of interstitial keratitis, no topical ophthalmic therapy is necessary.

Surgical

- The most common indication for ocular surgery is the development of cataracts that interfere with visual acuity. Cataracts may require interventions at an early stage secondary to the deafness commonly present and the resulting need to lip-read and use sign language.
- Cochlear implants have been used successfully in deaf patients with Cogan syndrome.
- Aortic valve replacement should be considered in patients with hemodynamically significant aortic insufficiency. Aortitis can make this technically challenging, and the cardiovascular surgeon should be made to understand the inflammatory nature of the problem. Ideally, the operation should occur after a period of treatment that is deemed effective.
- Vascular bypass procedures may be indicated to prevent ischemic tissue damage. Operating at a time of active inflammation can complicate such procedures; therefore, if possible, surgery should be postponed until effective treatment has been established.

Other

- Patients with progressive hearing loss should be strongly encouraged to learn lip-reading and sign language.
- Patients should be educated about the symptoms and signs of large-vessel inflammatory disease (e.g. limb claudication, pulse changes, new aortic insufficiency murmur and different blood pressure in each arm) and taught to seek medical attention if these signs and symptoms occur.

COMPLICATIONS

Corticosteroids are potentially dangerous medications, so patients must be closely supervised and given individualized dosages in accordance with the severity of the Cogan syndrome, the therapeutic response, the side effects evident (if any), and the anticipated duration of therapy. Corticosteroids should be given as a single morning dose except for a few days when starting therapy or in the case of an active inflammatory exacerbation of the disease. The lowest possible dose that controls the specific manifestation or manifestations being treated should be sought and used for the shortest amount of time possible. Alternate-day regimens can commonly provide therapeutic benefit while minimizing significant side effects. Tapering of corticosteroids should be performed gradually and cautiously while monitoring the clinical parameters of disease activity. The side effects of systemic corticosteroids are numerous and potentially serious, and they occur commonly in patients receiving prolonged therapy. Side effects include osteoporosis, susceptibility to infections, weight gain, rounded facies, cataracts, increased intraocular pressure, proximal muscle weakness, easy bruisability, striae and psychosis. Given the potential for side effects, trials of corticosteroid therapy should be administered only when therapeutic goals, therapeutic endpoints and criteria for monitoring have been established at the onset of the trial. The best indicators for corticosteroid therapy are hearing loss and the development of inflammatory vascular complications.

The most common side effects of hydrochlorothiazide and chlorthalidone are volume and potassium depletion. Potassium replacement therapy may be necessary. Unusual side effects of these drugs include leukopenia, allergic problems and rashes.

Cyclosporine is a potent immunosuppressive agent that profoundly inhibits normal T cell activation and function, in part through effects on interleukin-2. The primary clinically significant toxic manifestations of cyclosporin A are renal dysfunction and hypertension. Therefore, careful monitoring of both blood pressure and renal function is necessary. Baseline serum creatinine should be established prior to the institution of therapy, with monthly monitoring to follow. Serum creatinine should not be allowed to rise more than 30% above the baseline. If this occurs, the cyclosporin A dose should be decreased by 50 mg/day, and repeat monitoring should be undertaken in 2 weeks. The usual starting dose of cyclosporin A is 2.5 to 5.0 mg/kg/day in two equally divided doses 12 hours apart. Doses of ≤5.0 mg/kg/day and trough levels of ≤400 mg/mL may be associated with less renal dysfunction. Other potential cyclosporine side effects include hirsutism, infection, tremulousness, hypomagnesemia, hepatic dysfunction, nausea and lymphoreticular neoplasm.

Cyclophosphamide, an alkylating agent, is also a potent immunosuppressive drug. Potential side effects include bone marrow suppression, hemorrhagic cystitis, bladder cancer, nausea, infection (particularly herpetic), gonadal dysfunction, pulmonary and hepatic reactions, and lymphoreticular neoplasm. The drug is usually given each morning with breakfast and forced intake of 1 to 2 L of fluid between breakfast and lunch to minimize the risk of bladder irritation. Initial doses are 2 mg/kg/day unless severe inflammatory vascular disease is present; in that case, doses can begin at 4 mg/kg/day with careful monitoring. Blood counts are monitored every 1 to 2 weeks initially and drug doses are adjusted to keep the white blood cell count in the range of 3500 to 4000 cells/mm^3 with an absolute neutrophil count of ≥1000 cells/mm. Use of cyclophosphamide beyond 1 to 1$^1/_2$ years of continuous therapy should be undertaken only with the utmost care.

COMMENTS

Inflammatory vascular complications occur in 10% to 12% of patients. Periodic monitoring for signs and symptoms of systemic vasculitis is essential. This should include carefully palpating all pulses and listening for the murmur of aortic insufficiency. Periodic two-dimensional echocardiographic monitoring of the aortic valve could be considered.

If aortitis with aortic insufficiency or large-vessel (vasculitis-like Takayasu syndrome) develops, treatment should be instituted with prednisone at 1 to 2 mg/kg/day and immunosuppressive therapy. Cyclophosphamide at 2 mg/kg/day with appropriate monitoring of the white blood cell count has been used for aortitis. Cyclosporin A at 5 mg/kg/day with appropriate monitoring of blood pressure and renal function is chosen for large-vessel vasculitis. If one form of immunosuppressive therapy proves ineffective, the other should be tried. Prednisone is tapered to every-other-day therapy after 4 to 6 weeks, with subsequent tapering off corticosteroid in 2 to 3 months. Prolonged remissions of both aortitis and large-vessel vasculitis have been established by the judicious use of the above treatment protocols in patients with the inflammatory vascular complications of Cogan syndrome.

SUPPORT GROUPS

Cogan's Contact Network is a national network, founded in 1989, dedicated to the mutual support and sharing of experiences and strategies for persons with Cogan's syndrome. The network's aim is to help people understand Cogan's syndrome. Write to YUPPA/Cogan's Contact, P.O. Box 145, Freehold, NJ 07728-0145, call 732-761-9809 Anthony TDD/FAX, or E-MAIL: uscogans@juno.com.

REFERENCES

Allen NB, Cox CC, Cobo M, et al: Use of immunosuppressive agents in the treatment of severe ocular and vascular manifestations of Cogan's syndrome. Am J Med 88:296–301, 1990.

Cobo LM, Haynes BF: Early corneal findings in Cogan's syndrome. Ophthalmology 91:903–907, 1984.

Cogan DG: Syndrome of nonsyphilitic interstitial keratitis and vestibuloauditory symptoms. Arch Ophthalmol 33:144–149, 1945.

McCallum RM, Allen NB, Cobo CM, et al: Cogan's syndrome: clinical features and outcomes. Arthritis Rheum 35:S51, 1992.

McCallum RM, St Clair EW, Haynes BF: Cogan's syndrome. In: Hoffman GS, Weyland C, eds: Inflammatory diseases of blood vessels. New York, Marcel Dekker, 2001.

92 PSEUDOXANTHOMA ELASTICUM 757.39 (Grönblad–Strandberg Syndrome)

F. Hampton Roy, MD, FACS
Little Rock, Arkansas

ETIOLOGY/INCIDENCE

Pseudoxanthoma elasticum (PXE) is an inherited systemic disease characterized by changes in the elastic tissue of the skin. This disease is characterized by redundant folds of soft, wrinkled and lax skin typically located on the neck, lower abdomen, or perineum and in the flexures of the arms, the popliteal fossae, and the axillary and groin areas. Degeneration and calcium deposition occur in the elastic tissue of the skin, eyes, or cardiovascular system. In the eyes it can be associated with angioid streaks, choroidal neovascular membranes, macular hemorrhage and loss of central vision.

There are two autosomal dominant and two recessive forms of the disease; most patients have the autosomal recessive type. It usually appears by age 30, although it may appear in childhood or in old age. The rate of occurrence is 1 in 100,000 and the ratio of female to male incidence is 2.3 : 1.

DIAGNOSIS

Clinical signs and symptoms

Skin

- Xanthomatous eruptions, yellow, 1 to 3 mm, plucked-chicken appearance.
- Sagging skin folds of neck, axillae and groin.

Ocular

- Retina:
  - Angioid streaks, bilateral, radiating from the disk;
  - Choroidal neovascular membrane;
  - Hemorrhagic maculopathy and scar, central blindness;
  - Vitreous hemorrhage;
  - Retinal mottling or peau d'orange.
- Other:
  - Exophthalmos (orbital hematoma);
  - Optic disk drusen;
  - Optic atrophy, visual field defects, paralysis of extraocular muscles (secondary to vascular lesions of central nervous system).

Cardiovascular and other

- Hypertension, premature atherosclerosis, coronary insufficiency, angina pectoris, mitral valve prolapse, arterial insufficiency in the extremities, dilation of the aorta, vascular aneurysms and gastrointestinal or cerebral hemorrhages.

Laboratory findings

- Characteristic skin and retinal findings.
- Fluorescein angiography to detect early angioid streaks and choroidal neovascular membranes.

Differential diagnosis
- Skin: Marfan syndrome, Ehlers–Danlos syndrome, cutis laxa and epidermolysis bullosa.
- Eye (angioid streaks): Paget disease and hemoglobinopathies, calcium and phosphorus abnormalities, and connective tissue disorders such as Ehlers–Danlos syndrome.

PROPHYLAXIS

- Avoidance of minor head and eye trauma.
- Avoidance of heavy lifting and straining.
- Safety glasses.
- Genetic counseling.

TREATMENT

Systemic
- Treatment of hypertension.
- Arteriography for management of ischemic symptoms.
- Plastic surgery for skin changes.

Ocular
- Argon or krypton laser photocoagulation of choroidal neovascular membranes; prophylactic treatment of angioid streaks should be avoided because it may induce choroidal neovascular membranes.
- Low-vision aids.

Other
- Coordination among subspecialists.

COMPLICATIONS

- Eye: macular hemorrhage and loss of central vision.
- Cardiovascular and other: coronary artery insufficiency, arrhythmias and sudden death; gastrointestinal bleeding (may be precipitated by nasogastric tube), increased anesthesia risk.

COMMENTS

Patients with angioid streaks are at high risk, with many patients experiencing eventual deterioration of vision to 20/200 or worse.

REFERENCES

Albert DM, et al: Pseudoxanthoma elasticum (PXE)-angioid streaks/systemic associations. In: Principles and practice of ophthalmology clinical practice. Philadelphia: WB Saunders; 1994.

Brancato R, Menchini U, Pece A, et al: Laser treatment of macular subretinal neovascularization in angioid streaks. Ophthalmologica 195:84–87, 1987.

Gelisken O: A long-term follow-up study of laser coagulation of neovascular membranes in angioid streaks. Am J Ophthalmol 105:299–303, 1988.

Krechel SLW, Ramirez-Inawat RC, Fabian LW: Anesthetic considerations in pseudoxanthoma elasticum. Anesth Analg 60:344–347, 1981.

Neldner KH: Pseudoxanthoma elasticum. Int J Dermatol 27:98–100, 1988.

93 RELAPSING POLYCHONDRITIS 733.99

Peter G. Watson, MD, MBBChir, FRCS, FRCOphth, DO
Cambridge, England

Inflammation of cartilaginous structures occur throughout the body in relapsing polychondritis. The most commonly affected tissues are the nose, with collapse of the tip, and the ear which becomes swollen and tender. The sclera (especially the posterior sclera) the eustachian tubes, larynx, trachea, bronchi and costochondral cartilages are frequently involved. The laryngeal and tracheal cartilages may collapse causing death from bronchial obstruction. Migratory oligo- or poly-arthritis is commonly the presenting feature and is usually progressive but non-deforming and non-erosive. Other features include a seronegative arthropathy, intraocular inflammation, inner ear involvement, skin lesions, aortitis and fever.

ETIOLOGY/INCIDENCE

Relapsing polychondritis has all the characteristics of an autoimmune connective tissue disorder, directed at the collagen of cartilage. In the early stages of the disease all classes of glycosamino-glycans are lost from the interstitial tissue. Susceptibility to the condition is significantly associated with HLA-DR4 ($P < 001$). The extent of organ involvement is negatively associated with HLA-DR6. Antibodies to type II collagen have been found.

COURSE/PROGNOSIS

The onset is usually acute with fever and polyarthritis affecting wrists, ankles, hands and feet. Ocular complications usually follow within 2 to 3 months. Untreated, this disease is usually fatal because of the eventual collapse of the laryngeal and tracheal cartilage. Even adequately treated, the prognosis is uncertain. The 5- and 10-year survival rates are 74% and 55%, respectively, with death due mainly to infection, vasculitis, malignancy, and the complications of therapy. A patient under 50 years old with anaemia, deformity of the nose and systemic vasculitis has a poor prognosis.

Ocular involvement occurs in 50% to 65% of patients. Anterior and posterior scleritis and episcleritis are the most common ocular findings.

DIAGNOSIS

Clinical signs and symptoms
To diagnose relapsing polychondritis, three or more of the following symptoms should be present:
- Non-erosive inflammatory polyarthritis;
- Recurrent chondritis of both auricles;
- Chondritis of the nasal cartilage;
- Inflammation of ocular structures;
- Laryngo-tracheal chondritis;
- Vestibular or cochlear inflammation.

Ocular

- Episcleritis;
- Anterior scleritis and destructive peripheral keratitis that may lead to perforation of the cornea;
- Sclero-kerato-uveitis can occur with severe intractable secondary glaucoma;
- Posterior scleritis producing choroidal folds, loss of vision, optic neuropathy and exudative retinal detachment.

Laboratory findings

There are no specific serologic markers for relapsing polychondritis. Careful radiological evaluation of major airways and joints is of paramount importance. This may be supplemented by computed tomography and magnetic resonance imaging scans, as necessary.

Histology of affected tissue shows inflammation and a non specific vasculitis with immunoglobulin and immune complex deposition.

Differential diagnosis

Wegener's granulomatosis and systemic vasculitis are differential diagnoses. The nasal saddle deformity of Wegener granulomatosis affects the bone, not the cartilage. The antinuclear cytoplasmic autoantibody (ANCA) tests can be used for differentiation.

TREATMENT

Relapsing polychondritis is notoriously difficult to treat. Aggressive treatment even in the apparently benign early stages of the disease is essential. Multiple therapies are often required to obtain adequate suppression of the inflammation of the sclera, cartilage and other connective tissue.

Systemic

On diagnosis, particularly in patients with severe disease and those with acute onset, intravenous methylprednisolone should be used. Initially, 500 mg is given over a period of 1 hour; this may have to be repeated on two or more occasions during the subsequent days or weeks, depending on the clinical response. Prednisolone 80 mg orally, reduced rapidly to 10 mg, should be given from the start of treatment. If this fails to control the condition or if there is evidence of a raised level of circulating immune complexes, 500 mg IV cyclophosphamide will probably induce a remission of the disease. A second dose may have to be given intravenously after a week, and all therapy may have to be continued orally. Patients on cyclophosphamide must be well hydrated, so if the drug is given by intravenous infusion, it should be followed for 24 hours with intravenous fluids. Most patients can be maintained on low doses of oral steroids alone, (<12.5 mg prednisolone per day) although some will require the addition of an immunosuppressive drug, such as cyclophosphamide, methotrexate, or azathioprine. Colchicine and non steroidal anti-inflammatory drugs can be used for some patients in remission.

Recurrences should be treated in a similar fashion to the initial attack. This is particularly effective if given within 24 hours of the recurrence.

In those cases resistant to conventional immunosuppressive therapy biological response modifiers should be used, anti TNF alpha (infliximab) or etanecept. These are given parenterally with a loading dose (infliximab 3–5 mgm/kg at 0.2 weeks) or subcutaneously (etanercept) twice weekly. These agents may be used alone or with another disease modifying agent (DMARD)

Ocular

Topical ophthalmic corticosteroids alone will not suppress the inflammation but are occasionally helpful when the cornea is involved and for recurrent ocular problems when the systemic disease is quiescent. Prednisolone eyedrops or ointment may be applied on an hourly basis for acute episodes and then tapered. Synaechiae formation needs to be prevented if uveitis occurs.

Surgical

Elective surgical procedures for *any* condition should be avoided if at all possible and should be undertaken only during periods of remission and under immunosuppression. These patients tolerate anaesthesia very poorly, have laryngeal and tracheal disease, so active and expert anesthetic care is essential.

Supportive

Any sign of respiratory distress with tracheal inflammation should be observed closely and treated early by intubation. If perichondrial inflammatory masses narrow the airway, surgical removal of the masses and reconstruction of the airway may be indicated.

As collapse of the nasal cartilage or development of nasal-tip deformity usually worsens after surgery, cosmetic surgery is not recommended. In extreme cases of cardiovascular involvement, valvular replacement with prosthetic valves or aortic aneurysm resection may become necessary symptomatic treatment.

COMMENTS

Relapsing polychondritis should be considered not only in patients presenting with scleral disease but also in those who develop diffuse joint disease. When the diagnosis has been established, immunosuppressive therapy should be started as early as possible. However, it must be remembered that corticosteroids stop neither the disease's progression in the more aggressive cases nor the development of potentially lethal organ system involvement. There is some evidence that cyclophosphamide may induce a prolonged remission. The use of subconjunctival corticosteroids must be avoided, as diseased sclera may melt at the site of the injection.

Although relapsing polychondritis is more commonly a chronic, low-grade, episodic disease, it may be a fulminant disease with a rapid downhill course. The critical organ system involved in relapsing polychondritis is the respiratory tract. However, death from ruptured abdominal aneurysms and progressive heart failure secondary to aortic regurgitation, have also occurred. Because of the variation in severity and the episodic nature of the disease, careful and prolonged follow-up and individualised therapy are the keys to optimal treatment. Aggressive therapy is necessary during an acute attack.

REFERENCES

Buckner JH, Van Landeghen M, Kwok WW, et al: Identification of type II collagen peptide 261–273-specific T clones in a patient with relapsing polychondritis. Arthritis Rheum. 46(1):238–244, 2002.

Damian JM, Levine HL: Relapsing polychondritis and the anaesthetist. Anaesthesia 43:573–577, 1988.

Harada M, Yoshida H, Mimura Y, et al: Relapsing polychondritis associated with subclinical Sjogren's syndrome and phlegmon of the neck. Int Med 34:768–771, 1995.

Hoangh-Xuan T, Foster CS, Rice BA: Scleritis in relapsing polychondritis: response to therapy. Ophthalmology 97:892, 1990.

Hughes RA, Berry CL, Seirfert M, et al: Relapsing polychondritis. Three cases with clinicopathological study, and literature review. Quart J Med 41:363–380, 1972.

Kraus VB, Stabler T, Le ET, Saltarelli M, et al: Urinary type II collagen neopitope as an outcome measure f relapsing polychondritis. Arthritis Rheum 48(10):2942–2948, 2003.

Magargal LE, Donoso LA, Goldberg RE, et al: Ocular manifestations of relapsing polychondritis. Retina 1(2):96–99, 1981.

McAdam LP, O'Hanlan MA, Bluestone R, et al: Relapsing polychondritis: prospective study of 23 patients and a review of the literature. Medicine 55:193–215, 1976.

McKay DAR, Watson PG, Lyne AJ: Relapsing polychondritis and eye disease. Br J Ophthalmol 58:600–605, 1974.

Michet CJ, Gabriel SE, Beard CM, et al: Relapsing polychondritis: survival and predictive role of early disease manifestations. Ann Intern Med 104:74–78, 1986.

Richez C, Dumoulin C, Coutouly X, et al: Successful treatment of relapsing polychondritis with infliximab. Clin Exp Rheumatol 22(5):629–631, 2004.

Zeuner M, Straub RH, Rauh G, et al: Relapsing polychondritis: clinical and immunogenetic analysis of 62 patients. J Rheumatol 24:96–101, 1997.

94 RHEUMATOID ARTHRITIS 714.0

Sibel Kadayifçilar, MD
Ankara, Turkey

ETIOLOGY/INCIDENCE

Rheumatoid arthritis is a systemic inflammatory disease affecting 1–3% of the population. Persistent synovial inflammation leading to joint deformities via cartilage and bone destruction is the characteristic feature. The onset of the disease is usually in the fourth and fifth decades of life with a predilection for women. There is evidence to implicate autoimmune mechanisms in the pathogenesis of the disease. Family studies indicate a genetic predisposition. HLA-DR4 and related alleles are found to be major genetic risk factors.

COURSE/PROGNOSIS

The clinical course can be quite variable, from mild oligoarticular involvement to progressive, polyarticular and systemic disease. Most patients experience persistent but fluctuating disease activity accompanied by a variable degree of joint deformity.

DIAGNOSIS

Clinical signs and symptoms

Articular

All joints may be involved, but mainly the proximal interphalangeal joints of the hands and feet; the metacarpophalangeal joints; the metatarsophalangeal joints; the wrists, ankles, knees, hips and shoulders; and the temporomandibular joints are affected. The arthritis is usually symmetric. Initial articular manifestations may be poorly localized but include pain, tenderness, swelling and limitation of movement. Morning stiffness lasting more than 1 hour is a key feature in the diagnosis. Persistent inflammation leads to certain characteristic hand deformities: radial deviation of the wrist and ulnar deviation of the digits (Z-deformity) and hyperextension of the proximal interphalangeal joints and flexion of the distal interphalangeal joints (swan neck deformity). Deformities of the feet and knees can cause severe pain and prominent difficulty in walking.

Extra-articular

The extra-articular manifestations of rheumatoid arthritis are sometimes more prominent than the articular disease. Fever, weakness, fatigability, anorexia and weight loss may often be the presenting signs and symptoms. Rheumatoid nodules, mostly asymptomatic, are seen in 20 to 30% of patients. Vasculitis in rheumatoid arthritis can result in cutaneous ulceration, digital gangrene, peripheral neuropathy, myocardial infarction, and involvement of the lungs, bowel, liver, spleen and pancreas and, if severe, can be fatal. Usually asymptomatic pulmonary involvement includes pleuritis, interstitial fibrosis, or nodular infiltration. Pericarditis and myocarditis can occur but are often evident only at autopsy. Hematological manifestations include anemia, lymphoid hyperplasia, and Felty syndrome, characterized by lymphadenopathy and hypersplenism, resulting in neutropenia and less commonly in anemia and thrombocytopenia.

Ocular

Keratoconjunctivitis sicca is the most common ophthalmic manifestation of rheumatoid arthritis, with a reported prevalence of 15–25%. However, autopsy specimens of nearly all rheumatoid arthritis patients disclosed lymphocytic infiltration of the salivary glands as in Sjögren syndrome.

Corneal manifestations include filamentary keratitis, marginal furrowing or limbal guttering, sterile central ulceration, microbial keratitis, peripheral ulcerative keratitis, sclerosing keratitis, stromal keratitis and keratolysis.

Episcleritis and scleritis are classically described in patients with rheumatoid arthritis. Patients with episcleritis usually complain of discomfort rather than pain. Scleritis in rheumatoid arthritis is associated with a graver prognosis with regard to ocular complications and associated extra-articular findings when compared with episcleritis. Anterior scleritis is the most common form and generally responds well to therapy, but may be complicated by corneal involvement, glaucoma, exudative choroiditis and iritis. Recurrent scleritis may result in thinning of the sclera (Figure 94.1). Painful necrotizing scleritis should be differentiated from the more benign scleromalacia perforans, which is characterized by severe thinning of the sclera in an otherwise clinically noninflamed, nonpainful eye. Inflammatory necrotizing scleritis is often associated with wide spread visceral involvement. Necrotizing scleritis and peripheral ulcerative keratitis in rheumatoid arthritis are associated with high mortality when not treated with systemic immunosuppression. Posterior scleritis may occur less commonly and may be associated with proptosis, limited extra-ocular movements, retinal detachment and optic disc edema. In rheumatoid arthritis iritis may occur secondary to scleritis or vasculitis.

Tendinitis of the sheath of the superior oblique muscle which may result in Brown syndrome, venous stasis retinopathy as a

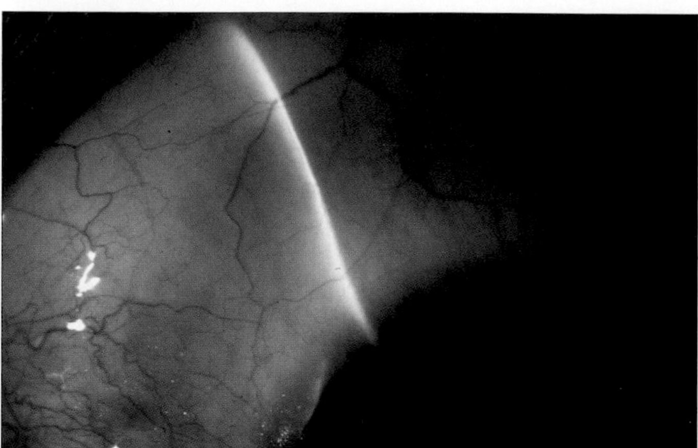

FIGURE 94.1. Thinning of the sclera in a case with recurrent scleritis.

result of polyclonal gammopathy, cranial nerve palsies, geniculocortical blindness and orbital apex syndrome due to orbital rheumatoid nodules have also been described in association with rheumatoid arthritis.

Laboratory findings

Approximately 80% of the patients are positive for rheumatoid factor, which is an IgM autoantibody directed against IgG. Rheumatoid factor is not useful in screening for rheumatoid arthritis, as it is also found in systemic lupus erythematosus, Sjögren syndrome, sarcoidosis, hepatitis B, tuberculosis and other various disorders, but can be used to confirm the diagnosis in patients with the appropriate clinical findings.

Elevated ESR, CRP levels and circulating immune complexes correlate with active systemic disease.

Evaluation of inflammatory synovial fluid and radiographic findings of juxta-articular bone demineralization and erosion of the affected joints support the diagnosis. Radiograms are employed to monitor the impact of therapy.

Patients with rheumatoid arthritis often have abnormal Schirmer tests and abnormal rose bengal staining of the conjunctiva.

Differential diagnosis

Other causes of arthritis such as other collagen vascular diseases, sarcoidosis, ankylosing spondylitis, Reiter syndrome, osteoarthritis, systemic-onset juvenile rheumatoid arthritis and gout should be considered in the differential diagnosis.

TREATMENT

Systemic

The therapeutic interventions are mostly palliative; aiming to relieve pain, reduce inflammation, stop or slow down joint damage and improve function. Exercise, periods of rest and physical therapy contribute to coping with rheumatoid arthritis.

Nonsteroidal anti-inflammatory drugs (NSAIDs)

The NSAIDs include aspirin, fenoprofen, ibuprofen, indometacin, naproxen, ketorolac, nabumetone, diclofenac, etodolac, meclofenamate, piroxicam, sulindac, tolmetin. These agents have analgesic, anti-inflammatory and antipyretic effect through blocking the activity of cyclooxygenase enzyme, hence the production of prostaglandins, prostacycline and thromboxanes. There are at least two isoforms of this enzyme. Recently developed COX-2 isoform inhibitors are found to have less gastrointestinal toxicity, but higher rate of myocardial infarctions for which one of them, rofecoxib has been withdrawn from the market. All NSAIDs appear to be equally effective, but the response of the individual patient may vary from one drug to another.

Disease modifying antirheumatic drugs (DMARDs)

Recent data have shown that early initiation of DMARDs can lead to significant improvement in disease and delay radiographic progression. These agents include methotrexate, leflunomide, sulfasalazine, hydroxychloroquine, D-penicillamine and gold (intramuscular or oral).

Injectable gold salts have been used in rheumatoid arthritis for more than 60 years. Aurothioglucose or gold sodium thiomalate up to 50 mg are injected IM weekly until a total dose of 1 g is reached. Then the medication is tapered to once every three to four weeks. Gold can also be taken orally as auranofin, at a dose of 3 mg b.i.d., but has not been found as efficient. The value of gold salts in rheumatoid arthritis is questioned recently. It does not work for all people and it may lose its effectiveness over time. Furthermore, it often takes three to six months to determine whether it is useful or not. Therefore, people beginning gold injections must continue other medications such as aspirin or NSAIDs. Urinalysis and complete blood count must be monitored frequently for potential toxicities including anemia, leukopenia, thrombocytopenia, rash, flushing, renal disease and deposition in cornea.

D-penicillamine is a slow-acting medication whose effect may not be seen until the forth month. Toxicity includes loss of taste, thrombocytopenia, nephrotic syndrome and a variety of immune-mediated side effects like optic neuropathy.

Since the mid-1980s methotrexate has become much more popular as a treatment for rheumatoid arthritis. It works more quickly than gold (2–3 weeks) and maintains control of the disease in a higher ratio over periods of five years or longer. Methotrexate is given weekly 7.5–30 mg orally or as an IM injection. Major toxicity includes gastrointestinal upset, oral ulceration, liver function abnormalities, hepatic fibrosis and pneumonitis.

The antimalarials, oral hydroxychloroqine 200 mg b.i.d.or chloroquine 250 mg qd do not have serious side effects except retinopathy with cumulative dose. The risk decreases if the daily dose does not exceed 6.5 mg/kg/day and may increase if therapy continues for more than 8 years. Major drawbacks are the late onset of benefit -as long as 3 months – and the response rate – 40%.

Sulfasalazine (2–3 g/day) is effective especially in recent onset disease.

Although corticosteroids are not considered traditional DMARDs, new data indicate that they actually do suppress the inflammatory and erosive course of rheumatoid arthritis. Low-dose (<7.5 mg/day) prednisone has been advocated as an additive therapy to control symptoms. However, the side effects preclude long term use alone for disease control.

Combination therapy rather than monotherapy with DMARDs is gaining popularity. Methotrexate, sulfasalazine, hydroxychloroquine and prednisolone combination has been demonstrated to be more beneficial in patients with early rheumatoid arthritis.

Immunosuppressive therapy

Immunosuppressant drugs azathioprine, cyclosporin A and cyclophosphamide have been shown to be effective in rheumatoid arthritis treatment with similar therapeutic effects to those of the DMARDs. Because of toxicity, they have been reserved for DMARD failure and extra-articular disease like rheumatoid vasculitis or necrotizing scleritis.

Biologic response modulators

These new and exciting agents include inhibitors of tumor necrosis factor (TNF) alpha (infliximab, etanercept, adalimumab) and interleukin -1 (anakinra). They have been shown to slow the rate of radiographic progression. In contrast to rapid action of anti-TNF therapy, the effect of anakinra is slower. Side effects include increased risk of serious opportunistic infections like tuberculosis.

Ocular

Symptomatic therapy for keratoconjunctivitis sicca is not different from that of primary Sjögren syndrome, i.e. artificial tears, acetylcysteine, punctal occlusion, slow-release inserts, topical cyclosporin A and occasionally tarsorraphy.

Simple diffuse scleritis associated with rheumatoid arthritis is treated with oral NSAIDs. In case of no response or recurrence, DMARDs like methotrexate or immunosuppressives need to be introduced. Alkylating immunosuppressive agents, such as cyclophosphamide in combination with methotrexate, are the treatment of choice in necrotizing scleritis.

Surgical

Surgery plays a role in the management of patients with severely damaged joints.

COMPLICATIONS

Major ocular complications due to medications are as follows:

- Gold: chrysiasis;
- Antimalarials: pigmentary retinopathy and/or corneal opacities;
- NSAIDs: reversible blurring of vision;
- Corticosteroids: posterior subcapsular cataracts and/or glaucoma.

COMMENTS

Rheumatoid arthritis is a disease characterized by usually symmetric inflammation of the peripheral joints, potentially resulting in progressive destruction of the articular structures. Extra-articular manifestations are frequently seen especially in patients with high rheumatoid factor titres. The rheumatoid process involves the eye in less than 1% of the patients in the form of episcleritis or scleritis but the prevalence of keratoconjunctivitis sicca is much higher. Treatment for scleritis in rheumatoid arthritis should include therapy for the systemic disease. During ocular examination of patients with rheumatoid arthritis, ocular toxicities of the systemic medications should also be kept in mind.

SUPPORT GROUPS

Web sites of some support groups:
www.arthritis.ca
www.arthritis.org
www.arthritissupport.com
www.rheumatoid.org.uk

REFERENCES

Foster CS, Forstot SL, Wilson LA: Mortality rate in rheumatoid arthritis patients developing necrotizing scleritis or peripheral ulcerative keratitis: effects of systemic immunosuppression. Ophthalmology 91:1253–1262, 1984.

Kwoh CK, Anderson LG, Greene JM, et al: Guidelines for the management of rheumatoid arthritis: 2002 update. Arthritis Rheum 46:328–346, 2002.

Lipsky PE, van der Heijde DM, St Clair EW, et al: Infliximab and methotrexate in the treatment of rheumatoid arthritis. N Engl J Med 343:1594–1602, 2000.

Möttönen T, Hannonen P, Leirisalo-Repo M, et al: Comparison of combination therapy with single drug therapy in early rheumatoid arthritis: a randomized trial. FIN-RACo trial group. Lancet 353:1568–1573, 1999.

Watson PG, Hayreh SS: Scleritis and episcleritis. Br J Ophthalmol 60:163–191, 1976.

95 SARCOIDOSIS 135

Daniel H. Gold, MD, FRCOphth
Herzliya, Israel
Ernesto I. Segal, MD
Boca Raton, Florida

Sarcoidosis is a systemic inflammatory disease characterized by the development of noncaseating epitheliod cell granulomas in tissues and organs throughout the body. It may take an acute or chronic course and is often a benign self-limited disorder. Its clinical manifestations are protean and depend upon the specific site(s) of inflammation in any given patient. Intrathoracic involvement occurs in close to 90% of cases, with granulomas in the lungs or intrathoracic lymphoid tissue. Ocular involvement occurs in about 25% of cases and produces some of the most serious complications of this disorder.

ETIOLOGY AND INCIDENCE

Although its etiology is unknown, sarcoidosis is associated with several immunologic abnormalities. Compartamentalization' of the T cells has been proven by immunohistopathologic studies that have demonstrated a high ratio of T-helper to T-suppressor lymphocytes in the lungs, lymph nodes and eyes of patients with active sarcoidosis, with simultaneous reduction of this ratio in blood. Interleukin-2 produced by these activated T-helper cells (CD4) may attract other inflammatory cells, resulting in the subsequent development of a typical granuloma. They may also affect the humoral immune system by stimulating B-lymphocytes to produce a polyclonal increase in circulating immunoglobulins, as well as a variety of autoantibodies.

The antigenic stimulus for the T-cell activation and initiation of the immunological cascade as well as the environmental or host factors that contribute to limit the course of the disease, are unknown.

Sarcoidosis occurs in the United States with an overall incidence of 6 to 10 cases per 100,000. It is far more common among the black population. More than 25 % of the patients with sarcoidosis have ocular involvement.

COURSE AND PROGNOSIS

Sarcoidosis can affect virtually every organ and tissue in the body. Most commonly it involves the lungs, lymph nodes, eyes, liver and skin.

The most common ocular findings are: keratoconjunctivitis sicca, conjunctival granulomas and uveitis.

- Sarcoidosis can involve all the segments of the eye or ocular adnexal:
  - Periocular region: granulomatous infiltration of the eyelids, ptosis (secondary to paralysis of the third nerve), eyelid paralysis (secondary to seventh nerve palsy). Granulomatous infiltration of the orbits, extraocular muscles, third, fourth and sixth cranial nerves, causing proptosis, paralysis and diplopia.
  - Lacrimal system: lacrimal gland infiltration and enlargement. More rarely dacryoadenitis, dacryocistitis or lacrimal drainage system obstruction.
  - Conjuctiva: granulomas, non-specific conjunctivitis, and phyctenules.
  - Cornea: keratoconjunctivitis sicca, band keratopathy, hypesthesia, (secondary to fifth nerve palsy), interstitial keratitis, inferior corneal thickening, keratitic precipitates.
  - Sclera: episcleritis, scleritis, scleral thinning, anterior stafiloma.
  - Iris and anterior chamber: anterior acute or chronic granulomatous or non-granulomatous uveitis, with cell and flare, anterior or posterior synechiae, iris nodules (Koeppe and Busacca), iris mass.
  - Lens: cataracts
  - Ciliary body: intermediate uveitis (snowbank).
  - Vitreous: granulomas (snowball or string of pearls configuration, usually inferior), vitritis, vitreous hemorrhages.
  - Retina and choroid: retinal periphlebitis, hemorrhages, edema, neovascularization, pigmentary loss, clumping or mottling, retinal vein occlusions, superficial exudative 'candle-wax' lesions, cystoid macular edema and detachments. RPE detachments, AMPPE-like and birdshot chorioretinopathy-like syndromes. At the level of the choroid: granulomas, punched-out lesions, chorioretinal scarring and neovascular membranes.
  - Optic nerve: papillitis, retrobulbar or optic neuritis, granulomas at any level of the optic nerve, papilledema secondary to increased intracranial pressure, neovascularization, atrophy.
- Other characteristic presentations are:
  - Heerfordt syndrome: uveitis, parotid enlargement, fever and facial or other cranial nerve palsies.
  - Lofgren syndrome: erythema nodosum, bilateral hillar adenopathy, acute iritis and parotitis.
  - Another chronic sarcoid syndrome: chronic uveitis, cutaneous sarcoidosis, bone cysts and pulmonary fibrosis.
  - Several forms of pediatric ocular sarcoidosis.
- Ocular prognosis: the majority of the patients preserve their baseline visual acuity, approximately 11% developed legal blindness (many due to macular edema and glaucoma).

Diagnosis/laboratory findings

- The diagnosis is made on the basis of three main criteria: compatible clinical and radiologic evidence, histopathologic demonstration of noncaseating epitheliod-cell granulomas in affected tissues, and negative results of bacterial and fungal studies of tissues or body fluids.
- Radiologic tests: chest x-rays, chest and brain CT scans, brain MRI.
- Gallium 67 head, neck and chest scan : elevated take in granulomatous tissue.
- Elevated serum levels of: angiotensin-converting-enzyme (ACE), lysozyme, calcium, gamma-globulines.
- Bronchoalveolar lavage: with an increased number of T-lymphocytes and elevated T-helper/T-suppressor ratio.
- Tissue biopsies: from superficial or palpable lesions in skin, lymph nodes, conjunctiva, lacrimal gland, any mucosa, lung tissue.
- Tears analysis: elevated ACE concentration and ACE/protein ratio.
- Skin tests: positive Kveim–Siltzbach and non reactive PPD and other delayed hypersensitivity tests.

TREATMENT

Local

Treatment of anterior uveitis

- Topical steroids like 1% prednisolone eyedrops every 1–2 hours during waking hours with gradual tapering of the dose as the inflammation subsides.
- Topical nonsteroidal anti-inflammatory agents, such as: diclofenac sodium 0.1% or flurbiprofen sodium 0.03% t.i.d. can be added as adjunctive therapy to the steroids.
- Mydriatic or cycloplegic drops to avoid pain and development of synechiae: cylopentolate 1%, homatropine (2–5%) or atropine 1% b.i.d. to q.i.d.
- A combination of 2.5%–10% phenylephrine may be considered on an attempt to break pre-existent posterior sycnechiae.
- When anterior segment inflammation is very severe or does not respond quickly to topical medication, this treatment should be supplemented by anterior sub-Tenon steroid injection: 40 mg of methylprednisolone, 40 mg of triamcinolone, 24 mg of dexamethasone or 20 mg of betamethasone may be used.

Treatment of posterior segment disease

- Posterior sub-Tenon injection of the above mentioned steroids.
- The use of intravitreal triamcinole (4 mg/0.1 cc) might be considered in cases of severe, persistent or recurrent CME after sub-Tenon injections have failed.
- Indication for the use of systemic steroids.
- Intralesional steroid injection can be used for the treatment of sarcoidosis lesions of the eyelid skin.
- If glaucoma develops as a result of the disease or in response to the steroid therapy a change to fluorometholone drops should be considered.
- Control of the IOP can be achieved with antiglaucoma medication, such as: timolol or any other beta-blocker, latanoprost, dorzolamide, iopidine, brimonidine or oral acetazolamide.

Systemic

- May require consultation with other physicians.
- Systemic corticosteroid therapy is indicated for control of posterior segment inflammation, orbital disease, eyelid lesions, and the neuro-ophthalmologic complications of

sarcoidosis, or anterior segment inflammation that is not responsive to topical or periocular steroids.

- Treatment should begin with 60–80 mg (0.5–1.0 mg/kg/day) of prednisone daily (or equivalent doses of prednisolone or dexamethasone). The drugs may given in a single daily dose before breakfast or divided doses q.i.d. The dosage should be slowly tapered as the inflammation subsides. Alternate-day therapy with twice the usual daily dose may avoid some of the complications of prolonged systemic steroid therapy.
- In patients requiring treatment and in whom strong contraindications to the use of systemic steroids are present, who are resistant to steroid therapy, or who develop intolerable side effects to them, immunosuppressive therapy with cyclophosphamide, chlorambucil, azathioprine, methotrexate or ciclosporin may be of value, either alone or in combination with systemic steroids. The drugs are given orally in daily doses. They should be considered only under unusual circumstances and given in consultation with physicians thoroughly familiar with their use.
- Non-steroidal anti-inflammatory agents, such as oxyphenbutazone or indometacin, may be of value in selected patients with ocular or systemic inflammation but are not widely used.
- Oral chloroquine phosphate has been used in the treatment of cutaneous sarcoidosis, including eyelid lesions or as adjunctive therapy for extracutaneous systemic sarcoidosis and to control hypercalcemia and hypercalcinuria associated with this disease.

Surgical

May be required in the management of late complications.

- Cataract surgery with IOL implantation.
- Surgical or laser iridectomy in cases of pupillary block glaucoma.
- Filtering surgery with or without antimetabolites for uncontrolled secondary glaucoma. And seton valve implantation in severe cases.
- Cyclophotocoagulation or cyclocryotherapy should be used as a last resort in end stage uveitic glaucoma.
- Argon laser photocoagulation in cases of disc or retinal neovascularization, neovascular glaucoma and choroidal neovascular membranes.
- Pars plana vitrectomy may be required for non-clearing vitreous opacities, specially when patients are resistant or intolerant of corticosteroid therapy, for vitreous hemorrhages or traction retinal detachment.

Radiation treatment

- High-voltage radiation therapy has been used in the treatment of anterior visual pathways sarcoidosis in patients who are intolerant to systemic steroid treatment. Temporary beneficial response was seen and subsequent immunosuppressive therapy was necessary.

COMPLICATIONS

Complications of the disease

- Phtisis.
- Secondary glaucoma: due to peripheral anterior synechiae, posterior synechiae and iris bombe, infiltration of the trabecular meshwork or rubeosis.
- Visual field defects: due to granulomatous involvement of the visual pathways.

Complications of the treatment

- Adverse effects of the systemic steroids: heart failure, hypertension, diabetes mellitus, peptic-ulcerative disease, infections, myopathy, osteoporosis, psychiatric problems, adrenal insufficiency, Cushing syndrome.
- Ocular complications of both systemic and topical steroids: posterior subcapsular cataracts, elevated intraocular pressure. The use of intralesional corticosteroids for eyelid lesions may create some degree of skin atrophy. And central retinal artery occlusion has been reported as well
- Chloroquine can produce macular pigmentary changes progressing to bull's eye maculopathy with loss of central vision. Also corneal deposits and cornea verticillata have been found.

PRECAUTIONS

- The major complications of the treatment of sarcoidosis are related to the adverse effects of steroid therapy, these are better prevented and handled by the patients' internist or immunologist.
- When chloroquine is used, a baseline ophthalmologic exam with subsequent follow-up, including visual acuity testing, fundus exam and central visual field test with an Amsler grid should be performed. Fluorescein and ICG-angiography, fundus photos, color vision tests and electro-oculogram may be useful in the following of these patients.

OVERVIEW ON MANAGEMENT

- The ocular complications of sarcoidosis are part of a systemic disorder, and a coordination of effort between the ophthalmologist and other physician caring for the patient is essential. Almost all the patients with ocular sarcoidosis have evidence of active disease elsewhere in the body. Although there has been widespread debate in the medical literature as to when sarcoidosis should be treated, the presence of ocular inflammatory disease is almost universally accepted as an absolute indication for initiating therapy.
- Sarcoid inflammatory disease tends to be recurrent, especially as therapy is decreased or withdrawn. Both the patient and the treating physician must be aware of this pattern, and careful follow-up evaluations are essential.
- Patients should be encouraged to seek attention at the first sign of a change in their ocular status. At the same time, the physician must not 'overtreat' the disease. Many uveitis patients develop a chronic 'breakdown' in their blood-ocular barrier, with mild flare and an occasional cell in the anterior chamber, which does not need to be treated.
- Every patient with anterior segment sarcoidosis, should be carefully evaluated for posterior segment disease. Care must be taken to avoid a situation in which topical therapy is producing a satisfactory regression of anterior uveitis while leaving a serious, progressive posterior inflammatory process untouched. Also both eyes should be always carefully monitored.

REFERENCES

Ciulla TA, et al: Corticosteroids in posterior segment disease: an update on new delivery systems and new indications. Curr Opin Ophthalmol 15(3):211–220, 2004.

Dev S, et al: Methotrexate treatment for sarcoid-associated panuveitis. Ophthalmology 106(1):111–118, 1999.

Ieki Y, et al: Pars plana vitrectomy for vitreous opacity associated with ocular sarcoidosis resistant to medical treatment. Ocul Immunol Inflamm 12(1):35–43, 2004.

Khalatbari D, et al: Demographic-related variations in posterior segment ocular sarcoidosis. Ophthalmology 111(2):357–362, 2004.

Maca SM, et al: Semicircular tumor of the iris and uveitis as unilocal manifestation of sarcoidosis. Ocul Immunol Inflamm 12(3):237–240, 2004.

Machida S, et al: Choroidal circulatory disturbances in ocular sarcoidosis without the appearance of retinal lesions or loss of visual function. Jpn J Ophthalmol 48(4):392–396, 2004.

96 SCLERODERMA 710.1
(Systemic Sclerosis, Progressive Systemic Sclerosis)

Larry P. Frohman, MD
Newark, New Jersey

INTRODUCTION

Scleroderma also goes by the names systemic sclerosis or progressive systemic sclerosis. In the diffuse systemic form, numerous organ systems may be targeted, including skin, the vascular system, synovium, the gastrointestinal tract, as well as the cardiac, renal and pulmonary systems. Perhaps the most classical manifestations are the common appearance of taut, smooth skin and of Raynaud phenomenon.

There is an overlap between Sjögren syndrome and scleroderma, patients with secondary Sjögren syndrome may have scleroderma as the underlying cause.

Sjögren syndrome consists of xerophthalmia (dry eye) and dry mouth (xerostomia). It is felt to be due to a lymphocytic infiltration of the lacrimal and salivary glands.

ETIOLOGY/INCIDENCE

Whereas there is no racial predilection, there is a strong female preponderance, 80% of cases are female. The incidence is said to be 20 cases/1 million.

In the skin in scleroderma, there is an exuberant deposition of collagen, leading to dysfunction from thickening, tightness and contracture. The trigger is presumably cytokine-mediated. Jimenez has indicated that there is an overproduction of collagen due to alteration in the regulation of the alpha1 (I) collagen gene. Shi-Wen has implicated the gene that codes for human connective tissue growth factor.

Another line of thought postulates that altered arteriolar responses to vasoconstrictors may play a role. Chemicals, foods, and other agents have been reported as potential causative factors of scleroderma or a scleroderma-like illness. These include silica dust, silicone breast implants, cocaine, l-tryptopahn, and the toxic rapeseed oil syndrome in Spain in the early 1980s which affected about 20,000 people.

Box 96.1 – A classification of scleroderma

Systemic scleroderma (SS)

- Limited cutaneous SS
- Diffuse cutaneous SS
- Scleroderma sine scleroderma

Localized scleroderma

- Morphea
- Linear
- En coup de sabre

DIAGNOSIS

Clinical signs and symptoms

The signs and symptoms depend upon which form of scleroderma is present. One classification is seen in Box 96.1. In general, the localized forms do not get vasospasm, structural vascular damage, or internal organ involvement, and localized forms may have a dermatome distribution.

Systemic findings

Many organ systems may be involved in scleroderma. The skin is the most frequently affected. The lungs may be involved; early on there is an interstitial inflammatory response with fibrotic changes appearing later in the course. Cardiac involvements (clinically apparent in 20–25% of cases) may include myocardial, pericardial, conduction system disease, or arrhythmias. Gastrointestinal motility disorders are a hallmark of scleroderma, with the esophagus being most commonly involved (90%) with rectal dysmotilty seen in 50–70%. It is said that 60–80% may have chronic myopathy. Neurological involvement may take the form of cranial neuropathy (especially the trigeminal nerve) or of peripheral polyneuropathy and mononeuropathy multiplex, with the most common form being distal mononeuropathy of the median nerve, manifesting as carpal tunnel syndrome. Renal disease and arthritis are less common.

Local involvement is typically divided into:

- Localized (with isolated patches that resolve over years without sequelae);
- Generalized (also called Morphea, more widespread distribution of patches) and linear forms (like morphea, but with deeper involvement.) A particular type of linear form is called 'coup de sabre,' because of its resembling a saber wound. It involves the face and the skull.

Ocular findings

It is said that keratoconjunctivitis sicca occurs in 70% of cases Kirkham reported the incidence of decreased tear production as 50%.

In a series of 38 patients with scleroderma without renal involvement, findings included stiffness or tightness of the eyelids (29% of cases), telangectasia of the eyelids (10%), insufficient tear production (37%), conjunctival injection (50%) and conjunctival vascular sludging (71%). Many other changes were seen, but were felt to be either age-related or secondary to corticosteroid therapy (e.g. posterior subcapsular cataract). Recently, pellucid marginal degeneration has been reported in systemic scleroderma.

Yet, in another series of 21 patients with generalized scleroderma studied by ophthalmic exams, fundus photography, and fluorscein angiography, none had anterior segment abnormalities. Aside from one case of macular degeneration (felt to be unrelated), none had fundus abnormalities, although fluroscein angiography was abnormal in seven (33%). The findings were hyper fluorescence of the retinal pigment epithelium, or of the retina. It was presumed that the cause was a vascular insult to the choroid. Retinal vessels were not affected. This was similar to what was reported by Grennan, who found that the choroidal bed was involved in 5/10 (50%) of patients with scleroderma when studied with fluorescein angiography. They also found that 1/10 (10%) had an abnormality of the retinal vasculature. A case of serous detachment of the retinal pigment epithelium in a patient with scleroderma has been described by Egerer.

Ocular involvement may occur in the coup de sabre form of scleroderma, which may have orbital or intracerebral involvement. Ramboer has reported a patient with this form of scleroderma who presented with loss of lashes and narrowing of the palpebral fissure of one side, and then developed enophthalmos (presumably due to atrophy of the orbital fat) with entropion of the right lower lid. This lesion ultimately was demonstrated to grow into the orbital apex via MRI scan, and the patient ultimately lost sight on the involved side.

There may be an association between the coup de sabre form of scleroderma and Parry Romberg syndrome (progressive hemifacial atrophy).

Obermoser et al have recently reported a case where the orbital lesions were successfully treated with interferon gamma. In this case, there was an intracerebral enhancing cystic-gliotic mass. Upon biopsy, it demonstrated a perivascular B and T-cell infiltration.

A patient with linear scleroderma developed a coloboma of the upper lid, blepharoptosis, enophthalmos and ophthalmoplegia.

Another association with local ocular atrophy was reported by Stone and Scheie, who described two patients with scleroderma associated with a pigmentary abnormality of the anterior segment. This may feature heterochromia iridis, upper eyelid atrophy, blepharoptosis, pigmentary glaucoma and paresis of extraocular muscles.

Another similar case of scleroderma en coup de sabre with local atrophic changes of ocular tissue developed a spontaneous filtering bleb.

Ocular motility may be involved in scleroderma. In a series of 13 cases, one patient had motility disturbances. When pathology was obtained, it showed massive increases in interstitial collagen with muscular atrophy. The author stated that this was similar to the pathology of scleroderma in the myocardium. Scleroderma and a similar less severe entity, lichen sclerosis and atrophicus, can cause a Brown superior oblique tendon syndrome.

The CREST syndrome (*C*alcinosis, *R*aynaud phenomenon, *E*sophageal motility disorder, *S*clerodactyly, and *T*elangectasias) will only be briefly mentioned here. Ocular manifestations have included keratomalacia, uveitis, parafoveal telangectasia, and optic neuropathy.

Laboratory findings

The diagnosis of scleroderma relies upon laboratory studies and clinical evaluation, as no one sign or test may establish the diagnosis. Fifty percent of cases have hypergammaglobulinemia, and the ANA is elevated in 40–70%, typically with a speckled pattern.

Anticentromere antibodies are present in 55% of cases of the CREST syndrome, but are not specific for this diagnosis, and titers do not correlate with disease actvity.

Anti-scl 70 antibodies (anti-topoisomerase-I) are associated with the presence of severe gastrointestinal, heart and lung involvement.

In children with scleroderma, up to 55% have elevated rheumatoid factor or anti-ss DNA.

Although not useful in the diagnosis of early cases, where it tends to be normal, anti-endothelial cell antibody (AECA) may correlate with disease activity.

Another assay, soluble cytotoxic T-lymphocyte associated molecule-4 (sCTLA-4), is elevated in the diffuse cutaneous form of scleroderma, but not in the limited cutaneous form.

Skin biopsy will help establish the diagnosis.

Angiography may play a role. Stuckler reported that 27/29 (93%) of scleroderma cases had stenosis on digital subtraction angiography, primarily in the upper extermeties.

Junger states that nearly all with diffuse or limited systemic scleroderma present with Raynaud phenomenon. Morphologic or functional abnormalities in fingernail capillary bed circulation as evidenced by nail bed fluroscein studies are present in nearly all cases.

Differential diagnosis

- Rheumatoid arthritis.
- Systemic lupus erythematosus.
- Raynaud phenomenon.
- Eosinophilic fasciitis.
- Eosinomyalgic syndromes.
- Mixed connective tissue disease.

PROPHYLAXIS

Aside from avoidance of inciting agents, none available.

TREATMENT

Ocular

Systemic

Ciclosporin has been of some uses in treating scleroderma, with 50% having improvement in cutaneous manifestations and 25% having resolution of digital vasculitis. The combination of cyclophosphamide and prednisone may be of value. Tissue plasminogen factor has been reported to be of benefit. Recently, a stabilized prostacycleine, iloprost, has been beneficial in a case of systemic sclerosis.

As no drug therapy has been satisfactory for diffuse systemic sclerosis, work is being done on using other modes of therapy. Farge et al have reported on a European collaborative study of autonomous stem cell transplantation as a therapy of systemic sclerosis, with about $^2/_3$ of patients showing a beneficial reponse. Szucs has reported on the effects of plasmaphereis, which in a small series, slowed the progression of the disease.

COMPLICATIONS

Whereas scleroderma typically follows a course of relentless slow progression, death may ensue from involvement of several organ systems.

SUPPORT GROUPS

For a comprehensive listing, see http://www.sclero.org/support/swa/listings/support-united-states.html

REFERENCES*

Frohman LP: Systemic disease and neuro-ophthalmology: annual update 2000 (Part II). J Neuro-Ophthalmol 21(2):74–82, 2001.

Serup L, Serup J, Hagdrup H: Fundus fluorescein angiography in generalized scleroderma. Ophthalmic Research 19(5):303–308, 1987.

Wilson D, Edworthy SM, Hart DA, et al: The safety and efficacy of low-dose tissue plasminogen activator in the treatment of sclerosis. J Dermatol 22:637, 1995.

*Note that selected references only are shown for further reading.

97 SYSTEMIC LUPUS ERYTHEMATOSUS 710.1

André Barkhuizen, MD
Portland, Oregon
James Todd Rosenbaum, MD
Portland, Oregon

ETIOLOGY/INCIDENCE

Systemic lupus erythematosus (SLE) is an immunologically mediated disease of uncertain etiology that has the potential to affect virtually any organ system. SLE is much more common in females than in males. The prognosis depends largely on the organ system involved.

DIAGNOSIS

Clinical signs and symptoms

The American College of Rheumatology has suggested 11 classification criteria for SLE. Patients are considered to have lupus if they meet four of the following criteria and have no alternative diagnostic explanation for the abnormalities:

- Malar rash;
- Discoid rash;
- Photosensitive rash;
- Oral ulcers;
- Nonerosive arthritis in two or more joints;
- Pleuritis or pericarditis;
- Glomerulonephritis or proteinuria;
- Seizures or psychosis;
- Hemolytic anemia, leukopenia, lymphopenia, or thrombocytopenia;
- Immunologic laboratory abnormality, such as antibodies to double-stranded DNA or the SM antigen or a false-positive serologic test for syphilis;
- Positive antinuclear antibody test that is not caused by a medication.

Ocular or periocular

- Conjunctiva: conjunctivitis.
- Cornea: keratoconjunctivitis sicca, the most common ocular manifestation of SLE; peripheral corneal infiltrates; marginal corneal ulcer or keratolysis.

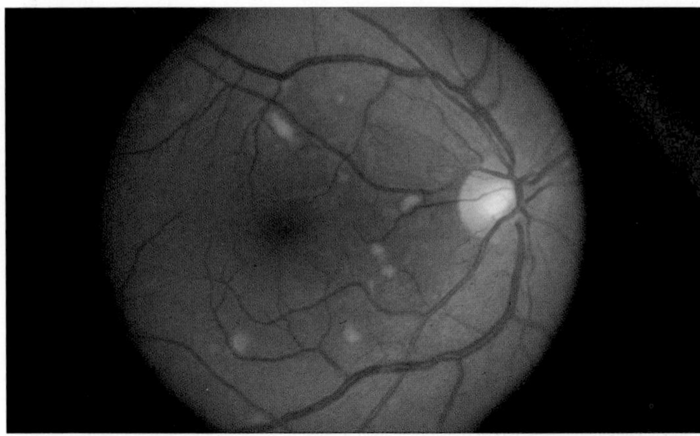

FIGURE 97.1. Fundus photograph demonstrates multiple cotton wool spots indicative of local retinal ischemia, a recognized association with systemic lupus.

- Eyelids: erythematous, hyperkeratotic rash; telangiectasia.
- Retina: cotton-wool spots (see Figure 97.1) or cytoid bodies, which occur in as many as 28% of patients with SLE and may correlate with disease of the central nervous system; retinal vasculitis; retinal vaso-occlusive disease including central or branch retinal artery or vein occlusions; secondary hypertensive retinopathy.
- Sclera: scleritis, episcleritis.
- Other: iritis; optic neuritis; changes secondary to central nervous system infarction, including cranial nerve palsies, homonymous hemianopsia, nystagmus and intranuclear ophthalmoplegia; papilledema may be present in association with pseudotumor cerebri.

Laboratory findings

In addition to criteria 10 and 11, as many as 50% to 60% of patients with SLE have antibodies to a phospholipid known as cardiolipin. These antibodies may prolong the partial thromboplastin time. Because of this laboratory property, antibodies to cardiolipin are sometimes referred to as the lupus anticoagulant, although they are rarely associated with clinical bleeding. In fact, paradoxically, antiphospholipid antibodies are frequently associated with thrombosis. Antibodies to the phospholipid may be responsible for false-positive serologic tests for syphilis. Antibodies to cardiolipin may be present without any manifestation of SLE or any other autoimmune disease.

Antibodies to cardiolipin are strongly associated with thrombosis, including deep venous thrombosis, pulmonary embolism, nonbacterial thrombotic endocarditis and central nervous system infarction. These antibodies may be causally related to spontaneous abortion. Antibodies to cardiolipin have been detected in association with an occlusive retinal vasculitis. The most severe complication caused by these antibodies which can be seen in SLE or in isolation, is the catastrophic antiphospholipid syndrome (CAPS), presenting with widespread thromboses and tissue ischemia. CAPS may be confused with a multisystem SLE flare.

TREATMENT

The treatment for SLE depends largely on the organ system that is involved and the severity of that involvement.

Systemic

- Arthritis and pleuropericarditis are generally improved by nonsteroidal anti-inflammatory drugs (NSAIDs), such as aspirin or indomethacin (75 to 200 mg qd).
- Antimalarials, including hydroxychloroquine (200 mg b.i.d.) or chloroquine (250 mg qd), are particularly effective for discoid rash and serositis.
- Anticoagulation drugs may be indicated for thrombosis secondary to antiphospholipid antibodies, which in the catastrophic antiphospholipid syndrome may need to be combined with plasmapheresis and/or immunosuppression.
- Immunosuppressive therapy is indicated for SLE when the disease involves a critical organ such as the kidney. For active lupus nephritis, monthly boluses of intravenous cyclophosphamide reduce the risk of end-stage renal failure. Intravenous cyclophosphamide is generally begun at 500 mg/m^2. The dose may be increased, depending largely on hematologic toxicity. Oral corticosteroids or intravenous methylprednisolone may be used to supplement cyclophosphamide. Intravenous cyclophosphamide is probably indicated to treat nonischemic optic neuritis in association with lupus. Corticosteroids alone are not as effective as cyclophosphamide for lupus-related renal disease. Other immunosuppressants such as daily oral azathioprine (1 to 2 mg/kg/day), daily oral mycophenolate mofetil (1000 to 1500 mg twice daily), daily oral cyclophosphamide (1 to 2 mg/kg/day), or weekly methotrexate (7.5 to 25 mg/wk) can be tried for patients who fail or who do not tolerate intravenous cyclophosphamide therapy. Pulse therapy with intravenous methylprednisolone and plasmapheresis are additional forms of immunosuppression that have been tried when more conventional therapy has not been efficacious. Sequential therapy with six months of pulsed intravenous cyclophosphamide followed by azathioprine or mycophenolate mofetil was as effective and less toxic than prolonged intravenous cyclophosphamide in proliferative lupus nephritis. A mild androgen, dehydroepiandrosterone (DHEA), was found to be slightly more effective than placebo for mild forms of lupus and many patients take it with modest symptomatic benefit.

(See Rheumatoid arthritis for additional discussion of therapy with NSAIDs, antimalarials and cytotoxics.)

Ocular

(See Sjögren's syndrome for discussion of the treatment for sicca.)

Topical

Dermatologic manifestations of lupus are usually treated by topical corticosteroid preparations, antimalarial drugs, or both.

PRECAUTIONS

(See Uveitis for a complete discussion of the adverse effects of corticosteroids.)

COMMENTS

SLE is a multisystem disease that may involve the eye. Although antinuclear antibodies are characteristic of this disease, a positive test for antinuclear antibodies does not establish a diagnosis in the absence of clinical findings.

The two most common ocular manifestations of SLE are dry eyes and cotton-wool spots.

Patients with lupus who experience retinal ischemic events have a greater likelihood of having central nervous system disease. The lupus anticoagulant or antiphospholipid antibodies such as those to cardiolipin may be causally related to some instances of retinal vascular occlusion. The treatment for retinal vasculitis may differ from the treatment of anticardiolipin-mediated retinal occlusive disease.

REFERENCES

Austin HA, Klippel JH, Balow JE, et al: Therapy of lupus nephritis: controlled trial of prednisone and cytotoxic drugs. N Engl J Med 314:614–619, 1986.

Boey ML, Colaco CB, Gharavi AE, et al: Thrombosis in systemic lupus erythematosus: striking association with the presence of circulating lupus anticoagulant. BMJ 287:1021–1023, 1983.

Contreras G, Pardo V, Leclercq B, et al: Sequential therapies for proliferative lupus nephritis. N Engl J Med 350:971–980, 2004.

Hochberg MC: Updating the American College of Rheumatology revised criteria for the classification of systemic lupus erythematosus. Arthritis Rheum 40:1725, 1997. Letter.

Jabs DA, Fine SL, Hochberg MC, et al: Severe retinal vaso-occlusive disease in systemic lupus erythematosus. Arch Ophthalmol 104:558–563, 1986.

Levine SR, Crofts JW, Lesser GR, et al: Visual symptoms associated with the presence of a lupus anticoagulant. Ophthalmology 95:686–692, 1988.

Petri MA, Lahita RG, Van Vollenhoven RF, et al: Effects of prasterone on corticosteroid requirements of women with systemic lupus erythematosus: a double-blind, randomized, placebo-controlled trial. Arthritis Rheum 46(7):1820–1829, 2002.

Reeves GEM: Update on the immunology, diagnosis and management of systemic lupus erythematosus. Intern Med J 34:338–347, 2004.

Rosenbaum JT, Simpson J, Neuwelt CM: Successful treatment of optic neuritis in association with systemic lupus erythematosus using intravenous cyclophosphamide. Br J Ophthalmol 81:130–132, 1997.

Stafford-Brady FJ, Urowitz MB, Gladman DD, Easterbrook M: Lupus retinopathy: patterns, associations, and prognosis. Arthritis Rheum, 31:1105–1110, 1988.

Van Vollenhoven RF, Engleman EG, McGuire JL: Dehydroepiandrosterone in systemic lupus erythematosus: results of a double-blind, placebo-controlled, randomized clinical trial. Arthritis Rheum 38:1826–1831, 1995.

98 GIANT CELL ARTERITIS 446.5
(Temporal Arteritis)

Sohan Singh Hayreh, MD, MS, PhD, DSc, FRCS(Edin), FRCS(Eng), FRCOphth

Iowa City, Iowa

Giant cell arteritis (GCA) is the prime medical emergency in ophthalmology because of its dreaded complication of visual loss in one or both eyes, which is preventable if these patients are diagnosed early and treated immediately and aggressively with systemic corticosteroids. This obviously raises two critical issues about management of GCA:

1. How can a definite diagnosis of GCA be quickly established? and
2. What is the proper treatment to prevent blindness?

ETIOLOGY/INCIDENCE

In GCA, the granulomatous inflammation produces marked narrowing of the lumen or thrombotic occlusion of medium-sized and larger arteries, with widespread arterial involvement in the body. From the ophthalmic perspective, it has a special predilection for posterior ciliary arteries, resulting in acute optic nerve head ischemia. The etiology of GCA is still unknown but there is evidence that it is an immunologic disorder. It is almost invariably a disease of persons aged 50 years and older, and its incidence increases with advancing age. It occurs about three times more often in women than men.

DIAGNOSIS

The key, crucial first step in management of GCA is early and accurate diagnosis to forestall the possibility of loss of vision. A patient with GCA presents to his/her physician with either systemic or ophthalmic manifestations of GCA, or both. Rheumatologists consider the criteria advocated by the American College of Rheumatologists as the 'gold standard' to diagnose GCA. According to that, a patient is considered to have GCA if at least 3 of the following 5 criteria are met:

1. Age ≥50 years;
2. New onset of localized headache;
3. Temporal artery tenderness or decreased temporal artery pulse;
4. Elevated erythrocyte sedimentation rate (ESR — Westergren) ≥50 mm/hour; and
5. Positive temporal artery biopsy for GCA.

It is invariably emphasized that GCA patients have constitutional symptoms and signs, including aches and pains, headache, jaw claudication, malaise, myalgia, anorexia, weight loss, anemia, scalp tenderness, tender temporal arteries, flu-like symptoms and fever of unknown etiology. Also, a high ESR is traditionally emphasized as a *sine qua non* for the diagnosis of GCA.

However, recent studies have revealed that those criteria are likely to result in some false-negative diagnoses of GCA, risking visual loss. The following important facts about the diagnosis of GCA must be considered, if visual loss is to be prevented.

- In a recent study, 21% of patients with visual loss and positive temporal artery biopsy for GCA had no systemic symptoms of any kind, at any time and visual loss was their sole complaint, i.e. they had *occult GCA;* therefore, most importantly, *absence of systemic symptoms and signs does not rule out GCA.* Lack of awareness of this important fact has resulted in missed diagnosis of GCA and consequent visual loss.
- Presence of jaw claudication has emerged as the most significant systemic diagnostic symptom of GCA, because patients with jaw claudication have 9 times the odds of having temporal artery biopsy positive GCA compared to those without it.
- Most importantly, contrary to the prevalent impression, *perfectly normal ESR does not rule out GCA,* because patients with ESR as low as 4–5 mm/hour Westergren have been found to have positive temporal artery biopsy.
- A much more sensitive and reliable hematologic benchmark is elevated level of C-reactive protein (CRP). Elevated ESR combined with elevated CRP gives the best specificity (97%) for diagnosis of GCA. Thrombocytosis and hematologic evidence of anemia may also provide additional help.

This shows that using the criteria advocated by the American College of Rheumatologists is going to result in missed diagnosis of GCA and consequent visual loss.

Visual symptoms of GCA include episodes of transient monocular or binocular visual loss, sudden loss of vision in one or both eyes and occasionally double vision. The incidence of visual loss depends upon how early the diagnosis of GCA is made and aggressively treated with high-dose steroid therapy. In one large study, 50% of the patients already had visual loss when first diagnosed with GCA. The visual loss most commonly is due to anterior ischemic optic neuropathy and much less commonly cilioretinal artery occlusion, central retinal artery occlusion, posterior ischemic optic neuropathy and cortical blindness. Other ophthalmic manifestations of GCA include retinal cotton-wool spots, choroidal infarcts, ocular ischemia, pupillary abnormalities and diplopia.

In conclusion, the combined information provided by systemic, hematologic and ophthalmic findings is highly useful for the diagnosis of GCA, although none of them individually is 100% sensitive and specific. Patients in whom the above findings strongly suggest GCA must have temporal artery biopsy to establish the diagnosis definitely. The biopsy should be performed as soon as convenient, but high-dose steroid therapy should be started immediately, because by the time the result of the biopsy is available, the patient may have lost further vision irreversibly in one or both eyes. Therefore, immediate starting of high-dose steroid therapy in suspected cases is the most crucial priority. Starting the steroid therapy does not interfere with the biopsy results. At least a one-inch-long piece of the artery should be excised and serially sectioned throughout its entire length. If a temporal artery biopsy is negative on one side but there is a high index of suspicion of GCA, the opposite temporal artery should be biopsied; in a recent study, 10% of second biopsies were positive. If biopsies on both sides are negative but there is still a strong index of suspicion of GCA from systemic, ophthalmic and hematologic evaluations, it is advisable to treat them as having GCA unless proven otherwise by a close follow-up and on steroid therapy (discussed below); the rare chance of a false negative temporal artery biopsy cannot be ruled out.

PROPHYLAXIS/TREATMENT

It is well established now that the only proven and effective treatment for GCA is high-dose systemic corticosteroids. The crucial fact is that visual loss from GCA is preventable if the patient is treated early and adequately. It is also universally agreed that if there is a reasonable index of suspicion of GCA, high doses of systemic corticosteroid therapy should be started *immediately,* as an *emergency measure* — even hours could make the difference between sight and blindness. However, the exact regimen of steroid therapy in GCA has become highly controversial. The main reason for this may be that rheumatologists and ophthalmologists differ in their perspective on GCA. The former see patients with rheumatologic manifestations (many of them with polymyalgia rheumatica), while the latter see only GCA patients with visual loss and occult GCA. The steroid therapy regimen advocated by rheumatologists may well be appropriate for polymyalgia rheumatica patients (with no risk of blindness), who usually require much lower doses of steroid therapy to control their disease than do those with GCA. Therefore, rheumatologists have quite different criteria and mode of management of GCA than do ophthalmologists — for rheumatologists the aim is essentially a control of rheumatologic symptoms but for ophthalmologists it is the prevention of visual loss. Hence the conflict and confusion on the dosage and duration of corticosteroid therapy required, and on how to regulate steroid therapy.

Initial steroid therapy

Patients without visual loss can be treated with prednisone in a dose of 1 to 2 mg/kg/day orally; however, it is recommended that the minimum dose should be not less than 80 mg daily. A recent study showed no evidence that intravenous megadose steroid therapy was more effective than high-dose oral therapy in improving vision or preventing visual deterioration due to GCA. In view of that new finding, in patients presenting with visual loss, it is recommended to give one initial intravenous loading dose of methylprednisolone (a dose of 1 g), followed by high-dose oral prednisone regimen. The initial intravenous loading dose is particularly indicated if there is a history of amaurosis fugax, visual loss and/or early signs of second eye involvement. To prevent visual loss and control GCA satisfactorily, all patients must be maintained at the initial high dose of prednisone till both the ESR and CRP have stabilized at low levels (that usually takes 2–3 weeks — CRP comes down much faster than ESR (see Figure 98.1); therefore, initially frequent estimation of ESR and CRP is essential. After that, very gradually and cautiously tapering of prednisone should be started.

Tapering regimen of steroid therapy

How to do this is the most controversial topic. *The most reliable and sensitive parameters to regulate and taper down steroid therapy are the levels of ESR and CRP, and not systemic symptoms or any other guide.* It is important to stress that no generalization at all is possible for tapering down of prednisone and there is no set formula because of the infinite variation between individuals. Therefore, the tapering regimen has to be individualized for each patient, depending upon his/her response, as judged by ESR and CRP levels only. The recommendation by rheumatologists to use systemic symptoms as the guide for tapering steroid therapy for patients with GCA can be dangerous, because they can lose vision irrevocably without developing any warning systemic symptoms at all; moreover, 21% of patients with visual loss have occult GCA. Also a common mistake made by physicians in these cases is to taper the steroids down rapidly to a very low dosage and then discontinue it. There is a common belief among rheumatologists that GCA burns itself out in a year or two and steroids can then be tapered off. This is a completely wrong notion and can prove disastrous for vision, because repeat temporal artery biopsy has shown evidence of active disease even after 9 years of steroid therapy

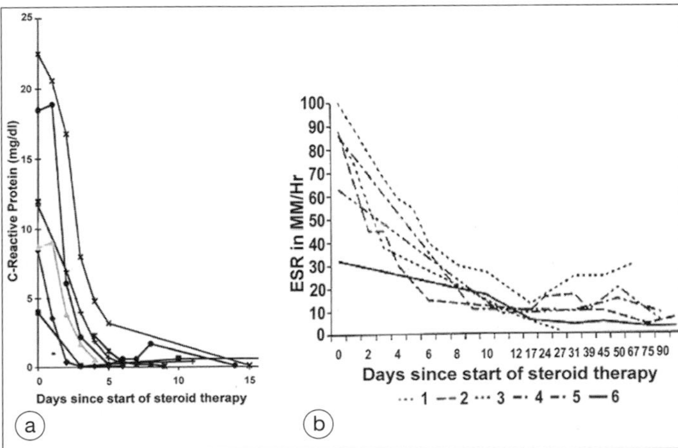

FIGURE 98.1. Graphs: (a) of C-reactive protein levels, and (b) of erythrocyte sedimentation rates (ESR) of 6 patients with GCA, showing their initial responses to high-dose corticosteroid steroid therapy. (Reproduced from Hayreh SS, Zimmerman B: Ophthalmologica 217:239–259, 2003.)

Maintenance dose and duration of steroid therapy

Determining the maintenance dose of steroid therapy is a slow, laborious, painstaking job, taking months or even years. *The only trustworthy and safe parameters to regulate the steroid therapy and to prevent visual loss are once again the levels of ESR and CRP, and nothing else.* Thus, the guiding principle, obviously, is to maintain *the lowest levels of ESR and CRP with the lowest dose of prednisone*. There are marked inter-individual variations among GCA patients in:

- The amount and duration of steroid required to control the active disease;
- The time needed to reach a maintenance dose;
- The maintenance dose required to keep the disease under control to prevent blindness and the total length of treatment.

Therefore, steroid therapy for GCA has to be individualized. Most GCA patients require a virtually life-long, very small maintenance dose, which has practically no systemic side-effects.

Recent studies have shown that in spite of aggressive high-dose steroid therapy, only 4% of the patients showed some visual improvement in the already involved eye; this fact makes early aggressive steroid therapy to prevent visual loss all the more crucial. It has also been found that in spite of the starting intensive corticosteroid treatment, 4% of the eyes can still suffer further visual loss during the first 5 days of treatment, but *none* after that; therefore it is important to warn the patient about that possibility and to stress that to maintain that vision, it is absolutely essential to be on adequate oral corticosteroids which is usually lifelong. Thus steroid therapy is most effective in preventing blindness. No significant difference in the time to reach the lowest maintenance dose has been found among patients with and without visual loss.

Complications of long-term steroid therapy

Systemic steroids usually produce a variety of systemic side-effects and complications. It is absolutely essential to discuss all those with the patients to make them aware of those, and they should be followed carefully by their internist to monitor them for the side-effects and their management.

Other advocated therapies for GCA

Alternate day steroid therapy

Some physicians tend to use this mode to reduce steroid side-effect. However, a prospective study showed that this type of therapy does not satisfactorily control the disease in most patients and is not recommended.

Use of steroid sparing agents in management of GCA

Various steroid sparing agents are often suggested to reduce the side-effects of prolonged steroid therapy in GCA. The most common agent considered is methotrexate. Randomized clinical trials have shown no real benefit in using methotrexate as a steroid sparing agent or to control GCA.

Overall, management of GCA is taxing and laborious, for both the patient and the physician, and it requires the trust and cooperation of all, including the patient's local physician, because of the systemic side-effects of the prolonged steroid therapy.

OCULAR OR PERIOCULAR MANIFESTATIONS

Optic nerve

Anterior ischemic optic neuropathy, posterior ischemic optic neuropathy.

Retina

Central retinal artery occlusion, cilioretinal artery occlusions, cotton wool spots.

Choroid

Infracts.

Extraocular muscles

Ischemic paresis or paralysis.

Pupil

Pupillary abnormalities.

Eye

Ocular ischemia.

Brain

Cortical blindness, internuclear ophthalmoplegia.

REFERENCES

Costello F, Zimmerman MB, Podhajsky PA, Hayreh SS: Role of thrombocytosis in diagnosis of giant cell arteritis and differentiation of arteritic from non-arteritic anterior ischemic optic neuropathy. Eur J Ophthalmol 14:245–257, 2004.

Hayreh SS: Steroid therapy for visual loss in patients with giant-cell arteritis. Lancet 355:1572–1573; 356:434, 2000.

Hayreh SS, Podhajsky PA, Raman R, Zimmerman B: Giant cell arteritis: validity and reliability of various diagnostic criteria. Am J Ophthalmol 123:285–296, 1997.

Hayreh SS, Podhajsky PA, Zimmerman B: Ocular manifestations of giant cell arteritis. Am J Ophthalmol 125:509–520, 1998.

Hayreh SS, Podhajsky PA, Zimmerman B: Occult giant cell arteritis: ocular manifestations. Am J Ophthalmol 125:521–526, 893, 1998.

Hayreh SS, Zimmerman B: Visual deterioration in giant cell arteritis patients while on high doses of corticosteroid therapy. Ophthalmology 110:1204–1215, 2003.

Hayreh SS, Zimmerman B: Management of giant cell arteritis. Ophthalmologica 217:239–259, 2003.

Hayreh SS, Zimmerman B, Kardon RH: Visual improvement with corticosteroid therapy in giant cell arteritis. Acta Ophthalmol Scand 80:355–367, 2002.

Hoffman GS, Cid MC, Hellmann DB, et al: International Network for the Study of Systemic Vasculitides: a multicenter, randomized, double-blind, placebo-controlled trial of adjuvant methotrexate treatment for giant cell arteritis. Arthritis Rheum 46:1309–1318, 2002.

Hunder GG, Bloch DA, Michel BA, et al: The American College of Rheumatology 1990 criteria for the classification of giant cell arteritis. Arthritis Rheum 33:1122–1128, 1990.

Hunder GG, Sheps SG, Allen GL, Joyce JW: Daily and alternate-day corticosteroid regimens in treatment of giant cell arteritis: comparison in a prospective study. Ann Intern Med 82:613–618, 1975.

Spiera RF, Mitnick HJ, Kupersmith M, et al: A prospective, double-blind, randomized, placebo controlled trial of methotrexate in the treatment of giant cell arteritis (GCA). Clin Exp Rheumatol 19:495–501, 2001.

99 UVEITIS ASSOCIATED WITH JUVENILE IDIOPATHIC ARTHRITIS
714.30

Quan Dong Nguyen, MD, MSc
Baltimore, Maryland
Diana V. Do, MD
Baltimore, Maryland

ETIOLOGY/INCIDENCE

Juvenile idiopathic arthritis (JIA) is the currently most widely accepted term to describe the formerly designated term of juvenile rheumatoid arthritis (JRA) or juvenile chronic arthritis. Therefore, in this chapter, the term *JIA* will be applied in lieu of *JRA*. Uveitis associated with JIA is the most common cause of chronic intraocular inflammation among children.

Approximately 6% of all cases of uveitis occur in children, and up to 80% of all cases of anterior uveitis in childhood are associated with JIA. Chronic uveitis is a serious complication of JIA: up to12% of children with uveitis associated with pauciarticular JIA develop permanent blindness as a result of low-grade chronic intraocular inflammation.

The prevalence of JIA in the United States has been estimated at 60,000 to 70,000 cases. JIA is more common in girls, with a female-to-male ratio of 3 : 2. There are 3 modes of JIA onset: systemic; polyarticular (5 or more joints); and pauciarticular (less than 5 joints). The peak age at onset of JIA is between 2 and 4 years. The incidence of iridocyclitis in patients with JIA ranges from 8% to 24%, and varies among subgroups of JIA. The uveitis is diagnosed an average of 18 months after the arthritis, although ocular manifestation may be the first sign of JIA in a child who has not yet begun to manifest evidence of systemic arthritis.

As with many other autoimmune conditions, where the targeted antigen is unknown.

The etiology for JIA or its associated uveitis is not known.

DISEASE COURSE/PROGNOSIS

Vision-threatening morbidities in JIA are mainly due to intraocular inflammation. The duration of the inflammation often correlates with the complications that cause vision impairment. The prognosis is dependent on the incidence and severity of the inflammatory disease, as well as the proper management of the patients. Overall, once the eye is affected with JIA uveitis, the prognosis is poor. Acute uveitis is often associated with persistent arthritis.

- Only one third of affected eyes retain visual acuity of >20/40 long-term.
- Approximately one third develop severe visual disability of <20/200.

Poor prognosticators include:
- Female sex;
- Young age of disease onset;
- Pauciarticular arthritis;
- Antinuclear antibody (ANA)-positivity;
- Posterior synechiae;
- Glaucomatous optic neuropathy.

DIAGNOSIS

Clinical signs and symptoms

JIA is not a precisely defined entity, but its presence is based on a clinical diagnosis.

- American Rheumatism Association defines JIA as clinical evidence of chronic arthritis (with duration of at least 3 months) of unknown cause in a child younger than 16 years.
- Patients with arthritis associated with a known etiology (see Differential diagnosis) are not classified to have JIA.
- ANA seropositivity is the chief laboratory risk factor for eye disease.
- Vast majority of JRA patients who develop eye disease are rheumatoid factor-negative.
- Three main subtypes of JIA:
    - Systemic 11% to 20%. Associated with fever, hepatosplenomegaly, lymphadenopathy, leukocytosis. Very low risk for eye disease;
    - Polyarticular 20% to 40%. Symmetric arthritis. Intermediate risk for eye disease: approximately 5% of patients with polyarticular-onset JIA develop uveitis;
    - Pauciarticular 40% to 70%. Four or fewer joints involved; often asymmetrically. High risk of developing uveitis: approximately 20% of patients with polyarticular-onset JIA develop uveitis.

Ocular

- Bilateral in 70% to 80%.
- Nongranulomatous uveitis (>90%).
- Chronic smoldering or recurrent course (>90%); rarely (<5%) acute monophasic.
- Mostly iridocyclitis (90%); rarely panuveitis or vitritis.

Differential diagnosis

- JIA.
- Juvenile arthropathies associated with HLA-B27.
    - Juvenile spondyloarthropathy;
    - Juvenile psoriatic arthritis;
    - Juvenile Reiter syndrome;
    - Juvenile enteritis (Crohn disease or ulcerative colitis).
- Juvenile sarcoidosis.
- Familial juvenile systemic granulomatosis.
- Infectious diseases (e.g. syphilis, herpetic keratouveitis, Lyme disease, tuberculosis).
- Masquerade syndromes:
    - Leukemia;
    - Retinoblastoma;
    - Other malignancies.

TREATMENT

JIA-associated uveitis may be silent; thus, the child may be asymptomatic and the eye may be normal in appearance until leukocoria secondary to cataract is detected or when the child fails a visual screening examination. Therefore, it is of significant importance that guidelines for ophthalmologic examinations, including slit-lamp biomicroscopy, be followed in all children diagnosed with JIA (Table 99.1).

Uveitis associated with JIA is often the most stubborn and most difficult to bring into durable remission. Leading authorities in the field of ocular immunology and uveitis have emphasized the need for ophthalmologist/ocular immunologist to 'stay in the hunt,' not quitting on the children with stubborn JIA-associated uveitis simply because the first NSAID or immunomodulatory agent that is tried does not successfully induce a durable remission. Rather, physicians should continue to search for a medication or combination of medications that will

TABLE 99.1 – **American Academy of Pediatrics guidelines for ophthalmologic examination in children with JIA**

Risk	Type	ANA	Age at Onset	Duration of Disease
High	Pauci or poly	+	≤7	≤4 years
Moderate	Pauci or poly	+	≤7	>4 years
	Pauci or poly	–	Any	≤4 years
	Pauci or poly	+	>7	>4 years
Low	Systemic	–	Any	Any
	Pauci or poly	(Rarely +)	≤7	After 7 years
	Pauci or poly	+ or –	>7	After 4 years

**American Academy of Pediatrics. Guidelines for examinations in children with Juvenile rheumatoid arthritis (RE9320). Pediatrics 92:295–296, 1993.*

High risk: ophthalmologic exam Q 3–4 months
Moderate risk: ophthalmologic exam Q 6 months
Low risk: ophthalmologic exam Q 12 months

Recommendations for low-risk follow-up continue into adulthood.

allow the patients to be completely free of all recurrences of inflammation, while at the same time being free of all steroid use at all times.

Systemic

- Systemic NSAIDs (e.g. naproxen at 10 to 15 mg/kg/day in divided doses) are used either as adjunctive therapy to help the steroid taper or as the sole systemic agent to supplement topical therapeutic measures.
- Long-term systemic treatment with corticosteroids is discouraged. A short course of systemic steroid therapy is occasionally used to supplement topical therapy in patients with significant inflammation. Systemic corticosteroid therapy retards linear growth in children, and most importantly, this effect can persist even after cessation of the corticosteroid therapy.
- Systemic steroid treatment (usually started at 0.5 to 1.0 mg/kg/day prednisone PO) is reserved for:
  - Severe uveitis;
  - Uveitis that is resistant to local treatment;
  - Uveitis that involves posterior segment.
- Systemic chemotherapy is reserved for very severe cases that prove steroid-resistant and is used to limit complications resulting from prolonged use of systemic corticosteroids.
- The immunomodulatory drug of choice is methotrexate, which is often administered weekly. A second immunosuppressive medication is used when the chronic or recurrent uveitis not controlled with methotrexate as monotherapy. An alkylating agent such as chlorambucil has been shown to be effective and safe in patients with JIA-associated uveitis. Biological agents (infliximab, daclizumab) may have a role in the management of JIA-associated uveitis. Studies suggest that cyclosporine A, either as monotherapy or as an add-on agent to methotrexate immunomodulatory therapy program, is not the ideal agent for induction of durable remission of JIA-associated uveitis. Etanercept, which has been found to be efficacious in managing rheumatoid arthritis, has not been shown to be effective in managing uveitis such as that associated with JIA.
- All systemic immunosuppressive agents should be used in consultation with experts in the use of these agents in the pediatric population. It is strongly recommended that management of patients with JIA-associated uveitis be conducted by ocular immunologists/uveitis specialists whenever possible.

Local

- Corticosteroids (e.g. prednisolone acetate 1%) are the mainstay of therapy for patients with mild to moderate disease. Once disease activity is controlled, the frequency and potency of the regimen is reduced (e.g. to fluorometholone 0.1%).
- About 20% of patients show little to no response to topical steroidal therapy.
- Periocular injections of corticosteroids (e.g. triamcinolone given as anterior sub-Tenon's injections) or intravitreal injections are reserved for:
  - More severe inflammation;
  - Patients with more posterior inflammation;
  - Patients with or at high risk for cystoid macular edema (CME).
- Prolonged therapy with steroids is associated with cataracts and glaucoma.
- Mydriatics (cycloplegics; e.g. scopolamine 0.25%) are used as adjunctive therapy to minimize posterior synechiae formation, maintain blood-aqueous barrier, and minimize visual disability from posterior subcapsular cataracts.
- Topical nonsteroidal anti-inflammatory drugs (NSAIDs) are employed as adjunctive therapy in patients at high risk for CME.
- Antiglaucoma therapy is necessary for patients with secondary ocular hypertension or glaucoma.

Surgical

- Cataract surgery.
- Glaucoma surgery.
- Ethylenediaminetetraacetic acid (EDTA) chelation for band keratopathy.
- Core vitrectomy for clearing inflammatory debris.
- Pars plana vitrectomy and membrane peeling for cyclitic and epiretinal membranes.

COMPLICATIONS

- Cataracts: 40% to 80%.
- Band keratopathy: 30% to 80%.
- Macular edema or epiretinal membrane formation: 30% to 50% in chronic cases.
- Vitreous haze/debris: 25%.
- Glaucoma: 15% to 30%.
- Chronic hypotony (ciliary body atrophy) and phthisis: 5% to 17%.
- Other posterior pole complications (disk neovascularization, ischemic optic neuropathy, macular hole): rare but can occur in chronic cases.
- Complications of treatments:
  - Ocular hypertension caused by steroids;
  - Growth stunting caused by oral corticosteroids;
  - Infectious disease and organ toxicity in patients receiving immunosuppressive chemotherapy.

SUMMARY

JIA-associated uveitis — the most common type of pediatric ocular inflammation — is, ironically, often asymptomatic in children with JIA, leading to insidious but progressive morbidity in a significant number of children with this serious disease:

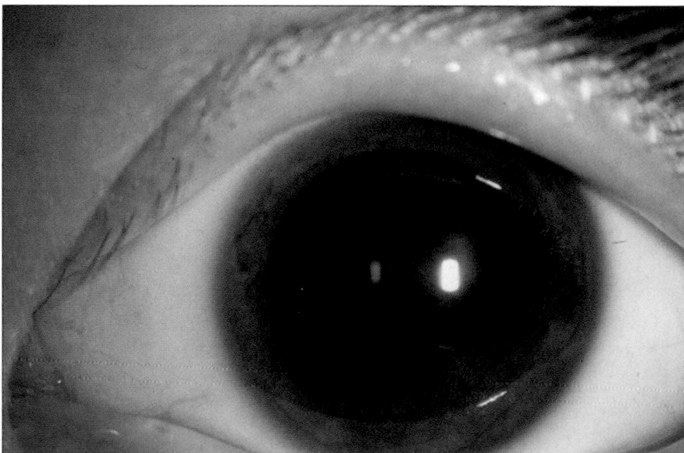

FIGURE 99.1. Chronic JIA-associated uveitis, with low grade inflammation and synnechiae, often presented as a 'white, quiet-appearing' eye.

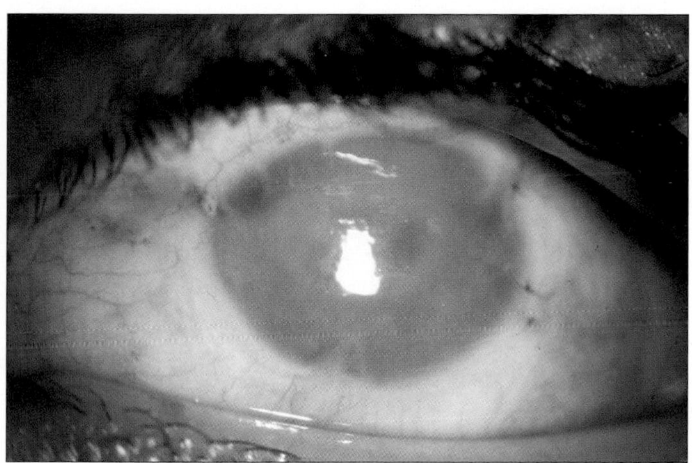

FIGURE 99.2. Improper management of JIA-associated uveitis may lead to formation of cataract, development of glaucoma, band keratopathy, among others, and eventual phthisis.

JIA-associated uveitis still blinds children. It is imperative that JIA patients with a high risk of developing eye disease (ANA-positive girls with pauciarticular disease) be identified, screened, and followed closely. Similarly, once the diagnosis of JIA uveitis is made, every attempt should be made to eradicate the inflammation so as to minimize the chance of irreversible loss of vision (Figures 99.1 and 99.2).

REFERENCES

Brewer EJ, Bass J, Baum J, et al: Current proposed revision of JRA criteria. Arthritis Rheum 20:195–199, 1977.

Chen CS, Roberton D, Hammerton ME: Juvenile arthritis-associated uveitis: visual outcomes and prognosis. Can J Ophthalmol 39:614–620, 2004.

Dana MR, Merayo-Lloves J, Schaumberg DA, Foster CS. Visual outcomes prognosticators in juvenile rheumatoid arthritis-associated uveitis. Ophthalmology 104:236–244, 1997.

Efthimiou P, Markenson JA: Role of biological agents in immune mediated inflammatory diseases. South Med J 98:192–204, 2005.

Foster CS: Diagnosis and treatment of juvenile idiopathic arthritis-associated uveitis. Current Opinion in Ophthalmology 14:395–398, 2003.

Giannini EH, Brower EJ, Kuzmind N, et al: Methotrexate in resistant juvenile rheumatoid arthritis: results of the U.S.A.-U.S.S.R. double-blind, placebo-controlled trial. N Engl J Med 326:1043–1049, 1992.

Kanski JJ, Shun-Shin A: Systemic uveitis syndromes in childhood: an analysis of 340 cases. Ophthalmology 91:1247–1252, 1984.

Kanski JJ: Uveitis in juvenile chronic arthritis: incidence, clinical features and prognosis. Eye 2:641–645, 1988.

Kanski JJ: Juvenile arthritis and uveitis. Surv Ophthalmol 34:253–267, 1990.

Kimura SJ, Hogan MJ, Thygeson P: Uveitis in children. Arch Ophthalmol 51:80–88, 1954.

Nguyen QD, Foster CS: Saving the vision of children with juvenile rheumatoid arthritis-associated uveitis. JAMA 280:1133–1134, 1998.

Olson NY, Lindsley CB, Godfrey WA: Nonsteroidal anti-inflammatory drug therapy in chronic childhood iridocyclitis. Am J Dis Child 142:1289–1292, 1988.

Rosenberg AM: Uveitis associated with juvenile rheumatoid arthritis. Semin Arthritis Rheum 16:158–173, 1987.

Smith JA, Thompson DJ, Whitcup SM, et al: A randomized, placebo-controlled, double-masked clinical trial of etanercept for the treatment of uveitis associated with juvenile idiopathic arthritis. Arthritis Rheum 53:18–23, 2005.

Wolf MD, Lichter PR, Ragsdale CG: Prognostic factors in the uveitis of juvenile rheumatoid arthritis. Ophthalmology 94:1242–1247, 1987.

100 WEGENER GRANULOMATOSIS 446.4

James L. Kinyoun, MD
Seattle, Washington

ETIOLOGY/INCIDENCE

Wegener granulomatosis is a necrotizing, granulomatous vasculitis of the sinuses (upper respiratory tract), lungs (lower respiratory tract), and kidneys. A limited form of the disease exists in which renal lesions are not present. All age groups can be affected, and symptoms include rhinorrhea, sinus pain, cough, malaise and weight loss. There is no gender predilection; almost all affected patients are white. Although the etiology remains unknown, available evidence (deposition of immune complexes) indicates that immunopathogenic mechanisms are responsible.

COURSE/PROGNOSIS

Most patients with Wegener granulomatosis initially have signs of upper respiratory tract inflammation that do not respond to treatment for commonly diagnosed conditions such as infection. Once the diagnosis has been established by biopsy, most affected patients have a relatively good prognosis with treatment; however, even with successful treatment, the disease is chronic, relapses occur and treatment complications are common.

DIAGNOSIS

Clinical signs and symptoms

Because eye symptoms can be the initial manifestation of Wegener granulomatosis, ophthalmologists should be aware of this disorder. Ophthalmic manifestations include proptosis due to orbital involvement usually via extension from adjacent sinuses; dry eyes; conjunctivitis; superficial corneal infection and ulceration (secondary to proptosis) Figure 100.1; scleritis or episcleritis; and uveitis. Other reported eye or periocular abnormalities include obstruction of the nasolacrimal duct, optic neuritis, papilledema, central retinal artery occlusion, retinal vasculitis and choriocapillariitis.

Laboratory findings

- Clinical findings: sinus and lung inflammation with or without renal involvement (e.g. proteinuria, hematuria, urinary casts).
- Histopathology: necrotizing, granulomatous vasculitis with infiltrative neutrophils, lymphocytes, plasma cells, histiocytes and giant cells.
- Antineutrophil cytoplasmic antibody (cANCA).

Differential diagnosis

- Upper respiratory infection (e.g. pulmonary infiltrates, sinusitis).

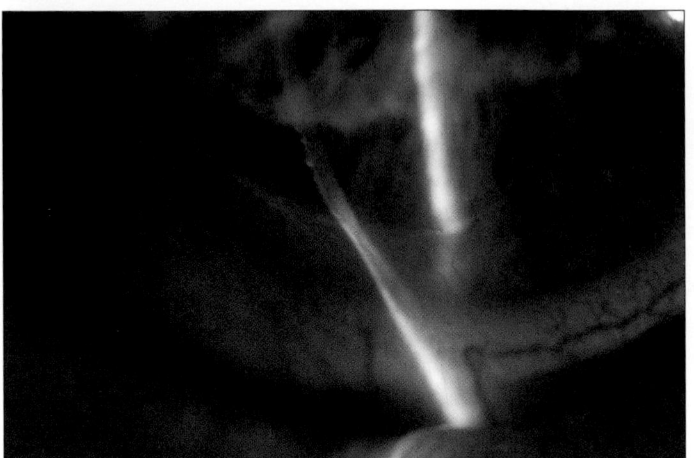

FIGURE 100.1. Wegener granulomatosis-corneal thinning.

- Glomerulonephritis.
- Otitis media.
- Orbital pseudotumor.
- Other small-vessel vasculitis (Churg–Strauss syndrome, microscopic polyangiitis, Henoch–Schönlein purpura, and essential cryoglobulinemic vasculitis).

TREATMENT

Systemic

- Cyclophosphamide 2 mg/kg PO qd and continuing for 1 year after active disease has subsided.
- Prednisone 1 mg/kg PO qd for 4 weeks, followed by a tapered dose and discontinuation.

Ocular

- Topical eye lubricants (e.g. carboxymethylcellulose sodium 0.5%) every 30 minutes to 4 hours.
- Topical ophthalmic antibiotic solution or ointment (e.g. trimethoprim sulfate and polymyxin B sulfate) every 3 to 4 hours.
- Topical ophthalmic corticosteroid drops (e.g. prednisolone 1%) every 3 to 4 hours; cycloplegic eyedrops (e.g. tropicamide 1%) every 4 hours.

Surgical

- Orbital decompression in patients with optic nerve compression that is unresponsive to medical treatment.
- Grafts (e.g. severe corneal ulceration).

Other

- Methotrexate or azathioprine (may be useful for patients in remission who have serious side effects due to cyclophosphamide).

COMPLICATIONS

Disease-related complications include vision loss, renal insufficiency, subglottic stenosis, and decreased hearing. Permanent morbidity occurs in a majority of patients.

Complications of treatment with cyclophosphamide include bone marrow suppression, hemorrhagic cystitis, azoospermia, bladder carcinoma, nausea, vomiting and hair loss. The leukocyte count should be followed closely during therapy (initially every other day and weekly during maintenance therapy) and should not decrease below 3000 cells/mm^3. Granulocyte count below 1500 cells/mm^3 increases the risk of infection. Dosages must be decreased at the first sign of bone marrow suppression because the full effect of the present dose will not manifest in the white blood cell count until 1 week later. Hemorrhagic cystitis can be minimized by adequate hydration to prevent concentrated urine. Fortunately, hair regrows in most patients who experience hair loss while taking cyclophosphamide.

Complications of systemic corticosteroids include fluid retention, weight gain, moon face, hyperglycemia, osteoporosis, bone fractures, psychologic disturbances, peptic ulcers and infections. Side effects can be minimized by switching to treatment every other day and discontinuing steroids as soon as inflammation has been controlled.

COMMENTS

Ophthalmologists' awareness of Wegener granulomatosis will lead to prompt referral to internists and early treatment with cytotoxic and immunosuppressant drugs. The promptness of diagnosis and successful treatment may not only save lives but also preserve useful vision. Affected patients will have to be followed by internists and ophthalmologists to monitor treatment effectiveness and the side effects of cytotoxic and immunosuppressive drugs. Depending on disease activity, follow-up examinations daily or at intervals of several months are appropriate.

REFERENCES

Harper SL, Letko E, Samson CM, et al: Wegener's granulomatosis: the relationship between ocular and systemic disease. J Rheumatol 28:1025–1032, 2001.

Hoffman GS, Kerr GS, Leavitt RY, et al: Wegener's granulomatosis: an analysis of 158 patients. Ann Int Med 116:488–498, 1992.

Jayne D, Rasmussen N, Andrassy K, et al: A randomized trial of maintenance therapy for vasculitis associated with antineutrophil cytoplasmic autoantibodies. N Engl J Med 349:36–44, 2003.

Kinyoun JL, Kalina RE, Klein ML: Choroidal involvement in systemic necrotizing vasculitis. Arch Ophthalmol 105:939–942, 1987.

Seo P, Stone JH: The antineutrophil cytoplasmic antibody-associated vasculitides. Am J Med 117:39–50, 2004

101 WEILL–MARCHESANI SYNDROME 759.8

(Marchesani Syndrome, Spherophakia–Brachymorphia Syndrome)

Teresa C. Chen, MD
Boston, Massachusetts
David Sellers Walton, MD
Boston, Massachusetts

ETIOLOGY/INCIDENCE

The Weill–Marchesani syndrome (WMS) is a very rare hereditary disorder that is manifested by microspherophakia, subluxated lenses, high myopia, glaucoma, short stature, joint stiffness, and brachydactyly. It demonstrates both autosomal recessive and autosomal dominant transmission.

COURSE/PROGNOSIS

- Adult dwarfism.
- Occasional heart defects.
- Glaucoma, the most serious ocular complication.

DIAGNOSIS

Clinical signs and symptoms

Diagnosis is made by recognizing ocular and systemic abnormalities. The affected lenses are small in diameter, are thickened, and often become dislocated anteriorly or inferiorly. Following shallowing of the anterior chamber, glaucoma may occur secondary to the pupillary block mechanism and appositional crowding of the angle due to a forward position of the lens iris diaphragm. The small stature of patients with this disorder can be striking and is associated with marked extremity abnormalities.

Laboratory findings

Delayed carpal ossification is revealed by radiography.

Differential diagnosis

- Other causes of dwarfism.
- Mucopolysaccharidoses.
- Isolated hereditary lens subluxation and myopia.
- Hereditary microspherophakia.

PROPHYLAXIS

Laser iridotomy may be performed in cases in which there is threatened pupillary block and associated angle closure.

TREATMENT

Ocular

- Optical correction for myopia and astigmatism.
- Glaucoma treatment: When glaucoma is present, topical β-blockers, alpha adrenergics, carbonic anhydrase inhibitors, and prostaglandin agents may be helpful.
- Pupillary block glaucoma: In the absence of lens subluxation, miotics may induce or exacerbate pupillary block. Cycloplegics/mydriatics may relieve pupillary block but may also increase the risk of spontaneous lens dislocation into the anterior chamber.

Surgical

Patients at risk for pupillary block glaucoma should be followed regularly with gonioscopy. Iridotomy is indicated to prevent and relieve pupillary block. Following iridotomy, laser iridoplasty may be helpful to further open the angle.

Goniosynechialysis may be necessary to remove an iris that is adherent to the trabecular meshwork so as to restore trabecular function. Early operation following angle closure is desirable.

Other surgeries that may ultimately be needed for the treatment of glaucoma may include the following: pars plana lensectomy, anterior vitrectomy, sutured posterior chamber intraocular lens (PCIOL) placement and/or tube shunt surgery. Phacoemulsification with in-the-bag (modified or unmodified) capsular tension ring and PCIOL has also been performed.

COMPLICATIONS

- Blindness secondary to glaucoma.
- Dwarfism.
- Clumsiness secondary to hand deformities.

COMMENTS

Genetic counseling is indicated. There is evidence of clinical homogeneity despite genetic heterogeneity in autosomal recessive (AR) and autosomal dominant (AD) families. These results underscore the difficulties for genetic counseling in supposed sporadic cases.

Loci have been mapped in AR WMS (19p13.3-p13.2) and AD WMS (15q21.1).

Systemic and ophthalmic screening should be performed to detect any previously unappreciated defects.

REFERENCES

Cionni RJ, Osher RH, Marques DM, et al: Modified capsular tension ring for patients with congenital loss of zonular support. J Cataract Refract Surg 29:1668–1673, 2003.

Faivre L, Dollfus H, Lyonnet S, et al: Clinical homogeneity and genetic heterogeneity in Weill-Marchesani syndrome. Am J Med Genet 123A:204–207, 2003.

Harasymowycz P, Wilson R: Surgical treatment of advanced chronic angle closure glaucoma in Weill-Marchesani syndrome. J Pediatr Ophthalmol Strabismus 41:295–299, 2004.

Jensen AD, Cross HE, Paton D: Ocular complications in the Weill-Marchesani syndrome. Am J Ophthalmol 77:261–269, 1974.

Ritch R, Wand M: Treatment of the Weill-Marchesani syndrome. Ann Ophthalmol 13:665–667, 1981.

SECTION

10 Skeletal Disorders

102 DOWN SYNDROME 758.0

(Trisomy 21)

Natalio J. Izquierdo, MD
San Juan, Puerto Rico

ETIOLOGY/INCIDENCE

Various chromosomal abnormalities may lead to the Down syndrome including: a free trisomy 21 (94% of patients), translocation (4% of patients), and mosaicism (2% of patients).

- Free trisomy 21 results from nondisjunction during meiosis in one of the parents. This occurrence is correlated with advanced maternal and paternal age. The most common type of nondisjunction occurs in the maternal first meiotic division. The percentage of errors during maternal second meiotic division is lower. The incidence of nondisjunction in the first and second meiotic division of the paternal gametogenesis is nearly equal.
- Translocation may occur de novo or be transmitted by one of the parents. Translocations are usually of the centric fusion type. They frequently involve chromosome 14 (14/21 translocation), 21 (21/21 translocation), or 22 (22/21 translocation).
- Mosaicism is considered a postzygotic event (following fertilization). Two cell lines are found; one with a free trisomy, and the other with a normal karyotype. This finding leads to patients with a great phenotypic variability, ranging from near normal to the classic trisomy 21 phenotype.

Occurrence strongly depends on maternal age. For young mothers, the risk of a free trisomy is 1–2%. For mothers aged 20 years or younger, the occurrence is 1 per 2500 births. The risk increases considerably for mothers aged 35 years. For mothers aged 45 years or older, the occurrence is 1 per 55 live births.The risk for recurrence of Down syndrome in a patient's siblings is also related to maternal age.

Down syndrome occurs once in every 600–700 live births in the United States and Japanese populations.

COURSE/PROGNOSIS

A primary care provider should lead and coordinate the multisystemic evaluation of patients with Down syndrome. Awareness of systemic and ocular findings is essential for managing patients with trisomy 21.

- Because of frequent congenital heart malformations, which occur in up to 60% of these patients, early cardiology consultation is desirable.
- Due to recurrent respiratory tract infections, a pediatric pneumologist should co-manage patients with Down syndrome.
- A child psychiatrist should lead liaison interventions, family therapies, and psychometric evaluations. Mental retardation is common in patients with trisomy 21; however, patients with mosaicism tend to have higher IQs.
- Up to 10% of patients with Down syndrome have epilepsy; therefore, neurological evaluation may be needed.
- Genetic counseling is indicated.
- Ophthalmic medical care for blepharitis, refractive errors, strabismus, corneal ectasias and cataracts is needed.
- Ophthalmic surgical indications used for non-handicapped patients are used for patients with Down syndrome. General anesthesia is desirable for patients with the syndrome who undergo surgery.

Patients with Down syndrome have a shortened life expectancy. Early evaluation, diagnosis and intervention may prevent deaths due to congenital heart defects.

DIAGNOSIS

Clinical signs and symptoms

Eight or more of the characteristic clinical findings lead to a definite diagnosis. In doubtful cases, chromosomal analysis may be necessary.

- General physical features in patients with Down syndrome include shortened extremities, short limbs, short and broad hands, short fifth middle phalanx, simian palmar creases, joint hyperextensibility or hyperflexibility, neuromuscular hypotonia, dry skin, premature aging, a wide range of intelligence quotients and congenital heart defects.
- Patients with the syndrome have characteristic craniofacial findings, such as flat occiput, a flattened facial appearance, anteriorly and posteriorly flattened head, dysplastic ears, small nose, depressed nasal bridge, protruding tongue, high-arched palate, dental abnormalities, and a short and broad neck.
- Ocular signs in patients with the Down syndrome include:
    - Lid anomalies such as prominent epicanthal folds, upward slanting of the palpebral fissures and congenital ectropion (rare) occur;

- Lid infections, including blepharitis, blepharoconjunctivitis, chalazion, and hordeola. Because of recurrent external infections, inspect lids for collarettes, foamy secretions, Meibomian plugging, marginal erythema and scurf;
- Nasolacrimal duct obstruction;
- Amblyopia associated to strabismus, refractive errors, or media opacities;
- Strabismus occurs in up to 20% of patients;
- Evaluate corneas carefully for keratoconus or keratoglobus. Scissoring of the retinoscopic reflex is an early finding in patients with keratoconus. Use Placido disks, keratometers, or topographies to evaluate patients with Down syndrome who have keratoconus. Rizzuti and Munson signs appear later;
- Up to 90% of patients with the syndrome may have iris' Brushfield spots. These spots are focal areas of iris stromal hyperplasia, surrounded by relative hypoplasia. These are more common in patients with lightly pigmented irides;
- Cataracts occur in patients with the syndrome. Lens opacities may be sutural, zonular, or complete. These may be congenital or may occur later in life;
- Glaucoma usually appears during infancy. Therefore, patients must be examined for corneal edema, megalocornea, increased intraocular pressure, progressive myopia, and optic nerve cupping;
- Retinal findings include: an increased number of retinal vessels crossing the disk margin, and retinal detachments;
- Patients with the syndrome may have refractive errors.

(Figure 102.1)

Laboratory findings

Previous studies discuss the benefits of amniocentesis during pregnancy in mothers with low α-fetoprotein serum values during the beginning of the second trimester.

Further, trisomy 21 may be diagnosed in the second and third trimester of pregnancy using prenatal echography. The following prenatal echographic findings are suggestive of Down syndrome and may be followed with amniocentesis and fetal chromosome analysis:

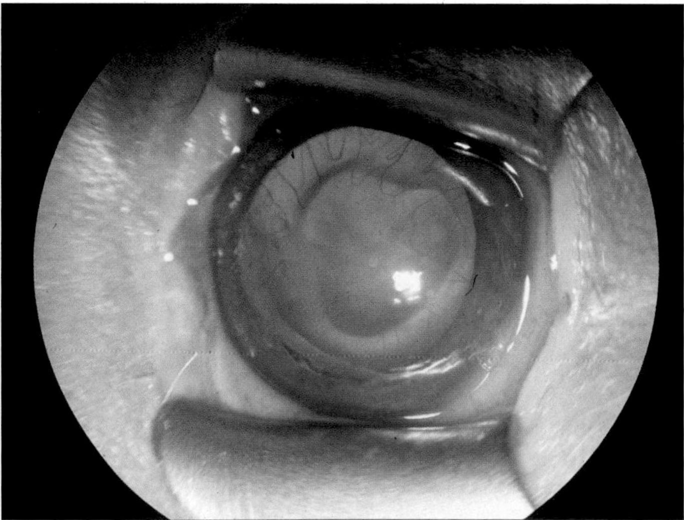

FIGURE 102.1. Cataract in patient with Down syndrome.

- Cystic hygroma colli;
- Cardiac defects;
- Duodenal obstruction;
- Hydrops fetalis;
- Prune belly anomaly.

Craniofacial radiographic findings in children with the syndrome may include: flattened facial features (including small or absent nasal bones), occiput, and brachycephaly.

Echocardiography is advisable in patients with the syndrome.

TREATMENT

Medical

A primary care provider should lead and coordinate the multisystemic evaluation of patients with Down syndrome. Awareness of systemic and ocular findings is essential for managing patients with trisomy 21.

- Medical therapy for blepharitis includes lid scrubs and topical antibiotics.
- Indications used for eyeglass prescription in nonhandicapped patients are used for patients with the syndrome. Glasses should be prescribed for patients at risk for amblyopia due to refractive errors, accommodative esotropia, aphakia, and pseudophakia.

Surgical

Surgical indications used for nonhandicapped patients are used for patients with the syndrome. General anesthesia is advisable during surgical interventions.

- Systemic surgery: patients with congenital cardiac malformations as part of the syndrome may require early cardiovascular surgery.
- Ocular surgery: systemic evaluation, including a cardiovascular evaluation, is desirable prior to eye surgery.
- Patients with strabismus as part of the Down syndrome may benefit from strabismus surgery.
- Patients with corneal pathologies as part of the syndrome may develop corneal hydrops and perforation. Corneal transplants are indicated for severe scarring.
- Patients with trisomy 21 have a high incidence of cataracts. Cataract extraction is indicated when decreased vision affects quality of life. Extracapsular cataract extraction with intraocular lens implantation facilitates visual rehabilitation. Phacoemulsification offers the advantage of a small incision.
- Patients with the syndrome who develop keratoglobus are at increased risk of traumatic eye injuries. Traumatic ocular injuries are treated when required.

REFERENCES

Berk AT, Saatci AO, Ercal MD: Ocular findings in 55 patients with Down's syndrome. Ophthalmic Genet 17(1):15–19, 1996.

Caputo AR, Wagner RS, Reynolds DR: Down syndrome. Clinical review of ocular features. Clin Pediatr (Phila) 28(8):355–358, 1989.

Copin H, Bremond-Gignac D: Ocular manifestations of Down syndrome and cytogenic aspects. J Fr Ophtalmol 27(8):958–959, 2004.

da Cunha RP, Moreira JB: Ocular findings in Down syndrome. Am J Ophthalmol 122(2):236–244, 1996.

Frantz JM, Insler MS, Hagenah M: Penetrating keratoplasty for keratoconus in Down's syndrome. Am J Ophthalmol 109(2):143–147, 1990.

Goto S, Yo M, Hayashi T: Intraocular lens implantation in severely mentally and physically handicapped patients. Jpn J Ophthalmol 39(2):187–192, 1995.

Haddow JE, Palomaki GE, Knight GJ: Prenatal screening for Down's syndrome with use of maternal serum markers. N Engl J Med 327(9):588–593, 1992.

Jaeger EA: Ocular findings in Down's syndrome. Trans Am Ophthalmol Soc 78:808–845, 1980.

Roizen NJ, Mets MB, Blondis TA: Ophthalmic disorders in children with Down syndrome. Dev Med Child Neurol 36(7):594–600, 1994.

Shapiro MB, France TD: The ocular features of Down's syndrome. Am J Ophthalmol 99(6):659–663, 1985.

Volker-Dieben HJ, Odenthal MT, D'Amaro J: Surgical treatment of corneal pathology in patients with Down's syndrome. J Intellect Disabil Res 37(2):169–175, 1993.

SECTION

11 Phakomatoses

103 ANGIOMATOSIS RETINAE 759.6

(Angiomatosis of the Retina and Central Nervous System, Retinal and Optic Disk Capillary Hemangiomas, Retinal Capillary Hamartoma, Retinal Hemangioblastoma, von Hippel–Lindau Disease, von Hippel's Disease)

Shiyoung Roh, MD
Boston, Massachusetts
John J. Weiter, MD, PhD
Boston, Massachusetts

ETIOLOGY/INCIDENCE

Angiomatosis retinae (von Hippel's disease) is characterized by congenital capillary angiomatous hamartomas of the retina and optic nerve. The retinal angiomas usually are diagnosed when the patient is between 10 and 30 years of age. Central nervous system (CNS) and visceral tumors are commonly noted after the ocular symptoms become manifest; if the CNS and viscera are involved, the condition is termed von Hippel–Lindau disease.

The disorder is transmitted by autosomal dominant inheritance with incomplete penetrance and variable expressivity; there is no well-established predilection for gender or race. The retinal tumors often are multiple and are bilateral in more than 50% of cases; about 20% of patients with retinal angiomas develop CNS tumors.

DIAGNOSIS

Clinical signs and symptoms

Ocular

- Angiomas of retina or optic nerve or both.
- Disk edema.
- Retinal or optic disk exudates, circinate exudative retinopathy.
- Epiretinal membranes.
- Dilated, tortuous retinal vessels.
- Macular star exudation.
- Retinal hemorrhage.
- Retinal detachment.
- Vitreous hemorrhage.
- Proliferative vitreoretinopathy.
- Phthisis bulbi.
- Secondary glaucoma.
- Vision loss.

The ocular angiomas may develop in the retina (usually from the inner layers, as discrete angiomas – endophytic angiomas), in the optic nerve head, in the peripapillary retina (frequently from the outer layers – exophytic angiomas) where they are diffuse, or in the retrobulbar portion of the optic nerve.

Histologic findings

- Masses of capillaries exhibit an embryonic appearance (hemangioblastoma), often with abnormal fenestrations.
- Glial proliferation (of astrocytes) separates the vascular channels.
- Vascular channels frequently contain large lipid-filled vacuoles, most likely representing astrocytic phagocytosis of leaking plasma.

CLINICAL COURSE/PROGNOSIS

Retinal tumors are usually at the equator or in the periphery, with a propensity for the temporal side. The tumor typically remains stable or grows very slowly. With gradual tumor growth, arteriovenous shunting occurs within the mass, resulting in an increasingly dilated, tortuous feeding artery and draining vein. With time, subretinal fluid and yellow exudate accumulate around the lesion and very often in the macula. Visual change resulting from the macular pooling of exudates often is the presenting sign.

Endophytic tumors often produce vitreous traction that may lead to vitreous hemorrhage or tractional retinal detachment (rhegmatogenous or nonrhegmatogenous).

Peripapillary angiomas tend to be exophytic and relatively flat, without feeding and draining vessels, resembling outer retinal telangiectasia.

Multiple tumors tend to occur in the same retinal quadrant. The earliest endophytic tumors tend to be in the peripheral retina, with subsequent tumors appearing proximally in the same quadrant, having the same feeding and draining vessels. Fluorescein angiography shows arteriovenous shunting of blood through the tumor or tumors with an associated relative hypoperfusion of the retina peripheral to the tumor, suggestive of a vascular steal syndrome. Although not proven, the subsequent, more proximal angiomas may well represent a 'neovascular angiomatous' reaction in a susceptible vascular bed.

Hemangiomas of the optic disk often mimic papilledema or disk edema; untreated retinal angiomatosis often leads to vitreous hemorrhage, total retinal detachment, secondary glaucoma, and phthisis bulbi.

TREATMENT

Surgical

Angiomatosis retinae is usually a progressive disease, so therapy should begin as soon as diagnosis is made. The treatment selected depends on the size and location of the tumor or tumors, the clarity of the ocular media, and the associated ocular complications. In treating smaller tumors with a clear medium, argon laser photocoagulation has proven effective; treatment should consist of a large spot size and low-intensity and long-duration burns directed at the angioma itself. Multiple treatment sessions should be planned for all but the smallest tumors. The endpoint should be the obliteration of the tumor both by clinical observation and by fluorescein angiography. Once the tumor becomes yellowish (secondary to gliosis and lipid ingestion), photocoagulation becomes difficult because of poor penetration of the laser light.

Anterior angiomas and larger posterior angiomas may be treated successfully with cryotherapy using a repetitive freeze-thaw technique. Only two or three freeze-thaw cycles should be used at each therapy session to minimize the risk of hemorrhage. Multiple treatment sessions usually are required. Eradication of the tumor or tumors by cryotherapy or photocoagulation usually results in resolution of the macular edema and improved visual acuity.

For larger angiomas, angiomas unresponsive to cryotherapy or photocoagulation, and those associated with retinal detachment, penetrating diathermy under a lamellar scleral bed has proven effective. If there is extensive subretinal exudation, the fluid should be drained and a scleral buckling procedure considered. Frequently, large tumors develop surface membranes and vitreous traction that can lead to vitreous hemorrhage or rhegmatogenous retinal detachment; these complications may be amenable to treatment using the following:

- Vitreous surgery techniques;
- Endodiathermy;
- Scleral buckling procedures.

The peripapillary and optic disk angiomas are difficult to treat without destroying useful central vision; diffuse exophytic peripapillary hemangiomas with associated visual loss may be considered for laser photocoagulation, using a wavelength that spares the inner retina and is well absorbed by blood; treatment should be conservative and aimed at the foci of greatest leakage.

PRECAUTIONS

Because these tumors are highly vascular, any form of treatment may cause further leakage or hemorrhage before the vascular channels are obliterated. This may result in further visual loss from macular exudation, vitreous hemorrhage and retinal detachment. Proliferative vitreoretinopathy frequently occurs after treatment of large tumors. Most of these complications are only exacerbations of the normal course of the disease process; however, many complications can be minimized by treating the angioma in multiple sessions rather than performing an aggressive single-session treatment.

Treatment is best accomplished when the tumor is small. Prognosis for vision is related to the size and location of the tumor and to associated complications at the time therapy is initiated. Early detection of a peripheral tumor results in a good prognosis, whereas large tumors with an associated retinal detachment or angiomas of the optic nerve have a less favorable prognosis.

These tumors are often multiple or bilateral or both, so close follow-up is important. Furthermore, because there is a familial tendency, other family members should be evaluated. The retinal angioma is the earliest and most common manifestation detected in screening examinations of families documented to have von Hippel–Lindau disease.

COMMENTS

About 20% of patients presenting with retinal angiomas develop multiple systemic involvement (von Hippel–Lindau disease), so patients with angiomatosis retinae should have a thorough systemic evaluation. Cerebellar hemangioma is the typical CNS tumor in von Hippel–Lindau disease and it tends to occur somewhat later than the retinal angioma. The cerebellar tumor is similar to the retinal angioma in histologic appearance and in having large feeding and draining vessels.

In von Hippel–Lindau disease, angiomas also may be found in the medulla oblongata, spinal cord, liver, or kidney. Cysts of the liver, pancreas, kidney, and epididymis occasionally are found as well, as is an elevated incidence of pheochromocytoma and renal cell carcinoma. In patients with von Hippel–Lindau disease, renal cell carcinoma is the most common cause of death, followed closely by cerebellar hemangioblastoma.

Vasoproliferative angiomatous lesions are not infrequently found in the peripheral retina and can mimic von Hippel's angiomas. There is evidence that both are related to upregulation of vascular endothelial growth factor (VEGF), and both may be amenable to treatment in the future with anti-VEGF agents.

The gene for von Hippel–Lindau disease recently has been mapped to the short arm of chromosome 3 (3p25-p26) and appears to function at the molecular level as does the retinoblastoma gene-that is, as a recessive tumor-suppressor gene. Early detection is important for genetic counseling, and it improves the visual prognosis by allowing early treatment of retinal angiomas. Diagnosis using DNA markers allows relatives at low risk to be screened less often, thus enabling a focus on affected individuals and high-risk relatives.

SUPPORT GROUPS

See internet *www.vhl.org* or email at info@vhl.org.

REFERENCES

Annesley WJ, Jr, Leonard BC, Shields JA, et al: Fifteen-year review of treated cases of retinal angiomatosis. Trans Am Acad Ophthalmol Otolaryngol 83:446–453, 1977.

Filling-Katz MR, Choyke PL, Oldfield E, et al: Central nervous system involvement in von Hippel-Lindau disease. Neurology 41:41–46, 1991.

Gass JDM, Braunstein R: Sessile and exophytic capillary angiomas of the juxtapapillary retina and optic nerve head. Arch Ophthalmol 98:1790–1797, 1980.

Hardwig P, Robertson DM: von Hippel-Lindau disease: a familial, often lethal, multi-system phakomatosis. Ophthalmology 91:263–270, 1984.

Lindau A: Zur Frage der Angiomatosis Retinae und ihrer Hirnkomplikationen. Acta Ophthalmol 4:193–209, 1926.

Machemer R, Williams JM, Sr: Pathogenesis and therapy of traction detachment in various retinal vascular diseases. Am J Ophthalmol 105:170–181, 1988.

Machmichael IM: von Hippel-Lindau's disease of the optic disc. Trans Ophthalmol Soc UK 90:877–885, 1970.

Maher ER, Bentley E, Yates JRW, et al: Localization of the gene for von Hippel-Lindau disease to a small region of chromosome 3 confirmed by genetic linkage analysis. Genomics 10:957–960, 1991.

Maher ER, Yates JRW, Harries R, et al: Clinical features and natural history of von Hippel-Lindau disease. QJ Med 77.1151–1163, 1990.

Miyagawa Y, Nakazawa, M, Noda Y, et al: von Hippel-Lindau disease type 2A in a family with a duplicated 21-base-pair-in frame insertion mutation in the VHL gene. Graefes Arch Clin Exp Ophthalmol 241:241–244, 2003.

Moore AT, Maher ER, Rosen P, et al: Ophthalmological screening for von Hippel-Lindau disease. Eye 5:723–728, 1991.

Neumann HP, Wiestler OD: Clustering of features of von Hippel-Lindau syndrome: Evidence for a complex genetic locus. Lancet 337:1052–1054, 1991.

Nicholson DH, Green WR, Kenyon KR: Light and electron microscopic study of early lesions in angiomatosis retinae. Am J Ophthalmol 82:193–204, 1976.

Shields JA: Diagnosis and management of intraocular tumors. St Louis, CV Mosby, 1983:534–556.

von Hippel E: Uber eine sehr seltene Erkrankung der Netzhaut; Klinische Beobachtungen. Graefes Arch Clin Exp Ophthalmol 59:83–97, 1904.

Welch RB: von Hippel-Lindau disease: The recognition and treatment of early angiomatosis retinae and the use of cyrosurgery as an adjunct to therapy. Trans Am Ophthalmol Soc 68:367–424, 1970.

Wing GL, Weiter JJ, Kelly PJ, et al: von Hippel-Lindau disease angiomatosis of the retina and central nervous system. Ophthalmology 88:1311–1314, 1981.

104 NEUROFIBROMATOSIS TYPE 1

237.7

(NF1, von Recklinghausen's Disease, Peripheral Variant of Neurofibromatosis)

Nastaran Rafiei, MD
Baltimore, Maryland
Cameron F. Parsa, MD
Baltimore, Maryland

ETIOLOGY/INCIDENCE

Neurofibromatosis (NF) is an autosomal dominant disorder predominantly affecting neuroectodermal derived tissue. It is characterized, thus, by the development of hamartomas of the skin and nervous system, increasing in number and size throughout life. In 1988, neurofibromatosis was reclassified into two distinct variants, NF1 and NF2.

NF1 occurs in approximately 1 in 4000 individuals and generally features multiple café-au-lait spots, cutaneous neurofibromas and iris hamartomas (Sakurai–Lisch nodules). Half of affected individuals inherit the disease, while the others have novel mutations of predominantly paternal origin (with no apparent relation to paternal age).

The genetic mutation responsible for NF1 is in a tumor suppressor gene has been mapped to chromosome 17q11.2. The protein encoded by the gene, neurofibromin, is expressed at reduced levels in NF1, resulting in down-regulation of the ras protein (a protein that is involved in cell growth and differentiation) and dysregulated cell growth. Deletion of a second copy of this tumor-suppressing gene is necessary for development of malignancies.

COURSE AND PROGNOSIS

Expressivity is highly variable and many patients with NF1 lead a normal life. Others, however, may have tumors of the central nervous system, structural abnormalities, or secondary malignancies. Visual prognosis depends on the presence or absence of optic pathway gliomas and orbital plexiform neurofibromas.

DIAGNOSIS

Clinical signs and symptoms

The 1988 National Institute of Health Consensus Development Statement has suggested the presence of two or more of the following criteria for the diagnosis of NF1:

- Six or more café-au-lait spots, 5 mm or larger in prepubertal children, 15 mm or larger after puberty;
- Two or more neurofibromas of any type (e.g. placoid, nodular, pedunculated), or one plexiform neurofibroma;
- 'Freckles' in intertriginous areas;
- Glioma involving the anterior visual pathways;
- Two or more Sakurai–Lisch nodules;
- A distinctive osseous lesion such as sphenoid dysplasia or thinning of the cortex of the long bone (with or without pseudoarthrosis);
- A first-degree relative who has NF1 by these criteria.

Cutaneous manifestations

Cutaneous manifestations include café-au-lait spots, neurofibromas and plexiform neurofibromas. Although over 10% of the general population may have one to three café-au-lait spots, nearly 99% of individuals with NF1 have multiple café-au-lait spots increasing in number and size with age. Neurofibromas are benign tumors consisting of Schwann cells admixed with nerve fibers, perineural cells and fibroblasts in various ratios accounting for differences in morphology. They grow around the time of puberty, continuing to enlarge throughout life. They contain increased numbers of mast cells and may be associated with pain, tenderness, or itchiness. Plexiform neurofibromas have markedly enlarged nerves surrounded by a thickened perineural sheath, and possess a 'bag of worms' consistency. Malignant degeneration of neurofibromas occurs in 5% of individuals.

Nervous system

Juvenile pilocytic astrocytomas are common. While MRI studies have demonstrated the presence of gliomas in over 25% of patients with NF1, clinical symptoms occur in only a fraction of these. Occasionally, ependymomas, meningiomas and primitive neuroectodermal tumors may develop.

Occasionally, mild cognitive impairment may result in various learning disabilities.

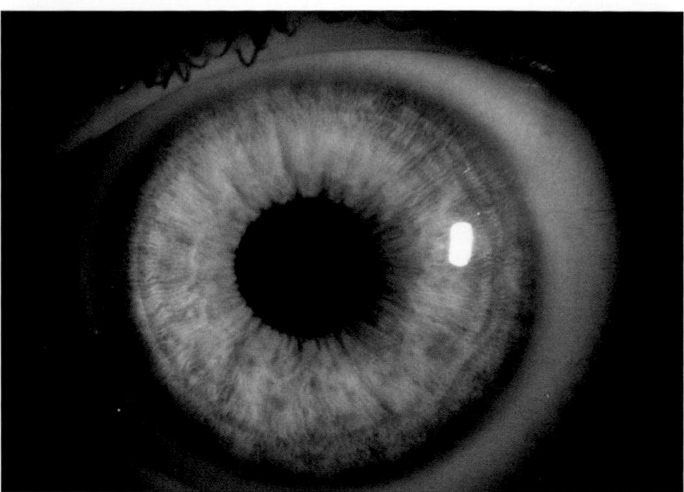

FIGURE 104.1. Multiple tan-colored and dome-shaped melanocytic hamartomas, Lisch–Sakurai nodules, are highly suggestive of NF1. They increase in number with age and may develop more commonly on the inferior aspect of the iris. The morphologic appearance, however, varies widely.

Ophthalmic involvement

Sakurai–Lisch nodules, smooth, dome-shaped pigmented hamartomas of the iris, are not noted at birth, but are usually seen by age 10 years, and by age 30, are present in essentially all individuals with NF1. Although not pathognomonic, the presence of Sakurai–Lisch nodules is highly suggestive of NF1 and screening of family members is often warranted (Figure 104.1).

Hamartomas of the conjunctiva, uveal tract or retina, and corkscrew retinal vascular abnormalities may be present. Indocyanine green angiography reveals hypofluorescent areas of the choroid.

Proptosis may be present due to optic nerve glioma, orbital neurofibroma, or sphenoid bone defects. Periocular plexiform neurofibromas may cause glaucoma, ptosis and amblyopia.

Musculoskeletal involvement

Musculoskeletal abnormalities include progressive kyphoscoliosis, pseudoarthrosis (often of the tibia), and hypoplasia of the sphenoid bone.

Other manifestations

Other tumors of neural-crest origin such as pheochromocytoma and neuroblastoma also occur with increased frequency. However, as for the musculoskeletal manifestations of NF1 and for reasons not yet well understood, non-neural crest derived conditions such as rhabdomyosarcoma and myelogenous leukemia are also associated. Neurofibromin is expressed in endothelial cells and the NF1 gene plays an essential role in endothelial development with an increased incidence of congenital heart disease in those who harbor a mutation. Secondary hypertension occasionally develops from pheochromocytoma or renal artery stenosis.

Laboratory findings

T2-weighted MRI images demonstrate multiple 'bright lesions' in the basal ganglia, cerebellum and brain stem in up to 80% of affected children — these decrease with age. Although a quarter of children imaged may also have gliomas, routine MR imaging for screening purposes is not recommended since the findings may not assist in management.

Optic nerve gliomas associated with NF1 often develop a perineural arachnoidal hyperplasia. The high water content of this tissue produces an image on T2-weighted MR imagery that looks like an expanded CSF space around the nerve. This so-called 'pseudo-CSF signal' is a specific marker of NF1.

Although the NF1 gene has been cloned and characterized, its high mutation rate has limited the sensitivity and diagnostic value of laboratory-based genetic testing.

Differential diagnosis

Ten times less frequent than NF1, NF2 ('central' or 'acoustic' neurofibromatosis) is characterized by vestibular schwannomas (acoustic neuromas) and the development of tumors typically involving neural coverings (meningiomas, schwannomas and ependymomas). Combined hamartomas of the retinal pigment epithelium and retina may be present. Sakurai–Lisch nodules are generally absent, but most affected individuals have presenile posterior lens opacities. Optic disc gliomas are rare, but highly suggestive of NF2. There is a relative lack of cutaneous findings. The genetic mutation has been mapped to the long arm of chromosome 22.

TREATMENT

Observation with supportive treatment is generally recommended for optic pathway gliomas, which can regress spontaneously. Due to germline tumor-suppressor gene haploinsufficiency, treatment of NF1-associated tumors with alkylating agent chemotherapy and irradiation can produce somatic mutations throughout the body leading to subsequent malignant neoplasms.

Plexiform neurofibromas affecting the orbit are generally diffuse and not fully excisable, with residua often leading to recurrences. Despite the cosmetic disfigurement, such tumors are often best left alone.

Mast cell stabilizers such as oral ketotifen may reduce the itchiness, tenderness and pain associated with neurofibromas, and retard their growth. Occasionally, excision may be required. Anticipation and management of NF1 associated conditions such as secondary hypertension and malignancies is an important aspect of care, as is family counseling.

REFERENCES

Arun D, Gutmann DH: Recent advances in neurofibromatosis type 1. Curr Opin Neurol 17:101–105, 2004.

Beauchamp GR: Neurofibromatosis type 1 in children. Trans Am Ophthalmol Soc 93:445–472, 1995.

Brodsky MC: The 'pseudo-CSF' signal of orbital optic glioma on magnetic resonance imaging: a signature of neurofibromatosis. Surv Ophthalmol 38:213–218, 1993.

Critler AD, Zhu Y, Ismat FA, et al: NF1 has an essential role in endothelial cells. Nat Genet 33:75–79, 2003.

DiMario FJ Jr, Ramsby G, Greenstein R, et al: Neurofibromatosis type 1: magnetic resonance imaging findings. J Child Neurol 8:32–39, 1993.

Jadayel D, Fain P, Upadhyaya M, et al: Paternal origin of new mutations in von Recklinghausen neurofibromatosis. Nature 343:558–559, 1990.

Muci-Mendoza R, Ramella M, Fuenmayor-Rivera D: Corkscrew retinal vessels in neurofibromatosis type 1: report of 12 cases. Br J Ophthalmol 86:282–284, 2002.

Riccardi VM: A controlled multiphase trial of ketotifen to minimize neurofibroma-associated pain and itching. Arch Dermatol 129:577–581, 1993.

Sakurai T: Multiple neurofibroma patient showing multiple flecks on the anterior surface of the iris. Acta Soc Ophthal Jpn 39:87–93, 1935.

Yasunari T, Shiraki K, Hattori H, Miki T: Frequency of choroidal abnormalities in neurofibromatosis type 1. Lancet 356:988–992, 2000.

105 STURGE–WEBER SYNDROME
759.6
(Encephalotrigeminal Angiomatosis Syndrome)

Monte A. Del Monte, MD
Ann Arbor, Michigan

Sturge–Weber syndrome (SWS) belongs to a group of disorders collectively known as phakomatoses ('mother-spot' diseases). It consists of congenital hamartomatous malformations that may affect the eyes, skin, and central nervous system at different times. SWS is classified into three categories:

1. Complete trisymptomatic SWS, in which all three organ systems are involved;
2. Incomplete bisymptomatic SWS, in which the involvement is either oculocutaneous or neurocutaneous;
3. Incomplete monosymptomatic SWS, in which there is only neural or cutaneous involvement.

Patients without cutaneous involvement appear to be spared the ocular manifestations of the syndrome.

ETIOLOGY/INCIDENCE

The clinical manifestations of SWS have a common embryologic basis, the primary defect being a developmental insult affecting precursors of tissues that originate in the pro- and mesencephalic neural crest. These affected precursors then give rise to vascular and other tissue malformations in the meninges, the eyes and the dermis. Sources of the insult have been suggested to be:

- A somatic mutation in the precursors that may result in overproduction of an angiogenic factor; or
- A lethal gene, surviving by mosaicism.

Incomplete SWS results from the same developmental defect but affects only those cells whose progeny are destined for the affected tissues.

Unlike the other phakomatoses, which often have clear-cut hereditary patterns, the role of heredity in SWS has not been documented; to date, no gene defect has been associated with the syndrome. Several types of chromosomal abnormalities have been reported, but most SWS patients have normal karyotypes. The majority of SWS patients have a sporadic, nonfamilial disease.

The syndrome occurs in all races, with no significant predilection for either sex. The incidence of SWS in the general population is unknown.

DIAGNOSIS

Clinical signs and symptoms

Systemic

The hallmark of SWS is a facial cutaneous venous dilation, also referred to as nevus flammeus or port-wine stain, that occurs in as many as 96% of patients and is visible at birth. The nevus appears as one or more dull red patches of irregular outline, usually in the areas of the trigeminal nerve branches. Although it does not increase in size and is not medically threatening, the nevus does darken with age, and as a cosmetic blemish, it may carry psychologic impact.

A leptomeningeal congenital venous angiomatosis, usually ipsilateral to the facial lesion and located most commonly in the meninges overlying the occipital and posterior parietal lobes, results in involvement of the central nervous system (CNS). Characteristic progressive calcifications in the external layers of the cerebral cortex beneath the angiomatosis are associated with cortical atrophy; occasionally, they extend anteriorly to the frontal and temporal lobes.

Focal or generalized motor seizures occur in up to 85% of patients; they usually begin in the first year of life and may become profound, resulting in further neurologic and developmental deterioration. Early diagnosis and treatment are necessary to minimize permanent brain damage.

Some degree of mental retardation is seen in about 60% of patients, as well as neurologic deficits such as:

- Hemiplegia;
- Homonymous hemianopsia.

Ocular

- Eyelid hemangioma-like superficial changes that show, on histology, only venous dilation.
- Glaucoma, which is a significant cause of morbidity because of its early onset and resistance to conventional forms of treatment.
- Conjunctival and episcleral hemangiomas.
- Prominent, tortuous conjunctival and episcleral vascular plexi.
- Diffuse choroidal hemangiomas.
- Iris heterochromia.
- Tortuous retinal vessels, with occasional arteriovenous communications.

Glaucoma is estimated to occur in 30% to 70% of patients, with early onset (at birth or in early infancy) the rule, although it may present at any time. The glaucoma is almost always unilateral and ipsilateral to the port-wine stain, although contralateral or bilateral glaucoma with unilateral skin lesions have been reported. Occurrence of glaucoma has been noted especially when the facial skin changes involve both the upper and lower eyelids.

As soon as SWS is suspected, a complete ophthalmic evaluation is essential to rule out glaucoma or to institute effective measures to control it, as the infant eye is quickly damaged by increased intraocular pressure (IOP). The earlier glaucoma can be detected and controlled, the less likely the patient is to suffer the secondary glaucomatous changes, including buphthalmos, increased corneal diameter, tears in Descemet's membrane, corneal edema, and optic nerve damage that results in myopia, anisometropia, amblyopia, strabismus and visual field defects. All SWS patients require regular ophthalmic examination throughout life, even when no ocular abnormalities are initially detected, to avoid vision loss secondary to later-onset glaucoma.

Amblyopia is an important cause of poor vision in patients with infantile glaucoma. It is usually anisometropic because of glaucoma-induced myopia or secondary to unilateral or bilateral pattern deprivation caused by cloudy corneas. Even when glaucomatous optic nerve damage is present, amblyopia may be superimposed on the organic damage and a trial of amblyopia therapy is indicated.

Prominent tortuous conjunctival and episcleral vascular plexi affect up to 70% of SWS patients and often correlate with increased episcleral venous pressure, probably resulting from arteriovenous shunts within the episcleral hemangiomas.

Diffuse choroidal hemangioma (which appears as a circumscribed, isolated form in otherwise normal adults) is present in up to 50% of patients with SWS. Almost always unilateral, and ipsilateral to the port-wine stain, choroidal hemangiomas also have been reported as bilateral in association with bilateral nevus flammeus. These hemangiomas:

- Are flat;
- Commonly cover more than half the fundus;
- Involve the posterior pole;
- Extend into the equatorial zone;
- May show diffuse involvement of the entire uvea;
- Can have a striking reddish 'tomato ketchup fundus' appearance.

Often a focal, perimacular area of the angioma is thickened and elevated, with dilation and tortuosity of the overlying retinal vessels and peripheral arteriovenous communications.

Choroidal angiomatosis grows slowly and is usually asymptomatic in childhood, but during adolescence or adulthood a marked thickening of the choroid may become evident, with secondary changes to overlying ocular structures. These changes can range from mild atrophy of retinal pigment epithelium (RPE) and focal RPE proliferation with drusen formation to severe fibrous transformation and focal ossification of the RPE.

The retina over the hemangioma may be attached and well preserved, attached but degenerated, or detached. Early-stage choroidal thickening and lifting of the retina may produce an increasing ipsilateral hyperopia. Degenerative retinal changes include focal chorioretinal adhesions, loss of photoreceptors, severe cystoid degeneration of the outer layers, and marked gliosis. Widespread serous detachment, retinal leakage, and edema may occur. Subretinal fibrosis near the macula and cystoid macular edema are associated with the most severe visual loss.

Glaucomatous damage, degenerative changes in the outer retinal layers, and vascular abnormalities in the occipital lobe may cause visual field defects; careful examination with visual field perimetry is indicated.

Iris heterochromia occurs in about 10% of SWS patients; the more deeply pigmented iris usually is ipsilateral to the port-wine stain, indicating an increase in melanocyte numbers or activity.

Laboratory findings

The three forms of SWS are generally diagnosed on clinical grounds by the association of the typical cutaneous, CNS, and ocular abnormalities.

When a typical facial vascular skin lesion is found in a newborn, it should alert the physician to perform a complete ophthalmologic and systemic assessment for the potentially serious associated disorders. Neonates with bisymptomatic or trisymptomatic SWS may initially seem neurologically normal, without symptoms of glaucoma or other ocular problems; thus, in some instances the diagnosis may not become clear for some time.

In young patients with suspected glaucoma, examination under anesthesia or deep sedation is necessary to confirm the diagnosis; careful assessment in each eye of intraocular pressure, corneal diameter, cycloplegic refraction, axial length, gonioscopy, and optic nerve cupping is mandatory.

Ocular signs of infantile glaucoma associated with SWS include:

- Corneal diameter >12.0 mm during the first year of life;
- Corneal edema;
- Tears in Descemet's membrane (Haab's striae);
- Unilateral or bilateral myopic shift;
- Optic nerve cupping >0.3 or any cup asymmetry;
- Intraocular pressure >18 or 19 mm Hg.

Increased conjunctival vascularity can be observed on a slit-lamp examination or can be seen by the naked eye as a pinkish discoloration. However, the abnormal plexus of episcleral vessels may be hidden by the overlying tissue of Tenon's capsule in infancy and appreciated clinically only in later childhood.

Diagnosis of diffuse choroidal hemangioma is based on:

- Tumor appearance on binocular indirect ophthalmoscopy;
- A- and B-scan ultrasonography; A-scan shows high internal reflectivity, whereas B-scan typically shows a solid echogenic mass;
- Fluorescein angiography may reveal;
- Only a heightened background choroidal fluorescence early in the disease;
- Widespread irregular hyperfluorescence as dye leaks from the surface of a progressing tumor;
- A diffuse multilocalized pattern of fluorescein accumulation in the outer retina characteristic of polycystic degeneration and edema in more advanced disease.

Diffuse choroidal hemangioma may easily be missed on ophthalmoscopic examination, especially in children, because the color of the hemangioma resembles that of the normal fundus, and the elevation may be minimal; comparison of the red reflex with the normal opposite eye can help in confirming the diagnosis.

Central nervous system involvement can be confirmed by various neuroimaging methods:

- Plain skull radiographs are often adequate for diagnosis.
- Magnetic resonance imaging (MRI) allows detection of malformations affecting the CNS, including abnormal venous drainage and abnormal pial contrast enhancement associated with SWS angiomatous malformations, and it can detect cerebral volume reduction and ipsilateral choroid plexus enlargement; in addition, the technique can demonstrate the curvilinear posterior contrast enhancement of ocular choroidal angiomas, using intravenous contrast.
- Computed tomography (CT) is superior to MRI in detecting the characteristic double-lined gyroform pattern of calcifications paralleling cerebral convolutions, which are known to radiologists as the 'railroad track' sign; however, these calcifications usually are not detectable before 1 year of age and may not be seen until several years of age.

Differential diagnosis

Disorders with clinical presentations similar to those of SWS must be included in differential diagnosis. They include the following:

- Klippel–Trenaunay–Weber (KTW) syndrome consists of port-wine stains of the extremities and face and hemihypertrophy of soft and bony tissues, as well as all the characteristics of SWS; KTW syndrome is sporadic, as is SWS. There is also an association in KTW syndrome between hemi-

hypertrophy and solid visceral tumors that most commonly affect the kidney, adrenal gland, or liver.
- Beckwith–Wiedemann syndrome consists of a facial port-wine stain, macroglossia, omphalocele, and visceral hyperplasia; note that there is also some associated risk of visceral neoplasia. Also, severe hypoglycemia resulting from pancreatic islet cell hyperplasia is very common and may be life threatening.

Neuroimaging findings similar to those of SWS may be found in several other conditions and should also be considered in the differential diagnosis:
- In Dyke–Davidoff–Masson syndrome, one cerebral hemisphere is partially or completely atrophic as a result of an intrauterine or perinatal carotid artery infarction; because the cerebral atrophy in SWS also occurs during infancy, changes similar to those of Dyke–Davidoff–Masson syndrome may be seen, including cerebral hemiatrophy with ipsilateral calvarial diploic space enlargement.
- Severe siderosis, prior to injection of contrast material, has MRI findings similar to those in SWS with cerebral hemiatrophy. The typical contrast enhancement and the abnormal veins seen with contrast injection easily differentiate the two conditions.
- Calcification secondary to intrathecal methotrexate therapy and meningitis also must be included in the CT differential diagnosis of cortical pattern calcification; neither of these, however, would demonstrate the specific unilateral geographic localization.

When assessing the status of a uveal mass in a patient with SWS, the ophthalmologist must consider the possibility that the lesion may be something other than a choroidal hemangioma.
- The major clinical difficulty can be distinguishing a choroidal hemangioma from a choroidal melanoma. There are a few reports of patients with SWS who developed a choroidal tumor in the eye ipsilateral to the port-wine stain, and it eventually proved to be a malignant melanoma rather than a hemangioma. Simultaneous occurrence of uveal melanoma and choroidal hemangioma in a patient with SWS also has been described. The reddish-orange color of choroidal hemangiomas as viewed by binocular indirect ophthalmoscopy is an important diagnostic sign that differentiates them from metastatic carcinomas and amelanotic melanomas which have a white or creamy appearance. When uveal melanoma is suspected, both fluorescein angiography and A- and B-scan ultrasonography are essential.
- Other orange-colored fundus tumors that must be considered in a differential diagnosis of a diffuse choroidal hemangioma include.
- Serous or partly organized detachment of the retinal pigment epithelium.
- Osteoma of the choroids.
- Nodular scleritis.
- Exophytic retinal capillary hemangioma.

TREATMENT

Ocular

For small degrees of anisometropia, full optical correction of both eyes or at least full correction of the refractive difference between the eyes is desirable. In higher degrees of anisometropia or if the child develops strabismus, treatment to prevent *amblyopia* and treat the strabismus should be initiated. Anisometropic amblyopia may require occlusion therapy along with correction of the refractive error; in some patients, a contact lens may be required to treat fusion difficulty due to aniseikonia.

Medical treatment for SWS *glaucoma* usually fails with time but may be tried initially, as significant (albeit temporary) reduction in IOP may be achieved. Reduced IOP may clear the cornea and permit surgery to proceed or, in younger patients, delay the need for filtration surgery. This is especially important considering the excessive difficulties of operating on a small eye, as well as the tendency of the younger patient to scar at the site of the scleral flap, which may reduce long-term success.

Medical therapy can also be used as an adjunct to surgery. Topical antiglaucoma therapy for extended periods is sometimes helpful postoperatively to further reduce borderline elevations in IOP without the need to reoperate. Initial medical therapy with a:
- Topical β-blocker, followed sequentially by the addition of a carbonic anhydrase inhibitor (systemic in infants and topical in older children), and an α-adrenergic agonist (brimonidine), or a topical prostaglandin receptor agonist (latanoprost) is a reasonable protocol in SWS patients.

In recent years, few patients with *diffuse choroidal hemangiomas* associated with a bullous nonrhegmatogenous retinal detachment have been treated with radiation therapy such as:
- Brachytherapy; or
- External beam irradiation.

Preliminary reports suggest that radiation therapy may be a reasonable alternative to the currently preferred photocoagulation in selected patients, but the ultimate risk-to-benefit ratio of this form of therapy is still unknown, as are its precise indications and contraindications.

Surgical

Surgery, rather than medical therapy, is still considered by most ophthalmologists to be the mainstay for *glaucoma* therapy in SWS, with antiglaucoma medications being used primarily as adjuncts. The selection of surgical technique remains controversial, however, because the long-term results are often disappointing with any of the procedures, and none of them enjoys the success with SWS glaucoma that it may have when initially performed for primary infantile glaucoma.

Because of the rarity of SWS, the published accounts of surgically treated cases have been uncontrolled, and no standard guidelines exist. *The objective of therapy is rapid and permanent lowering of the IOP* into the normal range (generally, <20 mm Hg) or to a level slightly higher but without progression of other signs, such as corneal enlargement, increased myopia, or increased optic nerve cupping.

Postoperative care for infants and young children commonly requires repeated examinations under anesthesia to assess surgical success. If continued borderline IOP elevation is found, then a trial of medical therapy with close follow-up may be safely continued as long as no progression of glaucoma damage is observed. However, if IOP remains clearly elevated or progressive glaucomatous damage is detected, repeat glaucoma surgery should be performed.

The anesthesiologist should be made aware that the patient has SWS, because the presence of a spinal cord or brain hemangioma may increase the risk of intracerebral bleeding or disseminated intravascular coagulation with anesthesia. In addition, an anesthesia protocol should be planned to prevent the development of hypertension that could result in hemorrhage.

- *Goniotomy* or *trabeculotomy* is believed by some to be the treatment of choice for early-onset glaucoma in infancy, when the probable mechanism for pressure elevation is an abnormal outflow angle. However, these procedures often are unsuccessful in infants with SWS, or they succeed only after being repeated several times and with the addition of adjunct medical therapy; in patients over the age of 4, an even shorter duration of pressure control is the rule. Nevertheless, some physicians prefer to perform these procedures initially because they are occasionally successful and goniotomy is also thought to be less likely to cause the complications (especially expulsive choroidal hemorrhage or choroidal effusion) that are associated with a precipitous drop in IOP.
- *Trabeculectomy* (either full- or partial-thickness) is more likely to be successful in treating glaucoma of later onset, when the outflow angle appears clinically normal, as it bypasses any component of the glaucoma possibly caused by elevated episcleral venous pressure. *Combined trabeculotomy-trabeculectomy* may be a reasonable compromise in the older patient with SWS, in view of the possible combination of angle abnormality and raised episcleral pressure in causing SWS glaucoma.
- *Adjunctive antimetabolites,* used in conjunction with a filtering surgery, may achieve a more satisfactory degree of IOP control in this patient population by slowing wound healing and scar formation. The most commonly used clinical agents are 5-fluorouracil (5-FU), given as a series of subconjunctival injections postoperatively, and mitomycin C, usually applied intraoperatively using a sponge saturated with the solution. Postoperative subconjunctival injections are usually impossible in very young patients, so the intraoperative application of mitomycin C is frequently required for these cases.

Both 5-fluorouracil and mitomycin C are associated with thinner, more cystic blebs and may carry a higher rate of complications such as wound leak, chronic hypotony, and possibly late endophthalmitis.

- *Corticosteroids* should be used after filtration surgery to minimize postoperative inflammation and scarring of the bleb. A sub-Tenon's injection of a short-acting corticosteroid such as dexamethasone or triamcinolone at the completion of surgery and the use of topical corticosteroid drops or ointment after surgery are recommended.
- *Cyclocryotherapy* is difficult to control and has a high complication rate; therefore, it should be used to save useful vision or to prevent or relieve severe pain only when all other procedures have failed or are not feasible. New types of cyclodestructive procedures, such as Nd : YAG transscleral laser and therapeutic ultrasound, have had only limited trial in pediatric and SWS glaucoma, and their potential for long-term success as well as the complications they may cause in the young patient is not yet fully understood.
- *Seton devices* also are being used when routine filtration surgery has failed. Encouraging initial results have been reported using various posterior tube shunt implant devices, but long-term follow-up results are not yet available.
- *Neodymium-YAG laser goniotomy* and *argon laser trabeculoplasty* have been used only to a limited extent in pediatric glaucoma, but favorable results in some SWS patients have been reported.
- *Eye muscle surgery* is the best treatment for any significant strabismus still present after completion of amblyopia therapy, refractive lens correction, and orthoptics. Avoidance or careful cauterization of the dilated subconjunctival and episcleral vessels during strabismus surgery is important in order to prevent bleeding and scarring so that the conjunctiva and anterior sclera can be preserved for future glaucoma procedures.

Unfortunately, no treatment has yet been shown to be effective in preventing or reversing the visual deterioration associated with the secondary changes of ocular structures overlying a *diffuse choroidal hemangioma.* Management of affected eyes emphasizes the reduction of subretinal fluid as the main therapeutic aim in an attempt to stabilize or reverse, if possible, visual impairment caused by nonrhegmatogenous retinal detachment. However, no reliable treatment for the retinal detachment that develops in these patients has been found, and even in the exceptional case in which the retina can be reattached, fibrous metaplasia of the retinal pigment epithelium and cystoid degeneration of the retina overlying the choroidal hemangioma prevent good visual results. Many such eyes eventually become blind and painful and must be enucleated. Attempts to repair the nonrhegmatogenous retinal detachment involve:

- Cryotherapy and diathermy;
- Xenon arc or argon laser photocoagulation;
- Draining of the subretinal fluid;
- Radiation therapy.

A factor critical to a successful outcome appears to be early initiation of treatment.

- Laser photocoagulation is generally considered to be the preferred therapeutic intervention. Light photocoagulation scars are placed over the entire tumor in an attempt to strengthen the adhesion of the retina to the underlying pigment epithelium and thus prevent the spread of the retinal detachment; this form of treatment has afforded limited success. However, retinal detachment often recurs even after photocoagulation therapy, and in some patients it is not possible to attain complete reattachment of the retina. Furthermore, with large hemangiomas and diffuse infiltrating tumors of the macula, treatment success is limited.
- External drainage of subretinal fluid, with or without scleral buckling in conjunction with xenon photocoagulation, has been used to treat diffuse choroidal hemangiomas associated with large exudative retinal detachments in SWS.
- Pars plana vitrectomy, endolaser and internal drainage of subretinal fluid can be performed.
- Cryotherapy and penetrating diathermy are of limited use because of the posterior location of the tumor.
- Dye laser photocoagulation has been very helpful in reducing the cosmetic blemish of the cutaneous port-wine stain.

PRECAUTIONS

Surgical management of secondary open-angle glaucoma in SWS using filtering surgery and Seton procedures bears an increased risk for a number of surgical complications, the most sight-threatening and feared being *expulsive choroidal hemorrhage* and *intraoperative massive choroidal effusion*.

- Sudden change in the IOP gradient when the eye is opened may result in expulsive choroidal hemorrhage from the choroidal hemangioma. Treatment involves rapid closure of all scleral incisions, with restoration of IOP. Transscleral drainage of suprachoroidal blood also may be indicated.
- The intraoperative formation of a massive choroidal effusion without hemorrhage also occurs frequently during filtering surgery in SWS patients. It is assumed that the increased episcleral venous pressure in these patients causes a similar increase in the venous pressure within the ciliary body and choroid. During surgery, when the eye is opened and IOP falls, rapid transudation of fluid from the intravascular to the extravascular space results. This extravasation of fluid may be massive enough to cause choroidal detachment instantaneously, as well as later serous retinal detachment; however, it seems that once the intraoperative effusion is managed with immediate drainage, the postoperative prognosis becomes excellent despite the persistence of some degree of choroidal and serous retinal detachment.
- Postoperatively, smaller serous choroidal detachment may develop.
- Serous retinal detachment often occurs in association with choroidal effusion and hypotony; it is possible that a choroidal effusion temporarily interferes with the metabolic transport systems of the retinal pigment epithelium. These serous retinal detachments usually resolve spontaneously as the IOP normalizes.

Various preoperative and perioperative measures have been suggested to counteract or prevent these complications, including hyperosmotics, maximum antiglaucoma therapy preoperatively, prophylactic posterior sclerotomy, prophylactic radiotherapy or laser photocoagulation of the choroidal hemangioma, and electrocautery of the anterior episcleral vascular anomaly.

Suggested steps to minimize the intraoperative and postoperative hypotony are preplacement of scleral flap sutures, injection of a viscoelastic prior to excision of the trabecular meshwork, and tight suturing of the scleral flap with a releasable suture that could be lysed after surgery with an argon laser or removed using a slit lamp or at the time of examination under anesthesia.

Any intraocular surgery predisposes the eye to the risk of *bacterial endophthalmitis*. Patients with filtering blebs, especially the thin avascular blebs seen with the use of mitomycin C, are at increased risk for developing bacterial endophthalmitis months or even years after surgery. Because this risk is intensified by contact lens wear, the use of any type of contact lenses by these patients is discouraged. Other potential sources of infection include normal conjunctival flora, episodes of bacterial conjunctivitis, and contaminated medication dropper-bottle tips.

SUPPORT GROUP

Sturge–Weber Foundation
P.O. Box 460931
Aurora, CO 80046
(303) 690-9735

REFERENCES

Akabane N, Hamanaka T: Histopathological study of a case with glaucoma due to Sturge-Weber syndrome. Jpn J Ophthalmol 47:151–157, 2003.

Board MJ, Shields MB: Combined trabeculotomy-trabeculectomy for the management of glaucoma associated with Sturge-Weber syndrome. Ophthalmic Surg 12:813–817.

Cibis GW, Tripathi RC, Tripathi BJ: Glaucoma in Sturge-Weber syndrome. Ophthalmology 91:1061–1071, 1984.

Eibschitz-Tsimhoni M, Lichter PR, Del Monte MA, et al: Assessing the need for posterior sclerotomy at the time of filtering surgery in patients with Sturge-Weber syndrome. Ophthalmology 110:1361–1363, 2003.

Iwach AG, Hoskins HD, Hetherington J, Shaffer RN: Analysis of surgical and medical management of glaucoma in Sturge-Weber syndrome. Ophthalmology 97:904–909, 1990.

MacDonald IM, Bech-Hansen NT, Britton WA, Jr, et al: The phakomatoses: recent advances in genetics. Can J Ophthalmol 32:4–11, 1997.

Ritch R: Serous retinal detachment after glaucoma filtration surgery in Sturge-Weber syndrome. J Glaucoma 1:58–62, 1992.

Sakai H, Sakima N, Nakamura Y, et al: Ciliochoroidal effusion induced by topical latanoprost in a patient with Sturge-Weber syndrome. Jpn J Ophthalmolol 46:553–555, 2002.

Schirmer R: Ein fall von telangiektasie. Graefe's Arch Clin Exp Ophthalmol 7:119–121, 1860.

Singh AD, Kaiser PK, Sears JE: Choroidal hemangioma. Ophthalmol Clin North Am 18:151–161, 2005.

Sturge WA: A case of partial epilepsy, apparently due to a lesion of one of the vaso-motor centers of the brain. Trans Clin Soc Lond 12:162–167, 1897.

Sullivan TJ, Clarke MP, Morin JD: The ocular manifestations of the Sturge-Weber syndrome. J Pediatr Ophthalmol Strabismus 29:349–356, 1996.

Susac JO, Smith JL, Scelfo RJ: The 'tomato catsup' fundus in Sturge-Weber syndrome. Arch Ophthalmol 92:69–70, 1974.

Weber FP: Right-sided hemi-hypotrophy resulting from right-sided congenital spastic hemiplegia with a morbid condition of the left side of the brain, revealed by radiograms. J Neurol Psychopathol 3:134–139, 1922.

Weiss DI: Dual origin of glaucoma in encephalotrigeminal hemangiomatosis. A pathogenetic concept based upon histopathologic and hemodynamic considerations. Trans Ophthalmol Soc UK 93:477–491, 1973.

Witschel H, Font RL: Hemangioma of the choroid: A clinicopathologic study of 71 cases and a review of the literature. Surv Ophthalmol 20:415–431, 1976.

SECTION

12 Neurologic Disorders

106 ACQUIRED INFLAMMATORY DEMYELINATING NEUROPATHIES 355.9

(Guillain–Barré Syndrome or Acute Inflammatory Demyelinating Polyradiculoneuropathy [AIDP], Chronic Inflammatory Demyelinating Polyradiculoneuropathy [CIDP], and Fisher Syndrome)

Paul W. Brazis, MD
Jacksonville, Florida
Andrew G. Lee, MD
Iowa City, Iowa

ETIOLOGY/INCIDENCE

Guillain–Barré syndrome (GBS) (acute inflammatory demyelinating polyradiculoneuropathy, or AIDP) can occur at any age and has an estimated annual incidence of approximately 1 to 2 cases in 100,000.

In at least two thirds of patients with GBS, a history of premonitory illness, usually viral, can be elicited by taking a careful history. Cytomegalovirus, Epstein–Barr virus, and human immunodeficiency virus (HIV) have been most closely associated with the condition. Infection by organisms of the *Campylobacter* genus has drawn much attention, with some reports suggesting that enteritis caused by species of *Campylobacter* occurs in as many as 15% to 20% of GBS patients. In addition to antecedent infections, Hodgkin's disease and recent surgery are well-recognized premonitory events.

COURSE/PROGNOSIS

The initial symptoms are almost invariably sensory-numbness and tingling in the fingers and toes and, occasionally, even on the trunk. Subsequently, weakness develops in the legs, with later involvement of the upper extremities. Weakness is the predominant clinical feature of GBS; it is the manifestation that results in hospitalization for most patients, and it is usually both proximal and distal and involves the facial muscles in 30% to 40% of patients. Muscle stretch reflexes are absent or depressed. Although approximately 90% of cases reach their nadir by 4 weeks, the tempo of progression is variable. In rapidly evolving cases, respiratory paralysis can occur within the first few days. About one third of hospitalized GBS patients eventually develop respiratory insufficiency. The diagnostic criteria for typical GBS require:

- Weakness that is symmetric in all limbs;
- Paresthesias in the hands and feet;
- Hyporeflexia or areflexia in all limbs by the end of the first week; and
- Progression of the weakness, paresthesias, and reflex abnormalities over several days to one month.

Guillain–Barré syndrome

- The overall prognosis for the majority of GBS patients is good, but 5% to 10% develop significant clinical impairment that precludes routine activities of daily living.
- Vedeler and colleagues reported the long-term outcome of 52 patients reexamined over a mean of 7 years. Of the 52 patients, 38 (73%) were free of symptoms. Neurologic examination revealed motor abnormalities in 21%, sensory signs in 31%, cranial neuropathy in 2%, and areflexia in 29%. Treatment with plasma exchange did not influence disability grade.
- In a retrospective questionnaire study of 175 patients with GBS, at the peak of disease 26% remained able to walk and 16% had to be artificially ventilated. The median time from onset of symptoms to ability to walk unaided was 37 days, and from onset to freedom from symptoms, 66 days. At long-term follow-up, 98 of 106 patients were symptom free.
- Mortality rate remains 2% to 5%, with most patients dying from pulmonary infections, sepsis, pulmonary emboli, or complications of autonomic instability.
- Risk factors for poor outcome include older age, ventilator dependence on admission, a rapid rate of disease progression (e.g. reaching nadir of weakness in less than 1 week), and low-amplitude motor responses on nerve conduction studies.

Chronic inflammatory demyelinating polyradiculoneuropathy

- CIDP is a chronic and serious disorder.
- Approximately 95% of patients with CIDP initially improve with prednisone treatment, but the relapse rate is very high. In one series, 50% of patients relapsed after a mean follow-up period of 49 months; only 51% made a complete recovery. Two patients who initially responded later died from complications of the disease.
- In the studies of Dyck and colleagues, 64% of 53 patients were improved or in remission and able to return to work, 8% were ambulatory but unable to work, 11% were bedrid-

den or wheelchair-bound, and 11% died of the disease; 6% died of other diseases.

DIAGNOSIS

Fisher syndrome is a variant of GBS and represents about 5% of GBS cases. The major criteria for the diagnosis are external ophthalmoplegia, ataxia and areflexia without significant muscle weakness. The disease is usually self-limited and relatively benign. Its course and the frequent (10% to 20%) occurrence of ophthalmoplegia in typical cases of GBS are the main reasons for its acceptance as a subtype of GBS. Anti-GQ1b antibodies may be identified in the serum in approximately 95% of patients with Fisher syndrome. Eye movement abnormalities that occur with GBS include palsies of cranial nerves III, IV, VI, or all three, complete ophthalmoplegia, pseudo-internuclear ophthalmoplegia, rebound nystagmus and preserved Bell's phenomenon with absence of upgaze. Other ocular complications of GBS include ptosis, lid lag, pupillary abnormalities (e.g. asymmetrically dilated and nonreactive pupils, light-near dissociation), impaired accommodation, impaired lacrimal secretions, reduced corneal sensation, trigeminal impairment, facial nerve palsies, unilateral or bilateral optic neuritis and papilledema.

Chronic inflammatory demyelinating polyradiculoneuropathy (CIDP) is a polyneuropathy whose course differs from GBS in that its progression is measured in months or years and it is generally not self-limited. CIDP can occur at any age but the ages of peak onset are between 40 and 60 years. Patients typically present with progressive, stepwise or relapsing muscle weakness. To fulfill the diagnostic criteria for CIDP, weakness must have been present for at least 2 months. Weakness varies from mild to severe, and some patients require assisted ambulation or wheelchairs. Sensory complaints are variable, usually consisting of numbness and tingling. Cranial nerve involvement includes facial weakness in 15% of cases; occasionally, patients have swollen optic disks or extraocular muscle impairment.

TREATMENT

Guillain–Barré syndrome

Systemic

- Steroids are probably of no benefit, although a small uncontrolled series suggested that a combination of intravenous immune globulins (IVIG) and high-dose methylprednisolone may be better than IVIG alone.
- Two specific forms of therapy that have been shown to alter the natural history of GBS are plasma exchange and intravenous immune globulin.
- Plasma exchange: prospective, controlled studies involving more than 500 patients have shown definite evidence that plasma exchange benefits patients with GBS. Plasmapheresis significantly improves muscle strength by 4 weeks and decreases the number of days required to achieve assisted ambulation. In addition, patients with respiratory failure have significantly fewer days of ventilator dependence following plasma exchange. A standard regimen for plasma exchange in GBS patients involves removing 200 to 250 mL of plasma per kilogram of body weight over a 7- to 14-day period. Therapy should be instituted as soon as possible following diagnosis. The role of plasma exchange in mild cases is still uncertain. Enough data have not been generated on ambulatory patients to be certain that the expense and discomfort can be justified.
- Considering the fact that plasma exchange and intravenous immune globulins are of equal benefit, final decisions regarding treatment of GBS relate more to individual patient considerations. For example, in an ICU setting in patients with poor venous access, cardiovascular instability, or concurrent infections, infusions of immune globulins may be indicated.

Ocular

- In patients with facial or trigeminal involvement, the cornea is threatened by the development of exposure and neuroparalytic keratitis. Thus, artificial tears, moisture chambers and lateral tarsorrhaphies may be warranted.
- Diplopia is treated with patching or prisms.
- Decreased accommodation may require reading glasses.
- Papilledema resolves spontaneously.

Supportive

- Careful monitoring of pulmonary function is critical; patients with a forced vital capacity below 12 to 15 mL/kg usually require endotracheal intubation.
- Chest physical therapy and prompt treatment of chest infections are important.
- Swings in blood pressure are common. In general, hypertension is manageable without medication, but hypotension may require pressor agents and fluid. Vagally mediated arrhythmias may require cardiac treatment.
- Heparin, 5000 units SC b.i.d., is indicated for the prevention of pulmonary emboli.
- GBS patients in an ICU setting are, of course, at high risk of acquiring nosocomial infections that must be treated promptly.
- Pain can be a significant practical problem, and narcotic analgesics are often required.
- Physical therapy is essential to ensure proper positioning; passive and active exercises maintain joint flexibility and minimize the likelihood of contractures.

CIDP

Systemic

- Randomized controlled studies have documented the effectiveness of prednisone plasma exchange, and IVIG. These forms of therapy represent the mainstay of treatment for CIDP.
- Following diagnosis of CIDP, high-dose daily prednisone is maintained until the patient shows significant improvement. The mean time for initial response to treatment is 2 months; by 3 months, 88% improve. Following improvement, the dose is changed to an alternate-day, single-dose regimen that is maintained until the patient reaches a maximum therapeutic response-that is, return to normal or reach a plateau.
- After the patient has attained maximum benefit from it, prednisone is slowly tapered. Plasma exchange added to the initial prednisone treatment regimen significantly diminishes the time necessary for improvement.
- Intravenous immune globulin appears to produce clinical improvement in some patients with CIDP.
- Other immunosuppressing drugs are often considered for refractory disease. They include azathioprine, cyclophosphamide, methotrexate, ciclosporin, mycophenolate mofetil,

pulse methylprednisolone, interferon-alpha 2a, and total lymphoid radiation but the potential toxicity of these agents must be carefully considered.

Supportive

- Patients with CIDP are rarely ventilator-dependent, seldom have bulbar impairment, and are usually ambulatory, although they may need assistance.
- The major problem is rehabilitation. Physical therapy is important, especially during steroid treatment, to preserve and improve muscle strength. Bracing and other aids may be necessary.
- As CIDP is a chronic and often debilitating disease, psychologic support is essential.

REFERENCES

Dalakas MC: Intravenous immune globulin therapy for neurologic diseases. Ann Int Med 126:721–730, 1997.

Donofrio PD: Immunotherapy of idiopathic inflammatory neuropathies. Muscle Nerve 28:273–292, 2003.

The Dutch Guillain-Barré Study Group: Treatment of Guillain-Barré syndrome with high-dose immune globulins combined with methylprednisolone: a pilot study. Ann Neurol 35:749–752, 1994.

Dyck PJ, Daube J, O'Brien P, et al: Plasma exchange in chronic inflammatory demyelinating polyradiculopathy. N Engl J Med 314:461–465, 1986.

Dyck PJ, Lais AC, Ohta M, et al: Chronic inflammatory demyelinating polyradiculoneuropathy. Mayo Clin Proc 50:621–637, 1975.

Dyck PJ, O'Brien PC, Oviatt KF, et al: Prednisone improves chronic inflammatory demyelinating polyradiculoneuropathy more than no treatment. Ann Neurol 11:136–141, 1982.

Gorson KC, Ropper AH, Clark BD, et al: Treatment of chronic inflammatory demyelinating polyneuropathy with interferon alpha-2a. Neurology 50:84–87, 1998.

Korinthenberg R, Monting JS: Natural history and treatment effects in Guillain-Barré syndrome: Multicentre study. Arch Dis Child 74:281–287, 1996.

McKhann GM, Griffin JW, Cornblath DR, et al: Plasmapheresis and Guillain-Barré syndrome: analysis of prognostic factors and the effect of plasmapheresis. Ann Neurol 23:347–353, 1988.

Plasma Exchange/Sandoglobulin Guillain-Barré Syndrome Trial Group: Randomized trial of plasma exchange, intravenous immunoglobulin, and combined treatments in Guillain-Barré syndrome. Lancet 349:225–230, 1997.

Ropper RH: The Guillain-Barré syndrome. N Engl J Med 326:1130–1136, 1992.

Van Doorn PA, Brand A, Strengers PFW, et al: High-dose intravenous immunoglobulin treatment in chronic inflammatory demyelinating polyneuropathy: a double-blind, placebo-controlled, crossover study. Neurology 40:209–212, 1990.

Van der Meché FG, Schmitz PIM, the Dutch Guillain-Barré Study Group: a randomized trial comparing intravenous immune globulin and plasma exchange in Guillain-Barré syndrome. N Engl J Med 326:1123–1129, 1992.

Vedeler CA, Wik E, Nyland H, et al: The long-term prognosis of Guillain-Barré syndrome: Evaluation of prognostic factors including plasma exchange. Acta Neurol Scand 95:298–302, 1997.

107 BELL'S PALSY 351.0
(Idiopathic Facial Paralysis)

Michael S. Harney, MD, MB, FRCSI (ORL)
Dublin, Ireland
Rory McConn Walsh, MD, MB FRCSI (ORL)
Dublin, Ireland

ETIOLOGY/INCIDENCE

The facial nerve is the most commonly paralyzed nerve in the body (Figure 107.1). The most common cause is Bell's palsy occurring at a rate of 20/100,000 per year. Though sometimes termed 'idiopathic facial nerve palsy', this is probably a herpetic induced neuritis, resulting in inflammation, subsequent entrapment in the tight confines of the temporal bone, causing ischemia and finally degeneration. Optimum management of this condition requires attention to three key principles:

- A correct diagnosis; It is important to ensure a more serious diagnosis of cerebrovascular accident, acoustic neuroma, middle ear disease or a parotid tumor is not missed.
- Minimizing the number of patients left with a residual nerve deficit.
- Anticipation and management of secondary ocular complications.

COURSE/PROGNOSIS

This condition classically occurs in otherwise healthy individuals. Patients will present to the health professional with a facial nerve weakness that has developed over a period of several hours to days. The history will often yield a recent viral illness. Occasionally, otalgia and a perception of some sensory change on the affected side will be present. The patient may complain of decreased tearing, epiphoria, dysgeusia or hyperacusis.

Most patients will show signs of recovery of facial function within 3 weeks, though in some remission may occur up to 6 months later. Eighty-three percent of patients will have full recovery, but 17% will be left with some residual neurological sequelae. A complete palsy carries a worse prognosis. Permanent sequelae result from abnormal weakness of the facial musculature (cosmetic deformity, lagopthalmus, ectropion) or from abnormal reinnervation of damaged nerve fibers (synkinesis, crocodile tears [tearing on eating], hemifacial spasm).

DIAGNOSIS

The first step in making a correct diagnosis of Bell's palsy is ensuring the palsy is a lower motor lesion. This is done by asking them to raise their eyebrows, to tightly close their eyes and to show their teeth. Patients with a lower motor lesion will demonstrate weakness in performing all three maneuvers. Those with an upper motor lesion will only display impairment of function with the last of these commands, due to contralateral innervation of the upper facial musculature. The most common cause of an upper motor facial nerve weakness is a cerebrovascular accident.

Having determined the palsy is lower motor, the second step is to ensure that there is not another cause for the palsy. Bell's

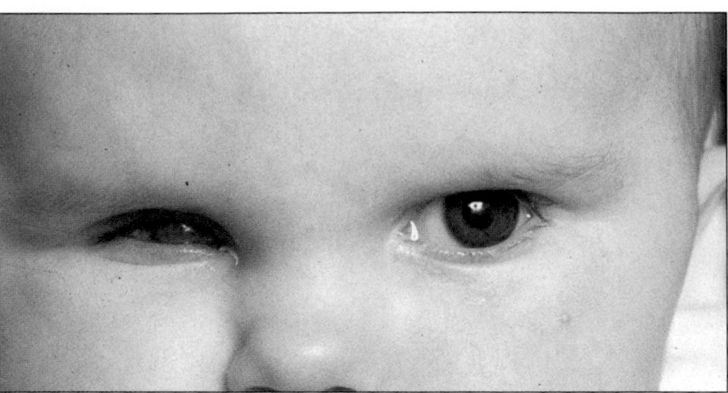

FIGURE 107.1. Seventh nerve palsy.

palsy remains a diagnosis of exclusion. Examination should include:

- Otoscopy to out rule many of the reversible causes of facial nerve palsy; acute otitis media, chronic suppurative otitis media, cholesteatoma and Ramsay–Hunt syndrome. Ear discharge (otorrhoea) should prompt urgent referral to an otolaryngologist as this strongly suggests an otological cause requiring surgery. Ramsay–Hunt syndrome (herpes zoster oticus) is diagnosed by the presence of vesicular eruptions on the pinna or in the ear canal.
- Parotid gland examination. The presence of a facial nerve palsy in the presence of a parotid mass indicates the mass is malignant.
- Examination of the cranial nerves particularly the trigeminal nerve and the vestibulocochlear nerve with tuning fork tests and audiometry if possible. These may be involved by an acoustic neuroma (or other cerebellopontine angle [CPA] lesions)
- The skin for the presence of erythema migrans in areas where Lyme disease is endemic.

If the above examinations are normal and the palsy is confirmed to be lower motor then the diagnosis is Bell's palsy. No further investigations are necessary at this stage except for lyme titres in endemic areas. An MRI should be done if the palsy fails to resolve at 6 weeks or if atypical symptoms are present to out rule a more sinister underlying cause.

TREATMENT

Systemic

Most clinicians would treat bells palsy with both steroids and aciclovir though neither have been shown to be clearly effective. Oral steroids may reduce inflammation in the facial nerve with a reduction in subsequent ischemia and degeneration. Antiviral agents may be useful if the disease is caused by a herpetic virus.

Local

The immediate aim of local treatment should be to prevent corneal exposure and subsequent ulceration.

- In most cases, topical ocular lubrication is sufficient (artificial tears frequently during the day and lubricating ophthalmic ointment at night; occasionally, ointment must be used around the clock).
- The eye may be taped at night using tape or adhesive strips (Steristrips). Caution must be exercised with patches as the eye may remain open underneath. Occasionally, a lid mattress suture in the skin of the upper lid, taping the ends firmly to the upper cheek, can be performed to close the eyelid.
- Punctal plugs might be helpful if dryness of the cornea is a persistent problem.
- Rarely, clear plastic wrap, cut to 8 × 10 cm and applied with generous amounts of ointment, can be used as an occlusive bandage at night.

Failure of Bell's palsy to resolve may require *local* treatment of its sequelae:

- Lower lid ectropion, or droop, can be temporarily helped by using tape applied below the lid margin in the center of the lower lid, pulling the lid laterally and upward to anchor it on the orbital rim;
- Botulinum toxin injected in to the levator palpebrae superioris muscle through the eyelid can produce a protective ptosis, possibly avoiding the need for a lateral tarrsorraphy.

Surgical

The theory of nerve dysfunction as a result of entrapment in the fallopian canal in the temporal bone, secondary to edema, gave rise to the practice of surgically decompressing the facial nerve. Serious complications such as permanent hearing loss may occur and the role for surgery in a virally induced neuritis is contentious. Restoration of facial nerve function may be considered using a hypoglossal to facial nerve anastomosis. Regional muscle transfers may also be attempted using temporalis muscle. A period of twelve months to allow for spontaneous recovery should be observed prior to undertaking these procedures.

Surgical treatment of the eye is required in the unusual instance of a Bell's palsy that fails to recover. It is more often required in facial nerve injury following acoustic neuroma surgery (or other CPA surgery), parotid tumour removal, or following trauma with a temporal bone fracture. Surgery for CPA lesions is of particular importance as there is often associated trigeminal paresis with corneal anesthesia.

- *Lagopthalmus* can be treated with lateral tarsorrhaphy. This decreases horizontal lid opening, provides better support of the precorneal lake of tears, and provides better coverage of the eye during sleep. This can be reversed if recovery occurs. To restore dynamic lid closure in cases of severe, symptomatic lagophthalmos, a variety of ingenuous devices have been invented. All overcome the elevator action of the levator palpebrae muscle. Weight-adjustable magnets, gold weights, palpebral springs, or silicone encircling bands can be inserted into the eyelids. These devices require close observation because they can extrude.
- *Lower lid ectropion* can be managed by a horizontal lid wedge shortening.
- *Punctal ectropion causing epiphoria* may be repaired with removal of a horizontal tarsoconjunctival ellipse of tissue inferior to the lower lid punctum (protecting the canaliculus with a probe), suturing the edges of the ellipse together.
- *Medial ectropion with punctual eversion* may benefit from a medial canthoplasty combined with horizontal shortening of the lower lid and a tarsoconjunctival ellipse.

COMMENTS

Bell's palsy is a diagnosis of exclusion. It is important to examine the ear to exclude many of the reversible causes of facial nerve palsy. No treatments have shown to be clearly effective though most clinicians will treat with both oral steroids and aciclovir. A clinician can be reassured that if the palsy is incomplete, 94% recover completely within months. Electrophysiological testing does not have a role to play in routine cases. Exercises may be useful and can give the patient the feeling that they are taking an active role in their own recovery. An MRI scan should be performed if the patient fails to recover, or demonstrates atypical signs, to exclude the remote possibility of a more sinister underlying cause. Topical ocular therapy is sufficient in the majority of cases of Bell's palsy.

REFERENCES

Ellis MF, Daniell M: An evaluation of the safety and efficacy of botulinum toxin type A (BOTOX) when used to produce a protective ptosis. Clin Experiment Ophthalmol 29(6):394–399, 2001.

Fisch U: Surgery for Bell's palsy. Arch Otolaryngol 107(1):1–11, 1981.

Peiterson E: Bell's palsy: the spontaneous course of 2500 peripheral facial nerve palsies of different etiologies. Acta Otolaryngol Suppl 549:4–30, 2002.

Salinas RA, Alvarez G, Alvarez MI, Ferreira J: Corticosteroids for Bell's palsy (idiopathic facial paralysis). Cochrane Database Syst Rev 1: CD001942, 2002.

Schirm J, Mulkens PS: Bell's palsy and herpes simplex virus. APMIS 105:815–823, 1997.

Sipe J, Dunn L: Aciclovir for Bell's palsy (idiopathic facial paralysis). Cochrane Database Syst Rev 4:CD001869, 2001. Update in: Cochrane Database Syst. Rev. 3:CD001869, 2004.

108 CEREBRAL PALSY 343.9

(Brain Damage Syndrome, Perinatal Encephalopathy)

F. Hampton Roy, MD, FACS

Little Rock, Arkansas

ETIOLOGY/INCIDENCE

Cerebral palsy is a group of conditions with widely diverse etiologies; these conditions arise as a result of brain damage that occurs before, during, or shortly after birth. *In utero* exposure to rubella or cytomegalovirus or placental insufficiency may result in brain damage and cerebral palsy; prematurity, precipitate labor, neonatal asphyxia and hypoxia, hypoglycemia, hyperbilirubinemia, and accidents during labor and delivery also are known to cause the condition. Neonatal meningitis, encephalitis, and trauma also have been implicated as causative. In addition, in about 10% of children with cerebral palsy there is no known cause, despite extensive investigation. It appears to be familial in a very small number of cases.

DIAGNOSIS

Clinical signs and symptoms

The disorders cerebral palsy comprises are not progressive but are not unchanging. They are dominated by motor abnormalities. Associated with the motor dysfunction are varying degrees of:

- Mental subnormalities;
- Emotional instability;
- Convulsive disorders;
- Abnormalities of hearing;
- Speech defects;
- Visual abnormalities.

Cerebral palsy is usually classified according to the motor abnormality and its topography; spastic, ataxic and athetoid forms are most common, appearing in isolation or, less commonly, in combination. Except in athetoid cerebral palsy, it is rarely possible to localize the site of the causative lesion in the brain; the broad array of associated disabilities reflects the diffuse and widespread nature of the nervous system lesions.

Ocular

Abnormalities of the visual apparatus are common in cerebral palsy; the incidence of ocular changes has been reported to be between 50% and 80% of cases. The range of disorders is wide and can include:

- Esophorias and exophorias;
- Hypertropia, esotropias, and exotropias;
- Paralysis of third, fourth and sixth cranial nerves;
- Gaze palsies;
- Epicanthus, ptosis;
- Refractive errors;
- Amblyopia;
- Leukomas;
- Nystagmus;
- Cataracts;
- Iris coloboma, heterochromias;
- Visual field defects;
- Microphthalmos;
- Chorioretinal scars, coloboma, pigmentary degeneration;
- Retinopathy of prematurity;
- Optic nerve hypoplasia, coloboma, atrophy;
- Cortical visual impairment.

Spastic types of cerebral palsy are most likely to have associated ocular abnormalities, whereas purely athetoid types are the least likely. There is some evidence that the incidence of ocular abnormality rises with the degree of mental subnormality; however, an ocular abnormality rate of 70% has been reported in children with cerebral palsy who have normal or near-normal intelligence. Problems caused by the ocular abnormalities are compounded by visuospatial and perceptual difficulties that result from the underlying brain damage.

TREATMENT

Ocular

Refractive errors are common.

- Myopia: associated with prematurity.
- Hyperopia: most often found in those children whose cerebral palsy is not due to prematurity.

If possible, children with normal or near-normal intelligence should have full correction of any refractive errors detected by a subjective refraction; this is frequently impossible, however, and in these cases an objective refraction should be carried out after instillation of a cycloplegic agent such as atropine (1.0%) or cyclopentolate (1.0%), depending on the child's age.

The level at which refractive errors should be corrected in those who are severely subnormal has been a matter of some discussion in the literature. Small refractive errors should be corrected only in those who are likely to benefit from such corrections; larger refractive errors should be corrected in all children with cerebral palsy, in whom the acceptance of spectacle correction is usually very good.

Those children at risk of amblyopia due to anisometropia or squint should be identified at an early age so that appropriate therapy for amblyopia can be carried out. Some infants appear to have an isolated deficit of accommodation that may require correction. At the same time, a thorough examination of the fundus and the optic nerve can be performed, particularly with the indirect ophthalmoscope.

Strabismus is detected in the usual manner in patients with cerebral palsy; there is a far higher incidence of divergent and incomitant strabismus in children with cerebral palsy than in children who are neurologically normal. Moreover, a variable strabismus angle is common and, in some cases, the deviation may be divergent or convergent at varying times. In addition, approximately 25% of children with concomitant squint have a retinal or optic nerve abnormality that precludes an improvement in visual acuity.

Full correction of any refractive error based on a cycloplegic refraction must be made, followed by:
- Occlusion of the squinting eye;
- Orthoptic treatment, if appropriate.

Rarely, treatment may involve the use of:
- Prisms;
- Anticholinesterase eyedrops (occasionally).

It is important, however, to guard against adverse reactions that may occur with the use of anticholinesterase compounds in this group of children. The aim of treatment is to give the child binocularity or at least good vision in both eyes before surgery, if surgery is indicated. There is some evidence that successful treatment of strabismus may improve a child's coordination.

Surgical

For nonaccommodative esotropia and exotropia, recession and resection of the appropriate muscles are usually adequate treatments. The degree to which the horizontal muscles are weakened or strengthened must be determined by repeated observation because of the variable angles often found in strabismus in these children. Particularly when squint presents a purely cosmetic problem and one eye has very poor vision that cannot be improved, the aim should be to undercorrect the deviation, to counteract the tendency to overcorrect.

Vertical deviations are fairly common; most of them manifest as overaction of the inferior oblique muscles, for which there may be several causes. In these cases, simple recession or myotomy of the inferior oblique muscle is satisfactory treatment.

In very young children, bilateral cataract/lens aspiration or lensectomy/vitrectomy may be carried out; subsequent optical correction with contact lenses or spectacles may pose special problems and difficulties, however. In older children in whom cataracts develop, appropriate cataract surgery can be carried out with the insertion of a posterior chamber lens implant. Although the use of intraocular lenses in children remains controversial, there may be a special place for their use in young patients who have severe behavioral or emotional problems or motor disabilities.

Rarely, other abnormalities amenable to surgical correction such as congenital glaucoma may be seen and should be treated along conventional lines.

Supportive

The aim of examination is to identify at an early age those defects that are treatable and to undertake treatment for them as if the child were otherwise normal. Many studies have shown that ocular disabilities in children with cerebral palsy are detected much later than in children who are normal.

It is equally important to identify children with severe visual impairment that is not amenable to treatment; the ophthalmologist is then in a position to counsel parents on the placement of their children in the correct educational environment. Those who will be responsible for assessing the children's intellectual abilities and those who will educate them have to be aware of each one's visual status. Teachers, in particular, have to understand the visual acuity, the size of the visual field, and the ability to match colors of the children in their care. Many of these children are deaf and their education relies heavily on visual stimulation.

The ophthalmologic findings in cerebral palsy cannot be taken in isolation; assessment and treatment must be coordinated with many other disciplines. To this end, the ophthalmologist should be part of a multidisciplinary team that includes psychologists, teachers and other physicians concerned with the welfare of the children. There is continual need for reassessment as the children grow and parents and teachers need constant reassurance. The aim of the ophthalmologist must be to provide the children with the best possible chance of attaining independence, or at least to minimize the amount of institutional care required when they leave the shelter of school.

PRECAUTIONS

Examination of children with cerebral palsy is often difficult, particularly when there is mental subnormality. Subjective tests, such as those for visual acuity, are unreliable and the examination may have to be repeated on several occasions before the ophthalmologist can be sure of the findings.

Newer methods of assessing visual acuity, such as the use of visual evoked potentials and the techniques of forced preferential looking, may be particularly useful in those patients who are mentally subnormal. It is easy to underestimate a child's visual capabilities, especially in those with gross disturbances of motility such as athetosis and in those with hemianoptic field defects.

Young, severely handicapped children should be examined in familiar surroundings, preferably with someone they know and trust alongside them. Doing so allays their fears and is imperative in cases in which deafness or speech impairment requires their responses to be interpreted.

Topical drugs with known systemic side effects should be used with caution; there are reports (largely anecdotal) that these children are unusually prone to developing adverse reactions to some types of eyedrops. It is important that surgical therapy, usually for strabismus, be planned in consultation with the other disciplines concerned with the medical care of such children, as these patients often are subjected to multiple surgical procedures, particularly for musculoskeletal problems. Few guidelines exist on the management of strabismus in these children, but the information that is available suggests that squints should be treated as they would be if the child were otherwise normal.

COMMENTS

It is apparent from the literature that visual problems in children with cerebral palsy are commonly overlooked or ignored because they are overshadowed by the more dramatic musculoskeletal and intellectual deficits. Diagnosis of cerebral palsy usually has been made by the time children are 12 months old, however, and the initial ophthalmologic examination also should have been made by this time. Prompt initiation of treatment for probable amblyopia, or at least a plan for such therapy, should be made; continued reassessment is necessary, particularly before these children start school; so that appropriate decisions regarding training can be made at the earliest opportunity.

The ultimate aim for medical care and training is to enable children with cerebral palsy to become independent; this aim is not feasible in severely affected patients, but such severity may not be apparent until the second decade of life. All possible help is required by the children before then. To this end, every treatable defect should be identified at a sufficiently early age to allow appropriate measures to be carried out.

REFERENCES

Black PD: Visual disorders associated with cerebral palsy. Br J Ophthalmol 66:46–52, 1982.

Case-Smith J: Fine motor outcomes in preschool children who receive occupational therapy services. Am J Occup Ther 50:52–61, 1996.

Coltarello J, LeGare M, Terdiman J: Eye movements in a small sample of cerebral palsied adults. Percep Mot Skills 80:355–369, 1995.

Crofts BJ, King R, Johnson A: The contribution of low birth weight to severe vision loss in a geographically defined population. Br J Ophthalmol 82:9–13, 1998.

Dowdeswell HJ, Slater AM, Broomhall J, Tripp J: Visual deficits in children born at less than 32 weeks' gestation with and without major ocular pathology and cerebral damage. Br J Ophthalmol 79:447–452, 1995.

Gormezano SR, Kaminski JE: The eye care profile and outcomes of multi-handicapped adults residing in Wayne County, Michigan group homes. Optometry 76(1):19–29, 2005.

Jacobson L, Ygge J, Flodmark O, Ek U: Visual and perceptual characteristics, ocular motility and strabismus in children with periventricular leukomalacia. Strabismus 10(2):179–183, 2002.

Lee SK, LeGare M, Zhang HP: Conjugate eye movements: comparison of cerebral palsied and normal adults. Percep Mot Skills 81:575–591, 1995.

O'Keefe M, Kafil-Hussain N, Flitcroft I, Lanigan B: Ocular significance of intraventricular haemorrhage in premature infants. Br J Ophthalmol 85(3):357–359, 2001.

Orel-Bixler D, Haagerstrom-Portnoy G, Hall A: A visual assessment of the multiply handicapped patient. Optom Vis Sci 66:530–536, 1989.

Schiemann MM: Optometric findings in children with cerebral palsy. Am J Optom Physiol Optics 61:321–323, 1984.

109 CHRONIC PROGRESSIVE EXTERNAL OPHTHALMOPLEGIA (CPEO) 359.1

(Abiotrophic Ophthalmoplegia, CPEO with Ragged Red Fibres, Oculocraniosomatic Neuromuscular Disease, Ocular Myopathy, Olson's Disease, Kearns–Sayre–Daroff Syndrome, Kearns–Sayre Syndrome, Progressive External Ophthalmoplegia Plus)

Judith A.M. van Everdingen, MD
Rotterdam, The Netherlands
Jan-Tjeerd de Faber, MD
Rotterdam, The Netherlands

ETIOLOGY/INCIDENCE

Chronic progressive external ophthalmoplegia (CPEO) includes a spectrum of clinical findings that usually becomes apparent between the second and fourth decades as a syndrome of bilateral, painless, and pupil sparing, slowly progressive ptosis and ophthalmoplegia of the extraocular muscles. CPEO may be isolated or associated with other ocular, neurological or systemic disease.

There is no known specific etiology. Most cases of CPEO arise sporadically and are associated with rearrangements (e.g. deletions and duplications) of mitochondrial transfer DNA (mtDNA) segments. There are a few pedigrees with maternal inheritance, suggesting an underlying mtDNA point mutation. Autosomal dominant or recessive inheritance, suggesting underlying nuclear DNA abnormalities, also has been reported. Only recently, mutations in at least three different genes, *ANT1* (4q34–35), *Twinkle* (10q24) and *POLG* (15q22–26) have been found in patients with autosomal dominant inheritance.

Kearns–Sayre syndrome (KSS) is regarded as a specific and severe form of CPEO, with more signs of mitochondrial disease. Patients with KSS tend to have more mutant mtDNA than individuals with less severe, isolated CPEO. Still, patients with similar phenotypes may have different mtDNA patterns and patients with different clinical presentations may appear to have the same mtDNA rearrangements. Even classical mitochondrial phenotypes without mtDNA mutations have been described.

CPEO is one of the four most common neuro-ophthalmic abnormalities seen in mitochondrial disease. The other three being bilateral optic neuropathy, pigmentary retinopathy and retrochiasmal visual loss. Pathogenic mtDNA mutations are found in at least one in 8000 individuals. There often is only one pathogenic mtDNA deletion involved in mtDNA disease. Maternal age does not seem to influence the incidence of mtDNA deletion disorders. Affected woman were previously thought to have a negligible chance of having clinically affected offspring, but the actual risk is on average about one in 24 births. Heteroplasmy, the co-existence of both mutant and normal mtDNA may play an important role in the variability in clinical expression: Different proportions of mutant mtDNA may be present in different tissues in the same person. Still the pathogenesis is only partly understood.

COURSE/PROGNOSIS

The development of ptosis usually proceeds the ophthalmoplegia. Both features usually develop insidiously and symmetrically but can become complete. Patients tend to remain sub-clinical for a long period as most patients experience no diplopia and gradually adjust to ptosis by a chin-up head position and by using the frontalis muscle. Partial sparing of down gaze may contribute to the chin-up head tilt. Ptosis treatment should be undertaken with caution as patients may be prone to develop corneal exposure due to poor Bell's phenomenon.

DIAGNOSIS

Clinical signs and symptoms

The first symptom of CPEO usually is symmetrical slowly progressive myopathic ptosis. Slowed saccadic velocity can be the first sign of extraocular muscle involvement, and may contribute to the diagnosis in the early stages of the disease. Ptosis and ophthalmoplegia usually develop insidiously and symmetrically and can become complete over time. Pupillary involvement, pain and proptosis are not symptoms of CPEO and warrant further investigation (Figure 109.1).

CPEO is not one distinct diagnosis but a spectrum of diseases ranging from clinically isolated CPEO to symptoms of more widespread mitochondrial disease including myopathy, retinopathy, endocrinopathy, cardiomyopathy, or a combination of symptoms. In 1968, Drachman introduced the term 'CPEO plus' for CPEO associated with neurodegenerative disorders.

Kearns–Sayre syndrome (KSS) is characterized by external ophthalmoplegia, pigmentary retinopathy, often referred to as 'salt and pepper fundus' and one of either cardiac conduction defect, ataxia or raised CSF protein. KSS typically presents in the second decade of life.

Deafness, and endocrine abnormalities (e.g. hypoparathyreoidism, gonodal dysfunction, and diabetes mellitus) may be present as well. The cardiac conduction defect usually is preceeded by the features of CPEO and can be treated with a pacemaker. Complete heart block resulting in sudden death in these patients, may be associated with long QT syndrome.

Recently, neuropsychological testing in patients with CPEO and KSS revealed specific cognitive deficits suggesting impairment of the visuospatial perception (like visual construction) associated with the parieto-occipital lobes and executive deficits associated to the prefrontal region. No general intellectual deterioration was found. There was no difference in outcome between patients with or without mtDNA deletions.

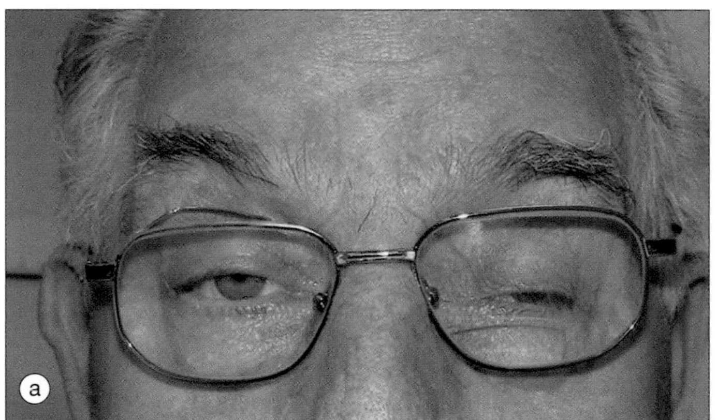

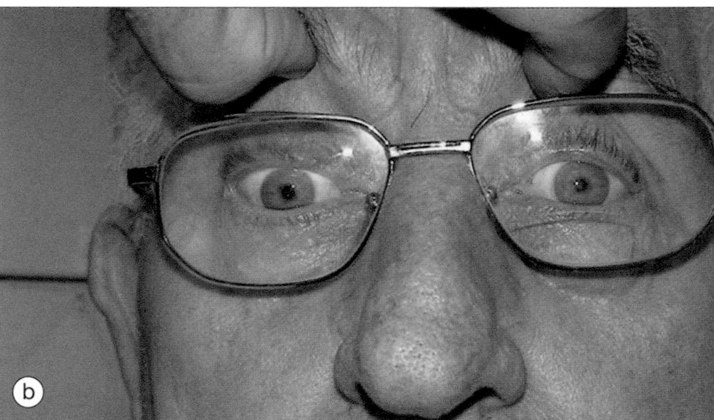

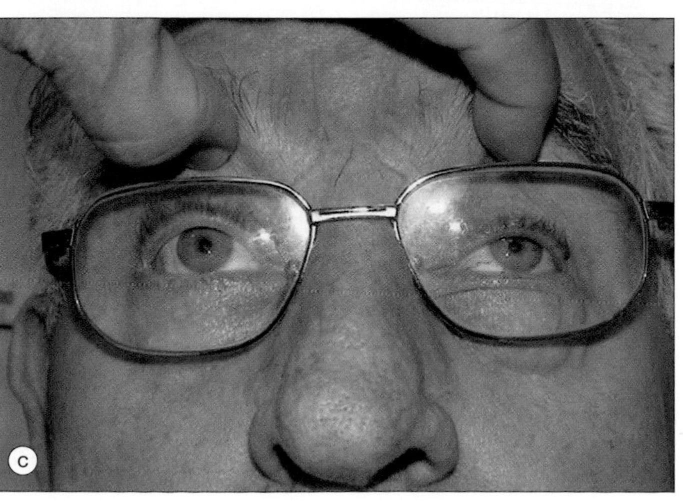

FIGURE 109.1. a) Notice the ptosis in the left eye. The right eye seems less ptotic but this eyelid is pulled up by a stainless steel crutch attached to the frame. b) In primary position with the eyelids pulled up the left eye is exotropic. c) Attempted upgaze shows restriction of elevation as a sign of ophthalmoplegia more in the left than in the right eye.

Awareness that mitochondrial POLG (polymerase gamma) mutations can underlie parkinsonism is important in patients with CPEO with muscle weakness and neuropathy, as the parkinsonism can be easily masked.

Laboratory findings

The diagnosis must be made on clinical grounds. There is no specific laboratory test for CPEO or KSS. Aim should be focused on ruling out any other underlying disease that could mimic CPEO, like thyroid ophthalmopathy and myasthenia gravis, and on the extent of multisystem involvement in case of mitochondrial disease. Laboratory findings that may aid to the diagnosis are:

- Elevated lactate on serum and CSF measurements as well as on magnetic resonance spectroscopy;
- Elevated pyruvic acid, creatine phosphokinase and aldolase;
- Elevated protein levels in CSF;
- Cytochrome c oxidase deficiency, low magnesium and parathyroid hormone levels also have been reported.

Limb and extraocular muscles of CPEO patients show ragged red fibres on light microscopy using modified Gomori trichrome strain. On electron abnormal paracrystalline inclusion bodies in only some of the muscle fibres, sparing all others, producing 'selective vacuolization' have been demonstrated. The selectiveness of the damage resembles that occurring in Leber hereditary optic neuropathy, another mitochondrial disease.

Differential diagnosis

- Neuromuscular junction disease, e.g. myasthenia gravis, botulism.
- Lambert–Eaton syndrome.
- Inflammatory disease, e.g. thyroid associated or idiopathic orbital myositis.
- Neoplasm, primary or metastatic.
- Infiltrative myopathy, e.g. sarcoidosis, amyloidosis.
- Neurologic disorders, e.g. progressive supranuclear palsy.
- Metabolic disease.

Simple and cost-effective tests may be helpful in differentiating CPEO from other diseases:

- The progressive course will rule out congenital deficits;
- Forced duction testing can rule out restrictive myopathies;
- The symmetry of the ophthalmoplegia makes these patients appear to have multidirectional gaze palsies. Full ocular rotations on oculocephalic manoeuvres differentiates supranuclear palsy from CPEO.

PROPHYLAXIS

No effective treatment for mtDNA disorders is available, making prevention important. Informed genetic counseling may be offered.

TREATMENT

Systemic

- Multidisciplinary approach in general, e.g. pacemaker in cases of KSS with serious cardiac conduction defect or heart block.

Ocular

- Adhesive tape or lid crutches for ptosis.
- Lubricants (e.g. artificial tears, gel, ointment).
- Eye patch, goggles and punctum plugs to prevent from exposure keratitis.
- Antibiotic drops or ointment in case of infection and ulceration.
- Fresnel- prisms to correct diplopia or head-tilt.

Medical

There is no proven medical therapy. Although various treatments (e.g. coenzyme Q10, riboflavin, ketogenic diets) have anecdotal success.

Surgical

- Levator resection only for ptosis with good levator muscle function.
- Frontalis sling or brow suspension if levator function is poor.
- Diplopia or head-tilt may be corrected with strabismus surgery in which cases muscle resections seem to be more successful than recessions.
- Punctum occlusion can be considered in cases of exposure keratitis.

COMPLICATIONS

Because poor Bell's phenomenon, these patients are prone to develop corneal exposure from inadequate lid closure due to ptosis treatment, with subsequent exposure keratitis, corneal ulceration and visual loss.

COMMENTS

CPEO is not a specific diagnosis. Mitochondrial DNA mutations, with or without a nuclear-mitochondrial interaction, are increasingly being recognized as the etiology for CPEO and CPEO syndromes.

SUPPORT GROUPS

United Mitochondrial Disease Foundation
P.O. Box 1151
Monroeville, PA 15146-1151
U.S.A.

REFERENCES

Biousse V, Newman NJ: Neuro-ophthalmology of mitochondrial diseases. Current Opinion in Neurology 16(1):35–43, 2003.

Bosbach S, Kornblum C, Schroder R, et al: Executive and visuospatial deficits in patients with chronic progressive external ophthalmoplegia and Kearns-Sayre syndrome. Brain 126(Pt 5):1231–1240, 2003.

Carta A, D'Adda T, Carrara F, et al: Ultrastructural analysis of extraocular muscle in chronic progressive external ophthalmoplegia. Arch Ophthalmol 118(10):1441–1445, 2000.

Chinnery PF, DiMauro S, Shanske S, et al: Risk of developing a mitochondrial DNA deletion disorder. Lancet 364(9434):592–596, 2004.

Lee AG, Brazis PW. Chronic progressive external ophthalmoplegia. Current Neurol Neuroscience Reports 2:413–417, 2002.

Luoma P, Melberg A, Rinne JO, et al: Parkinsonism, premature menopause, and mitochondrial DNA polymerase gamma mutations: clinical and molecular genetic study. Lancet 364(9437):875–882, 2004.

Odoari F, Rana M, Broccolini A, et al: Pathogenic role of mtDNA duplications in mitochondrial disease associated with mtDNA deletions. Am J Med Genet A 118(3):247–254, 2003.

Pulkes T, Liolitsa D, Nelson IP, et al: Classical mitochondrial phenotypes without mtDNA mutations; the possible role of nuclear genes. Neurology 61(8):1144–1147, 2003.

Rashid A, Kim MH: Kearns-Sayre syndrome: association with long QT syndrome. J Cardiovasc Electrophysiol 13(2):184–185, 2002.

110 CLUSTER HEADACHE 346.2

(Trigeminal Autonomic Cephalalgia, Cluster Headache Episodic or Chronic, Horton's Syndrome, Paroxysmal Hemicrania, Migrainous Neuralgia, Histaminic Cephalalgia)

Marijke Wefers Bettink-Remeijer, MD
Rotterdam, The Netherlands
Jan-Tjeerd de Faber, MD,
Rotterdam, The Netherlands

ETIOLOGY/INCIDENCE

Cluster headache is a rare primary headache with an incidence of 1–2 per thousand.

There is a male preponderance, but the male/female ratio is decreasing attributed to a different lifestyle of modern women. (tobacco smoking, alcohol and jobs).

Previously described as a neurovascular disorder, it now seems to be of central origin.

A recent report describes a patient with a complete surgical section of the left trigeminal sensory root who continued to have attacks.

Family studies show an increased risk for first and second degree relatives, but no precise mode of inheritance. Genetic studies suggest an autosomal dominant gene but with low penetrance in some families.

COURSE/PROGNOSIS

Cluster headache usually starts from the second decade to the third and fourth decade.

It has a strong circadian rhythm. It starts often as episodic but can turn into an chronic headache. Patients can have a chronic pattern from onset and some switch from chronic to episodic and vice versa.

Sleep deprivation occurs often, because severe attacks occur often during sleep.

DIAGNOSIS

Clinical signs and symptoms

Cluster headache is a (very) severe unilateral orbital, supraorbital and/or temporal pain lasting if left untreated 15–80 minutes. The headache is accompanied by one or more of the following ipsilateral autonomic signs: conjunctival injection and/or lacrimation, nasal congestion and/or rhinorrhoe, eyelid oedema, forehead and facial sweating, reversible miosis and ptosis and can be accompanied by a sense of restlessness.

Time between first attack and diagnosis can be very long (1 week to 48 years, median 3 years in one of the studies) 34% had consulted a dentist before diagnosis and 33% a ENT specialist before the diagnosis was established.

Diagnosis is often missed or delayed although circumscript and recognizable criteria are available.

The International Headache Society has put up new criteria.

Paroxysmal hemicrania was previously only recognized as chronic, but has a episodic as well as a chronic form. The main difference with cluster headache is the duration of the attacks and the good reaction to indometacine.

A new entrance in the TACs (trigeminal autonomic cephalalgias) is SUNCT (short-lasting unilateral neuralgiform headaches with conjunctival injection and tearing).

This syndrome consists of at least 20 attacks of unilateral orbital, supraorbital or temporal stabbing or pulsating pain, lasting 5–240 sec accompanied by conjunctival injection and tearing and occur frequent (3–200 per day).

Differential diagnosis

Structural lesions, as meningeoma and basilar artery aneurysm, have been reported with headache and unilateral autonomic symptoms, but in general clinical symptoms and course make the diagnosis clear. In general, scanning is wise to exclude structural lesions and to reassure the patient and family that there is no other pathological cause for the extreme painful headache.

TREATMENT

Acute attack

Oxygen inhalation and sumatriptan subcutaneous. Oral application is still not effective for aborting attacks. Sham therapy had a higher than expected effect comparing with hyperbaric oxygen sessions.

PROFYLAXIS

Verapamil is the first choice as maintenance prophylaxis, but other agents as lithium, methysergide and valproic acid may be effective as well. Cortisone therapy in a brief tapering course provides temporary relief . Topiramate, gabapentine, naratriptan , melatonine have all been reported effective in trials.

Therapy-resistant cases

Recent reports show effectivity of deep brain stimulation of the hypothalamus. PET scans showed activation of the inferior posterior hypothalamus, stimulation of this region aborts attacks in refractive cases. Cessation of the stimulation brought back the pains.

REFERENCES

Ekbom K, Hardebo JE: Cluster headache: aetiology, diagnosis and management. Drugs 62:61–69, 2002.

International Headache Society guidelines: Online. Available at: www.HIS.org.

Leone M, Franzini A, Bussone G: Stereotactic stimulation of posterior hypothalamic gray matter in a patient with intractable cluster headache. N Engl J Med 345:1428–1429, 2001.

Mathura MS, Goadsby PJ: Persistence of attacks of cluster headache after trigeminal root section. Brain 125:976–984, 2002.

May A, Leone M: Update on cluster headache. Current Opinion in Neurology 16(3):333–340, 2003.

111 CREUTZFELDT–JAKOB DISEASE 046.1

Catherine Creuzot-Garcher, MD, PhD
Dijon, France

ETIOLOGY/INCIDENCE

Creuztfeldt–Jacob disease (CJD) is a rare and fatal neurodegenerative disorder belonging to a larger family called 'prion disease' or subacute spongiform encephalopathies (SSEs) caused by a proteinaceous particle discovered by Prusiner in 1997. The agent responsible for the infection is an altered form PrPsc of a normal host-encoded glycoprotein (PrPc).

It can be divided as sporadic (85%) (sCJD), familial (10%) and acquired (5%). The former is the commonest SSE with an incidence of 1 per million per year and primarily affects the elderly. The latter includes iatrogenic CJD (iCJD) resulting from medical exposure. Recently, a form coined new-variant CJD (nwCJD) was described; it could be related to the same strain as bovine spongiform encephalopathy with strong concerns about cross-species transmission. Genetic predisposition could enhance transmission susceptibility.

The risk factors include a familial history of CJD, a treatment with native growth hormone before 1985, dura mater graft that first risk was recognized in the mid-1980s. There is emerging evidence about the potential transmission owing to ophthalmic surgery involving the retina, the optic nerve and the cornea as well.

COURSE/PROGNOSIS

The disease duration sCJD is about 4 months and mainly occurs at a median age onset of 60 years. The minimal incubation period for iCJD has been shown to range from 5 months to as long as 30 years. However the death usually occurred between 8 months to 2 years after the onset of the symptoms. NwCJD lasts longer (12 months) and involves younger patients (median 29 years).

DIAGNOSIS

Diagnosing CJD is a challenging task as presumptive diagnosis is based on clinical and biological tests but there are no available methods for reliable laboratory findings of CJD.

Clinical diagnosis

Clinical features of CJD are due to the progressive neuronal loss and gliosis of the brain. Some patients report on a vague prodrome of fatigue, improper sleep or vertigo. Cognitive impairment made of change in personality, behavioral change, disorientation and memory loss will occur during the course of the illness in 100% of cases. Cerebellar abnormalities are present in about $^2/_3$ of the patients in the later stages as well as myoclonus. Motor dysfunction and visual impairment are frequent. Visual loss is a revealing symptom reported in about $^1/_5$ of the patients. Heidenhain's variant is characterized by early cortical blindness and visual apraxia. On the contrary, lower neuron dysfunction and seizures are rare. All these data confirmed that the distinctive quadrate findings of cognitive change, myoclonus, cerebellar dysfunction and akinetic mutism occurring in a patient over the age of 60 indicate high risk of having CJD.

NwCJD differs from sCJD with the prominent psychiatric disturbance occurring in a younger patient presenting with painful dysesthesia and cerebellar symptoms. Genetic predisposition seems to be essential.

Laboratory findings

Biological detection

Serum S-protein is considered as a marker of activated glial cells seen in all stages of CJD.

CSF proteins are often moderately elevated but without any specific alteration: Neuron specific enolase, a non specific marker of neuronal degeneration is found in the early and middle stages of the disease. Increased amounts of 14-3-3 family of proteins, a marker of neuronal death, are detected by electrophoresis as two spots designed as p130 and 131.

MRI

Areas of symmetrical hyperintensities denoting the extent of the spongiosis are considered as nearly specific whereas cortical atrophy is not. Diffusion-weighted MRI is highly sensitive showing bilateral symmetrical hyperintense signals. PET and SPECT scan can guide the site of brain biopsy showing areas of abnormal metabolism and perfusion.

Electroencephalography findings

Characterized by a progressive slowing of the waveforms with disorganization of background rhythms, periodic sharp-wave complexes, triphasic sharp waves and giant responses to flash stimuli are present in about $^2/_3$ of patients.

Brain biopsy

Brain biopsy is interesting to detect the altered PrPsc form which is a marker of infectivity but lacks sensitivity. Neuropathology is the only definitive test for the diagnosis of CJD. It reveals a spongiform change with a fine-vacuole-like appearance involving all the cerebral cortex accompanied by gliosis and atrophy.

Differential diagnosis

Alzheimer's disease

Other SSEs: Kuru, Gerstmann–Straussler–Schneiker disease, fatal familial insomnia. Abnormal neurodegenerative changes (metabolic encephalopathies, toxicity, stroke, etc.).

TREATMENT

There is no curative treatment but symptomatic one can be proposed (neurological trouble).

PREVENTION

Treatment of the devices

Any tissue being discarded from a CJ suspect should be incinerated. Fully effective decontamination methods are steam autoclaving for one hour at 132°C and immersion in 1 N sodium hydroxide for 1 hour at room temperature. However, some devices cannot endure such procedures and methods such as steam autoclaving for a shorter period of time or lower temperature, or immersion in diluted solution of sodium chloride have to be considered as partially effective. All other methods (quaternary ammonium, ultraviolet, ethanol, etc.) are ineffective. The procedure according to the risk sub-groups has to be clearly defined before the situation raises (destruction, quarantining, declaration). Changes to improve the traceability of instruments and devices are needed. This point emphasizes the need to develop a full range of single-use devices that could be used, at least, in patients at risk of CJD and routinely in all circumstances increasing the risk of transmission (for instance retinal surgery or involvement of optic nerve).

Screening to prevent contamination

Screening before eye surgery is mandatory to minimize the risk of nosocomial spread of any form of prion-related disease. It should be based on both historical queries and clinical exam to detect the main clinical signs.

REFERENCES

Billette de Villemeur T, Deslys JP, Pradel A, et al: Creutzfeldt-Jakob disease from contaminated growth hormone extracts in France. Neurology 47:690–695, 1996.

Brown P, Brandel J-P, Sato T, et al: Iatrogenic Creutzfeldt-Jakob disease at the millennium. Neurology 55:1075–1081, 2000.

Creuzot-Garcher C, Lafontaine PO, Zabee L, et al: A screening questionnaire for determining risk of Creuzfeldt-Jacob disease transmission during ophthalmic examination. J Fr Ophtalmol 27:19–23, 2004.

Head MW, Nothcott V, Rennison, et al: Prion protein accumulation in eyes of patients with sporadic and variant Creuztfeldt-Jacob disease. Invest Ophthalmol Vis Sci 44:342–346, 2003.

Head MW, Peden AH, Yull HM: Abnormal prion protein in the retina of the most commonly occurring subtype of sporadic Creutzfeldt-Jakob disease. Br J Ophthalmol 89:1131–1133, 2005.

Hogan RN, Brown P, Heck E, et al: Risk of prion disease transmission from ocular tissue transplantation. Cornea 18:2–11, 1999.

Kennedy RH, Hogan RN, Brown P, et al: Eye banking and screening for Creutzfeldt-Jakob disease. Arch Ophthalmol 119:721–726, 2001.

S-Juan P, Ward HJT, de Silva R, et al: Ophthalmic surgery and Creutzfeldt-Jakob disease. Br J Ophthalmol 88:446–449, 2004.

Pedersen NS, Smith E: Prion diseases: epidemiology in man. APMIS 110:14–22, 2002.

Prabhakar S, Bhatia R: Diagnosis of Creutzfeldt-Jakob disease. Neurol India 49:325–328, 2001.

Shroter A, Zerr I, Henkel K, et al: Magnetic resonance imaging in the clinical diagnosis of Creutzfeldt-Jakob disease. Arch Neurol 57:1751–1757, 2000.

Ward HJ, Everington D, Croes EA: Sporadic Creutzfeldt-Jakob disease and surgery: a case-control study using community controls. Neurology 59:543–548, 2002.

112 DYSLEXIA 784.61

Marshall P. Keys, MD, PA

Rockville, Maryland

Dyslexia is a congenital difficulty in learning to read despite intact senses, normal intelligence, appropriate instruction and adequate motivation. Dyslexia must be differentiated from secondary learning disorders such as mental retardation, emotional disorders, seizure states, environmental deprivation, poor teaching and physical handicaps (including eye and ear defects).

ETIOLOGY/INCIDENCE

Anatomic research and functional magnetic resonance imaging studies have delineated focal aberrations in areas of the brain that are associated with the ability to relate letters with appropriate sounds. The genetic basis of dyslexia is evidenced by the high incidence of the problem among family members.

The lack of specific diagnostic criteria confuses the figures, but it is estimated that between 4% and 6% of school-age children in the United States are dyslexic. Other forms of learning failure account for problems in 10% to 20% of children.

COURSE/PROGNOSIS

- Dyslexia is noted when a child has difficulty learning letters and performing well in school during the early years.
- The dyslexic child has problems in relating letters and groups of letters with appropriate sounds (phonologic coding).
- Dyslexia may be associated with attention deficit disorder (ADD) and attention deficit hyperactivity disorder (ADHD).
- Dyslexic children usually have normal or superior intelligence.
- Secondary emotional problems may result from poor school performance.
- In true dyslexia, the reading difficulties are permanent but remedial education techniques can help the patient to compensate.

DIAGNOSIS

A multidisciplinary team that can provide diagnostic and prescriptive services may involve some or all of the following:

- A specialist in learning disabilities to classify various areas of strengths and weaknesses and offer plans for appropriate instruction;
- A primary care physician to screen for auditory and visual disorders and rule out any physical or emotional factors that may be contributing to poor school performance;
- An ophthalmologist, who is experienced in the care of children to screen for any contributory oculomotor, optical, or organic eye problems;
- A neurologist to rule out any problems in the central nervous system that may contribute to learning disabilities;

- A psychologist or a psychiatrist to assist in management and diagnosis.

TREATMENT

- Appropriate instruction rendered by learning disability specialists helps youngsters to cope with the disability and compensate for limitations.
- Medications, including psychostimulants, tranquilizers and antidepressants that are used in the therapy of ADD and ADHD, should be prescribed only by physicians who are familiar with their effects. These drugs are used in specific cases to enhance attention so that acceptable educational techniques may be utilized.
- Some youngsters with dyslexia have visual-perceptual difficulties in addition to phonologic coding problems. These youngsters may benefit from the use of talking books and enlarged print.

COMMENTS

The treatment of a patient with dyslexia goes beyond evaluating ocular motility and refractive errors. A simple statement by the ophthalmologist that 'the eyes are normal' is not sufficient. Parents who leave a medical office with insufficient information are likely to wander into a setting that promises an easy cure for a complex problem. Over the years, many magic cures for learning disabilities have been promoted, including perceptual motor training, laterality training, special diets, megavitamins, eye exercises, vision training, vestibular drugs, chiropractic skull manipulation and colored lenses. Although many of the controversial treatments have fallen into disrepute, eye-related therapies seem to linger on. It is important that families be directed to appropriate specialists in learning disability who can deal with a particular child's specific needs. In defining the role of the ophthalmologist in dealing with learning disabilities and dyslexia, the joint statement by the American Association for Pediatric Ophthalmology and Strabismus, the American Academy of Ophthalmology and the American Academy of Pediatrics emphasizes that:

> Ocular defects in young children should be identified as early as possible, and when they are correctable, they should be managed by an ophthalmologist, who is experienced in the care of children. Treatable ocular conditions among others include refractive errors, focusing deficiencies, eye muscle imbalances, and motor fusion deficiencies . . .

> Eye defects, subtle or severe, do not cause the patient to experience reversal of letters, words, or numbers. No scientific evidence supports claims that the academic abilities of children with learning disabilities can be improved with treatments that are based on 1) visual training, including muscle exercises, ocular pursuit tracking exercises, or 'training' glasses (with or without bifocals or prisms); 2) neurological organizational training (laterality training, crawling, balance board, perceptual training); or 3) colored lenses . . .

SUPPORT GROUPS

International Dyslexia Association (formerly The Orton Dyslexia Society)
Suite 382
8600 La Salle Road
Baltimore, MD 21286-2044
1(800)ABCD-123, www.interdys.org

National Center for Learning Disabilities (NCLD)
Suite 1401
381 Park Avenue South
New York, NY 10016
1(888)575-7373, www.ncld.org

Recording for the Blind and Dyslexic
20 Roszel Rd
Princeton, NJ 08540
1(866)732-3585, www.rfbd.org

REFERENCES

Committee on Children With Disabilities: American Academy of Pediatrics, American Association for Pediatric Ophthalmology and Strabismus, American Academy of Ophthalmology: Learning disabilities, dyslexia, and vision. Pediatrics 102:1217–1219, 1998.

Hall S, Wick B: The relationship between ocular functions and reading achievement. J Pediatr Ophthalmol Strabismus 28:17–19, 1991.

Helveston E, Weber D, Miller K, et al: Visual function and academic performance. Am J Ophthalmol 99:346–355, 1985.

Hoyt C: Visual training and reading. Am Orthopt J 49:23–25, 1999.

Keys M, Silver L: Learning disabilities and vision problems: Are they related? Pediatrician 17:194–201, 1990.

Metzger R, Werner D: Use of visual training for reading disabilities: a review. Pediatrics 73:824–829, 1984.

Shaywitz S, Shaywitz B: The science of reading and dyslexia. J Am Assoc Ped Oph Strabismus 7:158–166, 2003.

Shaywitz S, Shaywitz B, Pugh K, et al: Functional disruption in the organization of the brain for reading in dyslexia. Proc Natl Acad Sci USA 95:2636–2641, 1998.

Silver L: The magic cure: a review of the current controversial approaches for treating learning disabilities. J Learning Disabil 20:498–512, 1987.

Silver L: The misunderstood child. A guide for parents of children with learning disabilities. 3rd edn. Times Books/Random House, 1998.

113 FUNCTIONAL AMBLYOPIA 368.0

Huban Atilla, MD
Ankara, Turkey

Amblyopia is defined as a reduction of best-corrected visual acuity that cannot be explained by structural abnormalities, mostly with the onset in childhood, at the visual maturation or development stages. Von Graefe defined amblyopia as the condition in which the observer sees nothing and the patient very little. It is commonly known as 'lazy eye.'

ETIOLOGY/INCIDENCE

Amblyopia is commonly divided into three subtypes: strabismic, anisometropic and deprivation. Although the vast majority of cases is unilateral with the contalateral eye being normal, bilateral deprivation amblyopia can be seen in bilateral infantile cataracts and bilateral high hypermetropia/astigmatism cases.

Amblyopia is the most common cause of monocular visual impairment in both children and young to middle-aged adults with a prevalence about 1–4%, surpassing trauma, diabetic retinopathy, glaucoma, macular degeneration and cataract.

COURSE/PROGNOSIS

The organization of the central nervous system pathways is not complete at birth and continues into early life as a developmental progression from immature to adult axonal patterns. For normal visual development to occur, an infant's visual system requires proper stimulation. During fetal development, differentiation and organization of the visual system are likely guided by intrinsic control mechanisms. Unlike the prenatal period, environmental factors and visual experience influence the process in postnatal life. During this development, blurred retinal image (pattern distortion), cortical suppression or combination of these two mechanisms can interrupt normal visual development. Lack of formed or clear images on the retina of one eye early in life may lead to profound long-lasting defects in cortical function. Timing and duration of this lack is very important, causing intensive effects early and tapering off at later ages. This can be called as critical or sensitive period, starting and ending points of this period is poorly defined. It has been suggested that it may extend to anywhere between 6 to 12 years of age. The concept of the critical period in normal visual development in humans is important in the treatment of visually immature children. There are few case reports with an improved visual acuity in the amblyopic eye after loss of the sound eye after visual maturation.

About 25% of patients have a visual acuity in the amblyopic eye worse than 20/100, and about 75% have an acuity 20/100 or better. Success rates for treatment of moderate amblyopia in children have ranged from 30% to 90% for both patching and atropine. Deprivational amblyopia or amblyopia associated with an organic pathology such as retinal or optic nerve disease may be treated with occlusion therapy and visual acuity may be improved to 20/40 or better. The combination of anisometropia and strabismus have a lower rate of success with treatment when compared with pure anisometropia. Poor initial visual acuity in the amblyopic eye is associated with a poor outcome for final visual acuity in spite of an improvement with treatment.

DIAGNOSIS

Diagnosis of amblyopia can be made with exclusion of the structural abnormalities and correctable causes of low vision. A thorough fundus examination to rule out optic nerve and retina pathologies must be performed. Associated strabismus and anisometropia are accepted as the main risk factors for alerting the physician.

Clinical signs and symptoms

Visual acuity difference between two eyes can be diagnosed by fixation testing in children who are too young to cooperate with optotype acuity tests such as Allen cards, illiterate E and Snellen acuity. Teller acuity cards and the pattern visual evoked potential are useful for estimating visual acuity with low sensitivity. Crowding phenomenon should be kept in mind for optotype tests. Also Snellen acuity is affected to a greater degree than grating acuity in strabismic amblyopes.

Presence of brisk, large afferent pupillary defect must be accepted as a sign of optic nerve disease, however mild APD may be detected especially in severe amblyopia cases.

Laboratory findings

VEP and ERG can be performed to detect underlying organic causes however amplitude and latency changes that are usually nonreproducible have been reported in amblyopia too. Amblyopia is generally defined as a decrease in central visual acuity, but in fact this represents only one aspect of the distorted visual capacity, i.e. the smallest, high contrast stimulus which can be detected. It is well established that strabismic and anisometropic amblyopia result in marked losses of threshold contrast sensitivity especially in high spatial frequencies. The reduced contrast sensitivity function of the amblyopic eye represents a neural loss of foveal function. Neutral density filters reduce vision in eyes with organic lesions but there is no change of visual acuity in amblyopic eyes.

Differential diagnosis

Any associated pathology of the visual and central nervous system must be excluded with a detailed ophthalmic examination is a must before reaching the diagnosis of amblyopia. In amblyopia cases with a slow or no response to treatment, an organic pathology must be considered as well as the reliability of the compliance of the patient. Refractive error must be rechecked after institution of patching therapy if no improvement has been achieved.

PROPHYLAXIS

Nearly all amblyopic visual loss is preventable or reversible with timely, appropriate intervention. Children with amblyopia or at risk for developing it at a young age, when the prognosis for successful treatment is best, can be identified with screening methods such as photorefraction. Every child should have an eye examination at the age of three for measurement of visual acuity. If there are suspected eye diseases or associated risk factors such as family history, an earlier examination is needed.

TREATMENT

There may be two mechanisms for loss of vision in amblyopia: an anatomic decrease in the number of fibers from the deprived eye that is nonreversible and active suppression of afferent activity from the deprived eye that is reversible. The aim of treatment is to provide a clear retinal image in both eyes and to extend the sensitive period as long as to increase the treatment period. If there is any obstacle to vision such as cataract, corneal opacity or ptosis, it must be eliminated, refractive errors must be corrected and the vision in the poorer eye is enhanced by occluding or blurring the better eye. Blurring the vision in the better eye may be achieved with spherical lenses (or plano lens if there is a refractive error) or diffusing filters as well as pharmacological agents and potential side effects of pharmacological penalization can be avoided in this way.

Systemic

- Levodopa can be used to improve visual acuity and functional ability to increase compliance especially in severe amblyopia cases and older patients to extend critical period. However, the use of it is limited due to the uncertainty in the dose and duration of treatment in older patients, and possible side effects in younger patients.
- Citicoline and thyroid hormones are other agents for systemic therapy but further studies are needed for clinical use of these agents.

Ocular

- For more than 200 years, occlusion of the sound eye is the mainstay of treatment. However, opinions vary on the number of hours that should be prescribed for daily patching. In clinical practice, part-time patching (6–8 hours daily) is more commonly used as an initial therapy. The Pediatric Eye Disease Investigator Group compared patching treatment in a prospective, randomized study and reported that two hours of daily patching appears to be as effective as six hours in treating moderate amblyopia. Patching should be done according to the age of the patient and the severity of the visual loss. The occlusion must be applied directly on the eye instead of the spectacles in order to avoid peeking. Opaque contact lenses can be used as an occluder in selected patients.
- Full-time occlusion is preferred in severe amblyopia cases or in cases with no fusion potential. Near visual tasks such as reading or video games during a portion of the occlusion time may contribute to the improvement in visual acuity. Treatment is continued until visual acuity is same in both eyes or no improvement is achieved after 6 months with a reliable compliance. The success of occlusion therapy is dependent on compliance mainly.

Medical

- Penalization with atropine aims to blur the image in the preferred eye so that the fixation can be switched to the amblyopic eye. Pharmacologic penalization has generally been advocated only for mild and moderate amblyopia (20/100 or better) because the blurring effect on the sound eye may be insufficient when visual acuity in the amblyopic eye is worse than 20/100. Recent reports of randomized clinical trials showed that substantial improvement in the visual acuity of the amblyopic eye occurred with either daily patching or atropine treatment regimens and the difference between the patching and daily atropine regimens was clinically insignificant after 6 months. After a randomized trial of atropine regimens in moderate amblyopia cases, it was found that weekend atropine can provide an improvement in visual acuity of a magnitude similar to that of the improvement provided by daily atropine.

Surgical

- Surgery for the underlying causes such as cataract, corneal opacities or ptosis is an essential part of the treatment.
- In strabismic amblyopia cases, correction of the misalignment will be a part of the treatment, however strabismus surgery is usually performed after improvement in vision of the amblyopic eye.
- Patients with unilateral high myopia can be a candidate for refractive surgery after 9–10 years of age.

COMPLICATIONS

- Amblyopia in the occluded eye is the most expected complication of treatment. Fortunately this is rare and easily reversible after cessation of occlusion. In children under one year of age, part time occlusion and close follow up are recommended.
- In patients with limited fusion capacity, occlusion may deteriorate the compensated heterotropia and induce strabismus. This must be mentioned to the parents in order to increase compliance. Switching the fixation preference must be explained to the parents as a desired result. After discontinuation of patching therapy some degree of recurrence can be seen but this can be prevented with maintenance therapy.
- Skin irritation during patching therapy and light sensitivity, lid or conjunctival irritation, eye pain or headache and facial flushing during atropine penalization are the other main adverse effects of the therapy.

COMMENTS

Amblyopia is a developmental anomaly of spatial vision, occurring as optically uncorrectable subnormal visual acuity in an otherwise normal eye. Early detection and early treatment are critical in treatment. Patching has the potential advantages of a more rapid improvement in visual acuity and possibly a slightly better acuity outcome, whereas atropine has the potential advantages of easier administration and lower cost.

REFERENCES

Flynn JT: Amblyopia revisited. 17th Annual Frank Costenbader Lecture. J Pediatr Ophthalmol Strabismus 28(4):183–200, 1991.

Holmes MJ, Beck RW, Repka MX: Amblyopia: current clinical studies. Ophthalmol Clinics N Am, Pediatric Ophthalmol 14(3):393–398, 2001.

Hussein MAW, Coats DK, Muthialu A, et al: Risk factors for treatment failure of anisometropic amblyopia. J AAPOS 8:429–434, 2004.

Leguire LE, Rogers GL, Brmer DL, et al: Levodopa/carbidopa for childhood amblyopia. Invest Ophthalmol Vis Sci 34:3090–3095, 1993.

Nucci P, Drack AV: Refractive surgery for unilateral high myopia in children. J AAPOS 5:348–351, 2001.

Olitsky SE, Nelson BA, Brooks S: The sensitive period of visual development in humans. J Pediatr Ophthalmol Strabismus 39(2):69–72, 2002.

Pediatric Eye Disease Investigator Group: A randomized trial of atropine vs patching for treatment of moderate amblyopia in children. Arch Ophthalmol 120:268–278, 2002.

Pediatric Eye Disease Investigator Group: A randomized trial of patching regimens for treatment of moderate amblyopia in children. Arch Ophthalmol 121:603–611, 2003.

Pediatric Eye Disease Investigator Group: A randomized trial of atropine regimens for treatment of moderate amblyopia in children. Ophthalmology 111:2076–2085, 2004.

114 HYSTERIA, MALINGERING AND ANXIETY STATES 300.10

August L. Reader, III, MD, FACS
San Francisco, California

ETIOLOGY

Psychogenic ocular disease can be confounding to the ophthalmologist, as psychologic factors of stress and anxiety commonly accompany any disease state. Differentiating ocular disease that is totally psychogenic is essential so that serious problems that may be masked are not overlooked. *Hysteria* is the feigning of disease or injury on an unconscious level in order to satisfy unmet psychologic needs. It probably springs from early psychosexual conflict or from significant emotional trauma that occurred at any age. *Malingering* is the conscious exaggeration or simulation of symptoms in order to obtain some gain, such as financial reward in a lawsuit or avoidance of military duty. It is usually based on a history of compensable injuries or on fear of injury. *Anxiety states* are common and exist to a greater or lesser degree in the majority of patients who have serious disease or injury; however, they may be abnormally intense in certain patients who have relatively minor ailments. Their presence in excess indicates the existence of strong dependency issues and excessive fear. Occasionally, *dissimulation* occurs when patients claim to be normal when disease or disability is present in order to obtain a goal, for example, to qualify for a specific occupation such as pilot or truck driver.

COURSE/PROGNOSIS

- Symptoms persist and sometimes worsen unless intervention occurs.
- Prognosis varies with the responsiveness of the patient, but generally, it is excellent.

DIAGNOSIS

Laboratory findings

- Extensive ophthalmologic examination is necessary to rule out pathology.
- Special clinical tests should be run to pinpoint hysteria or malingering.
- Electrophysiology tests should be performed-visual evoked responses, electroretinography, and electro-oculography-looking for normal responses.

TREATMENT

Therapy for hysteria usually requires psychiatric intervention in severe cases; mild cases can be handled by emphasizing the normal findings of the examination and suggesting that the symptoms will resolve in a short time. Malingerers should be confronted cautiously, for they could feel accused and have been known to react with hostility. Anxious patients can be treated with calm reassurance and explanations of the findings. Temporary relief is usually obtained with benzodiazepines, which may be helpful in more severe cases.

Patients subject to panic attacks gain security with the use of rapidly acting anxiolytics. Patients with depression or sleep disorders can be helped with any of the new serotonin reuptake inhibitors, but these are best prescribed by a psychiatrist or neurologist rather than by an ophthalmologist. Patients with an organic disease that is worsened by anxiety, such as blepharospasm, may be helped by biofeedback therapy or hypnotherapy before contemplating botulinum injections or surgery.

Moralizing about hysterical disease and exhorting patients to stop imagining symptoms should be avoided. The examination of a presumed hysteric should be ended quickly to avoid reinforcement of secondary gain. The examination of a suspected malingerer should be extended and resumed on subsequent days and should include repetition of tests to uncover inconsistencies and to allow the patient to 'recover' in order to save face. The most difficult cases are those with real ocular disease plus secondary psychosomatic or psychogenic symptoms.

COMMENTS

Extensive and well-documented examinations are essential to explain all discrepancies between complaints and examination results. Many of these cases involve litigation, and the practitioner must be on guard to protect against being drawn into a lawsuit because of a hostile or psychiatrically unbalanced patient.

REFERENCES

Catalano RA, Simon JW, Krobel GB, et al: Functional visual loss in children. Ophthalmology 93:385–390, 1986.

Keltner JL, May WN, Johnson CA, et al: The California syndrome: functional visual complaints with potential economic impact. Ophthalmology 92:427–435, 1985.

Miller BW: A review of practical tests for ocular malingering and hysteria. Surv Ophthal 17:241–146, 1973.

Smith CH, Beck RW, Mills RP: Functional disease in neuro-ophthalmology. Neurol Clin 1:955–971, 1983.

Thompson HS: Functional visual loss. Am J Ophthal 100:209–213, 1985.

115 IDIOPATHIC INTRACRANIAL HYPERTENSION AND PSEUDOTUMOR CEREBRI 348.2

(Benign Intracranial Hypertension)

Eric Lowell Singman, MD, PhD
Lancaster, Pennsylvania

Pseudotumor cerebri (PTC) is intracranial hypertension in the absence of intracranial mass or hemorrhage. The primary form has also been referred to as benign intracranial hypertension (BIH), a term that should be discarded because it is inaccurate. The active disease can be disabling and even patients in remission may suffer further visual loss and recrudescence. Primary PTC must be a diagnosis of careful exclusion as the list of etiologies grows.

ETIOLOGY/INCIDENCE

A number of studies from different countries have agreed that the annual incidence rate of primary PTC in the general population is somewhere between 0.5–1.0/100,000/year, while in the population of obese women of childbearing age, the incidence is between 2.5–3.0/100,000/year. There is no question that obesity and female gender are among the key risk factors. Problematically, the definition of PTC is not uniformly accepted.

The mechanism through which obesity is associated with PTC is unclear. Obese patients more commonly have elevated markers of inflammation and prothrombotic states, both of which are associated with PTC. Perhaps these patients suffer infarction or obstruction of the arachnoid granulations or venous sinuses limiting cerebrospinal fluid (CSF) outflow. The osteopathic literature describes a craniosacral pump which fails because of alterations in spinal configuration of markedly obese patients, leading to increased intracranial pressure (ICP). This information is not widely available in allopathic journals but should not be simply dismissed.

Inflammatory and prothrombotic disease states associated with PTC include systemic lupus erythematosis (SLE), periarteritis nodosa, uremia, antiphospholipid antibody (APA) syndrome, anticardiolipin antibody syndrome (ACA), sarcoidosis, inflammatory bowel disease, Lyme disease, protein C and S deficiencies, multiple sclerosis and meningitis. Pregnancy is a significant risk factor for PTC, possibly because of weight gain or increased risk of thrombosis.

PTC can accompany post-concussion syndrome, Chiari malformation, sleep apnea, anemia, sickle cell disease, polycystic ovary syndrome (PCOS), mastoiditis (via secondary venous sinus thrombosis), hypoparathyroidism (from hypocalcemia) and thoracic outlet syndrome.

Drugs implicated in PTC include the tetracycline class antibiotics, nalidixic acid, growth hormone, vitamin A congeners, Synthroid, Norplant, oral contraceptives, danazol, lithium, cyclosporin A, cytarabine, nitrofurantoin, prednisone, thiazide diuretics and nonsteroidal anti-inflammatory drugs. Some of these drugs have a dual effect. Prednisone can both cause and treat PTC, and PTC sometimes accompanies prednisone tapering regimens. Hyper- and hypo-vitaminosis A both have been associated with PTC. Thiazide diuretics that can be used to treat PTC might also cause it through the side effect of hypocalcemia.

Drug-disease combinations often make for a confusing clinical picture regarding the etiology of PTC. For example, PTC can be seen with Lyme disease, hypothyroidism and sarcoid and also with the treatments therein (i.e. tetracyclines, thyroid replacement and steroids, respectively). Patients often have multiple risk factors. It would not be unusual for an obese woman with sleep apnea and anemia (from the menorrhagia associated with PCOS) to use tetracyclines or vitamin A products for acne (associated with PCOS).

COURSE/PROGNOSIS

Pseudotumor cerebri can develop acutely, such as with use of tetracyclines or after head trauma, or can be chronic, as with obesity or sleep apnea. Response to therapy is usually rapid but may be short-lived. Papilledema can linger for years however. It has been reported that long term vision loss can occur even after the apparent resolution of papilledema.

Acute vision loss can occur from breaks in Bruch's membrane and secondary subretinal hemorrhage. This predisposes patients to develop subretinal neovascularization. Papilledematous nerves are at risk for central retinal vein occlusion and nonarteritic anterior ischemic optic neuropathy.

Recurrence does occur and patients might have different symptoms and signs than they did at initial presentation.

DIAGNOSIS

Clinical signs and symptoms

Symptoms of PTC include head-, neck- or ear-ache, diplopia, tinnitus or pulsatile whooshing, transient visual obscurations (TVOs), peripheral vision loss, severe acute reduction of visual acuity, photophobia, vomiting and dizziness. Children may present with irritability, listlessness, somnolence or nervousness. Back pain and loss of bladder control can be seen with PTC due to a low spinal tumor. Depression often accompanies patients with PTC. While it is likely that PTC can cause or even present as depression, it must be remembered that some patients with bipolar disorder develop PTC from lithium therapy.

We have noted an extremely high frequency of convergence insufficiency in all age groups and a higher-than-expected frequency of attention deficit disorder (ADD) in our pediatric patients.

Headache is the most common presenting sign. Headache can range from disablingly severe to mild; it is usually constant although it fluctuates in severity. Many of our patients report that headache severity is altered in response to atmospheric barometric changes. Headache is usually worse in the morning, and is aggravated with Valsalva or bending. Visual obscurations occur with bending as well. Dizziness seems to be worsened by rapid head turns. Headache may not accompany PTC at all; this phenomenon may be more common in pediatric patients. In patients with headache, we often employ a 3 day therapeutic trial of acetazolamide (0.5–1.5gm qd) as part of our evaluation.

Signs of PTC include papilledema, esotropia from unilateral or bilateral sixth cranial palsy, convergence and accommodative insufficiency, hypertropia from fourth cranial nerve palsy, seventh cranial nerve palsy and hemifacial spasm.

Although papilledema facilitates the diagnosis, many patients do not show display this. The loss of spontaneous venous pulsations (SVPs) at the optic nerve head is also imperfectly correlated with PTC. Twenty percent of normal patients do not have SVPs and some confirmed PTC patients have normal SVPs. The absence of papilledema (i.e. *PTC sine papilledema*) is likely a significant risk factor for diagnostic delay.

Other ophthalmic findings include retinal hemorrhages, cotton wool spots (infarcts in the nerve fiber layer), macular exudate, choroidal breaks, and retinal folds concentric about the disc (Paton's lines).

Laboratory findings

Imaging studies are key to making the diagnosis of PTC. Magnetic resonance imaging (MRI) is particularly useful when looking for tumors of the brain and spinal cord (particularly ependymoma); magnetic resonance venogram (MRV) can detect venous sinus thrombosis. Common MRI findings in PTC include a flattened pituitary (pancake sign), empty sella, optic nerves bathed in CSF, slit-like ventricles and prominence of the temporal horns of the lateral ventricles. It is common to find cerebellar tonsillar herniation in patients with PTC, strongly suggesting that Chiari malformation and pseudotumor cerebri are related. Hyperintense white matter lesions on MRI are more common in patients with vasculitidies such as Lyme disease, MS, SLE and sarcoid.

Lumbar puncture (LP) is a crucial diagnostic test, as well as a potentially curative one. We recommend measuring the opening pressure with the patient lying prone or on the side. Radiographic guidance during LP is a safety measure for larger patients to help avoid injury. The ICP should be measured in every patient; if the pressure is elevated (above 250 mm water), 30cc should be drawn off for tests and to provide headache relief. The CSF should be sent for laboratory evaluation of markers of MS (oligoclonal banding, immunoglobulin synthesis rate and myelin basic protein) and Lyme disease (preferably by both Western blot and PCR), as well as for analysis of cells, protein and glucose.

Many patients will have an opening pressure within normal range. Regardless of the ICP, PTC should lead the differential list if a patient enjoys symptom relief after LP. Studies using continuous lumbar and intracranial pressure monitoring have proven that the ICP can vary diurnally and continuous monitoring is therefore critically useful in confirming atypical cases, e.g. normotensive PTC or PTC sine papilledema. It has been shown that many patients successfully treated with programmable shunts need the ICP set far below what would be considered normal.

Serum studies looking for evidence of inflammation associated with PTC include a Lyme PCR, Lyme Western blot and Lyme C6 peptide, serum protein electrophoresis, serum muramidase (for sarcoid), calcium, ACA, ANA, CBC, ESR, CRP, thyroid function tests and vitamin A level.

Visual field testing is necessary to follow optic nerve health. An enlarged blind spot is invariably associated with papilledema. Constriction of the peripheral field with a high false negative rate, a finding commonly seen in malingering patients, is also common with PTC; the physician must give the patient the benefit of doubt. Nerve fiber bundle defects, particularly in the nasal field, are also common. Visual field loss can occur even after apparently successful therapy so long-term follow-up is necessary.

We follow the appearance of the optic nerves with the Heidelberg retinal tomograph. This device allows 3-d viewing of the nerve (Figures 115.1 and 115.2) and measurements of nerve elevation. Fluorescein angiography can help differentiate papilledema from the pseudopapilledema of optic nerve drusen or hypertropia. High resolution sonography of the nerve provides only confirmation of optic nerve engorgement using the 30-degree turn test. During this test, the nerve width is compared at rest in primary gaze and under stretch in extreme lateral gaze, where a significant reduction in nerve caliber indicates edema.

Visual evoked potential (VEP) testing may be particularly useful to monitor optic nerve health in patients for whom the visual field might be suboptimally reliable or in patients who continue to lose vision despite the absence of papilledema.

Differential diagnosis

Pseudotumor cerebri must be differentiated from a true tumor as well as other constant headache syndromes such as chronic daily headache, converted migraine, cerebral aneurysm, mastoiditis, rhinosinusitis and temporal arteritis.

The differential diagnosis of papilledema is wide; when papilledema accompanies headache, one must consider malignant hypertension, Graves' disease and optic neuritis. It is important to differentiate between papilledema from pseudopapilledema, although patients could certainly have both conditions. On the other hand, high resolution ultrasonography has shown that perfectly healthy patients can have fluid-engorged, edematous optic nerves.

Patients with PTC can present with neither papilledema nor headache. Therefore, one should still include PTC in the differential list for any patient with even isolated findings of depression, double vision, refractory convergence insufficiency, dizziness, tinnitus or focal cranial neurologic findings.

TREATMENT

Systemic

Short term medical therapies include diuretics, particularly carbonic anhydrase inhibitors (CAIs) such as acetazolamide (500 mg PO up to q.i.d.), and furosemide (20 to 40 mg PO b.i.d.). One should generally avoid offering steroid therapy, especially prior to a CSF analysis confirming the absence of infection. Thereafter, a 2 week course of prednisone (60 mg PO qd) with a week long taper might be attempted if necessary. Short term surgical therapy includes multiple lumbar punctures. We have documented a few patients reporting significant short term relief with osteopathic manipulation. Many patients can achieve a cure with short term therapies.

Long term treatment of PTC requires removing inciting chemicals, treating sleep apnea, correcting metabolic disturbances and controlling weight. Bariatric surgery is a necessary option for many patients. Patients with intractable headaches or with continuing visual loss despite optic nerve sheath fenestration are candidates for ventriculo- or lumbo-peritoneal shunting. Some patients will need surgical therapy for concomitant Chiari malformation. Programmable shunts are now available to titrate ICP to the patient's reported comfort level

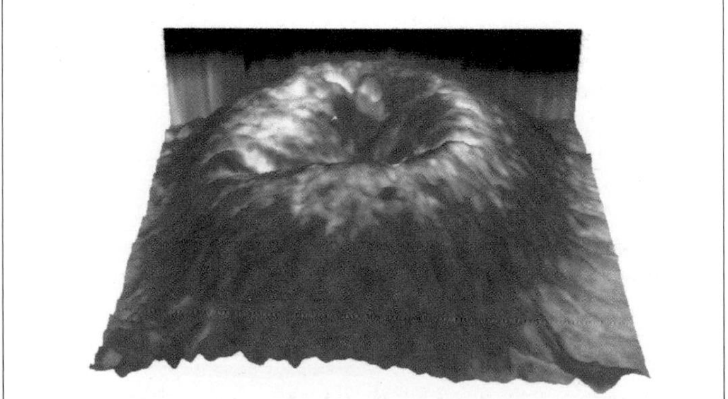

FIGURE 115.1. The right optic nerve of a 17 year old girl who was being treated for Lyme disease with tetracycline. She presented with severe headache and esotropia. The HRT 3-D view of 08/11/04 was captured at the patient's first visit.

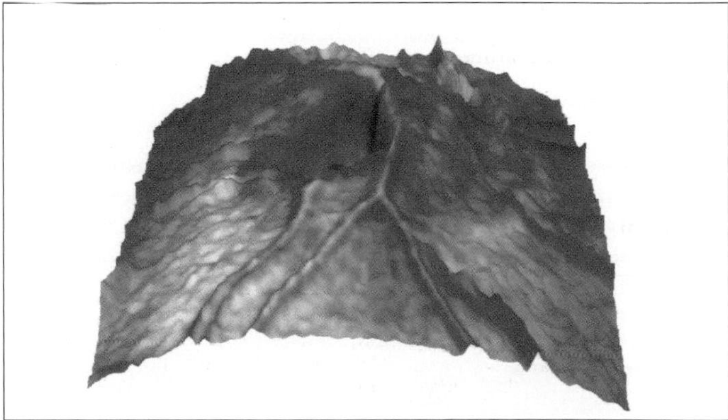

FIGURE 115.2. This view from 01/10/05 was captured after Diamox therapy and substitution of the antibiotic. The headache and esotropia resolved within two weeks.

in the clinic setting. Endoscopic third ventriculostomy is currently being studied as a treatment option.

Ocular

Optic nerve sheath fenestration is the only periocular therapy for PTC and is recommended where visual loss is predominant over headache. During this procedure, the surgeon cuts a window from the meningeal sheath of the optic nerve, preferably through a medial orbital approach to avoid the ophthalmic artery. The medial rectus must be surgically disinserted to gain sufficient exposure.

COMPLICATIONS

Acetazolamide can cause hypokalemia, acidosis and secondary calcium oxylate nephrolithiasis. Invariable but sometimes intolerable side effects also include dysgeusia, fatigue, anorexia and paresthesias. Because CAIs are sulfonamides, there is risk of allergy and bone marrow suppression. We recommend a baseline serum potassium and CBC prior to long-term therapy. Corticosteroids, even in short term dose, cause hyperglycemia and immunosuppression.

Aside from the usual complications associated with any surgery done under general anesthesia, blindness and double vision might follow optic nerve sheath fenestration. The unique concerns of even completely successful shunting procedures are blockage (with an estimated risk of 80% at 12 years postoperative), and migration of the shunt tip.

COMMENTS

For many, PTC is vision threatening and disabling. The protean manifestations demand that physicians consider this diagnosis much more often. Considering that patients suffering from this condition, i.e. women, obese individuals and chronic headache sufferers, have been reported to receive suboptimal care, it must be assumed that PTC is significantly underdiagnosed.

Support groups and patient registries are available to help both patients and caregivers cope with PTC. With further research into therapies and etiologies, it is hoped that the idiopathic form will disappear.

REFERENCES

Johnson S: The PTC primer . . . living with pseudotumor cerebri. Pseudotumor Cerebri Support Network, Powell, Ohio, 2000. Online. Available at: www.findmemyhouse.com/ptc/ptc_book/book_index.html.

Krishna R, Kosmorsky GS, Wright KW: Pseudotumor cerebri sine papilledema with unilateral sixth nerve palsy. J Neuroophthalmol 18:53–55, 1998.

McGirt MJ, Woodworth G, Thomas G, et al: Cerebrospinal fluid shunt placement for pseudotumor cerebri-associated intractable headache: predictors of treatment response and an analysis of long-term outcomes. J Neurosurg 101:627–632, 2004.

Milhorat TH, Chou MW, Trinidad EM, et al: Chiari I malformation redefined: clinical and radiographic findings for 364 symptomatic patients. Neurosurgery 44:1005–1017, 1999.

Nord JA, Karter D: Epub 2003 Lyme disease complicated with pseudotumor cerebri. Clin Infect Dis 37:e25–e26, 2003.

Spoor TC, McHenry JG: Long-term effectiveness of optic nerve sheath decompression for pseudotumor cerebri. Arch Ophthalmol 111:623–635, 1993.

Sussman J, Leach M, Greaves M, et al: Potentially prothrombotic abnormalities of coagulation in benign intracranial hypertension. J Neurol Neurosurg Psychiatry 62:229–233, 1997.

116 MULTIPLE SCLEROSIS 340
(Sclérose en Plaques Disseminées, Disseminated Sclerosis)

Amit Kumar Ghosh, MD, FACP
Rochester, Minnesota

Multiple sclerosis (MS) is the most common cause of disabling nontraumatic neurological disorder in the young adults. MS is a clinical disorder characterized with neurological attacks followed by remissions. Pathologically MS is characterized by multiple sharply delineated plaques reflective of demyelination in the CNS white matter affecting the optic nerves, periventricular areas, brain stem and spinal cord. The plaques are areas of active demyelination with loss of oligodendrocytes and astroglial scarring. Recent studies on active MS lesions also indicate the presence of substantial axonal injury with axonal transactions. The mean lifetime cost per case of MS is around $2.2 million.

ETIOLOGY/INCIDENCE

The risk of developing MS is around 0.1% in US. It is estimated that the prevalence in USA is approximately 350,000 with an annual incidence of about 12,000. The prevalence varies geographically reaching as high as 60 per 100,000 in North America and Europe and is lowest among Eskimos, Native Americans and Africans. Onset of the disease is between 20 and 50 years with the female to male ratio of 2 : 1. The peak onset is around 5 years earlier in women.

The exact pathogenesis of MS is unclear. Most cases are sporadic, though first degree relatives of a person with MS have a 20 to 40 times increased risk than general population of developing MS. The presence of HLA-DR2 allele is associated with an increased risk. Recent studies have dispelled the belief, that immunization with hepatitis B or other vaccines increase the risk of developing MS. Other theories have suggested Epstein–Barr virus reactivation, and smoking as possible risk factors. Migration from a high to low risk area during earlier childhood might confer lower risk of MS and vice-versa. Migration from higher to lower risk areas after reaching puberty seems to mitigate this advantage.

COURSE/PROGNOSIS

MS could present in several different courses. Around 85% of patients start out as *relapsing and remitting* (RRMS), characterized by self-limited attacks with complete or partial recovery and the patient is neurologically stable between attacks. The RRMS is followed in 50% of cases by *secondary-progressive* (SPMS) which is marked by gradual neurological deterioration between relapses. Approximately 15% patient begin with *primary-progressive* (PPMS) form that is characterized by gradual disease progression from onset with plateaus and minor fluctuations but no distinct relapses. A rarer form of MS is the *progressive-relapsing* (PRMS) that presents initially as PPMS with clear relapses with or without complete recovery. Progression continues between relapses.

Relapse is often referred to as acute or subacute worsening of clinical function that might peak in days to weeks and maybe followed by remissions where the symptoms and signs might resolve partially or completely. Relapse tend to occur frequently in the initial years (average 0.4 to 0.6/year) and decrease with time.

The course of MS is highly variable even in the same individual. Factors that might suggest a worse prognosis include, frequent relapse in the first 2 years, progressive type of MS, male sex, early motor and cerebellar disorder. Patient with optic neuritis, women, early age of onset, and predominantly sensory signs may have a better prognosis. Patients with no neurological disability after 15 years of the disease are often referred to have benign MS.

DIAGNOSIS

Clinical signs and symptoms

Common symptoms and signs include numbness, weakness, visual lose, diplopia, limb weakness, ataxia, Lhermitte's phenomenon, cognitive and affective disorder and bowel and bladder problems. Neurological symptoms maybe acute, chronic or progressive. These signs indicate involvement of corticospinal tract, posterior columns, brain stem, anterior visual pathways and cerebellum. The symptoms should last more than 24 hours and occur as discrete episodes separated by over a month or more.

Optic neuritis (ON) is the most common inflammatory condition involving the visual pathways. The presentation maybe acute or subacute unilateral eye pain with decrease in visual acuity, central field scotomas, relative afferent pupillary defect (Marcus Gunn pupil), normal fundus examination (retrobulbar neuritis) and less frequently optic disk edema (papillitis). Uveitis, retinitis and retinal periphlebitis are less frequent. Diplopia result from intranuclear ophthalmoplegia (INO), and is the most common eye movement disorder in MS, with loss or delayed adduction and nystagmus of the abducting eye on lateral gaze, due to lesion of the medial longitudinal fasciculus (MLS) on the side of adducting eye. Diplopia could also occur due to cranial nerve palsies (usually 6th cranial nerve, rarely 3rd and 4th cranial nerve palsy). Other visual disorders include pendular nystagmus with oscillopsia and defective ocular saccades and pursuits, Uhthoff's symptom (transient visual blurring after hot shower of physical exercise). The risk of development of MS after an episode of ON varies from 15 to 75%.

Laboratory findings

MS is a clinical diagnosis that includes demonstrating evidence of multiple neurological events (two or more symptoms and signs) separated in space (different anatomical location) and time. Several laboratory testing have been approved to support the diagnosis including, Brain MRI, cerebrospinal fluid (CSF) oligoclonal band, CSF albumin and IgG index, visual evoked response(VER), Brainstem auditory evoked response (BAER) and somatosensory evoked potentials (SEP).

Magnetic resonance imaging (MRI) demonstration of the characteristic brain and spinal cord plaque remains the test of choice to support the diagnosis of MS. These plaques are seen in the periventricular region, deep white matter, corpus callosum, brain stem, cerebellum, optic pathways. The plaques are located perpendicular to ventricular surface and appear hyperintense on proton density and T2-weighted studies. Gadolinium (Gd) enhancement usually suggest new or active plaques in MS.

Cerebrospinal fluid abnormalities in MS includes mononuclear cell pleocytosis, increased CSF IgG index, increased IgG synthesis rate and oligoclonal banding.

In 2001, The International Panel on MS proposed guidelines for diagnosis based on the objective demonstration of dissemination of lesion in time and space. Patients with two or more clinical attacks and 2 objective signs do not need any further tests to confirm the diagnosis of MS. In all other cases diagnosis of MS is made by a combination of clinical history and MRI, CSF evaluation and/or other ancillary testing (VER, BAER, VES). Patients should be classified as MS, 'possible' MS (those at risk for MS, but evaluations are equivocal) or 'not' MS.

TREATMENT

The treatment of MS involves:

- Treatment of acute attacks;
- Treatment to reduce the activity of MS using disease modifying therapy; and
- Symptomatic treatment.

The Kurtzke Expanded Disability Status Score (EDSS) are commonly used to measure clinical disability in MS. Most patients with RRMS have EDSS scores of <3.5 and can walk normally as opposed to patients with progressive MS (SPMS , PPMS) who have gait impairment with EDSS scores of >5.5.

Treatment of acute attacks

Corticosteroids are typically used to treat first episode or acute attacks of MS. They help in the short term by reducing the severity and duration of these attacks, however long term benefits on the course of MS is unclear. Mild attacks should not be treated.

Treatment for acute monosymptomatic optic neuritis (ON) is based on the results of two studies; the Optic Neuritis Treatment Trial (ONTT) with methylprednisolone and more recently the Controlled High-Risk Avonex MS Prevention Study (CHAMPS) with interferon β-1a (Avonex). Current recommendations for patients with ON with high risk of developing MS (two or more white matter lesions) include the use of intravenous methylprednisolone 1000 mg daily for 3 days , followed by oral prednisone (1 mg/kg per day for 11 days followed by a 4 day taper, [MP+ prednisone]) , and interferon β-1a (Avonex 30 μg intramuscular once weekly). Patients with less than two MRI white matter lesions can be treated with IV MP+ prednisone. Oral prednisone alone without prior treatment with methylprednisolone should not be used as the findings in ONTT showed an increase in the risk of recurrent ON in the group that received oral prednisone only.

Rapidly progressive disability in MS often have to be treated with IV cyclophosphamide with corticosteroid and in rare instances with plasma exchanges (every other day for 2 weeks).

Disease modifying agents used in MS

Disease modifying agents are used in RRMS and SPMS with exacerbations. Five agents have been approved in United States

TABLE 116.1 Side-effects of disease modifying agents for multiple sclerosis

Medication	Side Effects
Interferon beta 1α (Avonex)	Flu like symptoms, local injection site
	Reactions, abnormal liver tests, leucopenia, worsening depression
Interferon beta 1α (Rebif)	Similar to Avonex
Interferon beta 1β (Betaseron)	Similar to Avonex
Glatiramer acetate	Local injection site erythema, idiosyncratic reaction (shortness of breath, chest tightness, anxiety)
Mitoxantrone	Nausea, vomiting, cardiotoxicity, hair thinning, drug induced malignancy

for the treatment of RRMS. These include interferon β-1a (IFN-β1a , Avonex) , interferon β-1b (IFN β1b, Betaseron), interferon β-1a(IFN-β1a, Rebif), Glatiramer acetate (Copaxone) and Mitoxantrone (Novantrone).

These medications have also been tried in patients with SPMS with exacerbations. Patients receiving IFN-β1a, IFN-β1b, and glatiramer acetate have 30% fewer clinical episodes (measured by EDSS progression) and fewer MRI lesions. Patients with stable RRMS or SPMS without relapses should not treated. This group of patients need be observed by clinical examination and MRI every 6 months.

IFN-β1a (Avonex) is administered 30 μg intramuscular once weekly. IFN-B1b (Betaseron) is administered 250 μg subcutaneously every other day and IFN-β1a (Rebif), 44 μg subcutaneously three times a week. Common side-effects of interferons is outlined in Table 116.1. All interferons stimulate the development of neutralizing antibody that reduce the bioavailability of interferon. The rate of development of neutralizing antibodies after 18 months of treatment with Avonex, Rebif and Betaseron is around 2, 15 and 31 percent respectively. High dose of IFN-β can be tried in patients with SPMS with acute relapses, though this increases the risk of developing neutralizing antibody.

Glatiramer acetate/copolymer 1 (Copaxone) is administered 20 mg subcutaneous injection daily. The side effects include, local site reactions and systemic reactions such as flushing, chest tightness, dyspnea and anxiety after injections occur in around 15% of patients.

Mitoxantrone is given at a dose of 12 mg/m^2 every 3 months for a maximum of 2 to 3 years. Mitoxantrone is not a first line medication as its use has been associated with cardiotoxicity. Hence it is reserved for patients with SPMS, PRMS and RRMS with progressive disability who have failed other treatment. The maximum cumulative dose of Mitoxantrone allowed is 140 mg/m^2.

There is currently no effective treatment for PPMS despite numerous trails.

Other medications that has be tried in rapidly progressing MS, or RRMS and SPMS with inadequate response to the above disease modifying agents are, Azathioprine, Methotrexate, Cyclophosphamide, Cladribine, intravenous immunoglobulin (IVIg), and monthly high dose methylprednisolone.

Symptomatic treatment

Symptomatic therapy for MS is indicated for management of fatigue, spasticity, pain, bladder dysfunction, tremors, depression, paroxysmal motor symptoms (spasms, myoclonus, dystonia, dysarthria) and cognitive impairment. Eye movement disorders in MS is usually transient and does not need treatment. Bilateral INO may be treated with alternate compression or temporary press-in prisms. No effective treatment exists for unilateral INO. Oscillopsia arising from primary position nystagmus can arise form cerebellar or brain stem disorder . This can be treated with baclofen 20 mg PO t.i.d., and/or clonazepam 0.5 mg b.i.d.or t.i.d.

Currently several trials with experimental therapies are in progess, including monoclonal antibodies against a_4 – integrin, statins, estriol, Schwann cell transplants and bone marrow transplants.

Healthcare providers need to discuss the various aspects of treatment modalities and options with their patients and incorporate their patients values and opinions in making a treatment plan. Finally, a team approach with a primary care provider or neurologist well versed with numerous aspects in the care of MS is paramount for overall successful management.

REFERENCES

Arnold DL, Matthews PM: MRI in the diagnosis and management of multiple sclerosis. Neurology 58(Suppl 4):S23–S31, 2002.

Beck RW, Cleary PA, Anderson MM, Jr, et al: A randomized, controlled trial of corticosteroids in the treatment of acute optic neuritis. The Optic Neuritis Study Group. N Engl J Med 326:581–588, 1992.

Goodin DS, Frohman EM, Garmany GP, Jr, et al: Disease modifying therapies in multiple sclerosis: report of the Therapeutics and Technology Assessment Subcommittee of the American Academy of Neurology and the MS Council for Clinical Practice Guidelines. Neurology 58:169–178, 2002.

Jacobs LD, Beck RW, Simon JH, et al: Intramuscular interferon beta-1a therapy initiated during a first demyelinating event in multiple sclerosis. CHAMPS Study Group. N Engl J Med 343:898–904, 2000.

Krupp LB, Rizvi SA: Symptomatic therapy for underrecognized manifestations of multiple sclerosis. Neurology 58(8 Suppl 4):S32–S39, 2002.

McDonald WI, Compston A, Edan G, et al: Recommended diagnostic criteria for multiple sclerosis: guidelines from the International Panel on the diagnosis of multiple sclerosis. Ann Neurol 50:121–127, 2001.

Noseworthy JH, Lucchinetti C, Rodriguez M, Weinshenker BG: Multiple sclerosis. N Engl J Med 343:938–952, 2000.

Optic Neuritis Study Group: The 5-year risk of MS after optic neuritis. Experience of the optic neuritis treatment trial. Optic Neuritis Study Group. Neurology 49:1404–1413, 1997.

Whetten-Goldstein KFA, Sloan L, Goldstein B, et al: A comprehensive assessment of cost and compensation: the case of multiple sclerosis. Mult Scler 4:419–425, 1998.

Yong VW: Differential mechanisms of action of interferon- beta and glatiramer acetate in MS. Neurology 59:802–808, 2002.

117 MYASTHENIA GRAVIS 358.0

Jared J. B. Mee, MBBS
Melbourne, Australia
A. Justin O'Day, MBBS, FRANZCO
Melbourne, Australia

Myasthenia gravis is an autoimmune disease characterized by weakness and fatigability of voluntary muscles.

ETIOLOGY/INCIDENCE

- Myasthenia is caused by autoantibodies against acetylcholine receptors at the neuromuscular junction.
- Ten percent of patients with MG have a thymic tumor and 70% have hyperplastic germinal centers. It may be a breakdown in thymus generated immune self-tolerance that leads to myasthenia.
- Myasthenia may also be precipitated or worsened by a variety of drugs, including quinine, quinidine, procainamide, and aminoglycosides.
- Family history present in about 5% of cases
- Associated autoimmune disorders, particularly dysthyroidism, may be present concurrently.
- Occurs in 1 in 5000 people.
- Can develop at any age but reaches peak incidence in the third decade in women and in the fifth and sixth decades in men. It is probably underdiagnosed in the very old population.

COURSE/PROGNOSIS

- Diplopia or ptosis are commonly the initial presenting symptoms of myasthenia.
- A history of fluctuating symptoms that worsen towards the end of the day or with fatigue increases the likelihood of myasthenia. Without treatment, all symptoms gradually worsen over time.
- Ptosis maybe unilateral or bilateral. Characteristic features include Cogan's lid twitch on saccade from downgaze to upgaze and fatigability on sustained upgaze for 1 minute.
- Weakness of the orbicularis oculi muscle is a common early manifestation but occurs in other myopathies.
- Myasthenia may mimic any disorder of eye movement including myopathies, oculomotor nerve pareses, supranuclear gaze pareses, internuclear ophthalmoplegia or nystagmus. Vertical misalignments are common.
- About 60% of patients who present with purely ocular myasthenia progress to develop generalized manifestations. If this going to occur it will usually do so within 18 months. Early immunosuppression may reduce the risk of generalised myasthenia.
- Systemic involvement may cause proximal limb weakness or difficulties with breathing, speaking, chewing and swallowing.
- The disorder can cause death due to paralysis of the respiratory muscles.

DIAGNOSIS

Clinical signs and symptoms

- Myasthenia should be suspected in any patient with acquired ptosis or diplopia even if the physical examination is normal.
- Fluctuating symptoms, weak orbicularis oculi, Cogan's lid twitch and upgaze fatigue increase the likelihood of myasthenia.

Laboratory findings

- The 'ice test,' involves holding crushed ice in a surgical glove, over the ptotic eyelids for 2 minutes and then watching for a brief elevation of the eyelid.
- The 'rest' and 'sleep' tests are useful in patients with ptosis or disordered motility.
- The 'Tensilon test' (edrophonium chloride), and the 'Prostigmin test' (neostigmine bromide) may result in brief elevation of a ptotic eyelid, improved strabismus on prism measurement or improved motility on Hess test. Intravenous access, cardiac monitoring, atropine for bradycardia and equipment for cardiorespiratory arrest are essential.
- All of the above tests are generally about 90% sensitive and specific but probably less so in patients with atypical clinical features.
- Single-fiber electromyography 'SFEMG' shows blocking or increased jitter in myasthenia. If SFEMG is performed on a clinically weak orbicularis oris, the sensitivity is 99% and a normal test makes myasthenia highly unlikely. False positives occur in other motor unit diseases.
- About 65% of patients have serum antibodies to acetylcholine receptors and this test is 99% specific. Rare false positives may occur in dysthyroid patients or those with a family history of myasthenia. Repeat testing, looking for blocking and modulating antibodies or muscle-specific kinase (MuSK) antibodies can improve sensitivity.
- Striated muscle antibodies are associated with thymoma or older onset myasthenia.
- Cat scan of the chest may detect thymoma.
- Quantitative tests of systemic muscle function and fatigue, such as the arm abduction time and the vital capacity, may be useful.

Differential diagnosis

- When ocular findings are prominent, ocular motor palsies, intracranial lesions CPEO, oculopharyngeal dystrophy, and myotonic dystrophy may need to be considered.
- It may be difficult to diagnose myasthenia when thyroid eye disease or levator dehiscence are also present.
- When symptoms are generalized, muscular dystrophy, Eaton Lambert, botulinum toxicity, penicillamine and organophosphate poisoning may be considered.

TREATMENT

Ocular

- Prisms or occlusion of one eye may be helpful in selected cases of double vision.
- If strabismus is stable for 1 year then surgery is possible, but recurrent misalignment is common.

Systemic

- Anticholinesterase agents (pyridostigmine, Mestinon) are the first line of treatment but are commonly ineffective. The drug is used four times per day. This may increased to 180 mg four times per day unless there are side effects such as gastric upset or diarrhea. High doses may cause bronchospasm and weakness that mimics myasthenic crisis.
- Adrenal corticosteroids (prednisolone) are frequently used in myasthenia. The dose is progressively increased as high as 1–1.5 mg/kg. When symptoms are adequately controlled the drug is shifted to an alternate-day schedule and then gradually tapered. Blood pressure and blood glucose need to be monitored and H_2 antagaonists may be prescribed to prevent peptic ulcer.
- Azathioprine (Imuran) can be used in refractory myasthenia. It may not take effect for 6 months and its potential hematologic and liver toxicity requires monitoring of the blood count and liver function.
- Other immunosuppressive drugs such as mycophenolate mofetil, ciclosporin and cyclophosphamide may be useful in selected cases.
- Plasmapheresis may be temporarily beneficial in acute myasthenia or myasthenic crisis.
- Intravenous immune globulin may be beneficial in acute myasthenia, in patients with refractory myasthenia, and in the perioperative setting.

Surgical

- Thymectomy is usually performed in patients younger than 50 years who have a thymoma on CT. Its role in nonthymomatous ocular myasthenia is controversial.

REFERENCES

Barton J, Fouladvand M: Ocular aspects of myasthenia gravis. Seminars in neurology 20:7–20, 2000.

Ertas M, Arac N, Kumral K, et al: Ice test as a simple diagnostic aid for myasthenia gravis. Acta Neurol Scand 89:227–229, 1994.

Jaretzki A, Steinglass KM, Sonett JR: Thymectomy in the management of myasthenia gravis. Seminars in Neurology 24(1):49–62, 2004.

Mee M, Paine E, Byrne J, et al: Immunotherapy of ocular myasthenia gravis reduces conversion to generalized myasthenia gravis. J Neuroophthalmol 23(4):251–255, 2003.

Phillips LH, 2nd, Melnick PA: Diagnosis of myasthenia gravis in the 1990s. Semin Neurol 10:62–69, 1990.

Vincent A, Bowen J, Newsom-Davis J, McConville J: Seronegative generalised myasthenia gravis: clinical features, antibodies, and their targets. Lancet Neurology 2(2):99–106, 2003.

118 PARKINSON'S DISEASE 332.0

Stephen Gancher, MD, FAAN
Portland, Oregon

ETIOLOGY/INCIDENCE

Parkinson's disease is a degenerative neurological illness which results in the loss of dopaminergic neurons in the brain. It is rare before age 40 but is more common in older individuals, affecting up to 1% of the population over age 60. The cause is unknown, although genetic causes are implicated.

COURSE/PROGNOSIS

Parkinson's disease begins with subtle symptoms and signs, commonly affecting one side of the body initially. It is steadily progressive in all individuals but the rate of progression varies widely. With prolonged drug treatment, involuntary movements become especially prominent. In latter stages, mild dementia is very common.

Clinical signs and symptoms

Neurological signs include tremor, rigidity, bradykinesia, postural deformities and disturbances of gait. Associated symptoms include fatigue, depression, memory loss, constipation, speech and swallowing difficulties, pain, stiffness and seborrhea.

Biochemically, tremor, bradykinesia and rigidity result from dopamine deficiency and improve with levodopa, dopamine agonists, anticholinergics and other medications. Although levodopa is a mainstay of therapy, choreiform and dystonic involuntary movements develop in most patients after long-term treatment and produce difficulties in symptom control. Adverse mental effects, such as hallucinations and confusion, are common side effects of drug treatment and may limit therapy.

Parkinson's disease may affect eyelid function and produce reduced blinking, blepharoclonus, seborrheic blepharitis, hordeolum, and rarely, blepharospasm and apraxia of eye opening. Ocular motility disturbances include decreased convergence, hypometric saccades and saccadic pursuit. Although impaired contrast sensitivity can be demonstrated by specialized studies, papillary and retinal function is clinically unaffected, and prominent visual complaints should suggest an alternative diagnosis.

Laboratory findings

None in Parkinson's disease. Workup in a younger patient to exclude other conditions should include MRI or CT scan, calcium and ceruloplasmin. A screen for the *parkin* mutation can be a helpful confirmatory test in younger individuals.

Differential diagnosis

- Progressive supranuclear palsy (PSP): the hallmark is supranuclear vertical ophthalmoplegia, although it may not appear initially. Preserved vertical eye movements, produced by passive neck movement in a patient who cannot voluntarily generate vertical gaze is characteristic. A staring expression, lid retraction, slow saccades, impairment in voluntary vertical gaze and neck rigidity are characteristic signs. Visual complaints are more common than in other forms of parkinsonism.
- Multiple system atrophy (MSA, Shy–Drager syndrome): dysautonomia (hypotension, bowel and bladder dysfunction), dysarthria, dysphagia and facial grimacing as a result of levodopa therapy are common manifestations. Tonic pupils may be seen.
- Drug induced parkinsonism: dopamine antagonists such as antiemetics (metoclopramide and prochlorperazine) and neuroleptics (trifluoperazine, haloperidol) can produced drug-induced pakrinsonism. Oculogyric crisis and other dystonic reactions are common, particularly in younger patients.

- Vascular parkinsonism: multiple subcortical infarcts may produce bradykinesia and rigidity. Stroke risk factors, such as diabetes and hypertension, are usually present. A history of stroke or TIA may or may not be present. Multiple white-matter lesions on MRI are present. Vascular parkinsonism is resistant to drug therapy.
- Rare causes include Wilson's disease, Huntington's disease, sequelae of viral encephalitis, HIV infection, hypoparathyroidism and structural abnormalities such as communicating hydrocephalus or basal ganglia tumor.

TREATMENT

- Anticholinergics are used early in the course of the disease but commonly produce memory loss and accommodative paralysis.
- Levodopa (sold as a combination of levodopa and carbidopa [Sinemet] in the United States; sold as a combination of levodopa and benzerazide [Madopar] in Europe) is used for treatment of tremor, bradykinesia, rigidity and gait abnormalities and is useful in all stages of disease. Various formulations are available. It is a mainstay of treatment but commonly produces involuntary movements, especially in patients under age 50.
- Dopamine agonists available in the United States include pramipexole (sold as Mirapex), ropinirole (sold as Requip), pergolide (sold as Permax) and bromocriptine (sold as Parlodel). They are used as initial therapy or as an adjunct to levodopa.
- Other drugs include amantadine, the MAO-B inhibitors selegiline and rasagiline (sold as Azilect), and the COMT inhibitors entacapone (sold as Comtan and Stalevo) and tolcapone (sold as Tasmar). These latter four drugs inhibit the metabolism and clearance of levodopa or dopamine and prolong its actions.
- Axial motor symptoms, such as dysarthria, dysphagia, imbalance and freezing gait, do not consistently respond to drug treatment.

Ocular

- Lid hygiene is important for the prevention of seborrheic blepharitis and hordeolum.
- Eyes are lubricated with artificial tears or methylcellulose eyedrops.
- Botulinum toxin is used to treat blepharospasm and eyelid apraxia complicating parkinsonism.
- Side effects of drugs, such as visual hallucinations, diplopia and blurred vision, are very common; visual hallucinations may serve as a harbinger of psychotic reactions.
- Diagnosis of narrow-angle glaucoma and the risks of anticholinergic treatment should be discussed in detail with the patient and with other physicians.
- Refraction may vary depending on the dosage and the timing of drug therapy.
- Tremor and bradykinesia may interfere with ocular self-care.
- Ophthalmic evaluation and treatment, such as slit-lamp examination or surgical procedures, may be difficult because of tremor and dyskinesia, and may have to be timed with drug treatment.
- Narcotics and benzodiazepines do not markedly reduce tremor but may suppress both tremor and dyskinesia at sedating doses.
- Intravenous diphenhydramine, administered in 25-mg increments, is useful to achieve partial sedation and reduce tremor.
- Levodopa and dopamine agonists should be withheld for 4 to 6 hours before surgery to reduce risk of cardiac arrhythmia.
- The combination of selegiline and meperidine is contraindicated.
- Ocular anticholinergics may produce confusion in demented patients.

COMMENTS

The treatment of Parkinson's disease is challenging and may require input from a variety of specialists. Ocular signs and symptoms, such as slow saccades, difficulty initiating vertical gaze, or saccadic pursuit may precede other neurological manifestations and indicate the possibility that early Parkinson's disease is the diagnosis. However, prominent ocular or visual complaints, other than accommodative paralysis and drug-induced hallucinations, are not part of the spectrum of symptoms of Parkinson's disease, and their presence suggests that another diagnosis should be considered.

SUPPORT GROUPS

National Parkinson Foundation, Inc.
1501 NW 9th Ave/Bob Hope Road
Miami, FL 33136-1494
1-800-327-4545
www.parkinson.org

American Parkinson Disease Association, Inc
1250 Hylan Blvd, Suite 4B
Staten Island, NY 10305
1-800-223-2732
apdaparkinson.org

REFERENCES

Biousse V, Skibell BC, Watts RL, et al: Ophthalmologic features of Parkinson's disease. Neurology 62:177–180, 2004.

Nutt JG, Hammerstad JP, Gancher ST: Parkinson's disease: 100 maxims. London, Edward Arnold, 1992.

119 TOLOSA–HUNT SYNDROME 378.9

Russell M. LeBoyer, MD
Houston, TX
Rod Foroozan, MD
Houston, TX

ETIOLOGY

The Tolosa–Hunt syndrome is an idiopathic chronic granulomatous inflammation of the cavernous sinus causing episodic unilateral periorbital pain that is often self-limiting, lasting up to 8 weeks without intervention. The pain is often described as 'gnawing.' Inflammation of adjacent cranial nerves within the cavernous sinus often causes painful ophthalmoplegia. Contiguous structures, the orbital apex and superior orbital fissure, are often simultaneously affected, and if the optic nerve is affected within the orbital apex visual loss may occur.

COURSE/PROGNOSIS

- Variable involvement of the ipsilateral third, fourth and sixth cranial nerves may occur depending on the extent of infiltration.
- Ophthalmoplegia typically occurs within 2 weeks after the onset of pain, however the pain may begin after the onset of ophthalmoplegia.
- The maxillary and mandibular branches of the trigeminal nerve and periarterial sympathetic involvement may also occur.
- There is no predilection to gender, age or ethnicity.
- Spontaneous remission has been reported in 85% of patients.
- Recurrences are common, occurring in 40% of treated patients at intervals of months to years.

DIAGNOSIS

Clinical signs and symptoms

- Diagnostic criteria for Tolosa–Hunt syndrome include episodic unilateral orbital pain, lasting weeks if left untreated, that is associated with paralysis of one or more of the third, fourth or sixth cranial nerves and/or demonstration of a granuloma on magnetic resonance imaging (MRI) or tissue biopsy.

Differential diagnosis

- Other causes of cavernous sinus pathology must be excluded such as aneurysm, neoplasia, vasculitis and inflammation.

Laboratory findings

- Initial diagnostic studies should include MRI with axial and coronal views of the brain, which typically show thickening and enhancement of the involved cavernous sinus.
- Cerebral angiography can be performed if aneurysm, arteriovenous malformation, or arteriovenous fistula are suspected.
- Hematological testing should be considered for other inflammatory causes. Testing may include complete blood count, erythrocyte sedimentation rate, antinuclear antibody, antineutrophil cytoplasmic antibody and angiotensin-converting enzyme levels.
- Cerebrospinal fluid consistency should be normal.
- Tissue biopsy should be considered in patients with progressive deficits, persistent abnormal neuroimaging studies or lack of corticosteroid response.

TREATMENT

- A prompt response to corticosteroids is often considered to be a hallmark of Tolosa–Hunt syndrome.
- Systemic corticosteroid therapy is the mainstay of treatment with starting doses typically in the range of 1 mg/kg of prednisone.
- Some improvement of the pain and other symptoms should occur within 72 hours after the initiation of treatment.
- Periorbital pain often responds before the improvement of the ophthalmoplegia.
- Corticosteroids can be tapered after the first few weeks of therapy in most cases.
- Long-term corticosteroid therapy may be necessary for recurrent disease.
- Low-dose radiotherapy has demonstrated long-term efficacy and safety for patients with corticosteroid resistance or intolerance.
- Immunosuppressive therapy with corticosteroid sparing agents such as cyclophosphamide and azathioprine can be helpful for some patients.

COMPLICATIONS

Typical side effects from long-term corticosteroid use are common. Although neurologic symptoms typically resolve with treatment, residual deficits, including diplopia, may persist.

COMMENTS

Patients with Tolosa–Hunt syndrome have symptoms and neuroimaging that are not specific to this disorder. Other disorders including meningioma, lymphoma and sarcoidosis may have a similar appearance on MRI. In addition, various parasellar neoplasms such as lymphoma, giant cell tumors and epidermoid tumors, have shown responses to corticosteroid treatment. Therefore, careful follow-up is necessary to ensure adequate response to therapy and the exclusion of these other conditions.

Histopathologic specimens from patients with Tolosa–Hunt syndrome show similar findings to those of idiopathic orbital inflammation (orbital pseudotumor), and some investigators have suggested that these conditions have a similar pathophysiology.

REFERENCES

Foubert Samier A, Sibon I, Maire J, Tison F: Long-term cure of Tolosa-Hunt syndrome after low dose focal radiotherapy. Headache 45:389–391, 2005.

Hunt WE, Meagher JN: Painful ophthalmoplegia: its relation to indolent inflammation of the cavernous sinus. Neurology 11:56–62, 1961.

International Headache Society: The international classification of headache disorders. Cephalalgia 24(suppl 1):131, 2004.

Kline LB: The Tolosa-Hunt syndrome. Surv Ophthalmol 27:79–95, 1982.

Kline LB, Hoyt WF: The Tolosa-Hunt syndrome. J Neurol Neurosurg Psychiatry 71:577–582, 2001.

Mantia L, Erbetta A, Bussone G: Painful ophthalmoplegia: an unresolved clinical problem. Neurol Sci 26:579–582, 2005.

Pless MP: Cavernous sinus disorders. In: Levin LA, Arnold AC, eds: Neuro-ophthalmology the practical guide. New York, Thieme 2005:301–302.

Sargent JC: Nuclear and infranuclear ocular motility disorders. In: Miller NR, Newman NJ, eds: Walsh & Hoyt's clinical neuro-ophthalmology. 6th edn. Baltimore, Lippincott Williams & Wilkins, 2005:I:989.

Wasmeier C, Pfadenhauer K, Rosler A: Idiopathic inflammatory pseudotumor of the orbit and Tolosa-Hunt Syndrome — are they the same disease? J Neurol 249:1237–1241, 2002.

120 TRIGEMINAL NEURALGIA 350.1
(Tic Douloureux)

Baird S. Grimson, MD
Chapel Hill, North Carolina

ETIOLOGY/INCIDENCE

Trigeminal neuralgia is a brief, sharp, unilateral facial pain that usually occurs in the middle or lower face within the distribution of the second or third division of the trigeminal nerve. Occasionally, the first division of the trigeminal nerve is involved, with the cephalalgia occurring in or around the eye. This pain usually occurs in patients over 40 years old and is experienced more frequently by females than by males. The right side of the face is more often involved than the left.

Characteristically, this memorable pain is precipitated by mechanical stimulation of trigger zones in the ipsilateral face or mouth during such activities as chewing, swallowing, laughing, teeth brushing, hair combing or shaving. Each attack of trigeminal neuralgia usually lasts for only a few seconds or minutes, often presenting intermittently at first; however, the frequency can increase to many episodes per day.

Spontaneous exacerbations and remissions of tic douloureux are not uncommon and can complicate the evaluation of the efficacy of therapeutic measures taken to control the pain. If the pain presents bilaterally, or occurs in younger patients, the rare occurrence of multiple sclerosis as an underlying cause of trigeminal neuralgia should be suspected.

DIAGNOSIS

Clinical signs and symptoms

Characteristic signs and symptoms of trigeminal neuralgia include:

- Sharp facial or periorbital pain;
- Ipsilateral conjunctival hyperemia;
- Ipsilateral lacrimation during pain episodes.

The pain of tic douloureux has been described as 'stabbing,' 'searing,' 'lightning-like' or 'electrical.'

TREATMENT

Systemic

When begun shortly after the onset of tic douloureux, systemic (oral) medications such as carbamazepine (beginning at 100 mg PO b.i.d. after meals, up to 400 to 800 mg and not to exceed 1.2 g daily), or phenytoin 300 to 700 mg PO qd, are particularly useful.

Carbamazepine usually proves the more effective drug, but prolonged use of either carbamazepine or phenytoin is limited because of the toxic side effects involved and because trigeminal neuralgia has a tendency to become refractory to medical management.

Baclofen, and gabapentin are also useful in the management of trigeminal neuralgia; baclofen should be begun at 5 mg PO t.i.d. for 3 days, then increased to 10 mg t.i.d. for 3 days and then to 20 mg t.i.d. The total dosage of baclofen should not exceed 80 mg daily. Gabapentin is initiated using 300 mg once on day 1, then 300 mg twice on day 2 and 300 mg three times on day 3; total daily dosage of gabapentin should not exceed 1800 mg.

Surgical

Surgical intervention for tic douloureux is reserved for cases that have become refractory to medical management. Numerous surgical procedures have been tried in the past, but radiofrequency (thermal) trigeminal gangliolysis and microsurgical decompression of the trigeminal nerve rootlet gamma knife radiosurgery are the current procedures of choice, as they provide the best chance for permanent relief of pain and produce minimal postoperative complications.

Thermal trigeminal gangliolysis is performed by means of percutaneous insertion of the radiofrequency needle through the foramen ovale and directly into the trigeminal nerve. After radiofrequency stimulation locates the rootlets responsible for the trigeminal pain, the needle tip is heated for thermal coagulation. This procedure does not require a craniotomy but occasionally produces disagreeable subjective sensations within the trigeminal nerve distribution and sometimes produces objective trigeminal involvement (hypalgesia, neuroparalytic keratitis or weakness of the jaw muscles). A significant rate of recurrence of the trigeminal neuralgia does occur over time, but radiofrequency thermocoagulation can then be repeated without difficulty.

Microsurgical decompression of the trigeminal nerve root near the brain stem does require a suboccipital craniotomy, but this has proved to be a relatively safe procedure and is associated with a low incidence of postoperative trigeminal nerve dysfunction and moderate return of pain in the postoperative period.

Gamma knife radiosurgery targets the trigeminal nerve root near its exit from the brainstem and delivers a radiation dose usually between 70 to 90 Gy. Trigeminal nerve dysfunction is the major post-treatment complication, and the return of the trigeminal neuralgia following this procedure is not unusual.

PRECAUTIONS

Among the common side effects of carbamazepine therapy are lightheadedness, drowsiness, and lethargy; ataxia, nausea and vomiting, and skin rashes also can occur. Cardiac arrhythmias and congestive heart failure may develop, and carbamazepine should be used with caution in patients with heart disease. A rare but serious drug reaction is the development of leukopenia, thrombocytopenia or a plastic anemia. A complete blood and platelet count is recommended before starting carbamazepine, every week or two after its initiation for several months and then every 3 or 4 months during maintenance therapy.

Side effects of phenytoin include nystagmus, slurred speech, dizziness, nausea, vomiting, and epigastric pain; gingival hyperplasia, peripheral neuropathy, hirsutism, skin rashes and a generalized lymphadenopathy also may develop. Liver dysfunction occasionally occurs and rarely leukopenia, agranulocytopenia, thrombocytopenia, or pancytopenia has been observed.

Baclofen usually is well tolerated but can cause drowsiness, weakness, fatigue, headache, dizziness, nausea and hypotension.

Major side effects of gabapentin include fatigue, dizziness, ataxia, and somnolence; tremor, nystagmus and diplopia also can occur.

Although carbamazepine, phenytoin, baclofen, and gabapentin are very successful at first in controlling the pain, trigeminal neuralgia often becomes refractory to systemic treatment; when this happens, surgical management is successful and should not be delayed.

COMMENTS

Magnetic resonance imaging and magnetic resonance angiography can help document structural compression of the trigeminal nerve rootlet (usually from an aberrant loop of an artery or vein) as the cause of trigeminal neuralgia. Magnetic resonance imaging also is useful in the evaluation of multiple sclerosis that occasionally is the underlying etiology of trigeminal neuralgia.

If objective trigeminal nerve involvement is detected on the initial evaluation or if other parasellar cranial nerve palsies (third, fourth or sixth) are found, then the diagnosis of trigeminal neuralgia is in question, and an investigation for a parasellar mass lesion, including computed tomography, magnetic resonance imaging, and possible cerebral angiography, should be initiated.

REFERENCES

Irving GA: Contemporary assessment and management of neuropathic pain. Neurology 64:S21–S27, 2005.

Kanpolat Y, Savas A, Bekar A, Berk C: Percutaneous controlled radiofrequency trigeminal rhizotomy for the treatment of idiopathic trigeminal neuralgia: 25-year experience with 1600 patients. Neurosurgery 48:524–534, 2001.

Li S, Wang X, Pan Q, et al: Studies on the operative outcomes and mechanisms of microvascular decompression in treating typical and atypical trigeminal neuralgia. Clin J Pain 21:311–316, 2005.

Lopez BC, Hamlyn PJ, Zakrzewska JM: Systematic review of ablative neurosurgical techniques for the treatment of trigeminal neuralgia. Neurosurgery 54:973–983, 2004.

McNatt SA, Yu C, Giannotta SL, et al: Gamma knife radiosurgery for trigeminal neuralgia. Neurosurgery 56:1295–1303, 2005.

Sheehan J, Pan HC, Stroila M, Steiner L: Gamma knife surgery for trigeminal neuralgia: outcomes and prognostic factors. J Neurosurg 102:434–441, 2005.

Sindrup SH, Jensen TS: Pharmacotherapy of trigeminal neuralgia. Clin J Pain 18:22–27, 2002.

Tawk RG, Duffy-Fronckowiak M, Scott BE, et al: Stereotactic gamma knife surgery for trigeminal neuralgia: detailed analysis of treatment response. J Neurosurg 102:442–449, 2005.

SECTION

13 Neoplasms

121 ACTINIC AND SEBORRHEIC KERATOSIS 702

Ronald R. Lubritz, MD, FACP
New Orleans, Louisiana

ETIOLOGY/INCIDENCE

Actinic keratosis is a precancerous lesion that occurs most commonly on sunlight-exposed areas of the skin, such as the face, neck, and dorsa of the hands. It is more common in middle-aged or older individuals and is primarily noted in fair-complexioned individuals. Chronic sun exposure is a key element in the development of actinic keratoses. Severe, acute sunburns at an early age probably are as important as chronic exposure or causal factors.

Seborrheic keratosis is a benign epithelial tumor that appears predominantly on the trunk and head. It is rare in children but very common in adults older than 40 years. Heredity probably plays a role in cases where large numbers of keratoses are present.

COURSE/PROGNOSIS

Actinic keratosis

These premalignant lesions can progress to squamous cell carcinomas. Possible imminent or future malignant transformation can be suspected when lesions bleed, ulcerate, or become painful or pruritic or when the lesions begin to show changes that include, but are not limited to, increased erythema, pigmentation, scaling, hyperkeratosis or irritation.

Seborrheic keratosis

Some lesions can grow to several centimeters, but most remain much smaller-several millimeters to 1 cm. Although a small percentage can transform into carcinomas, most remain benign.

DIAGNOSIS

Clinical signs and symptoms

Seborrheic keratoses can occur on both the eyebrows and the eyelids. The upper lids are more often involved than the lower lids. When located on the lids, seborrheic keratoses can occasionally be somewhat pedunculated. Actinic keratoses most often involve the eyebrows. Although they can occur on the eyelids, this is uncommon because the eyelids, especially the upper eyelids, are usually protected from sunlight.

Actinic keratoses usually occur as small, mildly erythematous patches with or without scaling.

Seborrheic keratoses usually occur as flat to moderately raised plaques that are somewhat verrucoid or velvety.

Differential diagnosis

Actinic keratosis

- Contact dermatitis.
- Lupus.
- Psoriasis.
- Seborrheic dermatitis.
- Seborrheic keratosis.
- Squamous cell carcinoma.
- Squamous papilloma.
- Tinea.
- Biopsy sometimes necessary.

Seborrheic keratosis

- Lentigo.
- Lentigo maligna and superficial melanoma.
- Nevus (intradermal, compound, or dysplastic).
- (Pigmented) actinic keratosis.
- (Pigmented) basal cell carcinoma.
- Squamous papilloma.
- Verruca.
- Biopsy sometimes necessary.

PROPHYLAXIS

Actinic keratosis

- Limit unprotected sun exposure, especially in children, teenagers, and persons in their early 20s.
- Sun exposure between 10 a.m. and 3 p.m. during summer is most harmful.
- Unprotected sun exposure on cloudy days can also provide harmful ultraviolet rays.
- Limit the use of tanning beds.
- Sunscreens and protective clothing are invaluable in decreasing harmful exposure.

TREATMENT

Surgical

Actinic keratosis

Cryosurgery is the treatment of choice. Usually, a small, portable cryosurgical unit is used, and no anesthetic agent is necessary. A spray tip is placed just above the target site and sprayed either in an ever-widening circle or in a back-and-forth 'paintbrush' pattern until the entire lesion is covered. Freezing should be carried just outside the border of the lesion. Total thaw time (the time from stopping freezing until all white frosted areas on the surface disappear or all hard areas resolve on palpation) is approximately 20 to 30 seconds.

A crusted/vesicular stage will occur, followed by eschar. This usually resolves or falls off around 14 days. A smooth, pinkish residual remains, which fades in time. Occasionally, hyperkeratotic or other lesions may need superficial shave excisions. When this occurs, usually no suturing is required, but local anesthetic is usually necessary.

Seborrheic keratosis

Flat lesions may be treated in a manner similar to the treatment of actinic keratoses. Raised or pedunculated lesions require light freezing. While frozen, a sharp curette or iris-type scissors are used to remove the lesion level to the skin; a local anesthetic agent is optional.

Electrodessication and curettage, along with a local anesthetic agent, can also be used to remove some lesions, especially those on loose periorbital skin.

COMPLICATIONS

Removal with curette or scissors generally requires routine measures for hemostasis, such as the use of Gelfoam dressing or the application of aluminum chloride (precautions should be taken around the eye for *any* chemical hemostasis). However, patients who receive anticoagulants must be observed and cautioned regarding prolonged bleeding.

COMMENTS

Care should be taken during cryosurgical procedures around the eye to avoid unnecessary harm to the global structures. When the technique described is used for raised seborrheic keratoses, the lesions should not be frozen too hard; if this happens, the operator must wait until the lesion is partially thawed before continuing. Clinical experience is necessary to judge the degree of freezing required for these techniques; too much freezing can result in scarring or pigmentary changes that are out of proportion to the tumor being treated. Patients should be informed of the possibility that pigmented lesions may not lose all their color after cryosurgical treatment. Occasionally, fissures occur within a lesion. Liquid nitrogen sprayed under too great a pressure into such an opening can lead to 'ballooning' of the eyelid. This is usually self-limited but can have an alarming appearance. The use of topical 5FU or imiquimod is also used for the selective treatment of multiple actinic keratoses. However, these treatments are usually not indicated for individual lesions and should not be used on the eyelids or above the inferior periorbital ridge.

REFERENCES

Kuflik EG: Cryosurgery updated. J Am Acad Dermatol 31:925–944, 1994.

Lubritz RR: Cryosurgery of benign lesions. Cutis 16:426–432, 1975.

Lubritz RR: Cryosurgery for benign and malignant skin lesions: Treatment with a new instrument. South Med J 69:1401–1405, 1976.

Lubritz RR: Cryosurgery of benign and premalignant cutaneous lesions. In: Zacarian SA, ed: Cryosurgical advances in dermatology and tumors of the head and neck. Springfield, IL, Charles C Thomas, 1977:55–73.

Lubritz RR: Cryosurgery of nonmalignancies. In: Zacarian SA, ed: Cryosurgery for skin cancer and cutaneous disorders. St Louis, CV Mosby, 1985:49–58.

Muriello JA, Napolitano J, McLean I: Actinic keratosis and dysplasia of the conjunctiva: clinicopathological study of 45 cases. Can J Ophthalmol 30:312–316, 1995.

Torre D, Lubritz RR, Kuflik E, eds: Practical cutaneous cryosurgery. East Norwalk, CT, Appleton & Lange, 1988:61–86.

Tseng SH, Chen YT, Huang FC, et al: Seborrheic keratosis of conjunctiva simulating a malignant melanoma: an immunocytochemical study with impression cytology. Ophthalmology 106:1516–1520, 1999.

122 BASAL CELL CARCINOMA 731

Hon-Vu Q. Duong, MD
Las Vegas, Nevada

ETIOLOGY/INCIDENCE

Basal cell carcinoma (Figure 122.1) accounts for 80–90% of eyelid malignancies and occurs more commonly in Caucasians. Prolong or significant unprotected exposure to UV radiation has proven to be tumorigenic. The tumor most commonly arises in the lower eyelids, followed by the medial canthus, the upper eyelids, and the lateral canthus. Basal cell carcinoma is slow growing, locally invasive, and rarely metastasizes. Prognosis is good with early detection and treatment with a cure rate of 95%.

DIAGNOSIS

Clinical signs and symptoms

Patients often present complaining of a painless, nonhealing ulcer. History may elicit a long history to sun exposure. Symptoms are: painless nodule with a shiny and waxy, indurated, firm and immobile, pearly, rolled border and with fine telangiectatic vessels on the surface (Figures 122.1 and 122.2).

Clinically, basal cell carcinoma can be grouped into three types: nodular, nodulo-ulcerative (rodent ulcer) and morpheaform or sclerosing.

Laboratory findings

Histology

Typical findings include nests of basaloid cells with a peripheral palisading pattern. Tumor cells have large, oval or elongated nuclei with scant cytoplasm, contraction artifact at the periphery of the tumor along with desmoplasia of the surrounding stroma.

Imaging studies

Imaging studies are often not necessary. However, radiological imaging of the facial and orbital bones and soft tissue may be helpful for an invading or deep tumor in the medial canthus.

The application of ultrasonography is producing controversy due to the inaccuracy in delineating malignant from benign lesions with a success rate of approximately 20%.

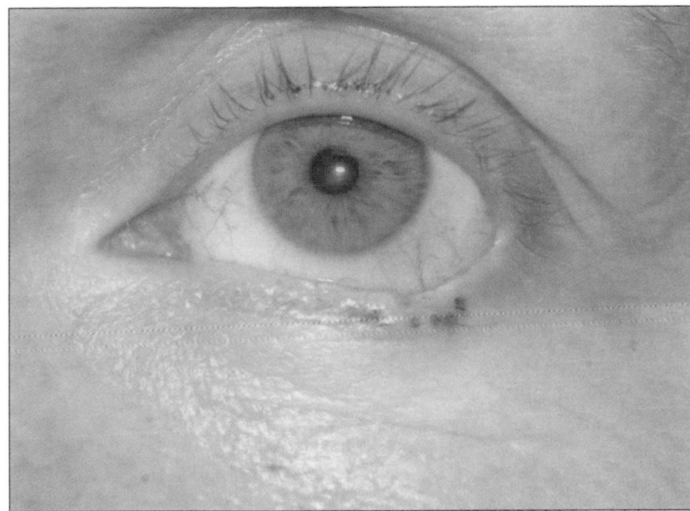

FIGURE 122.1. The lesion is located in the lateral one-third of the lower lid of the left eye. Note the indurated, whitish, raised border with a central ulceration. The purple dot was the marking made prior to Mohs surgery. The patient ultimately underwent a left lower lid reconstruction.

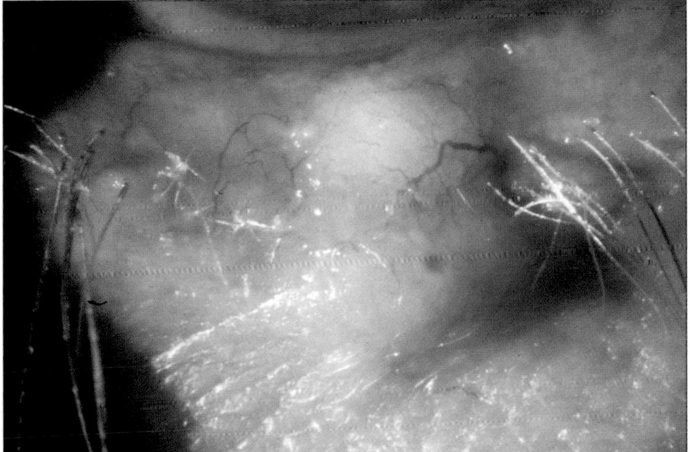

FIGURE 122.2. Basal cell carcinoma of lower lid.

Laser Doppler may be useful in delineating tumor margin. This instrument measures the rate of blood flow and it has been shown that cutaneous perfusion is significantly higher is affected area.

Cytology is another mean to diagnosed basal cell carcinoma. Although it is sufficiently accurate in diagnosis basal cell carcinoma, it is not sufficiently sensitive when planning surgical management.

Differential diagnosis

- Sebaceous gland carcinoma, eyelid.
- Squamous cell carcinoma, eyelid.
- Chronic chalazion.

TREATMENT

Medical

Radiation therapy is reserve for recurring tumors or tumors requiring difficult or extensive oculoplastic surgery. It eliminates skin grafting with good cosmetic results. Side effects include dermatitis, keratinization of the conjunctiva and chronic keratitis.

Chemotherapy (5-FU, cisplastin), although not curative, may be helpful in managing lesions located in the medial canthus, recurrent and invasive tumors, and large tumors where surgical resection may result in cosmetic deformity and functional defect.

Photodynamic therapy (PDT) with photosensitizers may be an effective treatment for superficial tumors. The success rate for PDT ranged from 50%–83%.

Systemic retinoid and alpha interferon have shown some efficacy but the long term toxicity of systemic retinoid agents generally excludes them as treatment of choices for most patients.

Surgical

Mohs micrographic surgery have gained wide acceptance among ophthalmologist. The 5-year recurrence rates for treated basal cell carcinoma after Mohs surgery was 1.0%, 7.5% after cryosurgery, 7.7% after desiccation and curettage, 8.7% after radiotherapy and 10.1% after surgical excision.

Electrodessication and curettage is a used method. Although quick to destroy tumor cells the surgeon cannot visually detect the depth of microscopic tumor invasion and surgical margin. Tumors lest than 5 mm in diameter have a 15% recurrence rate, while tumors with a diameter of 3 cm or greater have a 50% recurrence rate within 5 years when treated by electrodessication and curettage.

Cryosurgery may be considered for small, clinically well-defined primary tumors. It is reserve for patients who are debilitated with medical conditions that preclude other types of surgery. Cryosurgery is a viable alternative in tumors involving the inner canthus, thereby minimizing damage to the lacrimal system.

Carbon dioxide laser may be considered when a bleeding diathesis is present. This laser approach provides a bloodless field, minimal postoperative pain and good postoperative appearance without scar formation.

SUMMARY

Basal cell carcinoma is the most common eyelid tumor. Although surgical management is the treatment of choice, medical management may serve as an adjunct to surgery. Death from metastasis is highly unusual. Prevention for primary or recurrent should include the application of sunscreen, wearing long sleeve shirt and broad-brimmed hat, avoid sun exposure during midday and schedule regular follow-up after treatment. Although basal cell carcinoma is diagnosed in the sixth and seventh decade of life, basal cell carcinoma diagnosed in young adults should warrant a full workup to rule out other systemic disease.

REFERENCES

Cook BE, Jr, Bartley GB: Epidemiologic characteristics and clinical course of patients with malignant eyelid tumors in an incidence cohort in Olmstead County, Minnesota. Ophthalmology 106(4):746–750, 1999.

Eagle RC: Eyelid and lacrimal sac. In: Eye pathology-an atlas and basic text. Philadelphia: WB Saunders, 1999:223–224.

McLean IW: Tumors of the eyelid. Tumors of the eye and ocular adnexa. In: Atlas of tumor pathology. Washington, DC, Armed Forces Institute of Pathology, 1994:18–22.

Soparkar CN, Patrinely JR: Eyelid cancers. Curr Opin Ophthalmol 9(5):49–53, 1998.

Vaughn GJ, Dortzbach RK, Gayre GS: Eyelid malignancies. In: Yanoff M, Duker JS, eds. Ophthalmology. 2nd edn. Mosby, 2004:93:711–713.

123 CAPILLARY HEMANGIOMA 228.01 *(Angioblastic Hemangioma, Benign Hemangioendothelioma, Hemangioblastoma, Strawberry Hemangioma)*

Matthew W. Wilson, MD, FACS
Memphis, Tennessee
Roderick N. Hargrove, MD
Memphis, Tennessee

Capillary hemangiomas are among the most common orbital tumors that occur in the pediatric population. They are not true neoplasms but rather hamartomatous proliferations of primitive vasoformative tissues. Capillary hemangiomas consist of anastomosing blood-filled endothelium-lined channels that typically have an infiltrative growth pattern with no true encapsulation. Recent studies suggest that infantile hemangiomas may have a placental origin.

ETIOLOGY/INCIDENCE

There is a 3 : 2 female-to-male incidence ratio. These tumors follow a characteristic clinical course with a period of rapid hypertrophy for 3 to 12 months followed by a period of stabilization and then involution. The major degree of involution takes place by age 5 years, although lesser degrees of tumor regression may be noted until the end of the first decade. Involution is complete with no significant cosmetic sequelae in the majority of cases. In some larger lesions, however, especially those with a combined subcutaneous and superficial component, it is not uncommon to observe residual cosmetic defects. Ocular complications, such as amblyopia, have been noted in 50% to 75% of patients with orbital and adnexal hemangiomas. Rare dermatologic and systemic complications may occur.

COURSE/PROGNOSIS

Capillary hemangiomas usually present within the first 6 months of life, with one third of the lesions evident at birth. Rapid hypertrophy ensues for 3 to 12 months, followed by stabilization and then involution over the next 5 to 10 years. Clinically, these are benign tumors. Complications relate to amblyopia and cosmesis.

DIAGNOSIS

Clinical signs and symptoms

Clinical diagnosis is most often based on presentation. There are three clinical presentations of the disease:

1. Most commonly, a bluish-purple subcutaneous mass with normal overlying skin is noted in the anterior orbit.
2. Approximately one third of patients have an obvious overlying superficial component consisting of a strawberry hemangioma.
3. Five percent of patients present with a deep orbit mass and have no signs suggestive of the diagnosis.

Laboratory findings

- B-scan ultrasound reveals an irregular mass that blends into the surrounding orbital structures. A-scan demonstrates low internal reflectivity in areas of proliferating endothelial cells, some moderate reflectivity in regions of ectatic vascular channels and high reflectivity near fibrous septa that divide the tumor.
- Computed tomography reveals a well defined or infiltrating lesion that is isodense to the extra-ocular muscles and optic nerve. There may be enlargement of the orbit without evidence of bony erosion. Contrast material may help to delineate the tumor borders and major feeder vessels.
- Magnetic resonance imaging (MRI) reveals a hyperintense tumor on T2-weighted images against a hypointense background of orbital fat. The contrast on T1-weighted images is not as significant, but it is enhanced by the administration of gadolinium-DTPA and the implementation of fat-suppression protocols. Dynamic contrast MRI shows early focal enhancement, which helps differentiate hemangiomas from other orbital masses that diffusely enhance.
- Angiography is rarely diagnostic and is seldom used except before surgical manipulation.
- Biopsy is most often reserved for the infant with a rapidly expanding proptosis and an absence of superficial abnormalities or discoloration. Hemostasis control via compression, cauterization, or hemostatic agents is usually sufficient. Histopathologic findings are summarized as follows:
    - Masses of endothelial cells with increased mitotic figures have occasional vascular spaces characterized by small, irregular lumens;
    - Reticulin stain may delineate the vasculature nature of the tumor in questionable cases;
    - Weibel–Palade bodies occur within tumor cells in well differentiated hemangiomas.

Differential diagnosis

- Rhabdomyosarcoma.
- Lymphangioma.
- Choloroma.
- Neuroblastoma.
- Other neoplasms (Ewing's sarcoma, medulloblastoma and Wilms' tumor).
- Orbital cysts (dermoid).
- Cellulitis.

TREATMENT

Unless there are specific ocular, dermatologic, or systemic indications for rapid resolution, treatment should be withheld because all therapeutic modalities have significant real or theoretic risks. Ocular indications for treatment include occlusion of the visual axis, compression of the optic nerve or corneal exposure secondary to severe proptosis. When treatment is indicated, the use of intralesional steroids has assumed a prominent role.

Systemic

- Oral prednisone: 1 to 2 mg/kg/day prednisone or 2 to 4 mg/kg on alternate days. Tumor shrinkage is often dramatic and occurs within 2 weeks. There is a high incidence of rebound growth on the discontinuation of oral steroids. The use of oral steroids is limited by several adverse reactions, including adrenal suppression, growth retardation, increased susceptibility to infection and interruption of vaccination schedules.
- Interferon: subcutaneous injection of interferon alfa-2a (up to 3 million units/m^2 of body surface area) has demonstrated an ability to effectively induce hemangioma involution when administered over a period of weeks to months. Side effects include fever, neutropenia, nausea, vomiting, neurotoxicity and retinopathy; these usually are reversible and related to dosing and duration of therapy. Because of the seriousness of these side effects, interferon therapy is typical saved for the large, life threatening and refractory cases.

Local

- Intralesional steroids: triamcinolone 40 mg and a 6-mg preparation of betamethasone acetate and betamethasone phosphate injections are usually administered with the patient under general anesthesia without intubation, with separate 1- to 3-mL syringes on 25- to 27-gauge needles for each substance. Injection is made under low pressure while withdrawing the needle slowly to minimize the possibility of retrograde injection into the arterial channels. Tumor shrinkage may begin within several days and could be dramatic within 2 to 4 weeks. Additional treatment within 4 to 8 weeks usually is necessary to obtain a lasting response. Side effects include depigmentation of overlying skin, fat necrosis, adrenal suppression, retrobulbar hemorrhage and, rarely, central retinal artery occlusion. Live attenuated vaccines should be withheld secondary to patient immunosuppression.
- Irradiation: superficial or orthovoltage radiotherapy may be administered in a single treatment of 200 rads with appropriate shielding of the globe and adnexal tissues. Tumor shrinkage is usually noted within 1 to 2 weeks. Treatment may be repeated once or twice. Side effects of radiation include: cutaneous atrophy and scarring, dermatitis, radionecrosis, cataracts, cessation of bony development and neoplastic changes.
- Topical steroids: topical clobetasol has recently been reported to be successful when applied daily to superficial tumors.

Surgical

- Primary surgical excision is useful in a limited number of well-circumscribed, noninfiltrative lesions. The approach typically is through the upper eyelid crease. The meticulous dissection of overlying tissues and the judicious use of cauterization can result in superior cosmetic results. This can be done on an elective basis with directed-donor blood banking. A major risk is uncontrolled intraoperative hemorrhage.
- Various methods have historically been used in an attempt to occlude the feeder vessels, including surgical ligation and sclerosing solutions. The therapeutic benefit is questionable because of the incomplete nature of the intervention and the cosmetic deformities often associated with these interventions.
- Argon, Nd : YAG, and carbon dioxide lasers have been used with moderated success in attempts to ablate abnormal tumor blood vessels. The most promising results occur with the flash lamp-pumped pulsed-dye laser.

COMPLICATIONS

- Amblyopia affects as many as 60% of patients, usually resulting from anisometropia, visual deprivation or a combination.
- Strabismus may occur secondary to amblyopia or as a direct consequence of tumor infiltration into the extraocular muscles.
- Myopia is thought to be secondary to an axial elongation of the eye resulting from prolonged unilateral eyelid closure.
- Astigmatism can occur.
- Kasabach–Merritt syndrome is a coagulopathy that is caused by platelet or fibrinogen sequestration and consumption within the tumor. It is rarely reported in facial hemangiomas. Treatment includes corticosteroids and thrombocyte or platelet replacement. Radiotherapy and interferon have also been used successfully.
- High-output congestive heart failure is rarely reported as a complication of facial hemangiomas. A short circuit in the arteriovenous system leads to increased cardiac output in an attempt to maintain peripheral perfusion, cardiac dilatation, tachycardia, cardiac hypertrophy and, finally, heart failure.

COMMENTS

The most important factors governing the management of capillary hemangiomas are treatment indications. Children affected by this condition ultimately may not be helped cosmetically by treatment and indeed may be cosmetically disfigured by surgical scars or may develop systemic or local complications from the use of corticosteroids, radiotherapy or interferon. Treatment should be reserved for patients in whom the rapidity of tumor regression will significantly influence the clinical outcome. It is generally of great value to discuss the natural history of the tumor with the family and explain the advantages and disadvantages of administering or withholding therapy in any particular case. Likewise, parents of these patients often find it advantageous to study photographs of children who have undergone spontaneous regression and to speak with parents of children who have reached the stage of maximal tumor regression. Ocular indications for treatment include occlusion of the visual axis, amblyopia from anisometropia, compression of the optic nerve and corneal exposure secondary to severe proptosis. A high degree of both myopia and astigmatism is noted in the globe of the affected orbit and evidence exists that these changes are partially reversible if treated early. Systemic indications for treatment include oral or nasopharyngeal obstruction due to extensive hemangiomatous tissue, high-output congestive heart failure, thrombocytopenia, hemolytic anemia and disseminating intravascular coagulation. All forms of treatment must include periodic evaluation of refractive errors and amblyopia therapy, when indicated.

REFERENCES

Bilyk JR, Adamis AP, Mulliken JB: Treatment options for periorbital hemangioma of infancy. Int Ophthalmol Clin Orbital Dis 32:95–109, 1992.

Catillo BV, Jr, Kaufman L: Pediatric tumors of the eye and orbit. Pediatr Clin North Am 50:149–172, 2003.

Coats DK, O'Neil JW, D'Elia VJ, et al: SubTenon's infusion of steroids for treatment of orbital hemangiomas. Ophthalmology 110:1255–1259, 2003.

Deans RM, Harris GJ, Kivlin JD: Surgical dissection of capillary hemangiomas: an alternative to intralesional corticosteroids. Arch Ophthalmol 110:1743–1747, 1992.

DeVenecia G, Lobeck CC: Successful treatment of eyelid hemangioma with prednisone. Arch Ophthalmol 84:98–102, 1970.

Elsas FJ, Lewis AR: Topical treatment of periocular capillary hemangioma. J Pediatr Ophthalmol Strabismus 31:153–156, 1994.

Glassberg E, Lask G, Rabinowitz LG, Tunnessen WW: Capillary hemangiomas: case study of a novel laser treatment and a review of therapeutic options. J Dermatol Surg Oncol 15:1214–1223, 1989.

Guyer DR, Adamis AP, Gragoudas ES, et al: Systemic antiangiogenic therapy for choroidal neovascularization. Arch Ophthalmol 110:1383–1384, 1992.

Haik BG, Jakobiec FA, Ellsworth RM, Jones IS: Capillary hemangioma of the lids and orbit: an analysis of the clinical features and therapeutic results in 101 cases. Ophthalmology 86:760–789, 1979.

Haik BG, Jones IS, Ellsworth RM: Vascular tumors of the orbit. In: Hornblass A, ed. Ophthalmic and orbital plastic and reconstructive surgery. Baltimore, Williams & Wilkins, 1990:1018–1037.

Haik BG, Karcioglu ZA, Gordon RA, Pechous BP: Capillary hemangioma (infantile periocular hemangioma). Surv Ophthalmol 38:399–426, 1994.

Hobby LW: Further evaluation of the potential of the argon laser in the treatment of strawberry hemangiomas. Plast Reconstr Surg 74:481–489, 1991.

Loughnan MS, Elder J, Kemp A: Treatment of a massive orbital capillary hemangioma with interferon alfa-2b: short term results. Arch Ophthalmol 110:1366–1367, 1992.

North PE, Waner M, Brodsky MC: Are infantile hemangiomas of placental origin? Ophthalmology 109:633–634, 2002.

Tanaka A, Mihara F, Yoshiura T, et al: Differentiation of cavernous hemangioma from schwannoma of the orbit: a dynamic MRI study. AJR Am J Roentgenol 183:1799–1804, 2004.

Walker RS, Custer PL, Nerad JA: Surgical excision of periorbital capillary hemangiomas. Ophthalmology 101:1333–1340, 1994.

124 CONJUNCTIVAL OR CORNEAL INTRAEPITHELIAL NEOPLASIA AND SQUAMOUS CELL CARCINOMA 234

(Bowen's Disease of the Eye, Carcinoma In Situ, *Intraepithelial Epithelioma, Intraepithelioma, Intraepithelial Dysplasia, Invasive Neoplasm)*

Frederick W. Fraunfelder, MD
Portland, Oregon

Conjunctival or corneal intraepithelial neoplasia (CIN) varies from minimal to full-thickness dysplastic epithelial cells. Clinical and laboratory investigations have led to a simple classification of the intraepithelial process with CIN grades I-III, ranging from mild dysplasia (CIN I, partial-thickness intraepithelial neoplasia) to severe dysplasia (CIN III, full-thickness intraepithelial neoplasia). If the dysplasia process breaks through the basement membrane, squamous cell carcinoma has occurred.

ETIOLOGY/INCIDENCE

Altered regulatory mechanisms of limbal stem cell function can result from the following:

- Ultraviolet B light;
- Human papillomavirus type 16;
- Climatic extremes;
- Chemical exposure (such as to trifluridine, an arsenical, beryllium, or antiviral agents);
- Vitamin A deficiency;
- Exposure to petroleum products or cigarette smoke; and
- Herpes simplex virus type 1.

The incidence is 2 in 100,000 in the general population.

COURSE/PROGNOSIS

CIN is characterized by slow growth and a relatively low potential for malignancy. The clinical appearance of the lesions is that of an elevated, gelatinous, leukoplakic, or papilliform limbal mass (Figures 124.1, 124.2 and 124.3). The lesions are almost always unilateral and generally unifocal; they are primarily located at the nasal or temporal limbus. Squamous cell

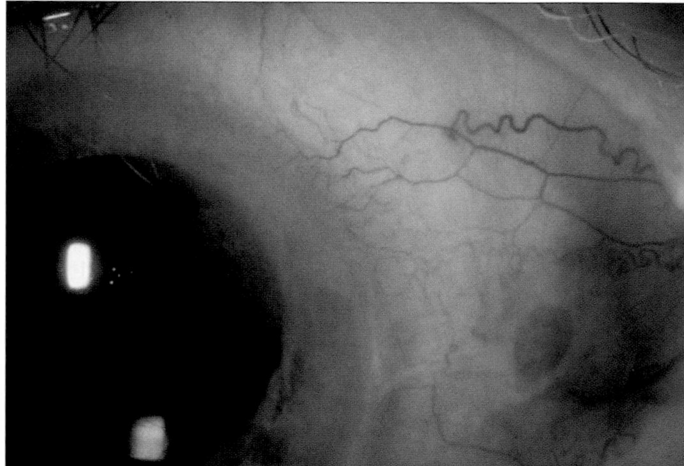

FIGURE 124.1. Corneal intraepithelial neoplasia.

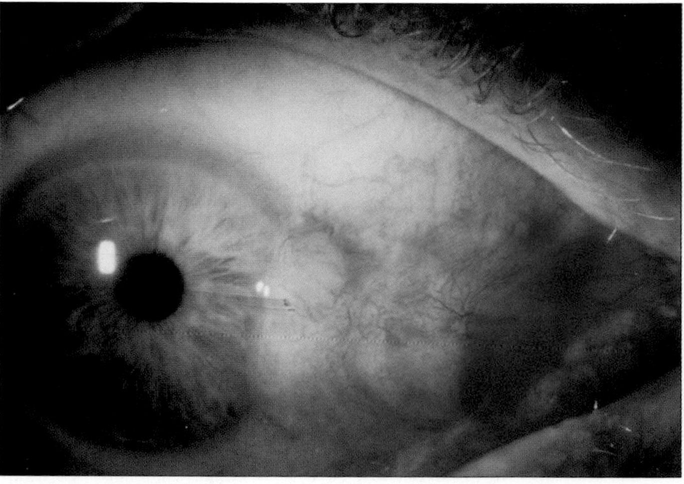

FIGURE 124.2. Conjunctival intraepithelial neoplasia.

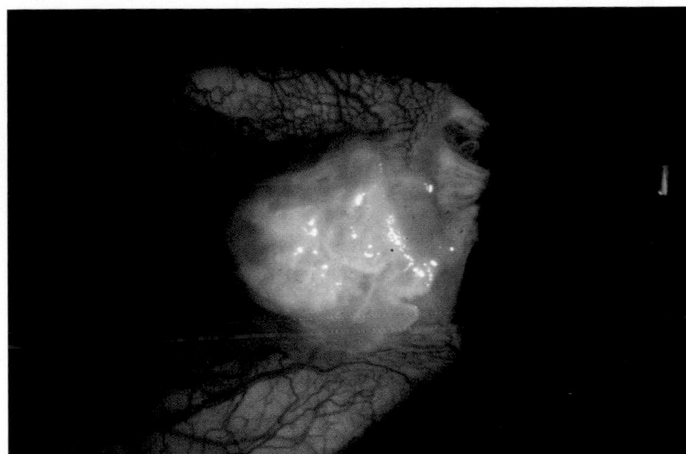

FIGURE 124.3. CIN with leukoplakia.

carcinoma seldom metastasizes until it grows to a considerable size. Its destruction primarily occurs through local invasion. CIN and squamous cell carcinoma affect men more often than women and are predominantly diseases of persons in the sixth and seventh decades of life.

If untreated, CIN may develop into squamous cell carcinoma over a period of many years. Cure rates for CIN with surgery alone range from 70% to 80%. Surgery plus cryotherapy achieves a cure rate of more than 90%. With early management, the prognosis for squamous cell carcinoma is similar to that for CIN. If untreated, intraocular or intraorbital extension, metastases and death may occur.

DIAGNOSIS

Laboratory findings

A full thickness conjunctival biopsy is the diagnostic method of choice and it must include the basement membrane. Papanicolaou's technique entails using a sterile platinum spatula or no. 15 Bard Parker blade, which may also be used on the conjunctiva to find the peripheral extent of the lesion when the biomicroscope exam is equivocal.

Rose Bengal staining is occasionally helpful to outline the lesion. Impression cytology and cytobrush techniques can be used as well.

Differential diagnosis

- CIN or squamous cell carcinoma.
- Papilloma.
- Amelanotic nevi.
- Amelanotic melanomas.
- Pingueculum.
- Pterygium.
- Pyogenic granuloma.
- Dermoid.

PROPHYLAXIS

- Ultraviolet light-blocking lenses.
- Broad-brimmed hat.
- Avoidance of chronic exposure to high-intensity sunlight and extreme environments.

TREATMENT

Conjunctival or corneal intraepithelial neoplasm

Simple excision

- Probably most commonly used method.
- Rarely used with frozen sections; then only if invasion is suspected.
- With microscopic tumor margin surveillance, excellent method but more costly.

Radiotherapy

- Seldom used.

Immunotherapy and chemotherapy

- Dinitrochlorobenzene.
- Urea.
- Mitomycin.
- Tretinoin.
- Thiotepa.

Surgery and cryotherapy

Local surgical excision of CIN lesions combined with cryotherapy involves the use of a double-cycle freeze-thaw-refreeze technique and has yielded the lowest recurrence rate. Topical ocular anesthetic agents, such as proparacaine or cocaine, are applied to the eye. The conjunctiva under and around the lesion is elevated with subconjunctival injection of 1% lidocaine with epinephrine. If the conjunctiva does not elevate in the eyes without prior surgery, the diagnosis of squamous cell carcinoma must be suspected. Multiple conjunctival cautery applications 1.5 to 2 mm from the suspected tumor margin are used to outline the area to be excised. An incision then is made through these marks down to the bare sclera. The conjunctival and episcleral tissues are surgically dissected to the limbus. In areas where the conjunctiva is adherent to the episcleral area, a superficial sclerectomy may be necessary. The area of corneal involvement must be identified by retroillumination before surgery. Multiple applications of a local anesthetic agent are used to soften the corneal epithelium. With a no. 64 Beaver blade, 1 mm of normal epithelium and the involved corneal epithelium are removed by simply 'bulldozing' the epithelium to the limbus. A superficial limbal keratectomy is not usually performed because a pannus may form after surgery, although areas that underwent prior surgical keratectomies or have suspected tumor invasion require a superficial keratectomy. Simple excision of the conjunctiva flush with the limbus is all that is required; however, if a squamous cell carcinoma is suspected, a superficial lamellar sclerokeratectomy is required.

A Brymill CryAc unit with a 2- or 4-mm liquid nitrogen cryoprobe tip is used to freeze the limbal area. The most important area in which to obtain adequate freezing is at the limbus because this is the site of most recurrences. The endpoint of the freeze is a 1-second application that, on removal of the probe, leaves a white circular imprint of the probe tip on the eye. Multiple overlapping imprints are made to cover the entire surgical limbus twice. If a scleral or limbal area of inadequate dissection is suspected, a triple freeze-thaw technique should be used; however, an attempt should be made not to freeze more than 1 mm of peripheral clear cornea. The conjunctiva is not sutured except over exposed rectus muscles. A topical antibiotic ointment is applied at the end of surgery and a pressure dressing should be worn for 24 to 48 hours.

Usually, no ocular medications are administered after surgery.

Other cryoprobes that involve the use of other cryogens are satisfactory; however, the contact time is doubled or tripled. This is a very superficial dysplasia and requires only a very superficial freeze.

Squamous cell carcinoma

Squamous cell carcinoma is treated in the same manner, but more aggressive cryotherapy (triple freeze-thaw) with wider margins around the tumor and deeper sclerectomy and keratectomy are necessary. Deep invasion of the sclera and cornea requires full eye wall resection. Lamellar transplants are seldom used because they cover the signs of an early recurrence. Small intraocular extension can be treated with iridocycletomy, whereas more extensive intraocular extensions may require enucleation.

COMPLICATIONS

Although deep cryotherapy may result in iritis, posterior synechiae and corneal scarring, the complications of superficial cryosurgery are minimal, even when the cornea is treated. To avoid adherence of the cryoprobe, it is of utmost importance to have the probe completely frozen before ocular application. If the probe is applied warm and then frozen, it will cause a tight ocular adherence that is not easily removed. The use of the thawing option with some cryoprobes markedly decreases the cytotoxic effects of cryotherapy.

COMMENTS

An obvious advantage of cryosurgery over other methods of treating CIN is that 'root tips' that are missed with surgery alone, especially at the limbus, can be treated. This procedure results in a higher cure rate and is more cost effective than most other procedures. The use of surgical excision combined with cryotherapy has almost tripled previous cure rates of the use of surgery alone.

Despite the low virulence rate of CIN, it can be difficult to cure. CIN recurrence is dependent more on how the treatment is performed than on the clinical appearance, presence of early invasion, degree of dysplasia, or cell type. However, not all incompletely excised lesions recur. Recurrence most often develops in the first 2 years after surgery but has been reported as late as 10 years. The highest recurrence rates occur with lesions that involve more than two thirds of the limbus and with repeat operations.

REFERENCES

Erie JC, Campbell RJ, Liesegant TJ: Conjunctival and corneal intraepithelial and invasive neoplasia. Ophthalmology 93:176–183, 1986.

Fraunfelder FT, Wingfield D: Management of intraepithelial conjunctival tumors and squamous cell carcinomas. Am J Ophthalmol 95:359–363, 1983.

Frucht-Pery J, Rozenman Y: Mitomycin C therapy for corneal intraepithelial neoplasia. Am J Ophthalmol 117:164–168, 1994.

Tabin G, Levin S, Snibson G, et al: Late recurrences and the necessity for long-term follow-up in corneal and conjunctival intraepithelial neoplasia. Ophthalmology 104:485–492, 1997.

Tsubota K, Kajiwara K, Ugjin S, Hasegawa T: Conjunctival brush cytology. Acta Cytol 34:233–235, 1990.

Waring GO III, Roth AM, Ekins MB: Clinical and pathologic description of 17 cases of corneal intraepithelial neoplasia. Am J Ophthalmol 97:547–559, 1984.

125 CRANIOPHARYNGIOMA 237.0

Mandeep S. Tamber, MD
Toronto, Ontario
Abhaya V. Kulkarni, MD, PhD, FRCSC
Toronto, Ontario

ETIOLOGY/INCIDENCE

Craniopharyngiomas are benign neuroepithelial tumors of the parasellar region that are believed to develop from squamous cell remnants of Rathke's pouch. Although histologically benign, their involvement of neural structures in the suprasellar region, vis-à-vis local invasion of the optic apparatus, hypothalamus and pituitary, greatly complicates their management.

Craniopharyngioma is the most common non-glial intracranial tumor of childhood, constituting 2.5–4% of pediatric brain tumors overall and fully 46% of childhood tumors of the sellar and parasellar region. That being said, craniopharyngioma remains a rare diagnosis, with an incidence of approximately 1.3 per million person-years.

COURSE/PROGNOSIS

Despite recent advances in treatment modalities, craniopharyngioma remains a challenging entity. Most studies quote a 90% 10-year survival. There is a 1–2% risk of perioperative mortality. Permanent endocrine replacements are required for 85–90% of patients, mostly for the correction of ADH, cortisol and thyroxine deficiencies. A significant proportion of patients suffer major non-endocrine morbidity, including visual deficits (13–38%), seizures (12–18%), stroke (2–4%) and hypothalamic dysfunction (obesity, hypersomnolence, neurobehavioral effects).

DIAGNOSIS

Clinical signs and symptoms

Clinical manifestations depend largely upon the origin, direction and degree of tumor extension and the consequent involvement of surrounding neurovascular structures. Localized *sellar tumors* compress the pituitary gland, producing *endocrine deficiency* states (diabetes insipidus, short stature). *Prechiasmatic tumors* emerge from the sella and grow forward along the optic nerves, resulting in often severe *visual compromise* (reduced acuity, hemianopsias, optic atrophy). *Retrochiasmatic tumors* protrude behind the chiasm, shifting it anteriorly and distorting the third ventricle and hypothalamus. Accordingly, retrochiasmatic tumors are known to produce *hydrocephalus* (headache, papilledema) and *hypothalamic dysfunction* (endocrine and neuropsychological disturbances).

Laboratory findings

Cranial computed tomography (CT) and magnetic resonance (MR) imaging are the current imaging standards. The presence of suprasellar calcification, best demonstrated by CT, is important information for the surgeon, for it signals potentially difficult surgical extirpation. Sellar enlargement may also be visualized.

MR imaging is essential for preoperative planning, for it provides exquisite detail regarding the precise configuration of the solid ± cystic components of the tumor, as well as its relationship to surrounding neurovascular structures (Figure 125.1).

Comprehensive neuro-ophthalmological and endocrine evaluations also form part of the preoperative assessment of the child with craniopharyngioma.

TREATMENT

Craniopharyngioma is a complex clinicopathological condition that requires a multidisciplinary approach to treatment. The surgeon must bear in mind the goals of treatment as well as the sequelae of therapy. Treatment should be individualized so as to achieve the best possible retention of quality of life.

The optimal management strategy for these lesions remains controversial. At some centers, the treatment philosophy includes an initial attempt at gross total resection, based on the premise that total resection offers the best opportunity for tumor free survival. However, this aggressive surgical position is associated with significant upfront risks to endocrine, hypothalamic, and visual function.

In an effort to avoid surgical injury to these critical structures, others have adopted a less aggressive surgical position, advocating safe partial resection followed by adjuvant radiotherapy, either in the form of conventional fractionated external beam radiation, or stereotactic radiosurgery. In terms of local tumor control, data appears to suggest that both treatment alternatives are equivalent. With respect to treatment complications, radiotherapy results in delayed endocrine and visual defects similar to those observed following surgery, but the severity of these complications, particularly with respect to hypothalamic dysfunction, appears to be reduced. It must be remembered, however, that radiotherapy has its own inherent risks (cognitive dysfunction, second malignancy).

A third treatment alternative, reserved for cystic tumors, is cyst drainage followed by intracystic instillation of bleomycin or phosphorus-32.

At time of writing, chemotherapy for craniopharyngioma remains investigational.

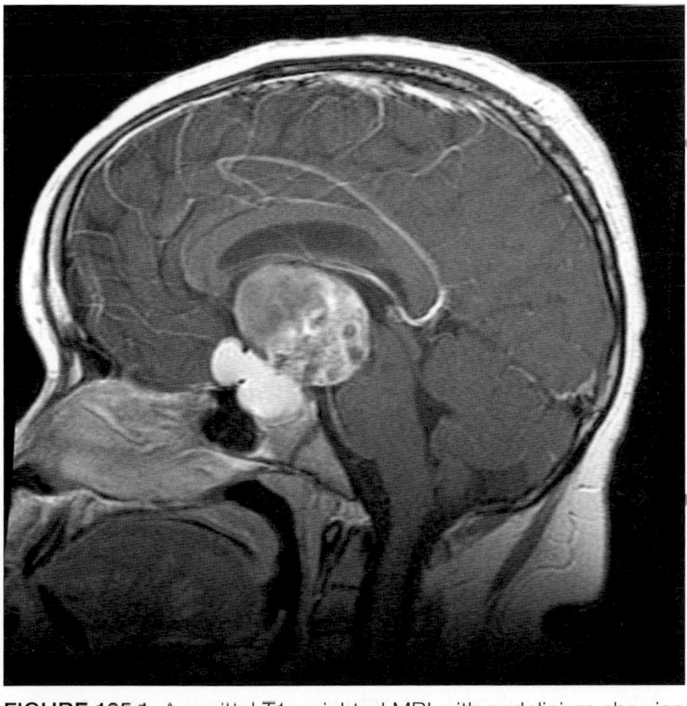

FIGURE 125.1. A sagittal T1-weighted MRI with gadolinium showing a typical large craniopharyngioma. The tumor is inhomogeneously enhancing and involves the sellar and suprasellar regions, with expansion into the third ventricle.

REFERENCES

Chiou SM, Lunsford LD, Niranjan A, et al: Stereotactic radiosurgery of residual or recurrent craniopharyngioma, after surgery, with or without radiation therapy. Neuro-oncol 3:159–166, 2001.

Duff JD, Meyer FB, Ilstrup DM, et al: Long-term outcomes for surgically resected craniopharyngiomas. Neurosurgery 46:291–305, 2000.

Hasegawa T, Kondziolka D, Hadjipanayis CG, et al: Management of cystic craniopharyngiomas with phosphorus-32 intracavitary irradiation. Neurosurgery 54:813–820, 2004.

van Effenterre R, Boch A-L: Craniopharyngioma in adults and children: a study of 122 surgical cases. J. Neurosurg. 97:3–11, 2002.

126 DERMOID 224.9

(Dermoid Cyst, Epidermoid Cyst, Epibulbar Dermoid, Limbal Dermoid, Lipodermoid, Dermolipoma)

Richard M. Robb, MD

Boston, Massachusetts

ETIOLOGY/INCIDENCE

Dermoids are choristomas that occur on or around the eye in two forms. One form is a cystic lesion with an inward-facing epidermal lining that surrounds a cavity filled with keratin, cholesterol clefts, oily sebum, and hairs. The wall of a true dermoid cyst contains dermal appendages, such as hair follicles and sweat glands. Epidermoid cyst walls lack these appendages. The other form of dermoid is a solid lesion at the corneal limbus or under the lateral bulbar conjunctiva.

DIAGNOSIS

Clinical signs and symptoms

Cystic dermoids most often occur at the superior orbital margin. If they are anterior to the orbital septum, they are usually recognized early in childhood. They have a soft rubbery consistency and are not attached to the overlying skin but may be bound to underlying periosteum. There often is a shallow crater in the orbital bone just under the lesion. Occasionally, the cysts have a dumbbell shape, with one end extending around the orbital margin and through the septum. Dermoid cysts that are located completely within the orbit behind the septum are usually discovered later. If they are relatively anterior and palpable, they may become apparent during the first two decades of life after a period of apparent growth. Such lesions are usually in the superior orbit and are not associated with propotosis, bone remodeling or diplopia. The more posterior cysts commonly present during the third and fourth decades and are nearly always heralded by proptosis and displacement of the eye. The lesions are extraconal. Diplopia and limitation of upward gaze are common. The cysts may grow beyond the confines of the orbit, sometimes superiorly through the frontal or sphenoid bone into the intracranial cavity and sometimes laterally into the temporal fossa, where mastication can induce a dynamic change in the degree of proptosis. Although these orbital dermoids are presumed to grow slowly and steadily from infancy, their clinical course suggests a long period of dormancy followed by rapid growth and symptoms over a period of about 1 year. What triggers this late growth is not known.

Solid dermoids at the corneal limbus are composed of dense connective tissue that contains hair follicles and sebaceous glands and is covered by keratinized squamous epithelium. Most of the lesions are temporal or inferior and straddle the limbus, but occasionally a dermoid will occur centrally on the cornea, completely occluding the visual axis. The limbal lesions exert their effect on vision by inducing corneal astigmatism that has a characteristic orientation with respect to the location of the dermoid. These limbal dermoids do not appear to grow with time. They may be isolated but can be associated with other anomalies. A common association is with the Goldenhar variant of hemifacial microsomia.

Conjunctival lipodermoids occasionally coexist with limbal dermoids, but usually they are isolated lesions. They are present temporally at the lateral canthus in the upper or lower quadrant or both. Their dense dermal-like connective tissue overlies a deposit of adipose tissue but usually contains no pilosebaceous units. The lesion extends back into the lateral orbit, but in the untreated form, it is not associated with abnormalities of ocular motility or displacement of the globe. Lipodermoids do not enlarge with time and are usually noticed only as a small fold of conjunctival tissue when the patient looks away from the side of the lesion.

There is little difficulty recognizing solid dermoids at the limbus, especially if there are hairs projecting from the lesion. Lipodermoids at the lateral canthus are also characteristic in form and location.

Laboratory findings

- Radiography is not usually helpful in the diagnosis of cystic dermoids anterior to the orbital rim, but plain films of the orbit reveal the deeper orbital cysts as radiolucent defects with polished sclerotic rims, where the bone adjacent to the cyst wall has been under pressure from the expanding mass.
- Computed tomography is commonly used to image orbital cysts. A simple cyst may appear as a smooth oval mass with a well-outlined border and a low-density homogeneous center. Larger posterior cysts may have a more heterogeneous appearance depending on the contents of the cyst and its pattern of growth. Calcium may be deposited in the wall of some cysts.
- Magnetic resonance imaging of dermoid cysts may be particularly useful in deeper orbital lesions because it distinguishes differences in soft tissue density and may help define the cystic nature and extent of the lesion.

TREATMENT

- Complete surgical excision is the treatment of choice for cystic dermoids. The lesions at the orbital rim anterior to the septum usually can be approached directly through a skin incision over the lesion. The same is true for upper orbital lesions just behind the septum. A transconjunctival approach may be appropriate for the infrequent cysts in the anterior orbital space just behind the orbital septum in the lower quadrants.
- Orbital cysts in the retrobulbar space are more difficult to remove completely and require a lateral orbitotomy. For lesions involving the sphenoid bone or showing a hiatal opening into the intracranial cavity, a transfrontal craniotomy is the better approach. The transfrontal approach is also preferred for a cyst in the orbital apex involving the optic canal and the superior orbital fissure.
- Limbal dermoids may be removed by shaving them off the underlying sclera and cornea to a depth sufficient to remove all grossly recognizable choristomatous tissue. Epithelium recovers the area of the excision spontaneously, leaving a flat gray corneal scar that is less conspicuous than the original white elevated dermoid. The astigmatic refractive error that frequently accompanies a limbal dermoid has not been eliminated by this surgery. Central corneal dermoids can be dissected off, but useful vision is rarely obtained. Corneal or corneoscleral grafts have occasionally been used for lesions that extend more deeply.
- Subconjunctival lipodermoids at the lateral canthus are not usually removed surgically because of the risk of scarring that might involve the underlying ocular muscles or the excretory ducts of the lacrimal gland. Limited excision of the anterior portion of the lesion has occasionally yielded a satisfactory cosmetic result.

COMPLICATIONS

- The main complication of dermoid cyst removal is a recurrent cyst due to incomplete removal. This is mostly a problem with posterior lesions, especially those that have ruptured in the course of removal. The recurrence may not become evident until many years after the initial surgery. Repeat operation may be required.
- The complications of an attempt to totally remove a lipodermoid at the lateral canthus include restricted ocular motility, strabismus, blepharoptosis and dry eye due to severing of the excretory ducts of the lacrimal gland.
- Limbal dermoids may involve the full thickness of the cornea or sclera, and perforation of the globe may result from attempting complete removal. It is better to remove only that portion that protrudes from the surface of the eye. In some cases, there may be regrowth of conjunctiva over the cornea after surgery, causing a more conspicuous postoperative scar. The use of postoperative topical corticosteroids helps to limit this regrowth.

REFERENCES

Elsas FJ, Green WR: Epibulbar tumors in childhood. Am J Ophthalmol 79:1001–1007, 1975.

Grove AS, Jr: Giant dermoid cysts of the orbit. Ophthalmology 86:1513–1520, 1979.

Henderson JW: Orbital tumors. 3rd edn. New York, Raven, 1993:53–61.

McNab AA, Wright JE, Caswell AG: Clinical features and surgical management of dermolipomas. Aust N Z J Ophthalmol 18:159–162, 1990.

Nevares RL, Mulliken JB, Robb RM: Ocular dermoids. Plast Reconstr Surg 82:959–964, 1988.

Pfeiffer RL, Nichol RJ: Dermoid and epidermoid tumors of the orbit. Arch Ophthalmol 40:639–664, 1948.

Robb RM: Astigmatic refractive errors associated with limbal dermoids. J Pediatr Ophthalmol Strabismus 33:241–243, 1996.

Sullivan GL: Caveat chirugicus. Trans Am Ophthalmol Soc 70:328–336, 1972.

Zaidman GW, Johnson B, Brown SI: Corneal transplantation in an infant with corneal dermoid. Am J Ophthalmol 93:78–83, 1982.

127 EWING'S SARCOMA 170

Terry D. Wood, MD
Portland, Oregon
Julie Falardeau, MD, FRCSC
Portland, Oregon

ETIOLOGY/INCIDENCE

Ewing's sarcoma belongs to a family of malignancies known as small, blue, round cell tumors of childhood. Sarcomas are generally thought of as deriving from mesoderm, but the embryological origin of Ewing's sarcoma is neuroectoderm. The underlying genetic defect is a chromosomal translocation. In greater than 95% of cases, the translocation is t(11;22)(q24;q12); the Ewing sarcoma gene (*EWS*) on chromosome 22, whose function is unknown, fuses with the *FLI-1* proto-oncogene on chromosome 11. The result is a chimeric protein with increased transcriptional activity and the ability to induce neoplastic transformation in fibroblasts.

Ewing's sarcoma can occur at any age, although it usually appears during the first or second decade of life with a peak incidence during the second decade. The male to female ration is 1.4 : 1. This tumor most often originates in bone, but it may also arise from soft tissue. The most common areas of origin are the femur, pelvis, tibia, humerus, fibula, scapula and ribs. The most common site of metastasis is to the lung. Only 2% to 3% of Ewing's sarcomas arise from the head and neck. Papilledema has been reported as a rare sign of intracranial involvement. Orbital involvement includes proptosis and swelling of orbital tissue, with or without decreased vision and is usually secondary to metastatic disease.

The cause is unknown; there is an increased incidence in patients with retinoblastoma and in areas of prior irradiation. The annual incidence is 0.6 to 0.8 in 1 million population.

COURSE/PROGNOSIS

- The most common presenting complaint is intermittent pain.
- A fever is present in 20% of cases.
- The prognosis has markedly improved during the past 25 years, with survival rates increasing from 10% to 70%.
- Prognosis improves if the site is distal (e.g. hands, feet), the tumor is small, and most importantly, if the tumor has not metastasized at the time of diagnosis.
- There is good pathologic response to chemotherapy.

DIAGNOSIS

Laboratory findings

- Current histologic testing requires more fresh tissue than previously required.
- The biopsy site should be in the area to be included in the radiation field.
- Biopsy should be done only by those with prior experience with this type of tumor because the long-term prognosis depends on where and how the biopsy is performed and how adjacent tissues are managed.

Differential diagnosis

- Primary lymphoma of bone.
- Embryonal rhabdomyosarcoma.
- Metastatic neuroblastoma.
- Small cell osteogenic sarcoma.

TREATMENT

The treatment of Ewing's sarcoma requires a multidisciplinary approach and the patient is best referred to a tertiary center with experience with this tumor. The management team usually includes a pediatric oncologist, a radiation therapist, an orthopedic oncologist and an orbital surgeon.

Systemic

- Multiagent chemotherapy agents include vincristine, cyclophosphamide, actinomycin D and doxorubicin. For resistant cases, ifosfamide has been advocated.
- Newer agents include granulocyte colony-stimulating factor and recombinant human cytokine glycoprotein.

Local

- Wide en bloc resection is performed.
- Most patients have postoperative radiation therapy with chemotherapy.

COMPLICATIONS

Radiation

- The usual local complications can occur.
- Pathologic fractures can occur.
- There is a long-term risk of secondary local malignancy (40× increase at 60-Gy dose).
- The risks of radiation have increased as the survival rates of patients have increased.

Chemotherapy

- As with all antimetabolite agents, multiple complications can occur.
- Alkylating chemotherapeutic agents have been associated with late secondary malignancies.

COMMENTS

Recent advances in molecular biology have shed light on the etiology of Ewing's sarcoma. Continued progress holds the promise of significant improvements in diagnosis and treatment.

REFERENCES

Bhatoe HS, Deshpande GU: Primary cranial Ewing's sarcoma. Br J Neurosurgery 12(2):165–169, 1998.

Gunduz K, Shields J, Shields CA, et al: Ewing sarcoma metastatic to the iris. Am J Ophthalmol 124:550–552, 1997.

Jakobiec FA, Rootman J, Jones IS: Secondary and metastatic tumors of the orbit. In: Duane TD, ed: Clinical ophthalmology. Hagerstown, MD, Harper & Row, 1982:II(46):1–67.

Jurgens H, Exner U, Gadner H, et al: Multidisciplinary treatment of primary Ewing's sarcoma of bone: a 6-year experience of a European Cooperative Trial. Cancer 61:23–32, 1988.

Kiratli H, Shields CL, Shields JA, DePotter P: Metastatic tumors to the conjunctiva: report of 10 cases. Br J Ophthalmol 80:5–8, 1996.

Smith LM, Donaldson SS: Incidence and management of secondary malignancies in patients with retinoblastoma in Ewing's sarcoma. Oncology (Huntingt) 5:135–141, 1991.

Thorner PS, Squire JA: Molecular genetics in the diagnosis and prognosis of solid pediatric tumors. Pediatrics and Developmental Pathology 1:337–365, 1998.

Woodruff G, Thorner P, Skarf B: Primary Ewing's sarcoma of the orbit presenting with visual loss. Br J Ophthalmol 72:786–792, 1988.

128 FIBROSARCOMA 171.9

Donna Siracuse-Lee, MD
Brooklyn, New York
Norman A. Saffra, MD
Brooklyn, New York

ETIOLOGY/INCIDENCE

Primary orbital fibrosarcoma is a rare malignant tumor of fibroblastic origin. Congenital, juvenile and adult forms have been described. It most commonly presents in adults aged 30 to 70 years. Primary orbital tumors usually present at 55 to 60 years of age. Pediatric occurrences are rare. Orbital radiation therapy may increase the incidence of secondary fibrosarcomas, usually in patients 30 to 50 years of age. Generally, most primary fibrosarcomas arise in the soft tissue or bone of the extremities.

Orbital fibrosarcomas often occur as a result of invasion from tumors in adjacent paranasal sinuses or bones. Extensive radiotherapy for prior malignancies of the eye or adnexa, most commonly retinoblastoma, may also cause secondary fibrosarcomas. In this clinical setting, fibrosarcoma is second in incidence only to osteosarcoma. Primary fibrosarcoma should be strongly considered in the differential diagnosis of mass lesions of the orbital soft tissue or the lacrimal sac. These lesions may also arise on the eyelid, canthus, sclera or conjunctiva.

DIAGNOSIS

Clinical signs and symptoms

Symptoms of fibrosarcoma may vary according to the age of presentation. Congenital and infantile forms are rapidly growing, with less than 8% metastasis. One series of five juvenile fibrosarcomas presented with proptosis and usually painless lid swelling. Most grew within weeks to months. Adult lesions have a 50% recurrence rate and are locally aggressive, causing neural and functional deficits at presentation. Signs may include exophthalmos, soft-tissue orbital mass, optic nerve edema, and extraocular muscle paralysis. History of prior radiation should be elicited.

Laboratory findings

Neuroimaging findings with CT and MR are usually nonspecific and not pathognomonic. Upon neuroimaging, adult tumors may be either circumscribed or infiltrative, although an aggressively infiltrating soft tissue mass is more common. Bone may be eroded on CT or MR. Infantile forms may be more circumscribed in appearance.

In an adult, the differential diagnosis should include fibromatosis, malignant fibrous histiocytoma (MFH), nodular fasciitis, schwannoma, hemangiopericytoma, meningioma, lymphoma and metastasis. The differential diagnosis in the pediatric population includes rhabdomyosarcoma, fibromatosis, and metastatic neuroblastoma. In all patients post radiation, the most common tumors include osteosarcoma and MFH.

Incisional or excisional biopsy is necessary, as histopathology is diagnostic. Fibroblasts differentiate into many connective tissue cells, therefore features of other mesenchymal cells may be found on pathology. Light microscopy typically demonstrates immature fibroblasts presenting as uniform spindle cells arranged in a characteristic interlacing fascicular or herringbone pattern, with little surrounding collagen. Abundant reticulin fibers may be seen.

EM findings may be used to confirm the diagnosis, with prominent Golgi apparatus and well developed rough endoplasmic reticulum.

TREATMENT

Complete excision is necessary for survival. Local excision with wide margins or exenteration is recommended in adults and children, particularly in fibrosarcomas of the head and neck. Frozen-tissue examinations are very useful in locating tumor borders. Chemotherapy and radiation are ineffective for cure but may be useful as palliation.

MANAGEMENT

Recurrences, metastases, or intracranial extensions of neoplasm usually develop within 6 to 8 years after the initial surgery. Prognosis in children less than ten years of age is generally good. In children less than 5, recurrence in one series was 43%, and death from metastases was 7.3%. Children older than ten have a 50% metastasis rate at 5 years. In adults, it is a highly malignant tumor. Non-orbital tumors have a 60% 5-year survival rate. A definite cure is considered to have occurred after 10 to 12 years if there are no recurrences, metastases, or extensions. Post irradiation tumors have a poor prognosis.

REFERENCES

Dalley RW: Fibrous histiocytoma and fibrous tissue tumors of the orbit. Radiol Clinics N Amer 37:1:185–194, 1999.

Jakobiec FA, Tannenbaum M: The ultrastructure of orbital fibrosarcoma. Amer J Ophthalmol 77:6:899–917, 1974.

Weiner JM, Hidayat AA: Juvenile fibrosarcoma of the orbit and eyelid. Arch Ophthalmol 101:253–259, 1983.

129 HODGKIN'S DISEASE 201.9

Warren L. Felton, III, MD
Richmond, Virginia

ETIOLOGY/INCIDENCE

Hodgkin's disease is a malignant lymphoma. Two entities are recognized. Classical Hodgkin's lymphoma comprises the majority (95%), while nodular lymphocyte-predominant Hodgkin's lymphoma (LPHL) is rare. Classical Hodgkin's lymphoma is distinguished from non-Hodgkin's lymphoma by the presence of Reed–Sternberg (RS) cells, predominantly B cell in origin (less than 2% derive from T cells). In LPHL, variants of RS cells termed lymphocytic and histiocytic (L&H) cells, are identified. In both forms, however, neoplastic cells make up only a small minority of the total cell population, which is primarily composed of reactive inflammatory cells.

The cause of Hodgkin's disease is not known. Infectious and genetic factors are thought to play roles. The involvement of the Epstein–Barr virus (EBV) is well established, but a causative role is not proved. Familial clustering and concordance in first-degree relatives, especially monozygotic twins, support a genetic predisposition to the disease in some patients.

Hodgkin's disease is uncommon. The incidence is 2.4 per 100,000 per year and appears to be stable. In North America and Europe combined, 20,000 patients are diagnosed annually, of which 7800 are found in the United States. In Western developed countries, there is a bimodal incidence from ages 15 to 30 years and after age 50 years. In some developing countries, the disease is more common in childhood.

The male-to-female ratio is approximately 3 : 2. Immunosuppressed patients, including those with acquired immunodeficiency syndromes, are at a higher risk.

COURSE/PROGNOSIS

In most patients the disease begins in one lymphoid site and then extends to contiguous lymphoid tissue. Extranodal involvement may occur through direct invasion or hematogenous spread. Prognosis is determined by the stage of the disease, the presence of systemic symptoms, and whether there is bulky involvement of the mediastinum. Patients with early-stage Hodgkin's disease are often asymptomatic and have a better prognosis, whereas those with systemic symptoms more typically have advanced-stage disease and a poorer prognosis, as do those with a bulky mediastinal mass. Other features indicating an adverse prognosis include male gender, age 45 years or older, elevated sedimentation rate, anemia, leukocytosis, lymphocytopenia and low serum albumin. If untreated, patients with Hodgkin's disease may die within two to three years of presentation. With treatment, Hodgkin's disease may be cured in more than 80% of patients.

DIAGNOSIS

Clinical signs and symptoms

Patients with Hodgkin's disease most often present with painless regional lymphadenopathy. The affected lymph nodes are located above the diaphragm in 80% of patients, including the neck, supraclavicular region, axilla, and anterior mediastinum. About one-third of patients present with systemic symptoms of fever, night sweats, or weight loss. Pruritis is also common. Pain at involved sites, including bone pain, induced by alcohol consumption is an uncommon but classic symptom. Extranodal involvement is uncommon.

Ocular

Ocular manifestations of Hodgkin's disease are rare and usually occur as a late complication or as a consequence of treatment; more rarely, ocular involvement is the initial presentation of the disease. Chorioretinitis, vitritis, and anterior uveitis are reported more often than other ocular findings.

- Anterior chamber: uveitis.
- Choroid: infiltration
- Conjunctiva: infiltration.
- Cornea: keratitis.
- Cortical visual loss: infiltration, tumor mass.
- Extraocular muscle: infiltration, Grave's disease.
- Horner's syndrome: cervical lymphadenopathy, infiltration.
- Iris: posterior synechiae.
- Lacrimal gland: infiltration.
- Lens: cataract.
- Lid: infiltration, ptosis.
- Ocular motor nerves: infiltration, tumor mass, increased intracranial pressure.
- Optic chiasm: infiltration.
- Optic nerve: infiltration, papilledema, paraneoplastic optic neuropathy, tumor mass.
- Orbit: infiltration, tumor mass, exophthalmos.
- Pupil: afferent papillary defect, parasympathetic dilatation, Horner's syndrome.
- Retina: exudates, hemorrhages, ischemia, perivascular sheathing, vasculitis, Roth's spots, central retinal artery occlusion, central retinal vein occlusion, serous macular detachment.
- Sclera: scleritis, episcleritis.
- Vitreous: infiltration.
- Other: visual field defects, visual hallucinations, gaze palsies, internuclear ophthalmoplegia, nystagmus, cavernous sinus syndrome, paraneoplastic cerebellar degeration, paraneoplastic myasthenia gravis syndrome, opsoclonus-myoclonus paraneoplastic syndrome, Sjögren's syndrome, Vogt–Koyanagi–Harada syndrome, opportunistic infections.

Laboratory findings

The diagnosis of Hodgkin's disease rests on the biopsy of lymph glands or other involved tissue. Immunophenotype studies aid in distinguishing Hodgkin's lymphomas from other pathologies (e.g. CD 15 and CD 30 in classical Hodgkin's disease). Based on the number of Reed–Sternberg cells and the inflammatory

milieu, classical Hodgkin's disease is divided into four subtypes:
1. Nodular sclerosing, which is the most common;
2. Mixed cellularity;
3. Lymphocyte-rich; and
4. Lymphocyte-depleted.

Less important to treatment than establishing the histopathologic subtype is the careful staging of the disease. Staging is based on the number of sites involved, whether one or both sides of the diaphragm is affected, tumor bulk (X), extranodal involvement (E sites), and the presence (B) or absence (A) of systemic symptoms. Stages I and II and stages III and IV are termed early-stage and advanced-stage Hodgkin's disease, respectively. Staging is accomplished by history; physical examination; serum hematologic and chemistry studies; radiographic imaging, including thoracic, abdominal and pelvic computed tomography scans; and, in selected patients, positron emission tomography, gallium scan, magnetic resonance imaging, laparotomy, bone marrow biopsy and other procedures.

- Hematologic findings include elevated sedimentation rate, anemia, lymphopenia, eosinophelia, leukocytosis, monocytosis and thrombocytopenia.
- Other labarotory abnormalities may include liver functions, lactic dehydrogenase, alkaline phosphatase, albumin and calcium.
- Biopsy of orbital structures, optic nerve, optic chiasm, cavernous sinus, meninges, brain parenchyma, or other related tissue may be necessary to establish the diagnosis when an ocular manifestation is the presenting sign and lymphadenopathy is not evident on physical examination.

Differential diagnosis

The differential diagnosis of Hodgkin's disease is that of lymphadenopathy, typically regional and less commonly generalized. When the presentation is extranodal, including ocular manifestations, the differential diagnosis is in part dependent on the site of involvement. In addition to non-Hodgkin's lymphoma, conditions that should be considered include the following:

- Mediastinal neoplasms, germ cell tumors, thymoma, infections, primarily tuberculosis and inflammations, especially sarcoidosis.
- Primary cancers of the head, neck, lung, breast, thyroid and rectum.
- Generalized lymphadenopathies, including viral, fungal, bacterial and mycobacterial infections; human immunodeficiency virus-associated lymphadenopathy; and autoimmune disorders.
- For certain ocular or ophthalmologically related manifestations, the following conditions should be considered:
  - Uveal tract infectious, inflammatory and neoplastic conditions;
  - Retinal ischemic, vasculitic, and inflammatory processes;
  - Orbital neoplastic, inflammatory, and autoimmune conditions;
  - Intracranial malignancies and inflammatory disease.

TREATMENT

The goal in the treatment of patients with Hodgkin's disease is to produce a cure and to minimize the side effects of the treatment. Chemotherapy and radiation are the mainstays of therapy. The primary determinant of the type, dose, and duration of treatment is the stage of the disease and, in early-stage disease, whether prognostic factors are favorable or unfavorable.

Systemic

Chemotherapy is increasingly used for all stages of the disease. Patients with early stage disease may be treated with combined chemotherapy followed by low-dose radiation to involved sites. Combined chemotherapy is the standard for patients with advanced-stage Hodgkin's disease. The ABVD regimen is most commonly used in the United States. Stanford V and BEACOPP are other chemotherapeutic combinations.

- ABVD: doxorubicin (Adriamycin), bleomycin, vinblastine, dacarbazine.
- Stanford V: doxobubicin, vinblastine, mechlorethamine, vincristine, bleomycin, etoposide, prednisone.
- BEACOPP: bleomycin, etoposide, doxorubicin (Adriamycin), cyclophosphamide, vincristine (Oncovin), procarbazine, prednisone.

Both intravenous and oral corticosteroids are used in a variety of settings, including those with ocular impact, to reduce inflammation.

Local

For patients with early-stage disease and favorable prognosis, local radiation to involved sites and to adjacent sites, without chemotherapy, is a traditional option. However, low dose radiation restricted to involved regions, combined with chemotherapy, is more commonly employed. The role of radiation therapy in advanced-stage Hodgkin's lymphoma is controversial and is most often directed at bulky sites of the disease. Radiation alone is not an option for patients with advanced stage disease. Radiotherapy, without or with chemotherapy, is used for the LPHL variant.

Local radiation therapy is directed to affected extranodal sites with ocular impact, including the orbit, optic nerve, optic chiasm, cavernous sinus and brain.

Surgical

The application of surgery is limited in Hodgkin's disease. Surgical biopsy of lymph nodes or other involved sites is essential to establish the diagnosis and is sometimes indicated to determine the response to treatment. Surgical decompression of the orbit, optic nerve, optic chiasm, or cavernous sinus may be required when visual function is compromised by the mass effect of an advancing tumor.

Other

Salvage treatment for patients with relapsed Hodgkin's disease includes chemotherapy for those initially receiving radiation alone, high-dose chemotherapy, bone marrow transplantation and autologous stem cell transplantation.

In pediatric patients, chemotherapy is the standard and radiation is applied selectively in low doses.

COMPLICATIONS

The side effects of radiation therapy are dependent on the dose and the region treated and include coronary artery disease, pericarditis, dry mouth, nausea, dermatitis, pneumonitis, Lhermitte's sign, herpes zoster infection, hypothyroidism and infertility.

Radiation therapy-induced complications with ocular impact include lid edema, loss of lid lashes, insufficient or excessive tearing, keratitis, conjunctivitis, iritis, lens edema, cataract, retinopathy, optic neuropathy and trigeminal sensory neuropathy.

Chemotherapeutic toxicities vary with the regimen and dose and include fatigue, hair loss, nausea, myelosuppression, pulmonary impairment, peripheral neuropathy and infertility.

Ocular complications of chemotherapy used in Hodgkin's disease include keratitis, conjunctivitis, uveitis, retinal hemorrhage, neuroretinitis, ocular motor nerve palsies, cortical visual loss and possibly optic neuropathy.

The most serious complication of radiation or chemotherapy is the development of a second malignancy. Secondary malignancies include acute leukemia or other myelodysplasias, which usually occur within 1 to 2 years after treatment, and a variety of solid carcinomas of the lung (the most common second malignancy), breast, thyroid, head, neck and stomach, sarcomas and melanoma, which may develop after a latency period of many years.

COMMENTS

The treatment of Hodgkin's disease is continuously progressing. A clear understanding of the pathogenesis remains a challenge. When ocular complications occur, close cooperation is required among the ophthalmologist, pathologist, medical oncologist and radiation oncologist to achieve the best result for the patient.

REFERENCES

Barkana Y, Zadok D, Herbert M, et al: Granulomatous kerato-conjunctivitis as a manifestation of Hodgkin lymphoma. Am J Ophthalmol 131:796–797, 2001.

Connors JM: State-of-the-art therapeutics: Hodgkin's lymphoma. J Clin Oncol 23:6400–6408, 2005.

Diehl V, Thomas RK, Re D: Part II: Hodgkin's lymphoma-diagnosis and treatment. Lancet Oncol 5:19–26, 2004.

Kasner SE, Galetta SL, Vaughn DJ: Cavernous sinus syndrome in Hodgkin's disease. J Neuroophthalmol 16:204–207, 1996.

Klapper SR, Jordan DR, McLeish W, et al: Unilateral proptosis in an immunocompetant man as the initial clinical manifestation of systemic Hodgkin disease. Ophthalmology 106:338–341, 1999.

Nasir MA, Jeffe GJ: Cytomegalovirus retinitis associated with Hodgkin's disease. Retina 16:324–327, 1996.

Thakker MM, Perez VL, Moulin A, et al: Multifocal nodular episcleritis and scleritis with undiagnosed Hodgkin's lymphoma. Ophthalmology 110:1057–1060, 2003.

To TW, Rankin GA, Jakobiec FA, Hidayat AA: Intraocular lymphoproliferations simulating uveitis. In: Albert DM, Jakobiec FA, eds. Principles and practices of ophthalmology. 2nd edn. WB. Saunders, 2000:2(98): 1315–1338.

Yung L, Linch D: Hodgkin's lymphoma. Lancet 361:943–951, 2003.

130 JUVENILE XANTHOGRANULOMA 224.0 (JXG)

Theodore H. Curtis, MD
Portland, Oregon
David T. Wheeler, MD
Portland, Oregon

Juvenile xanthogranuloma (JXG) is a rare, generally benign, skin disorder of uncertain etiology that typically affects infants and young children, and very rarely presents in adults. It was first described by Adamson in 1905 as 'congenital xanthoma multiplex' and the first case with intraocular involvement was a child reported by Blank in 1949. It is characterized by single or multiple discreet, firm, rubbery, yellowish-pink to tan papulonodules several millimeters in diameter, preferentially occurring on the head and neck but also seen on the trunk and extremities. Skin lesions often regress spontaneously and are not usually associated with systemic manifestations.

Extracutaneous manifestations have been described in eye, lung, liver, pericardium, myocardium, spleen, colon, retroperitoneum, kidney, adrenal gland, gonads, central nervous system, bone, periostium, muscle, mucous membranes, salivary glands and larynx. The eye is the most frequently affected extracutaneous site, with an incidence of 0.3% to 0.5% in cutaneous JXG. Approximately 40% of patients with ocular involvement have cutaneous lesions, usually multiple. In patients with visceral involvement, cutaneous lesions are always multiple and ocular involvement is rare.

Ocular involvement occurs most often during the first two years of life. Uveal JXG is the most common presentation and can include a localized or diffuse iris tumor (heterochromia iridis), spontaneous hyphema, secondary glaucoma, erythema and uveitis. Additional sites of ocular involvement are much less common and include eyelids, cornea, limbus, conjunctiva, sclera, orbit, retina, choroid and optic nerve. Epibulbar lesions have been known to extend into the anterior chamber. Orbital lesions are rare and may occur with or without bony destruction; most present in the perinatal period. Most cases are unilateral, but bilateral involvement has been reported. Spontaneous regression of ocular lesions without medical intervention has been described rarely. Skin lesions develop after those in the eye or orbit in up to 45% of affected patients.

Associations have been noted with neurofibromatosis, epilepsy, Niemann–Pick disease, urticaria pigmentosa, insul-independent diabetes mellitus, leukemic disorders and cytomegalovirus infections. All but the association with neurofibromatosis and some leukemias are probably coincidental. A triple association with neurofibromatosis (type 1), juvenile chronic myelogenous leukemia and JXG has been well described. No lipid abnormality or other metabolic disturbances have been reported.

ETIOLOGY/INCIDENCE

The pathogenesis of JXG is believed to be a reactive granulomatous response of histiocytes to local tissue injury. Histiocytes arise from stem cells in bone marrow and undergo differentiation along monocyte-macrophage (phagocytic) or

Langerhans-dendritic (antigen-presenting) pathways. JXG is thought to be a disorder of macrophages. Other benign proliferative macrophage disorders such as benign cephalic histiocytosis, papular xanthoma and progressive nodular histiocytosis are probably clinical variants of the same underlying process. These tumors usually do not stain with S100 and lack Birbeck granules, which are typical of the 'histiocytosis X' group of diseases such as Hand–Schuller–Christian, Letterer–Siwe and eosinophilic granuloma. JXG is a clinically distinct entity and not a member of this family of diseases, which have vastly different clinical and pathologic findings.

The incidence of JXG is unknown but may be higher than reported as it often occurs early in life, may be mistaken for a 'mole' and may spontaneously regress. In cutaneous JXG, a male predominance (1.5 : 1) has been noted in childhood but there is no reported sex predilection in adults. There is no known ethnic predisposition. Tumors are present at birth in 5% to 17% and occur during the first year of life in 40% to 70%. Adult onset is infrequent with a peak incidence in late twenties and early thirties. Familial cases have not been observed.

COURSE/PROGNOSIS

Spontaneous regression of skin lesions is well documented but the natural history of ocular lesions is less well understood. JXG is an important cause of spontaneous hyphema in childhood. Secondary glaucoma and blindness can occur. Visual prognosis of anterior uveal involvement depends on prompt recognition of the disease and early resolution of the lesion. With orbital lesions, prognosis varies with the extent of orbital and optic nerve involvement and the degree of secondary fibrosis.

DIAGNOSIS

Laboratory findings

- Diagnostic techniques include biomicroscopy, high frequency ultrasound and cytologic examination of anterior chamber material obtained with paracentesis (see Karcioglu for method).
- Routine hematologic and metabolic screening is not indicated.
- Zimmerman has described the lesion histologically as containing densely packed polyhedral histiocytes with abundant cytoplasm that exhibits varying degrees of vacuolization, occasional Touton multinucleated giant cells and a prominent network of thin-walled vessels.
- Perivascular edema, duplication of capillary basement membranes, and endothelial cell swelling and degeneration suggest an inflammatory process.

Differential diagnosis

- Many dermatologic diseases can be confused with JXG on clinical examination (see Tanz for a comprehensive listing).
- The ocular lesions of JXG must be differentiated from dermoid, dermolipoma, neurofibroma, fibrous histiocytoma, Langerhans' granulomatoses and xanthoma disseminatum (see Yanoff for a more complete listing).
- Spontaneous hyphema in infancy may also be caused by unsuspected or unreported trauma, any intraocular tumor involving the anterior segment (including retinoblastoma, medulloepithelioma, leukemia and lymphoma), diseases that cause iris neovascularization (such as juvenile retinoschisis) or diseases characterized by pupillary or retrolental membranes (like retinopathy of prematurity or persistent fetal vasculature).

TREATMENT

Ocular

- For patients with skin lesions only, careful ophthalmic follow-up but no active intervention is indicated.
- Ocular involvement limited to eyelids or epibulbar tissue also does not require specific treatment but close observation for uveal lesions is necessary.
- Topical, intralesional and systemic corticosteroids have been used successfully for intraocular and orbital JXG. Diffuse or localized uveal lesions should probably be treated initially with topical medication but systemic treatment should be added if there is no response in several weeks. Intralesional steroids may be effective in orbital lesions (dexamethasone 4 mg and betamethasone 6 mg).
- Radiotherapy is recommended for diffuse uveal lesions or those associated with glaucoma, and for any lesions that fail to respond to corticosteroids. Dramatic response can occur to low doses of 250 to 400 cGy, usually 100 to 200 cGy per dose spread over 2 or 3 weeks. Total dose of greater than 500 cGy may increase the risk of radiation damage to normal structures.
- Surgery is reserved for well-localized iris lesions less than one quadrant in size. The benefit of tissue diagnosis must be weighed against the risks of hyphema and lens damage, particularly as these lesions are often extremely sensitive to steroids and radiation.

COMPLICATIONS

Although cutaneous JXG is generally regarded as a self-limited condition, systemic disease in some children has led to serious symptoms and occasionally death. With ocular involvement, the risk of complications is high. Uveal lesions may invade the angle and produce hyphema or uncontrolled glaucoma; corneal blood staining, cataract and amblyopia may occur. Although posterior involvement is rare, when extensive it may produce obliteration of the central retinal vein and/or artery and retinal detachment leading to blindness.

COMMENTS

Screening for ocular involvement is controversial due to its relatively low incidence; however, over half the patients with both ocular and cutaneous involvement have skin lesions first. In addition, these patients nearly always have multiple skin lesions and are usually younger than 2 years of age (92%). It would therefore be reasonable and cost-effective to refer only this subgroup of higher risk patients, i.e. patients less than 2 years old with multiple cutaneous lesions, to an ophthalmologist.

REFERENCES

Blank H, Eglick P, Beerman H: Nevoxanthoendothelioma with ocular involvement. Pediatrics 4:349–354, 1949.

Cadera W, Silver MM, Burt L: Juvenile xanthogranuloma. Can J Ophthalmol 18:169–174, 1983.

DeBarge LR, Chan CC, Greenberg SC, et al: Chorioretinal, iris, and ciliary body infiltration by juvenile xanthogranuloma masquerading as uveitis. Surv Ophthalmol 39:65–71, 1994.

Harley RD, Romayananda N, Chan GH: Juvenile xanthogranuloma. J Pediatr Ophthalmol Strabismus 19:33–39, 1982.

Hernandez-Martin A, Baselga E, Drolet BA, et al: Juvenile xanthogranuloma. J Am Acad Dermatol 36:355–367, 1997.

Karcioglu Z, Mullaney PB: Diagnosis and management of iris juvenile xanthogranuloma. J Pediatr Ophthalmol Strabismus 34:44–51, 1997.

Tanz WS, Schwartz RA, Janniger CK: Juvenile xanthogranuloma. Cutis 54:241–245, 1994.

Yanoff M, Perry HD: Juvenile xanthogranuloma of the corneoscleral limbus. Arch Ophthalmol 113:915–917, 1995.

Zimmerman LE: Ocular lesions of juvenile xanthogranuloma. Am J Ophthalmol 60:1011–1035, 1965.

Zvulunov A, Barak Y, Metzker A: Juvenile xanthogranuloma, neurofibromatosis, and juvenile chronic myelogenous leukemia. Arch Dermatol 131:904–908, 1995.

131 KAPOSI'S SARCOMA 131.13

Hassane Souhail, MD
Rabat, Morocco
M. Maliki, MD
Rabat, Morocco
A. Naoumi, MD
Rabat, Morocco
H. Channa, MD
Rabat, Morocco
A. Therzaz, MD
Rabat, Morocco

ETIOLOGY/INCIDENCE

Kaposi's sarcoma (KS) is an aggressive endothelial tumor that typically presents cutaneous lesions and visceral manifestations. It was first described in 1872 by Moritz Caposi, a dermatology specialist from Hungry and named idiopathic multiple pigmented sarcoma. Four types of KS since been described:

1. Classic indolent: sporadically, but ruthlessly, attacks elderly people from the Mediterranean area. Incidence is 0.4/100000.
2. Endemic African: more aggressive and attacks younger people. Incidence unknown.
3. Iatrogenic: related to the immunodepression is observed essentially in patients with transplanted organs or under a long term corticotherapy. Incidence varies between 0.45% to 4% of the tumors observed in patients with transplanted organs.
4. Epidemic, associated with AIDS: the most common neoplasm in patients with acquired immunodeficiency syndrome (AIDS). Approximately 30 to 40 % of patients with AIDS are affected. Ocular involvement could be observed in 20% of cases, while orbital location remains exceptional.

In extremely rare cases the initial clinical manifestation of AIDS- related to KS can be recognized by ophthalmic examination. Two cases of conjunctival KS have been reported as the initial clinical manifestation of AIDS.

The cause of KS is still mysterious but the current concepts and epidemiological evidence suggest that the human herpes virus 8 (HHV8) might be a possible causative agent.

COURSE/PROGNOSIS

The neoplasm is frequently a multifocal progressive lesion. Some authors consider the ocular lesion a sign of poor prognosis.

The ophthalmic manifestations of KS are usually limited to the conjunctiva and eyelid. They start with a bluish-red macula that coalesces and eventually spreads to internal organs. In cases of conjunctiva involvement, it appears as a flat, reddish lesion most often located in the lower fornix.

DIAGNOSIS

The diagnosis of the KS is histopathologic. It is based on the simultaneous presence of the vascular structure, cell fusiforms or kaposi cells, inflammatory infiltration and hemosiderin stocks. In immunohistologic exam, the KS reveals certain factors to different degrees: VIII, CD31, CD34. All cases, irrespective of epidemiologic subgroup, are HHV8 positive.

Differential diagnosis

- Cavernous angioma.
- Pyogenic granuloma.
- Chronic sub-conjunctival haemorrhage.
- Foreign body granuloma.
- Metastatic tumor.

TREATMENT

The treatment should not be over-aggressive to avoid the risk of aggravating or inducing an immunodeficiency. It should respect and secure a comfortable life for the patients. It is usually indicated for:

- Cosmetic reasons;
- Obstruction of vision;
- Obstruction of lacrimal system; or
- The lesion is complicated by haemorrhage or infection.

Classical SK usually develops very slowly and is rarely lethal. Immunosuppressive treatment drugs are gradually reduced resulting in the maintenance of a satisfactory immune function. This often causes a partial or total regression of the illness.

In KS-AIDS, the treatment is effective in 25% of cases. The illness might remain stable or increase, but is not the cause of death. Treatment may not be required for localized and stable lesions but regular supervision is necessary.

Systemic

Monotherapy

- Vinblastin, etoposid, bleomycin, adriblastine, epirubicine, idarabicine and doxorubicin.

Polychemotherapy

- AVB protocol (doxorubicin 40mg/m2/j1, bleomycin 15 mg/m2/j1, vincristin 6 mg/m2/j1) — single or alternated with the ADV protocol (actinomycin D, dacaerbazin, vincristine) — is indicated in the rapidly extensive types.

These chemotherapeutic regimens are associated with a dismal prognosis, but the introduction of highly active antiretroviral therapy has changed the course of the disease.

Topical

Drugs suggested for intralesional chemotherapy are bleomycin, vinblastine, interferon and inteleukine 2.

Surgical

Smaller lesions may be treated by electrodessication and curettage or surgical excision.

Cryotherapy

This technique is indicated in cases of palpebral lesions less than 1 cm in diameter.

Radiation

The KS lesions are generally radio-sensitive. Radiotherapy is likely to lead to a cicatrizing course of the external eye (external beam radiation) and lacrimal outflow system. The total dose is between 2000 cGy to 3000 cGy divided into 200–300 cGy a time for 3 weeks.

COMPLICATIONS

The major complicating factor in local treatment of KS is the relatively high rate of tumor recurrence – 29%–66% cases. The most frequent complication of the systemic treatment is the aggravation of the immunodepression for the worse.

COMMENTS

The evolution of disease depends on the epidemiological-clinical type of KS and its clinical extent in general. It is a very slowly developing disease, and the treatment should aim first at correcting a potential functional or aesthetic gene. The treatment should avoid the development of dangerous immunosuppression in patients.

REFERENCES

Christopher DM, Fletcher K, Krishnan U, Fredrik M: Pathology and genetics of tumors of soft tissue and bone. International agency for research of cancer IARC Press, Lyon, 2002.

Collaco L, Goncalves M, Gomes L, Miranda R: Orbital Kaposi's sarcoma in acquired immunodeficiency syndrome. Eur J Ophthalmol 10(1):88–90, 2000.

Corti M, Solari R, de Carolis L, Corraro R: Eye involvement in AIDS-related Kaposi sarcoma. Enferm Infec Microbiol Clin 19(1):3–6, 2001.

Heimann H, Kreusel KM, Foerster MH, et al: Regression of conjunctival Kaposi's sarcoma under chemotherapy with bleomycin. Br J Ophthalmol 81(11):1019–1020, 1997.

Munteanu G, Munteanu M, Giuri S: Conjunctival-palpebral Kaposi's angiosarcoma: report of a case. J Fr Ophtalmol 26(10):1059–1062, 2003.

Schmid K, Wild T, Bolz M, et al: Kaposi's sarcoma of the conjunctiva leads to a diagnosis of acquired immunodeficiency syndrome. Acta Ophthalmol Scand 81(4):411–413, 2003.

Souhail H, Albouzidi A, Laktaoui A, et al: Orbital location of Kaposi's sarcoma. J Fr Ophtalmol 26(10):1071–1074, 2003.

132 KERATOACANTHOMA 238.2

F. Hampton Roy, MD, FACS

Little Rock, Arkansas

ETIOLOGY/INCIDENCE

Keratoacanthoma is a benign epithelial tumor that arises in hair follicles in exposed skin of white patients. The majority of these tumors are solitary, occur on the face (including the eyelids and rarely the conjunctiva), where they may become unusually aggressive.

Keratoacanthomas occur in several different subtypes.

- The *Ferguson Smith* type consists of multiple self-healing keratoacanthomas of the skin and may appear in childhood or early adolescence.
- The *Grzybowski*-type keratoacanthomas are smaller (2 to 3 mm in diameter) and do not appear until adulthood.
- The *Witten Zak* variant combines characteristics of both the larger self-healing Ferguson Smith type and the multiple miliary Grzybowski keratoacanthomas.
- A *giant, massive,* or *confluent keratoacanthoma* is believed to result from the fusion of small, closely spaced tumors.
- In *keratoacanthoma centrifugum marginatum,* multiple keratoacanthomas appear at the periphery of a progressively expanding lesion with central scar formation; unlike solitary keratoacanthomas, this variant has no tendency to involute spontaneously.
- *Muir–Torre syndrome* is an autosomal dominant genodermatosis consisting of multiple keratoacanthomas and sebaceous skin tumors associated with up to 40% incidence rate of internal malignancies, especially adenocarcinoma of the colon.

The etiology of keratoacanthoma is unknown. Most lesions occur on sun-exposed areas of light-skinned individuals. Keratoacanthomas may occur:

1. In patients with xeroderma pigmentosa;
2. In immunologically compromised patients (e.g. transplant recipients and patients with metastatic cancer, leukemia, lymphoma or acquired immune deficiency syndrome);
3. In industrial workers exposed to mineral oils, pitch or tar; and
4. In patients treated with psoralen plus ultraviolet A light therapy.

Exposure to chemical carcinogens, immunologic depression and a hereditary component have been suggested as possible causes in some patients.

DIAGNOSIS

Clinical signs and symptoms

The usual solitary keratoacanthoma has the following manifestations.

- The onset is sudden.
- Growth is rapid, possibly reaching 1 to 2 or more cm in diameter in 6 to 8 weeks.

- The tumor is raised and dome shaped with rolled lateral borders and a central keratin core.
- There is occasional pain, irritation or discomfort.

Nodules on the conjunctiva may result in foreign body sensation and tearing; keratoacanthomas on the face may grow larger and regress more slowly than those on other parts of the body and some do not spontaneously regress at all.

Laboratory findings

- Biopsy of keratoacanthomas is essential.
- These lesions can closely resemble squamous cell carcinomas.
- The ideal biopsy should include a spindle-shaped portion across the entire lesion (i.e. the center, subcutaneous tissue beneath the lesion) and normal tissue at both edges of the lesion.
- Nonexcisional biopsies may accelerate rate of involution.

TREATMENT

Surgical

Lesions of periocular or ocular tissue are best treated with wide excisional biopsy.

Other

- Curettage.
- Cryotherapy.
- Radiation.
- Intralesional injections: fluorouracil (5-FU), methotrexate, interferon.
- Topical: 5-FU.
- Oral: etretinate, isotretinoin.

PRECAUTIONS

Whenever there are multiple accepted forms of therapy, the entity can be difficult to treat. Early intervention around the eye is important for both diagnosis and management, so excisional biopsy is the treatment of choice.

Occasional progression and malignant change of keratoacanthomas, especially in immunosuppressed patients, have been reported; however, most of these benign tumors that underwent a change probably were carcinomas that were not recognized initially because of an inadequate biopsy.

Recurrence rates of these lesions require a repeat biopsy because basal cell or squamous cell carcinoma may have developed or may have been missed.

COMMENTS

Aggressive surgical treatment for periocular or ocular keratoacanthoma is necessary because lesions in this area are more aggressive, may be disfiguring and cosmetically unacceptable and are easier to treat when they are small. A diagnosis must be made because the lesions may be malignant or associated with a malignancy. It cannot be predicted when or if spontaneous involution will occur.

REFERENCES

Grossniklaus HE, Martin DF, Solomon AR: Invasive conjunctival tumor with keratoacanthoma features. Am J Ophthalmol 109:736–738, 1990.

Grossniklaus HE, Wojno TH, Yanoff M, Font RL: Invasive keratoacanthoma of the eyelid and ocular adnexa. Ophthalmology 103:937–941, 1996.

Hintschich CR, Stefani FH: Keratoacanthoma of the eyelid area: problems and risks in diagnosis and therapy. Klin Monatsbl Augenheilkd 210:219–224, 1997.

LoSchiavo A, Pinto F, Degener AM, et al: Keratoacanthoma centrifugum marginatum: possible etiological role of papillomavirus and therapeutic response to etretinate. Ann Dermatol Venereol 123:660–663, 1996.

Melton JL, Nelson BR, Stough DB, et al: Treatment of keratoacanthomas with intralesional methotrexate. J Am Acad Dermatol 25:1017–1023, 1991.

Neumann RA, Knobler RM: Argon laser treatment of small keratoacanthomas in difficult locations. Int J Dermatol 29:733–736, 1990.

Schellini SA, Marques ME, Milanezi MF, Bacchi CE: Conjunctival keratoacanthoma. Acta Ophthalmol Scand 75(3):335–337, 1997. Review.

133 LEIOMYOMA
(Iris Leiomyoma, Ciliary Body Leiomyoma, Orbital Leiomyoma, Ocular Leiomyoma)

Manolette R. Roque, MD
Manila, Philippines
Barbara L. Roque, MD
Manila, Philippines

ETIOLOGY/INCIDENCE

Leiomyoma is a rare, benign smooth muscle tumor representing 2.3% to 14.5% of all primary iris tumors. It may involve the sphincter and dilator muscles of the iris, ciliary muscle of the ciliary body, Müller's or capsulopalpebral muscle in the orbit.

Ocular leiomyoma is reported most frequently in Caucasian females and younger patients, with cases ranging from 10 to 77 years old.

COURSE/PROGNOSIS

Leiomyoma is usually well-circumscribed and has a tendency for slow growth. Although degeneration may occur within its substance, resulting in hemorrhage and local necrosis, spread by continuity, contiguity, or metastasis has not been recorded. The prognosis for vision depends on the location and size of the tumor and is usually excellent. Prognosis for life is excellent.

DIAGNOSIS

Clinical signs and symptoms

Iris

- Localized, flat to slightly elevated, nonpigmented, transparent, vascular tumor, often at the region of the sphincter muscle.

- Presents as distorted pupil, ectropion uveae, or hyphema.
- Vision is not affected unless there is a complication of glaucoma or cataract.

Ciliary body

- Pigmented mass that slowly increases in size and may distort the iris, compress the lens, or locally occlude the filtration angle.
- Asymptomatic until it grows large enough to affect neighboring ocular structures.

Orbit

- Extremely rare, well-encapsulated, vascular tumor that is usually located in an extraconal position.
- Presents as painless proptosis, sometimes with intermittent episodes of pain.

Laboratory findings

Regardless of the primary site of the tumor, the diagnosis of leiomyoma is only made on histologic examination.

Light microscopy

- A leiomyoma is composed of interlacing, densely packed, elongated, spindle-shaped cells, with long oval nuclei that tend to be arranged in a palisading manner, and granular eosinophilic cytoplasm of the cells and longitudinal myofibrils within the cells and are best seen with phosphotungstic acid hematoxylin stain.

Electron microscopy

- Characteristic features of a smooth muscle neoplasm (thin basement membrane; plasmalemmal vesicles; and numerous, longitudinally aligned cytoplasmic filaments with scattered associated densities).

Immunohistochemistry

- The findings are consistent with a myogenic tumor. Tumor cells are positive for smooth muscle actin, desmin and vimentin. The tumor cells are negative for S-100 and melanin.

Differential diagnosis

Iris amelanotic melanoma; intraocular or iris foreign body; juvenile xanthogranuloma; peripheral anterior synechiae; lymphoid hyperplasia; iridoschisis; iridic neovascularization; atypical vessels of the iris; hemangioma; siderosis; hemosiderosis; iridic abscess; ciliary body melanoma; fully encapsulated orbital tumors.

TREATMENT

Ocular

Repeated frequent examinations (every 6 months) should include photography of the tumor to aid in the assessment of the size, gonioscopy, and fluorescein iridography.

Surgical

Leiomyomas of the iris and ciliary body are excised only if the tumors increase in size, bleed, or cause complications, such as glaucoma or cataract. When the tumors are removed, they should be removed in toto because local recurrences may occur if the tumor is excised incompletely.

A tumor of the ciliary body is treated with an iridocyclectomy, which can involve as much as one fourth of the ciliary body circumference.

Orbital leiomyoma is well encapsulated and usually shells out without difficulty.

COMPLICATIONS

Hyphema, proptosis, glaucoma or localized cataract may result from leiomyoma.

COMMENTS

An iris or a ciliary body leiomyoma cannot be differentiated clinically from a malignant melanoma and is diagnosed on the basis of histologic examination.

Fluorescein iridography was used as a preoperative mapping procedure to determine the actual tumor size, which may extend beyond that noted on clinical observation. In addition, the blood supply of the tumor may be determined before surgery. Radioactive phosphorus uptake may be done before surgery to help assess the vascularity of the tumor. More significantly, the extension of the tumor in the anterior chamber angle can be determined so it can be determined whether an iridectomy or iridocyclectomy is required.

REFERENCES

de Buen S, Olivares ML, Charlin VC: Leiomyoma of the iris: report of a case. Br J Ophthalmol 55:353–356, 1971.

Grossniklaus HE: Fine-needle aspiration biopsy of the iris. Arch Ophthalmol 110:969–976, 1992.

Henderson JW, Harrison EG, Jr: Vascular leiomyoma of the orbit: report of a case. Trans Am Acad Ophthalmol Otolaryngol 74:970–974, 1970.

Meyer SL, Fine BS, Font RL, et al: Leiomyoma of the ciliary body: electron microscopic verification. Am J Ophthalmol 66:1061–1068, 1968.

Roque MR, Roque BL, Foster CS: Leiomyoma, iris. Emedicine 2005. Online. Available at: http://www.emedicine.com/oph/topic589.htm. Mar 16, 2005.

Sevel D, Tobias B: The value of fluorescein iridography with leiomyoma of the iris. Am J Ophthalmol 74:475–478, 1972.

Shields J, Shields C, Eagle R, DePotter P: Observations on seven cases of intraocular leiomyoma. Arch Ophthalmol 112:521–528, 1994.

134 LIPOSARCOMA 190.1

Alan A. McNab, MBBS, FRANZCO
Melbourne, Victoria

Liposarcoma of the orbit is a malignant proliferation of lipocytes.

ETIOLOGY/INCIDENCE

Despite the abundance of adipose tissue in the orbit, liposarcoma of the orbit is a very rare tumor. Lipomas, which are true benign proliferations of orbital fat, are even rarer. Only a few cases of orbital liposarcoma have been described, and much of the information on this soft-tissue tumor is derived from the experience gained in managing liposarcomas of other sites, such as the retroperitoneum and deep thigh. Liposarcoma probably is the most common soft-tissue malignancy, accounting for 16% to 18% of sarcomas.

Approximately 35 cases of primary orbital liposarcoma have been described in the literature. Only a few cases of metastatic orbital liposarcoma have been described.

Men and women are affected equally, although a slight male predilection has been noted for liposarcoma lesions elsewhere (55% to 61% males).

The age range of patients is 5 to 77 years, with a median in the 30s for orbital lesions. In childhood, the occurrence of liposarcomas in other parts of the body is extremely rare, but several cases of orbital liposarcoma have been described. The median age of occurrence is in the 50s for lesions outside the orbit; the thigh and retroperitoneum are the most common sites.

COURSE/PROGNOSIS

Enziger and Weiss have classified liposarcoma into the following types:

- Well-differentiated;
- Myxoid;
- Round cell;
- Pleomorphic.

These types have differing prognoses, with well-differentiated and myxoid types having the best prognosis and pleomorphic types having the worst prognosis. Most of the cases of orbital liposarcoma have been myxoid or well-differentiated.

Most cases are unsuspected before biopsy or excision. Symptoms relate to mass effect, and most patients do not have pain, although this has occasionally been described as a presenting feature.

Of 21 patients described in the literature up to 1990, six cases resulted in death during the period of follow-up, which was usually short. Jakobiec and colleagues reported five cases with a follow-up period of 1 to 7 years (mean, 5.2 years) who had no regional or distant metastases. Three required exenteration for local recurrence; two patients who refused exenteration had radiotherapy alone.

The most recent series reported from Moorfields (Cai et al) describes 7 cases, 5 of whom had exenteration. No patient died from their disease but one had multiple local recurrences following initial local excision. These authors suggested a good prognosis provided the lesion is well-differentiated or myxoid, and wide excision is performed.

In a series of 77 liposarcomas occurring elsewhere in the body, prognosis was related to histology, with 12 of 20 patients with myxoid tumors surviving 10 years but only 1 of 24 patients with a round cell or pleomorphic lesion surviving 10 years. Site, size, and adequacy of excision were important factors in survival.

DIAGNOSIS

Clinical signs and symptoms

Most patients present with symptoms that occur over months and occasionally over years. Symptoms include proptosis, diplopia, and blurred vision, although vision is usually well preserved. Pain is an uncommon feature.

If the mass is palpable, it may feel rubbery or soft, and it usually is nontender.

Laboratory findings

Findings on computed tomography (CT) are variable, with some lesions appearing as a well-defined homogeneous soft tissue mass, sometimes of low density with a denser outer 'capsule' that probably represents compressed normal orbital tissue. This may give the erroneous impression of a cyst. Other lesions are poorly defined and may invade extraocular muscles with tissue of fat density.

Magnetic resonance imaging (MRI) rarely has been reported but shows a high signal on T2-weighted images, indicating the presence of fat.

Ultrasonography is helpful in separating true orbital cysts from liposarcomas with this 'cystic' appearance on CT with internal reflectivity indicating the true solid nature of the tumor.

Diagnosis is nearly always made only after biopsy. The pathologic findings are well summarized by Enziger and Weiss.

Differential diagnosis

The clinical and imaging differential diagnosis includes a large number of orbital neoplasms, especially when the lesion is well circumscribed. Clues to the diagnosis include a relatively short history and the presence of fat-tissue density on CT or signal characteristics of fat on MRI. Pathologic differential diagnosis may include normal orbital fat for well-differentiated lesions and other sarcomas or spindle-cell lesions.

It should always be borne in mind that an orbital liposarcoma may be secondary to an occult tumor elsewhere, for example, in the retroperitoneum. A careful clinical examination should be performed along with CT or MRI of the abdomen and thighs.

TREATMENT

Once the diagnosis is established, usually on the basis of an incisional biopsy, and the possibility of the lesion's being metastatic has been excluded, the treatment usually is wide surgical excision.

For occasional well-circumscribed lesions that can be easily dissected with a rim of normal tissue, local excision only can be offered, but there is a significant risk of local recurrence.

For the majority of lesions, orbital exenteration is required to obtain an adequate margin of tissue and to minimize the risk of local recurrence and possibly distant metastasis.

Radiation therapy has a role in the management of liposarcoma, with better responses recorded in the more poorly differentiated tumors when used elsewhere in the body. For orbital liposarcomas, after wide local surgical excision, if feasible without causing excessive ocular complications, or if the patient refuses exenteration, orbital irradiation in high doses may 'sterilize' the field of tumor cells. Radiation alone can be used for poorly differentiated or metastatic orbital lesions.

Chemotherapy alone does not have a well-defined role in the management of liposarcoma, but it may be useful as an adjunctive measure.

REFERENCES

Abdalla MI, Ghaly AF, Hosni F: Liposarcoma with orbital metastases. Br J Ophthalmol 50:426–428, 1966.

Brown HH, Kersten RC, Kulwin DR: Lipomatous hamartoma of the orbit. Arch Ophthalmol 109:240–243, 1991.

Cai YC, McMenamin ME, Rose GE, et al: Primary liposarcoma of the orbit: a clinicopathological study of seven cases. Ann Diagn Pathol 5:255–266, 2001.

Enziger FM, Weiss SW: Soft tissue tumors. St Louis, CV Mosby, 1983:242–280.

Fezza J, Sinard J: Metastatic liposarcoma to the orbit. Am J Ophthalmol 123:271–272, 1997.

Kindblom LG, Baker LH, Svendsen P: Liposarcoma: a clinicopathological, radiographic and prognostic study. Acta Pathol Microbiol Immunol Scand 253(suppl.):1–71, 1975.

Lane CM, Wright JE: Primary myxoid liposarcoma of the orbit. Br J Ophthalmol 72:912–917, 1988.

McNab AA, Moseley I: Primary orbital liposarcoma: clinical and computed tomographic features. Br J Ophthalmol 74:437–439, 1990.

135 LYMPHANGIOMA 228.1

Michael Kazim, MD
New York, New York
Jennifer Scruggs, MD
New York, New York
Joseph D. Walrath, MD
New York, New York

ETIOLOGY/INCIDENCE

Lymphangioma is a benign vascular hamartoma commonly identified in the head and neck. Lymphangioma is likely derived from vascular mesenchyme that has inappropriately differentiated into isolated lymphatic-like spaces without connection to the systemic circulation. The incidence rate is low.

COURSE/PROGNOSIS

The majority of patients present in the first decade of life. There are two growth patterns. Slow enlargement occurs over decades, producing progressive proptosis. In contrast, explosive growth results from intralesional hemorrhage, likely from intrinsic nutrient vessels, or in association with an upper respiratory tract infection with proliferation of the lymphoid aggregates.

Sequelae include spontaneous resolution of the proptosis, usually over a period of weeks to months; persistent proptosis; cutaneous disfigurement; compressive optic neuropathy; and restrictive strabismus.

DIAGNOSIS

Histologically, there are nonencapsulated, thin-walled, endothelium lined channels and cystic vascular spaces which may contain lymph-like fluid. Scattered lymphoid aggregates or hemorrhage may be present. Clinically, the lesions may be located superficially in the orbit and are cystic. More commonly, they are infiltrative and diffuse in the orbit. Those located apically or with intracranial extension are more likely to be associated with submucosal oral lesions and noncontiguous intracranial vascular anomalies.

Authors disagree as to whether lymphangiomas actually represent a distinct clinical or histopathologic entity; some do not differentiate these lesions from a larger spectrum of orbital venous anomalies. Others stress that hemodynamic distinctions do exist and should be used to categorize these lesions as well as guide their management.

Clinical signs and symptoms

- Proptosis: slowly progressive or sudden and painful.
- Ptosis.
- Conjunctival chemosis or hemorrhage: if superficially located.
- Optic neuropathy: if orbital hemorrhage is severe.
- Strabismus: if the lesion is large and infiltrative.
- Cutaneous blood-filled cysts: if superficially located.
- Oral mucosal vascular lesions: in deeply located lesions, with frequent intracranial component.

Laboratory findings

Ultrasonography

A 10-MHz probe is used to image the anterior two thirds of orbit. The soft-tissue and cystic components of the lesion are identified. Ultrasonography lacks specificity and soft-tissue detail.

Computed tomography

Computed tomography is best for imaging the bone deformity produced by long-standing lesions. There is good soft-tissue detail with this method, but it lacks specificity.

Magnetic resonance imaging

Magnetic resonance imaging provides superior soft-tissue details. The identification of cystic structures and blood-serum interfaces is diagnostic of the lesion. This technique is most helpful in surgical planning.

Differential diagnosis

- Hemangioma.
- Varix.
- Orbital hemorrhage.
- Orbital cellulites.
- Rhabdomyosarcoma.
- Neuroblastoma.

TREATMENT

Supportive

Management of lymphangiomas is difficult and observation is preferred. Except in cases of optic neuropathy, await the spontaneous resolution of hemorrhagic cyst or lymphoid hyperplasia associated with upper respiratory infection. Oral corticosteroids may help in the acute phase to resolve the lymphoid infiltrate.

Surgical

Surgery is generally avoided because manipulation of the tumor may promote further spontaneous hemorrhages. In addition, complete surgical excision is difficult due to the infiltrative nature of the tumor and risk of damage to surrounding structures. Recurrence rate is high.

Indications for surgery include compressive optic neuropathy, disabling diplopia and disfigurement.

Procedures include cyst drainage, which may be accomplished by computed tomography or ultrasound-guided percutaneous needle or open orbitotomy. Debulking of the lesion, often with multiple partial resections, may achieve satisfactory results. The surgical approach is guided by the location of the tumor. Carbon dioxide laser may be a useful adjuvant in the more solid vascularized variant.

There have been recent reports of the successful use of OK-432 (Picibanil; a sclerosing agent) in the treatment of macrocystic lymphangiomas located elsewhere in the head and neck region. There are few reports of the use of OK-432 in orbital lymphangiomas. Anticipated side effects of OK-432, including a profound local inflammatory response with edema, may produce elevated orbital pressure resulting in acute glaucoma or compressive optic neuropathy. More data is needed to determine the efficacy and safety of this treatment for orbital lesions.

COMPLICATIONS

- Optic neuropathy: pressure from tumor growth or hemorrhagic cyst.
- Strabismus: due to infiltration of the tumor.
- Ptosis.
- Amblyopia: secondary to occlusion or astigmatism.
- Orbital bone asymmetry: due to pressure effect of the tumor mass.
- Disfigurement.

COMMENTS

Lymphangioma is a histologically benign but clinically aggressive lesion. It generally is first identified in childhood, when it can adversely affect vision development. In most cases, it cannot be safely extirpated and therefore may result in a lifelong series of hemorrhages that threaten visual acuity, produce severe pain, and ultimately result in disfigurement that is socially challenging. The role of the treating physician is supportive, knowing that the acute episodes are generally self-limited. Surgery should be reserved for the more severe cases of disfigurement, diplopia or optic neuropathy.

REFERENCES

Coll GE, Goldberg RA, Krauss H, et al: Concomitant lymphangioma and arteriovenous malformation of the orbit. Am J Ophthalmol 112:200, 1991.

Giguere CM, Bauman NM, Sato Y, et al: Treatment of lymphangiomas with OK-432 (Picibanil) sclerotherapy: a prospective multi-institutional trial. Arch Otolaryngol Head Neck Surg 128:1137–1144, 2002.

Harris GJ: Orbital vascular malformations: a consensus statement on terminology and its clinical implications. Am J Ophthalmol 127:453–455, 1999.

Harris GJ, Sakol PJ, Bonavolenta G, et al: An analysis of thirty cases of orbital lymphangioma. Ophthalmology 97:1583–1592, 1990.

Jackson IT, Carreno R: Hemangiomas, vascular malformations and lymphovenous malformations: classification and methods of treatment. Plast Reconstr Surg 91:1216, 1993.

Jones IS: Lymphangiomas of the ocular adnexa: an analysis of sixty-two cases. Am J Ophthalmol 51:481–509, 1961.

Katz SE, Rootman J, Vangveeravong S, et al: Combined venous lymphatic malformations of the orbit (so-called lymphangiomas): association with noncontiguous intracranial vascular anomalies. Ophthalmology 105:176–184, 1998.

Kazim M, Kennerdell JS, Rothfus W, et al: Orbital lymphangioma: correlation of magnetic resonance imaging and intraoperative findings. Ophthalmology 99:1588–1594, 1992.

Kennerdell JS, Maroon JC, Garrity JA, et al: Surgical management of orbital lymphangioma with carbon dioxide laser. Am J Ophthalmol 102:308–314, 1986.

Pitz S, Dittrich M: Orbital lymphangioma. Br J Ophthalmol 84:124–125, 2000.

Rootman J, Kao SCS, Graeb DA: Multidisciplinary approaches to complicated vascular lesions of the orbit. Ophthalmology 99:1588, 1992.

Skalka HW, Callahan MA: Ultrasonically-aided percutaneous orbital aspiration. Ophthalmic Surg 10:41–43, 1979.

Suzuki Y, Obana A, Gohto Y, et al: Management of orbital lymphangioma using intralesional injection of OK-432. Br J Ophthalmol 84:614–617, 2000.

Tunc M, Sadri E, Char DH: Orbital lymphangioma: an analysis of 26 patients. Br J Ophthalmol 83:76–80, 1999.

Wilson ME, Parker PL, Chavis RM: Conservative management of childhood orbital lymphangioma. Ophthalmology 96:484, 1989.

Wright JE, Sullivan TJ, Garner A, et al: Orbital venous anomalies. Ophthalmology 104:905–913, 1997.

136 LYMPHOID TUMORS 202.8
(Inflammatory Pseudotumor, Ocular Adnexal Lymphoma, Intraocular Lymphoma, Neoplastic Angioendotheliomatosis, Reactive Lymphoid Hyperplasia)

Michael D. Eichler, MD
St. Cloud, Minnesota

Ocular lymphoid tumors represent an intriguing and diverse area of ophthalmology. Our knowledge of the pathology, natural histories and treatment responses of these tumors continues to evolve. Areas of overlap in histology create diagnostic challenges, although immunohistochemistry and molecular genetic analysis have greatly aided this effort. Three main categories of ocular lymphoid tumors exist based on natural history: orbital inflammatory pseudotumor, ocular adnexal lymphoid tumors and intraocular lymphoid tumors.

ORBITAL INFLAMMATORY PSEUDOTUMOR

ETIOLOGY/INCIDENCE

Orbital inflammatory pseudotumor is a localized disease that mimics an orbital tumor in causing proptosis due to diffuse multifocal infiltration of inflammatory cells; only rarely does it form a discrete mass.

Orbital inflammatory pseudotumor accounts for approximately 10% of orbital lesions. The age of onset is earlier than that of lymphoma, most commonly occurring in the third to fifth decades of life. About 10% of patients present in the first two decades of life.

COURSE/PROGNOSIS

- Orbital inflammatory pseudotumor typically responds rapidly to treatment, with complete resolution of symptoms in 1 to 2 months.

- Pseudotumor usually occurs as a single episode, but recurrences have been reported after 7 years.
- Intracranial extension of chronic pseudotumor has been reported.
- Pseudotumor is a diagnosis of exclusion based on the clinical, radiologic, and occasional histopathologic data. Systemic disease is associated in 5–10% of cases; these associated diseases are endocrinopathy, neoplasm or vasculitis. Infection must be ruled out prior to treatment.
- Orbital inflammatory pseudotumor does not have the potential for malignant transformation, however, neoplasm may present with inflammation.
- When orbital pseudotumors are bilateral, the chance that a systemic disorder will be discovered is increased, especially in adults.

DIAGNOSIS

Clinical signs and symptoms

Orbital inflammatory pseudotumor is characterized by a wide spectrum of presentations including acute pain, hyperemia, chemosis, periocular edema and erythema, extraocular motility disturbances, ptosis and the rapid development of proptosis. Inflammatory involvement adjacent to the optic nerve may produce visual disturbances and papillitis. Orbital inflammatory pseudotumor frequently affects the lacrimal gland, creating diagnostic confusion. A chronic form of pseudotumor exists that can lead to unrelenting severe pain and ophthalmoplegia due to sclerosis of orbital tissues.

Laboratory findings

- Computed tomography (CT) aids in the diagnosis of orbital inflammatory pseudotumor with diffuse infiltration and enlargement of orbital fat, extraocular muscles, optic nerve, and/or lacrimal gland with blurring of the margins. Rarely a mass and/or infiltration of the orbital apex or cavernous sinus may be seen. Bone erosion does not occur.
- Orbital inflammatory pseudotumor with a common presentation typically does not require a biopsy. A full response to treatment without recurrence is diagnostic.
- Histologic features of pseudotumor are a light dispersal of lymphocytes, plasma cells, macrophages, neutrophils and occasional eosinophils (particularly in children) around blood vessels and interstitially within the orbital fat, extraocular muscles, Tenon's space, and lacrimal gland. The involved tissue is variably fibrotic and the lymphoid component is not hyperplastic or sheet-like.
- Histologic features of chronic pseudotumor are increasing amounts of fibrosis with bridging septa replacing orbital fat and encasing extraocular structures.
- Graves' disease mimics or produces the clinical picture of an orbital pseudotumor, and the histopathologic appearance is remarkably similar to that of inflammatory pseudotumor.
- Orbital cellulitis of bacterial origin can usually be differentiated by historical features, sinus involvement and resolution with intravenous antibiotics.

Differential diagnosis

- Grave's orbitopathy.
- Infection: bacterial, fungal, parasitic.
- Granulomatous disease: sarcoidosis, idiopathic noninfectious granulomatous inflammation, Erdheim–Chester disease, necrobiotic xanthogranulomatosis.
- Sjögren's syndrome.
- Vasculitis: Wegener's granulomatosis, polyarteritis nodosa, giant cell arteritis.
- Neoplasia.
- Vascular disorders: dural-cavernous sinus arteriovenous fistula, orbital varix.

TREATMENT

- Systemic steroids are most helpful in patients with acute or subacute lesions and least effective in those exhibiting the histologic features of a chronic sclerotic phase. Chronic pseudotumor typically requires adjuvant therapy with radiation or chemotherapy.
- High doses of prednisone (80–100 mg/day) should be continued for a total of 3 weeks and tapered over a 3- to 6-week period to prevent a rebound.
- Radiation may be necessary for steroid-resistant or steroid-dependent lesions, with 20 cGy over 10 days.
- Recalcitrant cases may respond to immunosuppression therapy with methotrexate, cyclosporine, azathioprine, or cyclophosphamide.
- Surgical debulking is rarely necessary.

OCULAR ADNEXAL LYMPHOID TUMOR

ETIOLOGY/INCIDENCE

Ocular adnexal lymphoid tumors encompass both reactive lymphoid hyperplasia (RLH) and lymphoma (OAL). These disorders have similar natural histories, histologic features, and responses to therapy. While the incidence of lymphoma is increasing, this is in part due to an aging population and an increase in AIDS-related lymphomatous diseases. Chronic antigenic stimulation of mucosa associated lymphoid tissue leading to hyperplasia and potential genetic aberrations and malignant transformation is a proposed etiologic mechanism. *Chlamydia psittaci* is associated with lymphoid tumor pathogenesis.

Ocular adnexal lymphoid tumors occur in 1.5% to 4.0% of systemic lymphomas and fewer than 1% of patients have ocular involvement as the initial presentation. Nearly all ocular adnexal lymphomas are non-Hodgkin's lymphomas (NHLs) of B-cell origin. The age of onset for lymphomas typically is the sixth or seventh decade of life.

COURSE/PROGNOSIS

- A continuum of disease from RLH to NHL has been supported by DNA analysis showing monoclonal cells within RLH lesions and progression to systemic lymphoma. Because of the potential dissemination of both lesions, they are evaluated and treated similarly.
- Ocular adnexal lymphoma is categorized according to the World Health Organization (WHO) Classification of Lymphoid Neoplasms.
- The most common histological subtype identified in OAL is extranodal marginal zone B-cell lymphoma of MALT type (EMZL). This type accounts for 60–75% of OAL. EMZL and follicular lymphoma (FL) comprise nearly all low grade lesions; FL occurs in approximately 10% of cases.

- High grade lesions include diffuse large B-cell lymphoma (DLBCL), in approximately 10%; Mantle cell lymphoma (MCL), in approximately 5%; and Burkitt's lymphoma (BL) and others rarely.
- Both RLH and NHL of the ocular adnexa have approximately 10–30% association with prior and/or concurrent systemic lymphoma.
- OAL, with no evidence of systemic lymphoma (Stage IE) carries a risk of future systemic lymphoma. This risk is most dependent on the lesion histology and site of involvement. For EMZL, studies estimate the risk to be 40–70% at 10 years.
- Characteristics associated with a greater risk of future systemic lymphoma include higher grade lesions (DLBCL) and molecular genetic markers such as BCL6, MIB1 and p53.
- Most authors agree that conjunctival lesions have a lower risk of future systemic lymphoma compared to orbital or eyelid lesions. The same being true for unilateral versus bilateral lesions.
- Lymphoma related death is dependent on the patient age, stage of disease and histology. Stage IE EMZL has a good prognosis with lymphoma related death near 10% at 10 years. Systemic recurrences tend to be localized and salvageable with local therapy. Advanced stages with non-EMZL may have poor survival rates.

DIAGNOSIS

Clinical signs and symptoms

RLH and NHL have varying presentations depending on the site of involvement. Conjunctival lesions may be asymptomatic, although patients often seek medical attention because of a mass, ptosis, irritation and/or epiphora. Flesh-colored or salmon-pink patches are typically found. The forniceal, bulbar and palpebral conjunctivae can be affected, with a predilection for the fornices. Involvement of the orbit may result in painless, slowly progressive proptosis with or without diplopia and visual impairment. There is a distinct propensity for anterior orbital involvement with a palpable rubbery mass.

Laboratory findings

- CT of ocular adnexal lymphoid tumors reveals a mass lesion that tends to conform to pre-existing anatomic structures or tissue planes without bone destruction.
- A biopsy is required for all lesions. The biopsy should not be overly aggressive; because of the radiosensitivity of these tumors, the mass does not have to be removed in total.
- A surgical pathologist should be consulted before performing the biopsy because most require fresh tissue and special fixatives and adequacy of samples can be ensured before closure.
- RLH lesions appear as polymorphic proliferations of small lymphocytes and intermixed plasma cells, immunoblasts, histiocytes and endothelial cell proliferations.
- Malignant lymphomas are composed of cytologically malignant and immature lymphocytic cells. Depending on the grade lesion, cellular characteristics may be uniform and hyperplastic or show a mixture of malignant cell types.
- Immunohistochemistry and molecular genetic studies have greatly improved diagnostic accuracy with immunologically heterogeneous (polyclonal) lesions as benign and immunologically homogeneous (monoclonal) lesions as malignant. Molecular genetic markers appear to have prognostic significance.

TREATMENT

- Radiation is considered the standard treatment for localized disease. Usual doses are near 30 Gy for RLH and low-grade lymphomas and 30 to 40 Gy for higher-grade lymphomas.
- Side effects of radiation vary from self-limited conjunctivitis and erythema to potentially severe dry eye syndrome, symblepharon, cataracts, retinopathy and optic neuropathy. Side effects are dose dependent and they are infrequent with the low doses required for lymphoid tumors.
- A single lesion near or at the limbus can be managed with local excision and cryotherapy. Side effects are self-limited and minimal. Patients need to be followed for local recurrence and systemic lymphoma.
- Chemotherapy should be entrusted to an oncologist and although periocular lesions can be expected to shrink during chemotherapy, adjuvant radiation or excision may be required, especially if visual impairment is present.

INTRAOCULAR LYMPHOID TUMOR

ETIOLOGY/INCIDENCE

Intraocular lymphoid tumors can be divided into three groups: primary intraocular lymphoma (PIOL), lymphoid tumors of the uvea, and neoplastic angioendotheliomatosis. *Primary intraocular lymphoma* (also known as reticulum cell sarcoma, microgliomatosis, or intraocular large cell lymphoma) is a subset of primary central nervous system lymphoma (PCNSL). PIOL involves the retina, vitreous, and/or optic nerve. In contrast, *Malignant lymphoma and lymphoid hyperplasia of the uvea* occurs most frequently in patients who have systemic lymphoma; rarely is the central nervous system affected. Lymphoid tumors of the uvea share similar clinical features and histopathology with ocular adnexal tumors. *Neoplastic angioendotheliomatosis* is a variant of large cell malignant lymphoma with widespread intravascular proliferation of malignant cells of endothelial origin.

Intraocular lymphoma occurs in 15% to 25% of PCNSL. The incidence of CNS lymphoma has risen from an estimated at 7.5 in 10 million persons in the 1970s to 1 in 100,000, primarily related to human immunodeficiency virus infection. The mean age of onset of PIOL is 60 years, with a broader range compared to ocular adnexal tumors.

COURSE/PROGNOSIS

- Vision-threatening intraocular lesions respond rapidly to systemic steroids and local radiation therapy.
- PIOL has a poor prognosis. Eighty-five percent of patients will develop CNS lymphoma despite treatment within 2–3 years.
- The median survival rate for PIOL/PCNSL has improved from 16 months to 3 years over the past decade.
- Uveal lymphoid tumors very rarely present without known systemic lymphoma.

DIAGNOSIS

Clinical signs and symptoms

Virtually all patients with PIOL eventually develop cerebral lesions, but systemic lymphoma is unlikely. A common presentation is painless visual loss, with the examination showing vitritis, yellow-white subretinal infiltrates, or disk edema or a combination. Relapsing idiopathic vitritis may be a presenting sign. Focal neurologic deficits may present related to cerebral lesions. Patients with lymphoid tumors of the uvea may present with painless decreased vision, visual field defects, or both; yellow-white choroidal elevations may be seen on examination. The most common signs and symptoms of neoplastic angioendotheliomatosis relate to skin and CNS involvement, although ophthalmic manifestations may be present.

Laboratory findings

- Ocular ultrasound is a valuable diagnostic tool in the setting of dense vitritis, and it is useful for following the size of lesions and treatment response.
- Magnetic resonance imaging with gadolinium is most sensitive for the early detection of CNS lymphomas.
- Intraocular lesions require closed vitrectomy with vitreous fluid sampling. Pars plana fine needle aspiration of subretinal lesions may be necessary. Occasionally a full thickness chorioretinal biopsy is utilized.
- Nearly all PIOL are diffuse large B-cell lymphoma (DLBCL). Rarely T-cell lymphoma is diagnosed. The histopathology of uveal tumors is the same as that of ocular adnexal lymphoid tumors.

Differential diagnosis

- Toxoplasmosis.
- Herpes zoster ophthalmicus.
- Frosted branch angiitis.
- Cytomegalovirus retinitis.
- Syphilis.
- Tuberculosis.
- Sarcoidosis.
- Acute posterior multifocal placoid pigment epitheliopathy.
- Acute retinal necrosis.
- Retinal vasculitis.
- Branch retinal artery obstruction with coexistent multifocal.
- Chorioretinal scars.
- Birdshot choroidopathy.

TREATMENT

- Radiation therapy traditionally has been the main form of therapy for intraocular lymphoid tumors with ocular and whole brain treatment. Unfortunately, toxicity and recurrent disease were high.
- Chemotherapy protocols have increased survival rates. High dose methotrexate and/or cytosine arabinoside (Ara-c) are typically given. Intrathecal and/or intravitreal methotrexate may be used. Bone marrow transplant is an option.
- Lesions may respond to systemic steroids but recur during or after treatment.
- Uveal lesions are typically treated with systemic chemotherapy, although adjuvant radiation therapy may be needed for visually threatening lesions.

COMMENTS

The ophthalmologist may see patients with a wide array of lymphoid tumors. Fortunately, inflammatory pseudotumor is most common and responds well to treatment. Lymphoma and lymphoid hyperplasia should be evaluated and treated similarly. The lesion histology, site of involvement and the patient age are the most influential factors related to the development of systemic disease and lymphoma related death. Similar to other mucosa-associated lymphoid tumors of the lung and gut, local therapy offers an excellent prognosis. Intraocular lymphoma is uncommon and has an ominous prognosis.

When the diagnosis of lymphoma or lymphoid hyperplasia is made, a thorough evaluation is required for systemic or CNS disease depending on the primary site of involvement. Staging evaluation should include consultation with an internist/oncologist with laboratory findings (complete blood count, serum protein electrophoresis, chemistry panels), CT scan of chest versus chest radiographs, CT scan of abdomen, bone marrow biopsy, and neuroimaging. After therapy, patients should be followed every 6 months by an ophthalmologist and internist/oncologist to evaluate for local recurrence or systemic/CNS lymphoma.

REFERENCES

Chan CC, Wallace DJ: Intraocular lymphoma: update on diagnosis and management. Cancer Control 11:285–295, 2004.

Coupland SE, Heimann H, Bechrakis NE: Primary intraocular lymphoma: a review of the clinical, histopathological and molecular biological features. Graefe's Arch Clin Exp Ophthalmol 240:901–913, 2004.

Coupland SE, Hellmich M, et al: Prognostic value of cell-cycle markers in ocular adnexal lymphoma: an assessment of 230 cases. Graefe's Arch Clinic Exp Ophthalmol 1–31, 2003.

Fung CY, Tarbell NJ, et al: Ocular adnexal lymphoma: clinical behavior of distinct World Health Organization classification subtypes. Int J Radiation Oncology Biol Phys 57:1382–1391, 2003.

Jakobiec FA, Font RL: Non-infectious orbital inflammation. In: Spencer WH, ed: Ophthalmic pathology: an atlas and textbook. Philadelphia, WB Saunders, 1986:3.

Jenkins C, Rose GE, et al: Clinical features associated with survival of patients with lymphoma of the ocular adnexa. Eye 17:809–820, 2003.

Knowles DM, Jakobiec FA, McNally L, et al: Lymphoid hyperplasia and malignant lymphoma occurring in the ocular adnexa (orbit, conjunctiva, and eyelids). Hum Pathol 21:959–973, 1990.

Shields CL, Shields JA, et al: Conjunctival lymphoid tumors: Clinical analysis of 117 cases and relationship to systemic lymphoma. Ophthalmology 108:979–984, 2001.

Yuen SJ, Rubin PA: Idiopathic orbital inflammation: distribution, clinical features, and treatment outcome. Arch Ophthalmol 121:491–499, 2003.

137 MEDULLOEPITHELIOMA 225.0
(Diktyoma)

Michael O'Keefe, MB, FRCS, FRCOphth
Dublin, Ireland
Caitriona Kirwan, MB, MRCOphth
Dublin, Ireland

ETIOLOGY/INCIDENCE

Medulloepithelioma is a rare embryonic ocular tumor that was first described in 1931. It usually arises from the primitive nonpigmented medullary epithelium of the ciliary body and less commonly affects the optic nerve, iris and retina. There are two main types of tumors:

1. Nonteratoid, or diktyoma, which contains multilayered sheets or cords of poorly differentiated neuroepithelial cells, with some having a netlike appearance that accounts for the term *diktyoma*; and
2. Teratoid, which contains neuroepithelial cells and demonstrates varying degrees of heteroplasia. The tumor usually occurs in children between the ages of 2 and 4 and rarely occurs in infants and older patients. It is usually unilateral and has no hereditary or sexual predilection.

COURSE/PROGNOSIS

Medulloepithelioma may present with loss of vision, pain, leukocoria, mass in the iris or ciliary body, rubeosis iridis, ectopia lentis, heterochromia, exophthalmos and hyphema. These tumors may be locally aggressive but rarely metastasize in the absence of extraocular extension. Broughton and Zimmerman established histologic criteria for the subclassification of tumors as benign or malignant. On the basis of cell differentiation and degree of spread, two thirds are classed as malignant. Medulloepitheliomas are slow growing and early diagnosis of an intraocular tumor with early enucleation results in a high survival rate. Death may occur secondary to intracranial extension.

DIAGNOSIS

Clinical signs and symptoms

The tumor appears as a white, gray or yellow to pink fleshy mass with a characteristic cystic appearance. It may be associated with a cyclitic membrane. Local invasion may result in the development secondary glaucoma, cataract or rubeosis iridis.

Laboratory findings

Indirect ophthalmoscopy, slit-lamp examination and echography aid in diagnosis. Computed tomography scanning and magnetic resonance imaging may also be helpful. The diagnosis is confirmed on histological examination.

Differential diagnosis

- Congenital, inflammatory, traumatic, or neoplastic conditions.
- Persistent hyperplastic primary vitreous.
- Congenital glaucoma.
- Pars planitis.
- Retinoblastoma.
- Malignant melanoma.
- Adenomas.
- Adenocarcinomas of the pigmented or nonpigmented ciliary epithelium.
- Juvenile xanthogranuloma.

TREATMENT

There is no well-established treatment. Iridocyclectomy is indicated for small tumors of the ciliary body. Enucleation is recommended for large tumors of the ciliary body, retina and optic nerve or in the presence of extraocular extension and in practice is required in the majority of cases.

The roles of radiation, chemotherapy and exenteration are not clearly defined. Local recurrence or metastasis to distant organs requires one or a combination of these treatment modalities.

REFERENCES

Broughton WI, Zimmerman LE: A clinicopathologic study of 56 cases of intraocular medulloepitheliomas. Am J Ophthalmol 85:407–418, 1978.

Canning CR, McCartney ACE, Hungerford J: Medulloepithelioma (diktyoma). Br J Ophthalmol 72:764–767, 1988.

Foster RE, Murray TG, Frazier Byrne S, et al: Echographic features of medulloepithelioma. Am J Ophthalmol 130:364–366, 2000.

Grinker RR: Gliomas of the retina including results of studies with silver impregnations. Arch Ophthalmol 5:920–935, 1931.

Hasain SE, Husain N, Boniuk M, et al: Malignant nonteratoid medulloepithelioma of the ciliary body in an adult. Ophthalmology 105:596–599, 1998.

O'Keefe M, Fulcher T, Kelly P, et al: Medulloepithelioma of the optic nerve head. Arch Ophthalmol 115:1325–1327, 1997.

Shields JA, Shields CL: Tumours of the nonpigmented ciliary epithelium: intraocular tumors: a text and atlas. Philadelphia, WB Saunders; 1992:465–481.

Zimmerman LE: The remarkable polymorphism of tumours of the ciliary epithelium. Trans Aust Coll Ophthalmol 2:114–125, 1970.

138 MENINGIOMA 225.2

Robert A. Egan, MD
Portland, Oregon

ETIOLOGY/INCIDENCE

Meningiomas are generally benign, slow-growing tumors that arise from the dura and they account for about 15–25% of intracranial tumors. Twice as common in females than in males, meningiomas reach a peak incidence in the seventh decade of life, although those that arise from the sphenoid bone and result in visual complaints usually present in the fifth to sixth decades. An estimated 2–3% of the population harbors an incidental meningioma. Most meningiomas are sporadic, but certain risk factors increase the prevalence of these tumors including neurofibromatosis type 2 (NF2). It is currently unclear if the risk of meningioma increases after cranial radiation.

CLINICAL PRESENTATION

Meningiomas are seldom invasive; they produce symptoms by compressing adjacent structures, and these symptoms depend on the site of origin. Because of the characteristic slow tumor growth, clinical findings may have been present for a long time before the correct diagnosis is made. Also, in this day and age of computed tomography (CT) and magnetic resonance imaging (MRI) many meningiomas are found incidentally. These tumors commonly present with seizures as well as increased intracranial pressure and papilledema. Occasionally, they may mimic transient ischemic attacks or present with intracranial hemorrhage.

Due to the myriad types of presentations that meningiomas can portray, it is beyond the scope of this chapter to describe all of them. However, the location of these tumors is typically the most important feature in relation to the clinical symptoms. Focal neurologic deficits are caused by direct local brain, cranial nerve, or spinal compression. These may include aphasia as well as psychomotor symptoms and behavioral disturbances. Cranial neuropathies causing visual symptoms are common with sphenoid wing and tuberculum sella meningiomas due to their relation to the cavernous sinus. Progressive monocular vision loss is the hallmark of the primary optic nerve sheath meningioma (ONSM) although it may also occur from secondary ONSMs that grow toward and compress the optic nerve and its sheath. The classic syndrome denoted as Foster-Kennedy is extremely rare and describes optic disc pallor in one eye and disc edema in the fellow eye in the presence of large anterior falcine, olfactory groove or orbitofrontal meningiomas. Petroclival meningiomas may compress the cerebellum causing ataxia as well as other cranial neuropathies. This may also occur with cerebellopontine region meningiomas in addition to hearing loss.

The natural history of intracranial and spinal meningiomas is unknown. Most neurosurgeons advocate near immediate removal of the tumor despite the typical pattern of slow growth. More is known about growth patterns of ONSM and these tumors may remain quiescent without progression of symptoms for years. The visual prognosis after removal of suprasellar meningiomas is excellent, but tumors tend to regrow even after 10 years following surgery.

MOLECULAR CONSIDERATIONS

Many meningiomas express progesterone and somatostatin receptors. The presence of these receptors may influence the grade of the tumor. These serve as markers of the tumors and offer some possible avenues for treatments in the future. There have been several case reports so far detailing success in treatment of meningiomas by modulating the cellular response at the receptor site.

Up to 60% of meningiomas contain a somatic mutation of the *NF2* gene on chromosome 22q12. These mutations cause abnormalities in merlin or schwannomin proteins. The type of mutations may also affect the grade of these tumors. A number of other mutations have been found on other chromosomes.

NEUROIMAGING

Imaging with either CT or MRI will denote a well-circumscribed mass with several features typical of these tumors. They are extra-axial and adherent to dura. They may be associated with compression of brain, spinal cord, or optic nerve depending on location. Some of the tumor may taper into normal appearing dura; this wisp of tissue is referred to the dural tail and is highly suggestive of the radiographic diagnosis of meningioma. These tumors are typically isointense or slightly hypointense to brain on T1-weighted imaging. These tumors enhance readily and uniformly after administration of gadolinium and are typically dark on T2-weighted imaging after fat suppression. Uncommonly, these tumors may be so large that their extra-axial distinction is difficult to discern. Some of these masses may be hyperdense on CT. When ONSMs are calcified, they may show tram tracking along each side of the optic nerve, which confirms the diagnosis. However, less than half of ONSMs are calcified at the time of diagnosis.

Several other diseases may give an appearance similar to meningiomas and these include, but are not limited to metastatic disease, sarcoidosis, Wegener's granulomatosis and tuberculosis.

Skull based meningiomas often cause some remodeling of underlying bone via reactive sclerosis, erosion or invasion although this less commonly occurs with convexity meningiomas. This may be difficult to distinguish from other diseases including Paget's disease, fibrous dysplasia, osteomas, hemolytic anemias and hyperparathyroid disorders. MRI is useful in these instances by revealing the soft tissue mass of the tumor near the affected bony tissue.

These tumors may also affect the great cerebral veins if they grow near them. Magnetic resonance venography may be helpful in assessing for venous occlusion in the patient with papilledema and suspected increased intracranial pressure.

MANAGEMENT

Before one can make generalizations about treatment of a medical problem it is most beneficial to know what the natural history of the disorder is. For most meningiomas, except ONSMs, this is not known. For ONSMs, there is recent data suggesting that these tumors are very slow growing and following an ONSM conservatively without treatment as long as vision is stable and not deteriorating is an acceptable form of management. With this said, it is known that some meningiomas may grow in more hazardous areas of the intracranial space and cause mischief to the optic chiasm, nerves in the cavernous sinus, superior sagittal sinus occlusion, as well as focal brain compression with edema. These tumors need treatment while others that are not causing any neurologic or ophthalmologic compromise may be watched conservatively with very close clinical and neuroradiographic follow up.

The degree of resection of the meningioma and surrounding dura dictates the chance of recurrence. The greater the resection, the less chance for recurrence. However, even in cases where apparent total resection was performed, recurrences uncommonly occur. The resection may be made larger when away from important neural and vascular structures, but may be impossible when located in regions such as the cavernous sinus.

The advent of modern interventional neuroradiology has allowed endovascular treatment of meningiomas to take place. The arterial supply may be safely interrupted using glue or coils so that the tumor is devascularized allowing less blood loss at the time of craniotomy and resection. The efficacy of these treatments is still not known, but shows some promise.

Surgical resection of ONSMs is not recommended unless the patient is already blind and concerned about intracranial extension. Removal usually interrupts feeding arterioles to the optic nerve resulting in ischemia and instantaneous loss of vision in the involved eye. Rarely, vision is improved in an eye with an ONSM after surgery, but this needs to be stressed as the exception and not the rule.

Suprasellar meningiomas can be resected with the knowledge that the long-term visual prognosis is very good. However, many patients suffer recurrences even more than 10 years following apparent gross total surgical resection. This suggests that these patients require long-term follow-up and should be considered for post-operative radiation therapy.

Radiation is reserved for patients who have undergone incomplete resection of their tumor, after recurrence, and when histology shows atypia or anaplasia. A number of case reports document a clinical benefit in patients treated with radiation. However, there are no randomized, controlled, prospective trials documenting a therapeutic advantage to radiation or whether specific varieties of delivering radiation are better than others. These include stereotactic radiotherapy, three-dimensional conformal radiation therapy and intensity-modulated radiation therapy.

Although case reports suggest a benefit to radiation, concerns continue about the risks of therapy. Necrosis to the optic nerve, retina and neighboring brain tissue are all known to occur as a complication of therapy. The risk of developing radiation optic neuropathy using gamma knife therapy for patients with a variety of suprasellar tumors receiving no more than 12 Gy is less than 2%. However, the risk of a variety of neurologic problems increases to 33% when delivered to ONSMs using a variety of standard procedures. Radiation therapy should therefore be used with caution and the patients counseled about the risks and benefits despite controlled randomized trials. In patients with ONSM, radiation should be reserved for those who are suffering from vision loss that is progressing; patients with normal vision should be followed conservatively with close monitoring clinically.

Meningiomas are largely resistant to standard chemotherapy, but hormonal therapy may provide some promise in future treatment. Progesterone and somatostatin receptors have been found in many meningiomas, which is why the tumor may rapidly progress during pregnancy, during the luteal phase of the menstrual cycle, and with breast feeding. Hormonal therapy using progesterone antagonists or somatostatin analogues may therefore inhibit tumor growth. This therapy is still in its infancy.

REFERENCES

Bhatia S, Sather HN, Pabustan OB, et al: Low incidence of second neoplasms among children diagnosed with acute lymphoblastic leukemia after 1983. Blood 99:4257–4264, 2002.

Blankenstein MA, Verheijen FM, Jacobs JM, et al: Occurrence, regulation, and significance of progesterone receptors in human meningioma. Steroids 65:795–800, 2000.

Boldrey E: The meningiomas. In: Minckler J, ed. Pathology of the nervous system. New York, McGraw-Hill, 1971:2125–2144.

Chicani CF, Miller NR: Visual outcome in surgically treated suprasellar meningiomas. J Neuroophthalmol 23:3–10, 2003.

Das A, Tan WL, Teo J, Smith DR: Overexpression of mdm2 and p53 and association with progesterone receptor expression in benign meningiomas. Neuropathology 22:194–199, 2002.

Egan RA, Lessell S: A contribution to the natural history of optic nerve sheath meningiomas. Arch Ophthalmol 120:1505–1508, 2002.

Gursan N, Gundogdu C, Albayrak A, Kabalar ME: Immunohistochemical detection of progesterone receptors and the correlation with Ki-67 labeling indices in paraffin embedded sections of meningiomas. Int J Neurosci 112:463–470, 2002.

Louis D, Scheithauer B, Budka H, et al: Meningiomas. In: Kleihues P, CAvenee W, eds. Pathology and genetics of tumours of the nervous system: World Health Organisation classification of tumours. Lyon, IARC, 2000:176–184.

Lumenta CB, Schirmer M: The incidence of brain tumors: a retrospective study. Clin Neuropharmacol 7:332–337, 1984.

Meewes C, Bohuslavizki KH, Krisch B, et al: Molecular biologic and scintigraphic analyses of somatostatin receptor-negative meningiomas. J Nucl Med 42:1338–1345, 2001.

Schulz S, Pauli SU, Handel M, et al: Immunohistochemical determination of five somatostatin receptors in meningioma reveals frequent overexpression of somatostatin receptor subtype sst2A. Clin Cancer Res 6:1865–1874, 2000.

Stafford SL, Pollock BE, Leavitt JA, et al: A study on the radiation tolerance of the optic nerves and chiasm after stereotactic radiosurgery. Int J Radiat Oncol Biol Phys 55:1177–1181, 2003.

Turbin RE, Thompson CR, Kennerdell JS, et al: A long-term visual outcome comparison in patients with optic nerve sheath meningioma managed with observation, surgery, radiotherapy, or surgery and radiotherapy. Ophthalmology 109:890–899, 2002, discussion 899–900.

Wahab M, Al-Azzawi F: Meningioma and hormonal influences. Climacteric 6:285–292, 2003.

Wellenreuther R, Kraus JA, Lenartz D, et al: Analysis of the neurofibromatosis 2 gene reveals molecular variants of meningioma. Am J Pathol 146:827–832, 1995.

139 METASTATIC TUMORS TO THE EYE AND ITS ADNEXA 198.89

Devron H. Char, MD
San Francisco, California

ETIOLOGY/INCIDENCE

Metastases to the eye and adnexa are not rare; unfortunately, in as many as 50% of cases, they may be the presenting sign of the primary malignancy, especially of lung, renal and gastrointestinal carcinomas. The posterior uvea is the most common site of metastases to the eye. Metastases to the orbit have an incidence of approximately one eighth of those to the choroid. Metastases to other ocular sites, including the optic nerve, eyelid, retina, conjunctiva, aqueous and vitreous spaces, are much less common.

Several subjective, clinical and laboratory findings are important to make the correct diagnosis in any patient with an ophthalmic neoplasm. All patients with a tumor involving the eye or orbit should provide a thorough history, past medical history and review of systems. Unfortunately, as many as 14% of patients who present with a primary uveal melanoma have previously had a systemic malignancy; sometimes, that historic fact can mislead the clinician into believing that a uveal melanoma is a metastasis. Conversely, in approximately 30% of patients with metastases to the eye or orbit, there is no evidence of disease elsewhere.

Ninety percent of patients with breast metastases to ophthalmic structures have a known history of breast carcinoma. The incidence of uveal metastases in nonterminal patients is uncertain. In most ocular oncology centers, these tumors are diagnosed about 10% to 50% as frequently as primary melanomas. Orbital metastases are found in approximately 5% of orbital biopsies.

COURSE/PROGNOSIS

The life expectancy in patients with metastases to the eye or ocular adnexa is less than 2 years.

In patients with intraocular metastases, if the vision is better than 20/200, visual acuity usually can be either retained or improved.

In patients with orbital metastases, local palliation often can be achieved.

DIAGNOSIS

Clinical signs and symptoms

A thorough systemic history and review of systems should be obtained, with an emphasis on previous carcinomas and symptoms consistent with metastatic disease (e.g. weight loss, lymphadenopathy, subcutaneous nodules, hematuria, pulmonary symptoms, or change in bowel habits).

Uveal

In the choroid, these usually are amelanotic lesions in the macular area (because dissemination occurs via a hematogenous route). Often, there is a disproportionately large amount of subretinal fluid, given the small size of the tumor compared with a uveal melanoma. Often, the lesion has an infiltrative pattern; in breast metastases, this may have a peau d'orange appearance. Metastases do not have intrinsic pigmentation or produce a 'collar button,' or mushroom-shaped configuration.

In cases with an unknown primary tumor, how important is it to identify the initial site and histologic type of neoplasm? A PET-CT scan will detect an unknown primary site in 33–45% of cases. A fine needle aspiration biopsy can delineate the cell of origin of most metastases (melanoma, epithelial cancers, carcoma, etc.) In a few metastatic cases, the histologic tumor types will alter therapy. Immunocytology (on FNAB) or immunohistology (on standard biopsies) should identify a possible breast, uterine, prostate, or lymphoma malignancy origin since those metastases will be managed differently.

Laboratory findings

Systemic laboratory studies include general studies of complete blood cell count, erythrocyte sedimentation rate and liver function tests and specific studies of plasma carcinoembryonic antigen, CA-125, prostate-specific antigen and others.

For intraocular tumors, ultrasound is accurate. On B-scan, no acoustic quiet zone or choroidal excavation is seen. On A-scan, there may be coarse to medium-high spikes with a 'climbing' posterior face.

Orbital metastases have a predilection to invade bone. Metastases should also be considered in the differential diagnosis of focal extraocular muscle masses or a diffuse, infiltrative intraconal lesion in older patients. Less commonly, they can simulate a focal intraconal benign tumor.

Orbital imaging with magnetic resonance imaging is diagnostic in approximately two thirds of cases.

In both ocular and adenexal tumors, a definitive diagnosis may be achieved in more than 98% of cases with fine needle aspiration biopsy with either standard cytopathology or special stains (estrogen receptors, progesterone receptors, keratin, lymphocyte markers, epithelial antigens, HMB 45 stains and others). Scirrhous carcinoma and very small apical lesions can yield a false-negative fine needle aspiration biopsy.

Differential diagnosis

Amelanotic nevi, amelanotic melanoma, choroidal hemangioma, extramacular disciform lesion and rare benign choroidal tumors should be considered.

TREATMENT

Approximately 33% of patients with ophthalmic metastases present without a known primary tumor. In more than 10% of patients with ophthalmic metastases, no primary tumor site is found. Several studies have shown that in such patients, it is important to determine whether the metastases are of lymphoid, breast or genitourinary tract origin. Because the management of these malignancies is sufficiently different from that of other metastases, they should be delineated in patients without a known primary tumor. If those sites of origin can be determined not to be involved, further studies to elucidate the primary lesion are neither necessary nor productive.

The evaluation of systemic status and possible contiguous central nervous system involvement is crucial. Repeat staging of metastatic disease and brain magnetic resonance gadolinium-enhanced imaging are important for optimum treatment planning. If widespread systemic disease is present and amenable to chemotherapy, ophthalmic lesions usually also respond because there is no blood-ocular barrier.

In patients with focal metastatic lesions isolated to the eye or orbit, management depends on symptoms, systemic status and size and numbers of metastases (up to 25% of patients will have either multifocal or bilateral lesions).

Enucleation or exenteration is very rarely indicated for metastatic disease because these patients have a very short life expectancy. Enucleation is indicated in rare patients with a painful blind eye.

Some patients with ocular metastases do not require therapy. We followed a few patients for as long as 15 years with ocular metastases that have not activated or altered vision due to either systemic therapy or spontaneous inactivation. Similarly, in a terminally ill, ocularly asymptomatic patient, observation is the treatment of choice.

Chemotherapy

Some intraocular and adnexal metastases will respond to systemic chemotherapy. Serial evaluation of such lesions is a good way to measure the patient's response to systemic therapy.

Radiation

Radiation with teletherapy (external beams of photons or electrons) to a dose of approximately 4000 cGy is the most common treatment for choroidal or orbital metastases. It is imperative to rule out contiguous central nervous system involvement before teletherapy because if a frontal lobe metastasis is present, it should be included in the treatment field. Failure to do so, with a subsequent need to include that area in a second radiation field, needlessly increases morbidity rates. Occasionally, a single tumor will be treated with brachytherapy (usually a ^{125}I plaque). In some cases, a focused form of radiation, Intensity-Modulated Conformal Therapy (IMRT), gamma knife, cyber knife, or protons, can be advantageous compared to other radiation delivery systems.

Surgical

In orbital tumors that are nonresponsive to radiation, surgical debulking is a reasonable option. Only very rarely are intraocular metastases locally resected.

COMMENTS

Metastases to the eye and adnexa are associated with poor prognosis for life. Fortunately, many patients' visual symptoms occurring as a result of these metastatic deposits can be ameliorated with local or systemic therapy.

REFERENCES

Char DH: Tumors of the eye and ocular adnexa: Toronto, Canada BC Decker, 2001.

Ferry AP, Font RL: Carcinoma metastatic to the eye and orbit. A clinicopathologic study of 227 cases. Arch Ophthalmol 92:276–286, 1974.

Gutzeit A, Antoch G, Kuhl H, et al: Unknown primary tumors: detection with dual-modality PET/CT — Initial experience. Radiology 234:227–234, 2005.

Shields CL, Shields JA, Gross NE, et al: Series of 520 eyes with uveal metastases. Ophthalmology 104:1265–1267, 1997.

140 MUCOCELE 376.81
(Pyocele, Mucopyocele)

Robert C. Kersten, MD
Cincinnati, Ohio

ETIOLOGY

A mucocele is a cystic lesion arising from the accumulation and retention of mucus secretions, usually from an obstructed, often chronically inflamed paranasal sinus. As the mucous accumulates the mucocele expands and can erode through the sinus wall into the orbit leading to ophthalmic signs and symptoms. If the mucoid material becomes secondarily infected, the lesion is termed a *pyocele* or *mucopyocele*. The most common form is the frontoethmoidal lesion, with the ethmoidal or sphenoidal varieties being less common. Maxillary sinus mucocele is rare.

Causes of a mucocele include chronic sinusitis, cystic fibrosis (in children), fractures involving the nasofrontal duct, sinus polyps, previous sinus or orbital decompression surgery, primary sinus tumors (squamous cell carcinoma of ethmoid sinus), metastatic tumors and allergies.

DIAGNOSIS

Clinical signs and symptoms

- Mucoceles usually occur in adults with a history of chronic sinusitis. They usually present with progressive proptosis or globe displacement.
- Chronic headache and visual disturbance are less common complaints.
- Frontoethmoidal lesions typically produce outward and downward displacement of the globe and proptosis. Ptosis and limited supraduction and adduction of the globe may occur. Acquired Browns syndrome has also been reported. A fluctuant mass may be palpable beneath the orbital rim superonasally. Posterior erosion may produce epidural or subdural abscess formation.
- Isolated frontal sinus lesions lead to downward and outward displacement with minimal proptosis; ptosis and limited elevation may occur.
- Sphenoid and posterior ethmoid lesions tend to present with functional abnormalities related to the optic nerve, cavernous sinus, or orbital apex. Patients may have visual symptoms, retrobulbar pain, nerve palsies and nasal symptoms. Disk edema or optic atrophy can be present. Extraocular palsies (often the third nerve) occur in approximately half of patients. Sphenoid sinus mucopyoceles may cause sudden visual loss due to compression or inflammation of the adjacent optic nerve. Patients often complain of headache radiating to the apex of the skull.
- Maxillary sinus lesions usually lead to upward displacement of the globe but have been reported to cause enophthalmos.

Mucopyoceles are usually associated with acute inflammatory signs and symptoms including pain, erythema and edema of overlying soft tissues and mucopurulent nasal drainage.

Laboratory findings

- An imaging study should be obtained to make the diagnosis and determine the extent and location of the lesion.
- Computed tomography scanning is helpful to outline bony changes, including the status of orbital walls and the cranial cavity.
- Magnetic resonance imaging with gadolinium may be helpful in differentiating mucoceles from neoplasms in the paranasal sinuses.

Differential diagnosis

The differential diagnosis includes retrobulbar tumor; paranasal sinus, nasal, or pharyngeal tumors; thyroid disease; retrobulbar neuritis; meningocele; meningoencephalocele; subperiosteal hematoma; orbital pseudotumor; acute or chronic sinusitis; and temporal arteritis.

TREATMENT

Surgical

- A multidisciplinary approach involving an orbital surgeon and an otorhinolaryngologist is usually necessary, with neurosurgical backup if indicated by intracranial invasion.
- Access to the mucocele can be approached via an anterior orbitotomy (lid-crease incision) or transcaruncular incision (for isolated ethmoid lesion). Exposure of the frontal sinus itself may also include the creation of an osteoplastic bone flap.
- Surgical goals may include re-establishment of normal sinus drainage or removal of all sinus mucosa and obliteration of the sinus with fat.
- An isolated mucocele may be treated with complete removal of the lining, removal of degenerated bone with the use of a high-speed drill and re-establishment of drainage between the exenterated sinus and the nose.
- Silastic tubing, a nasal flap, or silicone rubber sheeting can be used to reconstruct the frontal-nasal duct and provide drainage to the nose.
- Another option is obliteration of the sinus after complete removal of the cyst lining and degenerated bone. Fat from the abdominal wall can then be packed into the sinus space.
- Endoscopic decompression of sphenoidal and ethmoidal mucoceles is a newer method of dealing with these lesions. Recurrence rates may be higher when endoscopy is used as the sole intervention.

COMPLICATIONS

Recurrence can be due to incomplete excision of sinus lining or restenosis of the new osteum. Infection can occur, as can fistula formation between the sinus and skin, or the orbit or cranial cavity.

COMMENTS

Proper planning and a multidisciplinary approach are crucial to success in treating mucocele. Treatment for sphenoidal mucocele with compressive optic neuropathy is more urgent than that for other varieties. Future treatments will likely incorporate endoscopic approaches, although an emphasis on re-establishing proper drainage of the diseased sinus is crucial.

REFERENCES

Benninger MS, Marks S: The endoscopic management of sphenoid and ethmoid mucoceles with orbital and intranasal extension. Rhinology 33:157–161, 1995.

Bhola R, Rosenbaum AL: Ethmoidal sinus mucocele: an unusual cause of acquired Brown syndrome. Br J Ophthalmol 89(8):1069, 2005.

Feldman M, Lowry LD, Rao VM, et al: Mucoceles of the paranasal sinuses. Trans PA Acad Ophthalmol 39:614–617, 1987.

Friedman A, Batra PS, Fakhri S, et al: Isolated sphenoid sinus disease: etiology and management. Otolaryngol Head Neck Surg 133(4):544–550, 2005.

Levy J, Monos T, Putterman M: Bilateral consecutive blindness due to sphenoid sinus mucocele with unilateral partial recovery. Can J Ophthalmol 40:506–508, 2005.

Rootman J, ed: Diseases of the orbit: a multidisciplinary approach. Philadelphia, JB Lippincott, 1988.

Wang TJ, Liao SL, Jou JR, Lin LL: Clinical manifestations and management of orbital mucoceles: the role of ophthalmologists. Jpn J Ophthalmol. 49(3):239–245, 2005.

Yoshida K, Wataya T, Yamagata S: Mucocele in an Onodi cell responsible for acute optic neuropathy. Br J Neurosurg 19(1):55–56, 2005.

141 NEURILEMOMA 215.9
(Neurinoma, Schwannoma)

Norman S. Levy, MD, PhD, FACS
Gainesville, Florida

ETIOLOGY/INCIDENCE

Neurilemoma is a slow-growing encapsulated neoplasm arising from Schwann's cells of nerves. Some neurilemomas are malignant. These tumors have been found diffusely throughout the body in both the sensory and motor nerves, but their frequency in sensory nerves is several hundred-fold greater than that in motor nerves.

Neurilemomas have been documented as arising from each of the nerves within and around the eye. They have been reported within the perilimbal conjunctiva, the uveal tissues and the sclera. They account for 2% of orbital tumors and can mimick intrinsic brainstem tumors. The involvement of branches of the trigeminal nerve is the most common periocular presentation.

COURSE/PROGNOSIS

Retro-orbital headaches, facial numbness, progressive exophthalmos, lid swelling, intermittent pain, numbness or paresthesia in the distribution of the appropriate sensory nerve branch and atypical trigeminal neuralgia have been described as initial signs. The presenting findings in neurilemomas of the third, fourth and sixth cranial nerves include diplopia, ptosis, Horner's syndrome and blurring of vision. The proximity of the optic nerve to the expanding tumor within the orbit has occasionally resulted in amaurosis fugax or the loss of vision. Hyperventilation induced nystagmus can occur in patients with vestibular neurilemoma.

DIAGNOSIS

Examination may reveal a localized swelling or a discrete mass. Papilledema has been reported as the presenting manifestation of spinal neurilemoma.

Laboratory findings

Computed tomography scanning of the suspected tumor can be extremely helpful in characterizing its size and extent. Magnetic resonance imaging has high sensitivity in defining the nature and invasiveness of the tumor. In vivo differential diagnosis of the tumor type may be achieved with localized H-1 proton magnetic resonance spectroscopy. Positron-emission tomography has also been used to image malignant neurilemomas. Orbital and ocular echography can be helpful, characteristically showing a sharply outlined capsule, a well-defined central cystic space, slight compressibility and blood flow.

Differential diagnosis

A melanotic neurilemoma of the orbit, ocular uvea, or choroid can grossly mimic a malignant melanoma and can be difficult to clinically differentiate. Before surgery, fine needle aspiration may be diagnostically helpful by allowing immunocytochemical and electron microscopic evaluation of the specimen. The tumor may consist of spindle-shaped cells with twisted nuclei, positive immunoreactivity for S-100 protein, vimentin, glial fibrillary acidic protein and neural cell adhesion molecules. Immunostaining for laminin and type IV collagen will demonstrate a continuous basal lamina encompassing the tumor cells. Ultrastructually, the tumor cells may have delicate cytoplasmic processes and scant organelles.

TREATMENT

Systemic

Intravenous combination chemotherapy, consisting of 2 mg of vincristine, 100 mg of doxorubicin, 1 g of cyclophosphamide and 500 mg of dacarbazine has been used. This therapy should be undertaken over a 5-day intensive course, followed by the weekly administration of vincristine. Dactinomycin has also been used. Recurrent courses may be required based on clinical response. Such chemotherapy should be undertaken only by a physician trained in these procedures.

Surgical

The tumor must be anatomically defined through the use of appropriate radiographic studies. Dissection of the tumor from the adjacent tissues is facilitated by careful study of the radiographic findings, a thorough knowledge of the anatomy, preoperative planning and intraoperative microscopic surgical control. Complete surgical excision is the therapy of choice, with preservation of the nerve function frequently possible. Tumors are not highly vascular, so bleeding is rarely a problem.

Radiation

When histologic examination of the tissue confirms malignancy or radiographic recurrence has been documented, focal application of up to 6000 rads of 10-MeV photons may be used for local treatment.

COMPLICATIONS

Occasionally, the extent and location of the tumor prevent complete excision. Surgery can cause damage to the nerve, the eye and adjacent tissues. If growth continues, repeated excision, irradiation, chemotherapy, or a combination is indicated.

PRECAUTIONS

Accurate diagnosis of the tumor is only achieved histologically, although the results of radiographic studies can be suggestive. The histologic evaluation must be done by a pathologist who is extremely familiar with this type of tumor. Studies indicate that the morphology and histology of the collagen of such tumors can be useful in their differentiation. Electron microscopy often is useful when standard histologic techniques are not definitive. Human glia-specific proteins, S100 and GFA, have been useful in characterizing the malignant status of these tumors.

The importance of a surgically aggressive approach to patients with malignant neurilemomas cannot be overemphasized. The 5-year survival rate in one study was 48%. Even tumors initially classified as low grade histologically often eventually metastasize and cause death. Prognosis of any lesion is dependent on its location and size, the adequacy of excision and the malignant potential of that particular neurilemoma.

COMMENTS

The occurrence of multiple tumors usually implies hereditary disease, such as neurofibromatosis type 2. The increased incidence of malignant neurilemomas in association with neurofibromatosis type 2 and in sites of prior irradiation should be recognized.

REFERENCES

Bickler-Bluth ME, Custer PL, Smith ME: Neurilemoma as a presenting feature of neurofibromatosis. Arch Ophthalmol 106:665–667, 1988.

Byrne BM, van Heuven WAJ, Lawton AW: Echographic characteristics of benign orbital schwannomas (neurilemomas). Am J Ophthalmol 106:194–198, 1988.

Capps DH, Brodsky MC, Rice CD, et al: Orbital intramuscular schwannoma. Am J Ophthalmol 110:535–539, 1990.

Costello F, Kardon RH, Wall M, et al: Papilledema as the presenting manifestation of spinal schwannoma. J Neuroophthalmol 22:199–203, 2002.

Fan JT, Campbell RJ, Robertson DM: A survey of intraocular schwannoma with a case report. Can J Ophthalmol 30:37–41, 1995.

Jacque CM, Kujas M, Poreau A, et al: GFA and S100 protein levels as an index for malignancy in human gliomas and neurinomas. J Natl Cancer Inst 62:479–483, 1979.

Mafee MF, Putterman A, Valvassori GE, et al: Orbital space-occupying lesions: role of computed tomography and magnetic resonance imaging: an analysis of 145 cases. Radiol Clin North Am 25:529–559, 1987.

Matsuo T, Notohara K: Choroidal schwannoma: immunohistochemical and electron-microscopic study. Ophthalmologica 214:156–160, 2000.

Minor LB, Haslwanter T, Straumann D, Zee DS: Hyperventilation-induced nystagmus in patients with vestibular schwannoma. Neurology 53:2158–2168, 1999.

Rose GE, Wright JE: Isolated peripheral nerve sheath tumours of the orbit. Eye 5:668–673, 1991.

Santoreneos S, Hanieh A, Jorgensen RE: Trochlear nerve schwannomas occuring in patients without neurofibromatosis: case report and review of the literature. Neurosurgery 41:282–287, 1997.

Senoy SN, Raja A: Cystic trochlear nerve neurinoma mimicking intrinsic brainstem tumour. Br J Neurosurg 18:183–186, 2004.

Shields JA, Font RL, Eagle RC, Jr, et al: Melanotic schwannoma of the choroid: immunohistochemistry and electron microscopic observations. Ophthalmology 101:843–849, 1994.

Zbieranowski I, Bedard YC: Fine needle aspiration of schwannomas: value of electron microscopy and immunocytochemistry in the preoperative diagnosis. Acta Cytol 33:381–384, 1989.

142 NEUROBLASTOMA 194.0

Devron H. Char, MD
San Francisco, California

ETIOLOGY/INCIDENCE

Neuroblastoma is a neoplastic proliferation of immature sympathetic ganglion cells. This tumor is the most common pediatric extracranial solid tumor; approximately half of these patients present with metastases at diagnosis. There are approximately 650 new cases per year in this country, with half presenting in children younger than 2 years. In whites, the annual incidence is approximately 10.5 per 1 million. Most patients with neuroblastoma ophthalmic metastases present to the ophthalmologist before the discovery of a primary neoplasm.

In approximately 3% of all neuroblastomas, orbital involvement can be the initial manifestation of the disease. Neuroblastoma can also present with other ophthalmic findings not directly related to ocular or adnexal metastases.

COURSE/PROGNOSIS

Presentation can mimic that of a battered child syndrome and can be either unilateral or bilateral. Approximately 30% to 40% of treated patients have good long-term survival rates. With treatment, the local ophthalmic prognosis is good, however most of these patients die of systemic diseases.

DIAGNOSIS

Clinical signs and symptoms

The diagnosis of metastatic neuroblastoma to the ocular adnexa may be difficult. In a child younger than 2 years who presents with orbital proptosis, the possibility of metastases must be considered.

Differential diagnosis

The differential diagnosis includes hemangioma, cysts, lymphangioma, leukemia, lymphoma, rhabdomyosarcoma, orbital extension of retinoblastoma, and a breakthrough orbital cellulitis or abscess from a contiguous sinusitis.

Laboratory findings

Computed tomography (CT) scanning or magnetic resonance imaging (MRI) often is diagnostic; metastatic orbital bone involvement has a typical pattern. Diagnosis can be established with fine needle aspiration biopsy; ancillary studies can be performed on biopsy material, including cytogenetic studies, comparative genomic hybridization (CGH) studies, N-myc analysis, and microarray urine analysis shows elevations of vanillylmandelic acid (VMA) and homovanillic acid (HVA).

All patients require a complete metastatic evaluation including body CT/MRI bone scan, multiple bone marrow biopsies (including fluorescence for Gd2 cells), metaiodobenzylguanidine (I-131 MIBG) imaging studies, and cytogenetic analysis of the tumor, including ploidy analysis, N-myc amplification, alterations in the area of chromosome 1p, 3p, 11q, 17q, and studies of ferritin, NSE, CD 44, nerve growth factor expression, and mRNA expression of *trk*. Serum lactate dehydrogenase levels are helpful, as may be telomerase levels. All of these tests are correlative with survival rates.

TREATMENT

Multimodality evaluation and therapy are optimal with pediatric oncology, radiation oncology and ophthalmic oncology.

Systemic

In most centers, a combination of systemic consolidation chemotherapy and either autologous bone marrow transplantation or stem cell transplantation appears to be better than continuous chemotherapy. Approximately 35% of patients will have long-term regression with this approach. Newer molecular trials with anti-GD2 drugs and newer agents such as rebeccamycin are in phase II trials.

Local

Local therapy often can be deferred until response to systemic treatment is observed. Radiation is useful for orbital palliation. These tumors will respond to 2000 cGy of external-beam photon radiation.

Surgical

Surgery to remove gross residual disease may be helpful in some cases.

REFERENCES

Char DH: Tumors of the eye and ocular adnexa. Hamilton, BC Decker, 2001.

Goldsby RE, Matthay KK: Neuroblastoma. Evolving therapies for a disease with many faces. Pediatric Drugs 6:107–122, 2004.

Ladenstein R, Philip T, Gardner H: Autologous stem cell transplantation for solid tumors in children. Curr Opin Pediatr 9:55–69, 1997.

Maris JM: The biologic basis for neuroblastoma heterogeneity and risk stratification. Curr Opin Pediatr 17:7–13, 2005.

Stram DL, Mattha IKK, O'Leary M, et al: Consolidation chemoradiotherapy and autologous bone marrow transplantation versus continued chemotherapy for metastatic neuroblastoma: a report of two concurrent children cancer group studies. J Clin Oncol 14:2417–2426, 1996.

143 OPTIC GLIOMAS 225.1

Cameron F. Parsa, MD
Baltimore, Maryland

ETIOLOGY/INCIDENCE

Juvenile pilocytic astrocytoma type I tumors intrinsic to the optic nerve, chiasm, or tracts are termed optic gliomas. Because of the static or slow growth of the astrocytic (glial) cells surrounding the nerve axons, in many cases followed by spontaneous regression, prolonged survival is the rule. These tumors do not metastasize in the usual sense; during infancy, rarely 'drop' metastases, often asymptomatic in nature, may occur to the leptomeninges via the cerebrospinal fluid passageways, particularly after ventricular shunt placement for elevated intracranial pressure.

About half of patients who present with optic gliomas also have neurofibromatosis type 1 (NF1) which is due to a mutation and loss of function of a tumor suppressor gene. While over 25% of NF1 patients may have detectable gliomas in MRI surveillance studies, most remain asymptomatic. Optic gliomas should be considered hamartomas with growth potential during childhood.

COURSE/PROGNOSIS

Gliomas of the optic nerve can be unilateral or bilateral. They often present within the first decade of life with proptosis. Acuity loss may be mild or profound; visual function correlates poorly with tumor size. They can be left alone until proptosis becomes unsightly.

Gliomas affecting the chiasm more often present with visual loss. In patients with hypothalamic involvement, hormonal dysfunction may be present. Involvement and obstruction of the third ventricle can produce elevated intracranial pressure.

Tumor growth is slow and by the time the tumor is discovered, often no further growth is noted. While tumor can extend along optic pathways, cell growth can also be multicentric. Spontaneous regression can occur.

DIAGNOSIS

Clinical signs and symptoms

Glioma affecting the optic nerve

The diagnosis can be suggested by proptosis in a child. There may be an afferent pupil defect or a swollen or pale optic nerve with optociliary shunt vessels. For reasons still unclear, the elongated nerve within the orbit has a predisposition to kink downward, producing upward rotation of the posterior aspect of the globe. Thus, a hypotropia is often noted.

Glioma affecting the chiasm

Chiasmal gliomas may lack external signs. In some cases, there is an asymmetric rotary nystagmus mimicking spasmus nutans. Visual loss can be very mild or profound. The discs can remain relatively healthy or may become pale depending on the degree of axonal injury. If the third ventricle is obstructed, signs of increased intracranial pressure may be present.

An emaciated yet hyperactive child points to hypothalamic involvement causing diencephalic syndrome of Russell. More frequently, more subtle hormonal imbalances are present, producing signs such as delayed growth or precocious puberty.

Associated signs of possible neurofibromatosis, such as multiple café-au-lait spots, axillary freckling and Sakurai–Lisch iris nodules may be present.

Laboratory findings

Neuroimaging, particularly magnetic resonance imaging with gadolinium contrast, is essential. The tumors enhance variably.

When the nerve is involved, fusiform, tubular, intrinsic enlargement is noted which can also remodel and widen the optic canal. A pathognomonic 'kinking' of the nerve may be seen, indicating elongation of the nerve within the orbit.

A perineural arachnoidal hyperplasia often occurs in NF-1-associated optic nerve gliomas. This tissue's high water content produces an image on T2-weighted MR imagery that looks like an expanded CSF space around the nerve. This so-called 'pseudo-CSF sign' is highly suggestive of NF1 optic nerve gliomas.

If the chiasm is involved, it becomes smoothly enlarged, often obliterating the normal contours of the chiasm and extending into nerves and tracts. Growth, when large, may involve the hypothalamus.

Clinical and neuroimaging characteristics are sufficiently specific such that tissue biopsies are often contraindicated because of hazard to remaining vision. Where perineural arachnoidal hyperplasia exists, biopsy specimens have been misread as meningiomatosis growth.

Differential diagnosis

Differentiation from meningioma may be made by age and by the presence of calcifications which are typical in meningiomas, but less common in gliomas. The uniform appearance of the glioma contrasts with the meningioma tissue surrounding the nerve itself. Straightening of the nerve with proptosis of the globe is more often noted with the stiffer meningiomas, whereas kinking is more common with the softer, elongated, gliomas. CT imaging of the canal can be useful in the demonstration of irregular hyperostosis occurring with meningiomas. Though uncommon in childhood, orbital hemangiomas compressing the nerve can be differentiated by the para-dural origin of the hemangioma with its center offset from observed neural tissue.

When the tumor involves the chiasm, it has smooth contours and expands the chiasm. Most other tumors, such as craniopharyngioma, pituitary tumors, and meningiomas compress and displace the chiasm.

TREATMENT

Glioma involving optic nerve alone

Observation. No proven efficacy has been shown for excision of tumor to prevent contralateral eye involvement; cell growth may be multicentric. Moreover, resection of nerve near chiasm may interrupt the shared blood supply, causing spreading necrosis to chiasm. If nerve atrophy and visual loss are already severe and proptosis is disfiguring, limited orbital resection can be performed to resolve the cosmetic problem.

Glioma involving the chiasm

Observation. Since the tumors are intrinsic, resection of tumor also excises axons and produces permanent visual deficit. In rare cases, however, an exophytic extension may compound injury to the visual pathway via external compression and the culpable portion excised.

Since these tumors are slow growing with few cells undergoing mitotic division and proliferation, both radiation therapy and chemotherapy offer little theoretical benefit. No studies have shown statistically significant efficacy with either intervention. Anecdotal reports of success have likely encompassed cases with co-incident spontaneous regression, particularly when regression was reported years after therapy. It is conceivable that only rapidly growing tumors, or a morphologically stable tumor with high cellular turnover rate, could respond to such treatments. Such determination is not possible by standard MR imagery for a slowly growing or static-appearing tumor. Biopsies indicating the number of cells undergoing proliferation could be misleading due to sampling errors with inhomogeneous tumors. Future research may reveal MR spectroscopy or other modalities to indicate if any tumors might be suitable for anti-mitotic treatment regimens. Radiation therapy, nevertheless, should not be used in children under five years of age due to the secondary effects of excessive brain atrophy and mental retardation in the yet unmyelinated brain pathways. Chemotherapy has been advocated for such situations. Nonetheless, efficacy of either radiation treatment or chemotherapy has not been demonstrated. Irradiated tumors rarely can undergo malignant degeneration. More commonly observed adverse effects of radiation include degenerative vascular changes. In patients with NF1, an increased incidence of secondary tumor development occurs in both irradiated patients and those having undergone chemotherapy.

COMPLICATIONS

Complications from tumor involvement include loss of vision, hypothalamic dysfunction, and hydrocephalus. Complications of radiation therapy include mental retardation, cerebral vasculopathy, malignant tumor degeneration and, in patients with NF1, secondary malignant tumor development. Complications of chemotherapy may also include an increased incidence of secondary tumor formation in NF1 patients.

SUMMARY

Given their intrinsic nature and slow progression, occasionally followed by spontaneous regression, (Figure 143.1) in the vast majority of cases optic gliomas should be managed with observation alone, with supportive treatment such as hormone replacement or ventricular shunts provided as needed.

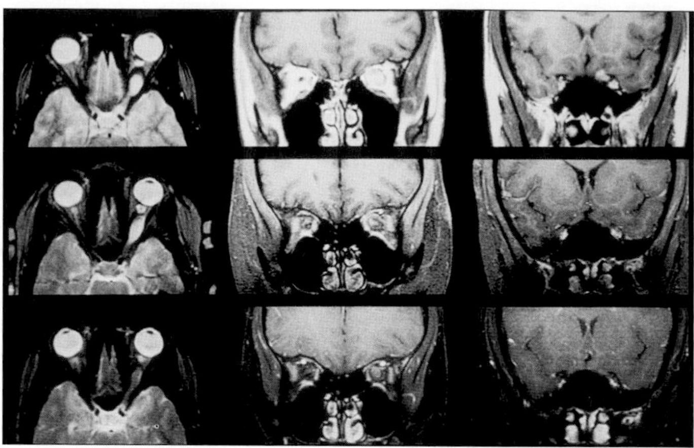

FIGURE 143.1. Spontaneous regression over the course of a year of an optic nerve glioma abutting the chiasm in a 14-year-old girl without neurofibromatosis.

REFERENCES

Brodsky MC: The 'pseudo-CSF' signal of orbital optic glioma on magnetic resonance imaging: a signature of neurofibromatosis. Surv Ophthalmol 38:213–218, 1993.

Fletcher WA, Imes RK, Hoyt WF: Chiasmal gliomas: appearance and long-term changes demonstrated by computerized tomography. J Neurosurg 65:154–159, 1986.

Glaser JS, Hoyt WF, Corbett J: Visual morbidity with chiasmal glioma: long-term studies of visual fields in untreated and irradiated cases. Arch Ophthalmol 85:3–12, 1971.

Hoyt WF, Baghdassarian SA: Optic glioma of childhood: natural history and rationale for conservative management. Br J Ophthalmol 53:793–798, 1969.

Imes RK, Hoyt WF: Childhood chiasmal gliomas: update on the fate of patients in the 1969 San Francisco study. Br J Ophthalmol 70:179–182, 1986.

Jakobiec FA, Depot MJ, Kennerdell J, et al: Combined clinical and computed tomographic diagnosis of orbital glioma and meningioma. Ophthalmology 91:137–155, 1984.

Parsa CF, Hoyt CS, Lesser RL, et al: Spontaneous regression of optic gliomas. Thirteen cases documented by serial neuroimaging. Arch Ophthalmol 119:516–529, 2001.

Russell A: A diencephalic syndrome of emaciation in infancy and childhood. Arch Dis Child 26:274, 1951.

Singh R, Trobe JD, Hayman JA, Deveikis JP: Ophthalmic artery occlusion secondary to radiation-induced vasculopathy. J Neuro-Ophthalmol 24:206–210, 2004.

Takeuchi H, Kabuto M, Sato K, Kubota T: Chiasmal gliomas with spontaneous regression: proliferation and apoptosis. Childs Nerv Syst 13:229–233, 1997.

144 ORBITAL RHABDOMYOSARCOMA 170.0 *(Malignant Rhabdomyoma, Myosarcoma, Rhabdomyoblastoma)*

Carol L. Shields, MD
Philadelphia, Pennsylvania
Jerry A. Shields, MD
Philadelphia, Pennsylvania

ETIOLOGY/INCIDENCE

Rhabdomyosarcoma is a highly malignant neoplasm that most often develops in the skeletal muscles of adults. The embryonal or alveolar varieties of this tumor have a tendency to affect the orbit and adjacent structures. The most characteristic presenting features of this orbital tumor include a fairly rapid onset of painless proptosis and inferotemporal displacement of the eye in a child. The mean age of presentation of orbital rhabdomyosarcoma is 8 years but this tumor can occur at birth and less often in adults. The tumor is generally unilateral and there is no racial predisposition. There is a slightly greater incidence in males. A palpable orbital mass is present in about 25% and ptosis in 33% of patients. The marked congestion and proptosis of the eye may cause diagnostic confusion with orbital trauma or inflammation.

Orbital rhabdomyosarcoma originates primarily in the orbital soft tissue but it can secondarily extend into the orbit from the adjacent ethmoid sinus or nasal cavity. Therefore some patients may have nasal congestion and epistaxis preceding the orbital findings. Rhabdomyosarcoma can occur anywhere in the orbit or adnexa, but it shows a tendency to involve the superonasal orbit. Occasionally it can arise inferiorly in the orbit or in the eyelids or conjunctiva. The clinical features tend to evolve rapidly over a few weeks due to the progressive growth of this neoplasm. When the disease is far advanced, facial and cervical lymph node metastases can occur. Regional lymph node metastasis is believed to be more common with the aggressive alveolar variant. Distant metastases of orbital rhabdomyosarcoma usually occurs through hematogeneous routes to various organs, particularly the lungs and bones.

- Etiology remains unclear but it is believed that this tumor arises from pluripotential mesenchyme in the orbit that normally differentiates into striated muscle.
- It is the most common soft tissue malignancy of childhood, accounting for approximately 4% of all childhood malignancies and 19% of all sarcomas.

COURSE/PROGNOSIS

Staging of rhabdomyosarcoma (Intergroup Rhabdomyosarcoma Study)

Group I — localized disease, completely resected.
Group II — regional disease (with or without lymph nodes involved) grossly resected.
Group III — incomplete resection or biopsy with gross residual disease.
Group IV — distant metastases (lung, bone marrow, brain, distant nodules).

The prognosis for life has improved over the past decades and is related to staging of the disease and histopathologic features. In an early series from the 1960s the survival was approximately 30%. More recent data indicates improved patient survival of 85% to 93%, using modern therapeutic modalities.

DIAGNOSIS

Clinical features

Clinical features include: proptosis, ptosis, ocular congestion, decreased extraocular motility.

Laboratory tests

- Blood tests:
  - Complete blood count to rule out pancytopenia from bone marrow infiltration;
  - Liver function tests to rule out liver metastases;
  - Renal function tests.
- Imaging tests:
  - Chest x-ray or computed tomography (CT) of the lung to rule out metastases;
  - Computed tomography or magnetic resonance imaging (MRI) of the orbit to assess the location and configuration of the tumor and plan the surgical approach. Both CT and MRI demonstrate an orbital mass that shows enhancement with contrast dye. It is uncommon to find bone erosion from this tumor.
- Pathology:
  - Gross features — firm yellow white tumor, often with hemorrhage;
  - Microscopic features — orbital rhabdomyosarcoma demonstrates tumor cells with cross striations within their cytoplasm. These striations are best appreciated with the Masson trichrome stain or the phosphotungstic acid-hematoxylin (PTAH) stain. Immunoperoxidase techniques assist in diagnosis by identifying desmin, myoglobulin, and actin. On electron microscopy the tumor cells can demonstrate thin (actin) myofilaments and thick (myosin) filaments. Characteristic muscle banding of A, I, and Z lines may be found.

Orbital rhabdomyosarcoma is classified into three histopathologic types as listed below, but often there is overlap of these types:

- Embryonal — found in nearly 70% cases and consists of loose and compact spindle cells; botryoid is a variant of embryonal pattern but located near the expandable conjunctival mucosa leading to a polypoid tumor;
- Alveolar — carries the worst prognosis and consists of loosely cohesive, poorly differentiated oval to round tumor cells arranged in a trabecular pattern resembling the alveoli of the lung;
- Pleomorphic — least common variant, consisting of variably sized, loosely arranged pleomorphic cells, often in association with muscles.

Clinical differential diagnosis

- Dermoid cyst.
- Orbital cellulites.
- Idiopathic orbital inflammation (pseudotumor).
- Capillary hemangioma.
- Lymphangioma.
- Orbital subperiosteal hematoma.
- Eosinophilic granuloma.
- Allergic fungal sinusitis.
- Metastatic neuroblastoma.
- Granulocytic sarcoma.
- Other rare conditions.

Pathologic differential diagnosis

- Fibrous histiocytoma.
- Fibrosarcoma.
- Nodular fasciitis.
- Malignant schwannoma.
- Leiomyosarcoma.
- Ewing's sarcoma.
- Metastatic neuroblastoma.
- Alveolar soft part sarcoma.
- Hemangiopericytoma.
- Granulocytic sarcoma.
- Lymphoma.
- Osteogenic sarcoma.
- Primitive neuroectodermal tumor (PNET).
- Other rare conditions.

PROPHYLAXIS

There is no known prevention of this disease. Rhabdomyosarcoma can occur as a second tumor in children with germinal mutation retinoblastoma.

TREATMENT

The treatment consists of local debulking of the orbital mass and adjuvant radiotherapy and chemotherapy. The combinations of various modalities must be individualized and depends on the specific extent of the disease. The disease progresses rapidly and treatment should be urgent. It is emphasized that the management of a child with rhabdomyosarcoma should be performed at a major oncology center with ocular oncologist and pediatric oncologist working in collaboration.

Local

Excisional biopsy — Orbital biopsy is performed with the intent to gently debulk as much tissue as possible for diagnostic and therapeutic purposes. The approach to the biopsy is dictated by the extent and accessibility of the tumor both clinically and on imaging studies.

Radiotherapy

- External beam radiotherapy — this is delivered to the orbit over 4 to 6 weeks for a total dose of 4000 cGy to 6000 cGy.
- Gamma knife radiotherapy — this new technique may have potential for orbital rhabdomyosarcoma but has not yet been reported.
- Orbital exenteration — This is reserved for aggressive recurrent disease. An eyelid sparing technique provides the most acceptable cosmetic appearance.

Systemic

Chemotherapy

- The most frequently used chemotherapy regimen is the VAC protocol:
  - Vincristine;

- Dactinomycin (Actinomycin-D);
- Cyclophosphamide.

COMPLICATIONS

The complications of uncontrolled rhabdomyosarcoma could cost the patient his or her life. However, the complications of treatment of this malignancy can be very destructive to the eye and orbit as well as the surrounding tissue. Excisional biopsy of the mass can lead to ptosis, diplopia, strabismus, and vision loss. Radiotherapy has side effects of cilia loss, cutaneous erythema, dry eye symptoms, cataract, retinopathy, papillopathy, neovascular glaucoma, orbital volume loss and visual loss. The orbital bones may be slowed in their growth due to radiotherapy. The systemic side effects of chemotherapy with bone marrow suppression, risk for infection and other short and long term effects should be realized.

COMMENTS

Orbital rhabdomyosarcoma is the most common primary orbital malignancy of childhood. It is characterized by rapid proptosis in an otherwise healthy child. Early diagnosis of the tumor is important to facilitate proper treatment and provide the best life prognosis. Management decisions are best approached by a coordination of multispecialists at major oncology centers.

REFERENCES

Abramson DH, Ellsworth RM, Tretter P, et al: The treatment of orbital rhabdomyosarcoma with irradiation and chemotherapy. Ophthalmology 86:1330–1335, 1979.

Fiorillo A, Migliorati R, Grimaldi M, et al: Multidisciplinary treatment of primary orbital rhabdomyosarcoma. Cancer 67:560–563, 1991.

Jones IS, Reese AB, Kraut J: Orbital rhabdomyosarcoma. An analysis of 62 cases. Am J Ophthalmol 61:721–736, 1966.

Shields CL, Shields JA, Honavar SG, Demirci H: The clinical spectrum of primary ophthalmic rhabdomyosarcoma. Ophthalmology 108:2284–2292, 2001.

Shields JA, Shields CL: Rhabdomyosarcoma: review for the ophthalmologist. Surv Ophthalmol 48:39–57, 2003.

Wharam M, Beltangady M, Hays D, et al: Localized orbital rhabdomyosarcoma. An interim report of the Intergroup Rhabdomyosarcoma Study Committee. Ophthalmology 94:251–254, 1987.

145 PAPILLOMA 078.1
(Wart, Verrucous Lesion)

Maristela Amaral Palazzi, MD, PhD

São Paulo, Brazil

ETIOLOGY/INCIDENCE

Papilloma is an acquired benign lesion that may affect the skin and mucous membranes especially those of genitourinary and respiratory tract, oral cavity and ocular surface.

Human papillomaviruses (HPVs) are a wide group of DNA viruses that have been recognized as the main cause or at least as an important cofactor in the genesis of benign and malignant epithelial neoplasm in humans, including the papilloma.

In the eye, HPV has been considereded as an important factor for the development of the conjunctival papilloma. Some oncogenic HPV types have been detected in carcinomas of the conjunctiva and lacrimal sac and in some sporadic retinoblastoma.

HPV is normally spread by contact, however, the transmission route of HPV to the conjunctiva is still object of investigation. Fetal contact with infected maternal tissue or fluids might be a way of direct transmission. Autoinoculation is another probable transmission mode and may result in multicentric infection.

There is no predilection for race, but a male preponderance has been found among patients with conjunctival papilloma.

The reported frequency of HPV DNA in conjunctival papilloma varies from 50% to 100%.

The HPV types found in papillomas of the conjunctiva are mainly HPV-6, 11, and less frequently HPVs 18, 33 and 16, considered a potent human carcinogen.

The lesions identified in children and young adults are always benign and often associated to HPV infection caused by HPV types 6 and 11. Papillomas seen in adults and older patients may also harbour HPV-16 or may not have a viral origin according to some authors.

PRESENTATION

Papillomas may affect one or both eyes and appear as isolated or multiple lesions of variable sizes. The main sites of involvement are the fornices (especially the inferior ones) followed by:

- Bulbar conjunctiva;
- Lacrimal caruncle;
- Lacrimal sac, puncta or canaliculus;
- Lid skin margin.

Lesions are redish (conjunctiva) or grayish (skin) and can be sessile or pedunculated with multiple tiny 'finger-like' projections (raspberry like).

Conjunctival papillomas tend to be sessile in adults and pedunculated in children. Although pedunculated papillomas most frequently are located in the fornix and sessile papillomas in the bulbar conjunctiva, both types may develop anywhere in the conjunctiva.

COURSE/PROGNOSIS

Some lesions may regress spontaneously without treatment, especially in children, while recurrences are often noted in many patients.

Papilloma should not be left untreated for many years in older patients once some lesions have shown malignant transformation.

DIAGNOSIS

The clinical appearence of a papilloma is very characteristic, however, the histologic evaluation is necessary to avoid misdiagnosis, especially in older patients.

Clinical signs and symptoms

Patients may be asymptomatic or may present mild to moderate symptoms, depending on the extent, location and size of the lesion(s). Among common signs and symptoms are:

- Tearing;
- Foreign body sensation;
- Mild to moderate itching;
- Mucous discharge;
- Hyperemia.

Sometimes the lesion may assume such a large volume that can interfere with the eyelid apposition breaking the integrity of the lacrimal film, causing:

- Punctata epithelial keratitis; or
- Diffuse conjunctivitis.

Large sessile papilloma may also spread onto the cornea and interfere with visual acuity.

Microscopically, these lesions are composed of multiple branching fronds emanating from a narrow base (pediculated) or a broad base (sessile). Each frond has a central vascularized core surrounded by connective tissue in which acute and chronic inflammatory cells are often found. In both types the fronds are covered by acanthotic, non-keratinizing, stratified squamous epithelium that is not atypical.

Differential diagnosis

Some benign and malignant lesions may present a papillomatous growth mimetizing a papilloma such as:

- Capillary hemangioma;
- Pyogenic granuloma;
- Squamous cell carcinoma (bulbar conjunctiva);
- Sebaceous cell carcinoma (caruncle, tarsal conjunctiva).

Laboratory findings

Various authors have analysed conjunctival papilloma for presence of HPV, and HPV types 6, 11, and less frequently HPV-16, 18 and 33 have been found.

Infection by multiple subtypes of HPV has also been described in papillomas.

The detection and typing of HPV has been done, nowadays, through PCR assays using consensus primers and techniques of molecular hybridization due to its high sensitivity and specificity for HPV types.

TREATMENT

Observation may be an option to treatment for asymptomatic or mildly symptomatic small lesions, once some viral papilloma may spontaneously regress over time, especially in children. However, when the lesion shows progressive growth or disturbing symptoms it should be treated.

Local treatment

- Surgical excision.
- Cryotherapy.

The association of both modalities offer advantages over the single procedure and is the technique of choice of many physicians, mainly for isolated primary lesions. It is associated with fewer recurrences and allows histopathologic diagnosis.

- Topical drugs.

Topical drugs have been used as adjunct or alternative therapy especially in cases of diffuse, large or recurrent lesions. Regression of lesions and reduction of recurrences have been observed after the use of topical antimetabolic agents such as mitomycin C (MMC) and topical immunotherapy with alfa-interferon (IFNα2b).

Treatment regimen and precautions may be similar to those employed to manage ocular surface squamous neoplasia.

- Mitomycin (MMC): A two-week course of topical mitomycin C (0.02mg/mL, 4 times daily at postoperative day 7) has proved to be useful as adjuvant treatment to avoid and manage recurrent conjunctival papillomas.

Reversible side effects include conjunctival discomfort, hyperemia, punctate epithelial keratopathy and blepharospasm. Superficial keratitis is a common and transitory early side effect. MMC is generally safe, but has the potential for causing serious ocular complications if not used as prescribed.

Overdose may cause side effects such as corneal toxicity, scleral thining, cataract and iritis. Sometimes complications can occur many years after its application.

Warnings and recommendations:

- Although successfull intraoperative application of MMC has been related in the literature, complications can develop when MMC is used with open conjunctival wounds or used excessively.
- Preplacement of punctual plugs to protect the nasopharyngeal tissue from exposure to this potentially toxic agent has been recommended.
  - Interferon alfa-2b (IFN α-2b)
- Topical interferon (IFN α-2b) has been used succesfully in the treatment of conjunctival papilloma and intraepithelial neoplasia (1–2.8 million IU/mL, 4 times daily until resolution is observed which and continued for a month thereafter). Long periods of treatment up to 1 year have been described. Interferon has been considered an effective nontoxic alternative therapy, especially useful for treating residual, diffuse, multifocal or recurrent lesions.
- The possible side effect of topical application of interferon is superficial keratitis. This drug has the advantage of having few side effects, no carcinogenic potential, and no corneal toxicity when applied topically. However, once interferon treatment is considered more suppressive than curative, long-term follow-up is required even after lesions have disappeared.

Systemic treatment

Oral cimetidine

Cimetidine is a histamine2 receptor antagonist used primarily to treat peptic ulcer disease. However, due to its immunemodulation properties it has been used succesfully to treat other disorders such as virally induced cutaneous warts and conjunctival papillomatosis. Authors have reported dramatic regression of a recurrent diffuse papillomatosis, employing oral cimetidine for 4 months (30 mg/kg/day in three divided doses), without local or systemic side effects and recurrences.

For those lesions that show recurrence, oral cimetidine for several months can resolve the papillomavirus-related tumor by boosting the patient's immune system and stimulating regression of the mass.

COMMENTS

Recurrences are common, so, all care must be taken to avoid seeding of viral particles during the surgical removal of a papilloma.

Histopathological analysis of lesions is always advisable in adults to avoid misdiagnosis with malignant tumors.

FUTURE PERSPECTIVES

HPV vaccines with both prophylatic and therapeutic potential are being developed and some are already being tested in gynecologic patients. This has been considered a promising perspective in the management of HPV associated tumors.

REFERENCES

Basti S, Macsai MS: Ocular surface squamous neoplasia — a review. Cornea 22(7):687–704, 2003.

Burnier MN, Jr, Correia CP, Mc Cartney ACE: Tumors of the eye and ocular adnexae, In: Fletcher CDM, ed: Diagnostic histopathology of tumors. London, Churchill Livingstone, 2001.

de Keizer RJW, de Wolff-Rouendaal D: Topical α-interferon in recurrent conjunctival papilloma. Acta Ophthalmologica Scandinavica 81:193–196, 2003.

IARC monographs on the evaluation of carcinogenic risks to human. Human papillomaviruses. Lyon, France: International Agency for Research on Cancer, 1995:64.

Koutsky LA, Ault KA, Wheeler CM, et al: A Controlled trial of a human papillomavirus type 16 vaccine. N Engl J Med 347(21):1645–1651, 2002.

Nakamura Y, Mashima Y, Kameyama K, et al: Detection of human papillomavirus infection in squamous tumours of the conjunctiva and lacrimal sac by immunohistochemistry, *in situ* hybridization, and polymerase chain reaction.Br J Ophthalmol 81:308–313, 1997.

Palazzi MA, Yunes JA, Cardinalli IA, et al: Detection of oncogenic human papillomavirus in sporadic retinoblastoma. Acta Ophthalmol Scand 81:396–398, 2003.

Parkarian F, Kaye J, Cason J, et al: Cancer associated human papillomaviruses: perinatal transmission and persistence. Br J Obst Gynecol 101:514–517, 1994.

Shields CL, Shields JA: Tumors of the conjunctiva and cornea. Surv Ophthalmol 49(1):3–24, 2004.

Sjö NC, Heegaard S, Prause JU, et al: Human papillomavirus in conjunctival papilloma. Br J Ophthalmol 85:785–787, 2001.

Wilson FM, Ostler HB: Conjunctival papilloma in siblings. Am J Ophthalmol 77:103–107, 1994.

Yuen HKL, Yeung EFY, Chan NR, et al: The use of postoperative topical Mitomycin C in the treatment of recurrent conjunctival papilloma. Cornea 21(8):838–839, 2002.

146 PERIOCULAR MERKEL CELL CARCINOMA 173.9

(Cutaneous Neuroendocrine Carcinoma, Endocrine Carcinoma of the Skin, Small Cell Skin Carcinoma, Trabecular Carcinoma)

Tero Kivelä, MD, FEBO
Helsinki, Finland

ETIOLOGY/INCIDENCE

Merkel cell carcinoma is an aggressive primary cutaneous neoplasm that frequently involves the eyelids and periocular region; tumors in these locations account for 10% of all cases. Since 1990, about 175 periocular Merkel cell carcinomas have been reported; however, this tumor is now well known and not all cases enter the literature.

Most periocular Merkel cell carcinomas develop in the eyelids and canthal region, preferentially in the upper eyelid; the remainder occur in the eyebrows. Merkel cell carcinoma metastatic to the eyelid, orbit, choroid and ciliary body has been described.

The median age of patients with eyelid tumors is 76 years, with an age range from 14 to 102 years, and two thirds are women. The tumor is extremely rare in Africans and Asians.

Human immunodeficiency virus infection, therapeutic immunosuppression (e.g. after renal and cardiac transplantation, in rheumatoid arthritis), chronic lymphocytic leukemia and chronic sunlight and arsenic exposure predispose also younger individuals and non-Caucasians to develop Merkel cell carcinoma.

Merkel cell carcinomas are ascribed to an epidermal stem cell common to keratocytes and Merkel's cells, specialized epidermal cells with neuroendocrine features associated with nerve endings in touch receptors.

- In the eyelids, single Merkel's cells occur in the epidermis, the outer root sheaths of hairs and eyelashes and the dermis.
- Aggregates of Merkel's cells, called *touch spots,* occur regularly at the palpebral margin between successive eyelashes.

COURSE/PROGNOSIS

A meta-analysis was performed of 112 patients with a Merkel cell carcinoma of the eyelid.

- The primary tumors grew rapidly, with a median history of 3 months; the range was from a few weeks to 3 years.
- Based on life-table analysis, a local recurrence in the eyelid or orbit developed in 30% of patients in 2 years; repeated recurrences were common.
- Regional metastases to ipsilateral preauricular, submandibular, cervical and jugulodigastric lymph nodes developed in 38% and 47% of patients in 2 and 5 years, respectively; systemic metastasis was often heralded by regional lymph node involvement.
- Systemic metastases most commonly affect the liver, bone, lungs, skin, and brain but may occur in any location.
- The cumulative 2- and 5-year survival rate was 81% and 68%, respectively. Survival was worse for patients who experienced a local relapse; mortality rates are decreasing with better recognition and more radical treatment of primary Merkel cell carcinoma.

These figures correlate closely both with those reported for Merkel cell carcinoma in general and with those of 28 patients who had eyebrow lesions. There is no firm evidence that periocular Merkel cell carcinoma has a better-than-average prognosis.

DIAGNOSIS

Clinical signs and symptoms

- A solitary, painless, nontender dermal skin nodule rapidly develops close to the lid margin or eyebrow. It is bulging or protuberant but may be pedunculated; it typically spares the eyelashes; and it rarely ulcerates the skin.

- Reddish or purplish erythematous skin and telangiectatic vessels from associated inflammation and possible invasion of local lymphatic vessels are highly characteristic and often imitate chalazion.
- Because of frequent lymph node metastasis, palpation and imaging of regional lymph nodes is mandatory; consideration should be given to sentinel node biopsy undertaken by an oculoplastic surgeon, plastic surgeon and pathologist familiar with this procedure.

Laboratory findings

- Histopathologic diagnosis is based on the presence of neuroendocrine granules and whorls of intermediate filaments by electron microscopy and on coexpression of cytokeratins, neurofilaments, and neuroendocrine markers by immunohistochemistry.

Differential diagnosis

Most periocular Merkel cell carcinomas are unidentified or misdiagnosed clinically.

- Chalazion is a frequent misdiagnosis.
- Other repeated clinical misdiagnoses include papilloma, hemangioma and basal cell carcinoma.
- Typical histopathologic misdiagnoses are large cell lymphoma and metastatic small cell lung carcinoma.

PROPHYLAXIS

- Protection of skin from excessive sunlight and burning; this will also reduce the incidence of other, more common skin cancers.
- Immunosuppressed patients can be cautioned about higher than average risk of skin cancer, including Merkel cell carcinoma, to expedite diagnosis.

TREATMENT

Prompt initial therapy is a prerequisite for a favorable outcome.

Systemic

- Chemotherapy is an effective treatment for extensive local or recurrent, as well as metastatic, Merkel cell carcinoma, but progressive disease after cessation of therapy is common.
- Chemotherapy regimens are continuously evolving, and the choice of treatment should be delegated to experts in cancer chemotherapy.
- Irradiation with or without chemotherapy is an effective palliative treatment for systemic metastases. It has fewer complications than chemotherapy and is likewise associated with risk of recurrence.

Ocular

- Uveal metastases respond well to radiation.

Medical

- In selected cases, irradiation may be successfully used as primary therapy to avoid extensive plastic surgery and chemotherapy in elderly or debilitated persons.

Surgical

- Full-thickness resection of eyelid tumors and wide resection of other periocular tumors with a 5-mm margin, followed by appropriate plastic surgical reconstruction, is recommended.
- Frozen section control is useful to ensure the deep margin of excision, but it does not guard against early lateral spread through lymphatic vessels.
- Because of very frequent lymphatic infiltration, prophylactic irradiation with 50 Gy in 20 to 25 fractions to the tissues between the tumor bed and local lymph nodes is recommended.
- Routine prophylactic lymph node dissection without sentinel node biopsy is not recommended.
- Radical neck dissection for proved regional lymph node metastases, with or without irradiation and chemotherapy, is recommended because it may result in a permanent cure.
- Consider exenteration for orbital recurrence in the absence of systemic metastases.

COMPLICATIONS

Some patients have died as a result of the chemotherapy regimens, and irradiation may be a better method of palliative therapy in selected cases.

COMMENTS

- Chalazia are rare in elderly people and should always undergo a biopsy to exclude Merkel cell or sebaceous carcinoma.
- A systemic workup is mandatory to exclude the possibility of a primary cancer elsewhere, especially to rule out metastatic Merkel cell or small cell lung carcinoma to the eyelid.
- Patients must be followed carefully for evidence of recurrent disease and regional or systemic metastases.

SUPPORT GROUPS

None identified. A general resource for skin cancer is provided by The Skin Cancer Foundation, New York, NY, URL www.skincancer.org

REFERENCES

Alexander E, 3rd, Rossitch E, Jr, Small K, et al: Merkel cell carcinoma. Long term survival in a patient with proven brain metastasis and presumed choroid metastasis. Clin Neurol Neurosurg 91:317–320, 1989.

Kivelä T, Tarkkanen A: The Merkel cell and associated neoplasms in the eyelids and periocular region. Surv Ophthalmol 35:171–187, 1990.

Mehrany K, Otley CC, Weenig RH, et al: A meta-analysis of the prognostic significance of sentinel lymph node status in Merkel cell carcinoma. Dermatol Surg 28:113–117, 2002.

Miller RW, Rabkin CS: Merkel cell carcinoma and melanoma: etiological similarities and differences. Cancer Epidemiol Biomarkers Prev 8:153–158, 1999.

Mortier L, Mirabel X, Fournier C, et al: Radiotherapy alone for primary Merkel cell carcinoma. Arch Dermatol 139:1587–1590, 2003.

Poulsen M: Merkel-cell carcinoma of the skin. Lancet Oncol 5:593–599, 2004.

Poulsen M, Rischin D, Walpole E, et al: High-risk Merkel cell carcinoma of the skin treated with synchronous carboplatin/etoposide and radiation: a Trans-Tasman Radiation Oncology Group Study — TROG 96:07. J Clin Oncol 21:4371–4376, 2003.

Veness MJ, Perera L, McCourt J, et al: Merkel cell carcinoma: improved outcome with adjuvant radiotherapy. Austr N Z J Surg 75:275–281, 2005.

147 RETINOBLASTOMA 190.5

F. Hampton Roy, MD, FACS
Little Rock, Arkansas

ETIOLOGY/INCIDENCE

Retinoblastoma is the most common intraocular malignancy of childhood. The incidence is 1 in 17,000 live births, which results in about 300 new cases in the United States each year. The overall survival rate is greater than 90%. The vast majority of patients present by the age of 2 years, and rarely affects older children.

The disease takes two distinct forms that have the same final common pathway: a malignant tumor arising from the retina. In approximately one third of affected patients, multifocal primary tumors form in both eyes. Children with the bilateral form of the disease harbor a germinal mutation, and this form of the disease is hereditable. In addition, these children are genetically prone to develop secondary nonocular carcinomas, most commonly osteosarcoma. The *RB* gene product is important in normal cell cycle control. The gene that is responsible for the *RB* protein has been cloned and is known to reside at band 14 on the long arm of chromosome 13. In the hereditary form of the disease, the affected child is born with one inactive allele of the *RB* gene in all cells of the body. A random second event inactivates the second allele and leads to the development of the tumor in the proliferating retina; thus, the children are prone to the development of multiple tumors in each eye. Of those with the germinal mutation, only 25% have a known positive family history. The vast majority of bilateral disease represents a new germline mutation.

Approximately 60% to 70% of cases are unifocal and unilateral. The vast majority of these children do not harbor the germinal mutation. In this population, a single carcinoma develops as the consequence of two spontaneous mutations in a single retinal cell that inactivate both alleles of the *RB* gene. These children will not pass the disease onto offspring and are not at any risk of developing second nonocular carcinomas. The genetic properties of this disease were accurately predicted by a statistician long before the gene was actually cloned (Knudson two-hit hypothesis).

Unfortunately, based on clinical presentation alone, it is not always possible to distinguish the two forms of retinoblastoma. From 10% to 15% of children with uniocular and unifocal disease secretly harbor the germinal mutation. A small percentage of individuals who carry the germinal mutation do not develop any intraocular cancers. The *RB* gene has been cloned and sequenced; it is very large, consisting of more than 200,000 base pairs. The functioning gene is an essential component of the normal regulation of cell growth. Many different mutations have been found that are known to cause disease. In many individuals, it is possible to identify the specific mutation and thus screen family members to determine who is at risk for developing retinoblastoma. Prenatal diagnosis is possible if the specific mutation has been identified within a family.

COURSE/PROGNOSIS

Retinoblastoma charactistically tends to remain intraocular until later stages, when it exits the eye either directly through invasion of the optic nerve or via blood-borne metastasis, most commonly to the bone marrow. Direct extension or metastasis is unlikely early in the course of the disease. Untreated, the tumors are almost uniformly fatal; successful treatment while the tumor is completely confined within the eye correlates with a very high survival rate.

The Reese–Ellsworth classification at this time is most commonly used to compare treatment results. Group I includes solitary (A) and multiple (B) tumors less than 4 disk diameters (dd) in size, located at or behind the equator. Group II includes solitary (A) and multiple (B) tumors of 4 to 10 dd, located at or behind the equator. Group III includes any tumor anterior to the equator (A) and solitary tumors of more than 10 dd behind the equator (B). Group IV includes multiple tumors of more than 10 dd (A) and any tumors extending to the ora serrata (B). Group V includes massive tumor involvement of more than half the retina (A) and vitreous seeding (B). A new classification system is being developed and may be in use in the near future.

DIAGNOSIS

Laboratory findings

The most common presenting sign of retinoblastoma is leukocoria (60%) and the second most common sign is strabismus (20%). Rarely, the tumor presents as a mimic of orbital cellulitis. Hyphema and tumor involvement of the anterior segment are also seen.

Any lesion in the posterior segment of a child's eye should raise the possibility of retinoblastoma. Characteristically, the tumor is creamy-white and nodular with vascularization and is easily identifiable based on appearance. However, the tumor can fragment into the vitreous cavity as isolated cells or masses of cells (vitreous seeds). In extreme cases, the tumor can appear as a diffuse vitritis or an inflammatory process, making the diagnosis difficult. In addition, the tumor may cause retinal detachment and complete distortion of the posterior pole. The term *exophytic* connotes a tumor growth pattern toward the subretinal space, and the term *endophytic* connotes growth toward the vitreous cavity. Intraocular biopsy for a diagnosis in an eye potentially harboring a retinoblastoma is contraindicated because this may lead to spread outside of the previously confined tumor.

In almost all suspected cases, a computed tomography (CT) scan of the head and orbit should be obtained. Calcification on the CT scan is a hallmark of the disease. Ultrasound may also be used for identifying calcification. Magnetic resonance imaging is useful in identifying the presence and extent of extraocular disease. A pinealoblastoma (trilateral retinoblastoma) is a rare secondary nonocular malignancy that may be found with central nervous system imaging. In cases in which the optic nerve is not easily visible or if metastatic disease is suspected, lumbar puncture and bone marrow aspiration and biopsy should be performed at the time of diagnosis.

A complete and detailed pedigree should be obtained to include a family history of eye disease and ocular and systemic cancer. Dysfunction of the *RB* gene has been noted to correlate with the development of other cancers, including osteosarcoma. Both parents should undergo dilated fundus examinations. Spontaneous regression is rare but does occur; therefore, an 'asymptomatic' parent may harbor signs of this spontaneously regressed disease. Siblings of an affected child should be examined. The frequency of these examinations depend on the statistical likelihood that a germinal mutation is present in the family.

Differential diagnosis

- Coats' disease.
- *Toxocara.*
- Toxoplasmosis.
- Norrie's disease.
- Medulloepithelioma.
- Leukemia.
- Malignant melanoma.
- Inflammatory lesion of posterior pole (cysticercosis).

TREATMENT

Medical therapy should be directed toward complete control of the tumor and the preservation of as much useful vision as possible. Treatment usually is individualized to the specific patient.

Unilateral retinoblastoma with a poor prognosis for vision usually is treated with enucleation. If the tumor has not invaded the optic nerve and there is no evidence of extraocular disease, then usually no further treatment is given (survival rate of greater than 90%). However, there is debate over the prognostic significance of histopathologic choroidal invasion. The patient with optic nerve invasion past the lamina cribrosa usually is treated with systemic chemotherapy after surgery; if the tumor is evident past the surgical line of transection, then orbital radiation is added to the regimen. Optic nerve involvement decreases the prognosis for survival to 60%, and disease past the line of transection decreases the survival rate to less than 20% even with additional treatments. Great care should be taken to avoid perforation of an eye harboring a retinoblastoma during enucleation (thus converting an intraocular retinoblastoma to extraocular disease). Efforts should be made to obtain the longest possible section of optic nerve at the time of enucleation.

Bilateral disease often presents a greater challenge in terms of preserving life and vision. These patients are genetically prone to second primary carcinomas; therefore, there is a great emphasis on treatment methods that will not enhance the lifelong risk of secondary carcinomas. Retinoblastomas are extremely sensitive to external beam radiation, but that treatment is associated with a lifelong increased risk of second primary carcinomas. For this reason, external beam radiation is no longer the initial treatment of choice of retinoblastoma.

Primary systemic chemotherapy (carboplatin, etoposide, and vincristine) to reduce tumor volume followed by local methods such as cryotherapy and laser photocoagulation, both hyperthermia and ablation, has been shown to be very effective in eradicating nondisseminated intraocular disease. The long-term effect of this regimen on the incidence of secondary carcinomas is unknown.

- Systemic chemotherapy plus local therapy (cryotherapy, laser, plaque).
- Enucleation.
- External-beam irradiation (4000 cGy); this is very effective for posterior tumors; increases the risk for second nonocular tumors.
- ^{125}I radioactive plaque.
- Locally directed; minimizes radiation to normal tissue; useful for small nondisseminated tumors.
- Cryotherapy.
- Especially effective for small anterior tumors.
- Laser photocoagulation.
- Directly over tumor.
- Ablative.
- Gentle heating (facilitates effect of chemotherapy).
- Hyperthermia.

COMPLICATIONS

Complications include secondary nonocular cancer, cataract (radiation), radiation retinopathy, radiation optic neuropathy, and bone marrow suppression (chemotherapy, increased risk of infection, and bleeding).

COMMENTS

Strategies for the treatment of bilateral disease are often complex and depend on the patient's age, tumor size and location, and vitreous involvement. Children with retinoblastomas should be managed by a team that includes an ophthalmologist, a pediatric oncologist, a radiation oncologist, a social worker, and a genetic counselor. This team should be composed of professionals who are familiar with this disease.

REFERENCES

Abramson DH, Greenfield DS, Ellsworth RM: Bilateral retinoblastoma: correlation between age at diagnosis and time course for new intraocular tumors. Ophthalmol Pediatr Genet 1:7, 1992.

Beck MN, Balmer A, Dessing C, et al: First-line chemotherapy with local treatment can prevent external-beam irradiation and enucleation in low-stage intraocular retinoblastoma. J Clin Oncol Aug 18(15):2881–2887, 2000.

DiCiommo D, Gallie BL, Bremner R: Retinoblastoma: the disease, gene and protein provide critical leads to understand cancer. Semin Cancer Biol 10(4):255–269, 2000.

Friedman DL, Himelstein B, Shields CL, et al: Chemoreduction and local ophthalmic therapy for intraocular retinoblastoma. J Clin Oncol 18(1):12–17, 2000.

Gallie BL, Budning A, Deboer G, et al: Chemotherapy with focal therapy can cure intraocular retinoblastomas without radiotherapy. Arch Ophthalmol 114:1321–1328, 1996.

Kingston JE, Hungerford JL, Madreperla SA, Plowman PN: Results of combined chemotherapy and radiotherapy for advanced intraocular retinoblastoma. Arch Ophthalmol 114:1339–1343, 1996.

MacDonald DJ, Lessick M: Hereditary cancers in children and ethical and psychosocial implications. J Pediatr Nurs 15(4):217–225, 2000.

Murphree AL, Villablanca JG, Deegan WF, et al: Chemotherapy plus local treatment in the management of intraocular retinoblastoma. Arch Ophthalmol 114:1348–1356, 1996.

Noorani HZ, Khan HN, Gallie BL, Detsky AS: Cost comparison of molecular versus conventional screening of relatives at risk for retinoblastoma. Am J Hum Genet 59:301–307, 1996.

Shields CL, Shields JA, Meadows AT: Chemoreduction for retinoblastoma may prevent trilateral retinoblastoma. J Clin Oncol 18(1):236–237, 2000.

148 SEBACEOUS GLAND CARCINOMA 173.9

Roger A. Dailey, MD
Portland, Oregon
John D. Ng, MD, MS, FACS
Portland, Oregon

ETIOLOGY/INCIDENCE

Sebaceous gland carcinoma is a rare epithelial tumor with a proclivity for occurring on the eyelids. It accounts for fewer than 1% of all eyelid tumors and 1.5% to 5% of malignant epithelial eyelid neoplasms in the United States. This low rate is in contrast to a 28% incidence rate of lid cancers that are sebaceous carcinomas in Shanghai and reports of sebaceous carcinomas being the second most common eyelid malignancy in Singapore. This tumor is 57% to 77% more common in women than in men.

Sebaceous gland carcinoma is life threatening and can be a diagnostic and management challenge to the ophthalmologist and pathologist. The 5-year tumor-related mortality rate has been reported to be as high as 30%.

Stepwise accumulation of genetic damage has been theorized to be the cause, and mutational inactivation of *p53* has been shown to be related to the progression of sebaceous carcinoma. DNA studies confirm that sebaceous tumors with pagetoid involvement demonstrate aneuploidy, which is characteristic of highly aggressive tumors.

This tumor is thought to arise from the Meibomian glands and glands of Zeiss of the eyelid, but it can also appear in the eyebrow, caruncle, conjunctiva, and lacrimal gland and in other areas of the face where tiny hair follicles are associated with sebaceous glands. It occurs twice as often on the upper as on the lower eyelid, which reflects the predominance of meibomian glands in the upper eyelid.

Unlike basal cell and squamous cell carcinomas, no link between ultraviolet light exposure and sebaceous cell carcinoma has been established.

Previous radiation therapy to the eyelids also is a risk factor for the development of sebaceous carcinoma.

COURSE/PROGNOSIS

- This tumor generally presents in women beyond the sixth decade of life as a localized nontender tumefaction of the eyelid or chronic unilateral blepharoconjunctivitis.
- Occasionally, there is history of treatment for one or more 'recurrent' chalazia.
- If not diagnosed early and cured with simple excision, these lesions can go on to involve multiple anterior orbital structures and the lacrimal drainage system.
- Sebaceous gland carcinoma tends to disseminate by way of the lymphatic vessels to the regional preauricular or cervical lymph nodes. If the tumor becomes very advanced, hematogenous spread to distant organs such as the lung, liver and brain has been reported.
- These tumors may be associated with Torre–Muir syndrome (sebaceous gland tumors and visceral malignancy).
- If diagnosed in a much younger population, human immunodeficiency virus infection should be suspected.
- The site of origin of the sebaceous carcinoma does not seem to be of prognostic significance in the periocular region; however, sebaceous gland carcinomas in non-eyelid skin have a much better prognosis.
- Tumors of the lower eyelid (low mortality rate) have a better prognosis than those of the upper lid (27% mortality rate). If both lids are involved, the mortality rate is as high as 83%.
- Poor prognostic factors include vascular or lymphatic invasion, orbital extension, poor differentiation, involvement of both the upper and lower eyelids, multicentric origin, duration of symptoms for longer than 6 months, highly infiltrative pattern, tumor diameter of greater than 10 mm, and involvement limited to the conjunctiva.
- Rao reported a 50% mortality rate in patients with pagetoid involvement and an 11% mortality rate in patients without pagetoid disease. In addition, there was a 7% mortality rate for well-differentiated tumors and a 60% mortality rate for poorly differentiated tumors.

DIAGNOSIS

Examination may show area of yellowish discoloration with loss of lashes (madarosis).

Definitive proof of this entity can be established by biopsy. A full-thickness biopsy probably should be performed on any patient with chronic, nonhealing chalazia or suspicious unresolving chronic blepharitis. The pathologist should be alerted to the suspected diagnosis.

Differential diagnosis

Differential diagnosis includes recurrent chalazia, carcinoma *in situ*, blepharoconjunctivitis, cutaneous horn, pyogenic granulomas, metastatic lesions, squamous cell carcinoma and basal cell carcinoma.

TREATMENT

- Tumor excision guided by frozen section or Mohs' technique appears to have the highest success rate.
- Because these tumors are often multicentric, conjunctival map biopsies may be used to determine pagetoid spread.
- Adjunctive cryotherapy may be useful in the treatment of residual intraepithelial pagetoid spread in the conjunctival sac.
- With significant orbital invasion, exenteration is recommended. If there is regional lymphadenopathy, other systemic evaluation is negative; then, radical neck lymph node dissection, parotidectomy, and postoperative radiation therapy should be considered.
- These tumors are generally considered radioresistant, and this method alone is generally reserved for palliative care in patients who are not surgical candidates. Occasional cures have been reported with the use of as much as 9800 cGy.
- Sentinel lymph node biopsy may be useful for prognostic purposes.

COMMENTS

Sebaceous gland carcinoma has the potential to produce significant morbidity and mortality rates. Early diagnosis facilitated by clinical suspicion is the key to successful surgical intervention at an early stage. Chronic unilateral blepharitis or recurrent chalazia should always trigger a histopathologic evaluation to ensure that a sebaceous cell carcinoma is not 'masquerading' as one of these benign entities.

REFERENCES

Doxanas MT, Green R: Sebaceous gland carcinoma. Arch Ophthalmol 102:245–249, 1984.

Gonzales-Fernandez F, Kaltreider SA, Patnaik BD, et al: Sebaceous carcinoma tumor progression through mutational inactivation of *p53*. Ophthalmology 105:497–506, 1998.

Khan JA, Grove AS, Joseph MP, Goodman M: Sebaceous carcinoma. Ophthalmic Plast Reconstr Surg 5:227–234, 1989.

Lisman RD, Jakobiec FA, Small P: Sebaceous carcinoma of the eyelids. Ophthalmology 96:1021–1026, 1989.

Nijhawan N, Ross MI, Diba R, et al: Experience with sentinel lymph node biopsy for eyelid and conjunctival malignancies at a cancer center. Ophthal Plast Reconstr Surg 20:291–295, 2004.

Nunery WR, Welsh MG, McCord CD: Recurrence of sebaceous carcinoma of the eyelid after radiation therapy. Am J Ophthalmol 96:10–15, 1983.

Putterman AM: Conjunctival map biopsy to determine pagetoid spread. Am J Ophthalmol 102:87–90, 1986.

Sakol PJ, Simons KB, McFadden PW, et al: DNA flow cytometry of sebaceous cell carcinomas of the ocular adnexa: introduction to the technique in the evaluation of periocular tumors. Ophthalmic Plast Reconstr Surg 8:77–87, 1992.

Yeatts RP, Waller RR: Sebaceous carcinoma of the eyelid: pitfalls in diagnosis. Ophthalmic Plast Reconstr Surg 1:35–42, 1985.

Yen MT, Tse DT: Sebaceous cell carcinoma of the eyelid and the human immunodeficiency virus. Ophthal Plast Reconst Surg 16:206–10, 2000.

149 SQUAMOUS CELL CARCINOMA 147

Frederick W. Fraunfelder, MD
Portland, Oregon

ETIOLOGY/INCIDENCE

Squamous cell carcinoma is a relatively rare periocular malignancy which usually occurs in the lower eyelid, with the lid margin being the preferential site of origin. In contrast, basal cell carcinoma accounts for 80% to 90% of eyelid malignancies with a ratio of lower lid involvement to upper lid involvement ranging from 3 : 1 to 5 : 1. Most periocular squamous cell carcinomas are of cutaneous origin; however, they may arise from the palpebral conjunctiva.

Squamous cell carcinoma is a malignant proliferation of well-differentiated keratinocytes in the epidermis. It occurs most often in fair-skinned, older individuals with a history of excessive cumulative sun exposure who are prone to develop actinic keratosis. It may arise from a precancerous solar (actinic) keratosis or *de novo*. There is a linear correlation between squamous cell carcinoma and ultraviolet light exposure, with a doubling of tumor incidence for each 8- to 10-degree decline in latitude. This tumor may also develop in individuals who have been exposed to radiation or chemicals (e.g. arsenic, hydrocarbons, tobacco), who have burn scars, or who have areas of repeated trauma. Immunocompromised persons are at a much greater risk, and the tumors tend to be more aggressive in these individuals.

The appearance of this tumor in children and adolescents may signify xeroderma pigmentosa, a hereditary disorder resulting in excessive actinic damage and multiple squamous and basal cell carcinomas by early adolescence.

COURSE/PROGNOSIS

The lesion initially appears discrete, flat, and indurated with overlying telangiectatic vessels and epidermal scaling. Clinically, the early tumor may be difficult to differentiate from an actinic keratosis, basal cell carcinoma, or other benign or malignant skin lesions. Over the course of a few months, a shallow ulcer develops surrounded by a wide, indurated, elevated border. The ulceration tends to occur more rapidly than with basal cell carcinoma. Cilia are frequently lost in the involved area, and bleeding occurs with minor trauma.

Prognosis depends on size, depth of invasion, histologic patterns and location. Depth of tumor invasion is the most important determinant of the tumor's metastatic potential. Lesions greater than 4 mm in depth have a 45.7% rate of metastasis. Metastasis rarely occurs in carcinoma arising from sun-damaged areas. Neglected lesions may metastasize to regional lymph nodes. Tumors arising in scars, irradiated areas, and immunocompromised hosts are more aggressive and have a higher metastatic rate. Death from squamous cell carcinoma rarely occurs from complications associated with intracranial extension or with extensive lymphatic and visceral metastasis.

DIAGNOSIS

Squamous cell carcinoma has more than 10 different subtypes, each of which has unique clinical features, etiology, and histopathology that influence the diagnosis, treatment and prognosis. The diagnosis must be confirmed before the appropriate management can be determined. The diagnosis of squamous cell carcinoma requires a high index of suspicion followed by careful biopsy and histologic examination. A shave biopsy is an efficient way to obtain a tumor specimen because surgical closure is unnecessary and reepithelialization occurs without scar formation. Occasionally, deeper excision may be required to obtain sufficient tissue for diagnosis. Histologically, this carcinoma is characterized by varying degrees of differentiation with hyperchromatic nuclei and abnormal keratinization invading the dermis.

Differential diagnosis

A differential diagnosis of squamous cell carcinoma should include basal cell carcinoma, keratoacanthoma, inverted follicular keratosis, senile keratosis and pseudoepitheliomatous hyperplasia. In addition, squamous cell carcinoma has been found at the base of cutaneous horns. During the histologic evaluation, it is important for the pathologist to closely examine the base of these tumors. Patients who have had one skin carcinoma are at a greater risk of having additional carcinomas and require regular follow-up examinations.

PROPHYLAXIS

Prevention is ideal; all individuals should be encouraged to avoid sunshine exposure and to use protective clothing and sun-blocking agents (SPF 50). The use of preventive methods should be particularly emphasized to those patients who are diagnosed with precancerous or cancerous skin lesions, who have a genetic history of skin cancers, or who have both.

TREATMENT

Systemic

Systemic or intralesional chemotherapy, or both, has been effective when used in conjunction with surgery or radiation. Topical 5-fluorouracil (5-FU) has proved to be efficacious in the treatment of solar keratosis, but 5-FU should not be used for the treatment of squamous cell carcinoma. Topical 5-FU may mask deep extension of the carcinoma.

Surgical

Surgical excision is the treatment of choice. The modified Mohs' fresh tissue technique provides the best chance of complete tumor resection by controlling the tumor margin with frozen sections. The modified Mohs' technique is modified when a pathologist, who is not the surgeon, performs the histologic evaluation of the frozen section specimens. With a standard Mohs' technique, the surgeon prepares and reads the specimens; the standard Mohs' technique is best reserved for those with special training in dermatopathology. Specimens are sectioned in a plane parallel to the outer painted edge so that the entire periphery is microscopically examined. Margins positive for the tumor are depicted on a map of the resected area, and additional peripheral sections are obtained until all margins are negative for the tumor. If removal of the lesion is other than a full-thickness eyelid resection, the deep base of the tumor must be carefully examined for deep extension. More generous tumor-free margins should be excised than those excised with basal cell carcinoma. The success rate of this method relates directly to the meticulous care taken by both the surgeon and pathologist. Mohs reports a 5-year cure rate of 98% of eyelid squamous cell carcinomas in the 213 patients he has treated. In cases in which the tumor is extensive and penetrates into the orbit, the treatment of choice is orbital exenteration. In cases of metastasis to regional lymph nodes, radical neck dissection should be considered in conjunction with adjunctive radiation or chemotherapy.

Cryotherapy

This is effective treatment for precancerous lesions (actinic keratosis) and as adjunctive treatment after excision of malignant squamous cell carcinoma. The technique requires freezing the tumor and a 5mm to 6mm margin of surrounding 'normal' tissue, with a liquid nitrogen cryotherapy probe or spray, and then allowing the tissue to thaw before refreezing. Complications include lacrimal obstruction, skin depigmentation, loss of eyelashes and development of eyelid deformities requiring surgical reconstruction.

Radiation

Squamous cell carcinoma is relatively radioresistant. Radiation is an inaccurate method of determining the extent of the tumor because treatment is based solely on the radiation oncologist's clinical impression. Radiation is generally reserved for extensive tumors that are surgically inaccessible, usually after tumor debulking. Large radiation doses in the range of 20 to 60 Gy are required, so proper shielding of the eye is imperative. A control rate of 93.3% at 5 years has been reported with radiation therapy.

COMMENTS

Squamous cell carcinoma is a malignancy arising from differentiated cells in the epidermis and must be diagnosed early and managed correctly to ensure a favorable outcome. The majority of periocular squamous cell carcinomas arise from ultraviolet light damage secondary to sun exposure. Older, fair-skinned individuals with previous extensive sun exposure are particularly prone to developing squamous cell carcinoma. Tumors arising from solar damage tend to have a lower rate of metastasis.

The clinical presentation of squamous cell carcinoma may mimic that of other skin tumors, so a high index of suspicion is required to establish an early diagnosis. All suspicious lesions require a biopsy with histologic evaluation. Surgical excision with a modified Mohs' fresh tissue technique followed by plastic reconstruction of the site provides the optimal opportunity for complete tumor elimination while maintaining acceptable function and cosmesis. Patients who have developed one skin carcinoma are at a greater risk of developing new carcinomas and recurrences and require periodic reevaluation for the remainder of their lives.

REFERENCES

Christenson LJ, Borrowman TA, Vachon CM, et al: Incidence of basal cell squamous cell carcinoma in a population younger than 40 years. JAMA 294:681–690, 2005.

Dryden RD, Engen TB: Squamous cell carcinoma. In: Fraunfelder FT, Roy FH, eds: Current ocular therapy. 5th edn. Philadelphia, WB Saunders, 2000.

Mohs FE: Micrographic surgery for the microscopically controlled excision of eyelid cancers. Arch Ophthalmol 104:901–909, 1986.

Reifler DM, Hornblass A: Squamous cell carcinoma of the eyelid. Surv Ophthalmol 30:349–365, 1986.

Wilkes TD, Fraunfelder FT: Principles of cryosurgery. Ophthalmic Surg 10:21–30, 1979.

SECTION

14 Mechanical and Nonmechanical Injuries

150 ACID BURNS 940.9

James P. McCulley, MD, FACS, FRCOphth
Dallas, Texas
Dipak N. Parmar, BSc(Hons), MBBS, FRCOphth
Dallas, Texas

Acid injuries of the eyes are characterized by protein coagulation and precipitation with the anion, with direct tissue damage produced by the hydrogen ion. These injuries tend to be less severe than alkali burns because the tissue proteins of the epithelium and superficial stroma serve as a buffer for the action of the acid, localizing its damage to the anterior cornea. In addition, most exposure to acids involves mild or moderate strength solutions. The prognosis for complete corneal epithelial healing is good in such cases, provided there is only limited damage to limbal stem cells. However, very strong acids penetrate the stroma just as quickly as alkalis, leading to a far worse prognosis with corneal opacification, anterior chamber pH alteration, and anterior segment destruction.

ETIOLOGY

Sulfuric acid, a widely used industrial chemical and acid for batteries, is the most common cause of acid injury. Hydrofluoric acid causes the most serious acid injuries because of the small size of the acid molecule and its low molecular weight, which allows easy tissue penetration of the toxic fluoride molecule. Other frequently encountered causes of acid injury include sulfurous, hydrochloric, chromic, acetic, and nitric acids (Figure 150.1).

COURSE/PROGNOSIS

Acute phase (0 to 3 days)

- Injection, chemosis, 'ground glass' corneal epithelium, corneal epithelial defects, limbal blanching, corneal clouding.
- Severe pain, photophobia, decreased visual acuity.

Intermediate phase (3 to 7 days)

- Anterior uveitis.
- Severe burns: corneal ulceration, perforation.

Chronic phase (severe burns)

- Corneal vascularization, symblepharon formation, limbal stem cell deficiency, scarring and pseudopterygia (Figure 150.2).
- Anterior segment damage: iris atrophy, cataract, glaucoma.

TREATMENT

Immediate

- Immediate copious irrigation of the eyes is of paramount importance, using either normal saline or water for at least 20 to 30 minutes. Both solutions are widely available, but their low osmolarity relative to the cornea leads to influx of fluid into the stroma, with possible diffusion of the corrosive into deeper corneal layers. Balanced saline solution is a better irrigation fluid in this regard, with an osmolarity equal to aqueous humor and enhanced buffering capacity (isotonic citrate and sodium acetate) that prevents corneal swelling and preserves the corneal endothelium.
- If possible, measure the pH of the inferior cul-de-sac prior to irrigation.
- After initial irrigation, allow 5 minutes for equilibration, then measure cul-de-sac pH. If the pH remains abnormally low, continue irrigation and check.
- Debride any necrotic corneal epithelium to allow normal tissue to re-epithelialize.
- Evert the upper lid to remove any trapped particles that can be associated with the acid.

Medical

- Antibiotic prophylaxis for bacterial infection, preferably with a broad-spectrum agent such as a fluoroquinolone, is necessary until corneal epithelialization is complete.
- Topical steroids decrease inflammation and reduce damage caused by proteolytic enzymes released by inflammatory cells. Prednisolone 1% or dexamethasone 0.1% eyedrops should be applied intensively for 10 days if the epithelium is not healed or for as long as the inflammatory process dictates, if the epithelium is intact.
- Cycloplegic agents, such as scopolamine, can be administered several times daily to reduce painful ciliary spasm and prevent posterior synechiae formation in the presence of anterior uveitis.
- A large therapeutic soft contact lens promotes re-epithelialization of the cornea under the lens.
- Lubrication with preservative-free tears and lubricating ointment is required, as there is usually damage to conjunctival goblet cells and accessory lacrimal glands, in addition to sensory nerve damage impairing the corneo-lacrimal reflex arc. Autologous serum drops have been shown to promote epithelial healing in difficult cases, but topical antibiotic should be used to cover the additional risk of infection.
- Collagenase inhibitors are indicated in cases with evidence of collagen breakdown (stromal melt), which usually appears at 7 to 14 days after injury. The only available topical agent

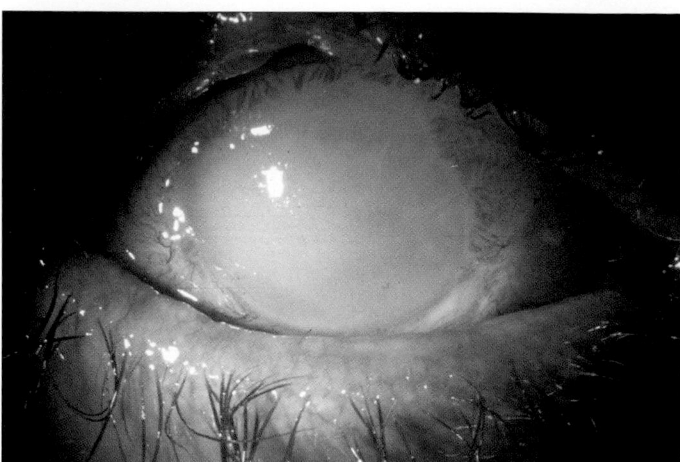

FIGURE 150.1. Acid chemical injury to cornea.

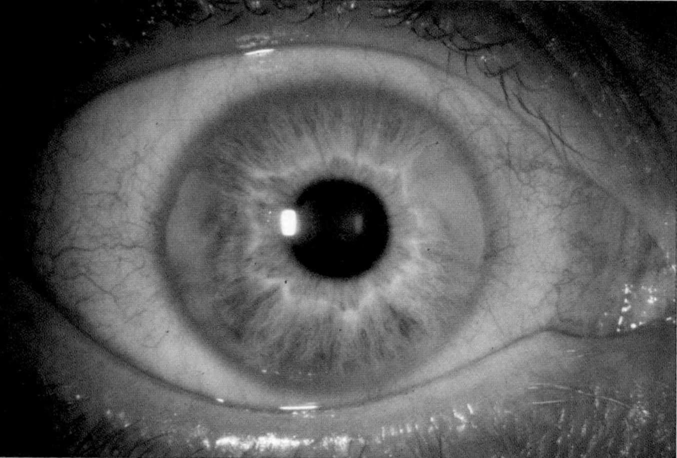

FIGURE 150.2. Nasal and temporal pseydopterygium from acid burn.

is acetylcysteine 10–20% (Mucomyst), which should be applied every 2 hours while the patient is awake. Oral tetracyclines may also be useful in this regard, as they can partly block metalloproteinase activity. Adjunctive therapy may also include topical citrate and ascorbate (inhibit leucocyte influx), topical aprotinin (inhibits proteinase activity) or topical heparin (re-opening of occluded vessels).

- Cyanoacrylate glue is used to prevent corneal perforation in the presence of severe thinning or actual perforations measuring less than 1 mm. A bandage soft contact lens is used adjunctively to improve comfort and to prevent displacement of the glue. The glue induces scarring and prevents further ulceration by providing a physical barrier to neutrophilic invasion.

Surgical

- Surgically debride any necrotic conjunctival tissue and maintain forniceal anatomy by ointment lubrication or by repeatedly opening them with a glass spatula or a special conformer.
- Conjunctival transplantation can assist in relieving mechanical restriction caused by cicatrisation.
- Tectonic penetrating keratoplasty may be necessary for the emergent management of a corneal perforation larger than 1 mm.
- Keratoplasty has a variable success rate, with a very poor prognosis in the presence of severe damage to limbal and conjunctival tissue as well as the eyelids, marked ocular surface dryness and extensive corneal vascularization. On occasion, a deep lamellar keratoplasty may be considered if the opacity is superficial and there is no deep stromal vascularization; otherwise a penetrating graft is required.
- Amniotic membrane transplantation can be useful in the initial period, as it inhibits inflammation and promotes healing of the ocular surface, preventing longterm complications such as corneal vascularization and conjunctivalization.
- Limbal stem cell (LSC) deficiency in unilateral cases can be treated with autologous LSC transplantation, harvested from the fellow healthy eye. In bilateral cases this is not possible and an allogeneic LSC transplant may be attempted; however, this would require long-term systemic immunosuppression — concomitant with the systemic risks incurred by such therapy — and is probably best avoided. *Ex-vivo* expansion of autologous LSC shows increasing promise, allowing harvesting of LSC while minimizing risk to the healthy fellow donor eye in unilateral cases. Particulary exciting is the development of tissue-engineered autologous oral mucosal epithelial sheets to successfully reconstruct the ocular surface in the presence of bilateral LSC deficiency secondary to chemical injury.
- Keratoprosthesis may be the only option in the most severe acid burns with bilateral involvement, as the prognosis for penetrating keratoplasty would be very poor. A through-and-through prosthesis, with the optical post protruding through the upper lid, has been used in limited cases. Perhaps the best approach in these cases may be the osteo-odonto-keratoprosthesis, which uses the patient's own tooth root and alveolar bone as biological support to an optical cylinder.

COMMENTS

Ocular burns caused by acids are generally not as severe as alkali burns due to the natural buffering capacity of the corneal stroma, the relatively weak strength of most acids, and the barrier to penetration formed by coagulating epithelial cells. As with alkali injuries, immediate copious irrigation is the most vital component of treatment following injury.

REFERENCES

Behndig A, Ehlers N, Stenevi U, et al: A case of unilateral acid burn. Acta Ophthalmol Scand 81(5):526–529, 2003.

Dua HS, Azuara-Blanco A: Autologous limbal transplantation in patients with unilateral corneal stem cell deficiency. Br J Ophthalmol 84(3):273–278, 2000.

Dua HS, Gomes JA, King AJ, Maharajan VS: The amniotic membrane in ophthalmology. Surv Ophthalmol 49(1):51–77, 2004.

Hille K, Landau H, Ruprecht KW: Os teo-odonto-keratoprosthesis. A summary of 6 years surgical experience. Ophthalmologe 99(2):90–95, 2002.

Kuckelkorn R, Schrage N, Keller G, Redbrake C: Emergency treatment of chemical and thermal eye burns. Acta Ophthalmol Scand 80(1):4–10, 2002.

McCulley JP: Chemical agents. In: Smolin G, Thoft RA, eds: The cornea. 3rd edn. Boston, Little, Brown, 1994:617–634.

Nishida K, Yamato M, Hayashida Y, et al: Corneal reconstruction with tissue-engineered cell sheets composed of autologous oral mucosal epithelium. N Engl J Med 351(12):1187–1196, 2004.

151 ALKALINE INJURY 940.9

F. Hampton Roy, MD, FACS
Little Rock, Arkansas

A splash of an alkaline solution into the eye causes an immediate rise in the pH that can result in the damage or death of the vital external ocular tissues (the corneal and conjunctival epithelium), the protective envelope (the cornea and sclera), and the intraocular tissues (the trabecular meshwork, iris, ciliary body, and lens). Alkali rapidly penetrates the cornea and sclera, causing saponification and lysis of cell membranes, denaturation of collagen, and hydrolysis of glycosaminoglycans. The severity of the injury is dependent on the anion concentration, the duration of exposure, and the pH of the solution. It is important to document exactly the degree of injury with respect to the extent of epithelial loss on the cornea and conjunctiva, as well as the corneal stromal opacity and perilimbal whitening. Accurate classification of the burn is the key to making the most probable prognosis.

ETIOLOGY/INCIDENCE

The most common cause of a severe alkali injury of the eye in the United States is an assault. Data gathered from a large urban hospital show that young black men are at greatest risk, usually in a domestic setting where there is low-income, high-density housing and a record of alcoholism and prior assaults. In the industrial sector, approximately 10% of 52,142 cases of ocular trauma reported from 16 states were chemical burns (1.6% acid and 0.6% alkali). Safety monitors have reduced the incidence of job-related eye injuries, but despite such programs, the storage and use of powerful alkalis, under extreme pressure and high temperature, continue to pose serious threats even to the properly attired worker wearing protective clothing and goggles. Farmers using liquid ammonia (ammonia causes the most serious alkaline injury) as fertilizer and homeowners using powerful cleansing agents, usually without eye protection, continue to be at special risk. The most common alkaline injury agent is lime.

COURSE/PROGNOSIS

The pain, lacrimation, and blepharospasm following an ocular alkali injury result from direct stimulation of free nerve endings located in the epithelium of the cornea, conjunctiva, and eyelids. With severe burns of the cornea and sclera, there is a sudden, spiking rise in the intraocular pressure that lasts about 10 minutes and is caused primarily by shrinkage of the collagenous envelope of the eye. A more prolonged rise in pressure quickly follows, secondary to prostaglandin release. Strong alkali rapidly penetrates into the eye, and the hydroxyl ions might remain for up to 2 hours, overcoming the poor buffering capacity of anterior segment tissues and the aqueous humor. Within 1 minute, the severe rise in aqueous humor pH causes lysis of corneal cells as well as of those lining and adjacent to the anterior chamber, compromising the blood-aqueous barrier and releasing necrotic debris into the aqueous humor. This leads to a severe fibrinous inflammatory reaction in the entire anterior segment of the eye.

Glaucoma may ensue because of inflammatory products accumulating in the aqueous humor and chamber angle, which promotes anterior synechial closure, especially inferiorly. The trabeculum and ciliary body may be injured directly by penetration of alkali through the sclera or by contact with alkalotic aqueous humor percolating through the meshwork. Ocular hypertension, hypotension, or both may occur at different times, depending on the aqueous dynamics occurring at that particular time. Chemical injury to the iris, crystalline lens, or ciliary body may produce mydriasis, cataract, or phthisis bulbi, respectively. Externally, this inflammatory reaction may be so profound as to lead to extensive symblephara and even ankyloblepharon caused by the apposition of raw conjunctival surfaces.

DIAGNOSIS

It may take 48 to 72 hours after the injury to correctly assess the degree of ocular damage and to offer an accurate prognosis. Classification of the degree of corneal opacification and of perilimbal whitening quantifies the extent of the injury and best projects the likely outcome:

- If mild corneal epithelial erosion and faint anterior stromal haziness are present and there is no ischemic necrosis of perilimbal conjunctiva or sclera, healing with little or no corneal scarring will result, and the visual loss will usually be no greater than one to two lines.
- When moderate corneal opacity and little or no significant ischemic necrosis of perilimbal conjunctiva have occurred, the epithelium will slowly heal, with moderate scarring and peripheral corneal vascularization, and a visual loss of two to seven lines may occur.
- Moderate to severe damage causes sufficient corneal opacity to blur iris details, and whitening of perilimbal conjunctiva is limited to less than one third. Corneal healing will be prolonged, and significant corneal vascularization and scarring will take place. The prognosis for visual acuity is usually limited to 20/200 or less.
- The blurring of the pupillary outline, ischemia of one third to two thirds of the perilimbal conjunctiva, and often a marbleized cornea indicate severe damage. Very prolonged corneal healing with inflammation and a high incidence of corneal ulceration and perforation are common. In the best cases, severe corneal vascularization and scarring result in counting-finger vision.
- When the pupil is not visible, more than two thirds of the perilimbal conjunctiva is ischemic, and the cornea is completely marbleized, only a very poor prognosis can be made. Corneal healing may be prolonged and show very severe corneal vascularization and scarring. The most severe cases show relatively rapid conversion of stroma into a necrotic sequestrum, with corneal perforation occurring through a thoroughly degraded corneal stroma. Phthisis bulbi is not uncommon.

TREATMENT

Ocular

The eyes should immediately be irrigated with copious volumes of an innocuous aqueous solution available at the scene of the injury and on the way to the hospital. Ocular irrigation with lactated Ringer's or other available intravenous solutions should be continued in the emergency facility for at least 2 hours or until the pH of the cul-de-sac has returned to neutrality. The intravenous tubing may be hand-held or, alternatively, a scleral shell with an inflow tube (Mediflow lens) may provide a more efficient method of delivering fluid to the eye.

- The sticky paste of lime (calcium hydroxide) may be removed from the conjunctiva with cotton-tipped applicators soaked in 0.01 M edetate calcium disodium.
- Mydriasis and cycloplegia should be induced with a 1% atropine instillation twice a day.
- Antibiosis is effected by topical application of a broad spectrum of antibiotics four times per day as long as an epithelial defect persists.
- Analgesics and sedatives are often required during the first several days for patients who have sustained severe burns.
- Glaucoma occurring after the injury commonly responds to carbonic anhydrase inhibitors such as 125 mg acetazolamide PO q.i.d. or topical 0.5% timolol b.i.d.
- Extensive destruction of the palpebral conjunctiva or eyelid skin may cause lagophthalmos and consequently exposure keratitis, a condition poorly tolerated by the damaged cornea. In these cases, use of an ointment and coverage of the affected eye with plastic wrap or a plastic bubble provide an immediate moist chamber to protect the cornea.
- Patching is only occasionally helpful in less severe injuries, when the redevelopment of epithelial defects simulates recurrent corneal erosions.
- The persistence of corneal epithelial defects correlates with the incidence of sterile ulcerations and increases the likelihood of infection.
- Soft contact lenses may facilitate re-epithelialization by acting as bandages to protect fresh epithelium from exposure to the air and by reducing the shearing stress of blinking. Disposable or extended-wear soft contact lenses are preferred. The use of 0.5 normal saline drops hourly and lubricants four times daily helps to maintain adequate hydration and lens mobility.
- If the epithelium can be encouraged to re-cover the cornea, stromal healing is accelerated and the incidence of corneal ulceration is reduced.
- In experimental animal studies, inhibitors of collagenase applied topically to the cornea reduced the incidence of corneal ulceration from 80% to 20%. Although both cysteine and acetylcysteine are effective inhibitors of collagenase, the latter is more desirable because of its stability, efficacy, and availability.
- In models of extreme injuries, acetylcysteine has not had any favorable effect. Although it is suspected that 20% acetylcysteine has a favorable effect in the human alkaline-injured cornea, this has not been proved by a randomized clinical trial.

Early insertion of a methylmethacrylate ring designed to fit into the cul-de-sacs might prevent fibrinous adhesions and reduce subsequent fibrotic contracture of the conjunctiva. An alternative approach has been to suture plastic wrap over the palpebral and fornix conjunctiva. Despite such treatments it is not unusual for severely injured eyes to undergo total ankyloblepharon. Later lysis of adhesions with or without mucous membrane grafts, insertion of a symblepharon ring, and placement of intermarginal lid adhesions can restore the cul-de-sacs, improve lid mobility, and reduce or eliminate corneal exposure.

Surgical

Animal studies by Grant have suggested that early paracentesis of the eye does not alter the outcome after an alkaline injury. However, the finding of a severely elevated pH in the aqueous humor of rabbits up to 2 hours after a 2 N sodium hydroxide injury does offer a compelling reason to remove aqueous humor and re-form the anterior chamber with a buffered solution.

- Paracentesis may be safely performed under topical anesthesia by an ophthalmologist.
- A No. 11 Bard–Parker blade can be used initially to facilitate the entry of a 27-gauge needle into the eye.
- If a significant proportion of the perilimbal palisades of Vogt (containing the corneal stem cells) has been destroyed, then a persistent epithelial defect is likely to occur.
- Transplantation of corneal limbal stem cells from the other eye is indicated to stabilize and renew the corneal surface after the episclera has revascularized. (The earliest recorded transplant was performed 2 weeks after injury.)
- To accomplish this, the residual epithelium and pannus, if present, must be removed (lamellar keratectomy), and peritomy with conjunctival recession must be performed to prepare the recipient eye.
- Two or three conjunctival autographs from the uninjured eye, spaced equidistantly around the eye, are delineated with a wet-field cautery 4 mm on a side and excised, including a narrow piece of cornea. The autographs are oriented around the recipient limbus the same way they were in the donor eye and sutured there with 9-0 vicryl.
- In binocular injuries, allografting of corneal stem cells from related or unrelated donors is necessary.
- Corneal stem cell transplantation is required 3 or 4 months before corneal transplantation.

In the acute phase, temporary amniotic membrane patching may be considered.

No medical way is known to reestablish corneal clarity after a moderately severe, severe, or very severe alkaline injury. Extensive scarring and vascularization of the cornea, without other complications, are the best possible outcomes. Corneal transplantation with fresh tissue may be considered no sooner than 12 to 18 months after injury. Such a transplant cannot survive without the normal blink mechanism and an adequate tear film. For this reason, operative procedures to lyse symblephara, expand cul-de-sacs, and eliminate lagophthalmos are often required to reestablish a more normal external anatomy and physiology before transplantation.

The success of corneal transplants in alkaline-injured eyes is steadily improving although they are still regarded as high-risk cases. The high incidence of secondary glaucoma, immunologic rejections, and recurrent epithelial erosions requires continued medical vigilance. Cataract extractions and multiple other procedures often complicate management.

COMPLICATIONS

- Conjunctiva: edema, ischemia, necrosis, scarring, symblepharon.
- Cornea: edema, infiltration, neovascularization, opacity, perforation, ulcer.
- Eyelids: lagophthalmos, scarring.
- Iris or ciliary body: chemical mydriasis, hypopyon, iridocyclitis, ischemic necrosis, phthisis bulbi.
- Other: cataract, secondary glaucoma.

PRECAUTIONS

Topical ophthalmic application of steroids after alkaline injury is extremely controversial. In mild or moderate ocular injuries, the anti-inflammatory effects may be beneficial throughout the acute phase without enhancing the chance of corneal ulceration. The use of topical steroids in these cases as well as in the more severe injuries for the first 7 days after injury might decrease the inflammatory reaction of the entire anterior segment, possibly reducing some of the late side effects such as glaucoma. The advantages of such treatment, however, must be weighed against the retardation of wound healing, a consequence of fibroblast inhibition. Topical steroids interfere with the repair process and result in corneal ulcerations and perforations when used for longer than 7 days after a severe injury. It seems most reasonable to avoid topical steroids if possible, but especially later than 7 to 10 days after the injury. The use of systemic steroids has certain theoretic advantages, but their efficacy is unproved.

COMMENTS

Promising new research focuses on orthomolecular approaches, including supplemental sodium ascorbate to stimulate collagen production from corneal fibroblasts and sodium citrate to inhibit the adherence of neutrophils to the vascular endothelium, chemotaxis, the respiratory burst, enzyme release, and superoxide radical production from the invading polymorphonuclear leukocytes. A randomized clinical trial of sodium ascorbate and sodium citrate in the treatment of the alkaline-burned eyes is currently in progress.

Recognition that inflammatory mediators act to chemically attract and activate neutrophils into the cornea is leading to the development of specifically designed inhibitors to interrupt this process.

REFERENCES

Dua HS, King AJ, Joseph A: A new classification of ocular surface burns. Br J Ophthalmol 85(11):1379–1383, 2001.

Kenyon KK, Tseng SCG: Limbal autograft transplantation for ocular surface disorders. Ophthalmology 96:709–723, 1989.

Kobayashi A, Shirao Y, Yoshita T: Temporary amniotic membrane patching for acute chemical burns. Eye 17(2):149–158, 2003.

Ozdemir O, Tekeli O, Ornek K: Limbal autograft and allograft transplantations in patients with corneal burns. Eye 18(3):241–248, 2004.

Pfister RR: Corneal stem cell disease: concepts, categorization and treatment by auto- and homotransplantation of limbal stem cells. CLAO J 20:64–72, 1993.

Pfister RR, Haddox J, Barr D: The combined effect of citrate/ascorbate treatment in alkali-injured rabbit eyes. Cornea 10:100–104, 1991.

152 CONJUNCTIVAL LACERATIONS AND CONTUSIONS 921.1

Larry F. Rich, MS, MD
Portland, Oregon

Traumatic injuries to the conjunctiva are usually not serious in themselves. However, they may mask an underlying ocular injury or retained foreign body. Puncture of the eyelid associated with a conjunctival laceration suggests the possibility of ocular penetration. Edema or hemorrhage may obscure the scleral or corneal entry site, so every conjunctival laceration must be explored for deeper trauma.

ETIOLOGY

Trauma, either blunt or sharp, is the usual cause of a laceration. A subconjunctival hemorrhage may be spontaneous or may be related to bleeding dyscrasias.

COURSE/PROGNOSIS

In most cases, the prognosis is excellent. If the laceration is extensive or if it is not repaired properly, necrosis, loss of fornices, or symblepharon may occur.

DIAGNOSIS

Laboratory findings

Surgical evaluation may be done under topical or local anesthesia if the patient is cooperative. Careful dissection of conjunctiva and Tenon's capsule from the sclera permits visualization of the sclera. Without direct visualization, vitreous, uveal, retinal, or even lens materials may be overlooked beneath conjunctival edema and associated blood. Complications may occur if a conjunctival laceration contains an embedded foreign body that goes unnoticed. Such an occurrence may result in corneal erosion, tissue reactions, conjunctival cysts or granuloma, and membrane formation.

In the exploration of conjunctival lacerations, care must be taken to eliminate any pressure on the globe, as it may cause prolapse of intraocular contents through an unsuspected scleral penetration. The wound should be examined carefully, usually under topical anesthesia, to determine the extent of injury and to search for retained foreign bodies. Any foreign bodies that are found and removed should be cultured for bacterial and fungal growth. Dental film is useful for detecting nonmetallic foreign bodies and a Berman metal locator is of value in selected instances. Echography may help to identify intraocular or intraorbital foreign bodies.

Differential diagnosis

A fracture of one of the paranasal sinuses allows air to be trapped within the conjunctival tissues; this can be diagnosed by crepitus as well as by radiography. Fractures involving the ethmoidal sinuses are probably the most common cause of traumatic conjunctival emphysema.

Injury from an air compressor hose may lacerate the conjunctiva and lead to subconjunctival emphysema. In this type of injury, air can dissect into the soft tissues of the eyelid or face, orbit or intracranial cavity without compromise of the skull or sinuses.

If laceration of the globe is detected at the time of exploration, it is desirable to proceed immediately with all necessary surgical repairs.

A prolonged course of conjunctival edema may be associated with an infectious process, a retained subconjunctival or orbital foreign body, or even a scleral rupture.

TREATMENT

Surgical

Surgical repair is rarely necessary if the laceration is less than 1 cm in length. If surgical reapproximation of a gaping wound is deemed necessary, interrupted or continuous 6-0 or 7-0 gut sutures are sufficient for this purpose. Careful attention should be given to reapproximation of lacerated conjunctival edges in order to exclude Tenon's capsule from the wound. If Tenon's fascia is included in a sutured conjunctival laceration, a chalky-white herniation will result. On rare occasions, extensive loss of conjunctiva may require a conjunctival graft from the other eye or a mucous membrane graft from the mouth. However, even injuries that have resulted in loss of a considerable amount of tissue can usually be closed satisfactorily because of the elasticity of the conjunctiva.

If tissue necrosis has resulted from a severe contusive injury, excision of the necrotic tissue will facilitate more rapid wound healing and will also decrease the possibility of infection.

Supportive

Because conjunctival hemorrhage and chemosis following contusions are usually not serious, treatment requires only supportive therapy such as ice packs to minimize swelling in the acute phase.

Subconjunctival hemorrhage following contusive injuries may at times result in chemosis so severe that the conjunctiva balloons out between the lids. In this situation, treatment does not relieve the edema but may be directed at relief of discomfort. The distended conjunctiva should be covered with ointment or a plastic sheet until the swelling subsides. At some point, the use of a muscle hook may allow an infolding of the conjunctiva into the fornices to a degree that will allow placement of a pressure patch.

Prophylactic use of topical antibiotic solutions is advisable for all conjunctival lacerations.

COMPLICATIONS

- Conjunctival cicatrisation.
- Conjunctival cysts.
- Granulation.
- Keratinization.
- Conjunctival necrosis.
- Pseudomembranous conjunctivitis.
- Symblepharon.

COMMENTS

Most conjunctival wounds involve the bulbar conjunctiva in the interpalpebral zone. Less frequently, the superior and inferior palpebral areas are lacerated, and in these instances, painstaking inspection must be performed. These tears are commonly seen in association with lid lacerations and perforations, and meticulous examination of the underlying sclera and a thorough fundus examination are essential. The possibility of scleral perforation always exists in these cases, and proper management depends on an immediate and accurate diagnosis.

REFERENCES

Norton AL, Green WR: Foreign bodies as a cause of conjunctival pseudomembrane formation. Br J Ophthalmol 55:312–316, 1971.

Paton D, Goldberg MF: Management of Ocular Injuries. Philadelphia, WB Saunders, 1976:181–190.

Rich LF: Conjunctival lacerations. In: Roy FH, ed: Master techniques in ophthalmic surgery. Baltimore, Williams & Wilkins, 1995:97–101.

Runyan TE: Concussive and penetrating injuries of the globe and optic nerve. St Louis, CV Mosby, 1975:1–7.

Williams T, Frankel N: Intracerebral air caused by conjunctival laceration with air hose. Arch Ophthalmol 117(8):1090–1091, 1999.

153 ELECTRICAL INJURY 940.1
(Electric Shock, Lightning)

Frederick T. Fraunfelder, MD
Portland, Oregon

ETIOLOGY/INCIDENCE

Voltages range from that of lightning-up to 100 million volts-to that of electricity. Burns may occur at potentials of less than 6 volts, but significant ocular injuries have not occurred at potentials of less than 200 volts.

The size of a cutaneous burn has a minimal relationship to the long-term outcome. Small skin burns may cause severe multisystem internal injury involving the cardiovascular, central nervous, and musculoskeletal systems. Extensive tissue necrosis and vascular injury can also result from small entry wounds.

Only rarely do lightning injuries cause ocular problems. It is estimated that between 800 and 1000 persons are hit by lightning each year in the United States. About 20% to 30% of these strikes are fatal. Most ocular injuries occur as a result of contact with an electric source. The contact or exit must be on the head, with the current passing through the eye, for ocular damage to occur.

COURSE/PROGNOSIS

Often, the ophthalmologist is not asked to see a patient until long after the injury has occurred because the patient may be severely injured and have ointments covering the face and eyes. Only after the patient improves and ointment is decreased will the patient have visual complaints.

Characteristics of lens changes

- The initial changes that occur in the formation of electricity-caused cataracts are multiple vacuoles beneath the anterior lens capsule.
- These vacuoles are replaced by anterior subcapsular 'streaks' in an irregular pattern.
- Scale-like gray opacities may appear in the subcapsular layer of the extreme anterior cortex.
- Vesicles and amorphous opacities, as well as crystalline formations, may also appear in the posterior subcapsular area.

- The lens changes may occur almost immediately or may take several years; the average time of onset is 2 to 6 months after injury.
- If only a few vacuoles are present in the anterior lens cortex within the first few weeks postinjury, there is a high probability that no significant cataract-one requiring surgery-will occur.

Part of the injury may be heat-related as much as it is true electrical damage secondary to contact between the iris and the lens. Retinal damage is more likely to be a thermal injury unless the exit point of the electrical injury indicated that the electrical current passed through the posterior segment of the eye.

DIAGNOSIS

Dilated-eye examination of both the lens and retina is necessary.

TREATMENT

Systemic

- Analgesics and tranquilizers are often required.
- Tetanus toxoid is administered if the patient has not had a booster within the past year.
- Antibiotics such as gentamicin 3 mg/kg or IM in three doses may be considered if necrotic tissue is present so as to decrease opportunistic bacteria.

Ocular

- Try to maintain a cool, dry, clean wound environment.
- Clean periocular tissue regularly with diluted soap solution or normal saline; this may have to be done b.i.d. to t.i.d.
- Apply periocular and ocular antibiotic ointments regularly.
- Try to keep burned areas open to the air if the lid can still cover the eye.
- Cycloplegics, such as 1% to 2% atropine qd to q.i.d. and dexamethasone 0.1% b.i.d. to q.i.d. may be necessary to control uveitis.
- As granulation tissue occurs, sterile dressings may be started.

Surgical

- If a cataract develops, lens extraction procedures are done as for nontraumatic cataracts.
- A split-thickness skin graft may be necessary for eyelid burns to protect the globe.

COMMENTS

Ocular injury secondary to electric shock or lightning may be thermal or electrical in its cause. Eyelid, conjunctiva, cornea, pupil, lens, retina, extraocular muscles, and central nervous system damage with secondary ocular effects may occur. Cataracts are the most common injury and usually appear within 3 to 6 months. Corneal and conjunctival injury are usually epithelial and subside after a few weeks. Usually, eyelid lesions are extensive only if the site of contact is close to the eye.

REFERENCES

Biro Z, Pamer Z: Electrical cataract and optic neuropathy. Int Ophthalmol 18:43–47, 1994.

Cooper MA: Treatment of lightning injury. In: Andrews CJ, Cooper MA, Darveniza M, Mackerras D, eds: Lightning injuries: electrical, medical, and legal aspects. Ann Arbor, MI, CRC, 1992:130–132, 1992.

Fraunfelder FT, Hanna C: Electric cataracts. I. Sequential changes, unusual and prognostic findings. Arch Ophthalmol 87:179, 1972.

Fraunfelder FT, Meyer SM: Treatment of lightning injury: special aspects of ocular management. In: Andrews CJ, et al: Lightning injuries: electrical, medical, and legal aspects. Boca Raton, CRC, 1992.

Grover S, Goodwin J: Lightning and electrical injuries: neuro-ophthalmologic aspects. Seminars in Neurology 15(4):335–341, 1995.

Hanna C, Fraunfelder FT, Johnston GC: Electrical-induced cataracts. Arch Ophthalmol 84:232, 1970.

Hanna C, Fraunfelder FT: Electric cataracts. II. Ultrastructural lens changes. Arch Ophthalmol 87:18, 1972.

Saffle JR, Crandall A, Warden GD: Cataracts: a long-term complication of electrical injury. J Trauma 25:17–21, 1985.

154 MANAGEMENT OF SCLERAL RUPTURES 871.4 AND LACERATIONS 871.2

Ferenc Kuhn, MD, PhD
Birmingham, Alabama

ETIOLOGY

Ruptures are caused by large, blunt objects that exert pressure on the eye upon contact. As a result, the intraocular pressure (IOP) is raised, and eventually the eyewall's resistance is overcome: the eye suffers an open globe injury. The eyewall opens where it's the weakest, not necessarily at the point of contact. The most likely sites of rupture are at the limbus, at the insertion of the extraocular muscles and along previous (surgical or traumatic) wounds. Typically, there is no entry of the object into the eye. Consequently, the risk of endophthalmitis is very low while the risk of tissue prolapse is high.

Lacerations are, as opposed to ruptures, caused by a sharp object that enters the eye at the point of contact. If the object remains inside the eye, it is an *intraocular foreign body* (IOFB) injury; if it leaves the eye via the same route it entered, it is a *penetrating* injury; if it leaves the eye via a different (exit) wound, it is a *perforating* injury.

Tissue prolapse is also common with lacerations, although a little less so than with ruptures. Endophthalmitis, on the other hand, is much more of a danger. The roughly 5% risk with penetrating trauma approximately doubles if it is an IOFB injury.

COURSE/PROGNOSIS

An open globe injury is likely to have a better prognosis if:

- The initial visual acuity is good;
- The wound is located anteriorly;
- The wound is small;
- The injury is caused by a sharp, rather than blunt, object;
- The object is not a missile.

DIAGNOSIS

Clinical signs and symptoms

The diagnosis of an open-globe injury should always be considered in the setting of ocular trauma. A detailed history is paramount as is a thorough ophthalmic examination. Some presentations may be obvious, with uvea prolapsed into the wound, but in other situations the diagnosis may not be as apparent. The following findings should raise suspicion of an occult scleral rupture:

Findings on clinical examination:

- A suspicious history;
- Decreased visual acuity/afferent pupillary defect;
- Hemorrhagic chemosis;
- Peaked pupil;
- Abnormally deep or shallow anterior chamber;
- Decreased intraocular pressure (although may also be elevated);
- Media opacity: hyphema, cataract and vitreous hemorrhage.

Laboratory findings

Based on the history and clinical findings, additional studies may be required:

- Axial and coronal computed tomography (for confirming/excluding intraocular and orbital foreign bodies, orbital fractures, and occult scleral ruptures).
- Ultrasound (rarely needed for retinal detachment or intraocular foreign bodies; may carefully be applied in experienced hands preoperatively, although intraoperative or postoperative use is more common).
- Surgical exploration may be necessary if presence of an open-globe injury cannot otherwise be excluded.

Differential diagnosis

Most signs and symptoms can occur in other conditions; history should help determine the traumatic origin.

PROPHYLAXIS

Although great strides have been made in the surgical instrumentation and techniques for the management of open-globe injuries, prevention would be the ideal situation. Reduction of ocular morbidity may be accomplished by educating patients about protective polycarbonate eyewear. This is especially important for patients who are at high risk, including those who are involved in certain recreational and occupational activities, and those who are monocular such as those who have already lost vision in the fellow eye because of previous ocular trauma.

TREATMENT

If risk factors for infection (soil contamination, an object of organic matter, and the presence of lens injury in persons over 50 years of age) are present, prophylactic intravitreal antibiotic injection is warranted; clinical signs of endophthalmitis demands immediate surgical intervention (typically complete vitrectomy with intravitreal as well as systemic and local antibiotic therapy). Otherwise, the following describes the 'typical' surgical approach.

Surgical treatment for ruptures

Management is primarily determined by the location of the wound. If the wound is *anterior* (i.e. easily accessible to the surgeon), the prolapsed tissue must be dealt with first. If it is *iris*, it is usually cleaned – using forceps, microsponge (e.g. Weck Spears), or irrigation – and then reposited. Only iris that cannot be adequately cleaned of contamination or debris (e.g. epithelial cells), or that is necrotic should be excised. If the wound is at the limbus, iris reposition should be done via 'pulling' rather than 'pushing': through a paracentesis created at 90 degrees or more away for increased maneuverability, and using a blunt tool such as a spatula. Prolapse of the *ciliary body* or *choroid* is much rarer as these tissues are quite elastic; in general, they should be reposited, not excised, to decrease the risk of hemorrhage and inflammation. If *vitreous* has prolapsed, it must always be excised. Conversely, *retina* is never excised but should be gently reposited. Viscoelastics can be used both for reposition and as a prevention against reprolapse.

Once there is no tissue between the wound lips, suturing can start. The order of suture placement primarily depends on convenience. Ideally and if the entire wound can be visualized (requiring careful dissection of the conjunctiva to ensure that the scleral wound does not continue beyond what appears to be its termination), the '50% rule' applies: the first suture is in the middle of the wound, the next two in the middle of each of the now two sections (at 25% and 75%), etc. An absorbable suture such as vicryl suffices: by the time of suture absorption in a few weeks, the wound is firmly closed by scar formation.

If the wound is *posterior*, the entire approach changes. It may be impossible, even dangerous, to inspect the wound in its entirety before suture placement, as this threatens with additional tissue prolapse and expulsive choroidal hemorrhage. The 'close-as-you-go' technique is recommended: the scleral wound is closed anteriorly, before another section of the conjunctiva is opened posteriorly; the sclera is closed again and the process can be repeated as needed. An assistant may be needed to ensure gentle but adequate exposure using traction sutures or retractor (e.g. Schepens). On rare occasions, an extraocular muscle may have to be temporarily taken off to increase access to the wound and ease of suturing.

The wound may be so posterior that accessing it is not only difficult but dangerous, threatening with (further) tissue prolapse/hemorrhage. The significance of this complication is greater than the benefit offered by suture-closure. In such cases, the wound is to be left open; by an outside-in process, proliferative cells will enter the site and close the wound within hours or days. Conversely, while this process ensures timely wound closure of acceptable firmness, it usually involves instant or eventual *retinal incarceration* that must be dealt with secondarily.

Surgical treatment of lacerations

If infection is not present or its risk is not elevated, management of the injured eye can be staged. The wound is dealt with in a similar fashion as described above: wound toilette, management of tissue prolapse, and suture-closure. If the wound is corneoscleral, the limbus is closed first, followed by the corneal part (typically using 10-0 nylon sutures), while the scleral aspect comes last.

If an IOFB is present, it is usually removed through a surgical, not the traumatic, wound: this provides for more control and less iatrogenic trauma. Again, whether IOFB removal and vitrectomy in eyes with posterior segment IOFB are performed in the same sitting is determined by the threat of infection versus the risk of intraoperative hemorrhage. In eyes with increased endophthalmitis risk or in a hostile medicolegal environment, comprehensive initial intervention is preferred; otherwise, the experience of the surgeon and the availability of the proper infrastructure (equipment/expertise/staff) should be weighted. Haste in IOFB removal does not compensate for inadequate or inappropriate surgery. Moreover, extraction of a posterior segment IOFB alone does not reduce the risk of infection: a complete vitrectomy must also be performed with (removal of the infected medium).

If the injury is perforating, management of the exit wound requires considerations similar to those mentioned with a posterior rupture. Surgical closure is advised only if it can be done without exerting so much extra pressure on the globe that would threaten with expulsive hemorrhage or tissue prolapse. If this cannot be avoided, the surgeon is better off leaving the wound open and wait for spontaneous closure.

This chapter does not describe the secondary management (often vitrectomy) of eyes with open globe injury.

Medical treatment

Regardless of injury type, the inflammation and the intraocular pressure must be aggressively controlled postoperatively.

COMPLICATIONS

Virtually any complication that exists may occur either as the result of the injury or of the intervention itself; the list of the most severe complications includes, among others, sympathetic ophthalmia, endophthalmitis, retinal detachment, and proliferative vitreoretinopathy. The treatment of these complications is beyond the scope of this chapter.

REFERENCES

Dalma J: Extrabulbar tissue prolapse. In: Kuhn F, Pieramici D, eds: Ocular trauma: principles and practice. New York, Thieme, 2002.

Kuhn F, Mester V, Morris R: A proactive treatment approach for eyes with perforating injury. Klin Monatsbl Augenheilk 221:622–628, 2004.

Kuhn F, Morris R, Witherspoon CD, et al: A standardized classification of ocular trauma terminology. Ophthalmology 103:240–243, 1996.

Lindsey JL, Hamill B: Scleral and corneoscleral injuries. In: Kuhn F, Pieramici D, eds: Ocular trauma: principles and practice. New York, Thieme, 2002.

155 INTRAOCULAR FOREIGN BODY: COPPER 871.6

Fleming D. Wertz, III, MD

Burlington, Massachusetts

ETIOLOGY/INCIDENCE

The increased incidence of intraocular copper-containing foreign bodies reflects the vocations and avocations of modern societies. Prior to the Industrial Revolution, before the changes in the engineering of weapons of war and the changes in the hobbies practiced by those with increased leisure time, the incidence of intraocular copper-containing foreign bodies was understandably low. During the past 150 years, the advent of sophisticated machinery in the workplace, on the battlefield, and in the hobbyist's workshop has produced an environment in which the number of penetrating injuries caused by copper-containing compounds has risen. During the United States Civil War, 1861 to 1865, the incidence of penetrating ocular injuries was 0.5%. This incidence rose slightly during World War I to between 3% and 4%. Thirty years later, statistics from World War II and the Korean War indicate the rate of penetrating ocular injuries had risen to 5% to 6%. The Vietnam War and the Israeli conflict resulted in a rate approaching 9% to 10%. These statistics reflect the effects of modern weapons designed to inflict maximum injury to combatants' anatomy above the level of the waist.

In plants and mills, copper and copper alloys are commonly used in the manufacture and repair of numerous devices. Copper wire and electromechanical devices containing copper alloys are routinely found in the workshops used for hobbies and home repairs. Therefore, the potential for penetrating injuries involving copper compounds is widespread. The true incidence of copper-containing retained foreign bodies is lower during times of peace than times of war, directly reflecting the nature of the military-industrial process.

The presence of intraocular copper-containing foreign bodies can result in one or more of the following:

- Suppurative endophthalmitis;
- Recurrent nongranulomatous inflammation;
- Fibrous encapsulation;
- Local or widespread dissemination of copper in the eye.

These ocular responses result from the chemistry of the copper ion within the eye. A copper ion participates in two processes. The first is oxidation-reduction reactions. Because of a moderately low redox potential, a copper ion is a reagent for and catalyst of electron transfer from organic donors. Ascorbic acid is oxidized by a cuprous ion to produce hydrogen peroxide. This has been associated with vitreous syneresis and collapse. A copper ion participates in the formation of free radicals. The resultant superoxide and hydroxyl radicals attack polyunsaturated fatty acids, which results in lipid peroxidation and the formation of alkoxy and peroxy radicals. This may lead to:

1. The initiation of arachidonic acid metabolism that produces prostaglandins and leukotrienes, creating inflammation; and
2. The incapacitation and death of cells, which results from the radicals' attack on lipid-containing cell membranes.

The latter contributes to progressive ocular dysfunction.

The second process of the ion occurs when copper complexes with key enzymes. The copper ion either displaces metal ions or alters the stereo configuration of the molecule, which generates altered intracellular metabolism. For example, copper inactivates carbonic anhydrase, and this results in decreased intraocular pressure.

COURSE/PROGNOSIS

The clinical course can be highly variable. It is dependent on the size, location and copper content of the foreign body. Larger foreign bodies offer more surface area from which to liberate copper ion. In theory, the greater the surface area the greater the reaction should be. However, if the foreign body is located in the mid vitreous, away from vascularized tissue with a high oxygen tension, it may sit intact without inciting inflammation, or it may be quietly encapsulated. Locations near the retina and ciliary body are more prone to be associated with inflammation or copper dissemination or both. If the foreign body is an alloy containing less than 85% copper, there may be no reaction. The most intense reactions are associated with a copper content greater than 85%. Apart from the damage caused by the penetrating injury, acute chalcosis will present rapidly with inflammation, hypotony and deteriorating visual function. Without intervention, this may progress to visual loss from the sequela of intraocular inflammation or intraocular fibrosis and result in inoperable retinal detachment. Chronic chalcosis may present with low-grade intraocular inflammation, variable degrees of intraocular copper dissemination, and highly variable changes or no changes in visual function. However, the tendency is toward gradual diminution of vision and for the clinical picture of chalcosis to appear over months or years. Surgical intervention is the most direct therapy, and recent advances in techniques and instrumentation ensure the best possible outcome, even in complex cases.

DIAGNOSIS

Clinical signs and symptoms

Ocular

- Anterior chamber: cells and flare, hypopyon, hyphema, copper-colored metallic particles.
- Cornea: deep stromal deposits, Kayser–Fleischer ring (usually superior and/or inferior, but may be circumferential).
- Globe: endophthalmitis, phthisis.
- Iris: greenish tinge, poor response to mydriatics.
- Lens: brownish-red, small, round deposits on zonules, subluxation, sunflower cataract, yellow or copper tinge.
- Optic nerve: papillitis.
- Retina: copper-colored macular sheen, detachment, edema, gliosis, 'gold-leaf' granular deposits in macula or adjacent vessels in the posterior pole, hemorrhages.
- Sclera: abscess, softening.
- Vitreous: abscess, fibrillar degeneration, greenish-brown or reddish-brown deposits, opacity, organization.
- Other: decreased visual acuity, nonspecific color vision defects, variable isopter constriction in visual field testing, variable disturbance in the rod and cone amplitudes in the electroretinogram, variable elevation in rod and cone thresholds in dark adaptometry, ocular hypotension, secondary glaucoma, subconjunctival foreign body resulting from intraocular extrusion (rare), sympathetic ophthalmia (rare), encapsulation of the foreign body with possible simulation of growing intraocular tumor without evidence of chalcosis.

Laboratory findings

- Computed tomography to define and localize the presence of an intraocular foreign body.
- B-scan ultrasonography to define the status of the vitreous and retina as dictated by the clinical situation.
- Visual field, color vision, electroretinogram, dark adaptometry, as required.
- Radiographic spectrometry to define the presence of intraocular copper ions.

PROPHYLAXIS

Use of protective eyewear designed to reduce ocular injuries would nearly eliminate penetrating ocular injuries in the workplace, on the field of battle, and in the home workshop.

TREATMENT

Systemic

Endophthalmitis prophylaxis should be employed on a routine basis in the presence of acute penetrating wounds and retained foreign bodies.

Oral prednisone suppresses the general inflammatory response and inhibits the migration of polymorphonuclear leukocytes as well as the release of inflammatory modulating factors. It can be used to stem the intraocular inflammation in preparation for a surgical procedure.

Local

After the appropriate diagnostic tests, in cases of recent trauma, the first maneuvers are directed to the closure of an open globe. The closure of anterior or posterior segment lacerations is accomplished with standard techniques and equipment.

Surgical

Vitrectomy, with or without lensectomy and scleral buckle, and immediate removal of the retained foreign body are the two initial options of a surgeon; the choice will be determined according to the associated ocular injuries and the type of surgical repair required. Copper alloys with a copper content of 85% or greater may incite an acute inflammatory response, including fibrosis and foreign body encapsulation, particularly when sited adjacent to the ciliary body and retina. Prompt surgical removal may be necessary.

Other

Local steroids may be effective in suppressing the eye's response to copper. Peribulbar dexamethasone has been shown to suppress both inflammation and the encapsulation of intraocular copper.

COMPLICATIONS

- Small, shiny retained foreign bodies may be observed.
- Corrosion of the foreign body's surface may herald the appearance of inflammation and/or the deposition of intraocular copper; this may necessitate removal of the foreign body.
- Serial visual acuities, color vision, visual fields, dark adaptometry, and electroretinography, if needed, may be used to follow small retained foreign bodies. Foreign body removal would be indicated in cases of progressive deterioration in the monitored visual parameters.
- The potential exists for the development of cataract, hypotony, uveitis, and altered visual function.
- Late surgical repair may be associated with cataract, aphakia, retinal breaks and/or detachment, intraocular hemorrhage and infection.

REFERENCES

Gorodetsky R, Weinreb A, Zeimer R, et al: Noninvasive copper measurement in chalcosis, comparison with electroretinography and ophthalmoscopy. Arch Ophthalmol 95:1059–1064, 1977.

McGahan MC, Bito LZ, Myers BM: The pathophysiology of the ocular microenvironment. II. Copper-induced ocular inflammation and hypotony. Exp Eye Res 42:595–605, 1986.

Mittag T: Role of oxygen radicals in ocular inflammation and cellular damage. Exp Eye Res 39:759–769, 1984.

Neubauer H: Ocular metallosis. Trans Ophthalmol Soc UK 99:502–510, 1979. The Montgomery Lecture.

Rosenthal AR, Eckhert C: Copper and zinc in ophthalmology. In: Karcioglu ZA, Sarper RM, eds: Zinc and copper in medicine. Springfield, IL, Charles C Thomas, 1980:595–609.

Rosenthal AR, Marmor MF, Leuenberger P, et al: Chalcosis: a study of natural history. Ophthalmology 86:1956–1959, 1979.

Sternberg P: Trauma: principles and techniques of treatment. In: Ryan S, Glaser B, eds: Retina. 2nd edn. St Louis, CV Mosby, 1994:3:2351–2378.

Zeimer R, Gorodetsky R, Lahav M, et al: Experimental chalcosis: a comparison between in vivo and in vitro findings. Arch Ophthalmol 96:115–119, 1978.

156 INTRAOCULAR FOREIGN BODY: NONMAGNETIC, CHEMICALLY INERT 871.6

Howard Shann-Cherng Ying, MD, PhD
Baltimore, Maryland
Peter L. Gehlbach, MD, PhD
Baltimore, Maryland

Intraocular foreign bodies are often associated with severely injured eyes. The subset of penetrating ocular trauma involving nonmagnetic, chemically inert foreign bodies may, in selected cases, present an opportunity to avoid the additional damage of foreign body removal. When an intraocular foreign body is suspected, basic surgical principles apply, and all open globes should be closed. If the foreign body is chemically inert, inorganic, does not interfere with the visual axis, and is not in a place to cause ongoing mechanical injury, then the most prudent course of management may be to leave it in the globe. A diagnosis of inert foreign body is always tentative, pending observation over several years. Careful attention during this interval is required for early detection of the significant sequelae associated with these injuries. If at the time of injury doubt exists as to the nature of the foreign body and removal seems to be straightforward, then surgical removal is appropriate.

ETIOLOGY/INCIDENCE

- The National Eye Trauma System Registry estimates that the annual number of reported ocular and orbital injuries in the United States is 2.4 million, 20,000 to 68,000 of which are vision-threatening injuries. In a report from this registry, of 492 eyes with intraocular foreign bodies, 92% were in male patients, 50% of injuries occurred in the occupational setting, 94% of persons wore no protective eyewear, and 44 (8.9%) had nonmetallic foreign bodies. In contrast, a review of hospital records from three centers in Tehran during the Iran-Iraq War (1980–1988) found 767 eyes with intraocular foreign bodies and 90% non-magnetic foreign bodies, suggesting that occupational and combat eye trauma may not be comparable.
- If intracorneal foreign bodies are excluded, roughly one fifth of intraocular foreign bodies are confined to the anterior segment, with a greater percentage of metallic foreign bodies having the energy to penetrate into the posterior segment.
- In the occupational setting, glass is the most common nonmetallic inert intraocular foreign body; however, in the combat setting, stone and sand are more common. Penetrating injuries secondary to glass differ from those caused by the more common foreign body, steel, in a number of ways. They tend to occur in a younger age group, are more commonly bilateral, and frequently involve multiple foreign bodies. These injuries present unique challenges with regard to direct visualization, detection, and surgical removal.

DIAGNOSIS

History

- Injuries associated with the shattering of glass, hammering, high-speed machinery, explosions and blasts, projectile weapons, release of materials under pressure, and so forth may lead one to suspect that an intraocular foreign body is present.
- Pediatric patients more often present with injuries from projectile weapons or explosions, leading to a higher proportion of multiple nonmetallic IOFBs, and greater incidence of retinal damage.
- Once a foreign body has been discovered and localized, preliminary assessment of its potential to cause toxic damage must be made.
- In most instances this determination can be made based on the historical account of the injury. If a fragment of an object has entered the eye, analysis of the remaining portion reveals its chemical composition.
- Materials such as gold, silver, aluminum, platinum, tantalum, glass, stone, porcelain, pottery fragments, gunpowder, silicone, rubber and plastics are generally considered nonreactive.
- Iron, copper, cobalt, lead, nickel and zinc are considered reactive and may require immediate removal in order to prevent additional toxic injury, e.g. acute chalcosis.
- Photochromic glass is not inert in the eye.

Physical examination

- In some instances a foreign body may be visualized directly, and no ancillary studies are necessary. If visualization of any portion of the globe is obscured and a foreign body is suspected, then imaging studies must be performed.
- Plain radiography of the globe and orbit is the traditional technique for screening purposes and will determine the presence of most metallic and many nonmetallic foreign bodies; however the sensitivity may be as low as 40%.
- Ultrasonography is sensitive in locating foreign bodies but requires a skilled examiner as well as caution if an open globe is suspected. Open globes do not necessarily preclude ultrasonography, as stand-off techniques that transmit minimal pressure to the eye may be employed.
- Magnet-assisted ultrasonography is performed when the examiner advances a strong magnet toward the globe during ultrasonography. Movement of the foreign body indicates that it is magnetic.
- Computed tomography (CT) is an important diagnostic modality for detection and localization of suspected IOFBs. It is atraumatic and provides valuable information about the

integrity of intraocular structures. It is also useful in cases involving multiple foreign bodies. Modern spiral CT scanning using 3-mm image sections may detect 0.5mm glass or stone IOFBs with excellent sensitivity. Certain nonmetallic foreign bodies, such as wood, are nearly isodense to intravitreal blood and may be difficult to detect with CT. Sensitivity in detection as well as accuracy in localization are increased when ultrasonography and CT are used concurrently.

- Magnetic resonance imaging (MRI) is now widely available and may detect and localize some nonmetallic, radiolucent (<600 Hounsfield units) IOFB not visualized by CT. If there is any possibility that the foreign body may be metallic, MRI should not be performed because of possible movement or heating of the object. MRI, in the setting of penetrating ocular trauma, has had limited application because of the potential for secondary injury.

COURSE/PROGNOSIS

- Visual outcomes correlate with the presenting visual acuity and mechanism of injury. Globe perforations secondary to lacerations or blunt trauma tend to do poorly compared to perforations caused by small, sharp-edged intraocular foreign bodies that may cause less direct mechanical damage when entering the eye. Foreign bodies that are larger, toxic, and of higher energy, e.g. gunshot or air rifle, at impact tend to do poorly. Recent series have verified these findings and add the presence of retinal lesions or vitreous hemorrhage as additional predictors of poor outcome.
- Endophthalmitis is reported to occur in 6.8% of eyes containing nonmetallic foreign bodies, in 7.2% of eyes containing metallic foreign bodies and, surprisingly, in only 5.9% of eyes containing vegetative material. A delay in primary closure of the globe beyond 24 hours results in a 4-fold increase in the incidence of the development of endophthalmitis overall and a 6-fold increase in patients older than 50 years. Mulivariate analysis has shown that delay in primary repair, ruptured lens capsule, and dirty wound are the major predictors of post-traumatic endophthalmitis.

PROPHYLAXIS

Prophylaxis remains the best approach to all penetrating ocular injury. It can be promoted through:

- Public education;
- Identification and avoidance of high-risk activities or situations;
- The wearing of protective goggles.

TREATMENT

Ocular

- Prophylactic topical antibiotics are indicated in all patients. Gram-positive and gram-negative coverage is appropriate.
- Most patients with IOFB have an accompanying traumatic uveitis that requires treatment with topical steroids and cycloplegics. Although steroids may increase the risk of infection, the potential sequelae of the inflammation that accompanies these injuries generally requires their use.
- Topical cycloplegics are also beneficial, as they reduce discomfort by placing the ciliary body at rest, and they may decrease vascular permeability.

Surgical

- Attempts at removal should be undertaken only under conditions that provide excellent visualization. Removal is normally easier during a secondary procedure when hemorrhage has cleared and hemostasis has improved.
- Anterior segment foreign bodies are generally managed through limbal incisions. Intralenticular foreign bodies associated with cataract formation are managed with lensectomy. Occasionally, small intralenticular inert foreign bodies do not cause cataract formation and can be observed.
- If a decision is made to remove a foreign body that is embedded in either the vitreous or retina or is lying on the retinal surface, then a pars plana vitrectomy is performed and the foreign body is grasped with an appropriate forceps. The object is then carefully removed through an incision in the pars plana or, for certain large foreign bodies, through the original entry site.
- Removal of nonmagnetic subretinal foreign bodies may require retinotomy or gentle expression through the entry site with a forceps. If the foreign body is thought to be inert and there is concern about causing further tissue damage during its removal, it should be left in place and the patient's status monitored for toxic or mechanical damage.
- Inert foreign bodies may become encapsulated when left in the globe. If secondary removal is attempted, the foreign body is first carefully dissected free from its encasement. This releases tractional forces that could result in iatrogenic injury to adjacent structures.

COMPLICATIONS

- Although in 26% of eyes containing IOFB, the vitreous has been reported to be culture-positive for bacteria, clinically manifest endophthalmitis following penetrating ocular injury is relatively uncommon. In eight studies published between 1984 and 1989, the incidence of endophthalmitis ranged from 2.9% to 13.3%. The largest of these (n = 492), from the National Eye Trauma System Registry, reported an incidence of 6.9%, consistent with the average incidence in the combined studies (n = 1420) of 6.8%.
- Presumably, the failure of culture-positive eyes to manifest clinically significant endophthalmitis is in part a result of current management.
- Even with ideal management, endophthalmitis remains a constant threat in the initial period of treatment. Increasing inflammation may be an indicator of incipient endophthalmitis. Fibrin, vitreous organization, and hypopyon are suggestive. The first posterior signs include a slight whitening of the retina and a subtle vasculitis.
- Even though the incidence of endophthalmitis is low, when it is present, its effects are often devastating. Therefore, a high index of suspicion must be maintained in all cases. When signs of endophthalmitis are present at the time of primary closure, cultures should be taken.
- Taking routine intraoperative bacterial cultures in patients without clinical indicators of endophthalmitis has not been shown to identify patients who will go on to develop

clinically significant endophthalmitis. The results of these cultures do not ordinarily serve to direct management decisions.

- All foreign bodies that are removed from the globe should be sent for culture and identification.
- Prophylactic intravitreal antibiotics in a prospective, double-masked randomized study failed to show a statistical benefit for intraocular antibiotics although all 4 eyes (6.6%) with endophthalmitis were in the control group; however, some authors feel that they are indicated if the wound is particularly dirty or the foreign body originated in the soil or in a farm environment.
- In this setting, antibiotic coverage must include organisms of the *Bacillus* genus, which are commonly β-lactamase-positive. This virulent pathogen is usually sensitive to vancomycin and is often sensitive to aminoglycosides and clindamycin.
- It should be noted that intravitreal agents are themselves potentially toxic and the procedure is not without complications. Intravitreal injection should not be administered unless there is excellent visualization of the needle tip during the procedure. A slow injection, with the stream directed away from the macula, is recommended.
- Vigilant observation for the possible development of endophthalmitis is mandatory. Ongoing evaluation for possible late sequelae of IOFB injuries, including but not limited to cataract, retinal detachment, and unexpected toxicity from a foreign body, is essential. Secondary retinal detachment with proliferative vitreoretinopathy was associated with poor initial visual acuity (<20/200) or vitreous hemorrhage and occurred in 11–13% of IOFB patients at 3.1–4.6 months after primary repair in two large cohorts. Prophylactic scleral buckling in a prospective, randomized study failed to show a statistical reduction in risk of secondary retinal detachment.

SUMMARY

Successful management of nonmagnetic, chemically inert intraocular foreign bodies requires a complete and comprehensive evaluation directed at:

- Assessing the extent of mechanical injury to the globe;
- Identifying and localizing all intraocular foreign bodies;
- Accurately assessing the foreign body's potential for toxicity.

These cases demand a combination of conservatism and vigilance. Because removal may entail high-risk surgery without the advantage of magnetic extraction techniques, early management should be biased toward leaving small inert (both chemically nonreactive and mechanically bengin) foreign bodies undisturbed-with the following cautions:

- All open globes require closure;
- Long-term follow-up to monitor for late sequelae is required;
- Inert objects may still cause fibrous tissue proliferation with late contraction, resulting in epimacular proliferation or retinal detachment;
- Endophthalmitis can cause devastating destruction as a result of a seemingly minor wound;
- A diagnosis of inert foreign body is always tentative until it has been observed for several years.

REFERENCES

Azad RV, Kumar N, Sharma YR, Vohra R: Role of prophylactic scleral buckling in the management of retained intraocular foreign bodies. Clin Experiment Ophthalmol 32:58–61, 2004.

Brinton GS, Aaberg TM, Reeser FH, et al: Surgical results in ocular trauma involving the posterior segment. Am J Ophthalmol 93:271–278, 1982.

Bryden FM, Pyott AA, Bailey M, McGhee CN: Real time ultrasound in the assessment of intraocular foreign bodies. Eye 4(Pt 5):727–731, 1990.

Cardillo JA, Farah ME, Mitre J, et al: An intravitreal biodegradable sustained release naproxen and 5-fluorouracil system for the treatment of experimental post-traumatic proliferative vitreoretinopathy. Br J Ophthalmol 88:1201–1205, 2004.

Chiquet C, Gain P, Zech JC, et al: Risk factors for secondary retinal detachment after extraction of intraocular foreign bodies. Can J Ophthalmol 37:168–176, 2002.

Dass AB, Ferrone PJ, Chu YR, et al: Sensitivity of spiral computed tomography scanning for detecting intraocular foreign bodies. Ophthalmology 108:2326–2328, 2001.

de Juan E, Jr, Sternberg P, Jr, Michels RG: Penetrating ocular injuries. Types of injuries and visual results. Ophthalmology 90:1318–1322, 1983.

Essex RW, Yi Q, Charles PG, Allen PJ. Post-traumatic endophthalmitis. Ophthalmology 111:2015–2022, 2004.

Foster RE, Martinez JA, Murray TG, et al: Useful visual outcomes after treatment of *Bacillus cereus endophthalmitis*. Ophthalmology 103:390–397, 1996.

Gopal L, Banker AS, Deb N, et al: Management of glass intraocular foreign bodies. Retina 18:213–220, 1998.

Greven CM, Engelbrecht NE, Slusher MM, Nagy SS: Intraocular foreign bodies: management, prognostic factors, and visual outcomes. Ophthalmology 107:608–612, 2000.

Cunene U, Maden A, Kaynak S, Pirnar T: Magnetic resonance imaging and computed tomography in the detection and localization of intraocular foreign bodies. Doc Ophthalmol 81:369–378, 1992.

Heimann K, Paulmann H, Tavakolian U: The intraocular foreign body. Principles and problems in the management of complicated cases by pars plana vitrectomy. Int Ophthalmol 6:235–242, 1983.

Jonas JB, Knorr HL, Budde WM: Prognostic factors in ocular injuries caused by intraocular or retrobulbar foreign bodies. Ophthalmology 107:823–828, 2000.

Khosla PK, Murthy KS, Tewari HK: Retinal toxicity of trace elements. Indian J Ophthalmol 35:311–314, 1987.

Mieler WF, Ellis MK, Williams DF, Han DP: Retained intraocular foreign bodies and endophthalmitis. Ophthalmology 97:1532–1538, 1990.

Neubauer H: The Montgomery Lecture, 1979. Ocular metallosis. Trans Ophthalmol Soc U K 99:502–510, 1979.

New PF, Rosen BR, Brady TJ, et al: Potential hazards and artifacts of ferromagnetic and nonferromagnetic surgical and dental materials and devices in nuclear magnetic resonance imaging. Radiology 147:139–148, 1983.

Nguyen QD, Kruger EF, Kim AJ, et al: Combat eye trauma: intraocular foreign body injuries during the Iran-Iraq war (1980–1988). Int Ophthalmol Clin 42:167–177, 2002.

Parver LM, Dannenberg AL, Blacklow B, et al: Characteristics and causes of penetrating eye injuries reported to the National Eye Trauma System Registry, 1985–91. Public Health Rep 108:625–632, 1993.

Penner R, Passmore JW: Magnetic vs nonmagnetic intraocular foreign bodies. An ultrasonic determination. Arch Ophthalmol 76:676–677, 1966.

Pieramici DJ, MacCumber MW, Humayun MU, et al: Open-globe injury. Update on types of injuries and visual results. Ophthalmology 103:1798–1803, 1996.

Rao NA, Tso MO, Rosenthal AR: Chalcosis in the human eye. A clinicopathologic study. Arch Ophthalmol 94:1379–1384, 1976.

Rubsamen PE, Cousins SW, Martinez JA: Impact of cultures on management decisions following surgical repair of penetrating ocular trauma. Ophthalmic Surg Lasers 28:43–49, 1997.

Rubsamen PE, Cousins SW, Winward KE, Byrne SF: Diagnostic ultrasound and pars plana vitrectomy in penetrating ocular trauma. Ophthalmology 101:809–814, 1994.

Soheilian M, Rafati N, Peyman GA: Prophylaxis of acute posttraumatic bacterial endophthalmitis with or without combined intraocular antibiotics: a prospective, double-masked randomized pilot study. Int Ophthalmol 24:323–330, 2001.

Thompson JT, Parver LM, Enger CL, et al: Infectious endophthalmitis after penetrating injuries with retained intraocular foreign bodies. National Eye Trauma System. Ophthalmology 100:1468–1474, 1993.

Williams DF, Mieler WF, Abrams GW: Intraocular foreign bodies in young people. Retina 10(Suppl 1):S45–S49, 1990.

157 INTRAOCULAR FOREIGN BODY: STEEL OR IRON 871.5

Christophe Chiquet, MD, PhD
Grenoble, France
Gilles Thuret, MD, PhD
Saint-Etienne, France
Philippe Gain, MD, PhD
Saint-Etienne, France
Jean-Paul Romanet, MD
Grenoble, France

ETIOLOGY/INCIDENCE

Intraocular foreign bodies (IOFBs) are a major cause of ocular trauma (up to 40%) and of legal blindness. Young adults, especially men, are the most likely victims, as a result of industrial, agricultural or firearm injuries. IOFBs are most commonly steel or iron, and generally result from hammering metal-on-metal (up to 72%) or from injuries caused by machines. Between 55% and 80% of metallic IOFBs are magnetic.

DIAGNOSIS

- A history of a metal-on-metal or machine-related accident is suggestive of the presence of a foreign body.
- The most common perforation sites are the cornea (52%), the sclera (34%) and an association of cornea and sclera (15%). A scleral wound may be masked by a subconjunctival hemorrhage and thus unnoticed by the patient.
- The presence of an IOFB in the anterior segment is frequently associated with a corneal perforation, positive Seidel's test, conjunctival laceration, hemorrhage or edema, hyphema, iris defect, or lens disruption with or without cataract formation. Gonioscopy may reveal a foreign body lodged in the anterior chamber angle.
- A posterior segment IOFB must be suspected if there are vitreous strands or hemorrhage, air bubbles, retinal hemorrhage, inflammation, or edema related to a retinal impact site. A posterior IOFB is sometimes encapsulated.
- Computerized tomography (CT) scanning has become the standard method for imaging ruptured globes and remains the most sensitive method for detecting metallic foreign bodies. CT scanning allows detection of IOFBs with diameters of 0.5 mm or more, can distinguish metallic from nonmetallic foreign bodies, and can identify the composition of many nonmetallic IOFBs. Moreover, CT evaluation of penetrating ocular trauma can be used to predict functional and anatomic outcome in eyes with penetrating injuries.
- Ultrasonography is both sensitive and specific in evaluating traumatized eyes, in localizing the IOFB, and in identifying associated lesions (choroidal hemorrhage, posterior exit sites, retinal and posterior vitreous detachment).
- Magnetic resonance imaging is contraindicated, as it may cause a shift in the position of a magnetic IOFB.

TREATMENT

Infection prophylaxis

- Intravenous antibiotics are routinely recommended as prophylaxis against endophthalmitis. Broad-spectrum coverage with antibiotics (association of fluoroquinolones and fosfocine or piperilline) is commonly used.
- Intravitreal antibiotics may be used prophylactically, at the time of initial surgical repair or at admission if no surgery is required prior to vitrectomy (vancomycin 1 mg with either ceftazidime 2.25 mg or amikacin 200–400 μg). They are particularly indicated if signs of endophthalmitis are present at the time of surgical repair or if the nature of the injury suggests a high risk of endophthalmitis developing.

Surgical

Closure of the entrance wound to restore integrity of the globe, and repositioning or removal of prolapsed uvea, are the first concern during primary surgery. The method of removal involving the least surgical trauma and greatest control is determined.

ANTERIOR SEGMENT INTRAOCULAR FOREIGN BODY

- An IOFB anterior to the lens may be approached through a limbal incision over the area of the foreign body or 180 degrees away.
- An anterior segment IOFB may be dislodged with a bent needle, pick, or intraocular forceps or by using magnet extraction.

INTRALENTICULAR FOREIGN BODY

- Depending on location and composition of the IOFB, it may be well tolerated indefinitely with little secondary lens change or may be associated with toxicity or cataractous lens changes necessitating IOFB removal (Figure 157.1).
- If cataract formation and/or IOFB toxicity is present, extracapsular cataract extraction or phacoemulsification may be accomplished. Anterior vitrectomy may be performed as needed for posterior capsule rupture.
- Aphakia may be corrected using posterior chamber intraocular lens (IOL) implantation, scleral or iris suture fixation of IOL, anterior chamber IOL implantation or contact lens correction.

POSTERIOR SEGMENT INTRAOCULAR FOREIGN BODY

After a 360° conjunctival peritomy, the sclera is explored and any corneoscleral wounds are closed with multiple interrupted sutures.

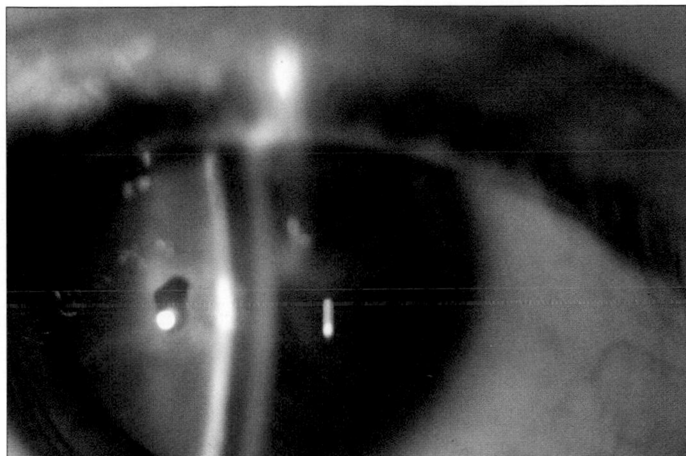

FIGURE 157.1. Intralenticular IOFB: this metal foreign body is located in the lens and was complicated by cataractous changes. There is no intraocular inflammation at this time.

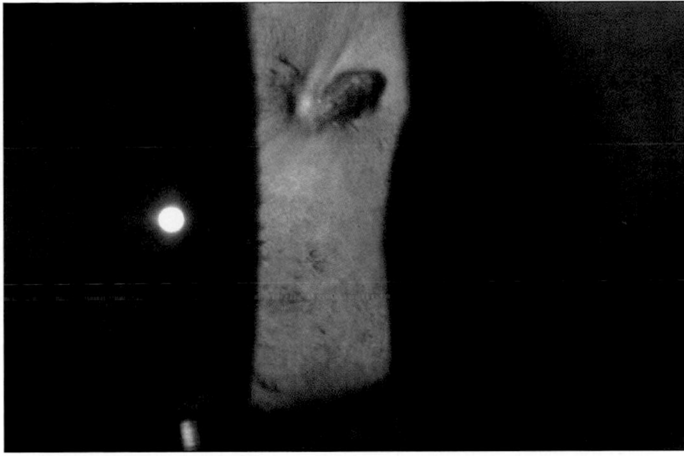

FIGURE 157.2. Siderosis: complicates ferric IOFB, located on the iris in this case. This complication must be suspected when IOFB is associated with discoloration of the cornea, iris, lens (note subanterior capsular deposits in this example). A prompt extraction of the IOFB is needed.

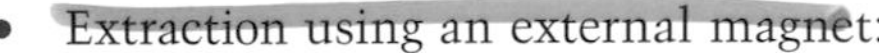

- Extraction using an external magnet:
  - Careful localization of the IOFB before extraction is critical;
  - A direct approach is possible for anteriorly located intra- or subretinal magnetic IOFBs via scleral cutdown (generally a T-shaped configuration) adjacent to the IOFB;
  - The indirect transvitreal approach may be attempted if the IOFB is magnetic, pre-retinal (without encapsulating fibrous material) or within the vitreous and small in size (<3 mm diameter). This technique consists of placing the electromagnet at an extraction site on the pars plana; the magnet should be directed so that, as the IOFB is removed, it does not inadvertently damage the lens or retina.
- Extraction using pars plana vitrectomy (PPV):
  - Vitreous surgery allows excellent visualization and removal of blood, lens materials, and organisms if present. It is the technique of choice for IOFB removal from the posterior segment, especially if the body is located in the retina, encapsulated, and/or associated with media opacities. Vitrectomy needs to be relatively complete. Attention to the removal of the posterior hyaloid to prevent later epiretinal membrane formation has been emphasized. However, in many young people, it may not be possible to remove a portion of the posterior vitreous cortex on the macula or the optic nerve;
  - Delaying vitrectomy (by 5–10 days) in eyes without evidence of infection decreases the chance of intraoperative bleeding and allows spontaneous separation of the posterior hyaloid;
  - Intraocular magnets can be used to pick up IOFBs for transfer to diamond-coated forceps and removal;
  - An intraretinal IOFB may be extracted using forceps or a 20-gauge rare-earth magnet. Subretinal IOFBs are removed with the foreign body forceps via a retinotomy;
  - For encapsulated IOFBs, after vitreous removal the fibrous capsule is incised with the MVR blade and removal of the top of the capsule with 20-gauge scissors allows the foreign body to be freed before removal;
  - Retinopexy around a retinal impact site is rarely necessary, and its benefit is debatable. Excessive and unnecessary retinopexy leads to greater wound-related cellular proliferation and inflammation;
  - Extraction may be accomplished via a limbal incision if lensectomy or phacoemulsification has been performed. Lens extraction may be necessary for the translimbal removal of a very large foreign body;
  - Secondary PPV is performed for postoperative complications, such as persistent vitreous hemorrhage, epiretinal membranes and RD.
- Other routes of extraction:
  - If the foreign body is in the choroid or sclera, extraction can be performed through a scleral trap door or a direct cutdown, using a forceps or magnet;
  - If corneal damage necessitates a penetrating keratoplasty, an open-sky vitrectomy with foreign body removal can also be effective.
- No surgery and frequent follow-up:
  - May be discussed for intralenticular IOFB;
  - Submacular and intraoptic nerve foreign bodies should be managed on an individual basis because of the hazards of removal.

COMPLICATIONS

Siderosis

- Is the process of chronic intracellular damage resulting from electrolytic dissociation or oxidation of elemental iron (Fe) to ferric (Fe^{3+}) and ferrous (Fe^{2+}) ions.
- Onset rapidity is determined by the location and iron content of the foreign body. Location has high prognostic significance, with a poorer visual outcome for posterior segment IOFBs (as compared to intralenticular or anterior segment IOFBs).
- May cause inflammation or hypopyon, rusty discoloration of the conjunctiva, the cornea (with corneal edema, Fleischer's ring, a Hudson–Stähli line, interstitial keratitis, or corneal neovascularization), the iris (with iridoplegia, or synechiae), the lens (with subanterior capsular deposits : see Figure 157.2, luxation, or subluxation), and/or the retina (with arteriolar narrowing).
- May be complicated by retinal detachment (RD), macular edema, pigmentary degeneration, secondary glaucoma,

dyschromatopsia, night blindness, visual loss, and phthisis bulbi.

- Electroretinography is a sensitive clinical measure of siderotic change and typically shows an initial supernormality with later slow decrease in b-wave amplitude. Abnormalities may be present before visual acuity is affected.
- Abnormalities in dark adaptation and electro-oculography have also been noted.

Endophthalmitis

Endophthalmitis remains a serious complication of IOFB injuries (2%–13%), and clinical signs (hypopyon, vitritis, retinal periphlebitis) may be masked in the acute phase after severe ocular injury, thereby making diagnosis difficult in some cases.

- The most organisms most commonly isolated are *Staphylococcus*, *Streptococcus* and *Bacillus* species.
- Risk factors include: a delay in primary repair, disruption of the crystalline lens, home or occupational injuries, contamination with organic matter.
- If diagnosis of endophthalmitis is probable, an injection of antibiotics in the vitreous must be performed at initial presentation, before early IOFB removal is then scheduled. This is combined with subconjunctival and fortified topical antibiotic administration and, in most cases, with at least a short course of systemic antibiotics as well.

Retinal detachment

- Preoperative RD is present in 5%–21% of patients.
- Postoperative RD occurs in 14%–37% of cases, mainly during the first four months after injury, and is a crucial factor in poor visual outcome after IOFB injury (final VA equal to or worse than 20/100 in 68%). Risk factors are firearm injury, size of IOFB, low initial visual acuity, vitreous prolapse and/or hemorrhage. Incidence of RD in patients with retinal IOFB is around 25%.
- Incidence of RD with proliferative vitreoretinopathy (PVR) is 20%. In patients with ocular trauma or IOFB, vitreous hemorrhage, persistent intraocular inflammation or a posteriorly located wound are independent predictive factors for the development of post-traumatic PVR. Severe vitreous hemorrhage is associated with intraocular fibroblastic proliferation and traction RD in experimental and clinical studies.
- To offset late vitreous base contraction, prophylactic scleral buckling has been suggested.

Others

Corneal decompensation (due to direct laceration or endothelial cell loss), glaucoma, pupillary membranes, ciliary body detachment (with subsequent hypotony), traumatic cataract, epiretinal membranes, choroidal hemorrhages (especially in eyes with IOFB lying deep within the choroid), focal granuloma formation in the choroid.

PROGNOSIS

Prognosis after IOFB removal is associated with:

- The nature of the injury: for example, prognosis is poor in the event of blunt injury, particularly when due to firearm accidents;
- IOFB characteristics, particularly size (the relative risk of poor visual outcome is multiplied by a factor of 1.21 with each IOFB size increase of 1 mm);
- Clinical data at initial presentation: poor visual acuity (VA), deficit of the pupil afferent reflex, presence of an hyphema, prolapse of intraocular tissue, lens injury, corneoscleral entry wound are indicators of poor final visual outcome;
- Post-operative RD.

Visual outcome is strongly influenced by the nature of the penetrating trauma and the extent of the initial wound(s). The percentage of patients with final VA better than or equal to 20/63 ranged from 39% to 66% in several studies.

COMMENTS

Steel or iron intraocular foreign bodies should be removed, particularly to prevent the possibility of siderotic damage. In recent decades microsurgical techniques have improved and IOFB management is better codified. Due to the magnetic nature of the foreign body, surgical removal may be performed using an external or a 20-gauge rare-earth magnet. Prognosis most often depends on the severity of the initial injury and on the development of secondary RD. Increased public awareness of the incidence of open-globe injuries in high-risk activities, and the promotion of safety glasses, should markedly decrease incidence of these injuries.

REFERENCES

Abu El-Asrar AM, Al-Amro SA, Khan NM, et al: Visual outcome and prognostic factors after vitrectomy for posterior segment foreign bodies. Eur J Ophthalmol 10:304–311, 2000.

Ahmadieh H, Sajjadi H, Azarmina M, et al: Surgical management of intraretinal foreign bodies. Retina 14:397–403, 1994.

Ambler JS, Meyers SM: Management of intraretinal metallic foreign bodies without retinopexy in the absence of retinal detachment. Ophthalmology 98:391–394, 1991.

Behrens-Baumann W, Praetorius G: Intraocular foreign bodies. 297 consecutive cases. Ophthalmologica 198:84–88, 1989.

Chiquet C, Gain P, Zech JC, et al: Risk factors for secondary retinal detachment after extraction of intraocular foreign bodies. Can J Ophthalmol 37:168–176, 2002.

Chiquet C, Zech JC, Denis P, et al: Intraocular foreign bodies. Factors influencing final visual outcome. Acta Ophthalmol Scand 77:321–325, 1999.

Chiquet C, Zech JC, Gain P, et al: Visual outcome and prognostic factors after magnetic extraction of posterior segment foreign bodies in 40 cases. Br J Ophthalmol 82:801–806, 1998.

Coleman DJ, Lucas BC, Rondeau MJ, et al: Management of intraocular foreign bodies. Ophthalmology 94:1647–1653, 1987.

De Juan E, Jr, Sternberg P, Jr, Michels RG: Penetrating ocular injuries. Types of injuries and visual results. Ophthalmology 90:1318–1322, 1983.

Essex RW, Yi Q, Charles PG, et al: Post-traumatic endophthalmitis. Ophthalmology 111:2015–2022, 2004.

Greven CM, Engelbrecht NE, Slusher MM, et al: Intraocular foreign bodies: management, prognostic factors, and visual outcomes. Ophthalmology 107:608–612, 2000.

Jonas JB, Knorr HL, Budde WM: Prognostic factors in ocular injuries caused by intraocular or retrobulbar foreign bodies. Ophthalmology 107:823–828, 2000.

Maguire AM, Enger C, Eliott D, et al: Computerized tomography in the evaluation of penetrating ocular injuries. Retina 11:405–411, 1991.

Mieler WF, Ellis MK, Williams DF, et al: Retained intraocular foreign bodies and endophthalmitis. Ophthalmology 97:1532–1538, 1990.

Mieler WF, Mittra RA: The role and timing of pars plana vitrectomy in penetrating ocular trauma. Arch Ophthalmol 115:1191–1192, 1997.

Punnonen E, Laatikainen L: Prognosis of perforating eye injuries with intraocular foreign bodies. Acta Ophthalmol (Copenh) 67:483–491, 1989.

Rubsamen PE, Cousins SW, Winward KE, et al: Diagnostic ultrasound and pars plana vitrectomy in penetrating ocular trauma. Ophthalmology 101:809–814, 1994.

Seal DV, Kirkness CM: Criteria for intravitreal antibiotics during surgical removal of intraocular foreign bodies. Eye 6(Pt 5):465–468, 1992.

Soheilian M, Abolhasani A, Ahmadieh H, et al: Management of magnetic intravitreal foreign bodies in 71 eyes. Ophthalmic Surg Lasers Imaging 35:372–378, 2004.

Wani VB, Al-Ajmi M, Thalib L, et al: Vitrectomy for posterior segment intraocular foreign bodies: visual results and prognostic factors. Retina 23:654–660, 2003.

Williams DF, Mieler WF, Abrams GW, et al: Results and prognostic factors in penetrating ocular injuries with retained intraocular foreign bodies. Ophthalmology 95:911–916, 1988.

158 IRIS LACERATIONS 364.74, IRIS HOLES 364.74, AND IRIDODIALYSIS 369.76

Richard A. Harper, MD
Little Rock, Arkansas

ETIOLOGY

Iris lacerations and holes are partial or full-thickness iris defects that are most often caused by trauma; the trauma can be surgical or nonsurgical.

An iridodialysis is a separation of the thin, weak iris root from its attachment to the ciliary body and scleral spur. This usually results in an irregular or D-shaped pupil. Iridodialysis is also most commonly caused by trauma to the globe, but may also be surgically induced.

COURSE/PROGNOSIS

An iris wound almost always results in a permanent defect because the healing abilities of the iris are minimal to absent unless the wound's edges are apposed.

Prognosis is good for small or isolated iris injuries. Symptoms and ocular morbidity are determined by the size of the iris defect and the damage to other ocular structures.

DIAGNOSIS

Small iris holes may be difficult to detect unless the pigment epithelium has been involved, resulting in transillumination defects. Larger defects and those that affect the pupillary sphincter often create abnormalities in pupil size (traumatic mydriasis), shape, or function. A common finding with sphincter injury is that of a small triangular defect in the pupillary border, oriented with the apex toward the peripheral iris. Extraneous light entering through iris defects may result in visual symptoms such as glare or monocular diplopia. Hyphema frequently coexists with iridodialysis because of the shearing of the vessel at the iris root. In these cases, the iridodialysis may not be noted until the hyphema clears. As with other iris injuries, an iridodialysis only infrequently results in visual symptoms such as monocular diplopia.

Differential diagnosis

All of the following entities present with iris atrophy or holes if iris trauma has not occurred:

- Iridocorneal endothelial (ICE) syndromes;
- Postinflammatory iris atrophy (e.g. herpes zoster);
- Ischemia (e.g. angle-closure glaucoma, anterior segment ischemia);
- Aging;
- Congenital defects (e.g. megalocornea, aniridia);
- Several ocular syndromes and systemic diseases (e.g. Axenfeld–Rieger syndrome).

TREATMENT

Ocular

- Topical cycloplegics and steroids for traumatic iritis.
- Rest and observation as supportive measures.
- Opaque contact lenses with clear pupillary zones for control of symptoms.

Surgical

- Not often required unless there is symptomatic glare or monocular diplopia.
- Normally deferred until intraocular inflammation has resolved; may be done in conjunction with traumatic cataract extraction or at the time of corneoscleral laceration repair.
- Lacerations without tissue loss may be directly closed with 10-0 polypropylene suture.

IRIDODIALYSIS

Symptomatic defects can be closed using a double-armed suture technique. A 10-0 polypropylene suture with straight needles is passed through the limbus, 180 degrees away from the iridodialysis. The needle continues across the anterior chamber, through the disinserted iris root, and out through the chamber angle and sclera. The other needle is then passed through the same entry site and through the iris root in a mattress fashion. The suture is then tied, drawing the iris back into place.

COMPLICATIONS

Associated ocular complications primarily reflect damage to other parts of the eye secondary to trauma:

- Corneal edema;
- Corneoscleral lacerations;
- Traumatic cataract, subluxed or dislocated lens;
- Hyphema;
- Angle-recession glaucoma;
- Cyclodialysis/ciliary body detachment with possible hypotony;
- Vitreous hemorrhage;
- Retinal tears, edema, or hemorrhage;
- Retinal detachment or dialysis;
- Choroidal rupture;
- Traumatic optic neuropathy.

COMMENTS

Iris injury due to blunt ocular trauma may result from one of two possible mechanisms. The first mechanism is that of direct corneal compression with resulting expansion of the globe in the coronal plane. This expansion directly stresses the area of the iris root and ciliary body. The second possible mechanism is that of a compression wave created in the aqueous as a result of blunt trauma. The subsequent posterior and lateral flow of the aqueous could cause sphincter or iris damage due to iris displacement.

Iris lacerations, holes, and iridodialyses by themselves do not commonly cause symptoms or ocular complications. Their primary significance lies in raising suspicions regarding injury to other ocular structures. Only if the iris defect creates significant symptoms should treatment be considered.

REFERENCES

Crouch ER, Williams PB: Trauma: ruptures and bleeding. In: Tasman W, Jaeger EA, eds: Duane's clinical ophthalmology. Philadelphia, Lippincott-Raven, 1997:IV:1–3.

Hanna C, Roy FH: Iris wound healing. Arch Ophthalmol 88:296–304, 1972.

Hersh PS, Zagelbaum BM, et al: Blunt iris injury. In: Albert DM, Jakobiec FA, eds: Principles and practice of ophthalmology. Philadelphia, WB Saunders, 2000:5208–5209.

Steinert RF: Iris trauma. In: Shingleton BJ, Hersh PS, Kenyon KR, eds: Eye trauma. St Louis, CV Mosby, 1991:95–103.

Wachler BB, Drueger RR: Double-armed McCannel suture for repair of traumatic iridodialysis. Am J Ophthalmol 122:109–110, 1996.

Waubke TN, Mellin KB: Treatment of iris injuries. In: Blodi F, Mackensen G, Neubauer H, eds: Surgical ophthalmology. Berlin, Springer, 1992: II:516–518.

159 ORBITAL IMPLANT EXTRUSION 996.59

Mark R. Levine, MD, FACS
Beechwood, Ohio
Amarpreet Singh, MD
Cleveland, Ohio

The loss of an eye because of enucleation or evisceration is emotionally traumatic, and is exacerbated by extrusion of an orbital implant. In general, the implant size used in enucleations is 18 to 22 mm. This (along with the prosthesis) maximally replaces the 6 mL of volume lost, prevents enophthalmos, superior tarsal sulcus deformity, and avoids the need for an oversized prosthesis and the complications associated with it. The implant in evisceration is as large as can be fit into the scleral envelope, which can be augmented with expansion sclerotomies or posterior placement of the implant.

There are three categories of implants used:

- Integrated: hydroxyapatite or porous polyethylene (Medpore);
- Non-integrated: silicone or acrylic spheres (methylmethacrylate);
- Biological: dermis fat grafts.

Problems formerly created by the rough surfaces of hydroxyapatite (HA) and porous polyethylene (PP) implants have been

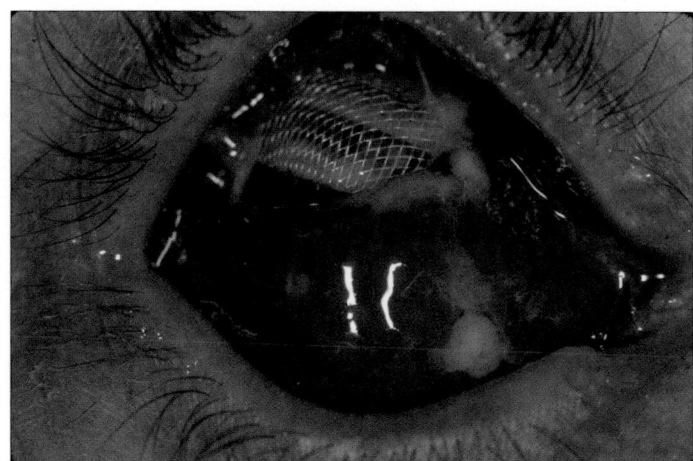

FIGURE 159.1. Extruding tantalum mesh from anophthalmic socket.

minimized by the recent refinement and smoothing of these surfaces as well as the use of wrapping materials. A secondary implant is always desirable to maintain orbital volume, minimize superior tarsal sulcus deformity, promote motility, and maximize cosmetic acceptability. It is important that the implant be centrally placed to facilitate the proper fit of a prosthesis.

ETIOLOGY

Extrusions may occur early in the postoperative period or many years after the initial implant (Figure 159.1). The causes of early extrusion are edema, hemorrhage, infection, too large an implant, and faulty surgical technique. Late extrusion is caused by erosion of the tissue covering the anterior surface of the implant. This erosion is a result of friction from a rough prosthesis or rough implant, such as hydroxyapatite, covered only by conjunctiva and Tenon's capsule. The erosion leads to extrusion either because of a secondary infection or because of epithelialization of the socket, with resulting contraction of the orbital tissues.

COURSE/PROGNOSIS

In evisceration, if the conjunctiva and Tenon's capsule have retracted but the scleral incision is intact, re-epithelialization may occur. If the sclera dehisces, exposing the implant, the likely course will be further wound dehiscence and extrusion. At this point, re-suturing the sclera is rarely effective.

In enucleation, retraction of the conjunctiva and Tenon's capsule with implant exposure leads to a natural course of extension of the exposure, with or without infection. If a porous implant is wrapped in fascia and the fascia is exposed, re-epithelialization and vascularization may occur. This is more likely if the defect is only 2 to 3 mm and the prosthesis is removed or vaulted. Larger defects of 10 to 15 mm will only occasionally re-epithelialize and vascularize.

Infection is another complication of orbital implant surgery. The fascial wrap may become infected or may resorb, during which time significant mucus production will be noted. An infection is more likely to develop from the combination of a moist socket, low-grade bacteria (usually *Staphylococcus epidermidis*), and the presence of a prosthesis. In the case of an infection, extrusion of the implant is usually inevitable.

DIAGNOSIS

The presence of a defect in the conjunctiva and Tenon's capsule and visualization of the implant require immediate attention. Significant muco-purulent discharge should alert the clinician to the possibility of socket infection and implant exposure, be it large or small.

TREATMENT

Systemic

- Systemic antibiotics when the socket is infected.

Local

- Good lid hygiene, using moist swabs as often as necessary.
- Observation for enlarging defects (keeping in mind that defects up to 3 mm usually resolve with conservative management).
- Removal or vaulting of the prosthesis to remove pressure from the affected area.
- Obtaining of a culture and sensitivity of any low-grade infection and use of appropriate topical antibiotics.

Surgical

Complete extrusion in cases of enucleation (no infection present)

- Immediate replacement with a fascia-enveloped sphere.
- Conjunctiva and Tenon's capsule are dissected from the rest of the orbital contents, taking care not to injure the recti muscles.
- A cavity may be present within the muscle cone if extrusion occurred within 2 to 3 weeks of placement of the implant. More commonly, the extraocular muscle and Tenon's capsule will have retracted into a small fibrotic mass.
- Sharp dissection is used to create a cavity in this mass.
- Excision of scar tissue posteriorly, or a posterior dissection, is carried out until Tenon's capsule and the muscles can stretch over the implant.
- A piece of autogenous fascia (either fascia lata, removed from the leg or temporalis fascia from the temple) is wrapped around an appropriately sized implant (16 to 20 mm), and sutured with 5-0 vicryl. Note that fascia as a wrap adds an additional 1 to 2 mm to the implant size.
- Sutures of 4-0 double-armed vicryl are placed in each of the four quadrants of the fascia-enveloped sphere.
- The implant is placed in the socket and the sutures are brought out from each socket quadrant between the recti muscles, through Tenon's capsule and the conjunctiva, and fixed externally to position the implant.
- Tenon's capsule posterior to the recti muscles is sutured over the fascial ball with interrupted 5-0 vicryl, taking bites of the fascia to create a barrier and centrally fix the implant.
- The recti muscles, if found, are gently approximated with 5-0 vicryl.
- Anterior Tenon's capsule is closed with 6-0 vicryl and the conjunctiva is closed with locking 6-0 chromic catgut suture.
- A small conformer is inserted so as not to place tension on the suture line.
- Two 4-0 silk tarsorrhaphies are performed, and a pressure patch is applied for 3–4 days.

Notes

- The choice of implant can be either PP, HA, silicone or acrylic sphere. The implant should be wrapped for added support and provide an additional barrier to extrusion.
- In the case of a porous implant, it too should be wrapped with fascia; however, multiple window defects are placed in the fascia to enhance vascular ingrowth.
- If the socket is infected, it is filled with antibiotic-impregnated gauze and replaced often until the infection is resolved (5 to 10 days); a secondary implant is placed at a later time.

Implant replacement in an evisceration

- The scleral pouch is irrigated with antibiotics.
- The implant of choice is placed in the scleral pouch so there is no tension on the scleral closure.
- If the scleral pouch is a too small, expansion sclerotomies are made with either radial or circumferential cuts. This is particularly important for vascular ingrowth if a HA or PP implant is being placed.
- The sclera is closed with running 5-0 vicryl, and Tenon's capsule and the conjunctiva are closed with locking 6-0 chromic catgut.
- Tarsorrhaphy is performed, and pressure patches are applied. A conformer is not needed, as the cul-de-sacs are formed and there will be no pressure on the suture line.

NOTES

- In the case where the volume of the scleral pouch is inadequate even after expansion sclerotomies, a posterior placement of the implant can be performed. The posterior sclera is cut from 3 to 9 o'clock and the implant placed within the muscle cone behind the posterior sclera. The posterior sclera is closed with running 5-0 vicryl and the anterior sclera is sutured to the posterior sclera with running 5-0 vicryl. The conjunctiva and Tenon's is closed with 6-0 chromic catgut. This permits a large enough sphere without placing tension on the sclera.

Large defects with implant exposure of 10 to 15 mm

- Immediate patch grafting with fascia.
- The conjunctiva and Tenon's capsule are dissected off the implant for several additional millimeters.
- The defect is irrigated with antibiotic solution copiously.
- Burr down the implant to reduce the size and remove areas of superficial infection.
- A piece of autogenous fascia (either fascia lata, removed from the leg or temporalis fascia from the temple) is placed over the implant, extending into all four quadrants of the socket.
- 5-0 vicryl sutures are placed into the fascia through Tenon's capsule, exiting through the conjunctiva in all four quadrants and tied.
- The conjunctiva and Tenon's capsule are closed over the fascia, taking bites of the fascia every third suture.
- If there are inadequate conjunctiva and Tenon's capsule, a bipedicle conjunctival flap is brought down from the upper fornix to cover the defect, and the upper fornix is allowed to heal by secondary intention.

NOTES

- A fornix based tarsoconjunctival flap from the upper eyelid also provides an excellent alternative approach in cases where recurrent exposure is an issue.

COMPLICATIONS

- Re-extrusion may occur, requiring either a dermis fat-graft repair, a delay of 6 months to a year prior to placing another secondary implant.
- A possibly infected porous implant must be removed and replaced with a new implant, either immediately or later.

COMMENTS

A dermis fat graft can always be substituted in implant extrusion. It must be of adequate size (25 mm × 25 mm) and must be placed in a non-infected orbit; otherwise it will become infected and will be absorbed. The complications of dermis fat grafts include atrophy and cyst or hair formation.

Autogenous fascia (as opposed to banked sclera) remains the safest and most convenient wrapping material. It is cost-effective and does not carry the risk of disease transmission. Topical antibiotic drops without steroid should be used to promote rapid wound healing.

REFERENCES

Levine MR, Older JJ: Enucleation surgery and treatment of the extruding orbital implant. In: Stewart WB, ed: Ophthalmic plastic surgery. A manual prepared for the use of graduates in medicine. 4th edn. San Francisco, American Academy of Ophthalmology, 1983:43–47.

Long JA, et al: Evisceration: a new technique of trans-scleral implant placement. Ophthal Plast Reconstr Surg 16(5):322–325, 2000.

Oberfeld S, Levine MR: Diagnosis and treatment of complications of enucleation and orbital implant surgery. Advan Ophthal Plast Reconstr Surg 8:107–117, 1990.

Soparkar CN, Patrinely JR: Tarsal patch-flap for obital implant exposure. Ophthal Plast Reconstr Surg 14(6):391–397, 1998.

160 SHAKEN BABY SYNDROME
995.55

William Barry Lee, MD
Atlanta, Georgia
Henry S. O'Halloran, MD, DOphth, FRCSI
San Diego, California

ETIOLOGY/INCIDENCE

Shaken baby syndrome, also known as whiplash shaken infant syndrome or shaken-impact syndrome, is a form of child abuse with an estimated annual incidence of 4000 cases per year. In the United States, one million children are severely abused annually. This syndrome includes nonaccidental head and body trauma with resulting intracranial hemorrhages, occult bone fractures, and retinal hemorrhages. The sustained injuries can result from violent shaking, direct impact, or compression injuries. The syndrome is commonly seen in infants under the age of two but can also be found in children up to five years of age. The underlying injuries are often hidden by the perpetrators and external findings of body or head trauma may be difficult to detect initially.

COURSE/PROGNOSIS

A high rate of mortality and morbidity is associated with shaken baby syndrome with mortality rates ranging from 15% to 40%. One third of identified patients with this syndrome die acutely with a significant proportion of survivors suffering severe neurological injury. Mortality was associated with extensive retinal injury, nonreactive pupils, and midline shifting of the brain. An additional one fifth of survivors have permanent visual impairment with cerebral injury accounting for the most common cause for profound vision loss. In addition, several studies have shown a correlation between the severity of retinal hemorrhage and the severity of head injury. The vast majority of intraocular injuries should be managed with observation in the acute phases with stabilization of life-threatening injuries including adequate ventilation and oxygenation by the primary care provider.

Shaken baby syndrome involves non-accidental injury exerted on a child by violent shaking and results in repetitive angular acceleration-deceleration motion similar to the force at the end of a whip. This motion creates high gravitational forces directed to the child's head. Brain injury can occur from compression or distention of the infant brain with direct axonal injury, direct trauma creating stress and tearing of blood vessels, and indirect damage from swelling, ischemia, hypoxia, and altered vasculature. Eye injuries are postulated to occur from either venous obstruction in the retina as a result of increased intracranial pressure or traction of the vitreous on the retina creating splitting or folds within the retinal layers.

DIAGNOSIS

Shaken baby presentations can vary dramatically from very mild and nonspecific complaints to severe and immediate life-threatening identifiable head injuries. The infants often present with lethargy, poor feeding, irritability, and/or vomiting and are often suspected of having an infection or intestinal/feeding disorders upon initial screening examinations because of lack of external findings of head or bodily injuries.

In the most severe situations, the infant can become immediately unconscious and exhibit impending central nervous system dysfunction including convulsions, comas, or respiratory failure.

A careful, yet expedient physical examination can display additional injuries such as bruises, rib or long-bone fractures, abdominal trauma and head trauma. Repeated physical examinations should be performed to find additional injuries that may have been missed on initial testing. Head trauma can range from skull fractures, subdural and subarachnoid hemorrhages to spinal cord trauma and brainstem injury. Physical examination must include a comprehensive ophthalmologic examination as up to 95% of cases of shaken baby syndrome have ocular findings. A dilated fundus examination must be included because retinal hemorrhages have been documented to occur in up to 50%–100% of nonaccidental head trauma cases. While retinal hemorrhages are not pathognomonic for

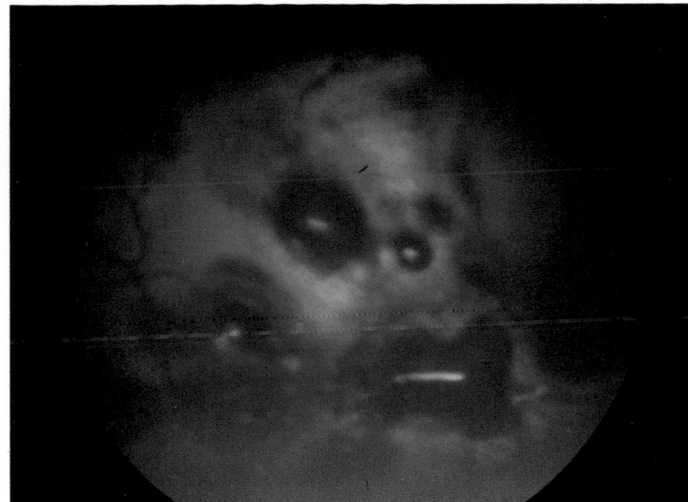

FIGURE 160.1. Shaken baby syndrome.

shaken baby syndrome, they are highly suggestive of a shaking or impact injury and several studies have shown that they are usually absent in pediatric accidental head trauma. Retinal hemorrhages often occur in all layers of the retina with no identifiable predominant location. Additional ocular findings include other forms of posterior segment injury such as vitreous hemorrhage, retinal detachment, retinoschisis, choroidal rupture, retinal folds, and optic nerve injury (Figure 160.1).

Laboratory findings

Diagnostic testing depends on the stability of the patient and may be limited for critically ill infants requiring life support. Neuroimaging should be performed in all cases of shaken baby syndrome to quantify the degree of head trauma. Computed tomography (CT) of the head should be the initial image of choice, preferably with intravenous contrast and bone and soft-tissue windows. CT is ideal for detection of subdural/subarachnoid hemorrhages and mass effect. Magnetic resonance imaging (MRI) of the head should be used as an adjunct to CT if patient stability is present and can be performed several days after initial testing. MRI can greater define intraparenchymal brain lesions and has a greater rate of detection for subdural hematomas. A skeletal survey should be performed once patient stability is achieved to evaluate for fractures of the hands, feet, long bones, skull, spine, and ribs. A repeat skeletal survey 2 weeks after the initial evaluation can demonstrate healing fractures that may have been missed on initial films.

Differential diagnosis

Retinal hemorrhages are an important clinical finding in diagnosis of shaken baby syndrome, but they are not pathognomonic for the syndrome. The most likely causes of retinal hemorrhages in an infant or young child include birth trauma, hematological disorders, Terson syndrome, severe accidental head trauma, infection, cardiopulmonary resuscitation, and child abuse. An estimated 15%–30% of infants have retinal hemorrhages from birth trauma, but they are often associated with a traumatic birth and resolve by 4 weeks of age. Hematologic testing can rule out coagulopathies such as hemophilia, von Willebrand disease, and vitamin K deficiency, and laboratory testing can help with confirmation of an infection. Several reports have shown that retinal hemorrhages are rare findings in accidental head trauma.

COMMENT

The wide variety of injuries that may occur in the syndrome require a multidisciplinary team approach in management and should include a pediatrician, neurologist, radiologist, ophthalmologist and/or a pediatric neurosurgeon. A child abuse specialist, social worker, law enforcement officer and child protection services must also work closely with the medical team. Appropriate documentation of injuries is imperative for future legal investigations with careful and detailed documentation of history, presentation, and examination as a high proportion of these cases develop into legal investigations.

Shaken baby syndrome is a leading cause of morbidity and mortality in infants and young children. All infants suspected of child abuse and shaken baby syndrome must have a careful evaluation with a complete physical exam including a dilated fundus examination. A multidisciplinary healthcare team is imperative in diagnosis and management of victims suffering from shaken baby syndrome. With an increasing incidence and high probability of underdiagnosed or unreported cases, a thorough physical and ophthalmologic examination can be critical in diagnosis of shaken baby syndrome. A greater understanding of this syndrome is important for the education of not only health care providers, but also the public, as prevention is the only method for alleviation of this abusive syndrome.

REFERENCES

Caffey J: The whiplash shaken infant syndrome: manual shaking by the extremities with whiplash-induced intracranial and intraocular bleedings, linked with residual permanent brain damage and mental retardation. Pediatrics 54:396–403, 1974.

Kivlin JD, Simons KB, Lazoritz S, Ruttum MS: Shaken baby syndrome. Ophthalmology 107:1246–1254, 2000.

Levin AV: Ophthalmology of shaken baby syndrome. Neurosurg Clin N Am 13:201–211, 2002.

Pierre-Kahn V, Roche O, Dureau P, et al: Ophthalmologic findings in suspected child abuse victims with subdural hematomas. Ophthalmology 110:1718–1723, 2003.

Tsao K, Kazlas M, Weiter JJ: Ocular injuries in shaken baby. Int Ophthalmol Clin 42:145–155, 2002.

161 THERMAL BURNS 940.9

F. Hampton Roy, MD, FACS

Little Rock, Arkansas

The thermally burned patient may present a challenging management problem for the ophthalmologist. Although many seriously burned individuals with total-body burns may initially escape direct damage to the globe of the eye, complications resulting from the overall injury can have a devastating effect on the ocular system.

ETIOLOGY

Many severely burned patients may escape direct injury to the cornea and conjunctiva because of Bell's phenomenon and the protection of the eyelids. On the other hand, many do suffer direct corneal and conjunctival injuries that are thermal in nature, caused by the flame itself or by hot gases. Some corneal injuries may also be toxic, caused by the combustion of toxic chemicals that are released when synthetic materials burn. Finally, severe corneal and ocular injuries may occur if hot liquids or molten metal explodes into the eyes. These more severe, direct ocular injuries behave much like toxic alkaline burns, with resultant avascular necrosis in some cases and symblepharon formation as well. They are managed much like toxic chemical injuries.

COURSE/PROGNOSIS

The course and the prognosis depend on the degree and extent of the burns, as well as on the status of the respiratory system. The ophthalmologist must assume that the patient will survive the injury, no matter how severe it appears.

DIAGNOSIS

The extent and degree of facial and eyelid burns should be established, although it may be difficult to determine the degree of the burns initially. The conjunctival and corneal injuries are then assessed. When the eyelids are swollen shut, the globes may be examined, after instillation of topical anesthetic, by opening the eyelids with Desmarres lid retractors. The extent of corneal and conjunctival burns is assessed with fluorescein. Foreign bodies, corneal lacerations, ruptured globe, and possible intraocular foreign bodies may be found, especially after injuries caused by explosion. The eyelids should be assessed for possible ectropion and entropion. It is imperative to analyze the extent of the ocular injury itself, and the extent and the degree of the total body burn must also be taken into account.

TREATMENT

Systemic

- Give intravenous antibiotics to avoid endogenous bacterial endophthalmitis.
- Give intravenous antifungal agents to prevent endogenous fungal endophthalmitis.
- Maintain fluid balance.
- Maintain nutritional status.

Ocular

- Remove foreign bodies.
- Debride necrotic tissue.
- Promote re-epithelialization of the cornea and conjunctiva and maintain intact epithelium throughout the course of the recuperation.
- Pressure-patch corneal and conjunctival injuries with antibiotic ointment daily until re-epithelialization is complete.
- Use bandage contact lenses when facial, brow, or eyelid burns preclude pressure patching.
- Use bandage contact lenses also to protect an uninjured cornea and to promote re-epithelization of a burned cornea when entropion is present.
- Use sterile wet compresses and topical antibiotic ointment for first- and second-degree burns of the eyelids.

Surgical

- Repair corneal lacerations and ruptured globe, if present.
- Remove intraocular foreign body, if present.
- Perform suture tarsorrhaphy if bandage contact lens fails to help re-epithelialize the cornea.
- The definitive treatment for third-degree eyelid burns is skin grafting; skin grafting will prevent cicatricial contractures of the eyelids and cicatricial ectropion, which in turn prevent exposure keratitis and potentially serious secondary corneal infection and ulceration. If eyelid contractures have already occurred, make relaxing incisions to release the contractures and then apply the skin grafts. Use split-thickness skin grafts or cultured skin on patients with large third-degree total-body burns.
- When the total-body burn is more than 50% to 60% and mostly third degree, there may not be enough normal skin to allow for early eyelid skin grafting, as the burned area must be replaced with skin from an unburned area. In such cases, a large, almost total tarsorrhaphy should be performed early to allow for healing time before the onset of contractures. If contractures occur before the tarsorrhaphy has healed, traction from the contractures may split the tarsorrhaphy open and cause it to fail. Leave a 5-mm opening medially for examination and to allow cross-fixation for children who may be in the amblyopic age group. If contractures have already developed before the tarsorrhaphy, sufficient relaxing incisions in the contracted tissue will allow the eyelid margins to come together without traction so that tarsorrhaphy may be performed successfully. Split-thickness skin grafts or cultured skin can be put into the tarsal bed thus created. If not enough skin is available from the patient to perform this lid grafting, time may be bought to allow the tarsorrhaphy to heal by placing donor skin, pigskin, or cultured skin onto the newly created subcutaneous bed. Later, during the reconstructive phase of therapy, the tarsorrhaphies may be released as the eyelids are rebuilt.

Supportive

- Maintain airway.
- Manage shock.
- Replace fluids.
- Prevent infection.

PRECAUTIONS

Scar tissue that may result from a burned cornea will not be prevented by corticosteroids. Furthermore, corticosteroids may delay the re-epithelialization and increase the chance of secondary infection.

COMPLICATIONS

It must be emphasized that although the corneas may not be injured initially, serious third-degree burns of the face and eyelids in the presence of a large third-degree total-body burn can lead to severe cicatricial contractures and ectropion of the eyelids. Exposure keratitis can ensue if tarsorrhaphy is not performed. Organisms of the *Pseudomonas* genus or other bacteria as well as fungi on the burned areas may find their way to the exposed cornea and cause serious corneal infection. This infection may be prevented by the use of aggressive early tarsorrhaphies. Prophylactic antibiotics do not always prevent corneal infections in such cases. This is especially true when the patient is upsidedown on a rotating bed and minimal therapy can be given to the eyes. A tarsorrhaphy protects the corneas during this phase of the therapy in a severely burned patient.

COMMENTS

For severe conjunctival burns caused by exploding liquids or molten metal, severe necrosis of the conjunctiva and cornea may occur. These injuries behave like severe acid or alkali burns. Local mucosal grafts may be applied in such cases, and the use of symblepharon rings may also help to prevent symblepharon. Because these injuries are similar to severe chemical burns, the articles on acid and alkali burns provide further information on the management of these cases.

In large, total-body burns, the acute phase of the injuries requires frequent operations for debridement as well as skin grafting. Until these patients are totally covered with skin, they are susceptible to infections both systemically and locally. These patients need frequent follow-up care after the application of large tarsorrhaphies. Once tarsorrhaphies are healed, examinations may be less frequent, provided that the blood cultures remain negative and signs of orbital cellulitis do not occur.

When the entire burned area is covered, the reconstructive phase of therapy can begin. When reconstruction of the eyelids with skin grafting is successful, tarsorrhaphies may be released.

Significant corneal complications such as corneal ulcers caused by *Pseudomonas* species may be prevented by tarsorrhaphies; this technique is preferable to treating such an infection, especially in combination with lid retraction and exposure keratitis. For this reason, the need for adequate and early tarsorrhaphies to protect the corneas in the severely burned patient cannot be overemphasized.

REFERENCES

Bloom SM, Gittinger JW, Jr, Kazarian EL: Management of corneal contact thermal burns. Am J Ophthalmol 102:536, 1986.

Children's Hospital Boston: Fire safety and burns. Online. Available at: Injury Statistics and Incidence Rates Children's Hospital Boston Web site. Accessed April 22, 2005.

Deutsch TA, Feller DB: Paton and Goldberg's management of ocular injuries. 2nd edn. Philadelphia, WB Saunders, 1985:99–103.

Guy RJ, Baldwin J, Kwedar S, Law EJ: Three-years' experience in a regional burn center with burns of the eyes and eyelids. Ophthalmic Surg 13:383–386, 1982.

Kulwin DR, Kersten RC: Management of eyelid burns. In: Focal points: clinical modules for ophthalmologists. San Francisco, American Academy of Ophthalmology, 1990:8:module 2:1–10.

Wibbenmeyer LA, Amelon MJ, Torner JC, et al: Population-based assessment of burn injury in southern Iowa: identification of children and young-adult at-risk groups and behaviors. J Burn Care Rehabil 24(4): 2003.

SECTION

15 Unclassified Diseases or Conditions

162 HYPERTENSION 365.04

Jeffrey R. Parnell, MD
Chicago, Illinois
Lee M. Jampol, MD
Chicago, Illinois

Systemic hypertension can be associated with vascular constriction, leakage, and arteriosclerosis, which can affect the function of many target organs throughout the body. The eye is the only target organ in which arteries and veins can be directly viewed *in vivo* with ease and by noninvasive techniques. Changes in the vasculature observed in the retina in hypertensive patients may reflect the status of the vascular system throughout the body.

The eye has a complex vascular system in which blood supplies to the optic nerve, choroid, and retina are derived from distinct sources, each having special anatomic and physiologic properties. Each vascular system has a unique response to systemic hypertension, and it is useful to separate into categories the different manifestations in the eye. Hypertensive eye disease can take the form of hypertensive retinopathy, hypertensive choroidopathy, hypertensive optic neuropathy, or all three.

ETIOLOGY/INCIDENCE

Systemic hypertension accounts for more visits to physicians than any other disease. As many as 58 million adults in the United States are estimated to have the disease. It is estimated up to 25% of adults and 60% of patients over 60 may be hypertensive. Blacks and males are more often affected.

Over 90% of cases of hypertension are due to essential hypertension for which there is no known cause. Heredity and environmental factors such as a high sodium diet and sedentary life style may play a role.

The remaining 10% of cases can be divided into the secondary causes of systolic and diastolic hypertension or isolated systolic hypertension.

One percent of patients may develop malignant hypertension, a particularly severe and often sudden onset of elevated blood pressure.

- Secondary causes of systolic and diastolic hypertension:
  - Renal vascular or parenchymal disease;
  - Endocrine disease;
  - Coarctation of the aorta;
  - Eclampsia or pre-eclampsia;
  - Neurologic disorders;
  - Increased intravascular volume;
- Isolated causes of systolic hypertension:
  - Increased cardiac output due to aortic valve insufficiency, arteriovenous fistula, patent ductus;
  - Arteriosus, thyrotoxicosis, beri-beri, hyperkinetic circulation;
  - Aortic rigidity.

COURSE/PROGNOSIS

In hypertensive retinopathy, acute elevations of blood pressure lead to retinal arterial vasoconstriction, an auto regulatory response. Persistent hypertension causes irreversible arteriolar narrowing. Chronically elevated pressure also causes sclerotic changes in the media of the arterial wall. Light-reflex changes observed on examination reflect the degree of sclerosis, which, in severe cases, may take on the appearance of burnished copper wire. Arteriolar occlusion may look like silver wire. At arteriovenous crossing sites, where the artery and vein share a common adventitial sheath, compression of the venule causes visible 'nicking' (Gunn's sign) of variable severity. Salus' sign refers to the abnormal deflection of the venule as it crosses the arteriole at an increasingly obtuse angle or even a right angle. Chronic hypertension may also cause occasional retinal microaneurysms. Arterial macroaneurysms are also seen in association with chronic hypertensive retinopathy. Sclerotic hypertensive vascular changes may contribute to branch or central vein occlusion and branch or central retinal artery occlusions.

Acute, malignant, or accelerated hypertension leads to leakage of the retinal arterioles, with decompensation of the inner blood-retina barrier. This may be manifested as extravasation of blood and lipoprotein into the retina in the form of superficial hemorrhages, cotton wool spots (infarcts), hard exudates (lipid), and capillary occlusions. Malignant hypertension also can cause hypertensive choroidopathy and hypertensive optic nerve changes. In hypertensive choroidopathy, fibrinoid changes in the choriocapillaris result in focal nonperfusion that leads to ischemia of the outer retina and the retinal pigment epithelium. Acute Elschnig's spots are white or yellow patches of ischemic retinal pigment epithelium overlying occluded choriocapillaris. Acute exudation through the injured retinal pigment epithelium layer can lead to neurosensory detachments. These spots 'heal' and become hyperpigmented over time. Linear hyperpigmentation overlying choroidal arteries is called Seigrist's streaks and represents hyperplastic retinal pigment epithelium. Elschnig's spots, after healing, are also hyperpigmented.

Disk edema is seen with severe hypertension. This swelling of the nerve head may be secondary to hypertensive encephalopathy with raised intracranial pressure, local ischemia, or vascular (venous) congestion within the nerve. Anterior ischemic optic neuropathy and optic nerve atrophy can be seen.

DIAGNOSIS

Systemic hypertension is diagnosed when the diastolic blood pressure is 90 mm Hg or above or the systolic pressure is 140 mm Hg or above on two or more separate examinations. A new category termed pre-hypertension has been created which encompasses patients with systolic readings between 120–139 mm Hg and diastolic pressures of 80–89. There has been a recent trend toward early diagnosis and treatment since 'high normal' readings may result in increased cardiovascular events. Malignant hypertension is diagnosed when systolic readings are above 200 mm Hg and/or the diastolic pressure is above 140 mm Hg.

The diagnosis of ocular changes associated with hypertension is largely a clinical one. Fluorescein angiography can be useful in some circumstances for delineating problems in the retinal and choroidal vasculature. Ocular coherence tomography may be useful in evaluating retinal edema and subretinal fluid. The scanning laser ophthalmoscope may be useful as a research tool in assessing vascular caliber and flow velocity.

The predictive value of diagnosing systemic hypertension based solely on retinal findings is only roughly 50%. People with poor blood pressure control are more likely to show retinal findings.

TREATMENT

- Early detection and treatment of systemic hypertension has led to dramatic reduction in the occurrence of severe hypertensive ocular disease.
- Diagnosis of hypertensive retinal vascular changes could provide guidance for systemic treatment and stratification of risk for development of clinical stroke, coronary artery disease and death.
- Co-management and early referral to an internist for prompt workup and institution of systemic antihypertensive therapy is essential. Blood pressure should be measured in all patients with retinal vascular occlusions.
- Aggressive treatment and hospitalization are required for malignant hypertension.
- Diuretics, β-blockers, vasodilators, angiotensin-converting enzyme inhibitors, and calcium channel blockers, alone or in combination therapy, are among the options for regulating blood pressure.
- Nonpharmacologic therapy may include a regimen of regular aerobic exercise, weight reduction, sodium restriction, potassium supplementation, and moderation of alcohol consumption.

COMPLICATIONS

- Central or branch retinal artery occlusion.
- Central or branch retinal vein occlusion.
- Macroaneurysm.
- Cotton-wool spots, lipid exudates, hemorrhages.
- Macular edema and exudate (macular star).
- Disk edema, optic atrophy, anterior ischemic optic neuropathy.
- Focal or widespread neurosensory detachment.

CLASSIFICATION SYSTEMS

Recent international management guidelines have implied an association between retinopathy grade with cardiovascular and cerebrovascular disease. Unfortunately, there is no universal or widely accepted classification system. The Keith, Wagner and Barker classification system is the oldest and most referenced system, but is not standardized.

A more clinically relevant classification system today may be the system developed by Tso and Jampol, which grades the retinal vasculature with reference photographs of the fundus.

1. Arterial narrowing:
   a. Mild;
   b. Moderate;
   c. Severe.
2. Arteriovenous nicking:
   a. Mild;
   b. Moderate;
   c. Branch venous occlusion.
3. Arteriosclerosis:
   a. Mild;
   b. Copper-wire appearance;
   c. Silver-wire appearance.
4. Arterial tortuosity:
   a. Mild;
   b. Moderate;
   c. Severe.
5. Branching angle of arteries:
   a. Mild = 45 to 60 degrees;
   b. Moderate = 60 to 90 degrees;
   c. Severe = >90 degrees.

COMMENTS

Ocular findings in systemic hypertension depend on the degree of arteriosclerosis already present from independent causes such as aging, trauma, inflammation, or other vascular diseases. It has been suggested that aged or arteriosclerotic arterioles are less affected by acute elevation of blood pressure than are normal blood vessels and may actually provide a 'protective' effect. Diabetic patients, on the other hand, may experience accelerated diabetic retinopathy in the presence of elevated blood pressure.

REFERENCES

Brown SM, Jampol LM: New concepts of regulation of retinal vessel tone. Arch Ophthalmol 114:199–204, 1996.

Chobonian AV, et al: Seventh Report of the Joint National Committee on prevention, detection, evaluation and treatment of high blood pressure. Hypertention 42:1206–1252, 2003.

Guidelines Committee: 2003 European Society of Hypertension/European Society of Cardiology guidelines for management of arterial hypertension. J Hypertens 21:1011–1053, 2003.

Klein R, et al: Hypertension and retinopathy, arteriolar narrowing, and arteriovenous nicking in a population. Arch Ophthalmol 112:92–98, 1994.

Morse PH: Elschnig's spots and hypertensive choroidopathy. Am J Ophthalmol 66:844–852, 1968.

Perkovich BT, Meyers SM: Systemic factors affecting diabetic macular edema. Am J Ophthalmol 105:211–212, 1988.

Puliafito CA, et al: Imaging macular diseases with ocular coherence tomography. Ophthalmology 102:217–229, 1995.

Tso MOM, Abrams GW, Jampol LM: Hypertensive retinopathy, choroidopathy, neuropathy. In: Singerman LJ, Jampol LM, eds: Retinal and choroidal manifestations of systemic disease. Baltimore, Williams & Wilkins, 1991:79–127.

Tso MOM, Jampol LM: Pathophysiology of hypertensive retinopathy. Ophthalmology 89:1132–1145, 1982.

Walsh JB: Hypertensive retinopathy: description, classification, and prognosis. Ophthalmology 89:1127–1131, 1982.

Wolf S, et al: Quatification of retinal capillary density and flow velocity in patients with essential hypertension. Hypertension 23:464–467, 1994.

Wong TY, et al: Atherosclerosis Risk in Communities Study. Retinal arteriolar diameter and hypertension. Ann Intern Med 140:248–255, 2004.

Wong TY, et al: Retinal microvascular abnormalities and ten-year cardiovascular mortality. A population-based case-control study. Ophthalmology 110:933–940, 2003.

163 PAPILLORENAL SYNDROME
743.57, 753.0
(Renal–Coloboma Syndrome)

Cameron F. Parsa, MD
Baltimore, Maryland

ETIOLOGY/INCIDENCE

Papillorenal syndrome (sometimes inaccurately called renal-coloboma syndrome) is an inherited condition often characterized by the association of bilateral, centrally excavated ('vacant') optic disks with multiple cilioretinal vessels (Figure 163.1) and dysplastic kidneys. Visual acuity is normal unless secondary serous retinal detachments develop. Kidneys may be small or normal in size, and vesicoureteral reflux can be an associated finding. Patients may be asymptomatic until renal failure is advanced. Not infrequently, both patient and physician are unaware that the ocular and renal findings are related.

Infrequently reported until recently, papillorenal syndrome remains underdiagnosed. Disk excavations may be misinterpreted as acquired due to glaucoma, or they may be thought to represent atypical bilateral morning glory anomaly or optic pit. Many are simply labeled colobomatous although they do not possess the features of true colobomas.

The syndrome is passed down in an autosomal dominant fashion with variable expressivity and de novo mutations also occur. It is important to examine family members whenever the condition is diagnosed and to provide family counseling.

Some affected families have a mutation in the homeobox gene *PAX2*. Often, however, no mutation can be found, implicating other genes to be involved as well.

COURSE/PROGNOSIS

The ocular course is highly variable; many patients have superonasal field defects but otherwise normal vision. Some patients develop nonrhegmatogenous serous retinal detachments, leading to severe visual loss. The propensity for retinal detachment is related to the degree of thinning of the neuroretinal rim which may allow cerebrospinal fluid (CSF) to seep into the subretinal space. Spontaneous reattachments may occur, leaving behind a characteristic pattern of retinal pigment epithelial changes. The small, or dysplastic kidneys, often lead to chronic glomerulonephropathy and proteinuria. Although some patients eventually require dialysis and renal transplantation, others remain entirely asymptomatic.

DIAGNOSIS

Laboratory findings

Diagnosis has been hampered in the past by the lack of clear nomenclature for disk anomalies. Often erroneously referred to as a coloboma, the disks in this syndrome present with characteristics distinct from actual colobomas, related to failure of

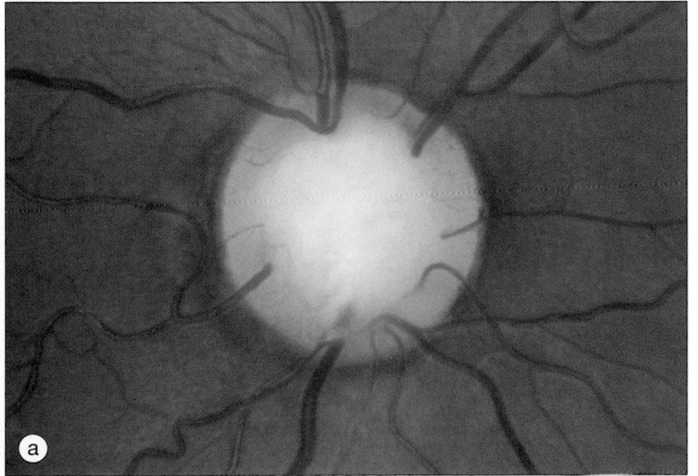

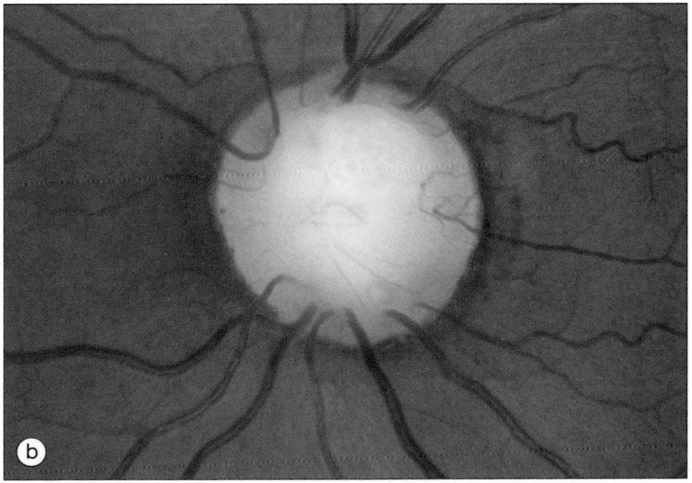

FIGURE 163.1. a) Fundus photos show vessels leaving and entering from the disc periphery. Note bending of vessels making hairpin turns over the rim of each disc. Near the center of the left disc (b), there is a very attenuated central vessel. The variable lack of persisting central vascular and glial structures may give the discs a 'vacant' appearance, as seen here.

the embryonic optic fissure to close, and from other optic disk anomalies.

- The most characteristic feature is the cilioretinal blood supply of the retina compensating for an attenuation or absence of central retinal vessels. A multiplicity of peripheral arteries and veins are visible that bend and make hairpin turns over and into the neural rim of the disk, indicating their cilioretinal origin. If present, the variably attenuated central retinal vein and artery remain centrally located in the disk (Figure 163.1b). Doppler ultrasonography often reveals extensive anastomoses between such centrally-placed vessels and the ciliary circulation deeper within the nerve.
- The disks may possess a broad, central excavation, with a variable amount of glial tissue centrally.
- The findings are bilateral. There may be asymmetry in the appearance of central vessels, though both eyes have an essentially cilioretinal origin of their blood supply.
- The disks are normal in size without peripapillary excavations or staphyloma.
- Superonasal field defects may be present.

The combined findings may sometimes create the appearance of centrally 'vacant' disks, which should hint to the underlying diagnosis.

- Ultrasonography may show bilateral, variably small or normal-sized, echogenic, dysplastic kidneys. In some cases, Doppler ultrasound may reveal high resistive indices to blood flow.
- Serum chemistry may indicate elevated blood urea nitrogen and creatinine levels, and urinalysis may reveal proteinuria. Microalbuminuria testing is a sensitive marker for disease.
- Blood can be drawn for *PAX2* mutation analysis which is positive in some families.

Note: Unlike true or 'typical' colobomas, the dysplastic, vacant disks noted in this syndrome do not have central vessels displaced superiorly, nor is the area of the disk excavation greatest inferonasally. Thus, the alternative appellation for this entity, 'renal-coloboma syndrome,' is a misnomer and should be avoided since it implies a failure of embryonic fissure closure rather than a genetic anomaly affecting angiogenesis-mediated (as opposed to vasculogenesis) vessel formation.

Differential diagnosis

- Unlike a *coloboma,* there is no superodisplacement of blood vessels, nor is the disk excavation centered inferonasally in association with retinal or choroidal defects.
- Unlike *morning glory anomaly,* the findings are essentially bilateral and associated with good central vision (unless a serous retinal detachment occurs secondarily). The disk size is normal, and the central excavation is broad based rather than funnel shaped. Both conditions, however, do share the common feature of multiplicity of cilioretinal vessels.
- Unlike *optic pits,* the excavations are broad and not located toward the temporal aspect of the disc. Multiple, if not all, vessels enter and leave the disk periphery, bending or making hairpin turns over the neural rim.
- The presence of a central glial tuft and the often extensive, and frequently exclusive, cilioretinal vascular supply should help to exclude *glaucoma.* Although superonasal field defects often are present, they are due to hypoplastic retinal development rather than to acquired nerve fiber defects.

PROPHYLAXIS

No prophylaxis is known other than the identification of affected individuals, examination of family members, and genetic counseling.

TREATMENT

Individuals with these findings generally have normal visual acuity. Those with large disc excavations and potential defects in Kuhnt intermediary tissue which allows subretinal CSF seepage are at risk for developing secondary serous retinal detachments. There have been reports of varying degrees of success in reattaching these retinas using methods such as optic nerve sheath fenestration or vitrectomy with gas bubble injection. Given the underlying etiology, lowering retrolaminar CSF pressure via sheath fenestration, or, alternatively, raising intraocular pressure, may be more effective approaches.

The most important role of the ophthalmologist in these cases is to refer the patient to a nephrologist for an evaluation and ultrasound examination of the kidneys (including Doppler scanning for resistive indices). Many individuals with ocular findings have undiagnosed chronic renal disease. Others may have normal kidney function at the time of their initial examination with abnormal anatomy, and develop premature renal failure years later. The identification of individuals at risk for renal failure may allow the timely institution of renal protective measures such as aggressive blood pressure control. Such measures are recognized to vastly improve renal potential in dysplastic kidneys and defer the need for dialysis and other procedures by many years.

COMPLICATIONS

Complications include serous retinal detachment and renal failure. Pronounced congenital disc excavations may predispose patients with otherwise 'normal' intraocular pressures to superimposed acquired glaucoma. Thus, careful evaluation for progressive visual field changes should be performed. Since the retina is congenitally hypoplastic, and the discs dysplastic, field changes are often atypical in form. Baseline stereo disc photos should be obtained for early detection of potential changes in disc morphology.

REFERENCES

Barroso LHL, Hoyt WF, Narahara M: Can the arterial supply of the retina in man be exclusively cilioretinal? J Neurol Ophthalmol 14:87–90, 1994.

Bron AJ, Burgess SEP, Awdry PN, et al: Papillo-renal syndrome: an inherited association of optic disc dysplasia and renal disease: report and review of the literature. Ophthalmic Paediatr Genet 10:185–198, 1989.

Chang S, Haik BG, Ellsworth RM, et al: Treatment of total retinal detachment in morning glory syndrome. Am J Ophthalmol 97:596–600, 1984.

Chen CS, Odel JG, Miller JS, Hood DC: Multifocal visual evoked potentials and multifocal electroretinograms in papillorenal syndrome. Arch Ophthalmol 120:870–871, 2002.

Dureau P, Attie-Bitach T, Salomon R, et al: Renal coloboma syndrome. Ophthalmology 108:1912–1916, 2001.

Ford B, Rupps R, Lirenman D, Van Allen MI, et al: Renal-coloboma syndrome: prenatal detection and clinical spectrum in a large family. Am J Med Genet 99:137–141, 2001.

Irvine AR, Crawford JB, Sullivan JH: The pathogenesis of retinal detachment with morning glory disc and optic pit. Retina 6:146–150, 1986.

Parsa CF, Cheeseman EW, Maumenee IH: Demonstration of exclusive cilioretinal vascular system supplying the retina in man: vacant discs. Trans Am Ophthalmol Soc 96:95–109, 1998.

Parsa CF, Silva ED, Sundin OH, et al: Redefining papillorenal syndrome: an underdiagnosed cause of ocular and visual morbidity. Ophthalmology 108:738–749, 2001.

Sanyanusin P, Schimmenti LA, McNoe LA, et al: Mutation of the PAX2 gene in a family with optic nerve colobomas, renal anomalies and vesicoureteral reflux. Nat Genet 9:358–363, 1995.

164 VOGT–KOYANAGI–HARADA DISEASE 364.24

(Harada's Disease; Uveomeningitis)

Russell W. Read, MD
Birmingham, Alabama

ETIOLOGY/INCIDENCE

Vogt–Koyanagi–Harada (VKH) disease is characterized by inflammation involving the eye, inner ear, skin, hair, and meninges of the central nervous system, but the exact cause remains unknown. Immunohistochemistry of ocular and skin specimens have shown an infiltration of CD4+ T-cells, epithelioid cells, and multinucleated giant cells, indicative of granulomatous inflammation. Evidence increasingly suggests that this attack is directed against an as of yet unidentified component of the melanocytes contained in the targeted tissues. This data includes studies revealing that immunization of rats or Akita dogs with tyrosinase family peptides produces a uveitis that is similar to human VKH disease. Human studies have shown that cerebrospinal fluid obtained from patients with VKH disease contains melanin-laden macrophages. This finding could be due to directed phagocytosis of melanin or to non-specific phagocytosis of melanin liberated during inflammation. However, peripheral blood lymphocytes from patients with VKH disease proliferate upon stimulation with tyrosinase-family peptides, suggesting that melanin-related components are an immunological target. The exact inciting event that leads to the autoimmune attack against melanin is unknown, but several possibilities exist. Occult trauma of melanocyte-containing tissues could lead to a sensitization to melanin. Viral infection could likewise cause a collateral sensitization to melanin components. While not conclusive proof, Epstein–Barr virus DNA has been isolated from the vitreous of patients with VKH disease. A genetic predisposition may contribute to disease, with numerous studies showing a strong association with the human leukocyte antigen (HLA) DR4 allele and specifically with HLA-DRB1*0405 and HLA-BRB1*0410 subtypes.

VKH disease is more common in Asians, Asian Indians, Middle Easterners, Hispanics, and American Indians. The condition is rare in Africans and Caucasians. Frequency of disease varies by study clinic, ranging from 1% to 7% of uveitis cases in United States studies to over 9% of uveitis cases in Japanese studies. VKH disease affects females more commonly than males. Average age of disease onset is the third to fifth decade of life, but patients as young as 4 years of age have been reported.

COURSE/PROGNOSIS

VKH disease is typically divided into four stages: prodromal, acute uveitic, convalescent, and chronic-recurrent stages. The prodromal stage manifests with predominately neurologic and auditory symptoms including headache, meningismus, tinnitus, and dysacousia. Patients may be diagnosed with aseptic meningitis if they seek medical care prior to the onset of ocular inflammation. The uveitic stage begins a variable time later, but typically within a week, with the onset of a diffuse choroiditis as the hallmark of disease. This may manifest as diffuse choroidal thickening (best demonstrated on ultrasonography), exudative retinal detachments, and papillitis. Vitreous and anterior chamber cell may be present. Fluorescein angiography reveals multiple pinpoint areas of subretinal leakage with eventual pooling in the subretinal space (Figure 164.1 and 164.2). Ciliary body edema and detachment may occur, with forward rotation of the lens-iris diaphragm and a resultant shallowed angle. As the inflammatory attack subsides, typically following

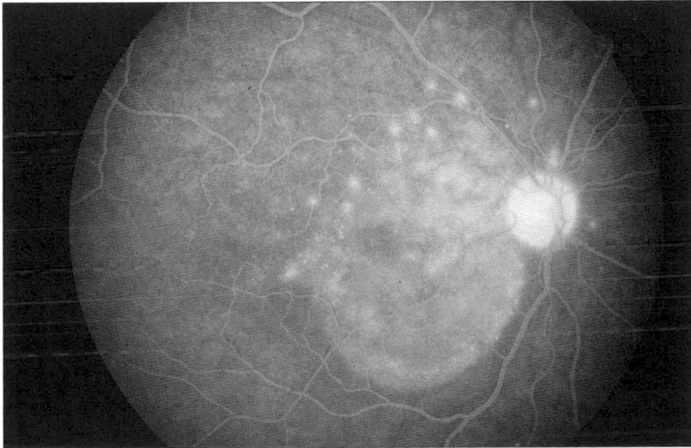

FIGURE 164.1. Vogt–Kayanagi–Harada syndrome (fluoroscein angiogram).

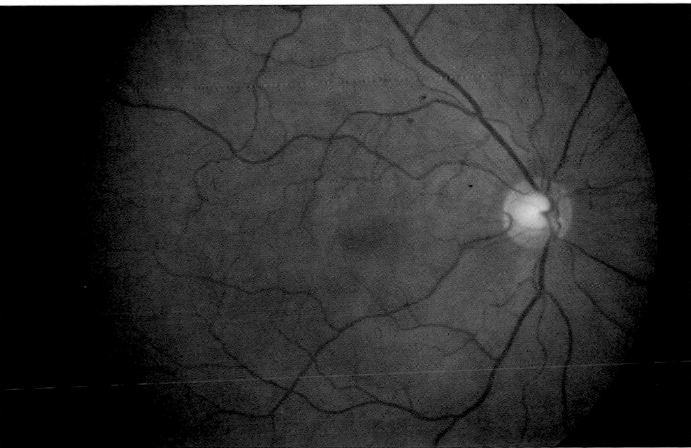

FIGURE 164.2. Vogt–Kayanagi–Harada syndrome.

treatment, the convalescent stage begins. It is during this stage that variable depigmentation of the eye, skin and hair may occur. Sugiura's sign, consisting of perilimbal pigment loss, most pronounced at the superior limbus, may develop. Loss of choroidal pigment produces the classic sunset-glow fundus. Areas of hyperpigmentation and pigment clumping in the fundus may develop. Multiple, well-defined yellow nummular chorioretinal scars may develop, primarily in the inferior peripheral fundus. Patients may experience chronic-recurrent disease at any point following resolution of the acute uveitic phase. This recurrent disease is interesting in that it is primarily an anterior uveitis, with a recurrence of posterior segment findings being very uncommon. The recurrent anterior uveitis may be very difficult to control. Anecdotal evidence suggests that early, aggressive treatment of the acute disease may reduce the incidence of both depigmentation and recurrent uveitis.

Ocular complications may develop in VKH disease as they do in other forms of uveitis and the development of complications appears to be a predictor for visual outcome, with those patients that develop fewer complications generally doing better than those who develop more. Cataract, glaucoma, choroidal neovascular membranes, or subretinal fibrosis may occur. Approximately half of patients will maintain vision of at least 20/40.

DIAGNOSIS

Diagnostic criteria exist for VKH disease and require documentation of an absence of prior ocular penetration; absence of evidence of another uveitic condition; presence of bilateral ocular inflammatory disease manifesting as a diffuse choroiditis acutely and ocular pigmentary disturbances late; presence of prodromal neurological or auditory findings; and depigmentation of the skin or hair or loss of hair. Varying combinations of these manifestations result in a diagnosis of probable, incomplete, or complete disease. The reader is referred to the original diagnostic criteria publication for complete details and an explanation of the application of the criteria.

Clinical signs and symptoms

Prodromal and acute uveitic stages

- Ocular findings:
  - Anterior segment: anterior chamber cells and flare with keratic precipitates (variably present); anterior chamber shallowing;
  - Choroid: diffuse choroiditis, which may be demonstrated as thickening on ultrasonography or multiple areas of dye leakage with subretinal pooling on fluorescein angiogram;
  - Retina: exudative retinal detachment; retinal folds or striae;
  - Optic nerve: swollen optic disc with hyperemia;
  - Vitreous: cells (variably present).
- Extraocular lesions:
  - Inner ear: sensorineural hearing loss, especially at high frequencies; tinnitus;
  - Neurologic manifestations: headache, meningismus.

Convalescent stage

- Ocular lesions:
  - Anterior segment: atrophy of iris stroma; perilimbal vitiligo;
  - Choroid: sunset-glow fundus; nummular chorioretinal scars; hyperpigmentation and pigment clumping;
  - Retina: choroidal neovascular membrane; subretinal fibrosis.
- Extraocular lesions:
  - Inner ear: persistent sensorineural hearing loss, especially at high frequencies;
  - Skin, hair: alopecia; vitiligo; poliosis.

Chronic-recurrent stage

- Ocular lesions:
  - Anterior segment: anterior chamber cells and flare; keratic precipitates; atrophy of iris stroma; iris nodules; perilimbal vitiligo;
  - Choroid: same as Convalescent stage above;
  - Retina: same as Convalescent stage above.
- Extraocular lesions:
  - Same as Convalescent stage above.

Laboratory findings (in prodromal or acute uveitic stages)

- Lymphocytic pleocytosis of cerebrospinal fluid.
- Diffuse choroidal thickening without evidence of posterior scleritis on ultrasonography.
- Multiple pinpoint areas of leakage with eventual pooling of dye in subretinal space on fluorescein angiography.
- High-frequency hearing deficit on audiometry.

Differential diagnosis

- Sympathetic ophthalmia.
- Posterior scleritis.
- Uveal effusion syndrome.
- Acute posterior multifocal placoid pigment epitheliopathy (APMPPE).
- Sarcoidosis.
- Primary central nervous system lymphoma with ocular involvement.

TREATMENT

Systemic

Common practice among uveitis specialists entails the use of high-dose corticosteroids as initial therapy. Oral or intravenous forms may be used, with recent data suggesting no difference in final visual acuity. Prednisone may be used at 1 mg/kg/day orally or methylprednisolone 500 mg to 1 g per day intravenously, either divided or in a single dose. Methylprednisolone is typically continued for 3 days with tapering accomplished with subsequent oral prednisone.

Similar to other uveitic conditions, if systemic corticosteroids at safe and tolerable doses are insufficient to bring the disease under control or the condition recurs with tapering to a dose less than 10 mg/day prednisone, then non-corticosteroid immunosuppressive agents should be considered. Selection of a specific agent should be based on individualized patient characteristics and comorbidities, as no agents have been shown to be of greater efficacy than any other in treating VKH disease. Use of immunosuppressive agents should be coordinated by an experienced specialist. Agents used to treat VKH disease include antimetabolites, T-cell specific agents, and alkylating agents. Newer biologic agents may be of benefit, but data is lacking at present regarding their use in VKH disease.

Ocular

Topical corticosteroids are adequate only as an adjunct in acute disease with posterior segment manifestations, but may be sufficient for a mild recurrent anterior uveitis. Prednisolone acetate 1% is commonly used with the same principles of corticosteroid use for other uveitic entities applying here as well, including frequent enough use to ensure control of disease. With active anterior segment inflammation, cycloplegia should be utilized to prevent posterior synechiae. An agent strong enough to keep the pupil moving should be employed, such as homatropine, scopolamine, or atropine.

Periocular corticosteroid injections via the sub-Tenon's or orbital floor routes may be used either as primary or adjunctive therapy in acute or recurrent disease, though typically its use as primary therapy occurs in mild cases or where systemic corticosteroid use is contraindicated. This route of administration is especially appealing for asymmetrical disease. Triamcinolone acetonide, triamcinolone diacetate or dexamethasone may be utilized.

Surgical

There is little, if any, role for surgery as a primary therapy for VKH disease. Some clinicians have attempted to drain subretinal fluid that was slow to resolve with medication alone, but this should be considered an exceptional situation. Surgery is primarily utilized to address the ocular complications that may occur and includes cataract extraction, glaucoma filtering or shunt surgery, and removal of choroidal neovascular membranes.

COMPLICATIONS

Ocular complications

Cataracts; posterior synechiae; glaucoma (angle-closure or open-angle); choroidal neovascular membranes; subretinal fibrosis; pigment disturbances; optic atrophy.

Extraocular complications

Vitiligo; poliosis; alopecia.

COMMENTS

Ocular complications have been shown to be associated with a longer duration of disease, and an increasing number of cumulative complications is associated with a worse final visual acuity. Anecdotal evidence suggests that early, aggressive therapy, typically with high-dose corticosteroids, reduces the occurrence of complications and recurrent disease. Non-corticosteroid immunosuppressive agents may be required to achieve and maintain adequate control.

SUPPORT GROUPS

While no VKH specific support groups exist in the United States, groups dedicated to uveitis in general do exist, as follows:

- American Uveitis Society, www.uveitissociety.org
- Immunology and Uveitis Service of the Massachusetts Eye and Ear Infirmary *www.uveitis.org*

REFERENCES

Hayakawa K, Ishikawa M, Yamaki K: Ultrastructural changes in rat eyes with experimental Vogt-Koyanagi-Harada disease. Jpn J Ophthalmol 48:222–227, 2004.

Moothy RS, Inomata H, Rao NA: Vogt-Koyanagi-Harada syndrome. Surv Ophthalmol 39:265–292, 1995.

Ohno S: Immunological aspects of Behçet's and Vogt-Koyanagi-Harada's disease. Trans Ophthalmol Soc UK 101:335–341, 1981.

Read RW: Vogt-Koyanagi-Harada disease. Ophthalmol Clin North Am 15:333–341, 2002.

Read RW, Rechodouni A, Butani N, et al: Complications and prognostic factors in Vogt-Koyanagi-Harada disease. Am J Ophthalmol 131:599–606, 2001.

Read RW, Holland GN, Rao NA, et al: Revised diagnostic criteria for Vogt-Koyanagi-Harada disease: report of an international committee on nomenclature. Am J Ophthalmol 131:647–652, 2001.

Rubsamen PE, Gass JD: Vogt-Koyanagi-Harada syndrome: clinical course, therapy, and long-term visual outcome. Arch Ophthalmol 109:682–687, 1991.

Yamaki K, Takiyama N, Itho N, et al: Experimentally induced Vogt-Koyanagi-Harada disease in two Akita dogs. Exp Eye Res 80:273–280, 2005.

SECTION

16 Anterior Chamber

165 EPITHELIAL INGROWTH 379.8
(Epithelial Downgrowth)

F. Hampton Roy, MD, FACS
Little Rock, Arkansas

ETIOLOGY/INCIDENCE

Epithelial ingrowth in a sheet-like fashion is a rare and problematic complication of ocular trauma or anterior segment surgery. Factors contributing to its presence include postoperative wound leak, hypotony, prolonged inflammation, and the presence of any external 'wick' into the eye. Fortunately, the incidence of epithelial ingrowth after surgery has decreased from 1% around 1960 to less than 0.1%.

DIAGNOSIS

The diagnosis of epithelial ingrowth, which is often delayed, is based on a constellation of signs and symptoms, together with awareness of the importance of early diagnosis; suspicion of the disease allows earlier diagnosis and attempt at surgical treatment.

Clinical signs and symptoms

- The onset is insidious, usually occurring within 3 years after surgery or trauma.
- The patient has tearing; dull, aching pain; photophobia; and blurred vision.
- Wound gape, bleb, or fistula may be revealed with 2% fluorescein and light pressure on the eye.
- On the posterior cornea, a translucent membrane is demarcated by a grayish, often scalloped edge, with focal pearly areas of thickening.
- Diminished corneal sensation, corneal vascularization, edema, or a combination may be present.
- Anterior chamber cells ('flaky') and flare often are present.
- Glaucoma is present in half of cases.
- Iris involvement, as indicated by areas of immobility, distortion, and obliteration of detail, can be delineated using argon laser (500-µm spot, 100 mW, 0.1 second); normal iris sustains a slight burn, whereas an epithelial sheet overlying the iris shows fluffy white lesions.
- Festoons of epithelial sheets over the pupil, lens implant, and vitreous face can be seen in advanced cases.
- Photocoagulation can confirm the diagnosis, but surgery should follow promptly because photocoagulation causes moderate anterior chamber inflammation.
- Iris biopsy or corneal endothelial curettage provides histologic confirmation.

Differential diagnosis

- Anteriorly shelved cataract incision, seen as a diagonal intrastromal line on slit-lamp examination.
- Fibrous ingrowth, distinguished by its slow growth and vascularity.
- Vitreocorneal adhesions, which can have a grayish color and cause overlying corneal edema.
- Detachment of Descemet's layer.
- Peripheral corneal edema due to endothelial cell loss from surgery or trauma.
- Reduplication of Descemet's layer, which can grow to involve the posterior cornea, angle, and iris; however, the photocoagulation test is negative.

TREATMENT

Before surgery, the site of incision, any fistula or bleb, and the exent of iris involvement are determined.

- Local excision consists of fistula repair, vitrector excision of involved iris and vitreous, and removal of the intraocular lens and capsular bag, if present. With an air bubble in the anterior chamber, a single freeze-thaw procedure is applied to areas of involved cornea, sufficient to form ice crystals on the posterior surface. Areas of ciliary body involvement are treated similarly.
- En bloc excision of epithelial sheets has been reported with variable success. A tectonic corneoscleral graft is necessary after this surgical approach.

COMPLICATIONS

- Closure of a leaking fistula in an otherwise inoperable eye can lead to intractable glaucoma.
- Corneal transplantation may be needed after cryotherapy to an extensively involved cornea.
- Epithelial involvement of the angle, iris, and ciliary body may progress while the extent of corneal involvement seems stable; therefore, observation alone with medical treatment is not advocated.
- Vitreous hemorrhage, retinal detachment, glaucoma, and recurrence may complicate excision of ingrowth.

REFERENCES

Ghaiy R, Meyer DR, Farber MA: Epithelial downgrowth complicating evisceration with orbital implant exposure. Arch Ophthalmol 123(9):1268–1270, 2005.

Giaconi JA, Coleman AL, Aldave AJ: Epithelial downgrowth following surgery for congenital glaucoma. Am J Ophthalmol 138(6):1075–1077, 2004.

Kim SK, Ibarra MS, Syed NA, et al: Development of epithelial downgrowth several decades after intraocular surgery. Cornea 24(1):108–109, 2005.

Kuchle M, Green WR: Epithelial ingrowth: a study of 207 histopathologically proven cases. Ger J Ophthalmol 5:211–223, 1996.

Rummelt V, Naumann GO: Block excision with tectonic corneoscleroplasty for cystic and/or diffuse epithelial invasion of the anterior eye segment. Report of 51 consecutive patients. Klin Monatsbl Augenheilkd 211:312–323, 1997.

Schaeffer AR, Nalbandian RW, Brigham DW, O'Donnell FE, Jr: Epithelial downgrowth following wound dehiscence after extracapsular cataract extraction and posterior chamber lens implantation: surgical management. J Cat Refr Surg 15:437–441, 1989.

Smith PW, Stark WJ, Maumenee AE: Epithelial, fibrous, and endothelial proliferation. In: Ritch R, Krupin T, Shields MB, eds: The glaucomas. 2nd edn. St Louis, CV Mosby, 1996:1325–1361.

Yu CS, Chiu SI, Tse RK: Treatment of cystic epithelial downgrowth with intralesional administration of mitomycin C. Cornea 24(7):884–886, 2005.

166 INTRAOCULAR EPITHELIAL CYSTS 379.8

Wen-Hsiang Lee, MD, PhD
Baltimore, Maryland
Julia A. Haller, MD
Baltimore, Maryland
Patricia W. Smith, MD
Raleigh, North Carolina
Walter J. Stark, MD
Baltimore, Maryland

ETIOLOGY

Anterior chamber epithelial cysts develop when implanted epithelial cells proliferate centripetally. Cysts have been reported after penetrating trauma, cataract surgery, penetrating keratoplasty, and perforating corneal ulcer, and they may be congenital in origin. Delayed or inadequate wound closure, especially with vitreous or iris incarceration, also contributes to epithelial cyst formation.

COURSE/PROGNOSIS

- Some cysts remain small and stable, others may grow and enlarge rapidly.
- Intervention is indicated if pupillary obstruction, iridocyclitis, secondary glaucoma, corneal decompensation, loss of vision, and intractable pain develop. Prognosis of cysts requiring surgical intervention is variable, depending on how much tissue is affected, choice of surgical technique, associated complications, and presence or absence of recurrence.

DIAGNOSIS

- A translucent, white or gray cyst in the anterior chamber that often connects at one end with the wound.
- The cyst transilluminates, trembles with eye movement, lacks vascularity, and may demonstrate a meniscus of epithelial cells.
- The epithelial cyst typically indents the iris surface, in contrast to the primary iris stromal cysts that arise from the iris stroma.

TREATMENT

- Small cysts may be observed, often for years, if they are stable and asymptomatic. Surgical intervention is required if complications such as visual axis obstruction, glaucoma, uveitis, and corneal edema arise. Numerous surgical approaches have been reported, including aspiration, radiation, electrolysis, diathermy, injection of sclerosing agents, laser photocoagulation, vitrectomy-assisted cyst excision combined with cryodestruction, and en bloc excision.
- Argon laser photocoagulation has been applied to the pigmented base or the surface of the cyst to shrink the cyst. Limitations of photocoagulation include recurrences requiring repeat treatment, difficulty with anterior cyst wall visualization and treatment, problem with treating some large cysts, and risk of cyst rupture, converting the cyst into sheet-like epithelial ingrowth.
- En bloc excision of large cysts followed by tectonic corneoscleral grafts has been reported and can be successful. However, a more conservative, tissue-preserving, surgical approach may avoid destruction of ocular structures and may lead to better visual outcome.
- A conservative surgical strategy consists of viscodissection of the cyst wall from adjacent ocular structures, aspiration of fluid-filled cyst contents, and endolaser photocoagulation of the collapsed cyst wall and base (Figure 166.1). This may be particularly useful in children in the amblyopia age group, where preservation of the crystalline lens is important.

COMPLICATIONS

- Recurrence of cystic ingrowth, or conversion to sheet-like form of ingrowth.
- Corneas treated with cryotherapy may opacify and require keratoplasty.
- Cataract, hemorrhage, retinal detachment, loss of vision, and loss of eye (especially with more extensive eye wall excisions).

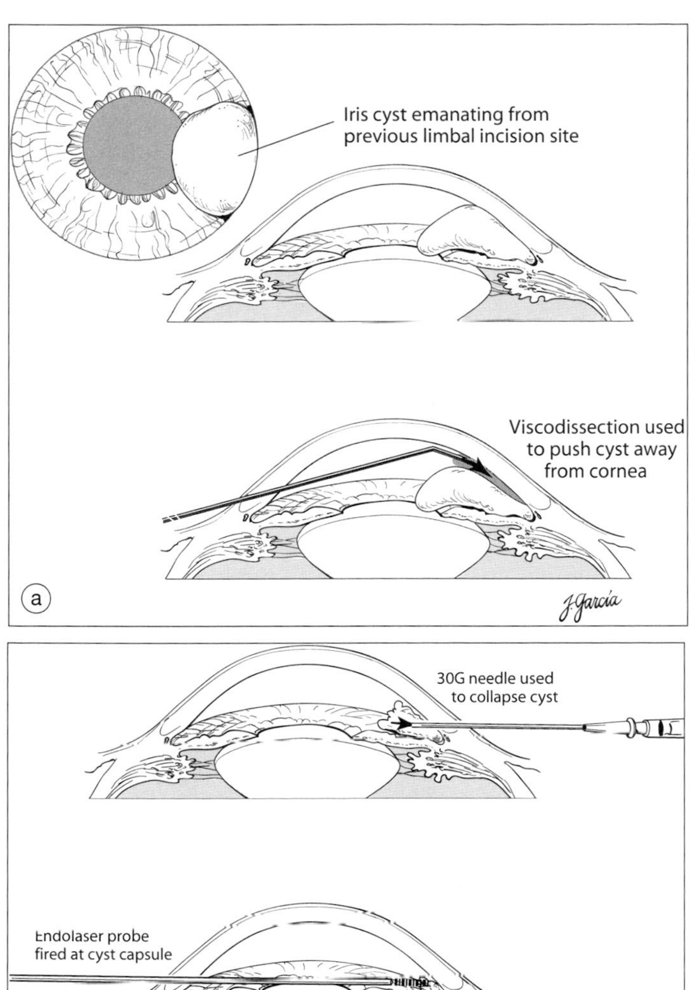

FIGURE 166.1. Conservative surgical strategy. a) The cyst is first viscodissected from the cornea and other structures. b) A 30-gauge needle is inserted into the apex of the cyst and its contents aspirated. The endolaser probe is then directed at the residual cyst wall, and the collapsed capsule is destroyed with photocoagulation. (From: Haller JA, Stark WJ, Azab A, et al: Surgical management of anterior chamber epithelial cysts. Am J Ophthalmol 135(3):309–313, 2003, with permission.)

REFERENCES

Haller JA, Stark WJ, Azab A, et al: Surgical management of anterior chamber epithelial cysts. Am J Ophthalmol 135:309–313, 2003.

Harbin TS, Jr, Maumenee AE: Epithelial downgrowth after surgery for epithelial cyst. Am J Ophthalmol 78:1–4, 1974.

Kuchle M, Green WR: Epithelial ingrowth: a study of 207 histopathologically proven cases. Ger J Ophthalmol 5:211–223, 1996.

Okun E, Mandell A: Photocoagulation treatment of epithelial implantation cysts following cataract surgery. Trans Am Ophthalmol Soc 72:170–183, 1974.

Roy FH, Hanna C: Spontaneous congenital iris cyst. Am J Ophthalmol 72:97–108, 1971.

Rummelt V, Naumann GO: Block excision with tectonic corneoscleroplasty for cystic and/or diffuse epithelial invasion of the anterior eye segment. Report of 51 consecutive patients. Klin Monatsbl Augenheilkd 21:312–323, 1997.

Scholz RT, Kelley JS: Argon laser photocoagulation treatment of iris cysts following penetrating keratoplasty. Arch Ophthalmol 100:926–927, 1982.

Solomon KD, Stark WJ, Smith P, et al: Epithelial, fibrous, and endothelial proliferation. In: Ritch R, Krupin T, Shields MB, eds: The glaucomas. 2nd edn. St Louis, CV Mosby, 1996:1325–1361.

167 POSTOPERATIVE FLAT ANTERIOR CHAMBER 360.34

F. Hampton Roy, MD, FACS
Little Rock, Arkansas

Collapse of the anterior chamber is a serious complication of anterior segment surgery that may lead to corneal decompensation, cataract, or intractable glaucoma due to peripheral anterior synechiae. The flat anterior chamber is characterized by apposition between the iris and peripheral cornea with little or no visible anterior chamber. Slight contact of the peripheral iris with peripheral cornea with formation of the central chamber is normally classified as a shallow anterior chamber, graded either by units of corneal thickness or by fraction of normal depth. Apposition of the lens surface to the central cornea constitutes the most severe form of flat chamber and usually mandates immediate intervention. It may immediately follow glaucoma or cataract surgery or may be delayed for days, weeks, or even months into the postoperative period. Shallowing of the anterior chamber is considerably more common after glaucoma-filtering surgery, particularly when the full-thickness procedures are chosen instead of the partial-thickness 'trabeculectomy' procedures. The latter technique reduces the incidence but does not eliminate the flat chamber as a complication. In an attempt to prevent flat anterior chamber, many surgeons now place multiple sutures in the split thickness scleral flap to achieve a watertight closure. These are then released or incised with the use of a laser during the early postoperative period in an attempt to establish filtration. Although this practice may reduce the frequency of immediate flat chamber, delay in release of the sutures may also lead to adhesion of the flap to the scleral bed over the fistula and a nonfunctional filtration bleb.

ETIOLOGY/INCIDENCE

The flat anterior chamber almost invariably results from one or a combination of the following events: excess aqueous humor runoff through an intact bleb, wound leak, serous or hemorrhagic choroidal detachment, pupillary block, and posterior misdirection or entrapment of aqueous humor (malignant glaucoma or ciliary-block glaucoma). With the advent of modern small-incision cataract surgical techniques and trabeculectomy, postoperative flat anterior chamber has become an exceedingly uncommon surgical complication.

COURSE/PROGNOSIS

The expected course of postoperative flat anterior chamber depends entirely on its cause. Moderate to severe shallowing of the chamber associated with a low intraocular pressure (less than 5 mm Hg), even with small choroidal detachment, nearly always resolves spontaneously within 7 to 10 days with no definitive intervention. Most important, activity and strain must be minimized to prevent suprachoroidal hemorrhage in the soft eye. On the other hand, flat anterior chamber associated with hypotony and a leaking conjunctiva or, alternatively, a high intraocular pressure with pupillary block or a massive hemorrhagic choroidal detachment or aqueous misdirection mandates intervention.

DIAGNOSIS

Identification of the pathogenesis is essential to plan the safest and most effective therapy. Occasionally, the appropriate etiologic diagnosis becomes clear only during surgical intervention, so the surgeon must be prepared to follow a logical series of surgical steps to do the least necessary to correct the problem and prevent its recurrence.

The wound should be examined carefully to identify any possible leak. In an eye that does not appear to be extremely soft, the intraocular pressure can be carefully measured with a sterilized applanation tonometer. A hypotonus eye suggests a wound leak or choroidal detachment, whereas a normotensive or firm eye is more suggestive of pupillary block or posterior aqueous misdirection. Pupillary block may also occur with a soft eye if wound leak or choroidal detachment coexists. Prolonged shallow or flat anterior chamber, initially arising from a wound leak or excess filtration, may eventually develop posterior aqueous misdirection as the associated inflammation blocks the access of aqueous humor to the anterior chamber.

Excess aqueous runoff through the filtration site most commonly occurs during the first few days after filtering procedures, resulting in shallowing of the anterior chamber and choroidal detachment, which in turn lead to further flattening of the anterior chamber. With the contemporary practice of 'no-stitch' cataract surgery, postoperative wound leaks, inadvertent filtering blebs, and their attendant flat anterior chambers occasionally occur. Pupillary block rarely follows filtration surgery if an adequate iridectomy has been performed. This condition occurs more commonly after cataract surgery, especially with anterior chamber intraocular lenses, when vitreous or lens material can block one or more iridectomies. In some cases, particularly when pupillary block has been allowed to persist, the aqueous humor may be misdirected into the vitreous cavity, driving the vitreous forward and blocking access to both the anterior and posterior chambers, leading to 'malignant glaucoma.'

Hemorrhagic choroidal detachment also occasionally follows any intraocular procedure, but it is more common in eyes that have had multiple intraocular procedures, especially vitrectomy. Such hemorrhages may occur intraoperatively and be heralded by rapid shallowing of the anterior chamber and prolapse of ocular contents into the wound site. Even patients under local and retrobulbar anesthesia will sometimes have pain. After filtration surgery, hemorrhagic choroidal detachment more commonly occurs during the early postoperative period rather than during surgery, and again it is heralded by severe pain and loss of vision with flattening of the anterior chamber. These postoperative suprachoroidal hemorrhages occur more frequently than in previous decades because with the availability of adjunctive chemotherapy or tube implants, more high-risk eyes are being subjected to filtration surgery. Aphakic eyes that have undergone vitrectomy are especially prone to suprachoroidal hemorrhage after filtration surgery. Although most suprachoroidal hemorrhages will absorb spontaneously, prompt diagnosis will permit the institution of appropriate therapy that can save vision.

Differential diagnosis

- Low intraocular pressure.
- Wound or bleb leak.
- Excess aqueous humor runoff.
- Serous choroidal hemorrhage.
- High/normal intraocular pressure.
- Massive serous or hemorrhagic choroidal detachment.
- Aqueous humor misdirection.

TREATMENT

Ocular

Appropriate therapy for the flat anterior chamber depends entirely on correct determination of its pathogenesis. Wound leaks usually require surgical repair, but very tiny wound leaks sometimes heal spontaneously with a pressure dressing and the administration of aqueous suppressants to reduce aqueous flow. Absorbable collagen shields or large-diameter soft contact lenses may also successfully tamponade a slowly leaking bleb until it heals with endogenous fibrosis.

When a flat anterior chamber results from excess filtration, tamponade with a Simmons scleral shell or hydrogel large-diameter contact lens applied with or without a pressure dressing often is useful if applied before extensive choroidal detachment is well established (see Surgical for management of choroidal detachment). The anterior chamber usually deepens within 2 to 3 hours, but the tamponade should then be left in place for at least 48 hours. Mydriasis and cycloplegia are also helpful to retrodisplace the lens-iris diaphragm and prevent complicating pupillary block.

Pupillary block rarely follows filtration surgery if an adequate iridectomy has been performed; it more commonly occurs after cataract surgery or after filtration in aphakic or pseudophakic eyes. These eyes invariably require a laser or surgical iridectomy, but the attack should initially be broken medically to reduce the intraocular pressure and to allow clearing of the cornea. Mydriasis should be achieved with 1% cyclopentolate plus 2.5% phenylephrine. Vitreous dehydration with osmotic agents, such as oral glycerin, oral isosorbide, or intravenous mannitol, is also useful in combination with ocular mydriatic/cycloplegic agents to reverse some cases of pupillary block and posterior entrapment of aqueous humor.

A flat anterior chamber, associated with visible patent iridectomy, a high intraocular pressure, and a visible red fundus reflex, should raise the specter of posteriorly entrapped aqueous humor (aqueous misdirection) or malignant glaucoma. In previous years, these cases required surgical intervention, and the diagnosis often was made with the patient on the operating table. Currently, eyes with malignant glaucoma, which are aphakic or pseudophakic, are more typically treated in the office with the neodymium-YAG laser. The vitreous face appears to be tightly adherent to the entire posterior surface of the posterior capsule, the intraocular lens, and the iris, and the vitreous appears to be bulging forward through a patent iridectomy. Careful slit-lamp examination of the vitreous cavity reveals vitreous fibrils pressed densely against the posterior capsule or anterior hyaloid face, with clear fluid-containing space entrapped posteriorly. In some cases, these findings can be confirmed by ultrasonic examination. Disruption of the anterior and posterior vitreous surface with the YAG laser allows a pathway for posteriorly entrapped aqueous humor to enter the anterior chamber and exit the eye. This neodymium-YAG laser 'vitrotomy' results in dramatic deepening of the anterior chamber and lowering of intraocular pressure. Malignant glaucoma in the phakic eye is more difficult to treat with YAG vitrotomy because of poor visibility; it usually requires surgical intervention with vitrectomy.

Vitreous dehydration with osmotic agents, such as oral glycerin, oral isosorbide, or intravenous mannitol, is useful in combination with ocular mydriatic/cycloplegic agents to reverse some cases of pupillary block and posterior aqueous entrapment.

Surgical

Wound leaks usually should be repaired surgically. Small focal or diffusely oozing leaks from filtering blebs may be tamponaded temporarily with the large soft contact lenses while natural wound-healing mechanisms fill in the offending defects. Filtration blebs leaking substantially associated with a flat anterior chamber usually must be repaired surgically. Tapered noncutting needles with 10-0 suture material permit surgical closure with minimal further disruption of delicate conjunctiva. Leaking cystic blebs at the limbus may be excised locally, sliding adjacent conjunctiva over to cover the resultant defect. To provide a smooth limbal area and to firmly anchor the new conjunctiva, a very small corneal-scleral groove can be prepared to recess the conjunctival flap edge for suturing.

In the absence of a wound leak, surgical anterior chamber reformation after filtering surgery almost always includes drainage of suprachoroidal fluid from a choroidal detachment. Most moderately shallow anterior chambers after filtering surgery will reform spontaneously without any intervention. Deepening the chamber at the slit-lamp examination is rarely necessary and subjects the patient to the risk of infection and lens injury.

If surgical intervention must be undertaken for suprachoroidal detachment, it is best performed with good anesthetic control and visibility in an operating room. After the anterior chamber is surgically reformed through a corneal paracentesis wound, suprachoroidal fluid should be drained completely from two inferior posterior sclerotomies. If no suprachoroidal fluid is present and the anterior chamber remains flat, especially with increased intraocular pressure, pupillary block or posterior misdirection of aqueous humor is likely to be present. In this case, an additional peripheral iridectomy should be performed. If the anterior chamber remains shallow even after peripheral iridectomy, malignant glaucoma from posterior diversion of aqueous humor is the most likely diagnosis. In this case, liquid vitreous may be aspirated through the pars plana as described by Chandler in 1949 and Simmons in 1972 or, even better, through a vitrectomy, performed via the pars plana in phakic eyes if visibility permits or through the limbus in the aphakic eye.

If pupillary block is strongly suspected, the safest procedure probably is laser iridotomy. An incomplete iridectomy is readily opened with an argon laser applied to the underlying intact iris pigment epithelium. An occluded iridectomy requires additional laser iridectomies to be placed. Two iridotomies, one on each side of the intraocular lens, should be performed in patients with pupillary block associated with anterior chamber intraocular lenses.

COMPLICATIONS

- Anterior synechia.
- Angle-closure glaucoma.
- Corneal decompensation.
- Cataract.
- Tractional retinal detachment.
- Hypotony.
- Cystoid macular edema.

REFERENCES

Arevalo JF, Garcia RA, Fernandez CF: Anterior segment inflammation and hypotony after posterior segment surgery. Ophthalmol Clin North Am 17(4):527–537, 2004.

Azuara-Blanco A, Dua HS: Malignant glaucoma after diode laser cyclophotocoagulation. Am J Ophthalmol 127(4):467–469, 1999.

Beigi B, O'Keefe M, Algawi K, et al: Sulphur hexafluoride in the treatment of flat anterior chamber following trabeculectomy. Eye 11(Pt 5):672–676, 1997.

Gressel MG, Parrish RK, II, Heurer DK: Delayed nonexpulsive suprachoroidal hemorrhage. Arch Ophthalmol 102:1757–1760, 1984.

Shields MB: Trabeculectomy vs. full-thickness filtering operation for control of glaucoma. Ophthalmic Surg 11:498–505, 1980.

168 TRAUMATIC HYPHEMA 921.3

Bahram Rahmani, MD, MPH
Chicago, Illinois

ETIOLOGY/EPIDEMIOLOGY

Hyphema is an accumulation of blood in the anterior chamber of the eye. Trauma is the most common cause of hyphema, although bleeding may occur spontaneously in conditions such as rubeosis iridis, leukemia, hemophilia, anticoagulation therapy, retinoblastoma or juvenile xanthogranuloma of the iris. Presence of hyphema can be a sign of associated damage to other intraocular tissues which is usually the cause of poor vision after the resolution of the hyphema.

Mean annual incidence of traumatic hyphema is about 17 per 100,000 population. Patients with traumatic hyphema are predominantly male with a median age below 20 years of age. The majority of traumatic hyphema occurs in the pediatric population. Direct injury resulting in traumatic hyphema in adults usually consists of a high-energy blow to the orbit or blunt trauma to the cornea and eyeball from a finger or a fist, while a low velocity missile such as a rock, a ball or a stick is commonly responsible for hyphema in children. Lack of protective eyewear in sports is a predisposing factor and the current literature suggests that further education of workers, athletes and parents, along with an increase in the use of polycarbonate safety lenses, may decrease the incidence rate of traumatic hyphema. Hyphema may also occur with penetrating injuries of the globe, but here we consider the management of hyphema that occurs after closed globe trauma.

COURSE/COMPLICATIONS

Sudden contusion and posterior displacement of the iris/lens complex results in a tear and bleeding from the iris and/or ciliary body and can damage the angle. The blood in the anterior chamber may settle inferiorly or form a clot and gradually exit via the trabecular meshwork. Lysis and contraction of the fibrin plug in the injured vessel may result in secondary bleeding. The days 2–5 after the trauma carry the highest risk of secondary hemorrhage and after day 7 the chance of rebleeding becomes negligible. The usual duration of an uncomplicated hyphema is 5–6 days.

Most hyphemas fill less than one third of the anterior chamber and less than 10% are total hyphemas. The size of the hyphema, is only weakly related to the general risk of secondary hemorrhage. Because prevention of rebleeding is the primary objective, in general all the subtotal hyphemas are initially treated the same regardless of their size. There probably are race-related differences in the rate of secondary hemorrhage. Rate of the rebleeding is lower in the Scandinavian patients compared to reports from centers in the United States with mostly African-American patients.

Corneal blood staining occurs with large hyphemas, secondary hemorrhage and persistently elevated intraocular pressure (IOP) above 25 mm Hg. Previous or concomitant corneal endothelial damage can increase the risk of blood staining. Corneal staining requires from several months to 1–2 years for resolution and has the potential for causing deep amblyopia and permanent vision loss in children.

Elevated IOP can occur in traumatic hyphema of any size, and approximately one third of all patients experience elevated IOP (above 24 mm Hg) during hospitalization. Intraocular hypertension can lead to secondary glaucoma and irreversible optic nerve atrophy resulting in permanent vision loss. The mean duration of elevated IOP is 6 days.

The prognosis for visual recovery is directly related to the associated damage to other ocular structures, secondary hemorrhage, development of glaucoma, corneal blood staining and optic atrophy. Prevention of the secondary hemorrhage is the primary objective of therapy because complications such as glaucoma, corneal blood staining, and visual loss are more likely to occur with recurrent rebleeding and indications for surgical intervention are more likely to arise. This risk appears to be greatest in patients with sickle cell trait or disease. Patients with traumatic hyphema need appropriate long term follow up to evaluate for anterior and posterior synechea, damage to iris, cataract, optic atrophy and angle recession glaucoma.

HISTORY/EXAMINATION

The ocular examination should begin with a complete history. Past medical and ocular history, current medications, and circumstances surrounding the event must be evaluated. Bleeding disorders such as hemophilia and von Willebrand's disease and hemoglobinopathies like sickle cell disease/trait, may affect the course of the hyphema and the long-term outcome. Thus, all African American patients with traumatic hyphema should be screened for sickle cell disorder. If several days have elapsed since the injury, the onset of diminished visual acuity or an increase in ocular pain may indicate a secondary hemorrhage.

Inspection for gross ocular injury, evaluation of the adnexa, and assessment of visual acuity, visual fields, pupillary function, ocular motility and the position of the globe should be undertaken. Significant conjuctival edema may indicate a scleral rupture, excessive proptosis may represent a retrobulbar hematoma, and restriction in ocular motility may suggest an orbital blowout fracture. Many patients diagnosed with traumatic hyphema may appear drowsy which should be differentiated from the effect of an associated head injury. Computed tomography and plain film radiography may reveal orbital and facial fractures. Most hyphemas are identified by gross inspection. Sitting the patient upright at an angle of 30° allows the hyphema to settle at a fluid level. A detailed drawing showing the size and shape of the hyphema should be recorded daily, so that its resolution can be assessed or a secondary hemorrhage can be quantified. Documenting visual acuity, extraocular movements, and pupillary function on a daily basis will also assess the progress of the medical management. In most studies, the size of the hyphema does not have significant correlation with chance of rebleeding.

The pupil should be dilated if one suspects an intraocular foreign body, rupture of the globe, or a retinal detachment. Otherwise, the fundus examination may be deferred till the media are clear following resolution of the hyphema. A B-scan should be considered if retinal detachment cannot be ruled out. Unless elevated IOP is suspected, applanation tonometry to record IOP after the initial diagnosis is discouraged to avoid additional trauma to the globe. One should avoid gonioscopy until after day 7 because of the risk of induction of a secondary hemorrhage.

MEDICAL MANAGEMENT

Proper communication of the current status and the serious nature of the injury to the eye is the first step of its management. Patients and their parents should be informed of the possible short and long term vision threatening complications of traumatic hyphema. Goal of the short term management is minimizing the chance of secondary hemorrhage, glaucoma and corneal blood staining.

There remains a significant diversity of opinion among practitioners regarding how to best manage the patients with traumatic hyphema. This diversity reflects the scientific literature, in which recommendations are based on low and often variable frequency of rebleeding in the test populations; difficulties in reproducing prior study results due to uncontrolled nature of many studies and the widespread use of a variety of topical medications.

Supportive therapy

Elevation of the patient's head helps in settling the hyphema, and clears the visual axis to improve the vision and allow funduscopy. Eye patching with metal shield may improve the patient's comfort and protects the eye. In very young patients, patching may carry the risk of occlusion amblyopia and should be avoided. A shield should be worn at all times, including night time, until the hyphema is absorbed. Most studies have found no significant difference between moderate activity and strict bed rest. However, limited activity is strongly encouraged.

Inpatient management of the hyphema has been the standard of care for many years. It enables easier monitoring of the patient and administration of medications, but is more costly. Some other recent studies have shown comparable outcomes with outpatient daily visits which is less expensive and is preferred by the patient and their family and may be recommended in compliant patients. Inpatient hospitalization should still be considered for those patients who may have an increased risk of rebleeding, have uncontrolled glaucoma, are suspected of child abuse or are noncompliant or unable to make frequent office visits.

Cycloplegia/NSAID

Most studies have shown that cycloplegia has no effect on the rate of rebleeding, but it dilates the pupil, relaxes the ciliary body and iris and prevents stress on their injured blood vessels. Cycloplegia decreases the inflammation and patient's discomfort from associated traumatic iritis. Instillation of one drop of atropine at the time of first encounter provides adequate cycoplegia while avoids the manipulation and trauma of regular application of short acting cycloplegics.

Numerous studies have suggested the deleterious effect of aspirin in increasing the rate of rebleeding and most practitioners discontinue aspirin and other nonsteroidal anti-inflammatory agents in the face of a hyphema.

Antiglaucoma drugs

Elevated IOP is common in post traumatic period and may lead to optic atrophy and corneal blood staining. The main cause is thought to be the blockage of the inflamed trabecular meshwork by the red blood cells and inflammatory debris. Sickled cells block the meshwork and elevate the pressure more than normal erythrocytes.

Topical beta-adrenergic antagonists are usually the first choice for controlling the IOP. Topical and oral carbonic anhydrase inhibitors (CAI), hyperosmotic agents and topical alpha adrenergic agonists are also used with caution. One should avoid systemic acidosis or excessive hemoconcentration in sickle cell disease. Prostaglandin analogs and miotics may worsen the inflammation and caution should be exercised in using them in patients with traumatic hyphema.

Corticosteroids

By stabilizing the blood–ocular barrier and inhibiting fibrinolysis, corticosteroids might reduce the risk of secondary hemorrhage. Some studies, many of them not randomized, have demonstrated the effectiveness of the oral prednisone in the reduction of the rate of rebleeding in traumatic hyphema using the Yasuna's protocol. This protocol uses 40 mg/day of oral prednisone for adults and corresponding 0.6 mg/kg/day in divided doses for children. However, the randomized clinical trials using oral prednisone have shown variable results. Although in most of the studies, the rate of rebleeding was less in the group treated with oral prednisone compared to the control; this difference has failed to reach a statistically significant level in some reports.

Topical corticosteroids have shown to reduce intraocular inflammation and may prevent the secondary hemorrhage. They may be recommended for adults with traumatic hyphema to reduce the associated iritis and prevent posterior synechiae, but in children, it is better to start them only on the fifth day of a retained hyphema or persistant iridocyclitis.

Antifibrinolytics

Topical and systemic antifibrinolytic agents such as aminocaproic acid (ACA) and tranexamic acid may be used in traumatic hyphema to reduce rebleeding. They inhibit fibrinolysis and stabilize the blood clot and allow the injured bleeding vessel more time to heal and prevent further bleeding. The current recommended dose for oral ACA is 50 mg/kg every 4 hours, up to 30 gm/day for 5 days. Topical ACA ointment is also applied to the affected eye every 4 hours for 5 days. Patient receiving oral ACA is usually admitted to the hospital, owing to the potential side effects which include nausea, muscle weakness, abdominal cramps and hypotension. Topical ACA does not appear to have the systemic side effects and seems as effective as the oral form in lowering secondary hemorrhage risk and may be appropriate for the outpatient management. Oral dosage of tranexamic acid is 75 mg/kg per day divided into 3 doses. Tranexamic acid is more potent and has less systemic side effects compared to the ACA but has not yet been approved for ophthalmic use in the United States. Both ACA and tranexamic acid should be avoided in pregnant patients, patients with renal or hepatic dysfunction, or those at risk of thromboembolic disease.

Special considerations

Patients with sickle cell anemia or trait require a much more aggressive treatment than other patients. The red blood cells can sickle in the anterior chamber and impede the outflow of the aqueous from the trabecular meshwork. This will elevate the IOP, worsen the hypoxia and sickling and may lead to a refractory glaucoma. These patients are at risk of vaso-occlusive disease and even mild elevation of the IOP can lead to optic atrophy and permanent visual loss. Medical management of glaucoma should be aggressive and keep the IOP below 25 mm Hg, otherwise surgical intervention may be indicated. A beta-adrenergic antagonist is the drug of choice, but carbonic anhydrase inhibitors and hyperosmotic agents can be used. Caution should be applied to avoid acidosis that can predispose to sickling.

In the past, admission to the hospital was indicated for all children with traumatic hyphema. Recently patients treated as outpatient have been reported to have final visual outcome comparable to the inpatient. Still the patients who are suspected of rebleeding or child abuse or being noncompliant, have large hyphema (>50%) or sickle cell hemoglobinopathy or uncontrolled elevation of IOP, have to be admitted and managed as inpatient.

SURGICAL MANAGEMENT

Medical management of total hyphemas is preferable for the initial 4 days if one can control the IOP satisfactorily with medications and there is no corneal blood staining. Hyphema evacuation is recommended in the following situations:

- Mean IOP greater than 24 mm Hg for more than 24 hours in a patient with sickle cell disease.
- IOP greater than 50 mm Hg for 5 days (to prevent optic atrophy).
- IOP greater than 25 mm Hg with a total hyphema for 5 days (to prevent corneal blood staining).
- Any corneal blood staining.
- The hyphema that fails to resolve to less than 50% of the anterior chamber volume by 8 days (to prevent peripheral anterior synechiae).

Definitive clot evacuation is done in the operating room and different techniques may be used to remove the clot and/or control the elevated IOP. Clot expression and delivery through a limbal incision is advocated after day 4, when clot lysis and retraction is at its peak. Vitrectomy probe with or with out viscoelastics may be used in the anterior chamber to remove the clot when dealing with a subtotal hyphema. Instruments should not be introduced to the anterior chamber with out good visualization and a clot that adheres firmly to the iris should not be removed. Intracameral tissue plasminogen activator injection may be considered as an adjuvant therapy in eyes with persistent elevated IOP and total hyphema, although it may increase the risk of bleeding.

Trabeculectomy combined with manual clot expression may be an effective alternative, particularly in patients with very high IOP and total hyphema, compromise in the view of the anterior chamber (e.g. corneal bloodstaining) and particular susceptibility to IOP-induced damage (e.g. sickle cell disease). Transcorneal oxygen therapy may reverse the sickling process and reduce the IOP in patients with sickle cell disease.

Corneal blood stain may take several months to years to clear, so penetrating keratoplasty may be considered in children who have significant staining and are at high risk of amblyopia.

SUMMARY

Initial bleeding

Initial encounter

- Complete medical and ocular history and medications, check for sickle cell disease/trait (patients with black ancestry), pregnancy, renal insufficiency, thromboembolic disease, bleeding disorder and anticoagulation history.
- Complete ocular examination; record the level and amount of hyphema, check for elevated pressure or corneal blood stain, avoid checking IOP of noncompliant children.
- Defer gonioscopy and scleral depression for 7 days.
- Outpatient daily examination for qualified patients; Patients who are noncompliant (e.g. late presentation), high risk (e.g. sickle cell disease, large hyphema or elevated IOP) or have associated ocular/systemic injuries and most of the children should be treated as inpatient.
- Elevate the patient's head 30 degrees.
- Replace clotting factors and platelets if indicated.
- Apply patch and metal shield to the injured eye (only shield in very young patient).
- Limited activity.
- Atropine 0.5–1% 1 drop in traumatized eye (only once).
- Stop aspirin or other NSAID medicine.
- Acetaminophen and antiemetics if indicated.
- Start:
    - Prednisone 40 mg/day for adults or 0.6 mg/kg/day PO for children in 2 divided doses for 5 days (not recommended in diabetes, peptic ulcer disease or systemic infection). Topical prednisolone acetate 1% Q4H for 5 days if oral prednisone is not used (not recommended in children).

  Or:
    - Aminocaproic acid 50 mg/kg PO Q4H (not to exceed 30 g/day) for 5 days (not recommended in total hyphema, pregnancy or renal insufficiency, contraindicated in hemophilia and thromboembolic disease).
    - Topical 30% Aminocaproic acid gel Q6H or oral Tranexamic acid 75 mg/kg per day divided into 3 doses for 5 days are the other alternatives but are not approved by the FDA.
- Treat elevated IOP with topical timolol and/or oral/topical CAI; may add hyperosmotic agents with caution.

Subsequent encounters

- Daily examination for rebleeding; record vision, level of hyphema and corneal clarity. Check IOP if clinically indicated or in high risk patients (e.g. sickle cell disease). Patients with sickle cell disease or elevated IOP may need frequent evaluation.
- Treat elevated IOP if indicated.
- Consider surgical removal of the hyphema if there is:
    - Any sign of corneal blood staining or high risk of its development (large hyphema >50% of the anterior chamber with pressure >25 mm Hg for 6 days or >4 days of total hyphema);
    - High risk of synechiae formation (large hyphema >50% of the anterior chamber for >8 days);
    - High risk of optic atrophy (IOP > 24 mm Hg for >24 hours in sickle cell disease, IOP > 60 mm Hg for >2 days or >50 mm Hg for 5 days).

Secondary bleeding

- Admit the patient to the hospital if not already admitted.
- Consider the rebleeding as a new hyphema and continue the daily examination and treatment for at least 5 more days.
- All of the criteria for initial management of the hyphema apply to the management of the secondary bleeding.

Follow up

- Long term follow up of the hyphema patient is indicated for the detection of the late onset complications such as cataract and secondary glaucoma.

REFERENCES

Crouch ER, Jr, Frenkel M: Aminocaproic acid in the treatment of traumatic hyphema. Am J Ophthalmol 81:355–360, 1976.

Farber MD, Fiscella R, Goldberg MF: Aminocaproic acid versus prednisone for the treatment of traumatic hyphema. Ophthalmology 98:279–286, 1991.

Goldberg MF: The diagnosis and treatment of sickled erythrocytes in human hyphema. Trans Am Ophthalmol Soc 76:481–501, 1978.

Nasrullah A, Kerr NC: Sickle cell trait as a risk factor for secondary hemorrhage in children with traumatic hyphema. Am J Ophthalmol 123:783–790, 1997.

Rahmani B, Jahadi HR: Comparison of tranexamic acid and prednisolone in the treatment of traumatic hyphema: a randomized clinical trial. Ophthalmology 106:375–379, 1999.

Rahmani B, Jahadi HR, Rajaeefard A: An analysis of risk for secondary hemorrhage in traumatic hyphema. Ophthalmology 106:380–385, 1999.

Read J: Traumatic hyphema: surgical vs medical management. Ann Ophthalmol 7(5):659–670, 1975.

Read J, Goldberg MF: Comparison of medical treatment for traumatic hyphema. Trans Am Acad Ophthalmol Otolaryngol 78:799–815, 1974.

Recchia FM, Saluja RK, Hammel K, Jeffers JB: Outpatient management of traumatic microhyphema. Ophthalmology 109:1465–1470, 2002.

Romano PE, Robinson JA: Traumatic hyphema: a comprehensive review of the past half century yields 8076 cases for which specific medical treatment reduces rebleeding 62%, from 13% to 5% (P < 0001). Binocul Vis Strabismus Q 15(2):175–186, 2000.

Rynne MV, Romano PE: Systemic corticosteroids in the treatment of traumatic hyphema. J Pediatr Ophthalmol Strabismus 17:141–143, 1980.

Sears ML: Surgical management of black ball hyphema. Trans Am Acad Ophthalmol Otolaryngol 74:820–826, 1970.

Walton W, Von Hagen S, Grigorian R, Zarbin M: Management of traumatic hyphema. Surv Ophthalmol. 47(4):297–334, 2002.

Yasuna E: Management of traumatic hyphema. Arch Ophthalmol 91:190–191, 1974.

SECTION

17 Choroid

169 ANGIOID STREAKS 363.43

Robert C. Kwun, MD
Park City, Utah

ETIOLOGY/INCIDENCE

Angioid streaks are irregular, jagged, curvilinear lines that radiate from the optic nerve in all directions. These lines were first described in 1889 by Doyne and later called *angioid streaks* by Knapp because of their resemblance to the branching pattern of blood vessels. The streaks lie beneath the retina and above the choroidal vasculature and are caused by breaks in the collagenous and elastic portion of Bruch's membrane. These reddish-brown lesions are almost always bilateral and usually do not go past the equator. The streaks may be wide or narrow and may vary in length and number. Often, these lesions are associated with peripapillary chorioretinal changes.

The clinical significance of angioid streaks is based on the common association with several systemic disorders, such as pseudoxanthoma elasticum (Gronblad–Strandberg syndrome), osteitis deformans (Paget's disease), sickle cell anemia, senile elastosis of skin, hypertensive cardiovascular disorders and, rarely, fibrodysplasia hyperelastica (Ehlers–Danlos syndrome). In addition, streaks are associated with choroidal neovascularization, retinal pigment epithelial detachment and macular degeneration. Other associated findings include peau d'orange fundus changes, disc drusen, peripheral focal salmon spots and pigmentary changes along the streaks.

COURSE/PROGNOSIS

The patient is usually asymptomatic early in the course of the disease. Visual loss with metamorphopsia occurs with time. Exudative macular degeneration develops. Minor trauma may cause subretinal hemorrhage.

DIAGNOSIS

Laboratory findings

Fluorescein angiography

- Usually, early hyperfluorescence of the streaks is revealed with late staining. See Figure 169.1.
- Occasionally, hypofluorescence of the streaks is seen with hyperfluorescence of margins.
- Streaks not seen clinically and associated choroidal neovascularization, retinal pigment epithelium detachments, and serous or hemorrhagic detachments may be demonstrated.

Indocyanine green angiography

- There is early hypofluorescence of the streaks with later hyperfluorescence and staining.
- Tiny hyperfluorescence spots are seen at the borders of the streaks.
- There is high resolution of choroidal neovascularization around the streaks.

Histopathology

- Angioid streaks are discrete linear breaks in Bruch's membrane that are often characterized by extensive calcific degeneration.
- Fibrovascular ingrowth may occur in some of these breaks.
- Salmon spots are isolated breaks in Bruch's membrane with fibrovascular ingrowth.
- Optic nerve drusen with streaks is usually associated with pseudoxanthoma elasticum.

Related systemic diagnosis in patients with angioid streaks

- Pseudoxanthoma elasticum (89%).
- Paget's disease of bone (5%).
- Hemoglobinopathy (2%).
- Ehlers–Danlos syndrome (2%).
- Other (2%).

Differential diagnosis

- Macular degeneration.
- Choroidal sclerosis.
- Myopia and lacquer cracks.
- Pigment lines of reticular dystrophy of retinal pigment epithelium.
- Traumatic hemorrhage.
- Choroidal rupture.
- Chorioretinal folds.

TREATMENT

The use of safety glasses can prevent direct ocular trauma, and contact sports should be avoided. Low vision aids can be used.

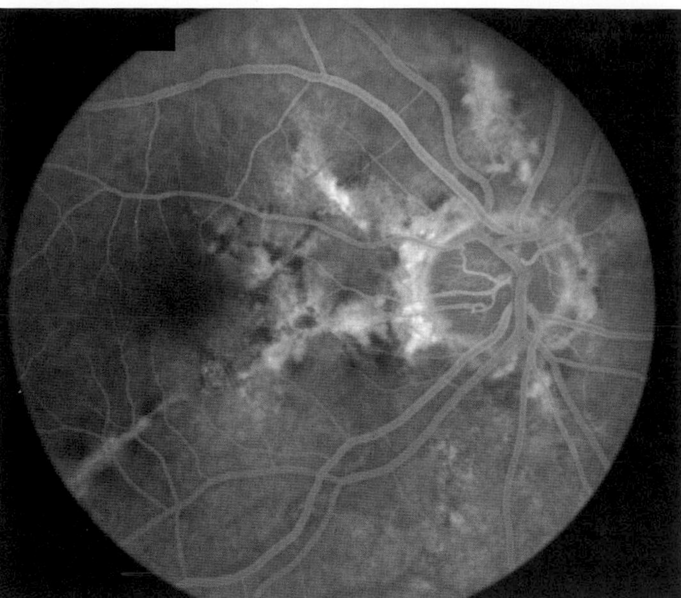

FIGURE 169.1. Angiography shows irregular hyperfluorescence along the course of the angioid streaks.

There is a possible role for laser photocoagulation in well-defined juxtafoveal choroidal neovascularization associated with angioid streaks.

Verteporfin photodynamic therapy of choroidal neovascularization in angioid streaks may limit visual loss.

REFERENCES

Browning AC, Chung AK, Ghanchi F, et al: Verteporfin photodynamic therapy of choroidal neovascularization in angioid streaks: one year results of a prospective case series. Ophthalmology 112:1227–1231, 2005.

Clarkson JG, Altman RD: Angioid streaks. Surv Ophthalmol 26:235–246, 1982.

Gelisken O, Hendrikse F, Deutmann AF: A long-term follow-up study of laser coagulation of neovascular membranes in angioid streaks. Am J Ophthalmol 195:299, 1988.

Groenblad E: Angioid streaks-pseudoxanthoma elasticum: vorlaeufige Mitteilung. Acta Ophthalmol 7:329, 1929.

Knapp H: On the formation of dark streaks as an unusual metamorphosis of retinal hemorrhage. Arch Ophthalmol 21:289–292, 1982.

Lebwohl M, Phelps R, Yannuzzi L, et al: Diagnosis of pseudoxanthoma elasticum by scar biopsy in patients without characteristic skin lesions. N Engl J Med 317:347–350, 1987.

Lim JI, Bressler NM, March MJ, Bressler SB: Laser treatment of choroidal neovascularization in patients with angioid streaks. Am J Ophthalmol 116:414–423, 1993

Paton D: The relation of angioid streaks to systemic disease. Springfield, Ill, Charles C Thomas, 1972.

Quaranta M, Cohen SY, Krott R, et al: Indocyanine green videoangiography of angioid streaks. Am J Ophthalmol 119:136–142, 1995.

Verhoeff FH: Histological findings in a case of angioid streaks. Br J Ophthalmol 32:531, 1948.

170 CHOROIDAL DETACHMENT 363.70
(Ciliochoroidal Detachment)

James W. Hung, MD
Boston, Massachusetts
A. Robert Bellows, MD
Boston, Massachusetts

ETIOLOGY/INCIDENCE

Choroidal detachment is a clinical term used to describe the separation of the choroid and sclera created by a fluid accumulation between the two layers. Anatomically the suprachoroidal space is a potential space, normally containing less than 10 microliters of fluid and is limited anteriorly by the scleral spur and posteriorly by the vortex veins. When fluid accumulates in this space, anterior displacement of the ciliary body and lens iris diaphragm often occurs and is associated with anterior chamber shallowing. The term *ciliochoroidal detachment* can be used interchangeably, since it implicates both the ciliary body and the choroid.

Although accumulation of any type of fluid can produce a choroidal detachment, the two most common forms are associated with the accumulation of serous and/or hemorrhagic fluids. The exact mechanism of any form of choroidal detachment is not fully understood, but intraocular hypotony is thought to be a primary contributor. When sufficient lowering of the intraocular pressure below episcleral venous pressure creates a pressure differential across the capillary bed, this gradient promotes the transudation of serous fluid from the choriocapillaris into the suprachoroidal space creating a detachment of the choroid and often retina from the sclera. Small and medium sized protein molecules move through intact cells with leaky junctions and accompanying the fluid into the suprachoroidal space. The drop in intraocular pressure creates a hydrostatic pressure gradient that can also produce mechanical traction on the arteries, veins and choroid when they emerge from the intrascleral canals. The rupture of these vessels is thought to be the etiology of hemorrhagic choroidal detachment referred to as a suprachoroidal hemorrhage. While there are many causes of hypotony it is most often found in the setting of ocular trauma, intraocular surgery, particularly glaucoma filtering surgery or tube shunt surgery, infrequently in cataract surgery and rarely in circumstances of aqueous suppressants or other pharmacologic agents.

Other specific entities associated with the development of choroidal detachment include inflammation, vascular abnormalities and malignancy. Inflammation as manifested in scleritis, choroiditis, Vogt–Koyanagi–Harada syndrome, Wegener's granulomatosis, orbital pseudotumor, and extensive panretinal photocoagulation frequently lead to the accumulation of serous fluid in the suprachoroidal space. Vascular malformations such as carotid-cavernous fistulas and Sturge Weber syndrome, as well as a unique ophthalmic syndrome associated with prominent episcleral vessels and elevated episcleral venous pressure. Thesc vascular entities are associated with an increase in resistance of blood flow through the episcleral vessels and result in accumulation of fluid in the suprachoroidal space. Additional unusual anatomic variants such as nanophthalmos and the uveal effusion syndromes are associated with choroidal detachment as are ocular tumors, primary and secondary, that can cause a choroidal detachment.

The risk factors of choroidal detachment include: advanced age, preoperative elevated intraocular pressure, high myopia, elevated episcleral venous pressure, severe hypertension, Valsalva maneuvers and aphakia. Choroidal detachments have also been documented to form spontaneously or related to medication. The risk factors of developing a suprachoroidal hemorrhage are many of the mentioned entities and, in addition, blood dyscrasias, anticoagulants, increased intraocular pressure that is lowered suddenly, filtering surgery and tube shunt procedures.

The reported incidence of choroidal detachments vary widely depending on the etiology and clinical setting. It must be emphasized that the incidence of choroidal detachment is far less since the advent of sutured flap closure of glaucoma filtering procedures and tight wound maintenance and closure following cataract surgery. The use of antimetabolites has resulted in more successful lowering of intraocular pressure and surprisingly enough has not been associated with an increase in the incidence of choroidal detachment. The entity of hypotony maculopathy is more prevalent with hypotony following antimetabolites than is the development of a choroidal detachment.

Serous choroidal detachments are more common following the postoperative periods of hypotony after glaucoma surgery. With the advent of phacoemulsification surgery the maintenance of intraocular pressure during surgery and tight wound closure following surgery has minimized postoperative hypotony with only the rare complication of choroidal detachment following cataract surgery. The more frequent use of glaucoma drainage implant surgery (tube shunt), both valve and non-valve, has been associated with a higher incidence of choroidal detachment, particularly hemorrhagic choroidal detachments. The entity of an expulsive suprachoroidal hemorrhage during surgery is now rare because of the small incision tight wound closure associated with most cataract and glaucoma surgery. The incidence of choroidal detachment has also diminished in penetrating keratoplasty and vitreoretinal procedures.

DIAGNOSIS

Clinical signs and symptoms

A serous choroidal detachment is usually painless unless associated with underlying inflammatory cause such as scleritis. However, a hemorrhagic choroidal detachment is often heralded by severe sudden pain that is often diagnostic.

Choroidal detachments appear as large, brown, quadratic intraocular dome-shaped balloons that often exist circumferentially, most prominent nasal and temporal.

Minimally elevated anterior choroidal detachments are often difficult to identify with an ophthalmoscope and are more often associated with shallowing of the anterior chamber. B-scan ultrasonography is helpful in documenting a posterior choroidal detachment but ultrasound biomicroscopy (UBM) is frequently necessary to identify anterior choroidal detachments. A recent study has utilized color Doppler imaging to identify choroidal detachments and distinguish them from retinal detachments. This distinction is often more accurately made during the clinical examination.

Large choroidal detachments can lead to direct apposition of opposing retinal surfaces frequently referred to as 'kissing' choroidals and often require drainage. In an effort to distinguish a choroidal detachment from an intraocular tumor, transilluminating (Hagen's sign) results in a transillumination of a choroidal detachment with no transillumination in solid tumors.

Suprachoroidal hemorrhages may develop suddenly and present as large, very dark balloon-like elevations of the choroid. Occasionally B-scan ultrasonography can distinguish blood in the suprachoroidal space.

Development of an intraocular hemorrhagic choroidal detachment is heralded by the patient expressing severe pain, often 'breaking through' apparent adequate local anesthesia. The surgeon may notice an alteration in the red reflex, often associated with shallowing of the anterior chamber and positive vitreous pressure in the presence of a large wound, extrusion of retina and the intraocular contents. Principal effort is directed to closing the wound to prevent egress of tissue.

Differential diagnosis

- Serous choroidal detachment.
- Hemorrhagic choroidal detachment.
- Retinal detachment.
- Primary metastatic tumors.

PROPHYLAXIS

The development of a serous or hemorrhagic choroidal detachment is difficult to predict and to prevent. However, meticulous preoperative evaluation of the patient as well as intraoperative efforts to minimize the degree of length of time of ocular hypotony can diminish the attendant risk. Preoperative systemic hypertension should be medically controlled. Administration of anticoagulants, aspirin containing medications or anything altering the blood clotting mechanism should be avoided if possible. Intraocular pressures should be lowered slowly with digital pressure or osmotic agents. The choice of anesthetic, general or local, is not usually associated with the development of a choroidal detachment. However, in patients with elevated venous pressure, alteration of the venous drainage system from the head during general anesthesia can cause elevation of pressure in the venous drainage system of the eye.

Intraoperative

A paracentesis should be created to very slowly lower the intraocular pressure in order to slowly reduce the pressure gradient. Microsurgical techniques are necessary for visualization and appropriate closure of ocular tissues with fine suture material. The tight suture closure of trabeculectomy flaps or corneal incision and ligature sutures in non-valve tube shunt procedures can be utilized. Antimetabolite agents are always used with caution.

Postoperative

The need to avoid prolonged hypotony is possible.

Attempts are made to minimize coughing, straining, vomiting, heavy lifting and aggressive physical activity. Stool softeners, laxatives and anti-emetic agents are frequently recommended.

TREATMENT

Ocular

Serous or small hemorrhagic suprachoroidal detachment

Serous and small hemorrhagic suprachoroidal detachments are usually self-limited. When the intraocular architecture is not significantly altered surgical therapy is not indicated. Medical therapy typically results in spontaneous absorption of fluid or blood products within a few postoperative days heralded by a gradual resolution of the choroidal detachment. Topical use of cycloplegic/mydriatic drops in addition to frequent topical steroids is necessary. A hemorrhagic choroidal detachment with blood in the suprachoroidal space is often associated with more significant inflammation and frequently dull, achy pain that persists for a week or longer. In this situation topical corticosteroid drops should be applied every 2–3 hours and extended cycloplegia is often helpful to minimize pain associated with inflammation and throughout the ciliary body spasm. Occasionally high dose systemic corticosteroids may be of value while the consideration of topical non-steroidal anti-inflammatory agents perhaps can be helpful.

Excessive filtration following the filtration surgery might be diminished with a firm pressure patch early in the course or a large bandage contact lens or compressive shell.

Surgical

Serous choroidal detachment and intraoperative serous choroidal detachment

If an active wound leak is discovered in the presence of choroidal detachment, the wound leak should be sutured.

The indications for surgical intervention (choroidal tap) in the presence of a serous choroidal detachment include:

- Lens-corneal touch;
- Progressive corneal edema or rapid cataract formation;
- A flat anterior chamber with inflammation and a failing filtration bleb;
- Hemorrhagic choroidal detachment with a flat anterior chamber;
- Intraocular inflammation, a flat anterior chamber and aphakia or pseudophakia with no improvement in 3 to 5 days;
- A large pronounced choroidal detachment with appositional (kissing) choroidals for longer than 48 hours;
- Wound leak with flat anterior chamber and prominent choroidal detachment.

Choroidal tap

The tap is performed under local or general anesthesia.

Paracentesis is necessary to reform the anterior chamber. The use of a preexisting paracentesis incision is often helpful since the eye may be soft and a new incision difficult to create.

The conjunctiva and Tenon's capsule are incised circumferentially approximately 3.5 mm from the visible limbus in the inferotemporal and inferonasal quadrants. Both quadrants should be tapped to remove fluid because one quadrant tap may not be sufficient to remove all of the fluid that usually extends to 360-degrees in the suprachoroidal space. Adequate hemostasis is established with cautery.

A radial incision is made with a scratch-down maneuver and carried carefully into the suprachoroidal space. When entering the suprachoroidal space a copious amount of suprachoroidal fluid escapes. It is important that the incision be at least 1.5 to 2 mm long in order to facilitate the egress of fluid. In the presence of a serous detachment the fluid is xanthochromic while with hemorrhagic detachments, serous and serosanguinous fluid is released and frequently followed by dark, unclotted blood ('crank case' oil) that has a more viscous character.

Alternating elevation and depression of each side of the incision facilitates the release of the suprachoroidal fluid. It is advised to use an anterior chamber infusion cannula connected to balanced salt solution so that a controlled, steady intraocular pressure is maintained and the anterior chamber depth is unaltered during the procedure. If a cannula is not available, alternating reformation of the anterior chamber with balanced salt solution with release of fluid from the suprachoroidal space can be utilized. The eye must not be allowed to remain soft during this procedure since fragile vessels may bleed with tissue deformation.

The drainage procedure continues until as much fluid as possible is released. When little or no fluid can be evacuated, the anterior chamber is reformed, the sclerostomy is left unsutured and the conjunctiva is closed with absorbable suture.

Complications of choroidal tap include exacerbation of intraocular inflammation, bacterial endophthalmitis, recurrence of suprachoroidal hemorrhage or serous choroidal detachment, anterior chamber shallowing and flattening, corneal decompensation, cataract progression and the possibility of creating a cyclodialysis cleft.

Postoperative delayed suprachoroidal hemorrhage

A small or moderate suprachoroidal hemorrhage is usually localized and will frequently resolve spontaneously. If the ocular architecture is not significantly disturbed, medical therapy and clinical observation are indicated.

Larger hemorrhagic choroidal detachments associated with ocular inflammation or flat anterior chamber and elevated intraocular pressure as well as the potential for unresolved apposition of retinal surfaces requires surgical intervention.

The management includes choroidal tap combined with pars plana vitrectomy and infusion of expansive gasses, perfluorocarbon liquids or even silicone oil. The surgery is best performed when maximum liquification of the suprachoroidal hemorrhage has occurred, usually in the 10–14 day period. Collaboration with a vitreoretinal surgeon is strongly advised since these techniques are a standard part of vitreoretinal surgery. The likelihood of recurrence of a hemorrhagic choroidal detachment following the use of intraocular gas is diminished significantly.

Intraoperative expulsive suprachoroidal hemorrhage

Intraoperatively, all efforts are directed to rapidly close the wound and prevent extrusion of intraocular contents. Once this is accomplished it is wise to wait for liquification of the hemorrhagic clot and then proceed with drainage of the suprachoroidal space and the use of intraocular gas or perfluorocarbon.

Aggressive management of intraocular pressure, pain control and inflammation is necessary. Given the guarded prognosis following the suprachoroidal hemorrhage a frank and sensitive discussion with the patient and the patient's family is necessary.

COURSE/PROGNOSIS

Serous choroidal detachment

Serous choroidal detachment occurs in the early postoperative period from 2 to 7 days following glaucoma surgery or combined cataract and glaucoma surgery. With contemporary phacoemulsification cataract surgery choroidal detachment is a rare event.

Intraoperative choroidal detachments occur most often in patients with prominent episcleral vessels and elevated venous pressure but can also occur in vascular anomalies such as

Sturge–Weber syndrome. Draining of the suprachoroidal space during the procedure is effective in minimizing the complications of an intraoperative choroidal detachment.

Postoperative detachments are significant for painless visual symptoms related to hypotony, anterior chamber shallowing or awareness of a visual field defect from a large choroidal detachment. The prognosis of a serous choroidal detachment with or without drainage is usually associated with no significant change in functional vision. The development of cataract following choroidal detachment, particularly if drainage is necessary, is a common complication and may require cataract surgery.

Hemorrhagic choroidal detachment

Hemorrhage occurs either intraoperatively or postoperatively. Intraoperative hemorrhage, as mentioned, is quite uncommon with the advent of small incision surgery. When it occurs, it is a dramatic event associated with arterial bleeding, shallowing of the anterior chamber and loss of the red reflex with acute pain and possible extrusion of intraocular contents.

A postoperative suprachoroidal hemorrhage is more common and characterized by the sudden onset of excruciating pain and vision loss during the early postoperative period. This most often occurs during some form of physical activity or Valsalva maneuvers associated with vomiting or coughing. It may be associated with flattening of the anterior chamber and elevation of the intraocular pressure. The prognosis of a hemorrhagic choroidal detachment is guarded and is dependent upon the functional status of the intraocular tissues following the event.

COMMENTS

Identification and management of serous choroidal detachment has changed minimally in the last three decades while recognition and aggressive management of hemorrhagic choroidal detachments that require surgery has improved as the technology of vitreoretinal surgery has made great strides. The incidence of both serous and hemorrhagic detachments has diminished due to surgical techniques that utilize small, seal sealing or sutured wounds with maintenance of the intraocular dynamics during surgery to reduce profound and prolonged hypotony. While a cautious guarded prognosis for a massive intra or postoperative hemorrhagic choroidal detachment remains, medical observation or current surgical techniques have resulted in a more favorable prognosis.

REFERENCES

Bellows AR, Chylack LT, Epstein DL, Hutchinson BT: Choroidal effusion during glaucoma surgery in patients with prominent episcleral vessels. Arch Ophthalmol 97:493–497, 1979.

Bellows AR, Chylack LT, Hutchinson BT: Choroidal detachment: clinical manifestations, therapy and mechanism of formation. Ophthalmology 88:1107–1115, 1981.

Brubaker RF, Pederson JE: Choroidal detachment. Surv Ophthalmol 27:281–289, 1983.

Capper SA, Leopold IH: Mechanism of serous choroidal detachment: a review and experimental study. Arch Ophthalmol 55:101–113, 1956.

Chylack LT, Bellows AR: Molecular sieving in suprachoroidal fluid formation in man. Invest Ophthalmol Vis Sci 17:240–247, 1978.

Kuhn F, Morris R, Mester V: Choroidal detachment and expulsive choroidal hemorrhage. Ophthalmol Clinics of North Amer 14:639–650, 2001.

Wu J, Zou L, Wu Z: High frequency color Doppler image of choroidal detachment. Yan Ke Xue Bao 16:61–64, 2000.

171 CHOROIDAL FOLDS 363.8

John D. Bullock, MD, MPH, MSc
Dayton, Ohio
Ronald F. Warwar, MD
Dayton, Ohio

Choroidal folds represent folds in Bruch's membrane and the anterior choroid with secondary folds in the overlying retina. They are a distinct and separate entity from retinal folds. Choroidal folds were first described by Nettleship in 1884 as alternating light and dark striae in the posterior pole. They typically radiate horizontally from the temporal optic disc, but may also be vertical or oblique. Choroidal folds are of varying number, length, and width, and never extend beyond the equator.

ETIOLOGY

- Intraocular.
- Hypotony (after fistulizing surgery, cyclodialysis cleft).
- Scleral inflammation (posterior scleritis/uveitis) (Figure 171.1).
- Choroidal edema.
- Intraocular neoplasms.
- Choroidal neovascularization.
  - Central serous choroidopathy.
  - Endolaser photocoagulation.
  - Previous scleral surgery.
  - Retinal or choroidal detachment.
  - Choroidal tumor.
  - Endophthalmitis.
  - Hyperopia.
  - Steroid induced.
  - Orbital.

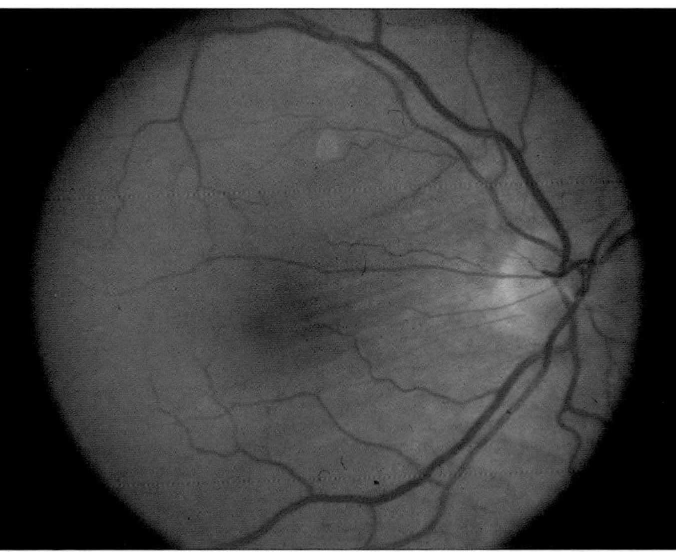

FIGURE 171.1. Choroidal folds in a patient with posterior scleritis.

- Traction on the optic nerve in the absence of scleral contact.
- Orbital tumors (hemangioma, meningioma).
- Thyroid orbitopathy.
- Orbital cellulitis/inflammation.
- Dural sinus fistula.
- Optic nerve edema/intracranial hypertension.
- Ethmoid sinus mucocele.
- Idiopathic.

COURSE/PROGNOSIS

- Can occur in normal eyes.
- May not affect visual function.
- Possible decreased visual acuity and/or metamorphopsia due to macular involvement.
- Possible permanent visual loss due to long-term macular involvement.
- Variable location of folds not predictive of the underlying pathology.
- Characteristic pigmentation patterns due to persistent or recurrent folds: typically bead-like pigmentation lines on the slope of the fold.

DIAGNOSIS

Laboratory findings

- Fluorescein angiogram.
- Early phase: alternating lines of hyperfluorescence and hypofluorescence corresponding to the density of the pigment epithelium at the peaks and valleys of the folds, respectively.
- Late phase: no leakage.
- Folds more visible angiographically than clinically.
- Computed tomography scanning or magnetic resonance imaging when orbital tumor or inflammation is suspected.
- Ultrasonography when posterior scleritis is suspected.

Differential diagnosis

- Retinal folds.
- Entirely separate entity rarely coinciding with choroidal folds.
- Appear finer on ophthalmoscopy.
- Associated with vitreoretinal disease and usually radiate from visible pathology in the retina.
- Fluorescein angiogram is normal (relative to the folds).

TREATMENT

When possible, treatment is reversal of the underlying cause.

REFERENCES

Bullock JD, Egbert PR: Experimental choroidal folds. Am J Ophthalmol 78:618–623, 1974.

Bullock JD, Egbert PR: The origin of choroidal folds: a clinical, histopathological, and experimental study. Documenta Ophthalmol 37:261–293, 1974.

Bullock JD, Waller RB: Choroidal folding in orbital disease. Proceedings of the Third International Symposium on Orbital Disorders, Amsterdam. 1977:483–488.

Cangemi FE, Trempe CL, Walsh JB: Choroidal folds. Am J Ophthalmol 86:380–387, 1978.

Friberg TR: The etiology of choroidal folds: a biomechanical explanation. Graefes Arch Clin Exp Ophthalmol 227:459–464, 1989.

Greibel SR, Kosmorsky GS: Choroidal folds associated with increased intracranial pressure. Am J Ophthalmol 129:513–516, 2000.

Newell FW: Choroidal folds. Am J Ophthalmol 75:930–939, 1973.

Newell FW: Fundus changes in persistent and recurrent choroidal folds. Br J Ophthalmol 68:32–35, 1984.

Norton EWD: A characteristic fluorescein angiographic pattern in choroidal folds. Proc R Soc Med 62:119, 1969.

Steuhl KP, Richard G, Weidle EG: Clinical observations concerning choroidal folds. Ophthalmologica 190:219–224, 1985.

172 CHOROIDAL RUPTURES 363.63

Scott D. Pendergast, MD
Beachwood, Ohio

ETIOLOGY/INCIDENCE

Choroidal rupture is characterized by tearing of Bruch's membrane and the closely associated choriocapillaris and retinal pigment epithelium (RPE) after contusive ocular injury. Direct choroidal rupture occurs at the site of injury and typically is located anterior to the equator and is oriented parallel to the ora serrata. Indirect choroidal ruptures are frequently crescent-shaped tears of the RPE-Bruch's membrane-choriocapillaris complex that are concentric to the optic disk and occur in the posterior pole remote from the site of impact. In the acute stages, choroidal ruptures often are associated with hemorrhagic detachment of the RPE, subretinal or intraretinal hemorrhage, and retinal edema, which may obscure the presence and extent of choroidal rupture. As the retina edema and hemorrhagic components resolve, a subretinal yellow-white scar develops that is frequently associated with hyperplasia of the RPE.

- Direct choroidal ruptures probably result from compression necrosis of ocular tissues at the site of contusive injury.
- Indirect choroidal ruptures have been attributed to contrecoup forces that result in rapid anteroposterior compression and horizontal expansion of the globe. Bruch's membrane is relatively inelastic and susceptible to rupture, whereas the relatively distensible retina and rigid sclera are less prone to rupture.
- The concentric configuration of most indirect choroidal ruptures may be due to a tethering effect of the optic nerve.
- Approximately 1% of patients evaluated at large eye clinics have choroidal rupture.
- The incidence of indirect choroidal rupture after blunt trauma is 5% to 10%.
- Multiple ruptures occur in approximately 25% of eyes.
- Rupture occurs temporal to the optic nerve in 80% of cases, with macular involvement in 66% of eyes.
- Indirect choroidal ruptures are more common than direct choroidal ruptures (80% versus 20%).

COURSE/PROGNOSIS

- Based on histologic studies, direct and indirect choroidal ruptures heal 14 to 21 days after injury.

- Retinal edema resolves in 2 to 3 weeks, whereas hemorrhage may persist for 2 to 3 months.
- A yellow-white subretinal scar develops that may be associated with hypopigmentation or hyperpigmentation of the surrounding RPE.
- Presenting visual acuity is frequently reduced to 20/200 or worse and ranges from 20/20 to light perception depending on the location of the choroidal rupture.
- Visual acuity improves in approximately 60% to 70% of cases, with mean final visual acuity ranging from 20/40 to 20/70 in recent series.
- Eyes with choroidal ruptures involving the fovea, the presence of dense subfoveal hemorrhage, and the development of extensive pigmentary changes in the macula portend a worse prognosis. However, a recent retrospective series found that eyes with foveal choroidal ruptures could maintain good central vision after 4 years of follow-up.

DIAGNOSIS

Laboratory findings

Diagnosis is based on the characteristic clinical appearance as well as a history of preceding ocular trauma.

- If retinal edema, hemorrhage, or both are present and obscure findings, serial examinations may be necessary to establish a diagnosis of choroidal rupture.
- Fluorescein angiography (FA) often is helpful in confirming the presence, location, and extent of choroidal ruptures and demonstrates a hypofluorescent curvilinear streak in the early transit phase followed by hyperfluorescence in the late transit phase with variable hyperfluorescence in the recirculation phase.
- Indocyanine green angiography (ICGA) is useful in localizing major and minor choroidal ruptures and is particularly useful in identifying ruptures obscured by dense hemorrhage. Initial ICGA typically shows hypofluorescent streaks that become more apparent over time and are often more numerous that hyperfluorescent streaks identified on FA.

PROPHYLAXIS

- Appropriate protective eyewear (e.g. polycarbonate lenses) worn while engaging in contact sports is the most effective prophylaxis.
- When Bruch's membrane is abnormal, as in angioid streaks, pathologic myopia, or pre-existing choroidal rupture, relatively minor trauma can result in extensive choroidal ruptures. High-risk patients should be advised of the hazards associated with blunt ocular trauma related to contact sports and other activities.

TREATMENT

- There is no treatment for choroidal ruptures, but a careful examination is important to exclude other ocular injuries associated with blunt ocular trauma, such as commotio retinae, retinal dialysis, hyphema, angle recession and traumatic iritis.
- Inflammation of the anterior segment can be treated with topical steroids and cycloplegics.
- Patients should be followed closely (e.g. monthly) for the first 6 months to detect complications such as retinal detachment and choroidal neovascularization (CNV).
- Retinal detachments that are progressive are usually repaired using standard scleral buckling techniques. In some instances, scar formation limits the detachment and may obviate the need for surgery.
- Choroidal neovascularization:
  - The incidence is unknown, but it appears to be relatively common.
  - This occurs 1 month to 4 years or more after injury and necessitates Amsler grid testing and long-term follow-up.
  - Patients may note decreased central visual acuity, metamorphopsia or scotoma.
  - Clinical signs include the presence of subretinal hemorrhage, fluid, or exudate or a pigmented subretinal lesion.
  - FA and/or ICGA should be performed to confirm the diagnosis and determine the extent and location of CNV relative to the fovea.
- No controlled studies are available and treatment remains somewhat controversial.
- Because choroidal rupture represents a focal abnormality of Bruch's membrane as in presumed ocular histoplasmosis syndrome (POHS), results of photocoagulation for CNV associated with POHS may provide useful treatment guidelines for CNV associated with choroidal ruptures.
- Laser photocoagulation is frequently used to treat CNV, particularly when the center of the fovea is not involved.
- Photodynamic therapy has been used successfully to treat subfoveal CNV associated with traumatic choroidal rupture.
- Submacular surgery with excision of subfoveal CNV improved visual acuity to 20/30 or better in 3 patients in a small series.
- Because CNV has been reported to spontaneously resolve, some investigators advocate observation of CNV.

COMPLICATIONS

- Choroidal neovascularization is the most frequent late complication of choroidal ruptures.
- Retinal detachment is occasionally observed in cases of anterior choroidal ruptures.
- A variety of visual field defects have been observed.
- Chorioretinal vascular anastomosis is a rare complication of choroidal ruptures.

REFERENCES

Bressler SB, Bressler NM: Traumatic maculopathies. In: Shingleton BJ, Hersh PS, Kenyon KR, eds: Eye trauma. St Louis, Mosby-Year Book, 1991:187–194.

Conrath J, Forzano O, Ridings B: Phtodynamic therapy for subfoveal CNV complicating traumatic choroidal rupture. Eye 18:946–947, 2004.

Gross JG, King LP, de Juan E, Jr, et al. Subfoveal neovascular membrane removal in patients with traumatic choroidal rupture. Ophthalmology 103:579–585, 1996.

Kohno T, Miki T, Shiraki K, et al: Indocyanine green angiographic features of choroidal rupture and choroidal vascular injury after contusion ocular injury. Am J ophthalmol 129:38–46, 2000.

Raman VR, Desai UR, Anderson S, et al: Visual prognosis in patients with traumatic choroidal rupture. Can J Ophthalmol 39:260–266, 2004.

173 EXPULSIVE HEMORRHAGE 363.62
(Suprachoroidal Expulsive Hemorrhage)

Fumiki Okamoto, MD, PhD
Ibaraki, Japan
Sachiko Hommura, MD, PhD
Ibaraki, Japan

Expulsive hemorrhage is one of the most serious and catastrophic complications of intraocular surgery. It occurs suddenly, as a localized or sometimes generalized suprachoroidal hemorrhage, breaking into the vitreous and then extruding the intraocular contents through the surgical wound. Early detection of the problem and prompt, aggressive treatment are essential to save the patient's vision; however, in many cases, even rapid remedial measures may fail to preserve useful vision. Prevention of the emergency by understanding the factors that may predispose a patient to experience an intraoperative expulsive hemorrhage is much preferable to attempting to deal with the after-effects.

ETIOLOGY/INCIDENCE

Expulsive hemorrhage is fortunately rare; according to Ling, it occurs in approximately 0.04% of cataract surgery. Among other ocular surgical procedures, expulsive hemorrhage occurs in 0.15% of glaucoma operations, 0.12% of pars plana vitrectomy, and 0.56% of penetrating keratoplasty. The incidence of this complication is higher in elderly patients who have arteriosclerosis or hypertension and glaucoma.

The exact cause of expulsive hemorrhage is unknown, but the immediate event occurs as a result of sudden drop in intraocular pressure gradient when the eye is opened. This sudden change may induce rupture of intraocular vessels if the vessel walls are fragile. The presence of necrotic artifacts in the walls of the short and long ciliary arteries is most important and contributes significantly to occurrence of expulsive hemorrhage.

Risk factors for expulsive hemorrhage fall into two categories: vascular factors and intraoperative risks. Vascular factors include:

- Older age;
- Elevated arterial pressure before surgery;
- Chronic systemic hypertension;
- Generalized arteriosclerosis;
- Hyperlipidemia;
- Diabetes;
- Use of anticoagulant agents;
- High myopia;
- Glaucoma (elevated preoperative intraocular pressure).

Many patients demonstrate combinations of two or more of these vascular factors; in our surgical experience, among 500 successful cataract procedures (controls) versus 5 cataract procedures that involved expulsive hemorrhage, the latter patients had higher numbers of vascular risk factors (four or five factors) compared with controls (only 3 in 500 had four risk factors and none had five factors).

Intraoperative risk factors include:

- Intraoperative systolic hypertension;
- Ocular pain;
- Urge to urinate;
- Cough reflex;
- Vitreous loss;
- Idiopathic (unknown) factors.

Among these factors, poorly controlled intraoperative pain, unsuppressed cough, or the urge to urinate indicates elevation of venous return pressure, which may be a contributing cause of expulsive hemorrhage.

Consideration also must be given to the type of surgical procedure; the procedure most commonly associated with expulsive hemorrhage is the penetrating keratoplasty, with vitreoretinal procedures, cataract extractions and glaucoma operations carrying somewhat lesser risk of expulsive hemorrhage. Penetrating keratoplasty is an 'open sky' procedure that induces prolonged hypotony, scleral collapse, and relative forward displacement of the intraocular contents; in retinal/vitreous operations, direct trauma to the choroid or the vortex vein may be responsible for precipitating expulsive hemorrhage. Glaucoma procedures carry a relatively low incidence of expulsive hemorrhage comparable with that of cataract surgery; in such cases, prolonged ocular hypotony probably results in rupture of the ciliary artery and subsequent massive bleeding.

There also may be *unknown factors* in the patient's medical background that increase the risk for expulsive hemorrhage during intraocular surgery. Wohlrab and associates report a recent case in which surgery was being performed for acute glaucoma and a mature cataract when expulsive hemorrhage occurred; after the operation, laboratory analysis of blood smears demonstrated a myelocytic proliferation, indicating the previously unsuspected presence of myelodysplastic syndrome. The operated eye was eventually enucleated due to extremely high intraocular pressure unresponsive to intensive antiglaucoma therapy; histopathologic examination revealed the retina and choroid were swollen due to leukemic cell infiltration and choroidal hemorrhages.

A second case, reported by Weissgold and coworkers, involved a penetrating keratoplasty being performed for delayed-onset fungal keratitis after fungal endophthalmitis; 3 months earlier, the patient had received aggressive therapy (vitrectomy and intraocular injection of antifungal drugs) for the endophthalmitis. Although the existing prosthetic intraocular lens was left in place after the vitrectomy, a posterior capsulectomy was performed. At the time of the penetrating keratoplasty and complicating expulsive hemorrhage, the eye could not be saved; histopathologic analysis of the eviscerated vitreous and the ulcerated cornea disclosed fungal elements of *Acremonium kiliense,* the causative organism of the original endophthalmitis. The authors conclude that despite aggressive therapy, fungal infections are particularly difficult to eradicate and may have exacerbated choroidal inflammation in this patient, perhaps increasing the risk of catastrophic expulsive hemorrhage.

COURSE/PROGNOSIS

Unfortunately, visual outcome after expulsive hemorrhage often is severely compromised, despite the most up-to-date vitreoretinal surgery. Welch and coworkers assessed visual outcome in 30 patients after massive suprachoroidal hemorrhage and reported that more than half (18) of the patients had a final visual acuity of 20/200 or better; in 1 patient, visual acuity returned to 20/20. The remaining 12 patients experienced immediate retinal detachment, an inoperable sequela that resulted in loss of vision. Fortunately, none of these patients required evisceration or enucleation. Ling et al reported visual outcome in 118 cases after suprachoroidal hemorrhage complicating cataract surgery; best corrected visual acuity was 6/12 or better in 40%, 6/18 to 6/60 in 20%, 6/60 or worse in 40%, after a median follow up interval of 185 days. These results strongly suggest that expulsive hemorrhage may be one of the most intractable conditions from a therapeutic standpoint.

DIAGNOSIS

Clinical signs and symptoms

Expulsive hemorrhage usually occurs during surgery, but it may occur as long as 24 hours after surgery; the patient typically complains of severe ocular pain at that time. When the complication occurs during a procedure, sometimes observed is:

- A dark, growing choroidal mass, visible through the pupil, if the hemorrhage begins slowly.

If this warning sign does not appear, the first indications of an imminent expulsive hemorrhage are:

- A sudden shallowing of the anterior chamber;
- Firmness of the globe;
- Forward displacement of the intraocular contents;
- Gaping of the surgical incision.

These events may be followed by:

- Iris prolapse;
- Spontaneous delivery of the lens, if present;
- Protrusion of the vitreous body and uveoretinal tissue;
- Profuse bleeding through the surgical wound.

If the suprachoroidal hemorrhage does not coagulate spontaneously. In the worst case, the entire intraocular contents may be lost.

TREATMENT

Surgical

The fundamental principle for response to an expulsive hemorrhage is to *close the globe as soon as possible;* this is most expeditiously done by suturing the corneoscleral incision.

- Interrupted sutures with 8-0 silk are the preferred technique to restore intraocular pressure, which serves as an effective tamponade to ruptured choroidal vessels.

In cases in which the surgical wound cannot be closed immediately:

- A prompt and adequate posterior sclerotomy should be performed to release the subchoroidal blood.

A scleral incision, T or Y shaped, should be made approximately 8 mm posterior to the limbus and, if possible, in the quadrant of the suspected source of bleeding. The subchoroidal blood, however, will find egress from a scleral opening at any quadrant, even if that quadrant does not correspond to the bleeding site; time should not be spent attempting to localize the burst vessel or vessels. It is advisable to keep the sclerotomy patent until subchoroidal bleeding ceases completely.

After the surgical incision has been closed:

- Sterile balanced saline solution may be injected carefully through a small limbal incision to re-form the anterior chamber.

When complete cessation of the subchoroidal hemorrhage has been confirmed, the surgical wound is reopened and:

- Anterior vitrectomy is performed to remove as much vitreous material as possible from the anterior chamber.

If vitreous hemorrhage or retinal detachment is involved:

- Posterior vitrectomy should be attempted, followed by:
  - SF6 or C3F8 gas injection;
  - Silicone oil tamponade.

If expulsive hemorrhage occurs during penetrating keratoplasty (the procedure with the highest incidence rate of this complication), it will typically occur after trephination of the host corneal button; in this circumstance, it is impossible to close the eye immediately. Taylor recommends having the assisting surgeon place a thumb over the corneal opening while the primary surgeon rapidly performs a posterior sclerotomy. After complete cessation of hemorrhage, it will be possible to suture the donor corneal button in place. Many eyes may be salvaged with this method.

Systemic

After surgical management of an expulsive hemorrhage, the patient is treated with systemic and topical corticosteroids to reduce intraocular inflammation:

- Prednisolone 30 to 40 mg/day PO; and
- Topical ophthalmic dexamethasone 0.1% or betamethasone 0.1% four to six times daily;
- Cycloplegic drops in addition.

To forestall massive suprachoroidal hemorrhage, Bequet and colleagues recommend high-dose corticosteroid prophylaxis *before* surgery; patients in their studies were administered:

- Methylprednisolone 500 mg/day IV for 3 days before surgery; followed by
- Prednisolone 1 mg/kg/day PO.

PRECAUTIONS

It is very difficult to prevent expulsive hemorrhage, whose pathogenesis is multifactorial. To avoid this complication and decrease its incidence, every reasonable effort should be made to control risk factors because the prediction of fragile intraocular vessels is similarly difficult.

First, special attention should be paid to patients with extensive vascular disease; such patients may routinely take hypotensive agents, vasodilators, anticoagulants, and so on. Insofar as is medically possible, these agents-especially anticoagulants-should be stopped several days before surgery.

In addition to hemostatic agents administered immediately before surgery, the use of a short-acting barbiturate sedative may be necessary for any patient who has anxiety in the operating room. Anxiety causes systolic hypertension and tachycardia, which increase the risk for expulsive hemorrhage. Careful monitoring of pulse rate and blood pressure is extremely important in these patients.

Reduction of intraocular pressure before surgery is fundamental and of utmost importance. Acetazolamide (250 mg PO) is administered the previous night and early on the morning of surgery. Intravenous hyperosmotic agents, such as 200 mL of 20% mannitol or 10% glycerol, also may be given; this infusion should be begun 1 hour before surgery. In addition, decompression of the globe and orbit by mercury bag or by massage is helpful.

At surgery, the intraocular pressure should be reduced to a minimum; it is equally necessary to prepare the patient properly for surgery, including voiding the urinary bladder, suppressing any cough reflex, and controlling the patient's pain, all of which will minimize any rise in venous return pressure.

COMMENTS

Recent improvements in surgical procedure, especially in cataract surgery, should reduce the occurrence of expulsive hemorrhage. The recent literature contains no case reports of expulsive hemorrhage during surgery when the smaller or self-sealing incisions for phacoemulsification are used. Blumenthal and colleagues reported a method in which constant infusion inflow through an anterior chamber maintainer was used to maintain positive intraocular pressure during cataract extraction through a self-sealing tunnel incision. With this technique, there were no expulsive hemorrhages in 5600 eyes.

The present closed-system techniques appear to be beneficial. Because of the risk of bilateral occurrence of this devastating complication, it is prudent to perform cataract extraction using the most current closed-eye technique for the fellow eye of any patient who has previously had an expulsive hemorrhage. Moreover, increased surgeon experience and shortened operation time may contribute to the elimination of intraoperative expulsive hemorrhage.

It is extremely difficult to completely prevent an expulsive hemorrhage and to manage it regardless of circumstances; although subsequent visual loss is too common, proper management can lessen the possibility of blindness.

REFERENCES

Bequet F, Caputo G, Mashhour B, et al: Management of delayed onset massive suprachoroidal hemorrhage: A clinical retrospective study. Eur J Ophthalmol 6:393–397, 1996.

Blumenthal M, Grinbaum A, Assis EI: Preventing expulsive hemorrhage using an anterior chamber maintainer to eliminate hypotony. J Cataract Refract Surg 23:476–479, 1997.

Ghoraba HH, Zayed AI: Suprachoroidal hemorrhage as a complication of vitrectomy. Ophthalmic Surg Lasers 32:281–288, 2001.

Ling R, Cole M, Shaw S, et al: Suprachoroidal haemorrhage complicating cataract surgery in the UK: epidemiology, clinical features, management, and outcomes. Br J Ophthalmol 88:478–480, 2004

Sekine S, Takei K, Hommura S, et al: Survey of risk factors for expulsive choroidal hemorrhage: Case reports. Ophthalmologica 210:344–347, 1996.

Speaker MG, Guerriero PN, Met JA, et al: A case-control study of risk factors for intraoperative suprachoroidal expulsive hemorrhage. Ophthalmology 98:202–210, 1991.

Taylor DM: Expulsive hemorrhage. In: Fraunfelder FT, Roy FH, eds: Current ocular therapy. 4th edn. Philadelphia, WB Saunders, 1995:448–450.

Weissgold DJ, Orlin SE, Sulewski ME, et al: Delayed-onset fungal keratitis after endophthalmitis. Ophthalmology 105:256–262, 1998.

Welch JC, Speath GL, Benson W: Massive suprachoroidal hemorrhage: follow-up and outcome of 30 cases. Ophthalmology 95:1202–1206, 1988.

Wohlrab TM, Pleyer U, Rohrbach JM, et al: Sudden increase in intraocular pressure as an initial manifestation of myelodysplastic syndrome. Am J Ophthalmol 119:370–372, 1995.

174 MALIGNANT MELANOMA OF THE POSTERIOR UVEA 190.6

(Choroidal Melanoma, Ciliary Body Melanoma, Uveal Melanoma, Intraocular Melanoma)

Paul A. Rundle, MBBS, FRCOphth

Sheffield, England

ETIOLOGY/INCIDENCE

Uveal melanoma represents the commonest primary intraocular tumor in adults. It may arise from the melanocyte in any part of the uveal tract, either anterior (iris) or posterior (ciliary body and choroid). The choroid is the most frequent site accounting for approximately 75% of cases. Annual incidence is approximately 6 per million with a median age of 55 years. Melanoma occurs almost exclusively in Caucasian populations. Bilateral disease is exceptionally rare. Risk factors for the development of uveal melanoma include pre-existing nevi and ocular melanosis however unlike cutaneous melanoma there is no direct relationship with UV exposure.

COURSE/PROGNOSIS

Whilst ocular treatment offers excellent rates of local control, ultimately many patients will succumb to metastatic disease. Despite this, at presentation only 2% patients will have detectable systemic metastases. Although metastasis from uveal melanoma usually presents within 5 years of enucleation, late-onset metastases have been recognized decades after treatment of the intraocular tumor. The liver, lung, and skin are the three most common sites for metastatic disease. Survival rates after enucleation of uveal melanoma have been reported to be 65% at 5-year, 52% at 10-year, and 46% at 15-year follow-up. In recent years the COMS study has compared brachytherapy and enucleation in the treatment of medium-sized melanomas and has shown comparable survival rates of approximately 81% at 5 years. Not surprisingly, overall survival rates correlate with tumor size and at 5-year follow-up, small melanoma has a mortality rate of approximately 16%; medium-sized melanoma, 32%; and large melanoma, 53%.

Clinical risk factors for metastases of posterior uveal melanoma include:

- Tumor location in the ciliary body;
- Largest tumor dimension of 15 mm or larger.

Histopathologic risk factors for metastasis of posterior uveal melanoma include:

- Large tumor size;
- Ciliary body involvement;
- Epithelioid cell type;
- Specific cytogenetic abnormalities;
- Extrascleral extension of tumor;
- Vascular patterns within tumor.

Clinical risk factors for growth of small uveal melanocytic tumors (3 mm thick or smaller) include:

- Tumor thickness of more than 2 mm;
- Tumor touching the optic disk;
- Presence of symptoms;
- Orange pigment;
- Subretinal fluid.

Clinical risk factors for metastasis of small uveal melanoma (3 mm thick or smaller) include:
- Tumor thickness of more than 2 mm;
- Documented growth;
- Tumor touching the optic disk;
- Presence of symptoms.

DIAGNOSIS

Clinical signs and symptoms

Uveal melanomas may give rise to symptoms (blurred vision, photopsia, metamorphopsia) or be detected during a routine eye examination. Melanomas tend to be dome-shaped but may appear flat and diffuse. Rupture of Bruch's membrane produces a 'collar-stud' appearance (Figure 174.1). Pigmentation is variable although surface orange-pigment (lipofuschin) is characteristic. The diagnosis is largely made on clinical appearance on indirect ophthalmoscopy or slit-lamp examination.

Laboratory findings

- Ultrasonography: acoustically hollow uveal mass on B-scan and medium to low internal reflectivity within the mass on A-scan.
- Intravenous fluorescein angiography: patchy early fluorescence and diffuse late staining of the choroidal mass, often with a double circulation pattern.
- Indocyanine green angiography: gradual hyperfluorescence over 20 minutes, but patterns can vary.
- Computed tomography: moderately dense, noncalcified intraocular mass.
- Magnetic resonance imaging: an intraocular mass that is hyperintense to vitreous on T1-weighted images, hypointense to vitreous on T2-weighted images, and moderate enhancement with gadolinium contrast.

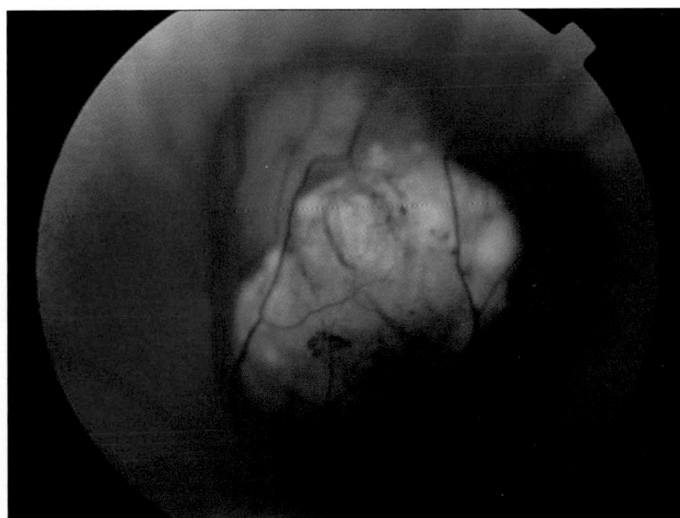

FIGURE 174.1. Typical 'collar-stud' melanoma. Note the amelanotic portion of the tumor that has breached Bruch's membrane.

- Microscopic histopathology: spindle or epithelioid cells according to the Callender classification.

Differential diagnosis

Common differential diagnoses include:
- Uveal neoplasms:
  - Nevus;
  - Metastasis;
  - Hemangioma;
  - Lymphoid tumor;
  - Osteoma.
- Retinal neoplasms:
  - Retinal astrocytic hamartoma;
  - Retinal capillary hemangioma;
  - Combined hamartoma retina and retinal pigment epithelium;
  - Vasoproliferative tumor of the fundus;
  - Retinoblastoma.
- Pigment epithelial neoplasms:
  - Pigment epithelial hypertrophy (CHRPE)/hyperplasia;
  - Pigment epithelial adenoma;
  - Medulloepithelioma.
- Non-neoplastic diseases:
  - Subretinal hemorrhage secondary to age-related macular/extramacular degeneration;
  - Retinal arterial macroaneurysm;
  - Choroidal hemorrhage/detachment;
  - Posterior scleritis;
  - Choroidal granuloma;
  - Retinal detachment.

TREATMENT

Systemic

A number of treatment options currently exist for metastatic melanoma, however, response rates are uniformly poor. Whilst patients with metastases to certain sites such as the skin may survive for several years, the majority of those with diffuse liver metastases die within 6 months. Owing to poor response rates intravenous therapy is often reserved for palliation of symptoms. Intrahepatic chemoembolization has been used for isolated liver metastases and similarly, focal metastases (in many organs) may be amenable to local surgical resection. Various groups have tried immunotherapy however a successful melanoma vaccine remains elusive.

Local

The aims of treatment of uveal melanoma are:
- To eradicate the tumor before metastasis occurs;
- Preserve the eye;
- Preserve vision.

The best form of treatment for any melanoma depends on many different variables including the size and apparent activity of the tumor, the health of the affected eye and it's fellow and the age and general health of the patient. What might be ideal for a 35 year old airline pilot might be wholly inappropriate for a 90 year old in residential care.

Observation

Periodic observation may be recommended to initially manage selected small melanomas that have dormant characteristics on ophthalmoscopic examination. Such a lesion should be carefully examined two or three times a year, and some form of active treatment should be instituted if growth of the tumor is subsequently documented.

The diagnostic tests and the frequency of follow-up examinations depend on the size and the apparent activity of the tumor. If a patient has a tumor that is classified as a suspicious nevus or dormant melanoma, then a repeat examination should be performed in 3 to 4 months, with fundus photography and ultrasonography for documentation. If no growth is detected, examination should be repeated every 4 to 6 months thereafter. If the lesion remains quiescent then these intervals may be increased. If however growth is documented, or the lesion shows increasing orange pigment, subretinal fluid or symptoms active treatment is advisable.

For those lesions that require treatment, the main therapeutic options consist of:

- Diode laser transpupillary thermotherapy;
- Brachytherapy (radioactive plaques);
- Charged particles (proton beam or Helium ion);
- Stereotactic radiosurgery;
- Local resection;
- Enucleation;
- Exenteration.

Transpupillary thermotherapy

Over the last decade transpupillary thermotherapy (TTT) has supplanted argon laser photocoagulation as the treatment for small uveal melanomas (<3.5mm in thickness) at the posterior pole. The technique utilizes an infrared diode laser to heat the tumour to a level that is cytotoxic without causing photocoagulation. Initial animal studies and subsequent clinical studies on enucleated eyes performed by Oosterhuis et al suggested that the technique could produce necrosis to a depth of 4 mm, ideal therefore for small melanomas. TTT is usually delivered via a slit-lamp-mounted diode laser and is performed under retrobulbar or sub-Tenons anesthesia. Laser is applied via a contact lens through a dilated pupil. Traditionally, a 3mm spot size has been used with a 1-minute application time per spot. Power levels vary from as little as 250 mW for deeply pigmented tumors to 1500 mW for amelanotic lesions. The aim of treatment is to produce a light gray burn at the end of the 1-minute application. A heavier burn results in photocoagulation which may impede the heating of the deeper portions of the tumor. Adjacent spots are applied to cover the entire surface of the tumor. The majority of melanomas require 3 (or more) treatments usually at 2 to 3 month intervals before ultimate regression to a (hopefully) flat chorioretinal scar.

Initial reports suggested excellent rates of local control as well as preservation of vision in patients treated with TTT. However as might be expected as follow-up continues, increasing numbers of local recurrences including cases of extraocular extension are now being reported. For this reason many authorities reserve TTT as an adjunct to plaque therapy (sandwich technique) rather than as a primary therapy.

Plaque radiotherapy

Plaque radiotherapy is the most widely used method in the management of melanoma of the choroid and ciliary body. Various isotopes have been used however the two main alternatives are ^{125}I (most popular in the USA) and ^{106}Ru (Europe). Each has its own advantages and disadvantages. Iodine is a potent gamma-emitter that may be used to treat tumors of essentially any size. Each plaque is tailor-made for the patient allowing unique flexibility. Half-life is short however at approximately 4 weeks. Ruthenium on the other hand is a low energy B-emitter with a half-life of 1 year, therefore Ruthenium plaques may be reused many times making them more economical. The main limitation of Ruthenium however is that it is only suitable for tumors up to 6mm in thickness. Regardless of the isotope used the majority of plaques are circular however notched plaques are available for the treatment of peripapillary lesions.

The current indications for treatment of a posterior uveal melanoma with an episcleral plaque are:

- Selected small melanomas that are documented to be growing;
- Most medium-sized and large choroidal and ciliary body melanomas that are less than 10 mm in thickness in an eye that has useful or salvageable vision; and
- Most medium-sized and large melanomas that occur in the patient's only useful eye, regardless of the visual acuity.

In the past extraocular extension of the melanoma has been considered a contraindication to plaque therapy, however small deposits can be easily covered by a plaque and respond as readily as the intraocular tumor.

Plaques may be inserted under general or local anesthesia. A peritomy is performed and the extraocular muscles are hooked with traction sutures to allow exposure of the tumor site. Extraocular muscles occasionally need to be disinserted to allow accurate placement of the plaque. Trans-scleral transillumination is performed to localize the tumor. The shadow of the tumor is outlined on the sclera with a sterile marking pencil, and a dummy plaque is used to align the scleral sutures. The dummy plaque is then removed, and the radioactive plaque is inserted and tied securely in position. The plaque is left in position long enough to deliver 80 to 100 Gy to the tumor apex, after which it is removed and the patient is discharged.

In general, brachytherapy offers excellent local control rates and preservation of the globe. Visual prognosis depends largely on the location of the tumor as some form of radiation retinopathy is inevitable.

Local resection

Theoretically, an ideal approach to the management of a melanoma of the ciliary body or choroid is to perform local resection to remove the tumor and salvage the eye, particularly if this can be achieved without worsening the patient's prognosis for life. In recent years, a technique of partial lamellar sclerouvectomy has been popular. This technique involves removing the tumor and inner sclera while leaving intact the retina and the outer sclera. A radioactive plaque may also be applied to the resection site for a brief period as a safeguard against local recurrence. The technique is lengthy and technically demanding requiring hypotensive anesthesia making case selection particularly important.

The relative indications for local resection of a posterior uveal melanoma are:

- A growing ciliary body melanoma or a ciliochoroidal melanoma that does not cover more than one third of the pars plicata; and
- A choroidal melanoma that is no greater than 15 mm in diameter, centered near the equator.

It should be stressed that melanomas that meet these criteria also can be managed with other conservative techniques such as radiotherapy in most instances. The preferred method of therapy is unresolved, and each case must be evaluated individually.

Proton beam

This technique utilizes protons produced by a cyclotron to kill the tumor. It is therefore limited to a handful of centers around the world. Tumors are localized with tantalum markers inserted in the operating theater. In theory, melanomas of any size may be treated with charged particles. Rates of local control and preservation of vision are similar to those with episcleral plaques however minor anterior segment complications are probably more frequent.

Stereotactic radiosurgery

This is a form of external radiotherapy delivered by means of a Leksell gamma knife. This unit consists of 201 individual cobalt sources that may be focused onto the tissue requiring treatment. It may therefore be used to treat inaccessible or complex lesions in the brain or for our purposes, the eye. The technique requires the application of a stereotactic frame to the skull and the use of MRI to localize the tumor with reference to the frame. Owing to the limited availability of the gamma knife unit, relatively few uveal melanoma patients have been treated with stereotactic radiosurgery.

Enucleation

Although a number of conservative therapeutic options now exist, enucleation remains a mainstay of treatment of uveal melanoma. There are definite indications for enucleation, although the indications for this procedure are fewer than they were in the past. Enucleation tends to be reserved for those melanomas that are too large to be managed with radiotherapy or local resection particularly if the vision has already been lost. Occasionally however patients request enucleation as they are unable to cope with the thought of a cancer in their eye and request that it be treated 'once and for all.'

The technique of enucleation for melanoma is no different than that for other conditions and a primary implant may almost always be inserted. The Collaborative Ocular Melanoma Study has shown that the use of pre-enucleation radiotherapy offers no survival advantage.

Orbital exenteration

Orbital exenteration is seldom necessary for uveal melanoma and is largely reserved for those with massive extraocular spread with no evidence of systemic metastases. With improved diagnostic techniques and earlier recognition of uveal melanomas, it has become uncommon for patients to present initially with extensive extraocular involvement.

COMPLICATIONS

There appears to be little or no danger in the close observation of small melanomas that show dormant features. Most of these tumors have little, if any, tendency to grow and a low potential to metastasize. Lesions located within 2 mm of the optic disk or foveola should be followed more frequently. If growth is documented, then plaque radiotherapy or transpupillary thermotherapy should be considered.

The complications of transpupillary thermotherapy appear to be fewer than those of photocoagulation and include retinal vascular obstruction, cystoid macular edema, preretinal membrane formation with retinal traction, choroidovitreal or retinal neovascularization, vitreous hemorrhage, and retinal detachment. Treatment with these methods is most often successful if the tumor is small, being less than 3 mm in thickness as measured by ultrasonography.

There are very early complications of episcleral plaque radiotherapy, including ocular irritation and diplopia. Diplopia can occur if a rectus muscle is disinserted to properly position the plaque. Later potential complications of episcleral plaque radiotherapy include radiation retinopathy, radiation papillopathy, neovascular glaucoma, vitreous hemorrhage, radiation cataract, keratoconjunctivitis sicca, radiation anterior uveitis, sclera necrosis, and persistent diplopia. Tumors treated with episcleral plaque radiotherapy may show a rather dramatic response to treatment however the majority show either stabilization or a gradual decrease in size during a follow-up period of 2 to 6 years. Depending on tumor location, visual results have been satisfactory, and complications relatively few.

The early complications of local tumor resection, however, are greater than those of plaque radiotherapy. The most important potential early surgical complications of local resection are hypotony, wound leak, vitreous bleeding, and retinal detachment. Potential late complications of local resection include vitreous fibrosis, cataract, and ischemic inflammation in the anterior segment. The vitreous fibrosis can lead to chronic traction on the retina and a delayed retinal detachment. In many cases, removal of a ciliochoroidal tumor necessitates removal of a large portion of the zonular support to the lens. This can lead to postoperative shifting of the lens, with inflammation, corneal edema, or glaucoma.

COMMENTS

The management of malignant melanoma of the posterior uvea is controversial. There is now little doubt that for comparable tumors the chances of survival are similar regardless of whether the eye is removed or another form of conservative therapy is used. Current management can range from periodic observation and fundus photography of selected small lesions that appear dormant to transpupillary thermotherapy, radiotherapy, or local resection for growing tumors in eyes with useful or salvageable vision. In cases in which the tumor is far advanced and there is no hope of useful vision, enucleation generally is advisable.

The choice of therapy is a complex issue, and each case must be considered individually. In selecting a therapeutic approach, certain factors must be carefully weighed; these include the size of the melanoma, its extent and location, its apparent activity, the status of the opposite eye, and the age, general health, and psychologic status of the patient.

Periodic observation can be cautiously used for selected small choroidal melanomas that have dormant characteristics. If such lesions are documented to grow or if they show substantial ophthalmoscopic risks for growth on the initial examination, then active treatment can be instituted. Transpupillary thermotherapy may be an option if the tumor is no more than 12 mm in diameter or 3.5 mm in thickness. For medium-sized or large tumors that are growing, the patient can be managed with either episcleral plaque radiotherapy or local resection of the tumor. Because radiotherapy has fewer immediate visual complications than local resection, more patients are managed with radiotherapy, most commonly in the form of a radioactive plaque.

Patients with large tumors that have produced severe visual loss are managed by enucleation. If there is significant extrascleral extension on initial examination or orbital recurrence after enucleation, orbital exenteration or one of its modifications may be advisable.

Patients who have known systemic metastases, either before or after enucleation or other treatment, have a poor prognosis. In such a case, local resection, palliative irradiation, chemotherapy, or immunotherapy may be used. The aim of the ocular oncologist at present is to reach an accurate diagnosis and achieve local control of the tumor prior to its dissemination. However an ultimate cure for this dreadful disease will require collaboration between ophthalmologists and researchers in the basic sciences, immunology and medical oncology.

REFERENCES

Cohen VM, Carter MJ, Kemeny A, et al: Metastasis-free survival following treatment for uveal melanoma with either stereotactic radiosurgery or enucleation. Acta Ophthalmol Scand 81:383–388, 2003.

Cree IA, Di Nicolantonio F, Neale MH: Chemotherapy of uveal melanoma. In: Jager MJ, Niederkorn JY, Ksander BR, eds: Uveal melanoma: a model for exploring fundamental cancer biology. London, Taylor & Francis, 2004.

Damato BE: Local resection of uveal melanoma. Bull Soc Belge Ophthalmol 248:11–17, 1993.

Gragoudas ES, Lane AM, Regan S, et al: A randomized controlled trial of varying radiation doses in the treatment of choroidal melanoma. Arch Ophthalmol 118:773–778, 2000.

Oosterhuis JA, Journee-De Korver HG, Kakebeeke-Kemme HM, et al: Transpupillary thermotherapy in choroidal melanomas. Arch Ophthalmol 113:315–321, 1995.

Shields CL, Shields JA, Kiratli H, et al: Risk factors for growth and metastasis of small choroidal melanocytic lesions. Ophthalmology 102:1351–1361, 1995.

Shields CL, Shields JA, Perez N, et al: Primary transpupillary thermotherapy for small choroidal melanoma in 256 consecutive cases: outcomes and limitations. Ophthalmology 109:225–234, 2002.

Singh AD, Rundle PA, Rennie IG: Uveal melanoma. In: Williams C, Chief ed: Evidence based oncology. London, BMJ, 2003.

175 SYMPATHETIC OPHTHALMIA
360.11
(Sympathetic Uveitis, Sympathetic Ophthalmitis)

F. Hampton Roy, MD, FACS
Little Rock, Arkansas

Sympathetic ophthalmia, is a rare, bilateral, granulomatous panuveitis that occurs a few days to many years after accidental penetrating ocular injury or ocular surgery. Both the injured, eye and the fellow, or 'sympathizing,' eye are affected. In nearly all cases, injury to and incarceration of uveal tissues are characteristic features in the exciting eye. It is potentially blinding and is the most feared of all ocular complications in ophthalmology.

ETIOLOGY/INCIDENCE

Most cases of sympathetic ophthalmia occur after penetrating ocular injuries (60%). The remainder occur after surgical procedures (30%) and perforated corneal ulcers (10%). Classically, inflammation develops as early as 4 to 8 weeks after the insult. The interval from trauma to onset of inflammation may be as short as 5 days or as long as 66 years. Most cases occur within 1 year after the injury (90%). Inflammation often is present in the injured eye at the time of the insult, but the uninjured eye develops sympathetic inflammation at a later date. Patients present with pain, photophobia, and decreased vision in the sympathizing eye. The inflammation is granulomatous with mutton-fat precipitates, iris nodules, anterior segment cell and flare, and Dalen–Fuchs nodules, representing aggregates of epithelioid cells at the level of Bruch's membrane. These Dalen–Fuchs nodules may be scattered throughout the fundus. Exudative retinal detachment, early optic disk edema, or late atrophy may be present. Occasionally, sympathetic ophthalmia may have systemic manifestations similar to those of Vogt–Koyanagi–Harada syndrome; these include cerebrospinal fluid pleocytosis; meningismus; skin manifestations such as alopecia, vitiligo, and poliosis; and dysacusis.

The cause of sympathetic ophthalmia is unknown. The common predisposing factor in the vast majority of cases is the presence of penetrating injury in which wound healing is complicated by incarceration of the iris, ciliary body or choroid. It is believed that a genetically predisposed host incites a cell-mediated immune response against some unknown uveal antigen or antigens. Experimental studies have shown that patients with sympathetic ophthalmia have lymphocytes that are sensitized to some component or components of uveal-retinal extracts. Retinal S-antigen, interphotoreceptor retinoid-binding protein, and retinal and choroidal melanocyte antigens have all been shown experimentally to produce uveitis similar to sympathetic ophthalmia in animal models. This immune response results in chronic granulomatous inflammation in both eyes.

The incidence of sympathetic ophthalmia is uncommon to rare, affecting 0.1% to 0.2% of patients with penetrating ocular injuries and 0.01% of patients who have undergone intraocular surgery. Sympathetic ophthalmia affects individuals of all ages. There is no race or gender predilection, although ocular trauma is much more common in men. Sympathetic ophthalmia can occur at any age, but cases tend to cluster in the first decade of life and in early adulthood, when trauma is more common, and in the sixth and seventh decades of life, when ocular surgical procedures become more common.

COURSE/PROGNOSIS

Untreated sympathetic ophthalmia runs a long, variable, and complicated course, with episodes of acute inflammation followed by long periods of quiescence lasting from several months to years. However, recurrent inflammation occurs in as many as 60% of patients with sympathetic ophthalmia. This chronic recurrent inflammation can lead to irreversible ocular damage and phthisis bulbi. With aggressive systemic corticosteroid or immunosuppressive therapy, or both, the prognosis improves, with more than 50% of eyes maintaining visual acuity of 20/60 or better.

DIAGNOSIS

Sympathetic ophthalmia is essentially a clinical diagnosis. Both the injured and sympathizing eyes demonstrate diffuse granulomatous inflammation of the uveal tract consisting of lymphocytes (predominantly T lymphocytes), epithelioid cells, and occasional giant cells. Pigment often is found within the epithelioid and giant cells. Nodular clusters of these epithelioid cells may be found between the retinal pigment epithelium and Bruch's membrane; these appear yellow-white clinically and are called Dalen–Fuchs nodules. In the majority of cases, the inflammation spares the choriocapillaris and retina. Necrosis of the inflamed tissues is characteristically absent.

Clinical signs and symptoms

- History of penetrating eye injury.
- Granulomatous panuveitis.
- Mutton-fat precipitates.
- Inflammatory iris nodules (Koeppe and Busacca).
- Vitritis.
- Dalen–Fuchs nodules in choroid (especially inferiorly).
- Creamy yellow-white lesions below the retinal pigment epithelium.
- Later may become punched-out chorioretinal lesions of one-fourth to one-half disk diameter.
- Exudative retinal detachments: shifting subretinal fluid.
- Early disk edema: late optic atrophy.

Laboratory findings

- Fluorescein angiography.
- Multiple pinpoint areas of choroidal hyperfluorescence in the posterior pole.
- Enlarge over time.
- Leak and coalesce late in subretinal fluid if there is exudative retinal detachment.
- Late disk leakage.
- Ophthalmic ultrasonography.
- Medium to high internal reflectivity thickening of choroid of posterior pole.
- Exudative retinal detachments with subretinal fluid.
- Laboratory testing.
- None.
- HLA: DR4/DQw3 associated but not helpful in diagnosis.

Differential diagnosis

- Vogt–Koyanagi–Harada syndrome.
- Phacoanaphylactic endophthalmitis.
- Infectious endophthalmitis.
- Multifocal choroiditis/panuveitis (idiopathic).
- Sarcoid panuveitis.

PROPHYLAXIS

Early enucleation of the severely injured eye with poor vision is the best way to prevent the onset of sympathetic ophthalmia. The decision to enucleate an eye that has been severely and irreversibly injured and has severe visual loss is an easy decision to make; however, in cases in which the eye has useful vision, has had minimal injury, and can be salvaged, most ophthalmologists do not advocate enucleation because of the extremely low incidence of sympathetic ophthalmia. It has been suggested by many that enucleation, if it is to be done, should be performed within 2 weeks of the injury. Once sympathetic ophthalmia begins, there does not appear to be a visual benefit to enucleation of the injured eye. In some cases, the exciting eye eventually provides better visual acuity, so enucleation could deprive the patient of visual potential.

TREATMENT

Aggressive systemic corticosteroid therapy is the cornerstone of the treatment of sympathetic ophthalmia.

Systemic

- Corticosteroids (mainstay of therapy for sympathetic ophthalmia).
- Prednisone 1 to 2.5 mg/kg/day with slow tapering over 6 months.
- Supplement with topical and periocular corticosteroids.
- Immunosuppressive therapy (if corticosteroids cannot be tolerated or fail).
- Cyclosporin A 5 mg/kg/day PO.
- Azathioprine 1 to 2.5 mg/kg/day PO.
- Methotrexate (low dose) 5 to 30 mg/week PO.
- Cyclophosphamide 1 to 2 mg/kg/day PO.

Local

Local therapy supplements systemic therapy.

- Topical therapy:
  - Prednisolone 1% (intensive; hourly, if necessary);
  - Mydriatics: cyclopentolate, homatropine, or atropine.
- Periocular therapy: corticosteroids.
  - Triamcinolone 40 mg. Repeat up to four times in first 4 to 8 weeks for severe inflammation. Supplements systemic therapy;
- Intravitreal steroid injection.

Surgical

- Enucleation of injured eye.
- Within 2 weeks after penetrating injury.
- If severely injured, unsalvageable eye with poor vision.
- May be helpful in the prevention of sympathetic ophthalmia.
- Enucleation of exciting eye after the onset of inflammation in the sympathizing eye probably not beneficial.

COMPLICATIONS

Complications are common. Cataracts can develop in 47% of patients, glaucoma in 43%, exudative retinal detachments in 25%, and severe chorioretinal scarring in 25%. Optic atrophy can also occur in late stages of the disease.

REFERENCES

Buller AJ, Doris JP, Bonshek R, et al: Sympathetic ophthalmia following severe fungal keratitis. Eye 12:261, 2006.

Chan CC: Relationship between sympathetic ophthalmia, phacoanaphylactic endophthalmitis, and Vogt-Koyanagi-Harada disease. Ophthalmology 95:619–624, 1988.

Chan CC, Roberge FG, Whitcup SM, Nussenblatt RB: 32 cases of sympathetic ophthalmia: a retrospective study at the National Eye Institute, Bethesda, Md, from 1982–1992. Arch Ophthalmol 113:597–600, 1995.

Chan RV, Seiff BD, Lincoff HA, et al: Rapid recovery of sympathetic ophthalmia with treatment augmented by intravitreal steroids. Retina 26:243–247, 2006.

Freidlin J, Pak J, Tessler, HH, et al: Sympathetic ophthalmia after injury in the Iraq war. Ophthal Plast Reconstr Surg 22:133–134, 2006

Jonas JB, Back W, Sauder G, et al: Sympathetic ophthalmia in vater association combined with persisting hyperplastic primary vitreous after cyclodestructive procedure. Eur J Ophthalmol 16:171–172, 2006.

Liddy BSL, Stuart J: Sympathetic ophthalmia in Canada. Can J Ophthalmol 7:757–759, 1972.

Lubin JR, Albert DM, Weinstein M: Sixty-five years of sympathetic ophthalmia: a clinicopathologic review of 105 cases (1913–1978). Ophthalmology 87:109–121, 1980.

Makley TA, Jr, Azar A: Sympathetic ophthalmia: a long-term follow-up. Arch Ophthalmol 96:257–262, 1978.

Rao NA, Robin J, Hartmann D, et al: The role of the penetrating wound in the development of sympathetic ophthalmia: Experimental observations. Arch Ophthalmol 101:102–104, 1983.

Rathinam SR, Rao NA: Sympathetic ophthalmia following postoperative bacterial endophthalmitis: a clinicopathologic study. Am J Ophthalmol 14:498–507, 2006

Reynard M, Riffenburgh RS, Maes EF: Effect of corticosteroid treatment and enucleation on the visual prognosis of sympathetic ophthalmia. Am J Ophthalmol 96:290–294, 1983.

SECTION

18 Conjunctiva

176 ALLERGIC CONJUNCTIVITIS
372.05
(Allergic Rhinoconjunctivitis, Hay Fever Conjunctivitis)

Russell Pokroy, MD
Rehovot, Israel

ETIOLOGY/INCIDENCE

This common conjunctivitis, caused by exposure of sensitive individuals to specific allergens, is recurrent: seasonal (spring and summer due to pollens) or perennial (house dust, animal dander). Airborne allergens presumably traverse the conjunctiva and cause cross-linking of mast cell-bound IgE antibody, resulting in mast cell degranulation, release of vasoactive mediators and allergic signs and symptoms.

COURSE/PROGNOSIS

Isolated conjunctivitis runs a milder course than cases with associated rhinitis or asthma. In children, seasonal allergic conjunctivitis often improves with age.

DIAGNOSIS

Clinical signs and symptoms

By far the most important symptom is itching: 'no itch, no allergy.' Erythema (pale pink), chemosis (milky edema), discharge (watery or mucoid) and swollen periorbita are common. The tarsal conjunctiva has milky papillary hypertrophy because of the conjunctival edema obscuring the blood vessels. The cornea is seldom involved (Figure 176.1).

Laboratory findings

Usually, the signs and symptoms are characteristic enough to make the diagnosis without laboratory tests. The conjunctival allergen challenge, which has proved useful in clinical trials, is more sensitive than skin challenge tests. Tear eosinophils, IgE and tryptase may be elevated.

TREATMENT

Although avoidance of the offending allergen is the most effective treatment, this is often impractical. Concurrent blepharitis and dry eye should be treated. Rhinitis may require nasopharyngeal referral. Topical treatment is usually adequate, a graded approach according to the severity and response is recommended as follows:

- Artificial tears (preferably nonpreserved);
- Cool compresses;
- Vasoconstrictors (chronic use should be avoided because of rebound hyperemia);
- Antihistamines (H1 receptor antagonists);
- Mast cell stabilizers;
- Nonsteroidal antiinflammatories;
- Steroids (fluorometholone is safer than prednisolone);
- Systemic antihistamines.

COMMENTS

Although allergic conjunctivitis is common, it is usually benign without ocular sequelae. Topical treatment is effective and should be used prudently to avoid side effects.

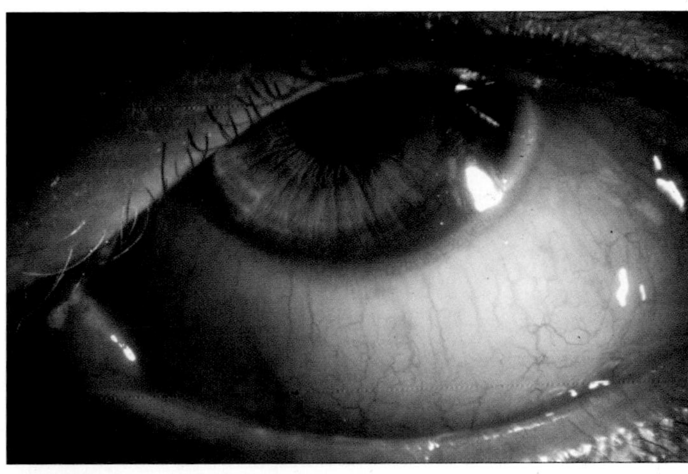

FIGURE 176.1. Allergic conjunctivitis.

REFERENCES

Abelson MB, Schaefer K: Conjunctivitis of allergic origin: immunologic mechanisms and current approaches to therapy. Surv Ophthalmol 38(suppl):115–126, 1993.

Friedlaender MH: Conjunctival provocation testing: overview of recent clinical trials in ocular allergy. Int Ophthalmol Clin 49:95–104, 2003.

Friedlaender MH, Ohashi Y, Kelley J: Diagnosis of allergic conjunctivitis. Arch Ophthalmol 102:1198, 1984.

Greiner JV, Mundorf T, Dubiner H, et al: Efficacy and safety of ketotifen fumarate 0.025% in the conjunctival antigen challenge model of ocular allergic conjunctivitis. Am J Ophthalmol 136:1097–1105, 2003.

177 BACTERIAL CONJUNCTIVITIS
372.05
(Infective Conjunctivitis, Mucopurulent Conjunctivitis, Purulent Conjunctivitis)

Aziz Sheikh, BSc, MBBS, MSc, MRCP, MRCGP, DCh, DRCOG, DFFP
Edinburgh, Scotland
Brian Hurwitz, MD, FRCP, FRCGP
London, England

ETIOLOGY/INCIDENCE

Community acquired bacterial infections of the conjunctiva are relatively common, generating an incident consultation rate in primary care of about 2% of all consultations per annum. These infections are more common in children and occasionally are seen in the elderly, but are relatively rare in younger and middle-aged adults; they affect both genders and all ethnic groups.

Most cases of infective conjunctivitis are caused by bacteria. The infective process is usually acute, but occasionally, a low-grade chronic infection may occur. This chapter concentrates on infection by bacteria other than *Chlamydia trachomatis*.

The most common mode of transmission is hand-to-eye spread of bacteria from the nasopharynx. For children, important risk factors include close contact with other children, superinfection after viral conjunctivitis, and bouts of otitis media, sinusitis and pharyngitis. In adults, chronic blepharitis, contact lens use, tear deficiency and lacrimal obstructions are important additional etiological and predisposing factors.

A number of different bacteria can infect the conjunctiva, the most important being *Streptococcus pneumoniae, Staphylococcal aureus* and *Hemophilus influenza*. Differentiating between these is not possible clinically. The only certain way to implicate a particular agent is to isolate it from swab material in the laboratory. There is considerable variation in causative organisms with the age of the patient, the locality and the season. Causative organisms include:

- Pathogenic gram-positive cocci, principally *Staphylococcus aureus, Streptococcus pneumoniae* and *Streptococcus pyogenes*.
- Aerobic gram-negative bacilli such as *Pseudomonas aeruginosa, Moraxella catarrhalis* and, particularly in children, *Hemophilus influenzae* and *Hemophilus parainfluenzae*.
- Overgrowth of normal skin flora, most commonly coagulase-negative staphylococci, and corynebacteria.
- Many enteric gram-negative bacilli.
- Genital infections that are transmitted to the eyes by hand or passed on to infants during birth, classically *Neisseria gonorrhoeae* and *Chlamydia trachomatis*.

COURSE/PROGNOSIS

Bacterial conjunctivitis is usually a mild affliction. Infection, which in only a minority of cases results in a mucopurulent discharge, typically begins in one eye, with the second eye becoming involved 2 or 3 days later. Infection is usually mild and resolves spontaneously in around 65% of cases within 2–5 days. Topical antibiotics do however significantly improve rates of clinical and microbiological remission (Figure 177.1).

A few organisms, particularly *N. gonorrhoeae*, can induce a profuse, purulent discharge with severe chemosis of the lids. Preauricular adenopathy is often present. The initial symptoms are similar to those of mucopurulent conjunctivitis but then rapidly worsen. Although very uncommon, prolonged exposure of the cornea to exudate containing hydrolytic enzymes can result in abscess formation and corneal perforation. Prompt diagnosis and therapy are essential in these cases.

DIAGNOSIS

Clinical signs and symptoms

Only about a half of patients presenting with conjunctivitis in primary care can be expected to have a demonstrable bacterial etiology. Patients with bacterial conjunctivitis typically present with rather non-specific features: redness, tearing, itching, periorbital edema and discharge; vision is generally normal.

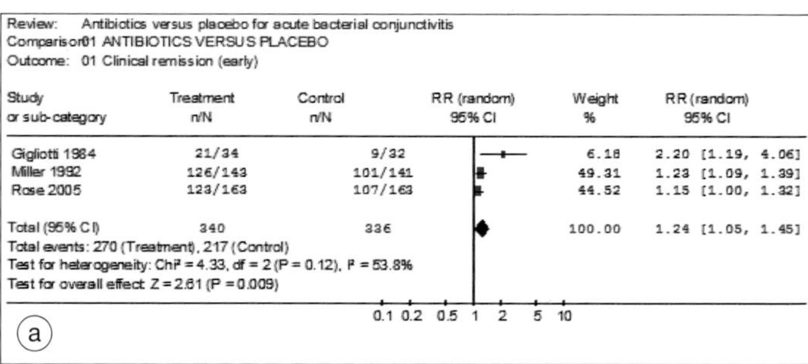

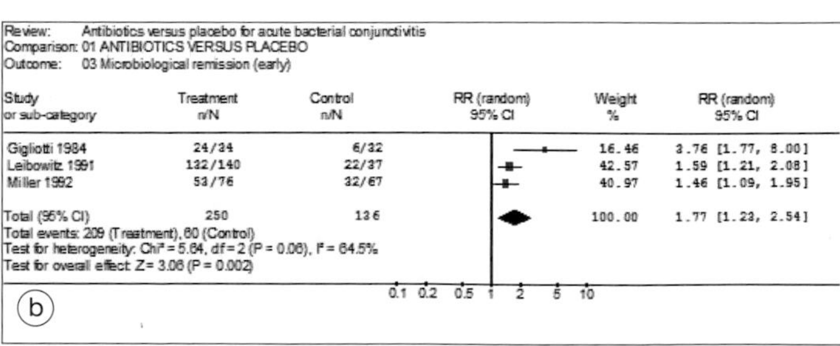

FIGURE 177.1. a) Random effects meta-analysis of efficacy of topical antibiotics vs. placebo in improving early (days 2–5) clinical remission (n = number of subjects in remission; N = number of subjects tested; CI = confidence intervals; RR = relative risk). b) Early microbiological remission. For abbreviations see above. (Reproduced with kind permission of British Journal of General Practice from: Sheikh A, Hurwitz B: Topical antibiotics for acute conjunctivitis: Cochrane systematic review and meta analysis update. Br J Gen Pract 5(521):962–964, 2005.)

Differentiating between bacterial and non-bacterial etiologies is however helped by asking three simple clinical questions:

- The number of glued eyes in the morning (0, 1 or 2)?
- Itchy eyes?
- History of conjunctivitis (i.e. has the patient suffered prior 'eye infections' with comparable symptoms)?

A positive response to the first question and negative responses to the second and third questions significantly increase the likelihood of identifying the presence of bacterial involvement.

Laboratory fndings

Patients to investigate

The following groups of patients should be investigated with swabs:

- Those with severe fulminating conjunctivitis;
- Patients not responding to initial therapy;
- All neonates with conjunctivitis.

Any patient with purulent conjunctivitis failing to respond to initial antibiotics should have medication withdrawn for 24 hours after which material should be collected for culture. Specific chemotherapy can then be initiated based on swab results.

Specimen collection

Pus is collected on a moist swab and sent to the laboratory. If plating out in the clinic, a swab or Kimura spatula is used to transfer material to a blood agar plate, a chocolate agar plate and a slide for a Gram's stain. One swab or scrape per medium is preferred. If local anesthesia is necessary in order to take a swab, preservative-free drops are recommended. Most laboratories will choose to incubate the blood agar plate under anaerobic conditions. Although obligate anaerobes are rarely cultured from the conjunctiva, the use of both an aerobic and an anaerobic plate can speed up the identification of isolates.

Culture interpretation

An obvious pathogen is isolated from around 30% of community conjunctival specimens. On other occasions, the cultures are negative or there is light growth of mixed skin flora only. In these cases, there is no specific indication for antibiotic treatment. In some instances, polymorphonuclear cells are seen in the Gram's stain, and there is a heavy growth of an organism of relatively low pathogenicity, such as one of the coagulase-negative staphylococci or viridans streptococci. Here, the isolate should be identified to at least genus level and reported to the clinician. Antibiotic treatment is then considered on a case-by-case basis.

Antimicrobial susceptibility testing

The need to test the susceptibility of an isolate depends on the proposed treatment and the likelihood of resistance for that species. Rates of resistance can vary markedly from community to community. Often, the pattern of antibiotic susceptibility of an isolate will depend on whether the infection was acquired in a hospital. Some laboratories do not routinely test conjunctival pathogens, and a specific request will have to be made in problem cases. Because high concentrations of antibiotics in the conjunctivae are achieved with topical treatment and susceptibility assays are traditionally based on levels attainable with systemic treatment, some laboratories are moving to increase the concentration at which conjunctival isolates are classified as resistant. This has particular relevance in automated, broth-dilution systems but is not yet accepted widely as an improvement over the traditional method.

Differential diagnosis

The main differential factors that need to be considered are:

- Conjunctivitis caused by *Chlamydia* or viruses such as herpes simplex, varicella zoster, adenovirus, or enterovirus;
- Allergic or toxic conjunctivitis, i.e. in response to local irritants such as chemicals or dust. Occupational history may be a helpful guide to the cause;
- Conjunctivitis associated with erythema multiforme or Reiter's syndrome;
- Obstruction of the lacrimal drainage system with a mucocele of the lacrimal sac;
- Malignancies such as sebaceous gland carcinoma and lacrimal gland tumors;
- Parinaud's oculoglandular syndrome, a unilateral chronic granulomatous conjunctivitis with regional adenopathy; most cases caused by *Bartonella henselae.*

TREATMENT

The management of bacterial conjunctivitis involves recognition of the disease at a clinical level, identification of the etiologic agent, appreciation of the importance of the case from a public health point of view, and considering the role of antimicrobial agents in the context of understanding that most cases will resolve spontaneously. A satisfactory antibiotic is one that is active against expected pathogens, has low local and systemic toxicity, and is nonallergenic.

Systemic

Systemic and local treatment is given for gonococcal conjunctivitis. Systemic treatment should be considered for children with *H. influenzae* type b (Hib) infection in whom the instillation of eyedrops is difficult. Hib is now less frequent due to the success of the immunization program.

- For gonococcal conjunctivitis, a single intramuscular injection of ceftriaxone is effective. The dose ranges from 125 mg in neonates to 250 mg in adults. The eye should be lavaged to remove pus.
- For Hib conjunctivitis, oral amoxicillin is recommended; the dosage for children less than 20 kg is 20 mg/kg/day every 8 hours. The dose for heavier children and adults is 250 mg every 8 hours. Continue the treatment for 2 to 3 days after symptoms have disappeared. If the strain is resistant to amoxicillin, a third-generation cephalosporin should be considered.

Local

Broad spectrum topical antibiotic therapy in specialist care patient settings results in significantly higher early (days 2 to 5) clinical remission rates, and in better early and late (days 6 to 10) microbiological remission rates. Most cases respond to a low dose of any broad-spectrum antibiotic applied locally. These agents are often used before laboratory results are known or, in most cases, without collection of material for microbiologic assessment. Ointments are useful with children or for overnight use in adults. Treatment should be given every 2 hours for 2 or 3 days until the process is controlled and then 4 times daily for another week.

Adverse effects from topically applied agents are uncommon; however, the prolonged use of bacitracin or polymyxin B may be toxic at the site of delivery, neomycin can induce hypersensitivity that typically presents as a periocular contact dermatitis. Chloramphenicol drops have been implicated in fatal aplastic anemia, although the risk is very low being estimated to be 1 in 220,000 prescriptions.

- Broad-spectrum single agents: chloramphenicol solution or ointment, fucidic acid, sulfacetamide solution or ointment, ciprofloxacin, norfloxacin, or ofloxacin solution.
- Broad-spectrum combinations: bacitracin-polymyxin B ointment, neomycin-polymyxin B-bacitracin ointment, neomycin-polymyxin B-gramicidin solution, or polymyxin B-trimethoprim solution. In cases of suspected infective conjunctivitis there is no place for antibiotic and steroid combination treatment.
- For most gram-positive infections: bacitracin ointment.
- For most gram-negative infections: gentamicin or tobramycin solution or ointment.
- For *Neisseria* or serious streptococcal infections, 100,000 units/ml penicillin G drops may be given; if the isolate is resistant or if the patient is allergic to penicillin, chloramphenicol 0.5% drops can be substituted.

PRECAUTIONS

A patient with purulent conjunctivitis may fail to respond to topical medication for a number of reasons. The disease may be due to an intracellular bacterial infection such as *C. trachomatis* or to one of the noninfective processes listed. If the condition is due to bacterial infection, the agent may be not be susceptible to the drug administered. Alternatively, the conjunctival sac may be full of organisms from the lacrimal sac or other nonocular sites under various circumstances. A persistent, uniocular, purulent discharge should alert the ophthalmologist to the possibility of a foreign body. Another reason for treatment failure is poor patient compliance with medication.

COMMENTS

The majority of cases are mild and will resolve spontaneously relatively quickly. Two broad approaches to management can be followed in primary care. A broad-spectrum antibiotic may be prescribed on the suspicion of bacterial infection for either immediate or 'delayed' use (i.e. in cases which do not spontaneously resolve within 3 days of onset) with laboratory investigations reserved for refractory cases (i.e. those with poor or no response to treatment), in which case treatment should ideally be discontinued for 24 hours before the swab is taken. Alternatively, more specific chemotherapy can be prescribed, based on the bacteria isolated if cultures are initiated as a first step. In favor of broad-spectrum therapy is the excellent response achieved in most patients with simple treatment. Against this approach are: the difficulty of distinguishing bacterial from non-bacterial etiologies at the clinical level, the fact that not all bacteria will respond to simple broad-spectrum therapy, and that when a patient has not responded to a trial of chemotherapy, the chance of achieving a microbiologic diagnosis may have been lost.

In most situations, broad-spectrum antibiotics are used based on a clinical diagnosis of bacterial conjunctivitis. Severe purulent conjunctivitis, however, requires initial laboratory investigation.

REFERENCES

Coster, DJ, Badenoch, PR: Bacterial conjunctivitis. In: Fraunfelder FT, Roy FH (eds): Current Ocular Therapy, 5th edn. Philadelphia, WB Saunders, 2000:323–325.

Donahue SP, Khoury JM, Kowalski RP: Common ocular infections: a prescriber's guide. Drugs 52:526–540, 1996.

Hwang DG: Bacterial conjunctivitis. In: Pepose JS, Holland GN, Wilhelmus KR, eds: Ocular infection and immunity. St Louis, Mosby, 1996: 99–817.

Laga M, Naamara W, Brunham RC, et al: Single-dose therapy of gonococcal ophthalmia neonatorum with ceftriaxone. N Engl J Med 315:1382–1385, 1986.

Lancaster T, Swart AM, Jick H: Risk of serious haematological toxicity with use of chloramphenicol eye drops in a British general practice database. BMJ 316:667, 1998.

Rietveld RP, van Weert HC, ter Riet G, Bindels PJ: Diagnostic impact of signs and symptoms in acute infectious conjunctivitis: systematic literature search. BMJ 327:789, 2003.

Rietveld RP, ter Riet G, Bindels PJ, Sloos JH, van Weert HC: Predicting bacterial cause in infectious conjunctivitis: cohort study on informativeness of combinations of signs and symptoms. BMJ 329:206–210, 2004.

Sheikh A, Hurwitz B: Topical antibiotics for acute bacterial conjunctivitis: Cochrane systematic review and meta-analysis update. Br J Gen Pract 55:962–964, 2005.

178 CONJUNCTIVAL MELANOTIC LESIONS 224.3

(Conjunctival Nevus, Conjunctival Junctional Nevus, Subepithelial Nevus, Compound Nevus, Blue Nevus, Melanosis Oculi, Conjunctival Melanosis, Epithelial Melanosis, Racial Melanosis, Subepithelial Melanocytosis, Congenital Melanocytosis, Primary Acquired Melanosis, Malignant Melanoma, Conjunctival Melanoma, Conjunctival Malignant Melanoma)

Manolette R. Roque, MD
Manila, Philippines
Barbara L. Roque, MD
Manila, Philippines

ETIOLOGY/INCIDENCE

Conjunctival melanotic lesions may be due to melanocytic or nonmelanocytic lesions. Conjunctival melanocytic lesions are secondary to disorders of melanocyte proliferation or of melanin production, may be primary or secondary, congenital or acquired, and benign or malignant, with unknown causes.

Suggested etiologic factors include light exposure, hormonal changes, racial pigmentation, and secondary pigment deposition.

Conjunctival malignant melanoma may begin from any of the following causes in decreasing order of frequency: primary acquired melanosis (PAM), pre-existing nevi, as *de novo* lesions, or occasionally, from a combination of any of the above.

Shields reported that tumors of the conjunctiva are melanocytic in origin in 53% of cases (52% benign nevi and ocular melanosis, 21% PAM, 25% malignant melanomas). The annual incidence in a Western population ranges from 0.02 to 0.05 cases per 100,000 population. These tumors are far more common in Caucasian patients, without any sex predilection.

COURSE/PROGNOSIS

The overall prognosis for epithelial melanosis, subepithelial melanocytosis and conjunctival nevi is good. The color of conjunctival nevi becomes either lighter or darker in 13% of cases, but it remains stable in 87%. Change in tumor size is seen in a small percentage of cases. Malignant transformation from compound and blue nevi is rare.

PAM can recur after surgical excision, and new lesions may develop elsewhere on the conjunctiva. Other than cosmetically, PAM is inconsequential without atypia. Biopsied elevated lesions usually have atypia. PAM is unlikely to progress to atypia if lesions have been stable for more than 10 years. 25% of cases are bilateral and 75% of cases of PAM have atypia. There is a 75% to 90% chance of malignant transformation to melanoma if atypia is present with a mean time frame of 2.5 years.

Conjunctival melanoma has an aggressive behavior characterized by a high tendency to develop recurrences and metastases. The prognosis is worse if it arises from PAM, is multifocal, involves the caruncle, fornix or palpebral conjunctiva, was incompletely excised initially and cryotherapy was not performed. Lesions of 1.5 mm or less in thickness do better and rarely metastasize while lesions beyond 2 mm in thickness are more likely to metastasize. Spread occurs through the lymphatic system, so regional nodes often are involved first. Local tumor recurrence, estimated to be 26% at 5 years, 51% at 10 years, and 65% at 15 years, may be the major risk factor for distant metastasis, which occurs in 16% at 5 years, 26% at 10 years, and 32% at 15 years. The 10-year survival rate is 70% to 80% and death from metastases may occur 25 years later.

DIAGNOSIS

Eliciting a good history regarding the growth characteristic of a lesion is very important. The keen patient would sometimes volunteer awareness of subtle changes in pigmented lesions. It is preferable that the diagnosis be made on examination and excisional biopsy results (Table 178.1).

Clinical signs and symptoms

Epithelial melanosis typically is bilateral flat patches of pigment scattered in the conjunctival epithelium, freely mobile over the globe, seen most commonly in the interpalpebral and perilimbal areas, fading near the fornices.

Conjunctival nevi are common benign lesions that are most often located (75%) at the nasal or temporal limbus, and rarely in the fornix, tarsus or cornea. About 65% are brown in color; the rest are tan or non-pigmented.

PAM consists of unilateral, multiple, flat, yellow to dark brown indistinct areas with irregular margins. It is usually freely mobile and may involve any part of the conjunctiva.

Conjunctival melanomas tend to be nodular and may invade the globe or extend posteriorly into the orbit. It may be pedunculated and multicentric. It is variably pigmented, and heavily vascularized. The bulbar conjunctiva and limbus are the most commonly involved sites.

Laboratory findings

Histopathology

Epithelial melanosis shows an increased deposition of melanin granules in the basal layer of the conjunctival epithelium.

Subepithelial melanocytosis reveals focal proliferation of subepithelial melanocytes that are more elongated and fusiform

TABLE 178.1 – **Classification of pigmented conjunctival lesions**

Type	Histology	Clinical Characteristics
Junctional nevus	Benign with more prominent branching process	Brown; clinically indistinguishable except in depth; moves with conjunctiva
Subepithelial nevus	Same	Same
Compound nevus	Same	Same
Blue nevus	Very cellular; increased malignant potential	Blue-gray; does not move with conjunctiva
Melanosis oculi *(Oculodermal melanosis, Nevus of Ota)*	Deep granules of melanin	Blue-gray; does not move with conjunctiva; rarely develops to malignant melanoma
Primary acquired melanosis	+/– melanocytic activity	Brown, speckled, flat; Nodularity suggests miotic activity 25% bilateral
Melanoma	Malignant changes	Slate-gray or black; usually elevated and vascular

(Modified from Fraunfelder FT: Conjunctival melanotic lesions. In: Fraunfelder FT, Roy FH, eds: Current ocular therapy. 5th edn. Philadelphia, WB Saunders 2000, 327–328.)

with more prominent branching processes than melanocytes found in nevi.

Conjunctival nevus shows spindle-shaped or multipolar dendritic cells full of fine melanin granules (nevus cells), the location of which determines if it is junctional, subepithelial, or compound.

PAM lesions without atypia may exhibit increased melanin production with or without melanocytosis usually restricted to the basilar regions of the conjunctival epithelium, absent nuclear hyperchromasia, and nonprominent nucleoli. PAM with atypia has five different patterns which include small polyhedral cells, spindle cells, large dendritiform melanocytes, epithelioid cells, or polymorphous (mixture). The degree of atypia increases with the size of the nucleus and nucleoli prominence. Lesions primarily composed of epithelioid cells or exhibiting pagetoid spread have the highest rate of malignant transformation. Immunohistostaining techniques with MIB-1 and PC-10 may help differentiate between PAM with or without atypia.

Conjunctival melanoma shows four different cell types: small polyhedral cells, spindle cells (lowest metastatic potential), balloon cells and round epithelioid cells.

Differential diagnosis

Secondary melanocytic lesions and nonmelanocytic pigmentary lesions of the conjunctiva; Addison's disease and pregnancy (hormone changes); drug toxicity (epinephrine, silver, phenothiazines); congenital blue sclera; iris, ciliary body, choroidal melanoma; conjunctival squamous cell carcinoma; conjunctival mycosis; conjunctival seborrheic keratosis; foreign body; conjunctival pseudomelanoma — iatrogenic; secondary to scleral tunnel.

TREATMENT

Ocular

The treatment for epithelial melanosis, subepithelial melanocytosis, and conjunctival nevi is repeated annual examinations which include photography of the lesion, applanation tonometry, and gonioscopy.

Medical

Glaucoma management may be needed in 10% of subepithelial melanocytosis.

Surgical

Complete excision, with tumor-free margins, of PAM with atypia should be the goal of treatment. Cryotherapy, radiotherapy, topical mitomycin C, or CO_2 laser are useful adjunctive therapies.

The treatment of conjunctival melanoma is surgical, with complete removal of the tumor. The Shields 'no touch' technique in the surgical management of circumscribed conjunctival melanomas is followed. No surgical instrument is used more than once in any area (addressing the concern of microscopically seeding tumor cells).

Treatment of primary conjunctival melanomas in the limbal region of the bulbar conjunctiva is with initial localized absolute alcohol epitheliectomy, followed with wide (2–3 mm clear zone) local excision by a partial lamellar scleroconjunctivectomy. The excision bed and adjacent conjunctiva or cornea away from the nodule, is treated with supplemental double freeze-thaw cryotherapy by a specific technique (lifting the conjunctiva).

If the tumors are located in the fornical or palpebral conjunctiva, wide surgical resection with alcohol treatment to the scleral base and cryotherapy to the surrounding conjunctiva is performed.

Exenteration of the orbit sometimes is necessary for large melanomas that have invaded the orbit and in patients in whom the objective is to do local debulking of a tumor, because this procedure does not improve the prognosis. The use of radical neck dissection at the period of exenteration may be useful.

COMPLICATIONS

Excessive freezing may result in synechiae.

COMMENTS

The poor survival rate, despite orbital exenteration, indicates that there is metastasis at the time of treatment and confirms that the stage of the disease at diagnosis is the most significant prognosticating factor. Extensive orbital involvement shows the need for exenteration. Subtotal exenteration can be performed if no evidence of radial extension of the lesion to the skin of the anterior lid exists. Nodal involvement suggests extensive metastatic disease, however, occasionally, cases in which lesions were limited to regional nodes and cured by node resection have occurred.

SUPPORT GROUPS

http://www.melanomasupport.org

REFERENCES

Baum TD, Adamis AP, Jakobiec FA: Primary acquired melanosis of the conjunctiva. In: Jakobiec FA, Colby KA, Gragoudas ES, eds: International ophthalmology clinics: recent advances in ocular oncology. Philadelphia, Lippincott-Raven, 1997:37:61–72.

Buckman G, Jakobiec FA, Folberg R, McNally LM: Melanocytic nevi of the palpebral conjunctiva. Ophthalmology 95:1053–1057, 1988.

Dutton JJ, Anderson RL, Tse DT: Combined surgery and cryotherapy for scleral invasion of epithelial malignancies. Ophthalmic Surg 15:289–294, 1984.

Finger PT, Czechonska G, Liarikos S: Topical mitomycin C chemotherapy for conjunctival melanoma and PAM with atypia. Br J Ophthalmol 82:476–479, 1998.

Frucht-Pery J, Pe'er J: Use of mitomycin C in the treatment of conjunctival primary acquired melanosis with atypia. Arch Ophthalmol 114:1261–1264, 1996.

Helm CJ: Melanoma and other pigmented lesions of the ocular surface. In: Focal points, clinical modules for ophthalmologists. San Francisco, American Academy of Ophthalmology, 1996:XIV(11):1–14.

Jakobiec FA, Folbert R, Iwamoto T: Clinicopathologic characteristics of premalignant and malignant melanocytic lesions of the conjunctiva. Ophthalmology 96:147–166, 1989.

Jakobiec FA, Rini FJ, Fraunfelder FT, et al: Cryotherapy for conjunctival primary acquired melanosis and malignant melanoma: experience with 62 cases. Ophthalmology 95:1058–1070, 1988.

Kurli M, Finger PT: Melanocytic conjunctival tumors. Ophthalmol Clin North Am 18(1):15–24, 2005.

Roque MR, Roque BL, Foster CS: Conjunctival melanoma. Emedicine 2005. Online. Available at: http://www.emedicine.com/oph/topic110.htm. Mar 17, 2005.

Shields CL, Shields JA: Tumors of the caruncle. In: Shields JA, ed: International ophthalmology clinics: Update on malignant ocular tumors. Boston, Little, Brown, 1993:33, III:31–36.

Shields CL, Demirci H, Karatza E, Shields JA: Clinical survey of 1643 melanocytic and nonmelanocytic conjunctival tumors. Ophthalmology 111(9):1747–1754, 2004.

179 CORNEAL AND CONJUNCTIVAL CALCIFICATIONS 371.43

F. Hampton Roy, MD, FACS
Little Rock, Arkansas

ETIOLOGY/INCIDENCE

Corneal and conjunctival calcifications may occur as isolated conditions or in association with a variety of disease entities. The corneal involvement is described as calcific band keratopathy because of the band-like distribution of the deposits across the interpalpebral zone. Clinically, calcific band keratopathy appears as a superficial corneal opacity resembling frosted or ground glass, with 'white flecks' and 'clear spots' interspersed within the band, giving it a 'Swiss cheese' appearance. The opacity is covered by clear epithelium and usually is localized to the area of exposed cornea in the interpalpebral fissure. The band is concentric with the limbus but is separated from it by a clear layer. Unlike calcific band keratopathy, calcareous degeneration usually spares the basement and Bowman's membranes and is characterized by clumps of calcium salts in the superficial and deep stroma. Conjunctival calcification appears as small, hard, white, or yellow elevated concretions in the palpebral conjunctiva.

Although the exact cause of calcific band keratopathy is not known, a combination of factors is thought to be responsible. Band keratopathy is the probably the result of precipitation of calcium salts on the corneal surface (directly under the epithelium). Serum and normal body fluids (e.g. tears, aqueous humor) contain calcium and phosphate in concentrations that approach their solubility product. Evaporation of tears tends to concentrate solutes and to increase the tonicity of tears; it is especially true in the intrapalpebral area where the greatest exposure of the corneal surface to ambient air occurs. Elevated serum calcium and phosphorus concentrations may also result in tissue deposition of calcium phosphate salts. Histologically, calcium salts are deposited in the extracellular space when the condition is secondary to local ocular disease and in the intracellular space when the condition is secondary to systemic alterations of calcium metabolism. The epithelial basement membrane, Bowman's layer and superficial stroma are involved.

Band keratopathy is associated with local ocular and systemic disease.

Chronic uveitis of any cause and ocular trauma, along with its accompanying chronic inflammation, are the most common ocular causes of band keratopathy. Systemic disease with altered calcium metabolism, such as hyperparathyroidism, vitamin D toxicity, and uremia, also are commonly associated with calcific band keratopathy. Calcific band keratopathy also has been described in persons treated with or exposed to organomercurials, such as phenylmercuric nitrate or thimerosal, and to intraocular silicone oil. Band keratopathy has been reported after the use of Viscoat (hyaluronate sodium and chondroitin sulfate sodium) during routine cataract extraction. Inborn errors of metabolism, such as hyperphosphatemia and hypophosphatemia, may also predispose patients to develop corneal and conjunctival calcification. Calcified deposits may occur within the palpebral conjunctiva; these generally represent chronic degenerative changes and often are observed in patients with chronic blepharitis or other external eye disease. Band keratopathy associated with hyperuricemia can occur and is differentiated based on historical data, the golden-brown color on examination and elevated uric acid levels.

The causes of calcific band keratopathy can be divided into five categories:

1. Chronic keratitis or uveitis (the most common causes);
2. Degenerative calcium deposition associated with chronic damage from mercurial preservatives in many ophthalmic preparations (e.g. phenylmercuric nitrate or thimerosal);
3. Hypercalcemia secondary to milk alkali syndrome, vitamin D toxicity, sarcoidosis, hyperparathyroidism, lytic lesions affecting the bones, and other systemic diseases;
4. Chronic renal failure, uremia, or other conditions that may cause a rise in serum phosphorus levels;
5. Heredity.

Calcareous degeneration occurs in severely diseased eyes with exposed stroma and vascular compromise or in eyes undergoing multiple operations. It also has been reported in a failed corneal graft. Conjunctival concretions are usually products of cellular degeneration, but they also may be associated with any chronic conjunctival inflammation.

COURSE/PROGNOSIS

As calcification progresses, fragmentation and even destruction of Bowman's membrane may ensue. Early in its course, before the calcific band approaches the pupillary area, there is no immediate effect on visual acuity. With progression, however, plaques composed of coalesced calcium replace the subepithelial layers of the cornea, resulting in epithelial erosions, accompanied by marked irritation and pain. Eventual involvement of the central cornea and pupillary axis results in decreased visual acuity. A limbus pannus may also develop. Calcareous degeneration can occur rapidly, especially with anterior segment ischemia. Conjunctival concretions may be accompanied by hyperemia and symptoms of irritation.

DIAGNOSIS

Patients should be questioned concerning excessive vitamin D ingestion. Although corneal and conjunctival calcification may be reversible with discontinuation of the vitamin, nephrocalcinosis may still develop. A general medical workup is advisable. Laboratory tests may include renal function test; serum calcium, phosphorus, uric acid, parathyroid hormone, and angiotensin-converting enzyme levels; and a search for lytic lesions affecting the bones.

TREATMENT

Surgical

Treatment of band keratopathy is indicated in patients with symptomatic irritation or decreased vision. The success of therapy in restoring vision may be limited if the underlying disease process has produced decreased acuity. In addition, unless the underlying disease process is controlled, calcium deposition may recur after therapy. In this situation, the treatment may need to be repeated. The surgical goal is to remove the opaque calcium deposits without producing stromal scarring. The initial approach is to attempt chelation of the calcium salt deposits with edetate disodium (EDTA).

A topical anesthetic agent instilled into the conjunctival cul-de-sac is sufficient to achieve intraoperative anesthesia; however, due to the frequent incidence of severe postoperative discomfort, many surgeons elect to use supplemental retrobulbar anesthesia with 0.5% bupivacaine HCl. Next, the epithelium is mechanically removed. The distal end of a Weck-cel sponge is saturated with 0.5% EDTA (prepared by mixing a 20% stock of NaEDTA with 0.9% sodium chloride) and held against the area of calcium deposition. A to-and-fro abrasive action is used to help remove the calcium deposits; this is best accomplished at the slit-lamp examination. If significant clearing has not occurred after 10 minutes of treatment, higher concentrations of EDTA (1.0% or 1.5%) should be used. Sometimes, the treatment must be continued for 20 to 30 minutes. In refractory cases, gentle curettage with a scalpel may be necessary. An antibiotic solution and weak cycloplegic then are instilled. A patch or bandage lens may be used for comfort and to facilitate epithelial healing.

If the opacification cannot be removed with chelation or curettage, lamellar keratoplasty should be considered. A technique using EDTA and a diamond bur on a Fisch drill has been shown to be effective in removing deposits without significant scarring. The excimer laser phototherapeutic keratectomy has also been shown to be effective for the removal of band keratopathy. Excimer keratectomy alters the corneal curvature with a shift toward hyperopia. In addition, the more peripheral deposits cannot be removed without inducing even greater changes in refraction.

Conjunctival concretions causing irritation and a foreign body sensation often can be shelled out with a sharp pointed knife or broad needle. On occasion, this procedure may be difficult; if so, it should be reserved for symptomatic lesions.

REFERENCES

Binder PS, Deg JK, Kohl FS: Calcific band keratopathy after intraocular chondroitin sulfate. Arch Ophthalmol 105:1243, 1987.

Bokosky JE, Meyer RK, Sugar A: Surgical treatment of calcific band keratopathy. Ophthalmic Surg 16:645–647, 1985.

Duffey RK, LoCascio JA: Calcium deposition in a corneal graft. Cornea 6:212–215, 1987.

O'Brart DPS, Gartry DS, Lohmann CP, et al: Treatment of band keratopathy by excimer laser phototherapeutic keratectomy: Surgical techniques and long term follow up. Br J Ophthalmol 77:702–708, 1993.

Pecorella I, McCartney AC, Lucas S, et al: Acquired immunodeficiency syndrome and ocular calcification. Cornea 15:305–311, 1996.

Sternberg P, Jr, Hatchell DL, Foulks GN, Landers MB, III: The effect of silicone oil on the cornea. Arch Ophthalmol 103:90, 1985.

Taravella MJ, Stulting RD, Mader TH, et al: Calcific band keratopathy associated with the use of topical steroid- phosphate preparations. Arch Ophthalmol 112(5):608, 1994.

180 FILTERING BLEBS AND ASSOCIATED PROBLEMS 997.9

Linda Her-Shyuan Lin, MD
Houston, Texas
Adam C. Reynolds, MD
Eagle, Idaho

FILTERING BLEB

A bleb is a blister-like elevation of conjunctiva and Tenon's capsule overlying a subconjunctival reservoir of aqueous fluid. This intraocular fluid comes from a fistula connecting the anterior or posterior chamber to the subconjunctival space. It is absorbed through veins and conjunctival lymphatics, and with thin conjunctiva, it may pass directly into the tear film.

Blebs are clinically described by their elevation, vascularity, extent in clock hours, microcyst presence, and wall thickness. Varying morphologic bleb appearances include being diffuse or localized, cystic (thin, localized, walled off at the edges) (Figure 180.1), or overhanging (extending onto the cornea). Scarring affects the function and morphology of a filtering bleb and can be modulated with topical steroids and antifibrosis agents.

Antimetabolite/antifibrotic usage in trabeculectomy

The antimetabolites mitomycin C (MMC) and 5-Fluorouracil (5FU) reduce fibroblast proliferation in the subconjunctival space and Tenon's capsule preventing episcleral fibrosis of the scleral flap. In trabeculectomy surgery, they are increasingly used to achieve lower intraocular pressures and to improve functional success of the surgeries in eyes at high risk for surgical failure.

The pyrimidine base analogue 5FU competitively inhibits the enzyme thymidylate synthase. Incorporated into the replicating nucleic acid strands, it is active only in the S (synthesis) phase of the cell cycle. This specificity makes 5FU more toxic to replicating cells. It is used intraoperatively over the scleral flap or as postoperative subconjunctival injections.

MMC is an alkylating agent secreted by the bacteria *Streptomyces caespitosus*. Independent of the cell cycle, it crosslinks DNA to inhibit cell synthesis. Its toxicity to the vascular

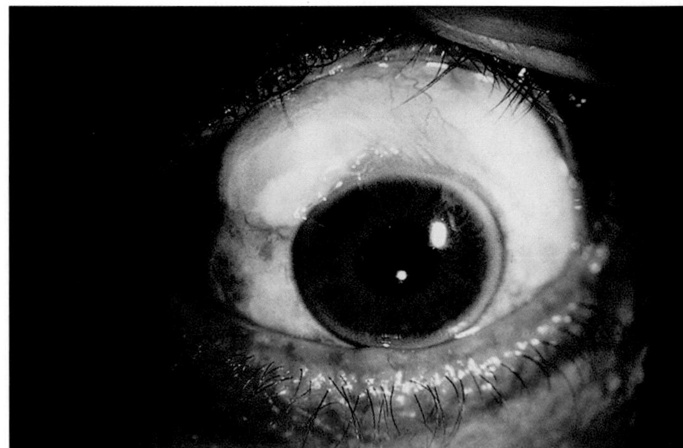

FIGURE 180.1. Thin polycystic filtration bleb (type 1) (From: Salmon JF, Kanski JJ: Glaucoma: a colour manual of diagnosis and treatment. 3rd edn. Butterworth Heinemann, 2004:144.)

endothelium makes it antiangiogenic. One hundred times more potent than 5FU, its direct cytotoxicity makes it more hazardous when exposed to intraocular structures. MMC is used intraoperatively over the scleral flap in concentrations of 0.2 to 0.5 mg/mL for 1 to 4 minutes and is tailored to the patient's tendency toward scar formation. It is generally avoided in young, white, myopic males who are at high risk for postoperative hypotony.

Antimetabolite-treated blebs have less fibrosis, a wider filtration area, and lower intraocular pressure IOP. However, they often create thin, focal, cystic, avascular blebs that are prone to leaks and infections. Given the higher success and complication rates associated with antimetabolites, the risk/benefit ratio should be assessed on a patient-by-patient basis.

The presence of a bleb inherently increases the risk of late complications. As a consequence, when confronted with bleb dysfunction, management issues come to the forefront. With regard to problems associated with filtering blebs, the following will be discussed in this chapter:

- Symptomatic blebs (dysesthesia, overhanging, large).
- Bleb overfiltration.
- Bleb leaks.
- Bleb infections (blebitis, endophthalmitis).
- Bleb encapsulation.
- Failing or failed blebs.

Bleb dysesthesia (symptomatic blebs), overhanging blebs

Filtering blebs are usually asymptomatic and well tolerated. Some patients experience dysesthesia, with symptoms of burning, foreign body sensation, tearing, pain, or vague discomfort. Predisposing factors include younger age, superonasal or nasal bleb location, large blebs, overhanging blebs, bubbles at the bleb-cornea junction, and poor eyelid coverage.

Bleb elevation interferes with blinking and tear film distribution causing superficial punctate keratopathy, ocular surface irregularities, corneal epithelial defects, dellen, and induced-astigmatism. Overhanging blebs have been associated with visual field changes, visual loss, and monocular diplopia. Dellen present in 2–9% of full-thickness glaucoma surgeries.

Conservative methods shrink and remodel blebs. Bleb–cornea junction bubbles and dellen are treated with aggressive lubrication. Compress sutures flatten high blebs that predispose to bubble formation. Failure to resolve symptoms conservatively requires surgical bleb excision or conjunctival flap reinforcement. Portions of overhanging blebs on the cornea are bluntly dissected and excised with little leakage. Although surgical results are generally good, bleb failure remains a risk.

Overfiltering blebs

Overfiltering blebs are very common early after surgery. Excessive aqueous outflow is more prevalent after full-thickness glaucoma procedures and with antifibrotic usage. These blebs are elevated. Most early postoperative cases resolve spontaneously or with aggressive cycloplegia. Activity restrictions of not bending over from the waist, not weightlifting, and avoiding Valsalva-inducing conditions are recommended.

Markedly shallow anterior chambers or large choroidal effusions require treatment. Flat anterior chambers with lens-corneal touch demand immediate anterior chamber reformation to prevent cataract development and irreversible corneal endothelial injury. Conservative therapeutic options are often ineffective with prior antimetabolite usage.

Hypotonous complications determine the timing of surgical interventions. Choroidals with persistent iridocorneal apposition and/or apposition of retinal surfaces (kissing choroidals) necessitate choroidal effusion drainage. Surgical revision involves resuturing the scleral flap, scleral reinforcement with a patch graft, bleb excision with conjunctivoplasty, or a combination of these procedures.

Bleb leaks

A bleb leak is a focal point of aqueous leakage from interrupted conjunctival tissue. Oozing is transconjunctival aqueous egress. A Seidel's test performed with 1% fluorescein solution or 2% fluorescein strip under slit-lamp magnification detects these phenomena and should be done whenever a bleb is examined.

Bleb leaks can occur any time. Early causes include conjunctival buttonholes or incisional wound leaks (especially in fornix-based filters). Test for conjunctival breaks prior to intraoperative antifibrotic agents. Carefully check for leaks at end of surgery to repair them intraoperatively. Most common in the first week, small leaks often resolve spontaneously or respond to conservative management. Surgically close early bleb leaks that cause marked bleb shallowing to avoid subconjunctival-to-episcleral fibrosis and bleb failure.

Spontaneous late bleb leaks occur more with avascular, thin, multilobulated blebs resulting from antimetabolite usage or full-thickness procedures. For full-thickness procedures the incidence of bleb leaks 3.3%. With antimetabolite-supplemented trabeculectomy, incidence is reported to be between 5% and 30%. Prevalence of bleb leaks with 5FU is 1.4% while for MMC it is 2.3% to 3.7%. Late antimetabolite-associated bleb leaks tend to occur in patients younger than age 40 and in patients with thin cystic avascular blebs or inferiorly located blebs. Contact lens and inferiorly positioned blebs predispose to trauma and bleb leaks.

Late bleb leaks without hypotonous complications can be observed for spontaneous closure. They may respond to medical management if no antimetabolites were involved. Bleb leaks in monocular patients and those with previous bleb-related infections should always be treated. Aqueous suppressants, discontinuation of topical steroids with or without patching, and topical tobramycin or gentamicin promote bleb leak closure.

Additional interventions include cyanoacrylate glue and autologous fibrin tissue glue. Additional treatments include cyanoacrylate glue and autologous fibrin tissue glue. Bleb tissue friability often makes surgical repair difficult. Autologous blood injection may be the best initial approach. Despite sealing with conservative management, late bleb leaks have a high likelihood of recurring especially if antimetabolite-associated.

Surgical repair becomes necessary for large complicated bleb leaks, imminent bleb failure, lack of response to conservative methods, and recurrent bleb leaks. Bleb leaks in adequately vascularized areas can be closed directly with a 10-0 nylon suture on a small tapered needle (BV75-3) placed in a figure-eight or horizontal mattress fashion.

Many surgical bleb leak repair techniques exist, but none is universally successful. Methods include partial or complete bleb excision buttressed by conjunctival flaps, autologous conjunctival grafts, or amniotic membrane. Conjunctival advancement or rotation without bleb removal for small bleb leaks and autologous conjunctival bleb resurfacing for large bleb leaks are recommended. For hypotony present preleak, the scleral flap is revised.

Surgical bleb revision complications include immediate postoperative IOP elevations, persistent or recurrent bleb leaks, conjunctival shrinkage and retraction, wound dehiscence, bleb dysesthesia, ptosis, and hyperopia. Decreased bleb function requires resuming glaucoma medications and possibly more glaucoma surgery.

Conservative treatment options for bleb dysesthesia, overfiltering bleb, and bleb leaks

Pressure patching, large diameter (20- or 22-mm) bandage contact lenses, collagen shields, symblepharon rings, and Simmons shells tamponade overfiltering blebs in the early postoperative period. Bandage contact lenses encourage epithelial migration to reepithelialize bleb defects.

Inflammation and scarring is a shared mechanism for chemical irritants, cryotherapy, laser thermotherapy, and autologous blood injection in the treatment of bleb dysesthesia, overfiltering blebs, and bleb leaks. For chemical cauterization, 0.25% to 1% silver nitrate or 50% trichloroacetic acid is applied to bleb surfaces and rinsed after drying. Cryotherapy is performed with the cryoprobe apposing the bleb surface to sclera at temperatures of –50°C to –80°C for 10–30 seconds. Argon laser treatment requires conjunctival painting with methylene blue or rose Bengal for laser energy absorption. Laser parameters are 200–500 micron spot size, 300–500 milliwatts power, and 0.2 seconds duration.

Autologous blood injection success rate has been reported to be 57–72%. Complications include hyphema, vitreous hemorrhage, severe visual loss, endophthalmitis, increased IOP requiring surgical intervention, bleb failure, corneal blood staining, corneal graft rejection, and reactivation of previously quiescent ocular toxoplasmosis.

Cyanoacrylate tissue adhesive is applied to dry conjunctiva to close bleb leaks. A bandage contact lens or collagen shield is placed to prevent dislodging of the adhesive, which spontaneously sloughs after epithelialization closes the defect. The most frequent complication is corneal abrasions at the application site.

Compression sutures remodel the bleb by walling off the leaking area from the main cavity when the leak is located away from the scleral flap. The suture is tied in an X compressing bleb to sclera. More than one suture can be placed. Epiphora, discomfort, and bleb erosion can occur.

Needling of thin, cystic blebs and late multifocal bleb leaks has been reported. Eliminating the physical barrier to posterior flow, the fibrotic 'ring of steel,' and decreasing hydrostatic pressure allows conjunctival epithelial cells to repopulate the bleb wall to heal the leak.

The effect of conservative treatment options in bleb leaks is usually not sustained. Consequently, these procedures often need to be repeated. They are less effective in thin avascular blebs and may even tear a hole or enlarge a previous break.

Bleb infections

Bleb-related ocular infection is a potentially devastating complication of glaucoma filtering surgery and can occur months to years after the initial surgery.

Blebitis is a limited anterior form of endophthalmitis. Presenting complaints include ocular pain, sudden redness and decreased vision, tearing, purulent discharge, photophobia, and foreign-body sensation. Examination reveals conjunctival and ciliary injection most intense around the bleb edge, mucopurulent discharge, periorbital chemosis, corneal edema, and anterior chamber reaction. A milky white bleb may contain a pseudohypopyon. A positive Seidel's test is common with possible hypotony. Increased IOP occurs when purulence and debris close the sclerostomy. Vitreous reaction is not evident early. After trabeculectomy with MMC, blebitis incidence is 5.7% per year.

Untreated blebitis rapidly spreads posteriorly causing bleb-associated endophthalmitis characterized by hypopyn, vitreous cells, and a guarded visual prognosis. Bleb-associated endophthalmitis after glaucoma filtering surgeries is reported to be 0.2% to 9.6%. Risk for endophthalmitis is estimated at 9% for full-thickness filtration blebs compared to 0.3% to 1.5% per year for partial-thickness filtration blebs. Incidence of bleb-associated endophthalmitis after MMC ranges from 0.8% to 2.6% per patient year and 1.7% per year with intraoperative 5FU. Most of the risk is concentrated in the first year, but the potential for infection lasts a lifetime. After trabeculectomy with MMC, blebitis incidence is 5.7% per year.

Numerous risk factors for bleb-associated infections exist. Surgical causes include antimetabolite use, full-thickness filtering surgery, releasable sutures, and silk conjunctival sutures. Chronic, episodic antibiotic use and early postoperative complications are associated with late-onset infections. Bleb leaks and postoperative bleb manipulations increase the likelihood of bleb-related infections with infections occurring 25 times more frequently in leaking blebs. Blepharitis, conjunctivitis, and nasolacrimal duct obstruction amplify the bacterial load. Patient characteristics for bleb-related infections include young age at surgery, male sex, a broken posterior capsule, and black race.

Streptococcus sp., *Staphylococcus* sp., and *Haemophilus influenzae* are the most common organisms associated with bleb-related infections. Conjunctival exudates are stained and cultured. The value of positive conjunctival cultures remains questionable since colonization and infection are not always differentiated. Anterior chamber tap and vitreous tap or vitrectomy with intraocular antibiotic injection is done depending on the areas involved.

Early intervention prevents progression to endophthalmitis. Blebitis without anterior chamber reaction is treated empirically with frequent topical broad-spectrum antibiotics, such as a fluoroquinolone, every half-hour to every hour until culture results are available.

Anterior chamber reaction with blebitis is treated with fortified topical antibiotics around the clock. Lack of clinical improvement or appearance of vitreous cells after 24–48 hours leads to intraocular antibiotic administration.

Bleb-related endophthalmitis is an emergency requiring aggressive management. More severe infection and poorer visual acuity prompt immediate pars plana vitrectomy. An oral fluoroquinolone and fortified topical antibiotics are used with intravitreal antibiotics. Intraocular and topical corticosteroid use is controversial.

Eyes successfully treated for bleb-related infection remain at risk for recurrent infection. Leaking or inferiorly located blebs are particularly vulnerable. Antibiotic prophylaxis may be used in high-risk blebs. Infected eyes retain good visual function if monitored closely and treated intensely. Good post-infection IOP control suggests that bleb function can survive blebitis episodes.

Encapsulated bleb

Also known as a Tenon's capsule cyst, an encapsulated bleb is a localized, high, tense, firm, 'tight-appearing' bleb with conjunctival vascular engorgement, thick connective tissue walls, and few microcysts. It appears 2–4 weeks after surgery. After initial pressure control, IOP rises with Tenon's cyst formation. IOP often decreases within several weeks to several months.

Long-term prognosis for IOP control is relatively good, although medical therapy is often required.

Encapsulated blebs occur commonly after trabeculectomy (10–14% of cases) with decreased incidence in trabeculectomy with MMC compared to 5FU. Associated factors include male sex, glove powder, topical steroids, prior sympathomimetic use, prior argon laser trabeculoplasty, and prior conjunctival surgery.

Initial management includes antiglaucoma medication, topical steroids, and digital ocular massage. Deciding between conservative medical management and a surgical approach depends on the severity of glaucomatous damage, the IOP level, and the response to conservative treatment.

Needling immediately lowers IOP. Cutting the fibrotic wall of the encapsulated bleb restores aqueous runoff to a larger subconjunctival area. Occasionally, there is no response to needling with multiloculated blebs. Even when successfully needled, Tenon's cysts can reform requiring another needling or more extensive surgical revision.

To surgically remove a Tenon's cyst, conjunctiva is bluntly dissected off the underlying fibrotic wall, and the fibrous capsule is excised. Subconjunctival 5FU injections after surgical revision increases success. If a Tenon's cyst recurs after surgical excision, repeat trabeculectomy (usually with tenonectomy) is indicated.

Failing and failed blebs

Failing blebs have uncontrolled IOP and impending or established obstruction of aqueous outflow. These blebs appear low or flat with minimal to no microcysts. Warning signs are increased bleb vascularization, bleb inflammation, and/or bleb thickening. These blebs should be recognized promptly to relieve aqueous outflow obstruction. Otherwise, permanent adhesions develop between conjunctiva and episclera making the bleb intractable to revision.

Bleb failure is usually a late occurrence. 'Early failing/failed blebs' occur within the first postoperative month mostly because of inadequate flow at the scleral flap site. Bleb failure is usually a late occurrence. 'Late failing/failed blebs' have a history of at least 1 month of good bleb function and adequate IOP control postoperatively. Subconjunctival and episcleral fibrosis cause most filtration failures. Factors accelerating subconjunctival fibrosis are black race, childhood, postoperative subconjunctival hemorrhage, reactive sutures, and inflammation.

In early bleb failure, 5FU enhances filtration. Subconjunctival 5FU in 5-mg aliquots is administered during the first 2 weeks after surgery. The frequency of administration is adjusted according to the occurrence of complications, which include corneal and conjunctival epithelial toxicity, corneal ulcers, conjunctival wound leaks, subconjunctival hemorrhage, and inadvertent intraocular spread of 5FU.

During the early postoperative period, sutures are removed when there is a high IOP, a flat filtration bleb, a deep anterior chamber, and an open sclerostomy. In a conservative stepwise manner, one suture is laser suture lysed or extracted at a time to avoid overfiltration. Releasable sutures are used when inflamed or hemorrhagic conjunctiva and thickened Tenon's tissue preclude suture lysis. Many different releasable suture techniques exist. Timing of suture release is critical. Without antimetabolites, this should be performed within 2–3 weeks. The time frame for successful suture release after trabeculectomy is 1–2 months with 5FU and several months with MMC.

Digital ocular compression/massage is directed through the eyelids to the inferior sclera or sclera posterior to the scleral flap to elevate the bleb and reduce IOP. Especially useful after suture release, it is less responsive with internal obstruction of the sclerostomy. Patients are instructed to massage several times a day during the early postoperative period. Potential complications include corneal abrasions, hypotony, flat anterior chamber, and choroidal effusion or hemorrhage.

Recombinant tissue plasminogen activator (tPA) is a serine protease with clot-specific fibrinolytic activity. TPA converts plasminogen to plasmin, which mediates fibrin degradation into fibrin-split products and fibrinogen-degradation products to lyse new clots. The most common dose is 7–10 micrograms. TPA is injected subconjunctivally or into the anterior chamber when hemorrhage or fibrin clots occlude the sclerostomy. Hyphema is the most frequent complication after glaucoma surgery (up to 36% of cases).

Management of late failing blebs depends on the site of aqueous resistance. Internal revision with Nd:YAG or Argon laser is useful early and late in the postoperative period when there is sclerostomy obstruction. Nd:YAG treats nonpigmented tissues (vitreous, lens capsule) while argon laser is effective for pigmented tissue (iris, ciliary body). A more favorable outcome occurs if the filtration bleb was well established before the fistula was occluded and if there is no significant subconjunctival scarring. Hemorrhage is a complication.

Laser external revision is directed to episcleral or subconjunctival fibrosis with or without simultaneous internal revision. To treat blebs transconjunctivally, a Nd:YAG Abraham iridotomy lens is placed over the bleb with 2% methylcellulose. Energies from 2.9–10.0 mJ in single pulse mode are used. The laser is retrofocused through the bleb onto episclera. Bubble formation indicates adequate power. After the procedure, Seidel to detect conjunctival breaks.

External revision by needling cuts the edge of the scleral flap to restore aqueous runoff. A short $^1/_4$ to $^5/_8$ inch 25–30 gauge needle penetrates conjunctiva 5–10 mm from the scleral fistula. Balanced saline solution or 1% lidocaine is injected to balloon up the conjunctiva. The needle is advanced into the bleb cavity beneath the scleral flap. A sweeping motion or to-and-fro movements lyse fibrotic strands at the bleb edges tearing a hole in the cyst wall. Avoid multiple punctures to prevent conjunctival buttonholes and excessive bleeding. An 'aggressive' alternative advances the needle through the internal ostium until visualized in the anterior chamber (use extreme caution in phakic eyes). Seidel for wound leaks. Pressure patch, cauterize, or suture with 10-0 nylon on a vascular needle if there is a brisk leak. Topical antibiotics and steroids are used postoperatively with or without additional subconjunctival 5FU.

Transient bleb leak is the most frequent complication. Other complications include endophthalmitis, choroidal hemorrhage, subconjunctival hemorrhage, choroidal detachment, and hypotony. The success rate is directly related to lower preneedling IOP and fewer previous surgical procedures. Use of 5FU or MMC with needling is controversial. A mixture of 0.02 mL of bupivacaine 0.75% with epinephrine and 0.01 mL of MMC (0.4 mg/mL) may be injected 20 minutes before needling.

If there is adequate conjunctiva elsewhere, it may be preferable to perform a MMC-augmented trabeculectomy in healthy tissue at another site or a glaucoma drainage implant rather than a bleb needling.

Potential bleb complications

- Hypotony (intraocular pressure less than 6 mm Hg).
  - From excessive filtration or a bleb leak.

- Hypotonous maculopathy with loss of vision (with chronic hypotony persisting for at least 3 months).
  - Risk factors include being young, white, male and myopic.
- Shallow to flat anterior chamber.
- Corneal edema with possible corneal decompensation.
- Choroidal effusions, ciliochoroidal detachments, possibly kissing choroidals.
- Endophthalmitis.
- Dellen with possible corneal ulceration or perforation.
- Uncontrolled glaucoma.
- Astigmatism.
- Cataract.
- Suprachoroidal hemorrhage.

REFERENCES

Azuara-Blanco A, Katz LJ: Dysfunctional filtering blebs. Surv Ophthalmology 43:93–126, Sept–Oct 1998.

Budenz DL, Hoffman K, Zacchei A: Glaucoma filtering bleb dysesthesia. Am J Ophthalmology 131:626–630, 2001.

Feldman RM, Altaher G: Management of late-onset bleb leaks. Curr Opin Ophthalmol 15:151–154, 2004.

Fine LC, Chen TC, Grosskreutz CL, et al: Management and prevention of thin, cystic blebs. Internat Ophthalmol 44:29–42, 2004.

Haynes WL, Alward WLM: Control of intraocular pressure after trabeculectomy. Surv Ophthalmology 43:345–355, 1999.

Mac I, Soltau JB: Glaucoma-filtering bleb infections. Curr Opin Ophthalmol 14:91–94, 2003.

Song A, Scott UI, Flynn HW, et al: Delayed-onset bleb-associated endophthalmitis clinical features and visual acuity outcomes. Ophthalmology 109:985–991, 2002.

Waheed S, Liebmann JM, Greenfield DS, et al: Recurrent bleb infections. Br J Ophthalmol 82:926–929, 1998.

181 GIANT PAPILLARY CONJUNCTIVITIS 372.12

Thomas L. Steinemann, MD
Cleveland, Ohio

ETIOLOGY/INCIDENCE

Giant papillary conjunctivitis (GPC) is a condition characterized by inflammation of the tarsal conjunctiva and is usually associated with soft contact lens wear. After the first report by Spring in 1974, Allansmith and coworkers described in 1977 a syndrome of contact lens intolerance, ocular itching, mucus discharge, hyperemia, blurred vision and eruption of giant papillae in the upper tarsal conjunctiva. These symptoms, which may resemble vernal conjunctivitis, are often seen in patients wearing soft, gas-permeable, or hard contact lenses. GPC is estimated to affect over 20% of the nearly 34 million contact lens wearers in the United States; contact lens wear clearly is the most common factor in the development of this syndrome. Identical findings may, however, be seen in other patients in conjunction with a variety of external ocular foreign bodies, including exposed monofilament suture ends, keratoprosthesis, artificial eyes, corneal-scleral shells, cyanoacrylate glue, and extruded scleral buckles. Filtering blebs and limbal dermoids are also associated with GPC.

The cause and pathogenesis of GPC are not fully understood. Evidence suggests that GPC may be the result of mechanical trauma combined with a hypersensitivity reaction to antigenic proteins trapped on the roughened surface of a worn contact lens, prosthesis, or suture ends. Because GPC occurs in wearers of soft, hard, and rigid contact lenses, it is unlikely that the lesions associated with contact lens wear are caused by a reaction to the lens material. In fact, contact lens-associated GPC develops as a response to prolonged contact of lens deposits (protein) with the tarsal conjunctiva. Factors which increase this contact (i.e. increased wear time, extended wear, increased lens deposits and increased contact lens surface area/size) would likely increase the severity of symptoms in the affected contact lens wearer.

Conversely, reducing the contact between lens deposits and the conjunctiva is a useful strategy in treatment and prophylaxis. Frequent replacement and disposable lenses offer some advantage over traditional soft lenses. Disposable lenses are replaced at 2–3 week intervals. Daily disposable lenses are also available. Donshik found a great incidence of GPC in those patients who replaced their lenses at intervals at 4 weeks or longer compared with those who replaced at intervals of 3 weeks or less. These findings support the assumption that the longer a lens is worn the more likely it will become coated with protein and thus trigger an antigenic challenge as well as mechanical trauma to the conjunctival surface.

Likewise, proper cleaning of contact lenses can remove the coating and deposits. Many eyecare professionals recommend manual rubbing of soft contact lenses in the palm of the hand despite the introduction of multipurpose 'no rub' cleaning solutions. Some wearers may benefit from separate enzymatic cleaning weekly or bi-weekly. Patients who continue to have significant protein deposition despite proper cleaning may find reduction of wear time or daily disposable wear advantageous. Others may require a refit in RGP lenses.

Donshik has acknowledged GPC can occur in patients wearing silicone hydrogel lenses: a diffuse (generalized) form across the entire palpebral conjunctiva and a localized version with patchy involvement near the lid margin. The generalized form is similar to that frequently seen in low-Dk hydrogel lenses, while the localized version is more frequent in wearers of high DK (silicone hydrogel) lenses. The overall prevalence of GPC is comparable in both low-Dk and high-Dk lenses. The observation that not all patients with contact lens deposits develop GPC indicates that an individual's immunologic response to protein deposits is a key factor in the development of GPC. A history of allergy to environmental allergens or systemic medication may be an important risk factor.

It is recognized that increased coatings on worn contact lenses exacerbate signs and symptoms of existing cases of GPC and may contribute to the onset of the disease. Conditions that favor the development or exacerbation of GPC include

- Wearing contact lenses for long periods (especially overnight wear).
- Continued use of worn contact lenses for months or years without replacing them with new lenses.
- Larger diameter contact lens (presenting a greater area to which adherent antigenic material can react with the conjunctival epithelium).
- Inadequate cleaning and enzyming of the lenses.

COURSE/PROGNOSIS

In early stages, GPC patients may note itching when the contact lenses are removed, mucus accumulation in the inner corners of the eyes upon awakening, and slight blurring of vision. These symptoms are so common that patients are not likely to report them. As GPC progresses, patients may report blurring of vision after wearing the contact lenses for several hours, excessive movement of the contact lenses, mucus discharge and contact lens awareness. The examination may reveal mucus strands and mild hyperemia of the upper tarsal conjunctiva. In early to moderate cases, the conjunctiva is usually translucent, but it may be somewhat thickened.

As inflammation increases, the conjunctiva may become opaque. In the late stages of GPC, patients develop contact lens intolerance and describe dryness, foreign body sensation or pain when wearing the lens. Sheets or ropes of mucus are usually present, contributing to sticking of the eyelids. Upon awakening, hyperemia is marked, and pseudoptosis may appear in some patients.

Concurrent with the opacification of the upper tarsal conjunctiva, enlarged collagen structures (papillae) begin to emerge from the tarsal plate. As they grow, they push aside the normal smaller papillae, and their apexes flatten gradually. The overlying conjunctiva may break down, resulting in fluorescein staining, which is critical sign of moderate-to-severe disease. In soft contact lens wearers, papillae appear on the upper tarsal conjunctiva and advance to the lid margin. In rigid gas-permeable contact lens wearers, papillae are fewer and smaller and appear first on the lid margin.

DIAGNOSIS

Clinical signs and symptoms

The syndrome includes a spectrum of clinical signs and symptoms. Abnormally large papillae (diameter of more than 0.3 mm) are diagnostic and best visualized with fluorescein and the cobalt-blue light. Giant papillae are classically described as 1 mm or larger in diameter and are concentrated in the superior tarsal conjunctiva (Figure 181.1). They are usually not seen except in advanced cases. Increased production of mucus results in strings or sheets that coat the contact lens may cloud vision.

Giant papillary conjunctivitis can resemble vernal conjunctivitis. In fact, similar immunologic process may be involved in both diseases. Both conditions present with ocular itching and mucoid discharge. However, the itching of GPC is usually milder than with vernal conjunctivitis. Also, unlike vernal conjunctivitis, GPC is not associated with atopy. GPC occurs in all age groups and both sexes, whereas vernal conjunctivitis is more common in young males. Vernal conjunctivitis usually displays seasonal variation, worsening in warm weather. Patients with GPC experience a rapid relief of symptoms upon discontinuation of contact lens wear, whereas vernal conjunctivitis patients do not have a dramatic response with any one treatment.

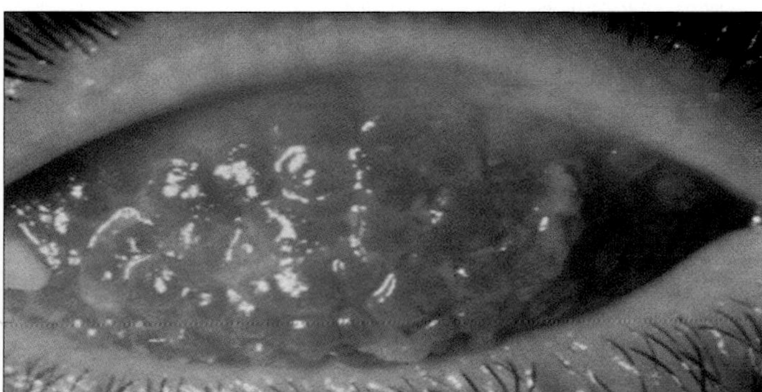

FIGURE 181.1. Giant papillary conjunctivitis.

Early symptoms include lens awareness, excessive lens movement, dryness, inner canthal mucus on awakening, redness, burnings, itching and blurring.

Later key signs include the following:

- Conjunctival injection;
- Upper tarsal papillae (at least 0.3 mm): macropapillae (0.3 to 1.0 mm), giant papillae (more than 1.0 mm). fluorescein staining of papillae, papillary flattening;
- Tarsal thickening/opacity;
- Mucus strands;
- Superficial punctate keratopathy;
- Eyelid: pseudoptosis (edema);
- Other: mucus coating/protein deposits on contact lenses.

Ocular or periocular

- Conjunctiva: macropapillae (0.3 to 1.0 mm diameter), giant papillae (more than 1.0 mm diameter), fluorescein staining of papillae, tarsal and bulbar conjunctival injection, tarsal conjunctival thickening and opacity, mucus strands, Horner–Trantas dots, gelatinous limbal nodules.
- Cornea: superficial punctate keratopathy.
- Eyelid: pseudoptosis.
- Other: mucus coating of contact lenses, protein deposits on contact lenses.

Differential diagnosis

- Vernal keratoconjunctivitis.

PROPHYLAXIS

- Consider more frequent replacement of disposable contact lenses (including daily disposable contact lenses) or reduce daily wear time.
- Encourage strict lens hygiene.
- Recommend preservation-free solution.
- Encourage enzymatic cleaning with papain preparations.
- Remove offending foreign body.

TREATMENT

The primary treatment of GPC involves removal of the foreign body and treatment of inflamed conjunctiva with pharmacotherapy. The removal of a prosthesis or contact lens or trimming of an offending suture barb usually results in prompt resolution of the problem. Most patients who wear contact lenses, however, wish to continue wearing their lenses.

Supportive

In severe cases, patients must stop wearing their contact lenses until symptoms such as hyperemia and mucus discharge resolve and the eye is 'quiet.' Fluorescein staining of the apexes of papillae, copious mucus discharge, tarsal hyperemia, and decentering of the contact lens are all indications for lens removal. Lenses should be discontinued for at least 4 weeks and may be reintroduced several days after the signs and symptoms have resolved. Patients should be free of injection, mucus discharge, and punctate keratopathy before being fitted with a new contact lens. Enlarged papillae may take months or year to regress.

Some patients will be able to continue contact lens wear without stopping, provided certain strategies are followed. First, lens replacement (with a new and preferably different type of contact lens) is recommended. A smaller-diameter, thinner-edge lens should be fitted. In addition, meticulous attention to lens hygiene is essential. Contact lens cleaners should be free of preservatives, such as thimerosol. Nonpreserved saline in an aerosol can is recommended. These steps will help minimize antigenic exposure. Sterilization with hydrogen peroxide has been found to be the best-tolerated disinfection method. Weekly enzymatic cleaning to remove deposits is necessary.

The patient should understand that regular replacement of traditional soft contact lenses should occur every 6 to 12 months or at the first sign of any significant lens coating or mucus discharge. In some soft contact lens wearers, a switch to a daily disposable or rigid gas-permeable contact lens may be the only alternative to increase contact lens tolerance.

Frequent-replacement (disposable) contact lenses are an important addition to the supportive treatment regimen for GPC patients. Disposable contact lenses may obviate the need for enzymatic cleaning; deposits are minimized because the contact lenses are discarded and replaced every 1 to 2 weeks. Daily disposable contact lenses may be indicated in some wearers. For patients with a history of GPC, disposable contact lenses should be worn on a daily basis with daily cleaning. Patients should not sleep in their lenses.

Ocular

After the discontinuation of contact lens wear, topical lubrication may be the only therapy required. In cases of advanced GPC in which inflammation is marked, a short course of topical corticosteroids may be appropriate to quiet the eye before initiating further treatment. However, corticosteroids have not proven particularly effective in the long-term management of GPC.

A recent double-blind, placebo-controlled study of loteprednol etabonate in 223 patients with GPC revealed a significant improvement in itching and lens intolerance, with only 7% showing a 10 mm Hg or greater increase in intraocular pressure. Pressure returned to normal after discontinuing of the drops. Other studies showed a significant reduction in papillae and symptoms for patients receiving loteprednol compared to placebo.

Cromolyn sodium, a mast cell stabilizer, has had a beneficial effect in the management of GPC. In conjunction with lens replacement and rigorous lens hygiene, 4% cromolyn sodium ophthalmic solution q.i.d. (even while the lens is in place) may help resolve early GPC before it progresses. More advanced cases of GPC are not amenable to treatment with cromolyn sodium alone. Once the signs and symptoms of GPC are brought under control with supportive therapy, cromolyn sodium may be introduced as part of regular maintenance therapy. Other agents (olopatadine 0.1%, ketotifen 0.025%) combine antihistamine (H_1 receptor) and mast cell stabilizer properties in the treatment of allergic conjunctivitis.

Both ketorolac tromethamine, a topical nonsterioidal anti-inflammatory drug and prostaglandin inhibitor, and lodoxamide tromethamine, a topical mast cell stabilizer, have been shown to improve contact lens tolerability in patients with GPC.

Levocabastine, a potent topical histamine (H_1 receptor) antagonist, has recently been extensively evaluated for allergic conjunctivitis. Results indicate that it has efficacy similar to or better than that of topical cromolyn sodium. Its safety and efficacy in patient with GPC remain to be determined.

A newer agent (epinastine hydrochloride 0.05%) has recently been introduced in the treatment of allergic conjunctivitis. It acts as a mast cell stabilizer and antihistamine, but blocks both short-term (H_1) and long-term (H_2) histamine receptors. Its utility in GPC patients remains to be determined.

- General:
  - Decreased contact lens coating (decreased antigen load/trauma to ocular surface);
  - Modulate immune response after the initiation of inflammation.
- Decrease contact lens coating:
  - Decrease wear time; consider the use of disposable contact lenses;
  - Improve the cleaning/enzyming regimen;
  - Change the lens material or design.
- Modulate the immune response:
  - Topical steroids can be used;
  - Topical nonsteroidal anti-inflammatory drugs can be used;
  - Topical mast cell stabilizers can be used.

There is no systemic or surgical treatment.

PRECAUTIONS

The successful treatment of GPC depends on the earliest possible recognition of the disease process and initiation of appropriate therapy. The symptoms of GPC usually precede the earliest subtle signs; therefore, the proper diagnosis requires careful examination and a high index of suspicion. Patient education regarding the nature of GPC is crucial to the successful continuation of resumption of contact lens wear. Patients should thoroughly understand the importance of meticulous lens care and frequent lens replacement as well as such alternatives as disposable contact lenses.

COMMENTS

To follow the progression of the clinical signs of PC with contact lens wear and therapy, it is necessary to accurately describe the appearance of the upper tarsal conjunctiva to each visit. A record should be made indicating the zone of involvement, the size and elevation of the papillae, the fluorescein-staining pattern of the tops of papillae, and the presence of mucus. The progression of these signs and symptoms in the initial disease state has some prognostic value. The earlier the GPC is treated, the more likely treatment will arrest progression of the disease while maintaining long-term tolerance of the contact lens.

REFERENCES

Allansmith ME, Ross RN: Giant papillary conjunctivitis. In: Duane TD, Jaeger EA, eds: Clinical ophthalmology. Philadelphia, Harper & Row, 1987:4:1–10.

Allansmith MR, Korb DR, Greiner JV: Giant papillary conjunctivitis in contact lens wearers. Am J Ophthalmol 83:697–708, 1977.

Allansmith MR, Ross RN: Ocular allergy and mast cell stabilizer. Surv Ophthalmol 20:229–244, 1986.

Donshik PC, Porazinski AD: Giant papillary conjunctivitis in frequent replacement. Trans Am Ophthalmol Soc 97:205–216, 1999.

Donshik PC: Contact lens chemistry and giant papillary conjunctivitis. Eye & Contact Lens 29:S37–S39, 2003.

Donshik PC: External wear contact lenses. Ophthalmol Clinic N Amer 16(3):305–309, 2003.

Donshik PC: Giant papillary conjunctivitis. Trans Am Ophthalmol Soc 92:687–744, 1994.

Driebe WT, Jr: Disposable contact lenses. Surv Ophthalmol 34:44–46, 1989.

Ehlers WH, Donshik PC, Suchecki JK: Disposable and frequent replacement contact lenses. Ophthalmol Clinic N Amer 16(3):341–352, 2003.

Ehlers WH, Donshik PC: Allergic ocular disorders: a spectrum of disease. CLAO J 18:117–124, 1992.

Friedlander MH, Howes J: A double-marked, placebo-controlled evaluation of the efficacy and safety of loteprednol etabonate in the treatment of giant papillary conjunctivitis. Am J Ophthalmol 123:455–464, 1997.

Suchecki JK, Donshik PC, Ehlers WH: Contact lens complications. Ophthalmol Clinic N Amer 116:471–484, 2003.

182 LIGNEOUS CONJUNCTIVITIS 372.10

Romain De Cock, MBChB, FRCS, FRCOphth
Canterbury, England

ETIOLOGY/INCIDENCE

Ligneous conjunctivitis is a rare form of recurrent conjunctival inflammation characterized by the formation of thick membranes and pseudomembranes leading to induration of the lids, which assume a woody or ligneous consistency. Usually bilateral, although often asymmetric, it generally affects infants and young children but may occur at any age. There is a slight female preponderance (1.4 : 1). A familial predisposition has been reported, but most cases are sporadic.

Deposition of membrane may also occur in extraocular mucosal sites such as the respiratory tract, vocal cords, gingiva, middle ear, vagina and cervix.

In several cases homozygous or compound heterozygous mutations in the plasminogen gene with decreased immunoreactive plasminogen antigen and decreased functional plasminogen activity (Type I plasminogen deficiency) have been described. In at least two reports tranexamic acid, an antifibrinolytic agent, has been implicated in the formation of conjunctival and/or gingival membranes. Both ocular and extraocular membranes consist of fibrin thus pointing to a failure of fibrinolysis at various mucosal sites of which the conjunctiva are the most common. Fibrin deposition is initiated by an inflammatory stimulus such as infection or trauma (including surgery to remove the membranes) with hypofibrinolysis leading to accumulation and persistence of the fibrinous membranes.

COURSE/PROGNOSIS

- Variable, with more profound decrease in functional and immunoreactive plasminogen levels possibly accounting for more severe disease.
- May persist for many years without severe discomfort or visual loss.
- Usually chronic irritation, redness, discharge and swelling of the lids.
- Mild secondary corneal involvement in 25% of cases; rarely, severe keratopathy.
- Spontaneous resolution in approximately 10% of patients.
- Possible relapse after a prolonged period of quiescence, often at a time of concurrent febrile systemic illness.

DIAGNOSIS

Clinical signs and symptoms

The condition presents most commonly in infancy or childhood as an acute or a subacute conjunctivitis with membrane and pseudomembrane deposition on the upper tarsal conjunctiva, although the lower tarsal and bulbar conjunctiva may also be affected. The membranes are firmly attached at their base and take on a flattened aspect on the surface due to lid movement and compression between the lid and the globe. A fibrinous pseudomembrane that can be readily removed often overlies the membrane. Excision or stripping of the membrane results in bleeding and rapid reformation of the membranous deposit leading to a chronic conjunctivitis. Corneal involvement with secondary neovascularization, scarring and thinning occurs in as many as 25% of patients, but severe keratopathy, including perforation, is rare now.

A systemic febrile illness, upper respiratory tract infection, or local trauma (including ocular surgery) often precedes the onset of the conjunctivitis and can be associated with relapses of the condition after periods of quiescence.

The deposition of membrane in extraocular mucosal sites may lead to life threatening respiratory obstruction. There is an association with occlusive hydrocephalus which in one case has been shown to be related to a craniocervical anomaly though obstruction of the acqueduct remains another possibility.

Laboratory findings

Histologically, the membranes consist of subepithelial deposits of amorphous hyaline material infiltrated to varying extents with lymphocytes, plasmacytes, neutrophils and eosinophils. The overlying epithelium is generally atrophic, and sometimes absent, with areas of epithelial downgrowth into the hyaline material containing goblet cells and mucus. The hyaline material consistently stains positive for fibrin.

Plasminogen activity and plasminogen antigen levels should be measured in all cases of suspected ligneous conjunctivitis.

Differential diagnosis

- Infective membranous and pseudomembranous conjunctivitis: bacterial, viral and chlamydial.
- Chemical burns.
- Stevens–Johnson syndrome.
- Lyell's syndrome.
- Synthetic fiber granulomatous conjunctivitis ('teddy bear conjunctivitis').
- Factitious conjunctivitis.

TREATMENT

Treatment remains difficult. Surgical excision of the conjunctival membranes and excision followed by cautery, cryopexy, irradiation or grafting with conjunctiva or sclera have proved generally disappointing in the absence of steps to prevent further fibrin deposition. Topical hyaluronidase and alpha-chymotrypsin have given inconsistent results because mucopolysaccharides are not a major feature of ligneous conjunctivitis.

Topical cyclosporin A used in combination with topical steroids has been used successfully in several cases.

The constant presence of fibrin in ligneous conjunctivitis has prompted the use of topical heparin after excision of the membrane to prevent fibrin reaccumulation, together with a topical steroid to reduce inflammation and a topical antibiotic as prophylaxis against infection until conjunctival epithelial cover has been regained. It is essential with this regimen to achieve complete hemostasis with very meticulous cautery after excision of the conjunctival membrane and to *immediately* initiate intensive topical heparin and steroid. Once the epithelium has been reestablished, both the concentration and the frequency of the heparin and steroid drops can be tapered, and the topical antibiotic can be stopped. This regimen is very demanding for both patients and medical staff but has been successful in approximately 75% of patients.

More recent treatment modalities have been directed towards re-establishing fibrinolytic activity after excision of membrane with the use of topical plasminogen derived from fresh frozen plasma initially every 2 hours reducing to four times daily after 3 weeks or when re-epithelialization could be confirmed. Alternatively subconjunctival injection of fresh frozen plasma (1 mL) after excision followed by topical fresh frozen plasma 2 hourly for 3 days then four times daily for 2 weeks has been successfully used in one case.

Intravenous administration of lys-plasminogen has proved to be effective in patients with severe systemic disease but is impractical due to the short half-life of lys-plasminogen.

Estrogen and progestrogen oral contraceptives can elevate plaminogen levels and have been associated with clinical improvement of ligneous conjunctivitis in two cases.

The severity and clinical course of this condition is probably related to the degree of underlying hypofibrinolysis and this may well account for the variable results that have been obtained with different forms of treatment. While the optimal treatment regimen remains to be identified a logical approach is to combine efforts to increase local fibrinolysis with steps to prevent fibrin reformation following excision of membranes.

1. Topical plasminogen (ca. 1 mg/mL) every 2 hours to soften membranes.
2. Excise membrane.
3. Achieve complete hemostasis with cautery.
4. Start 5000 IU/mL topical heparin, 1% prednisolone every 30 minutes to 1 hour, and an antibiotic four times daily.
5. When the epithelium is healed, reduce medications to 1000 IU/mL heparin and 0.5%, 0.3%, and 0.1% prednisolone in gradually decreasing frequency according to the degree of conjunctival inflammation. Reduce topical plasminogen to four times daily for 2–3 weeks.
5. Stop the antibiotic when the epithelium is healed.
6. Take special care to evert the lids for examination very gently so as to keep all microtrauma to a minimum.

Topical ciclosporin and cromoglycate have been successfully used in a few cases; it is possible that they may have a useful role in selected patients in whom the histologic examination confirms abundant lymphocytic or mast cell infiltration, respectively.

REFERENCES

De Cock R, Ficker LA, Dart JG, et al: Topical heparin in the treatment of ligneous conjunctivitis. Ophthalmology 102:1654–1659, 1995.

Heidemann DG, Williams GA, Hartzer M, et al: Treatment of ligneous conjunctvitis with topical plasmin and topical plasminogen. Cornea 22:760–762, 2003.

Hidayat AA, Riddle PJ: Ligneous conjunctivitis: a clinicopathologic study of 17 cases. Ophthalmology 94:949–959, 1987.

Holland EJ, Chan C-C, Kuwabara T, et al: Immunohistologic findings and results of treatment with cyclosporin in ligneous conjunctivitis. Am J Ophthalmol 107:160–166, 1989.

Martinovic E, Ells A: Ligneous conjunctivitis related to a defect in the fibrinolytic system. Can J Ophthalmol 36:147–149, 2001.

Mingers AM, Philapitsch A, Zeitler P, et al: Human homozygous type I plasminogen deficiency and ligneous conjunctivitis. APMIS 107:62–72, 1999.

Schott D, Dempfle C-E, Beck P, et al: Therapy with a purified plasminogen concentrate in an infant with ligneous conjunctivitis and homozygous plasminogen deficiency. NEJM 339:1679–1686, 1998.

Schuster V, Seregard S: Ligneous conjunctivitis. Surv Ophthalmol 48:369–388, 2003.

Schuster V, Zeitler P, Seregard S, et al: Homozygous and compound-heterozygous Type I plasminogen deficiency is a common cause of ligneous conjunctivitis. Thromb-Haemost 85:1004–1010, 2001.

Tabbara KF: Prevention of ligneous conjunctivitis by topical and subconjunctival fresh frozen plasma. Am J Ophthalmol 138:299–300, 2004.

Watts P, Suresh P, Mezer E, et al: Effective treatment of ligneous conjunctivitis with topical plasminogen. Am J Ophthalmol 133:451–455, 2002.

183 OPHTHALMIA NEONATORUM 771.6

William V. Good, MD
San Francisco, California
Irene T. Tung, BA
Houston, Texas

DEFINITION

Ophthalmia neonatorum is the traditional term used to indicate conjunctivitis in the newborn period. However, the World Health Organization prefers the more descriptive 'conjunctivitis of the newborn' in its communications. With an incidence perhaps as high as 18%, conjunctivitis of the newborn is one of the leading causes of infections in infants. In many cases, the etiology is viral or a low-grade bacterial pathogen, but in some cases, vision-threatening infections can occur. Many variables are responsible for the pathogen, including maternal infection (e.g. herpes simplex conjunctivitis, chlamydia and gonococcal conjunctivitis) and geographic location of the infant and family. In this chapter we describe clinical manifestations of various conjunctivitis entities, their timing of onset, laboratory investigations and treatment.

Signs and symptoms

In most cases, the signs and symptoms of conjunctivitis are non-specific. Timing of onset can offer a rough guide to possible etiologies. Signs of conjunctivitis in the first few days of life are often caused by antibiotic or silver nitrate toxicity. Both may be used to prevent conjunctivitis of the newborn. Gonococcal

(GC) disease appears in the first several days of life, and is often characterized by an extremely purulent discharge. *Chlamydia* infection appears between 5 and 20 days of life and manifests a less serious appearing presentation. Other pathogens can produce disease at any point in the first months of the infant's life.

Ophthalmic physical findings are often not helpful in distinguishing these various etiologies. The infant usually fails to develop a conjunctival follicular reaction, due to the immaturity of its immune system. Such a follicular reaction might otherwise be helpful in distinguishing viral and chlamydial infections from bacterial disease. Preauricular lymph nodes also fail to occur, for similar reasons. Such nodes are associated with viral and chlamydial pathogens, and occasionally with GC infections. As noted above, a strongly purulent reaction often indicates GC disease.

Laboratory studies

Since gonococcal disease can threaten vision, every case of conjunctivitis of the newborn should be investigated with lab studies. A Gram stain should be performed on a swab taken from the palpebral conjunctiva. When intracellular, gram-negative diplococci are noted, the infant should be treated for gonococcal disease. Gram-negative coccobacilli may indicate *Haemophilus influenzae*, but gram-positive cultures do not necessarily indicate the presence of *Staphylococcus* or *Streptococcus* species. Finding white blood cells on the smear is a general guide to the presence of an infection, since these are not normally present on the conjunctival surface.

Chlamydia infection can be identified with a McCoy cell culture, a Giemsa stain, or polymerase chain reaction (PCR). Cultures for chlamydia are negative frequently enough in the presence of disease, that additional tests are usually indicated. PCR is probably a more sensitive method for detecting *Chlamydia*. The Giemsa stain, which is highly sensitive and specific in adult chlamydial conjunctivitis, is not as sensitive in infants. In the Giemsa stain, intracytoplasmic inclusion bodies are identified in conjunctival swabs.

PCR becomes negative several weeks after systemic treatment for chlamydia, and can be used to monitor treatment response.

VIRAL CONJUNCTIVITIS

Viral pathogens such as adenovirus seen in adult conjunctivitis rarely occur in infants, with the exception of herpes simplex virus (HSV). HSV presents with vesicles around the eye. Culture of fluid from a vesicle will yield the virus, but the clinical presentation is typical enough, that systemic antiviral treatment is warranted to prevent or treat possible disseminated disease, and to treat local manifestations of the disease. We also advocate the use of topical antiviral treatment, even though there is no definitive evidence favoring its use. It is prudent to attempt to prevent infection of the infant's conjunctiva by administering viroptic.

CHLAMYDIAL CONJUNCTIVITIS

Chlamydia trachomatis is surprisingly common, occurring in close to 0.5% of all newborn children in the Western world. Left untreated, this pathogen can, over the course of many months, cause a micropannus and scarring of the palpebral conjunctiva. This, in turn, can lead to entropion with its potential risks to the ocular surface. Palpebral scarring and pannus formation are quite uncommon, but a more compelling reason for recognizing a chlamydial conjunctivitis is the fact that a significant number of infants develop chlamydial pneumonia in the months following birth. The presence of chlamydia conjunctivitis indicates risk for pneumonia infection.

Therefore, once the diagnosis is established, the infant should be treated with oral erythromycin. The dose is 50 mg/kg/day, given in four divided doses, for 2 weeks. Systemic treatment is more effective at eradicating conjunctivitis than topical treatment, although most infants should also be managed with topical erythromycin or tetracycline. In cases that relapse, an additional systemic course of erythromycin is warranted.

GONOCOCCAL CONJUNCTIVITIS (GC)

In developing countries, this pathogen is particularly common. In the Western world, cases of gonococcal conjunctivitis are very uncommon. GC can cause a significant keratitis in newborn children and adults, so prompt identification and treatment are paramount.

Once GC is identified, treatment consists of systemic, third-generation cephalosporins, because so many GC isolates are resistant to penicillin. A single dose of ceftriaxone (25–50 mg/kg) is sufficient to prevent GC conjunctivitis when maternal infection is known, but must be accompanied by topical treatment in known conjunctivitis. Topical treatment takes the form of lavaging the eyes on an hourly basis with sterile saline. Topical antibiotics are also indicated. If keratitis develops, very close monitoring of the corneal integrity is indicated, as perforations can occur. Opacification of the cornea, and even perforation managed successfully with keratoplasty, are highly amblyogenic, necessitating ongoing surveillance and treatment for amblyopia. Mothers and fathers should be screened for GC and treated when disease is present.

NASOLACRIMAL DUCT OBSTRUCTION

In any case of mild unilateral or bilateral eye discharge, nasolacrimal duct obstruction (NLDO) should be considered. Ironically, NLDO often presents several weeks after birth, because lacrimal gland function is less active in the days and weeks after birth. Thus, in the absence of significant aqueous tear production, signs of NLDO usually do not appear.

A number of signs and symptoms can be used to distinguish NLDO from conjunctivitis of the newborn. Later onset, persistent tearing without discharge, negative cultures and swabs, and refractory symptoms all point to NLDO. Most children with NLDO improve spontaneously, requiring topical treatment only when a conjunctivitis is superimposed on the problem of NLDO. After 9 months of age, when significant tearing and/or discharge is present, probing the tear duct should be considered.

OTHER CAUSES OF CONJUNCTIVITIS OF THE NEWBORN

The above more serious causes of conjunctivitis notwithstanding, most cases of conjunctivitis of the newborn are caused by less pathogenic organisms. *Staphylococcus aureus* is most common, but other species such as *Streptococcus pneumoniae*, *Staphylococcus epidermidis*, *Escherichia coli* and *Pseudomonas aeruginosa* may cause conjunctivitis. Cultures for conjunctivitis are negative in a significant number of cases. Given the array of possible pathogens, a broad-spectrum antibiotic should be used to manage conjunctivitis when an etiology cannot be ascertained.

PREVENTION OF CONJUNCTIVITIS OF THE NEWBORN

The best treatment for conjunctivitis of the newborn is prevention. Avoidance of inoculation is a mainstay of prevention, and takes the form of C-section when maternal infection with a sexually transmitted disease is identified. This is especially true in the case of maternal herpes simplex infection, where C-section should be performed. Ironically, the incidence of conjunctivitis of the newborn is the same in vaginal delivery compared to C-section. This fact indicates that most cases of conjunctivitis are mild and are acquired after birth.

Prophylactic treatment for conjunctivitis of the newborn is effective in preventing conjunctivitis, particularly GC. A drop of 2% silver nitrate placed on each eye was the mainstay of treatment until recently. This treatment was introduced by Crede in 1881 and frequently is referred to as 'Crede prophylaxis.' Silver nitrate has the disadvantage of occasionally causing a non-infectious (chemical) conjunctivitis.

Topical erythromycin or tetracycline is also effective at preventing conjunctivitis, and has replaced silver nitrate in many regions. Povidone-iodine (one drop in each eye) is also effective, and has the advantage of being inexpensive. This treatment has not been approved in the United States, but could assume importance in developing regions.

Other, milder, causes of conjunctivitis are not always prevented with prophylactic therapy. Chlamydia, too, may not be successfully managed with topical treatment. This raises the question: should prophylaxis be administered in infants whose mothers received good prenatal care? The assumption is that good prenatal care is associated with low risk of sexually transmitted disease, and remains an open question. In some areas, parents are offered the option of not having their infant receive prophylactic treatment, based on the above issues.

Use of other sterile prep solutions as prophylaxis should be avoided. Hibiclens (chlorhexidine) in particular is potentially toxic to the cornea, and can cause corneal ulceration and opacification.

REFERENCES

Crede C: Reports from the obstetrical clinic in Leipzig: prvention of eye infection in the newborn. Archives of Gynaekol 17:50–53, 1881.

Dannevig L, Straume B, Melby K: Ophthalmia neonatorum in northern Norway. II. Microbiology with emphasis on *Chlamydia trachomatis*. Acta Ophthalmol (Copenh) 70(1):19–25, 1992.

Fransen L, Klauss V: Neonatal ophthalmia in the developing world. Epidemiology, etiology, management and control. Int Ophthalmol 11(3):189–196, 1988.

Fredricks S: Hibiclens and eye damage. Plast Reconstr Surg 81(3):472, 1988.

Harrison HR, et al: *Chlamydia trachomatis* infant pneumonitis: comparison with matched controls and other infant pneumonitis. N Engl J Med 298(13):702–708, 1978.

Isenberg SJ, Apt L, Wood M: A controlled trial of povidone-iodine as prophylaxis against ophthalmia neonatorum. N Engl J Med 332(9):562–566, 1995.

Murthy S, Hawksworth NR, Cree I: Progressive ulcerative keratitis related to the use of topical chlorhexidine gluconate (0.02%). Cornea 21(2):237–239, 2002.

Schwab L, Tizazu T: Destructive epidemic *Neisseria gonorrheae* keratoconjunctivitis in African adults. Br J Ophthalmol 69(7):525–528, 1985.

Talley AR, et al: Comparative diagnosis of neonatal chlamydial conjunctivitis by polymerase chain reaction and McCoy cell culture. Am J Ophthalmol 117(1):50–57, 1994.

Zanoni D, Isenberg SJ, Apt L: A comparison of silver nitrate with erythromycin for prophylaxis against ophthalmia neonatorum. Clin Pediatr (Phila) 31(5):295–298, 1992.

184 PTERYGIUM AND PSEUDOPTERYGIUM 372.40

Larry F. Rich, MS, MD
Portland, Oregon

A pterygium is a triangular elevated mass of thickened bulbar conjunctiva that extends onto the cornea in the interpalpebral zone. Its name is derived from the Greek word for 'wing,' which describes its characteristic shape. Within the interpalpebral fissure, a pterygium is most commonly found on the nasal aspect of the globe and less often found on the temporal aspect. If present outside the interpalpebral fissure area, it is considered an atypical pterygium, and other diagnoses, such as phlyctenular keratoconjunctivitis or carcinoma, must be considered (Figure 184.1).

A pseudopterygium is similar in appearance to a true pterygium, but it bridges the limbus such that a probe can be passed beneath the lesion at the limbus. It often is the result of damage to the cornea from a chemical, thermal, or physical insult. Pseudopterygium is more likely to occur in atypical locations (e.g. outside the interpalpebral fissure area) than a true pterygium is. As with a true pterygium, recurrences are more aggressive than the primary lesion.

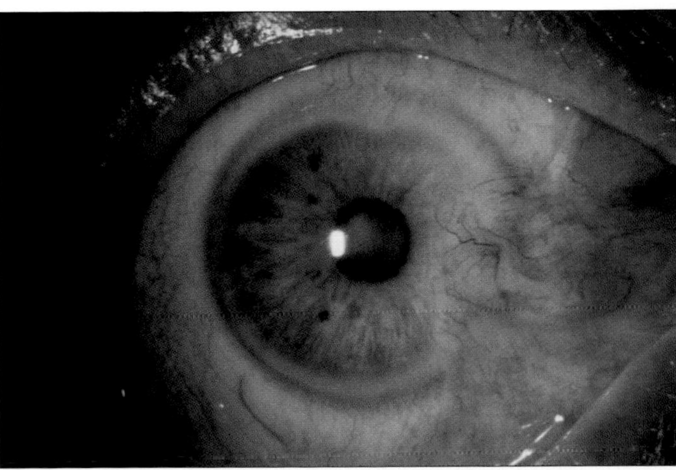

FIGURE 184.1. Pterygium extending 3 millimeters with moderate vascularity.

ETIOLOGY/INCIDENCE

Environment and heredity are thought to play important roles in the pathogenesis of pterygium. Its incidence is higher in tropical or subtropical areas of the world and in individuals frequently exposed to sunlight, airborne allergens, wind, dust, fumes, or other noxious stimuli. Frequently, a pinguecula precedes the pterygium. The elevated conjunctival tissue may lead to tear film defects and may form dellen (Fuchs' dimples) or an area of dryness in the adjacent tissue. Inflammation and vascularization are thereby initiated, and the patient may have symptoms of irritation or itching. Recurrent episodes of exposure may irritate the mass of tissue, enlarge it, and produce other dellen, which continue the advancement. Eventually, the lesion grows beyond the limbus, invades the cornea, grows into or beyond the visual axis, and may result in blindness.

There is evidence that basic fibroblast growth factor may play a role in pterygium growth. In addition, mutation of the *p53* gene, which is sensitive to ultraviolet radiation, has been found in pingueculae and pterygia.

COURSE/PROGNOSIS

- The rate of pterygium growth is variable.
- The size of the original lesion may play a role in the probability of recurrence. A large, fleshy, vascularized primary pterygium with inflammation indicates activity and should not be approached surgically until the inflammation has been minimized.
- Large pterygia require more extensive surgery, which produces greater injury to underlying and surrounding tissue than occurs when smaller lesions are removed.
- Serial photography is useful in following the course of growth.
- Primary excision of a pterygium is followed by recurrence in 40% to 50% of patients.
- Recurrent pterygium is more difficult to treat and is more likely to recur after a second excision than a primary pterygium.

DIAGNOSIS

- The history of growth of the mass is essential.
- Family history can be contributory.
- A history of exposure to sunlight without eye protection is common.
- Diagnosis is usually made on examination.
- Pterygia in the interpalpebral zone induce with-the-rule astigmatism.
- Corneal topography may reveal localized flattening central to the pterygium apex.

Differential diagnosis

- Pannus.
- Phlyctenule.
- Limbal tumors.
- Melanoma.
- Squamous cell carcinoma.
- Papilloma.
- Intraepithelial epithelioma.
- Fibrous histiocytoma.
- Dermoid.

PROPHYLAXIS

When outdoors, the patient should wear sunglasses or protective goggles with ultraviolet blocking tint. Occlusive goggles are of additional value in dusty, windy environments. If a patient has a known sensitivity to an airborne allergen and anticipates exposure, systemic antihistamines before exposure may prevent an allergic response. Once the response has occurred, however, antihistamines are of little value.

TREATMENT

Supportive

Unless the patient specifically requests surgery, it is best to avoid intervention and limit treatment to medical modalities. Advice can be given to help minimize the progression of the pterygium. Specifically, protection against sunlight and dryness is important. Episodes of irritation should be treated with topical lubricants, such as artificial tears or ointments; if inflammation and edema occur, a mild vasoconstrictor drop may prevent elevation and dellen formation. The patient must be warned, however, to use vasoconstrictor drops as infrequently as possible to avoid dependance. Punctal occlusion may ameliorate the symptoms of dryness, retard the progression of the pterygium, or both. Mild corticosteroids, such as medrysone, can be prescribed for short-term use. More potent steroids, particularly those with good ocular penetration, should be avoided if possible to minimize the complications associated with corticosteroid use. Topical nonsteroidal anti-inflammatory eyedrops may be useful for the treatment of inflamed pterygia.

Surgical

Surgical intervention is indicated when the patient requests removal of the pterygium for cosmetic reasons, the progression of the lesion threatens vision, or symblepharon limits ocular motility. If none of these indications exist, it is best to treat the pterygium medically because if the pterygium recurs after surgery, it often is worse than the primary lesion.

There are multiple surgical techniques for the removal of pterygium. Avulsion of the head of the pterygium from the cornea may be possible if the lesion is attached loosely. This technique has the advantage of being relatively noninvasive to corneal tissue. Leaving a smooth area with little or no removal of corneal and limbal tissue may lessen the chances of recurrence. Many surgeons smooth the base of the cornea where the pterygium had been removed by using a diamond bur or scalpel blade. If the pterygium is firmly attached and cannot be avulsed from the cornea, a delimiting keratotomy with partial lamellar keratectomy will aid in removal. This procedure is best done under an operating microscope to minimize removal of corneal tissue and to avoid perforation into the anterior chamber. Once the head of the pterygium has been removed from the cornea and dissection has been carried beyond the limbus, its body should be excised while avoiding the insertion of the medial rectus muscle. Some surgeons prefer to remove as little as possible of the body of the pterygium and attach the cut ends of conjunctiva to the sclera or to each other. Other surgeons prefer to leave the sclera bare. The control of bleeding is essential and all feeder vessels should be cauterized.

Local anesthesia is preferred over general anesthesia unless the patient is unable to cooperate or is extremely anxious about ocular surgery. Subconjunctival injection of lidocaine without hyaluronidase is preferred. Epinephrine may be added to the anesthetic agent to inhibit bleeding. A topical anesthetic, such as cocaine, also may be used to prevent pain when the eye is grasped in an area other than where the lidocaine had been injected. Occasionally, retrobulbar anesthesia is necessary if the patient is unable to control ocular movements; in such patients, akinesia of the eyelids may also be necessary.

After the lesion has been excised, it is wise to submit it to the pathologist for evaluation. Occasionally, malignancies may mimic a pterygium; in these cases, surgery may stimulate growth.

Several adjunctive measures lower the recurrence rate after pterygium excision, but each has significant drawbacks. Strontium-90 β-irradiation, applied to the limbus and the adjacent sclera in divided doses totaling 1800 to 2200 rads, decreases the rate of recurrence. However, significant complications may occur, including scleral necrosis, infection, and cataract. Triethylene thiophosphoramide (thiotepa) applied as eyedrops four to six times daily for 6 to 8 weeks after surgery also decreases the probability of recurrence, but depigmentation of the skin and eyelashes around the treated eye limits its use, particularly in dark-skinned individuals. More recently, mitomycin-C administered as 0.01% to 0.04% solution intraoperatively or 0.02% to 0.04% eyedrops b.i.d. for 5 to 14 days postoperatively has been advocated. Recurrence rates between 0% and 11% have been reported, but serious, potentially blinding complications such as scleral and corneal ulcers with perforation, glaucoma, sudden onset of cataract, corneal edema, and uveitis have occurred. If treatment with mitomycin-C is chose, it is best applied to the excision site with a sponge at the time of surgery rather than dispensing the drug as eyedrops postoperatively.

If symblepharon is present or the remaining conjunctiva is insufficient to permit adequate ocular motility, an amniotic membrane, mucous membrane or conjunctival graft may be needed to cover the bare area. Recurrence rates following the use of amniotic membrane transplantation, however, are disappointingly high. A conjunctival graft may be used from the same or the fellow eye and preferably is taken from a vicinity outside the interpalpebral fissure area. Autologous conjunctival grafting may be superior to adjunctive antimetabolite therapy at preventing recurrence and often provides a significantly better cosmetic result and a much lower incidence of complications. A conjunctival graft incorporating peripheral corneal epithelial stem cells may be of additional value toward prevention of recurrence. It is becoming the treatment of choice for recurrent pterygium.

Corneoscleral grafts with or without mucous membrane or conjunctival grafts have been advocated in cases of recurrent pterygium. Their use is advised in cases in which the limbal architecture has been disturbed by one or more surgical interventions. They are best accomplished with partial-thickness grafts incorporating corneal and scleral donor tissue in the same configuration as the tissue resected from the recipient eye. The grafted area can be trephined or cut freehanded, and the donor tissue is similarly dissected to fit the outline. If corneal and scleral tissue is used, it can be incorporated as a single graft to maintain the architecture of the limbal sulcus. A clear corneal graft that bridges the limbus has also been advocated, but it has the disadvantage of producing a single contour without providing a limbal sulcus. A corneal graft alone is likely to allow vascularization at the graft-host interface, so it is probably best to avoid leaving the edge of the graft at the limbus. Grafting is necessary if multiple excisions have left the corneal tissue thin and perforation or ocular weakness is imminent.

COMPLICATIONS

- The surgical process and the pterygium itself destroy limbal tissue and predispose the eye to recurrence of the lesion. In addition, the elevation of conjunctiva and the irregular corneal and limbal tissue resulting from surgery may reinitiate the pathologic process of localized dryness, vascularization, and regrowth. Furthermore, an acute inflammatory process after surgery may produce granulation tissue that can contract and stimulate conjunctivalization of the limbus and cornea. Excessive postoperative inflammation and irritation from exposure during the early postoperative period encourage regrowth. Recurrences may be seen as early as 2 weeks or several years after excision.
- Symblepharon formation can occur with or without surgical therapy.
- Temporal displacement of the semilunar fold can occur.
- Astigmatism (with-the-rule) can occur.
- Restriction of ocular motility can occur.
- Diplopia is a possible complication.

COMMENTS

Each surgical intervention can produce a greater cosmetic blemish and a more difficult management situation than the previous lesion. A pterygium is more likely to return after a recurrence than after removal of a primary lesion. Symblepharon is often a sequela of pterygium surgery; restriction of ocular motility and pain with extraocular movements, particularly abduction of the globe, may result.

REFERENCES

Bahrassa F, Datta R: Postoperative beta radiation treatment of pterygium. Int J Rad Oncol Biol Phys 9:679–684, 1983.

Chen PP, Ariyasu RG, Kaza V, et al: A randomized trial comparing mitomycin-C and conjunctival autograft after excision of primary pterygium. Am J Ophthalmol 120:151–160, 1995.

Ehrlich D: The management of pterygium. Ophthalmic Surg 8:23–30, 1977.

Gris O, Guell JL, delCampo Z: Limbal-conjunctival autograft transplantation for the treatment of recurrent pterygium. Ophthalmology 107(2):270–273, 2000.

Jurgenliemk-Schulz IM, Hartman LJC, Roesink JM, et al: Prevention of pterygium recurrence by postoperative single-dose β-irradiation: a prospective randomized clinical double-blind trial. Int J Rad Oncol Biol Phys 59:1138–1147, 2004.

Kleis W, Pico G: Thio-tepa therapy to prevent postoperative pterygium occurrence and neovascularization. Am J Ophthalmol 76:371–373, 1973.

Manning CA, Kloess PM, Diaz MD, et al: Intraoperative mitomycin in primary pterygium excision: a prospective, randomized trial. Ophthalmology 104:844–848, 1997.

Rubinfeld RS, Pfister RR, Stein RM, et al: Serious complications of topical mitomycin-C after pterygium surgery. Ophthalmology 99:1647–1654, 1992.

Singh G, Wilson MR, Foster CS: Long-term follow-up study of mitomycin eyedrops as adjunctive treatment for pterygia and its comparison with conjunctival autograft transplantation. Cornea 9:331–334, 1990.

Tananuvat N, Martin T: The results of amniotic membrane transplantation for primary pterygium compared with conjunctival autograft. Cornea 23(5):458–463, 2004.

Tarr KH, Constable IJ: Late complications of pterygium treatment. Br J Ophthalmol 64:496–505, 1980.

Vastine DW, Stewart WB, Schwab IR: Reconstruction of the periocular mucous membrane by autologous conjunctival transplantation. Ophthalmology 89:1072–1081, 1982.

Young AL, Leung GYS, Wong AKK, et al: A randomised trial comparing 0.02% mitomycin C and limbal conjunctival autograft after excision of primary pterygium. Br J Ophthalmol 88:995–997, 2004.

185 VERNAL KERATOCONJUNCTIVITIS 370.40

Russell Pokroy, MD
Rehovot, Israel

ETIOLOGY/INCIDENCE

Vernal keratoconjunctivitis (VKC) is a bilateral chronic and often severe allergic conjunctivitis. For many years, VKC was considered a classic type I hypersensitivity reaction (soley IgE-mediated) with an immunopathogenetic mechanism similar to seasonal allergic conjunctivitis (see Ch. 176). This was supported by the high prevalence of personal or family history of atopy (asthma, rhinitis and eczema), positive skin tests, positive radioallergosorbent tests and high serum IgE. However, Bonini and others have reported large patient series with almost 50% of VKC patients negative for the above IgE-related factors. Based on recent immune studies, non-IgE Th2-driven mechanisms were shown to be central to VKC. Today, VKC is considered a multifactorial disease with specific (IgE- and Th2-mediated) and non-specific (sun, dust and wind) immune mechanisms, manifesting as an allergic inflammatory disease of the conjunctiva and cornea.

Vernal means spring and youth, representing the usual age and season of presentation, although many cases continue into the summer and throughout the year. Typically, VKC begins in prepubertal boys (around 8 years) in warm dry climates like the Middle East, Mediterranean area, India and West Africa. Associated atopy is present in half to two-thirds of patients. Male predominance (around 75%) before age 10 is not evident at the age of 20.

COURSE/PROGNOSIS

The initial years often show seasonal variation, with signs and symptoms being more severe during the spring and summer. Patients suffering for longer than 3 years, especially those with giant papillae or fibrosis, tend to lose their seasonal variation. In 2000 Bonini et al, in a long-term follow-up study on 151 patients, showed that 16% of patients with a mean disease duration of 3 years, evolved into chronic, perennial VKC.

This study also showed that worsening or persistence of the disease could be predicted by the papillary size (>1 mm) and form (limbal worse than tarsal). These authors suggest that papillary size may be a reflection of the intensity and chronicity of the allergic reaction, with subsequent activation of conjunctival fibroblasts, resulting in disease persistence.

The prognosis of VKC is usually good, with >80%, especially boys, resolving by the late teens or early 20 s. Typically, there is no residual conjunctival scarring unless the disease was severe with persistent giant papillae or was treated with surgery or cryotherapy.

DIAGNOSIS

The diagnosis of VKC is usually clinical. Giant papillae on the upper tarsus or limbus in a young patient and itch are the hallmarks (Figures 185.1 and 185.2). Laboratory testing is seldom necessary for diagnosis.

Clinical signs and symptoms

The most common symptoms are itching, photophobia, mucous discharge and tearing. Conjunctival hyper-reactivity, manifesting as conjunctival redness on exposure to sun, dust and wind, is common.

The most common signs are giant cobblestone (flat-topped) papillae, usually on the upper tarsus (see Figure 185.1) marked conjunctival hyperemia and superficial keratopathy. Signs are bilateral, although they may be asymmetric. VKC does not cause preauricular lymphadenopathy.

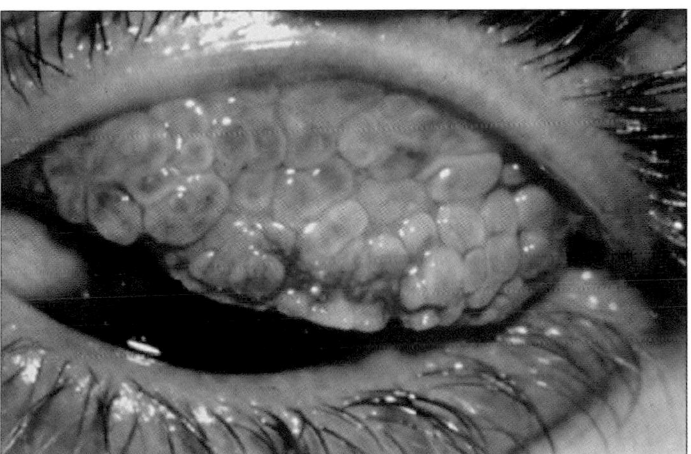

FIGURE 185.1. Giant papillae demonstrating the typical cobblestone (flat-topped) appearance of the upper tarsal conjunctiva.

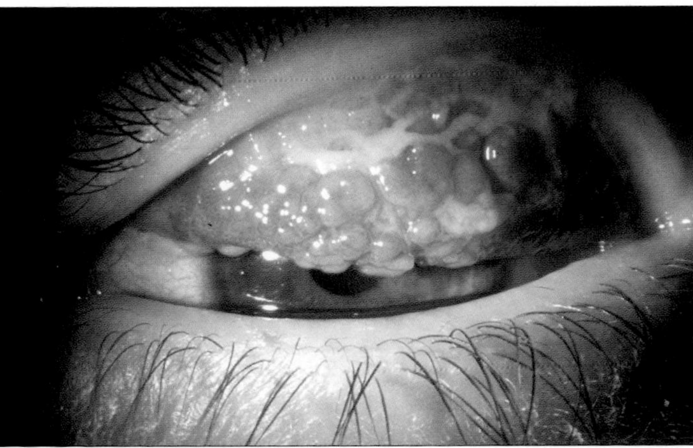

FIGURE 185.2. Maxwell–Lyons sign.

Eyelid signs include long and thick eyelashes, the mechanism of which is not fully understood. Ptosis may occur in active VKC. Blepharospasm suggests corneal involvement and potentially more severe disease.

Tarsal conjunctival signs, in addition to those mentioned above, include the Maxwell-Lyons sign, a milky coating of fibrinous exudate over the cobblestone papillae that is enhanced by the heat of the slit lamp. Tarsal conjunctival fibrosis is the natural evolution of severe giant papillae. Unlike atopic keratoconjunctivitis, most cases of VKC resolve without tarsal conjunctival scarring.

Bulbar or limbal VKC occurs in about 20% of Mediterranean series and is commoner in patients of African and Asian origin. Usually the superior limbus is more affected. Horner–Trantas' dots (aggregates of epithelial cells and eosinophils at the limbus) occur in approximately 15% of active VKC.

Epithelial keratopathy is very common and results from epithelial toxicity due to the release of eosinophilic major basic protein. Corneal shield ulcer, a vision threatening complication occurring in 3–11% of VKC, is characteristically a shallow, transversely oval, de-epithelialized area, located in the superior cornea. Mucous and epithelial cell plaque often cover the ulcer base. The surrounding epithelium is smooth and grayish. Superficial peripheral corneal vascularization is common in longstanding cases.

Laboratory findings

Usually, the signs and symptoms are characteristic enough to make the diagnosis without laboratory tests. Conjunctival cytology scrapings are usually positive for eosinophils and free eosinophilic granules. Other immune tests have low sensitivites (negative in >50%) and are therefore not clinically useful for diagnosis of VKC. These include activated eosinophils in conjunctival biopsies, total and specific serum IgE and skin tests. In 2003, Pucci et al showed a positive correlation between giant papillae score and serum eosinophil response, independent of IgE-sensitization, and found serum eosinophil cationic protein to be a useful laboratory marker of disease activity. Limbal VKC has an even lower prevalence of IgE-sensitization than tarsal forms.

Differential diagnosis

- Seasonal and perennial allergic conjunctivitis.
- Atopic keratoconjunctivitis.
- Giant papillary conjunctivitis associated with contact lens wear.
- Giant papillae on the tarsal conjunctiva secondary to an exposed ocular suture or ocular prosthesis.
- Ligneous conjunctivitis may occasionally be confused with large cobblestone papillae in young patients.
- Toxic conjunctivitis secondary to chronic use of ophthalmic preparations: may result in bulbar follicles that may mimic limbal changes. Unlike VKC, the signs are more pronounced inferiorly.

TREATMENT

Because VKC usually resolves without scarring or permanent loss of vision once the disease burns out, treatment should be as conservative as possible to achieve symptomatic relief, prevent structural damage to the ocular surface that may reduce vision, and minimize any iatrogenic complications.

Nonspecific

Although relocating to a cool moist climate is often effective, this is usually impractical. Concurrent blepharitis and dry eye should be treated.

Systemic

Oral antihistamines (e.g. loratidine) and oral nonsteroidal anti-inflammatory drugs (NSAIDs) may be useful in mild to moderate cases: the earlier for generalized hyper-reactivity and the latter for the inflammatory aspect of VKC. Oral prednisone 10 mg/day for 3–5 days in a 10-year-old child may be very useful in refractory VKC with corneal damage.

Ocular

Cold compresses decrease itching by reducing superficial vasodilatation and c-fiber stimulation. Artificial tears dilute antigens and immunogenic factors. Refrigerating artificial tears further improves their soothing effect.

Topical vasoconstrictors, such as naphazoline, should be restricted to t.i.d. for only a few days as rebound hyperemia is likely with longer use. Topical antihistamines and H_1 antagonists have a rapid onset but short duration. Levocabastine (Livostin) and emedastine (Emadine) may be used 1–4 times daily for long periods. Newer antihistamines (H_1 blockers) such as olopatadine (Patanol) also have mast cell-stabilizing properties. Topical NSAIDs, such as ketorolac (Acular), may provide symptomatic relief of itching. Their steroid sparing capability in VKC is yet to be determined. In the presence of any degree of keratitis, vasoconstrictors, antihistamines and NSAIDs alone are inadequate.

Mast cell stabilizers, such as cromolyn (Opticrom, Crolom), lodoxamide (Alomide), nedocromil (Alocril) and pemirolast (Alamast) are the mainstay of therapy for most cases of VKC. Although more severe cases require short courses of topical steroids to control the inflammation, mast cell stabilizers have prophylactic use during quieter phases of the disease and enable steroid sparing. Unpreserved solutions are preferable for long-term use.

Topical corticosteroids are the most effective therapy for VKC, especially with active keratopathy. Steroids inhibit epithelial toxic mediator biosynthesis by eosinophils and neutrophils, thus reversing corneal epithelial damage. Refractory symptoms, cobblestone papillae, limbal thickening, and shield ulcers are indications for steroid use. However, use should be strictly limited as prolonged use may cause cataract, increased intraocular pressure, and superinfection. High frequency intermittent (pulse) therapy (e.g. 2-hourly for 3–5 days) is effective and minimizes steroid complications. The steroid potency, such as 0.1% fluorometholone, 0.2% loteprednol or 1% prednisolone acetate, should be titrated against the severity of the inflammation. Patients and family members should be thoroughly educated regarding steroid complications.

Topical cyclosporin A 2% in olive oil was shown by Pucci et al in a randomized clinical trial to be effective in severe VKC. Most of the therapeutic effect was achieved within 2 weeks. Besides mild irritation on instillation, no ocular or systemic complications were seen. Cyclosporin A binds to cyclophilin, an intracellular protein, inhibiting interleukin-2 production and blocking Th2 lymphocyte proliferation. It also appears to decrease eosinophil recruitment and conjunctival fibroblast proliferation. Effective doses range from 2–4 times/day for 2–16 weeks. There is no need to check systemic blood levels.

Surgical

Supratarsal injection of steroids is useful in cases refractory to pulsed topical steroids, with non-healing shield ulcers. Dexamethasone, triamcinolone and hydrocortisone are equally effective. Surgical removal of a plaque in the base of a vernal ulcer preventing re-epithelialization, by scraping the base and margins, may promote healing.

Surgical excision, cryotherapy and beta-irradiation of giant papillae of the superior tarsus have been described. These procedures are not recommended as marked scarring and distortion of the upper eyelid often results.

COMPLICATIONS

Up to 6–10% of cases have a complication that causes visual impairment. Complications may be due to the disease itself (corneal vascularization and scarring after shield ulcers) or due to steroid use (cataract and glaucoma). In addition, keratoconus may be a late complication of VKC.

COMMENTS

Mild VKC responds well to topical antiallergics, especially mast cell stabilizers and usually resolves within 2–10 years with no ocular surface scarring. Severe VKC (giant papillae >1 mm or limbal forms) has fibrosis of the ocular surface, supposedly due to a Th2 lymphocyte driven mechanism, and requires steroid treatment. Continual effort to limit steroid side effects is necessary, such as mast cell stabilizers and cyclosporin A use.

REFERENCES

Bielory L: Update on ocular allergy therapy. Expert Opin Pharmacother 3:541–553, 2002.

Bonini S, Bonini S, Lambiase A, et al: Vernal keratoconjunctivitis revisited: a case series of 195 patients with long-term followup. Ophthalmology 107:1157–1163, 2000.

Bonini S, Coassin M, Aronni S, Lambiase A: Vernal keratoconjunctivitis. Eye 18:345–351, 2004.

Cameron JA: Shield ulcers and plaques of the cornea in vernal keratoconjunctivitis. Ophthalmology 103:985–993, 1995.

Holsclaw DS, Whitcher JP, Wong IG, Margolis TP: Supratarsal injection of corticosteroid in the treatment of refractory vernal keratoconjunctivitis. Am J Ophthalmol 121:243–249, 1996.

Pucci N, Novembre E, Cianferoni A, et al: Efficacy and safety of cyclosporine eyedrops in vernal keratoconjunctivitis.Ann Allergy Asthma Immunol 89:298–303, 2002.

Pucci N, Novembre E, Lombardi E, et al: Atopy and serum eosinophil cationic protein in 110 white children with vernal keratoconjunctivitis: differences between tarsal and limbal forms. Clin Exp Allergy 33:325–330, 2003.

SECTION

19 Cornea

186 BACTERIAL CORNEAL ULCERS 370.00 *(Bacterial Keratitis)*

Irina S. Barequet, MD
Tel Hashomer, Israel

Bacterial infection of the cornea is a sight-threatening process. Corneal ulceration, stromal abscess formation, and anterior segment inflammation are features of the disease. A particular feature of bacterial keratitis is its rapid progression; corneal destruction may be complete in 24 to 48 hours. Less pathogenic bacteria may induce a slower disease process than that induced by virulent fungi. The suspicion of an infective process demands careful microbiologic assessment. Commonly, predisposing factors exist, such as contact lens wear (especially overnight wear), trauma, contaminated ocular medications, impaired defense mechanism, or altered ocular surface.

ETIOLOGY/INCIDENCE

- Pathogenic gram-positive cocci, principally *Staphylococcus aureus* and *Streptococcus pneumoniae*.
- Aerobic gram-negative bacilli, principally *Pseudomonas aeruginosa*, *Haemophilus influenzae* and *Moraxella* spp.
- Various enteric gram-negative bacilli.
- Colonization by normal skin flora, most commonly coagulase-negative staphylococci, viridans streptococci, and corynebacteria.

About 30,000 (10 in 100,000) Americans develop bacterial keratitis annually. Bacterial keratitis is a leading cause of corneal blindness in developing countries, usually caused by trauma, but the incidence is unclear.

COURSE/PROGNOSIS

In many cases, bacterial infection of the cornea results in irreversible structural alteration. This compromises the visual outcome due to stromal scarring and irregular astigmatism. Infections caused by *P. aeruginosa* generally have a relatively poor outcome. Infections with *S. aureus* or *S. pneumoniae* typically leave a more focal, scarred area. About two thirds of patients retain vision of 20/200 or better after bacterial keratitis. In some cases, corneal transplantation for visual rehabilitation may be considered.

DIAGNOSIS

Clinical signs and symptoms

Patients with bacterial keratitis usually present with an abrupt onset of pain, redness, decreased vision and photophobia. Findings usually include stromal suppurative inflammation with indistinct edges, a defect in the overlying epithelium, and stromal edema around the infiltrate. An anterior chamber reaction or hypopyon can occur. Less virulent bacteria can cause a nonsuppurative infiltrate with intact epithelium.

Laboratory findings

When bacterial keratitis is suspected, microbiological diagnostic tests should be considered prior to treatment initiation. Large or progressive corneal ulcers, or ulcers not responding to treatment should always undergo laboratory investigation to identify and confirm the causal organism.

Specimen collection

Direct plating performed in a clinic with access to a microbiology service is preferred to sending a swab to an off-site facility. If local anesthesia is necessary, preservative-free drops are recommended. The advancing borders of the lesion are scraped with either a Kimura spatula, a needle, or rounded surgical blade. Inoculation onto microbiologic media (pre-warmed to room temperature) is immediately performed by small C-shaped streaks. One scrape per medium is preferred. A suggested protocol is to inoculate the following media in order: a chocolate agar plate; a slide for a Gram's stain; a blood agar plate; a supplemented brain-heart infusion broth ('special BHIB'); a cooked meat-glucose broth; and a slide for a Giemsa stain. A fungal medium (Sabouraud's dextrose agar) should also be included.

In addition, cultures of the contact lenses, cases, and solutions may add valuable information.

Culture interpretation

An obvious pathogen will be isolated from perhaps 40% of corneal specimens. Sometimes, skin flora only will be isolated; commensals such as coagulase-negative staphylococci, viridans streptococci, and corynebacteria can colonize defects in the corneal epithelium and contribute to the pathology. In these instances, the isolate should be identified to at least genus level and reported to the clinician. Antibiotic treatment is considered on a case-by-case basis. If there is no growth or growth of commensals only in the presence of a worsening condition, further investigations for nonbacterial pathogens must be considered.

Antimicrobial susceptibility testing

Susceptibility testing against particular antibiotics is normally performed on all significant bacterial isolates from the cornea.

Differential diagnosis

- Infectious keratitis due to other pathogens: yeasts, filamentous fungi, acanthamebae, parasites, viruses such as herpes simplex.
- Sterile corneal infiltrates with contact lens wear induced by endotoxin or other microbial components.
- Marginal subepithelial infiltrates associated with staphylococcal blepharitis or acute conjunctivitis.
- Toxic keratopathy associated with chemical injury or overuse of topical drugs.

PROPHYLAXIS

Prophylaxis with topical antibiotics is routinely given after traumatic injury to the cornea. An agent with a wide antimicrobial spectrum, such as a fluoroquinolone or chloramphenicol, is recommended. Antibiotic prophylaxis is also given before and/or after corneal surgery, such as transplantation or refractive procedures, but its value in reducing postoperative infection remains controversial.

TREATMENT

Systemic

Systemic administration of antibiotics is not indicated for bacterial keratitis unless structures beyond the cornea are directly involved.

Ocular

The principles of the treatment of bacterial keratitis are to eliminate the replicating etiologic agent with specific antibiotics, to suppress destructive inflammation, and then to withdraw therapy so as not to hinder repair of the cornea.

Subconjunctival injections are usually reserved for scleral and/or intraocular extension of the infection, or in cases with questionable compliance with the treatment regimen.

Initial topical broad-spectrum therapy is recommended until the microorganism is identified in culture. A combination of fortified antibiotic solutions effective against gram-positive and gram-negative bacteria is administered each hour, or even more frequently, for the first 24 hours: a first-generation cephalosporin (cefazolin 50 mg/mL) and gentamicin or tobramycin (9–14 mg/mL). The antibiotics chosen as initial therapy may be changed based on the clinical response. If the clinical response is favorable and the miroorganism has been identified, monotherapy may be considered.

Topical fluoroquinolones may also be used for bacterial keratitis. Early clinical trials have shown that second-generation fluoroquinolones (ofloxacin and ciprofloxacin) have low ocular toxicity and were as effective as a combination of fortified antibiotics. They have excellent activity against most strains of staphylococci, *P. aeruginosa*, and enteric gram-negative bacilli. *S. pneumoniae* and other streptococci are less sensitive, and based on in vitro susceptibility, cefazolin may be a better choice for these infections. Although quinolones are effective for most corneal infections in most parts of the world, it is unwise to assume that all keratitis is bacterial and will respond to these agents. Emerging resistance of various strains has been reported. The fourth-generation fluoroquinolones (gatifloxacin and moxifloxacin) possess an expanded spectrum of activity, greater potency, and resistance-thwarting capabilities.

Alternative agents according to culture result or the *in vitro* susceptibility profile are considered only if there is no favorable clinical response, or toxicity signs from the initial antibiotics (Table 186.1). If no organisms are cultured but the clinical picture suggests an active infection, the concomitant use of a cephalosporin and an aminoglycoside should be continued.

In addition, cycloplegic agents may be used to decrease synechiae formation, and reduce pain and ciliary spasm.

Surgical

Penetrating keratoplasty is indicated if corneal perforation occurs during the course of the disease and the area of necrosis is resectable, or the keratitis is unresponsive to antimicrobial therapy. The infected area should be included in the removed button. The success rate of corneal transplants made under these circumstances is low. When extensive peripheral corneal

TABLE 186.1 – Antibiotics used in the treatment of bacterial corneal ulcers

Organism	Antibiotic	Topical Concentration	Subconjunctival Dose in 0.5 mL
Gram-positive cocci	Cefazolin	50 mg/mL	100 mg
	Vancomycin	15–50 mg/mL	25 mg
	Fluoroquinolones	3 or 5 mg/mL	—
Gram-negative rods	Gentamicin/tobramycin	9–14 mg/mL	20 mg
	Ceftazidime	50 mg/mL	100 mg
	Fluoroquinolones	3 or 5 mg/mL	—
Gram-negative cocci	Ceftriaxone	50 mg/mL	100 mg
	Ceftazidime	50 mg/mL	100 mg
	Fluoroquinolones	3 mg/mL	—

necrosis occurs a conjunctival flap after a period of intensive chemotherapy often is the safest course of treatment.

Supportive

Close observation is mandatory. Progression of the condition may be rapid and blinding. Punctilious attention must be paid to treatment schedules. For these reasons, either hospital admission may be necessary or close follow-up is performed.

PRECAUTIONS

The use of topical corticosteroids in bacterial keratitis is controversial. Topical corticosteroids can suppress the inflammation and may reduce subsequent corneal scarring. Studies in animal models suggest that inflammation is inhibited without impairing the clearance of organisms provided an appropriate antibiotic is administered concurrently However, potential specific adverse effects include enhancement of bacterial growth by local immunosuppression, impairment of phagocytosis, or inhibition of collagen synthesis. It is probably safe to suppress anterior segment inflammation with topical steroids after the effectiveness of the antimicrobial therapy has been suggested by a nonprogressive clinical course.

COMMENTS

Continuation of the inflammation or the prolonged use of topical antibiotics can inhibit epithelial closure; thus, intensive medication should be maintained only until the clinical course suggests that bacterial growth is suppressed. Usually, only 2 or 3 days of intensive therapy are necessary, with careful reduction of medication over the next week. It often is possible for patients with a healing epithelial and stromal defect to be off the medication and under close supervision within 10 days.

Positive clinical response includes blunting of the perimeter of the infiltrate and reduction of its density, reduction of the anterior chamber inflammation, stabilization of the stromal thinning and re-epithelialization.

REFERENCES

Badenoch PR, Hay GJ, McDonald PJ, Coster DJ: A rat model of bacterial keratitis: effects of antibiotics and corticosteroid. Arch Ophthalmol 103:718–722, 1985.

Christy NE, Sommer A: Antibiotic prophylaxis of postoperative endophthalmitis. Ann Ophthalmol 11:1261–1265, 1979.

Huang AJW, Wichiensin P, Yang MC: Bacterial keratitis. In: Krachmer JH, Mannis MJ, Holland EJ, eds: Cornea. 2nd edn. Elevier Mosby, 2005:1005–1033.

Hyndiuk RA, Eiferman RA, Caldwell DR, et al: Comparison of ciprofloxacin ophthalmic solution 0.3% to fortified tobramycin-cefazolin in treating bacterial corneal ulcers: Ciprofloxacin Bacterial Keratitis Study Group. Ophthalmology 103:1854–1862, 1996.

McDonnell PJ: Empirical or culture-guided therapy for microbial keratitis? A plea for data. Arch Ophthalmol 114:84–87, 1996.

O'Brien TP, Maguire MG, Fink NE, et al: Efficacy of ofloxacin vs cefazolin and tobramycin in the therapy for bacterial keratitis: report from the Bacterial Keratitis Study Research Group. Arch Ophthalmol 113:1257–1265, 1995.

Stern GA, Schemmer GB, Farber RD, Gorovoy MS: Effect of topical antibiotic solutions on corneal epithelial wound healing. Arch Ophthalmol 101:644–647, 1983.

Wilhelmus KR: Bacterial keratitis. In: Pepose JS, Holland GN, Wilhelmus KR, eds: Ocular infection and immunity. St Louis, Mosby, 1996: 970–1031.

Williams KA, Muehlberg SM, Lewis RF, et al, eds: The Australian Corneal Graft Registry 1996 report. Adelaide, Mercury, 1997.

187 CONJUNCTIVAL, CORNEAL, OR SCLERAL CYSTS 371.23

(Epithelial Inclusion Cysts, Intrastromal Corneal Cysts)

James C. Liu, MD, MBA
San Jose, California

ETIOLOGY/INCIDENCE

Intracorneal cysts are rare lesions that have been described after trauma and congenitally. This is a slowly progressive condition in young patients. The eyes are usually quiet and uninflamed. Individual cases were presumed to be congenital in origin, but recent reports have overwhelmingly documented trauma as the most likely cause of corneal cysts. They usually appear after trauma to the cornea or sclera and probably develop from surface epithelium that was implanted in the stroma during the injury. The ectopic epithelium proliferates and enlarges to form a corneal or sclerocorneal cyst, depending on the location of trauma. The desquamated material within the cyst settles and gives the cyst its typical appearance, that of a pseudohypopyon. Therapeutic success and the procedure largely depend on the location of the cyst and the patient's visual impairment from the cystic lesion. Current discussion does not include epithelial cyst under the corneal flap following laser *in situ* keratomileusis (LASIK), reader should refer to a LASIK text for its treatment and management.

- The age of the patient at which the cyst is discovered varies significantly because the time of trauma varies.
- Most patients are young, in their first two decades of life. This finding may be attributed to the greater metabolic activity of corneal epithelial cells of young individuals. This enables the epithelium to survive and proliferate when implanted intrastromally.
- There is no gender predilection.
- Although in some cases there is no history of trauma, even minor corneal epithelial injury can cause implantation of epithelium in the stroma with subsequent development of intrastromal cyst, and these minor injuries can be easily forgotten or overlooked.

DIAGNOSIS

Clinical signs and symptoms

- Most patients present with a history of trauma or a previous surgical procedure.
- The vision of the affected eye varies widely on presentation from 20/20 to light perception, depending on the size and location of the cyst.
- The appearance of the cyst depends on the stage of development. In the early stages, the cyst may look like a small

nebulous opacity. In the advanced stages, the cyst becomes oval to round.

- The cyst may be single and round, or multiloculated. The color ranges from clear to opalescent; however, the majority of cysts have a hypopyon-like feature in which cloudy debris settles inferiorly and the top of the cyst is filled with clear fluid.
- The cyst may occupy different levels of stroma, but midstromal location appears most frequently in reports. It could extend horizontally into the limbus or sclera and posteriorly into the anterior chamber. Rarely, communication with the anterior chamber is formed.
- Isolated intrastromal cysts with no communication with anterior chamber is the hallmark.
- The size varies dramatically from a few millimeters in diameter to covering the entire cornea. The cysts tend to progressively enlarge at a slow pace, usually taking months to years to become noticeable.
- The surrounding tissue of the eye appears white and noninflamed.
- There may or may not be blood vessels around the cyst.
- The epithelial layer of the cornea above the cyst could be normal without fluorescein staining. In other patients, previous trauma may leave an obvious corneal scar over the cyst.
- The cysts typically do not cause significant pain or discomfort.
- Corneal cysts are usually unilateral, although Fox reported a bilateral corneal cyst in one patient.

Laboratory findings

The development of intrastromal corneal cysts represents an aberration of the normal wound-healing process. After the penetrating or perforating laceration to the cornea, edema of the corneal stroma and fibrin plug formation usually occur. Later, fibroplastic proliferation into the clot begins with the adjacent stromal cells. This fibrous reaction forms a linear scar, and posteriorly to the endothelium it extends across the wound and lays down a thin membrane. On the anterior surface, as the wound heals, the initial epithelial downgrowth between the wound edges is gradually pushed toward the surface by the fibrous scar. Occasionally, epithelium becomes sequestered and isolated within the corneal stroma. Early authors speculated on different congenital and embryonic causes of the development of these cysts. When more recent reports are examined, the concept of congenital origin appears doubtful. These cysts are usually unilateral and are not associated with other congenital anomalies. They are not inherited, and they have a similar appearance to cysts of known traumatic cause. Therefore, the congenital origin of corneal cysts is very unlikely. The inciting trauma in these cases may be relatively minor, such as a pencil, a pen, scissors, or other sharp objects. Minor injuries heal quickly, cause minimal symptoms, and may go unnoticed until the cysts reach a clinically significant size.

- In most recent reported cases, a history of corneal trauma is well documented, ranging from minor corneal ulceration to severe trauma causing hyphema and cataracts.
- Frequently, intracorneal cysts develop after surgical procedures, including cataract surgery, lamellar keratoplasty, keratomileusis, penetrating keratoplasty, epikeratoplasty, radial keratotomy and strabismus surgery.
- Trauma and surgery also may cause epithelial downgrowth into the anterior chamber, so coexistence of epithelial downgrowth should be suspected if the eye is irritated or inflamed or there are signs of corneal edema from endothelial cell damage.

Light microscopic examination of the cysts has been carried out by numerous authors, and the findings have been similar. The surface epithelium and Bowman's layer were normal. The stroma typically was nonvascularized and noninflamed. Occasional small vascular channels were observed. The epithelial cells lining the cysts varied in morphology, ranging from squamous to columnar and from one cell thick to multilaminar. The anterior cystic cells tend to be flattened or squamous, whereas the posterior cells are rounder or columnar. The epithelial cells were quiet without any signs of inflammation or malignant transformation. Desquamated cells were present in the cyst. There were no glandular structures or hair follicles.

TREATMENT

The treatment of intracorneal cysts depends on the depth, size, and location of the cyst at the time of diagnosis.

- The conservative approach is advised if the cyst does not involve the pupil or central cornea and if the patient still has good vision.
- Simple observation is prudent. These cysts are indolent and enlarge slowly or not at all over the years. Spontaneous reabsorption of the cysts has been reported; however, in these cases, the cysts most likely rupture into the anterior chamber. Others have reported very slow enlargement or no change in the size of the cyst for as long as 6 years.
- When the cyst has achieved a significant size or if it is near the pupillary axis and affects visual acuity, a definitive procedure should be considered.
- A simple incision and drainage procedure or needle aspiration has no permanent effect. These procedures have been tried repeatedly, and the result has been the same; the cysts invariably refill over time.
- Marsupialization through removal of a portion of the anterior wall of the cyst followed by destruction of the epithelial cell with chemical cautery is highly successful. Different chemical solutions have been used for the destruction of epithelial cells, including 10% acetic acid, 1% trichloroacetic acid, 1% iodine and cocaine.
- After chemical cauterization of the cavity, fine temporary sutures, such as 10-0 nylon, may be used to hold the walls of the cavity together until they have sealed. This suture is tied on the corneal surface and the knots are rotated into the stroma. This suture can be removed after 3 weeks with the marsupialization technique.

The marsupialization technique usually provides a high rate of success; in reported cases, the cysts either were destroyed completely or decreased significantly in size. Marsupialization could be difficult if the cyst is deep and centrally located; to provide visual rehabilitation in these cases, penetrating keratoplasty is the best procedure. During penetrating keratoplasty, the surgeon must avoid spilling the cyst contents into the anterior chamber. Copious irrigation should be performed. Cryotherapy can be applied to the cyst before penetrating keratoplasty to kill the epithelial cells. Anterior chamber cyst formation has been reported after penetrating keratoplasty for corneal cyst; in this case, the patient had a protracted and complicated course with poor visual outcome. No recurrence of corneal cysts has been reported after penetrating keratoplasty.

REFERENCES

Al-Rajhi A, Al-Kharashi S: Epithelial inclusion cyst following epikeratoplasty. J Refract Surg 12:516–519, 1996.

Avni I, Cahane M, Blumenthal M, Naveh N: Transformation of corneal epithelial cyst into anterior chamber implantation cyst and scleral cyst: A rare occurrence. J Pediatr Ophthalmol Strabismus 26:303–306, 1989.

Binder PS, Beale JP, Zavala EY: The histopathology of a case of keratophakia. Arch Ophthalmol 100:101–105, 1982.

Bloomfield SE, Jakobiec FA, Iwamoto T: Traumatic intrastromal corneal cyst. Ophthalmology 87:951–955, 1980.

Chan MY, Liao HR, Fong JC: Traumatic intracorneal cyst. Am J Ophthalmol 21:303–305, 1989.

Claiborne JH: Epithelial corneal cyst. Transam Ophthalmol 10:588–593, 1984.

Fox LW: Bilateral cysts of the cornea. Br J Ophthalmol 12:249–254, 1928.

Jester JV, Villasenor RA, Miyashiro J: Epithelial inclusion cysts following radial keratotomy. Arch Ophthalmol 101:611–615, 1983.

Liakos GM: Intracorneal and sclerocorneal cysts. Br J Ophthalmol 62:155–158, 1978.

Purcell J, Brady H: Intrastromal epithelial corneal cyst. Ophthalmic Surg 14:491–499, 1983.

Reed JW, Dahlman CH: Corneal cyst: a report of 8 cases. Arch Ophthalmol 86:648–652, 1971.

Vrolijk M: Corneoscleral cyst. Acta Ophthalmol 19:44–51, 1941.

Wood T: Corneal intrastromal cyst. Ann Ophthalmol 8:967–968, 1976.

Yee RD, Hit TH: Corneal intrastromal cyst following lamellar keratoplasty. Am J Ophthalmol 7:644–646, 1975.

188 CORNEAL ABRASIONS, CONTUSIONS, LACERATIONS 918.2, AND PERFORATIONS 370.06

Guruswami Arunagiri, MD, FRCSEd
Danville, Pennsylvania
Rupan Trikha, MD
Danville, Pennsylvania

Corneal abrasions

Corneal abrasion is the loss of part or all of the corneal epithelium, from direct or indirect injury. It is one of the most common reasons for new patient visits to the ophthalmic emergency room.

ETIOLOGY

- Mechanical: fingernail, paper, foreign body, curling iron, mascara brush, plant, and contact lens.
- Chemical: hair sprays, alkali and acid exposure.
- Iatrogenic: eye patching, tonometry, ocular surgery, general anesthesia.
- Others: heat, ultraviolet light.

DIAGNOSIS

Symptoms

- Tearing, eye pain, and foreign body sensation, photophobia, and blephrospasm.
- Symptoms may be delayed for several hours with ultraviolet keratitis or contact lens related injury.

Clinical signs

- Visual acuity is decreased due to excessive tearing or abrasion in the visual axis.
- Conjunctival erythema, chemosis and lid edema can occur in severe cases.
- Using a slit lamp, the edges of the abrasion can be visualized with direct illumination and scleral scatter techniques.
- Corneal light reflex is blunted due to surface irregularity.
- Initially, an epithelial defect is present with clear underlying stroma. A very mild stromal infilatrate may be present with minimal anterior chamber cell and flare reaction 12 to 24 hours later.
- Fluorescein dye with a cobalt-blue light filter will enhance visualization of the abrasion.
- Topical anesthetics may be used if pain and photophobia limit examination.
- Multiple, vertical, linear corneal abrasions are usually due to an upper lid palpebral foreign body and examination by lid eversion should be performed.
- Stromal abrasions are rare and due to trauma from a sharp or abrasive object. Most commonly seen with fingernail injury in sports. Often a corneal flap of varying thickness may be seen. These injuries take longer to heal, and are often associated with edema below the involved area.
- Atypical presentations or cases not involving trauma require consideration of other causes, especially herpes simplex epithelial keratitis.
- High velocity objects can penetrate the cornea and leave minimal evidence except a small epithelial defect.

TREATMENT

- Antibiotic prophylaxis with a broad-spectrum antibiotic (e.g. fluroquinolone, polysporin, erythromycin) is recommended in all cases, and may be in the form of an ointment or solution.
- For contact lens wearers, an antibiotic with pseudomonal coverage (e.g. fluroquinolone) should be used.
- Cycloplegic agents (e.g. cyclopentolate, homatropine) reduce discomfort from traumatic iritis. Topical nonsteroidal anti-inflammatory drug drops can also be used for pain control (e.g. diclofenac, ketorolac).
- Oral non-narcotic or narcotic analgesia is rarely required.
- Steroid use for iritis in this setting is not recommended as it can hinder epithelial healing and increase risk of infection.
- Eye patch use is controversial and should not be used in patients with history of contact lens use or injury involving vegetable matter.
- Bandage soft contact lenses (BSCL) are very effective in reducing pain, but should only be used with topical antibiotic coverage. BSCL use is contraindicated in cases involving vegetable matter or artificial fingernails.
- Follow up examination should be performed at every 2–5 days, and sooner for high-risk cases, until the epithelial defect has healed.

COMPLICATIONS

Most superficial corneal abrasions heal within a few days. Rare complications include:

- Infection.
- Corneal scaring.
- Recurrent corneal erosions:
    - Occur due to poor adhesion of epithelium to underlying basement membrane;
    - Treatment is the same as for any corneal abrasion;
    - Prevention involves long-term lubrication with ointment at bedtime;
    - In persistent cases, superficial keratectomy or micro-puncture may be necessary for resolution.

Corneal contusions

Corneal contusion results from blunt trauma to the cornea without penetration of the ocular surface.

ETIOLOGY

Common causes include injury with rubber bands, bungee cords, automobile airbags and BB gun pellets.

DIAGNOSIS

- Symptoms: pain, photophobia, and decreased vision.
- Signs:
    - Focal edema at the site of impact, or rarely diffuse corneal edema with severe endothelial damage;
    - Breaks in Descemet's membrane can occur from severe stretching and bending of the cornea;
    - Rarely, endothelial rings composed of damaged endothelial cells, fibrin, and leukocytes, surrounded by normal endothelium may be present. These resolve within a few days;
    - Other ocular injury includes iritis, hyphema, iridodialysis, angle recession, traumatic cataract, vitreous hemorrhage, choroidal rupture, retinal detachment, and commotio retina.

TREATMENT

Treatment of corneal contusions is initially conservative. In most cases the cornea regains its clarity in a few days, in spite of permanent endothelial cell loss.

- Topical steroid drops (e.g. Prednisolone Acetate) and hypertonic saline solutions (e.g. Hypertonic sodium chloride drops) have been used with little benefit.
- Penetrating keratoplasty is indicated for persistent corneal edema or stromal scar.
- Associated ocular injuries such as listed above should be managed appropriately.

Corneal laceration 918.2

ETIOLOGY

Corneal lacerations result from a sharp object that cuts through corneal tissue. A common cause includes high-speed pieces of material released when grinding or cutting metal, wood, glass, or plastic.

DIAGNOSIS

History is crucial in the diagnosis and for medical-legal reasons.

Information should be obtained of the time and place of injury, as well as the activity being done, uses of safety glasses, first aid measures undertaken, and additional injuries that occurred.

- Symptoms: eye pain, tearing, bleeding, foreign body sensation, photophobia, and decreased vision.
- Evaluation:
    - Visual acuity should be measured with pinhole or corrective lens when possible;
    - A wire lid speculum is useful when there is significant chemosis and ecchymosis;
    - External pressure or manipulation of foreign bodies at the site of laceration should be avoided;
    - Location, size, depth of the laceration, and prolapse of intraocular tissue should be noted. With prolapse of intraocular tissues, further examination is deferred until surgery;
    - Seidel test using fluorescein with cobalt blue light may be necessary to identify occult leakage of aqueous;
    - Further examination for lid laceration, hyphema, iritis, iridodialysis, disruption of the lens capsule and cataract, vitreous hemorrhage, intra-ocular foreign body must be done;
    - In suspected cases of intra-ocular foreign body, CT scan or ultrasound in expert hands is recommended.

TREATMENT

Treatment is dependent on whether the laceration is partial or full thickness.

- All patients require prophylaxis with broad-spectrum topical antibiotic (e.g. fluroquinolone) and a cycloplegic agent (e.g. homatropine, cyclopentolate).
- Partial thickness laceration:
    - Medically treated with topical broad-spectrum antibiotics with or without a cycloplegic agent;
    - Deep partial thickness lacerations may be sutured to reduce scaring, and risk of rupture.
- Full thickness lacerations:
    - For lacerations less than 2 mm and with minimal tissue loss, a bandage contact lens with or without cyanoacrylate glue (not FDA approved) may be used;
    - Lacerations larger than 2 mm or with tissue loss are repaired surgically. A shield is placed over the injured eye to prevent further damage, and the patient kept NPO.
- Use of systemic antibiotics is controversial. We give systemic antibiotics (ceftazidime and vancomycin) in the setting all full thickness corneal lacerations. Most agree with use of systemic prophylaxis in the presence of an intraocular foreign body.
- Antiemetic agents (e.g. promethazine, metaclopramide) should be used as needed to prevent Valsalva.
- Tetanus toxoid is recommended for all full thickness wounds.
- Postoperatively, patients are prescribed polycarbonate safety glasses for constant use to avoid injuries to either eye.

Surgical technique

Surgical repair in penetrating wounds should be performed in the operating room with general anesthesia. Depolarizing agents like succinylcholine, and retrobulbar anesthesia is avoided to prevent co-contraction of extraocular muscles and extrusion of intraocular contents.

A detailed description of surgical technique is beyond the scope of this chapter. The primary goal of surgery is to restore the anatomic integrity of the globe. Visual restoration is only secondary.

General principles for repair

- Use 10-0 nylon for suturing.
- Sutures are placed at 90% depth on both sides of the wound.
- Suturing should be watertight, and induce minimal scarring or astigmatism.
- Limbal or peripheral sutures are placed first. Wider spaced, long compressive sutures are applied peripherally to maintain flatter curvature.
- Suturing in the visual axis should be avoided, but if needed, short, minimally compressive sutures are applied to maintain steeper curvature.
- Knots should be trimmed and buried away from the visual axis.
- For perpendicular wounds, the length of each suture pass should be symmetrical from the anterior surface of the cornea.
- For oblique wounds, length of suture pass should be symmetrical from the posterior surface of the cornea. For combination wounds the perpendicular wounds are closed first.
- Watertight closure of the wound may be difficult in cases of tissue loss, puncture wounds, or unusual lacerations. In these cases, a X-shaped suture may be placed. Corneal patch or lamellar graft, or primary penetrating keratoplasty can be considered in severe or difficult cases.
- In traumas that are less than 24 to 36 hours with no signs of infection, viable uvea and retina are reposited through a paracentesis incision with viscoelastic device or cyclodialysis spatula. Nonviable tissue is excised.
- Vitreous prolapse is treated by vitrectomy with Wekcels and Wescott scissors or with automated vitrector. Surgery for cataract with an intact lens capsule is deferred for a later date.
- Cataract surgery is indicated for intumescent lens, anterior capsular rupture with release of lens material, but is performed after the corneal laceration is sutured. Intra ocular lens implantation is controversial.
- Vitreous hemorrhage, intraocular foreign body, retinal detachment should be managed by a retinal surgeon.

COMPLICATIONS

- The immediate injury can lead to iris prolapse, hyphema, cataract formation, lens disruption and vitreous loss.
- Secondary complications include infection, astigmatism, scarring, vascularization, chronic wound leak, epithelial ingrowth, iridocorneal adhesions and intraocular fibrous proliferation.
- Vitreous involvement predisposes to retinal detachment from direct traction or vitreal-fibrous proliferation and contraction.
- Direct damage to angle structures, or obstruction from inflammatory debris or cells can lead to glaucoma.

Corneal perforations 370.06

In addition to traumatic corneal injuries, corneal perforations can result from:

- Trauma;
- Corneal ulcers;
- Inflammatory diseases — connective tissue diseases, Mooren's ulcer;
- Exposure keratopathy, neurotrophic disease;
- Ectatic disorders — kerataconus, keratoglobus, pellucid marginal degeneration;
- Xerosis (vitamin A deficiency, cicatricial ocular surface diseases);
- Degenerative disease — Terrien's;
- Postsurgical.

- Symptoms: pain, decreased vision, tearing, photophobia.
- Signs:
  - Shallow or flat anterior chamber;
  - Radiating Descemet's folds;
  - Uveal tissue prolapse;
  - Seidel test positive for aqueous leak;
  - Central clear zone in area of infiltrate;
  - Hypotony.

TREATMENT

Treatment is guided by the etiology of the corneal perforation.

- Small, non-traumatic perforations can be treated with cyanoacrylate glue and a bandage contact lens.
- Larger perforations require patch grafting or penetrating keratoplasty (PKP) to restore ocular integrity.
- Infectious perforations have a better outcome with PKP instead of glue.
- Ocular surface or immunologic disorders are more effectively treated with glue to delay or prevent PKP.
- Amniotic membrane transplant can also be used for treating perforations. This is a multi-step procedure and involves wound debridement, filling of wound with pieces of amniotic membrane tissue, followed by suturing two layers of amniotic membrane over the effected area.
- Intravitreal or subtenon's antibiotics are highly recommended at the time of surgery in the setting of infectious causes.
- Treatment of the underlying medical condition, such as connective tissue disease or vitamin A deficiency, has to be addressed simultaneously.

COMPLICATIONS

- Wound leak or dehiscence.
- Recurrent perforation due persistent underlying disease.
- Astigmatism, scarring, vascularization, epithelial ingrowth, iridocorneal adhesions and intraocular fibrous proliferation.

REFERENCES

Arunagiri G: Corneoscleral laceration. emedicine. Ophthalmology 5:1–10, 2004.

Arunagiri G: Iris prolapse. emedicine. Ophthalmology 5:1–10, 2004.

Beatty RF, Beatty RL: The repair of corneal and scleral lacerations. Sem Ophthalmol 9(3):165–176, 1994.

Buzard KA: Compression sutures and penetrating corneal trauma. Ophthalmic Surgery 23(4):246–252, 1992.

Hamill MB: Corneal and scleral trauma. Ophthalmol Clin N Am 15(2):185–194, 2002.

Kaiser PK: The corneal abrasion patching study group. A comparison of pressure patching versus no patching for corneal abrasions due to trauma or foreign body removal. Ophthalmology 102(12):1936–1942, 1995.

Kunimoto DY, Kanitkar KD, Makar MS, eds: Corneal laceration. In: Wills eye manual. 4th edn. Pennsylvania, Lippincott Williams & Wilkins, 2004.

Macsai MS: Surgical management and rehabilitation of anterior segment trauma. In Surgical management and rehabilitation of anterior segment trauma. In: Krachmer JH, Mannis MJ, Holland E, eds: Cornea. 2nd edn. London, Elsevier, 2005.

Patrone G, Sacca SC, Macri A, Rolando M: Evaluation of the analgesic effect of 0.1% indomethacin solution on corneal abrasions. Ophthalmologica 213(6):350–354, 1999.

189 Corneal Edema 371.20
(Bullous Keratopathy, Epithelial Edema, Stromal Edema)

Joel Sugar, MD
Chicago, Illinois
Rashmi Kapur, MD, ECFMG
Chicago, Illinois

ETIOLOGY

Corneal edema is the condition of excess corneal hydration that is caused by altered fluid transport across the cornea. Epithelial edema is most troubling to visual acuity because it induces anterior irregular astigmatism. In epithelial edema, fluid accumulates initially within basal cells and then between epithelial cells, causing microbullae; ultimately, fluid accumulates beneath the basal cell layer, lifting up the corneal surface to form bullae.

Endothelial dysfunction, corneal hypoxia, and elevated intraocular pressure are the most common causes of corneal edema. Stromal infiltration and inflammation can also cause corneal edema. Endothelial dysfunction may be due to Fuchs' dystrophy, other endothelial disorders such as iridocorneal endothelial (ICE) syndrome, or endothelial damage from trauma, including cataract or other intraocular surgery. Endothelial dysfunction may also occur after uveitis, angle-closure glaucoma, prolonged contact with silicone oil, or with chronic hypotony and inadequate corneal endothelial nutrition. Herpetic disciform keratitis with endothelial inflammation can also produce corneal edema. Hypoxia from prolonged wear of contact lenses with poor oxygen transmissibility can lead to corneal edema. Acute or severe elevations in intraocular pressure (IOP) in the presence of endothelial dysfunction can lead to corneal edema. With high elevations of IOP in the presence of normal endothelial function, the stroma initially remains thin and clear, but there is the development of epithelial edema. Hypotony results in isolated stromal edema.

PATHOPHYSIOLOGY

Regardless of the inciting factor, endothelial cell loss results in migration of endothelial cells from neighboring areas to cover depleted areas. When these cells are not able to compensate, they enlarge and are irregular in shape (polymegathism and pleomorphism), resulting in stromal hydration and eventually leading to keratocyte loss, attenuation of Bowman's membrane and the epithelial basement membrane, and a decrease in glycosaminoglycans in the stroma. In response, epithelial cells, keratocytes, and fibroblasts produce βig-h3, tenascin-C, and fibrillin-1, which may contribute to the poor adhesive characteristics of the epithelium and the resulting epithelial bullae.

COURSE/PROGNOSIS

Because the corneal endothelial cell density diminishes over time, corneal endothelial damage added to the normal attrition of endothelial cells with advancing age can lead to progressive corneal edema. Initial mild corneal edema may over months to years become chronic, visually disabling corneal edema. Prolonged corneal edema may lead to corneal vascularization and subepithelial pannus formation, which can complicate future surgical treatments.

DIAGNOSIS

Clinical signs and symptoms

Stromal edema is less disturbing to visual acuity and is manifest as thickening and hazy opacification of the corneal stroma with folding of Descemet's membrane (Figure 189.1). Typically, the initial presentation of epithelial edema is blurred vision, which is most severe on awakening and decreases as the day progresses. As the severity increases, the visual acuity difficulty becomes persistent, and rupture of bullae may lead to recurrent pain, redness and photophobia. Anterior chamber inflammation may be seen as well, and secondary corneal infection can ensue.

Laboratory findings

- Epithelial edema and stromal edema are demonstrated at the slit-lamp examination or by pachymetry.
- Endothelial guttae or decreased endothelial cell density is demonstrated on slit-lamp evaluation, endothelial specular microscopy, or confocal microscopy.

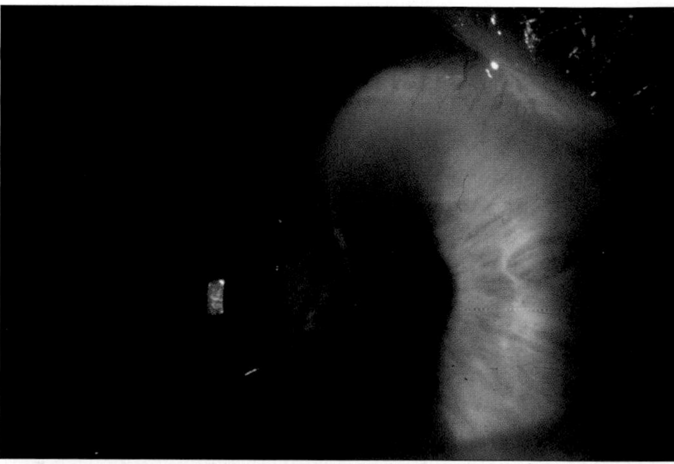

FIGURE 189.1. Corneal edema with Descemet membrane folds.

TREATMENT

- When elevated, intraocular pressure should be controlled.
- When inflammation is the source of the edema, it should be controlled.
- Corneal dehydration should be sought for patients with early or mild edema with hypertonic saline drops or ointments (usually drops as frequently as needed during the day and ointment at bedtime). A hairdryer held at arm's length for stimulation of tear evaporation on awakening in the morning may be helpful.
- Soft contact lenses should be used for painful recurrent bullae or for early mild irregular astigmatism.

Surgical

- Palliative anterior stromal puncture, corneal cautery, conjunctival flap placement, amniotic membrane transplantation, or phototherapeutic keratectomy (PTK) may be sufficient to provide comfort to patients with recurrent painful bullae in eyes with limited or no visual potential.
- Optical penetrating keratoplasty (PKP) may be combined with lens extraction in the face of cataract. Intraocular lens exchange and, if necessary, anterior vitrectomy may be indicated for corneal edema associated with intraocular lenses.
- Posterior lamellar keratoplasty (PLK) is an evolving procedure that involves surgical replacement of the endothelial cell layer with donor tissue, with minimal manipulation of the recipient corneal surface. Deep lamellar endothelial keratoplasty (DLEK) was initially described with instrument and procedural refinements over simple PLK and demonstrated successful results. However lamellar dissection of the recipient cornea still proved to be difficult for many surgeons. The current technique, Descemet's stripping endothelial keratoplasty (DSEK) or Desecmet's stripping automated endothelial keratoplasty (DSAEK) is a further technical advancement and involves scraping Descemet's membrane and endothelium from the recipient cornea. The advantage over a traditional PKP is that these variants of PLK can result in smoother surface topography with minimal astigmatism and decreased risk of wound dehiscence. Also the post-operative corneal power can be more stable and predictable, which allows for accurate calculations of intraocular lens power. Because of the lack of issues regarding sutures, wound stability, and topography, these techniques may result in more rapid visual rehabilitation.
- For patients who have undergone multiple PKPs or have a high risk of graft failure, keratoprosthesis can be offered as a treatment modality.
- Recent studies have shown that the corneal endothelium is arrested in the G1-phase of the cell cycle and retains the capacity to proliferate *in vivo*, but is inhibited by factors such as TGF-B and p27kip1. In the future, this information may help us to induce endothelial cell proliferation *in vivo* and create better procedures for repopulation of endothelial cells.

COMPLICATIONS

In addition to decreased vision and pain, patients may develop significant anterior segment inflammation when bullae rupture. This can lead to hypopyon formation in the absence of infection. Treatment with cycloplegic agents is very beneficial, in addition to the mentioned treatments. Secondary infection may also occur in the face of loss of epithelium due to the rupture of bullae and has been reported at a rate of 4.7% in bullous keratopathy patients.

REFERENCES

Adamis AP, Filatov V, Tripathi BJ, et al: Fuchs' endothelial dystrophy of the cornea. Surv Ophthalmol 38:149–168, 1993.

Akhtar S, Bron AJ, Hawksworth NR, et al: Ultrastructural morphology and expression of proteoglycans, βig-h3, tenascin-C, fibrillin-1, and fibronectin in bullous keratopathy. Br J Ophthalmol 85:720–731, 2001.

Cormier G, Brunette I, Boisjoly HM, et al: Anterior stromal punctures for bullous keratopathy. Arch Ophthalmol 114:654–658, 1996.

Flowers CW, Chang KY, McLeod SD, et al: Changing indications for penetrating keratoplasty, 1989–1993. Cornea 14:583–588, 1995.

Hatton MP, Perez VL, Dohlman CH: Corneal oedema in ocular hypotony. Experimental Eye Research 78:549–552, 2004.

Hicks CR, Crawford GJ, Lou X, et al. Corneal replacement using a synthetic hydrogel cornea, AlphaCor™: device, preliminary outcomes and complications. Eye 17:385–392, 2003.

Ishino Y, Sano Y, Nakamura T, et al: Amniotic membrane as a carrier for cultivated human corneal endothelial cell transplantation. Invest Ophthalmol Vis Sci 45:800–806, 2004.

Joyce NC: Proliferative capacity of the corneal endothelium Progress in Retinal and Eye Research 22:359–389, 2003.

Kangas TA, Edelhauser HF, Twining SS, et al: Loss of stromal glycosaminoglycans during corneal edema. Invest Ophthalmol Vis Sci 31:1994–2002, 1990.

Levenson JE: Corneal Edema: Cause and treatment. Surv Ophthalmol 20:190–204, 1975.

Luchs JI, Cohen EJ, Rapuano CJ, et al: Ulcerative keratitis in bullous keratopathy. Ophthalmology 104:816–822, 1997.

Maini R, Sullivan L, Snibson GR, et al: A comparison of different depth ablations in the treatment of painful bullous keratopathy with phototherapeutic keratectomy. Br J Ophthalmol 85:912–915, 2001.

McMahon TT, Polse KA, McNamara N, et al: Recovery from induced corneal edema and endothelial morphology after long-term PMMA contact lens wear. Optometry Vision Sci 73:184–188, 1996.

Mohay J, Lange DM, Soltau JB, et al: Transplantation of corneal endothelial cells using a cell carrier device. Cornea 13:173–182, 1994.

Pires RTF, Tseng SCG, Prabhasawat P, et al: Amniotic membrane transplantation for symptomatic bullous keratopathy. Arch Ophthalmol 117:1291–1297, 1999.

Terry MA, Ousley PJ: Replacing the endothelium without corneal surface incisions or sutures: The first United States clinical series using the deep lamellar endothelial keratoplasty procedure. Ophthalmology 110:755–764, 2003.

Waring GO, 3rd, Bourne WM, Edelhauser HF, et al: The corneal endothelium: normal and pathologic structure and function. Ophthalmology 89:531–590, 1982.

Melles GR. Posterior lamellar keratoplasty: DLEK to DSEK to DMEK. Cornea 25:879–881, 2006.

190 CORNEAL MUCOUS PLAQUES 371.44

Ramesh C. Tripathi, MD, PhD, FACS, FRCOphth
Columbia, South Carolina
Brenda J. Tripathi, PhD
Columbia, South Carolina
Richard M. Davis, MD
Columbia, South Carolina

Corneal mucous plaques are abnormal collections of a mixture of mucus, epithelial cells, and proteinaceous and lipoidal material that adhere firmly to the corneal surface. The plaques may

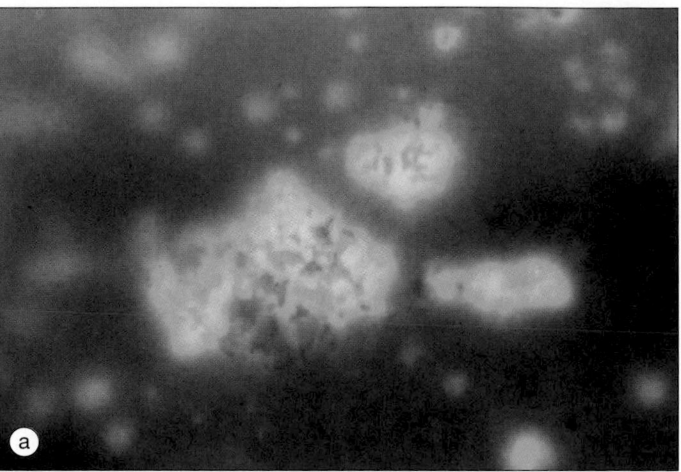

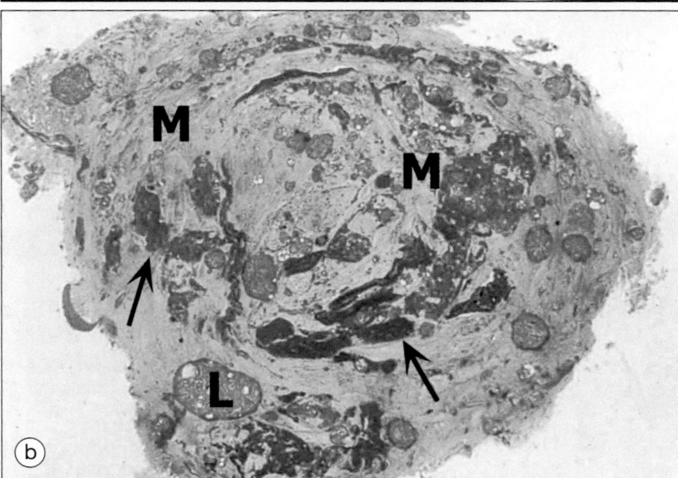

FIGURE 190.1. Corneal mucous plaques. a) Clinical photograph of multiple corneal mucous plaques of varying sizes and shapes in a patient with keratoconjunctivitis sicca. Fluorescein staining reveals breakup of the tear film over the plaques, which are slightly elevated from the corneal surface. b) Photomicrograph of 1 μm thick, toluidine blue stained section of a debrided mucous plaque that consists of desquamated degenerating epithelial cells (arrows), lipid globules (L), mucin (M) and foreign bodies. Original magnification × 160.

also enmesh calcareous granules and bacteria, as well as dust particles and other foreign bodies. The mucous plaques are translucent to opaque and may vary in size and shape from multiple small islands to bizarre patterns that may involve more than half the corneal surface (Figure 190.1).

ETIOLOGY/INCIDENCE

- An abnormality of the exposed surface of the superficial corneal epithelial cells and of tears with excessive mucus formation and the presence of epithelial receptor sites for the plaque elements predispose to this condition.
- The normal desquamation of epithelial cells beneath the plaque is retarded, and exfoliating surface cells become incorporated in the plaque. The plaque is formed when high-viscosity mucus and proteinaceous material adhere to the deeper squamous cells of the cornea or even to Bowman's layer through the intercellular spaces, as well as through abnormally formed transcellular aperture and epithelial defects; because of its physicochemical property, the mucous plaque enmeshes the desquamated epithelial cells.
- The viscosity of the mucus may increase due to dehydration or an increase in its sialomucin component, or secondarily because of infection with staphylococci, which liberate enzymes that can lyse the mucoprotein and glycosaminoglycan components of mucus produced normally by the conjunctival goblet cells.
- Corneal mucous plaques occur primarily in patients with keratoconjunctivitis sicca but may also occur with herpes zoster, vernal keratoconjunctivitis, and other forms of keratitis, especially in patients with neuroparalytic or neurotrophic keratitis or after local radiation exposure in whom corneal sensation is defective.
- Corneal mucous plaques and filamentary keratitis may coexist in the above conditions and also after Lasik, Lasek and, more frequently, penetrating keratoplasty at the donor-recipient interface.
- In filamentary keratitis, the corneal epithelial cells use the mucin strand as a substrate to grow along the filament, whereas, the cells are enmeshed in the corneal mucous plaque and the plaque remains flat and only slightly elevated from the corneal surface.
- Delayed plaques and pseudodendrites associated with herpes zoster may also be infectious, as they are positive for zoster DNA by polymerase chain reaction.
- Ciliary or conjunctival injection, mild iritis, with or without keratic precipitates, and epithelial and stromal edema are associated findings.

DIAGNOSIS

Clinical signs and symptoms

- Symptoms associated with the plaques vary from blurring of vision to foreign body sensation and marked pain; except when severe, they are often indistinguishable from the symptoms of keratoconjunctivitis sicca with or without Sjögren syndrome.
- These symptoms may also occur with herpes zoster keratitis and in patients using extended-wear soft contact lenses and in recurrent erosion syndrome.
- This entity is also associated with systemic disease, primarily rheumatoid arthritis or other collagen diseases.

TREATMENT

- Topically applied 10% to 20% acetylcysteine drops qd to q.i.d. can rapidly loosen the adherent plaque and dissolve its mucoid component and may prevent reformation.
- Mucous plaques causing severe symptoms may be removed surgically by debridment, scraping or pulled out with forceps or by rolling up with cotton swabs or Weck-cel sponge. A bandage gas permeable soft contact lens may be applied to the cornea. In some patients, a soft contact lens is also of therapeutic or preventive value. However, because of associated dry eye problems and deposit formation, the contact lenses may need frequent replacement or cleaning.
- Staphylococcal blepharitis may occur in association with corneal mucous plaques and may predispose patients to this condition. Treatment should also include the control of associated local microbial infections.

- Artificial tear preparations may be indicated for the treatment of dry eye. In the presence of filamentary keratitis and the formation of excessive mucus, hypotonic artificial tear substitutes (rather than the mucoid or viscous type of tear substitutes) may be combined with acetylcysteine.
- As cyclosporin A, non-steroidal anti-inflammatory agents and topical low-potency corticosteroids are used in the treatment of dry eye and filamentary keratitis, these agents could be another avenue for the medical management of corneal mucous plaques, which are often associated with a varying degree of inflammation.
- Delayed plaques and pseudodendrites associated with herpes zoster may be responsive to certain antiviral therapy.
- Because preservatives, such as benzylkonium chloride, chlorobutanol and thimerosol, adversely affect the corneal epithelium, the use of preservative-free tear substitutes or lubricants is preferable.
- Excimer laser phototherapeutic keratectomy may be a useful adjunct in the treatment of shield-shaped corneal ulcers and plaques in associated conditions such as vernal keratoconjunctivitis.

Ocular/Periocular

- Conjunctiva: conjunctivitis, fornix filaments, hyperemia, mucoid discharge.
- Cornea: filamentary keratitis, keratoconjunctivis sicca, mucous plaques, keratic precipitates associated with mild iritis.
- Eyelids: chronic blepharitis, blepharospasm.

PRECAUTIONS

- Because of variations in the frequency and severity of corneal mucous plaques, the use and concentration of topical mucolytic agents, such as acetylcysteine, should be individualized.
- Often, bandage soft contact lenses are subject to deposit formation and spoilage secondary to alterations in tear function (including rapid tear break-up time), associated necrosis of keratoconjunctival tissue and the plaque exposure. Therefore periodic cleaning or change of the soft contact lens may be required.
- Because treatment with topical steroids may delay healing and long-term use may induce or exacerbate open-angle glaucoma, these agents should be used with caution.

COMMENTS

- In some cases, corneal mucous plaques recur when the mucolytic agent is discontinued.
- Plaques may occur even in those patients receiving acetylcysteine, but usually they are smaller or remain on the corneal surface for shorter periods of time than those in patients who did not receive therapy.
- In some patients, plaques may recur if the soft contact lens is discontinued.
- Multiple plaques, which are frequently bilateral, are common.
- When a plaque has adhered to the cornea, it remains for a few days or weeks; recurrences may appear but seldom in the same location.
- Thickened plaques with a dry surface may appear elevated well above the tear film and may even cause dellen (Fuchs' dimples) formation.

REFERENCES

Avisar R, Robinson A, Appel I, Yassur Y, Weinberger D: Dicolfenac sodium, 0.1% (Voltaren Ophtha), versus sodium chloride, 5%, in the treatment of filamentary keratitis. Cornea 19:145–147, 2000.

Cameron JA, Antonios SR, Badr IA: Excimer laser phototherapeutic keratectomy for shield ulcers and corneal plaques in vernal keratoconjunctivitis. J Refract Surg 11:31–35, 1995.

Fraunfelder FT, Wright P, Tripathi RC: Corneal mucus plaques. Am J Ophthalmol 83:191–197, 1977.

Grinbaum A, Yassur I, Avni I: The beneficial effect of diclofenac sodium in the treatment of filamentary keratitis. Arch Ophthalmol 119:926–927, 2001.

Marsh RJ, Fraunfelder FT, McGill JI: Herpetic corneal epithelial disease. Arch Ophthalmol 6:1899–1902, 1976.

Pavan-Langston D, Yamamoto S, Dunkel EC: Delayed herpes zoster pseudodendrites: Polymerase chain reaction detection of viral DNA and a role for antiviral therapy. Arch Ophthalmol 113:1381–1385, 1995.

Perry HD, Doshi-Carneavale S, Donnenfeld ED: Topical cyclopsorin A 0.5% as a possible new treatment for superior limbic keratitis. Ophthalmology 110:1578–1581, 2003.

Rotkis WM, Chandler JW, Forstot SL: Filamentary keratitis following penetrating keratoplasty. Ophthalmology 89:946–949, 1982.

Shaw EL, Gasset AR: Management of an unusual case of keratitis mucosa with hydrophilic contact lenses and N-acetyl-cysteine. Ann Ophthalmol 6:1054–1056, 1974.

Tripathi BJ, Tripathi RC, Kolli SP: Cytotoxicity of ophthalmic preservatives on human corneal epithelium. Lens Eye Tox Res 9:361–374, 1993.

Tripathi RC, Tripathi BJ, Frankel RA: Corneal mucus plaques. In: FT Fraunfelder, FH Roy, eds: Current ocular therapy. 5th edn. WB Saunders, Philadelphia, 1999:352–353.

Tripathi RC, Tripathi BJ, Haggerty C: Drug-induced glaucomas: mechanism and management. Drug Safety 26:749–767, 2003.

Tripathi RC, Tripathi BJ, Silverman RA, Rao GN: Contact lens deposits and spoilage: Identification and management. Int Ophthalmol Clin 31:91–120, 1991.

191 CORNEAL NEOVASCULARIZATION 370.60

F. Hampton Roy, MD, FACS
Little Rock, Arkansas

ETIOLOGY

Corneal neovascularization can be defined as a pathologic state in which new blood vessels extend from the limbus into the superficial or deep areas of the cornea and is the result of various causes, including trauma, inflammation, infection, toxic insult, and underlying inherited corneal dystrophy or degeneration.

The normal cornea is a physiologically capillary-free and optically transparent tissue that supports optimal visual function. The normal cornea is devoid of blood vessels; this characteristic, combined with some other structural facts in the anatomy of the cornea, is responsible for the transparency of this tissue.

COURSE

Three potential mechanisms for the pathogenesis of corneal neovascularization have been proposed:

- A corneal injury inactivates a restraint that the normal cornea exerts on cell division and migration of the vascular cells of the pericorneal plexus.
- Corneal edema loosens corneal stromal tissue and therefore permits the ingrowth of vessels normally restrained by its composition.
- Corneal neovascularization is related to the production of locally generated angiogenic factors. The most noted of these angiogenic factors are epidermal growth factor, fibroblast growth factor, urokinase-like plasminogen activator, interleukin I, interleukin II, and many other angiogenic factors and cascades yet to be discovered. Increasing basic science research has been aimed at the identification of these angiogenic factors and the cells producing these substances in attempts to improve the prognosis of corneal neovascularization.

ANGIOGENESIS

Angiogenesis as a multistep process involving:

- Extravasation of plasma proteins;
- Degradation of extracellular matrix;
- Endothelial cell migration and proliferation;
- Capillary tube formation.

This angiogenic process is mediated by a wide array of cytokines and growth factors to which both the extracellular matrix and endothelial cells (and in inflammation, infiltrating inflammatory cells) contribute. Accumulating evidence suggests significant codependence between angiogenesis and inflammation in many models of neovascularization. Proinflammatory molecules can stimulate the production of collagenases and lead to degradation of basement membrane, as well as being directly mitogenic for endothelial cells. Furthermore, the chemotactic activity of proinflammatory cytokines can enhance migration (and activation) of inflammatory cells (e.g. neutrophils and macrophages), which can in turn stimulate more angiogenesis and the recruitment of yet more inflammatory cells to the site of inflammation. Corneal neovascularization leads to the loss of immune privilege in the anterior segment manifested as the inability to sustain anterior chamber-associated immune deviation. Moreover, topical angiostatic strategies can lead to the restoration of immune privilege when instituted sufficiently early in the course of the neovascular response.

DIAGNOSIS

Neovascularization can be as simple as a *micropannus*, which is a superficial fibrovascular proliferation that extends 1 to 2 mm beyond the normal vascular arcade. In contrast, a superficial vascular pannus that extends more than 2 mm beyond the normal vascular arcade is considered a *gross pannus*. New vessels can be made based on the phases of action. Initially, there is a stimulus. Then, there is localized fragmentation of the basal membrane and the extracellular matrix around the vessel involved. Endothelial cell migration occurs through the vessel wall, and lysis of the extracellular matrix continues, promoting new vessel growth. Multiple enzymes and blood products perpetuate the cycle and subsequent progression of corneal neovascularization.

Differential diagnosis

- Pterygium.
- Keratoconjunctivitis sicca (inflammatory).
- Vernal conjunctivitis (inflammatory).
- Pellagra (inflammatory).
- Vitamin B deficiency (inflammatory).
- Aphakic/pseudophakic bullous keratopathy (inflammatory).
- Fuchs' dystrophy (degenerative/inflammatory).
- Glaucoma (degenerative).
- Infectious keratoconjunctivitis (infectious/inflammatory).
- Contact lens use (infectious/inflammatory).
- Rosacea (infectious/inflammatory).
- Phlyctenular keratoconjunctivitis (infectious/inflammatory).
- Molluscum contagiosum (infectious).
- Lymphopathia venereum (infectious).
- Leishmaniasis (infectious).
- Onchocerciasis (infectious).
- Trachoma (infectious).
- Leprosy (infectious).
- Herpes simplex keratitis (infectious).
- Herpes zoster keratitis (infectious).
- Alkali burns (toxic).
- Acid burns (toxic).

TREATMENT

Supportive

Particularly in patients with a micropannus, observation rather than treatment of the underlying condition is indicated. When the micropannus proceeds to gross corneal neovascularization, treatments may be instituted other than simply treating the underlying disease process.

Ocular

The primary treatment of NV is eliminating the underlying cause. Various regimens have been proposed for the treatment of active, corneal vascularization. Sometimes just elimination of the inciting insult will lead to resolution, as is typically seen with contact lens wearers.

The mainstay of the ocular treatment is corticosteroid therapy. Topically applied prednisolone acetate may be administered liberally, except when used in cases with infectious causes. Its judicious use is indicated in infectious cases to prevent collagenase activation and the associated melting of the cornea. In severe cases, subconjunctival injections of corticosteroids may be considered, but their benefit beyond that of topical administration is limited, and complications associated with subconjunctival injections may be potentiated by this therapy. Vascularization that has been present for a long time, particularly when located in the deeper layers of the cornea, is usually resistant to any form of treatment.

Surgical

Various surgical procedures have been recommended in the treatment of corneal neovascularization. Initially, diathermy of large feeding vessels into the cornea has been advised by some clinicians. More recently, corneal laser photocoagulation for the treatment of neovascularization has included the use of the argon and the yellow dye laser. Both of these methods depend primarily on energy absorption by hemoglobin and oxyhemoglobin. Results from these studies show that many subsets of patients with corneal neovascularization can be treated effectively with laser photocoagulation; however, recurrence of the neovascularization has been an associated problem. Penetrating keratoplasty in vascularized corneas can be very difficult. Some authors have advised pretreatment of the recipient bed with diathermy of large feeder vessels into the cornea. In addition, diathermy of the inside graft edge must be done with extreme caution to prevent induced postoperative astigmatism. Early suture removal has been advocated because sutures have been implicated as a source of irritation and increased neovascularization with associated corneal graft rejection. In the past, the use of ß-irradiation was advocated; but this practice has been abandoned because the use of corticosteroids and immunosuppressive agents achieves better results. The suppression of corneal neovascularization with topical cyclosporin A has also been demonstrated. Investigators have treated corneal NV with argon laser obliteration of the vessel lumen. This can be achieved in the corneal part of the vessels (accessible to be lasered) but usually has a short-term effect, as the vessel lumen invariably reopens. Argon laser pannus obliteration is mainly a temporizing measure. Hyperbaric oxygen treatment has been used with limited success. This treatment modality aims to suppress angiogenesis by supplying the corneal tissue with redundant oxygen supply.

PRECAUTIONS

It is important to keep in mind that prolonged topical ophthalmic treatment with corticosteroids can increase intraocular pressure and cataract formation. It is essential to follow these patients closely. As mentioned, the treatment of certain infectious states with corticosteroids alone can potentiate collagenase activity and exacerbate corneal melting. Radiation, diathermy, and cryotherapy have all been used in an attempt to treat corneal neovascularization, but none of these methods has been found to be any more effective than corticosteroids. For deep, long-standing corneal neovascularization, most of these methods are unsuccessful.

COMPLICATIONS

- Tissue scarring.
- Opacification.
- Lipid keratopathy.
- Persistent inflammation.
- Immune corneal melting.
- Cicatrization.
- Edema.
- Exudates.
- Infiltration.
- Visual loss.
- Blindness.

COMMENTS

As knowledge of the biochemical pathogenesis of corneal neovascularization improves, so will treatment. Current research in arachidonic acid metabolism has shown that corticosteroids and cyclo-oxygenase inhibitors applied topically can significantly decrease the neovascular response to various insults. Attempts to use lipoxygenase and lipoxygenase inhibitors have not proved to be successful in decreasing the neovascular response in an animal model of corneal neovascularization. An understanding of interleukin and T cell associations has led to the use of cyclosporin A to suppress corneal neovascularization. Also, evaluation of collagenase inhibitors in alkali burns has shown that reducing the initial injury and the associated response of the body can limit the associated disruption of normal corneal architecture. The use of tissue-matched corneas in corneal transplantation has been successful in ABO-matched tissue but not with the HLA-associated markers. Finally, extended contact lens use, either the disposable or nondisposable form, will continue to cause corneal neovascularization via the mechanisms of hypoxia and lactic acid accumulation. Identification of these problems early can be rewarding when closer follow-up of the patients is implemented. In addition, contact lens technology continues to change rapidly, thereby reducing the problems.

The response of the cornea to injury or inflammation and the associated corneal neovascularization that may follow have plagued the ophthalmic surgeon and diagnostician for years. Continued research and the development of new topically applied agents and preventive mechanisms should reduce the prevalence of this potentially devastating ocular pathologic process.

REFERENCES

Baer JC, Foster S: Corneal laser photocoagulation for treatment of neovascularization: efficacy of 577 NM yellow dye laser. Ophthalmology 99:173–179, 1992.

Boyd BD, ed: Highlights of ophthalmology. New York, Arcata Book Group, 1998.

Collaborative Corneal Transplantation Studies: Effectiveness of histocompatibility matching in high risk corneal transplantation. Arch Ophthalmol 110:1392–1403, 1992.

Dana MR, Streilein JW: Loss and restoration of immune privilege in eyes with corneal neovascularization. Invest Ophthalmol Vis Sci 37:2485–2494, 1996.

Dana MR, Zhu SN, Yamada J: Topical modulation of interleukin-1 activity in corneal neovascularization. Cornea 17:403–409, 1998.

Folkman J, Shing Y: Angiogenesis. J Biol Chem 267:10931–10934, 1992.

Jackson JR, Seed MP, Kircher CH, et al: The codependence of angiogenesis and chronic inflammation. FASEB J 11:457–465, 1997.

Klintworth GK: Corneal angiogenesis: a comprehensive critical review. New York, Springer-Verlag, 1991.

Lipman RM, Epstein RJ, Hendricks RL: Suppression of corneal neovascularization with cyclosporine. Arch Ophthalmol 110:405–407, 1992.

192 DETACHMENT OF DESCEMET'S MEMBRANE 371.33

Alexandre S. Marcon, MD
Porto Alegre, Brazil
Italo M. Marcon, MD, PhD
Porto Alegre, Brazil
Christopher J. Rapuano, MD
Philadelphia, Pennsylvania

Descemet's membrane (DM), which is approximately 10 μm thick in adults, is the basement membrane of the corneal endothelium. Descemet's membrane detachment (DMD) is an uncommon but serious complication of intraocular surgery.

ETIOLOGY

- DMD has most often been reported after cataract extraction, surgical iridectomy, cyclodialisis, trabeculectomy, holmium laser sclerostomy, penetrating keratoplasty, lamellar keratoplasty, pars plana vitrectomy and viscocanalostomy. It can also be caused by external corneal trauma such as forceps delivery.
- The most important mechanisms implicated in causing DMD are probably the use of dull blades, engaging Descemet's during intraocular lens implantation or with the aspiration/irrigation device, injection of viscoelastic and insertion of instruments between Descemet's and stroma, and the creation of clear-corneal incisions.

COURSE/PROGNOSIS

- Small incidental DMDs near the surgical wound are common. The vast majority are self-limited and of little visual consequence.
- Nonscrolled and planar DMDs (DM separated from stroma by ≤1 mm) are most likely to spontaneously reattach in several weeks to months, in contrast to scrolled and nonplanar DMDs (DM separated from stroma by >1 mm).

DIAGNOSIS

The diagnosis of a DMD can be difficult to make due to corneal edema. Also, most detachments are self-limited and peripheral, only seen by gonioscopy. A high index of suspicion should be kept. High-magnification, high-light intensity slit-lamp examination can help. Ultrasound biomicroscopy can aid.

TREATMENT

Nonscrolled DMDs will often spontaneously reattach thus observation for several weeks to months is acceptable. Topical hyperosmotic agents can also be administered. In some cases, surgical intervention may be necessary.

Surgical

- Injection of air or viscoelastic in the anterior chamber can be performed if DMD is noticed during surgery and sulfur hexafluoride (SF_6) or perfluoropropane (C_3F_8) are not available. Air often reabsorbs too rapidly to work and big bubbles can cause pupilary block.
- Intracameral injection of 20% SF_6 or 14% C_3F_8 should be the treatment of choice and do not seem to expand or damage the endothelium.
- Full-thickness suturing of DM to the cornea can be tried for recalcitrant cases. Occasionally penetrating keratoplasty is needed.

COMPLICATIONS

- Persistent endothelial dysfunction and corneal edema with visual loss.
- Ocular discomfort/pain secondary to corneal edema or infection of ruptured corneal bullae.
- Anterior stromal haze may result from prolonged corneal edema.

COMMENTS

DMD appear to be increasing and this may be explained by clear-corneal cataract procedures. They do not require urgent surgical repair and waiting several months before attempting it is acceptable. The decision on when to intervene in DMDs must be made on a case-by-case basis after evaluating the configuration of the detachment, the risks of additional intervention, and the need for rapid rehabilitation of vision.

REFERENCES

Assia EI, Levkovich-Verbin H, Blumenthal M: Management of Descemet's membrane detachment. J Cataract Refract Surg 21:714–717, 1995.

Gault JA, Raber IM: Repair of Descemet's membrane detachment with intracameral injection of 20% sulfur hexafluoride gas. Cornea 15:483–489, 1996.

Macsai MS, Gainer KM, Chisholm L: Repair of Descemet's membrane detachment with perfluoropropane (C_3F_8). Cornea 17:129–134, 1998.

Mahmood MA, Teichmann KD, Tomey KF, et al: Detachment of Descemet's membrane. J Cataract Refract Surg 24:827–833, 1998.

Marcon AS, Rapuano CJ, Laibson PR, et al: Descemet's membrane detachment after cataract surgery: management and outcome. Ophthalmology 12:2325–2330, 2002.

193 EPITHELIAL BASEMENT MEMBRANE DYSTROPHY 371.52 *(Cogan's Microcystic Corneal Dystrophy; Map, Dot, Fingerprint Dystrophy)* AND RECURRENT EROSION 371.42 *(Recurrent Epithelial Erosion)*

Peter R. Laibson, MD
Philadelphia, Pennsylvania

ETIOLOGY/PROGNOSIS

Corneal erosion and recurrent corneal erosion are common ocular disorders that are sometimes preceded by trauma but may occur spontaneously. After trauma involving the epithelium and basement membrane, recurrent corneal erosion probably occurs as a result of inadequate basement membrane healing, either because the basal epithelial cells fail to produce proper basement membrane complexes to attach to Bowman's membrane and stroma or because of faulty basement membrane adherence. A traumatic cause has a better eventual prognosis for full recovery than does the spontaneous form.

In the case of spontaneous corneal erosion, the underlying disease process may be an epithelial basement membrane corneal dystrophy. Recent studies with electron microscopic analysis of adhesion mechanisms of the corneal epithelium during recurrent erosion episodes have shown separation of the anchoring system at the level of the epithelial cell membrane or below the level of the anchoring plaques. Normal and degenerate polymorphonuclear leukocytes (PMNs) were found within and between the epithelial cells and within the anchoring layer. The degenerate PMNs may secrete metalloproteinases that cleave Bowman's membrane below the anchoring system.

Epithelial basement membrane dystrophy and recurrent corneal erosions occur:

- In adults of each sex, although slightly more often in women;
- Usually after the fourth decade of life, although literature has associated recurrent corneal erosion with;
- Juvenile Alport's syndrome, an X-linked condition that also presents with anterior lenticonus and retinal flecks, as well as renal complications.

Epithelial basement membrane dystrophy is usually bilateral and characterized by:

- Various patterns of dots, parallel lines that mimic fingerprints, and random linear pattern that resemble maps, which usually appear in the epithelium of the central two-thirds of the cornea.

These intraepithelial cyst patterns are composed of opaque, putty-gray cysts, termed:

- Cogan's cysts, which are made up of cytoplasmic and nuclear debris and range in size from pinpoints to as much as 2 mm across.

Individual microcysts may be oval, oblong, or comma-shaped and rarely appear along but are usually associated with map and less often fingerprint patterns. The map and fingerprint patterns, on the other hand, frequently appear without 'dots,' or individual microcysts.

Map and fingerprint alterations in corneal epithelium are not rare and can be found in asymptomatic individuals without a prior history of trauma or ocular disease; in face, the literature suggests that these epithelial changes are more diffuse than previously recognized. They are frequently seen in conditions involving:

- Corneal edema. This localized edema may occur near a healing cataract surgical incision or in the central cornea associated with Fuchs' corneal dystrophy.

Epithelial basement membrane dystrophy, and recurrent erosion, are:

- Probably hereditary, with variable penetrance.

In a large study population, 6% of patient treated for a variety of other ocular non corneal conditions and diseases also demonstrated map, dot, and fingerprint changes in the epithelium.

Even when frank epithelial defects or opaque microcysts are absent or undetectable with biomicroscopy, computed videokeratography may reveal the presence of corneal epithelial 'lagoons,' or micro depressions, indicative of microscopic folding and redundancies in basement membrane, especially in post-traumatic recurrent erosion syndrome.

Fingerprint lines and map-like patterns are histologically similar, both have:

- An aberrant or a multilaminar basement membrane produced by the basal epithelial cells of the corneal epithelium. The literature suggests that especially in spontaneous (non traumatic) recurrent erosions, there may be an inherent structural weakness of the corneal basement membrane with respect to the synthesis and deposition of type IV collagen.

DIAGNOSIS

Clinical signs and symptoms

At least 80% to 90% of patients who have epithelial basement membrane dystrophy are asymptomatic. Symptoms, when they occur, consist of one or more of the following:

- Slightly blurred vision (when epithelial and basement membrane changes are in the visual axis);
- Visual acuity loss due to irregular astigmatism;
- Epithelial blebs;
- Foreign body sensation with recurrent erosion, when the epithelium loosens and detaches;
- Sudden sharp pain, often in the early morning during sleep or on awakening, when a frank epithelial defect occurs prompted by eyelid movement across loosened epithelium.

This commonly is the first symptom of a *recurrent* erosion, and in rare cases, a patient who has previously experienced this pain on awakening is so fearful of the pain that he or she is unable to sleep well. The pain is fleeting in most cases, lasting only seconds, but it may last for some minutes to 1 or 2 hours and is a warning that the epithelium is not healed.

Laboratory findings

In one study, patients with a history of recurrent corneal erosion (12 eyes) presented with signs suggestive of microbial keratitis. They had developed.

- An acute corneal stromal infiltrate beneath the epithelial defect and this was associated with, an intense anterior uveitis; and
- Hypopyon in three eyes.

Bacterial cultures of these corneas, however, revealed a positive isolate in just two eyes; treatment with topical antibiotics and topical corticosteroid rapidly resolved these episodes with good visual outcomes, frequently with a complete resolution of the recurrent erosion as well.

PROPHYLAXIS

Precautionary measure for patients with recurrent corneal erosion associated with epithelial basement membrane dystrophy include:

- Avoidance of rubbing the eyes through the eyelids, especially upon awakening;
- Liberal use of ointment medications at bedtime during an erosion episode.

Some times these measures must be followed for several months after resolution of the episode.

TREATMENT

Ocular

Of first importance for the patient with epithelial basement membrane dystrophy is minimization of the pain associated with recurrent corneal erosion. If the erosion is small, it will heal spontaneously or with the aid of:

- A pressure patch, placed on the eye for 1 or 2 days;
- An antibiotic ointment, such as bacitracin or erythromycin, which can be used beneath the patch.

The literature suggests that patching for longer than 2 days can introduce hypoxia or a lacrimal hyposecretion, or both, that may actually inhibit healing.

Minor corneal erosions can be treated with:

- Lubricating ointment alone, for several weeks to months, to control symptoms;
- Bandage soft contact lenses, which have been helpful in some cases of multiple recurrent erosion; however, concerns persist about overnight use of extended-wear soft contact lenses due to the risk of infectious keratitis.

In some cases, the recurrence of very mild corneal erosion may be prevented with:

- Sodium chloride drops 2% or 5% several times during the day; and
- Sodium chloride ointment 5% at bedtime.

Many patients believe that sodium chloride ointment is no more effective than a lubricant ointment or an ointment without preservatives. Each patient must establish a regimen of medication that seems to control his or her symptoms most effectively. This might involve using a medication only when symptoms recur, or in some instances, daily application for many months after the resolution of an erosion episode to prevent further recurrences.

Resistant case may require:

- Mechanical debridement, with or without chemical cautery, depending on the size of the defect and the amount of ocular irritation;
- Local cycloplegic agents;
- A diamond burr, which is used to 'polish' Bowman's membrane after mechanical debridement (has proved to be very effective in preventing recurrence).

With the more severe cases of recurrent corneal erosion that do not seem to respond to any of the above therapies, the use of:

- Anterior stromal puncture has been advocated. The procedure involves making 75 to 150 small punctures with a bent 23 needle through the epithelium and Bowman's membrane into the anterior stroma. The needle tip is inserted through the loosened epithelium, making momentary micro depressions in the cornea to enter the stroma; the bent tip limits the excursion of the needle tip and permits the micropunctures to affect only the anterior stroma.

Patients who have had multiple recurrent erosion episodes, unresponsive to debridement alone or debridement with cautery, have shown significant improvements with anterior stromal puncture. Used correctly, the technique is effective in 90% of cases with recalcitrant recurrent erosion with the first application; a few patients may require a second application of anterior stromal puncture.

Surgical

For spontaneous recurrent erosions and erosions secondary to corneal dystrophies such as Reis-Bücklers' dystrophy, lattice dystrophy, and the superficial variant of granular dystrophy, as well as epithelial basement membrane dystrophy.

- Excimer laser photoablation (phototherapeutic keratectomy, or PTK) of the epithelium, the basement membrane, and just into Bowman's membrane has been performed with some success, although it is more expensive that mechanical debridement.

PRECAUTIONS

Treatment should be as simple as possible with the use of as few drugs as necessary. Some drugs, such as local anesthetic agents, have been shown to delay epithelial wound healing. For this reason, it is imperative to never prescribe a topical anesthetic agent for the patient's own use, even when symptoms are severe; ointments, bandage soft contact lenses, or patching should suffice to manage pain while initiating healing.

Indications for chemical cautery or lamellar keratectomy for resistant erosions have become almost non existent with the advent of therapeutic soft contact lenses, anterior stromal puncture, and PTK. In fact, due to the cost of bandage contact lenses and the frequent follow-up visits required, as well as the potential for corneal infections with long-term use, contact lens therapy should be postponed until milder forms of treatment prove to be ineffective. Anterior stromal puncture or PTK is preferred for treatment of the most severe cases of recurrent corneal erosion that do not resolve with ointments and patching.

COMMENTS

Systemic disease does not seem to play a role in epithelial basement membrane dystrophy or recurrent corneal erosion.

REFERENCES

Baum JL: Prolonged eyelid closure is a risk to the cornea. The Castroviejo Lecture, 1997. Cornea 16:602–611, 1997.

Brunette I, Boisjoly HM: Should we patch corneal erosions?[letter] Arch Ophthalmology 115(12):1607, 1997.

Heyworth P, Morlet N, Rayner S, et al: Natural history of recurrent erosion syndrome-A 4-year review of 117 patients. Br J Ophthalmol. 82:537–540, 1998.

Ionides AC, Tuft SJ, Ferguson VM, et al: Corneal infiltration after recurrent corneal erosion. Br J Ophthalmol 81:537–540, 1997.

Laibson PR: Microcystic corneal dystrophy. Trans Am Ophthalmol Soc 74:488–531, 1976.

Liu C, Buckley R: The role of the therapeutic contact lens in the management of recurrent corneal erosions: a review of treatment strategies. CLAO 22:79–82, 1996.

Maine R, Loughman MS: Phototherapeutic keratectomy re-treatment for recurrent corneal erosion syndrome [letter]. BJ Ophthalmology 86(3):270–272, 2002.

McDonnell PJ, Seiler T: Phototherapeutic keratectomy with excimer laser for Reis-Buckler corneal dystrophy. Refract Corneal Surg 8:306–310, 1992.

McGhee CN, Bryce IG, Anastas CN: Corneal topographic lagoons: a potential new marker for post-traumatic recurrent corneal erosion syndrome. Aust NZ J Ophthalmol 24:27–31, 1996.

McLean EN, MacRae SM, Rich LP: Recurrent erosion: treatment by anterior stromal puncture. Ophthalmology 93:784–788, 1986.

Park AJ, Rapuano CJ: Diamond burr treatment of recurrent erosions. Techniques in Ophthalmology 2(3):114–117, 2004.

Rapuano CJ: Excimer laser phototherapeutic keratectomy: long-term results and practical considerations. Cornea 16:151–157, 1997.

Reidy JJ, Paulus MP, Suma G: Recurrent erosions of the cornea: epidemiology and treatment. Cornea 19(6):767–771, 2000.

Rhys C, Snyers B, Pirson Y: Recurrent corneal erosion associated with Alport's syndrome: Rapid communication. Kidney Int 52:208–211, 1997.

Soong H Kaz, Farjo E, Meyer RF, Sugar A: Diamond burr superficial keratectomy for recurrent corneal erosions. BJ Ophthalmology 86(3):296–298, 2002.

Trobe JD, Laibson PR: Dystrophic changes in the anterior cornea. Arch Ophthalmol 87:378–382, 1972.

194 FILAMENTARY KERATITIS 370.23

William R. Morris, MD
Memphis, Tennessee

DESCRIPTION

Filamentary keratitis is a condition in which fine filaments develop on the anterior surface of the cornea. These filaments are gelatinous and refractile, varying from 0.5 to 10.0 mm long. They move freely and twist with blinking while remaining attached to the cornea at their base. Gray subepithelial opacities may occur at the base of the filaments. The filaments are composed of degenerated epithelial cells and mucoid debris. There may be single or multiple filaments; the condition may be acute or chronic. Symptoms may include foreign body sensation, tearing, photophobia or blepharospasm.

ETIOLOGY

- Unknown.
- Possibly an increased ratio of mucus to aqueous tear components.
- Detachment of corneal epithelial basement membrane with elevation of epithelium, providing attachment points for mucus and degenerated epithelial cells.

ASSOCIATED CONDITIONS

- Keratoconjunctivitis sicca.
- Prolonged lid closure (patching or ptosis).
- Superior limbic keratoconjunctivitis.
- Post-operative states (intraocular or extraocular surgery).
- Brain stem injury or stroke.
- Radiation therapy.
- Atopic dermatitis.
- Sarcoidosis.
- Ocular pemphigoid.
- Recurrent corneal erosion.
- Soft contact lens wear.
- Corneal edema.
- Ligneous conjunctivitis.
- Carcinoma of conjunctiva.
- Epidemic keratoconjunctivitis (EKC).
- Nodular degeneration of cornea.
- Antihistamines.
- Topical antiviral medication.
- Large angle strabismus.
- Beta-irradiation.
- Ectodermal dysplasia.
- Psoriasis.
- Neurotrophic keratitis.
- Hereditary hemorrhagic telangiectasia (Rendu–Osler–Weber disease).
- Trachoma.
- Acquired nystagmus treated with retrobulbar botulinum toxin.
- Acquired strabismus after surgical correction.
- Anticardiolipin antibodies.

COURSE

- Most acute cases resolve within a few days.
- Most cases associated with keratoconjunctivitis sicca resolve within one month.
- Chronic cases may require continued therapy.

TREATMENT

Local

- Treat underlying disease.
- Debridement of filaments — fine forceps, cotton tip applicator or cellulose acetate filter paper.
- Sodium chloride 5% ophthalmic drops four times daily.
- Sodium chloride 5% ophthalmic ointment at bedtime.
- Diclofenac sodium 0.1% four times daily.
- Hypotonic artificial tears frequently.
- Soft contact lens for:
  - Post-operative cataract;
  - Post-operative penetrating keratoplasty;
  - Brain-stem injury or stroke.
- Surgical:
  - Punctal occlusion in patients with keratoconjunctivitis sicca.

REFERENCES

Arora I, Singhvi S: Impression debridement of corneal lesions. Ophthalmology 101(12):1935–1940, 1994.

Avisar R, Robinson A, Appel I, et al: Diclofenac sodium, 0.1% (Voltaren Ophtha), versus sodium chloride, 5%, in the treatment of filamentary keratitis. Cornea 19(2):145–147, 2000.

Baum JL: The Castroviejo Lecture. Prolonged eyelid closure is a risk to the cornea. Cornea 16:602–611, 1997.

Davis WG, Drewry RD, Wood TO: Filamentary keratitis and stromal neovascularization associated with brain-stem injury. Am J Ophthalmol 90:489–491, 1980.

Fakadej AF, Plotnik RD: Filamentary keratitis. In: Krachmer JH, Mannis MJ, Holland EJ, eds: Cornea. St Louis: Mosby; 1997:1327–1332.

Hamilton W, Wood TO: Filamentary keratitis. Am J Ophthalmol 93:466–469, 1982.

Lemp MA, Gold JB, Wong S, et al: An in vivo study of corneal surface morphologic features in patients with keratoconjunctivitis sicca. Am J Ophthalmol 98:426–428, 1984.

Lohman LE, Rao GN, Aquavella JV: In vivo microscopic observations of human corneal epithelial abnormalities. Am J Ophthalmol 93:210–217, 1982.

Miserocchi E, Baltatzis S, Foster CS: Ocular features associated with anticardiolipin antibodies: a descriptive study. Am J Ophthalmol 131(4):451–456, 2001.

Pons ME, Rosenberg SE: Filamentary keratitis occurring after strabismus surgery. JAAPOS 8:190–191, 2004.

Tomsak RL, Remler BF, Averbuch-Heller L, et al: Unsatisfactory treatment of acquired nystagmus with retrobulbar injection of botulinum toxin. Am J Ophthalmol 119(4):489–496, 1995.

Wolper J, Laibson PR: Hereditary hemorrhagic telangiectasis (Rendu-Osler-Weber disease). Arch Ophthalmol 81(2):272–277, 1969.

Zaidman GW, Geeraets R, Paylor RR, Ferry AP: The histopathology of filamentary keratitis. Arch Ophthalmol 103(8):1178–1181, 1985.

195 FUCHS' CORNEAL DYSTROPHY

371.57

(Fuchs' Endothelial Dystrophy of the Cornea, Combined Dystrophy of Fuchs, Endothelial Dystrophy of the Cornea, Epithelial Dystrophy of Fuchs, Fuchs' Epithelial-Endothelial Dystrophy)

Mark A. Terry, MD
Portland, Oregon

ETIOLOGY/INCIDENCE

Fuchs' dystrophy is a bilateral, slowly progressive, primary corneal disease which results in vision loss due to corneal edema. Often asymmetric, this genetic disease is autosomal dominant with a high degree of penetrance and variable expressivity. Females are more severely affected than males, but not more frequently. The primary physiologic defect is a gradual decline in the density of the ATPase pump sites of the diseased endothelium. This results in progressive stromal and, in advanced cases, epithelial edema which usually does not become clinically evident until the fourth or fifth decade of life. Associated conditions include keratoconus, axial hypermetropia, cardiovascular disease, glaucoma, and age-related macular degeneration. Due to the spectrum of disease severity and asymptomatic nature of most affected individuals, the incidence of Fuchs' dystrophy is unknown.

DIAGNOSIS

Endothelial dysfunction results in corneal edema and this is the basis of the signs and symptoms of the disease. The endothelium produces an abnormal, banded, posterior layer of Descemet's membrane with characteristic central guttae excrescences which are a hallmark of this disease. Progressive endothelial cell loss with endothelial polymegathism and pleomorphism can be documented by specular or by confocal microscopy. With the presence of stromal edema found by slit-lamp biomicroscopy or by sequential corneal ultrasonography, the diagnosis of Fuchs' dystrophy is made. Characteristically, initial visual loss is noted by the patient upon awakening with clearing of the vision during the day. As stromal edema spills over into epithelial edema, the patient may note a sudden dramatic decrease in vision. Untreated, epithelial edema leads to surface scarring and severe visual loss.

Clinical stages

Stage I

- Central corneal guttae, with or without pigment on the posterior cornea, with a gray and thickened appearance of Descemet's membrane.
- Asymptomatic.

Stage II

- Same as stage I, but with stromal edema.
- Painless.
- Mild decreased vision (20/25 to 20/50).
- Increased glare.
- Symptoms often worse on awakening.

Stage III

- Microcystic or bullous epithelial and subepithelial edema seen best with flourescein dye application.
- Irritation or pain.
- Vision worse (20/60 to 20/400).

Stage IV

- Severe vision loss (20/400 to hand motion).
- Subepithelial fibrous scarring.
- Often pain free.

Differential diagnosis

- Posterior polymorphous dystrophy.
- Peripheral Hassall–Henle warts.
- Pseudoguttae due to trauma, infection or toxins.
- Disciform keratitis.
- Pseudophakic bullous keratopathy.
- Chandler syndrome.
- Congenital hereditary endothelial dystrophy.

TREATMENT

Systemic

None.

Systemic oral carbonic anhydrase inhibitors are contraindicated due to their possible suppression of the Na-K ATPase pump and long term systemic risks.

Local

- Sodium choride 5% solution or ointment up to eight times a daily and tailored to the patients visual symptoms for osmotic dehydration of epithelial edema.
- Use of a hair dryer at arm's length with a low heat setting for tear film evaporation and corneal detergescence.
- Lower intraocular pressure with standard glaucoma topical medications.

Surgical

- Corneal transplantation.
- Traditional full thickness PK is highly successful (>90%) for clear grafts but often results in high irregular astigmatism and other refractive problems. Long term complications of wound dehiscence and globe rupture can occur between 5% and 17%.
- Endothelial Keratoplasty (EK) with Deep Lamellar Endothelial Keratoplasty (DLEK) or Descemet's Stripping Endothelial Keratoplasty (DSEK) represents a new surgical approach that avoids surface corneal incisions or sutures. EK has

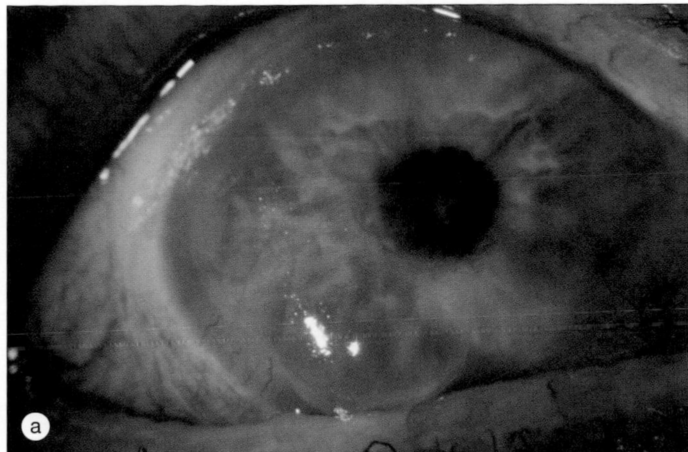

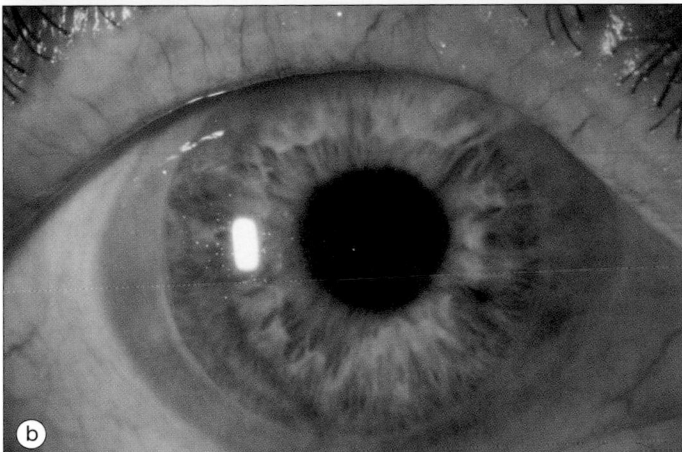

FIGURE 195.1. a) Cornea with Fuchs' dystrophy stage III corneal edema pre-operatively showing large surface bullae extending onto lower lid and painful red eye. b) Post-operatively at 6 months after deep lamellar endothelial keratoplasty (DLEK) the cornea is clear with no sutures, there are no bullae, and the eye is comfortable.

faster visual rehabilitation than PK and may avoid the short and long term complications.

Painful corneal epithelial bullae with no light perception vision

Cautery, Gunderson flap, and amniotic membrane surgery have all been useful for pain control.

COMMENTS

Fuchs' dystrophy is a slowly progressive disease which can be observed until the patients symptoms warrant treatment. Every effort should be made to reduce endothelial damage from episodes of intraocular inflammation (iritis) or surgical trauma (cataract surgery). Medical management is best until visual acuity is compromised to the point of interfering with activities essential to daily life. While PK is highly successful, new methods of selective corneal transplantation (DLEK and DSEK) may offer topographic, refractive and tectonic advantages.

REFERENCES

Bergmanson JP, Sheldon TM, Goosey JD: Fuchs' endothelial dystrophy: a fresh look at an aging disease. Ophthalmic Physiol Opt 19:210–222, 1999.

Borboli S, Colby K: Mechanisms of disease: Fuchs' endothelial dystrophy. Ophthalmol Clin N Am 15:17–25, 2002.

Chiou AG-Y, Kaufman SC, Beuerman RW, et al: Confocal microscopy in corneal guttata and Fuchs' endothelial dystrophy. Br J Ophthalmology 83:185–189, 1999.

Egan CA, Hodge DO, McLaren JW, Bourne WM: Effect of dorzolamide on corneal endothelial function in normal human eyes. Invest Ophthalmol Vis Sci 39:23–29, 1998.

Elder MJ, Stack RR: Globe rupture following penetrating keratoplasty: how often, why, and what can we do to prevent it? Cornea 23:776–780, 2004.

McCartney RK, Wood TO, McLaughin BJ: Moderate Fuchs' endothelial dystrophy ATPase pump site density. Invest Ophthalmol Vis Sci 30:1560–1564, 1989.

Terry MA, Ousley PJ: Small incision deep lamellar endothelial keratoplasty (DLEK): 6-month results in the first prospective clinical study. Cornea 2005 (in press).

Terry MA: Deep lamellar endothelial keratoplasty (DLEK): pursuing the ideal goals of endothelial replacement. Eye 17:982–988, 2003.

Terry MA, Ousley PJ: Deep lamellar endothelial keratoplasty (DLEK): Visual acvity, astigmatism, and endothelial survival in a large prospective series. Ophthalmology 112:1541–1549, 2005.

Terry MA: Endothelial keratoplasty (EK): History, Current State, and Future Directions. Cornea 25:873–878, 2006 (Editorial).

196 FUCHS' DELLEN 371.41
(Facets, Fuchs' Dimples)

F. Hampton Roy, MD, FACS
Little Rock, Arkansas

ETIOLOGY/INCIDENCE

Dellen are paralimbal corneal ulcerations that occur at the base of abnormal conjunctiva or corneal elevations. These ellipsoid depressions, or dells, in the cornea represent a common but not well known phenomenon. Dellen are usually elliptic and saucer shaped with clearly defined edges. Although transient dellen are superficial and purely epithelial, they may last several weeks and become deep. Cicatrization normally follows, often with reduction in corneal thickness (facets).

Abnormal paralimbic conjunctival elevation is associated with:

- Filtering bleb;
- Hematoma;
- Chemosis;
- Conjunctival tumor;
- Rectus muscle surgery;
- Conjunctival autograft;
- Pterygium.

Abnormal corneal elevations can be seen secondary to:

- Localized graft displacement or edema;
- Corneal sutures that are too tight;
- Corneal tumor.

Poor palpebral congruence prevents the lids from normally spreading the tears, which causes a break in the oily film. This break and the resulting desiccation can be aggravated by a trapped air bubble that sometimes bursts when the lids open.

COURSE/PROGNOSIS

- Possible perforation.
- Astigmatism.

TREATMENT

- Elimination of the cause.
- Pressure dressing to control any abnormal conjunctival elevation.
- Surgery rarely necessary to remove the elevation.
- Topical corticosteroids when the elevation is of inflammatory origin.
- Treatment of the ulceration.
- Ocular lubricants to avoid desiccation of the ulcer and to coat it.
- New anticollagenase eyedrops to reduce collagen necrosis.
- Antibiotic eyedrops to avoid secondary infections.

COMMENTS

Dellen are more common than is commonly thought. They are usually benign but occasionally present difficulties. In almost all cases, they heal well with the use of the simple techniques described.

REFERENCES

Fuchs A: Pathological dimples ('Dellen') of the cornea. Am J Ophthalmol 12:877–883, 1929.

Insler MS, Tauber S, Packer A: Descemetocele formation in a patient with a postoperative corneal dellen. Cornea 8:129–130, 1989.

Lagoutte F, Gauthier L, Comte P: A fibrin sealant for perforated and preperforated corneal ulcers. Br J Ophthalmol 73:757–761, 1989.

Soong HK, Quigley HA: Dellen associated with filtering blebs. Arch Ophthalmol;101:385–387, 1983.

197 FUNGAL KERATITIS 111.1

Denis M. O'Day, MD, FACS
Nashville, Tennessee

ETIOLOGY/INCIDENCE

Fungi invade the cornea as a result of a break in the natural host defenses of the eye. This occurs either after trauma or when there is a breakdown of local or general defense mechanisms. Unless the trauma has penetrated the deep layers of the cornea, infection is initially superficial. It progresses slowly to invade the deeper cornea and may involve the adjacent sclera, anterior chamber, and intraocular structures.

Fungal infections are most common in tropical and subtropical climates, where the most frequent isolates are the filamentous fungi *Fusarium solani* and *Aspergillus* spp. The majority of cases involve minor trauma, usually with vegetable material as the inciting event. In temperate and colder climates, the infectious agent most often is a yeast. Such infections, however, are rare and are usually associated with reduced immunocompetence, immunosuppression, or severe structural alteration of the cornea and adnexa. In tropical climates, fungal keratitis is a major cause of corneal blindness.

COURSE/PROGNOSIS

The onset of a fungal infection is slow. As the fungus invades corneal tissue, it establishes a progressive inflammation over a period of weeks. The clinical signs initially may be subtle. Infiltrate develops slowly, and the epithelium may heal over the superficial defect. As the infection becomes more severe, hypopyon may develop. Yeast infections tend to remain localized in the more superficial layers of the cornea; filamentous fungal infections steadily progress to invade the anterior chamber, cornea, and surrounding structures.

Untreated, the prognosis is poor, with blindness or loss of the eye as the usual outcome.

DIAGNOSIS

Laboratory findings

- Corneal smear: Giemsa, KOH, or Gomori's methenamine silver stains.
- Culture: Sabouraud dextrose agar, brain-heart infusion broth (no inhibitors).
- Prolonged incubation possibly necessary (weeks).
- Possible contamination of culture (use C streaks to identify inoculum).

Differential diagnosis

- Bacterial and protozoal infections, herpes simplex, or herpes zoster keratitis.

TREATMENT

Yeast infections

Topical 0.15% amphotericin every hour while awake for 48 hours and then every 2 hours (prolonged treatment necessary).

Filamentous fungi

Topical 5% natamycin suspension every hour while awake for 48 hours and then every 2 hours (prolonged treatment necessary).

Subconjunctival therapy

No evidence of efficacy.

Systemic therapy

- Yeasts: none indicated.
- Filamentous fungi: some evidence in deep corneal progressive infections for the efficacy of systemic itraconazole or fluconazole (especially for *Aspergillus* spp. infection).

Surgical

Excisional keratoplasty indicated when disease progresses despite medical treatment.

COMPLICATIONS

- Perforation.
- Anterior endophthalmitis.
- Fungal scleritis.
- Fungal glaucoma.

COMMENTS

The signs of disease progress or regress slowly. Antifungal agents can be toxic to the cornea and may mask response. Steroids have no place in treatment. If a patient is receiving topical steroids at the time of diagnosis, withdraw them slowly.

REFERENCES

Forster RK: Fungal keratitis and conjunctivitis: clinical disease. In: Smolin G, Thoft RD, eds: The cornea: scientific foundations and clinical practice. Boston, Little, Brown, 1994:228–240.

Killingsworth DW, Stern GA, Driebe WT, et al: Results of therapeutic penetrating keratoplasty. Ophthalmology 100:534–541, 1993.

O'Day DM: Fungal keratitis. In: Pepose JS, Holland GN, Wilhelmus KR, eds: Ocular infections and immunity. St Louis, Mosby, 1996:1048–1061.

O'Day DM, Ray WA, Head WS, et al: Influence of corticosteroids on experimentally induced keratomycosis. Arch Ophthalmol 109:1601–1604, 1991.

198 GRANULAR CORNEAL DYSTROPHY 371.53

Joseph D. Iuorno, MD
Minneapolis MN, USA
Jay H. Krachmer, MD
Minneapolis MN, USA

EITIOLOGY/GENETICS/INCIDENCE

Granular dystrophy is an autosomal dominant inherited dystrophy affecting the corneal stroma. First named Groenouw type I in 1890, the etiology of granular corneal dystrophy (GCD) is still evolving. Recent understandings of molecular genetics have organized GCD into four subtypes. Each subtype has been associated with mutations (Table 198.1) in beta transforming growth factor induced gene in human clone 3 (*βIG H3*) also known as transforming growth factor beta induced gene (*TGFβI*). This gene produces an abnormal protein called TGFβI protein (kerato-epithelin) in all four types of granular dystrophy.

Classic GCD type I is characterized by the deposition of small, grayish-white, sharply demarcated opacities mostly in the anterior corneal stroma that can resemble breadcrumb, snowflake or popcorn shapes (Figure 198.1). Characteristic clear intervening spaces are noted between these corneal deposits. Throughout life, these deposits increase in size and number eventually coalescing to obliterate the clear intervening areas. Initially, these deposits appear in the central anterior stroma, however, over time, they extend posterior and peripherally. Despite their outward expansion, the outlying peripheral corneal stroma remains clear at least 2 mm in from the limbus.

On light microscopy, eosinophilic hyaline deposits appear bright red with Masson's trichrome stain. Electron microscopy (EM) reveals 100 μm to 500 μm sized rod-shaped extracellular phospholipid structures surrounded by microfibrillar proteins. Proposed etiologic theories suggest an epithelial genesis of GCD based on the prominent epithelial-like whirl pattern noted in corneal transplant graft recurrence.

COURSE/PROGNOSIS

- Onset is early in the first decade of life.
- Visual acuity is minimally affected until the second decade.

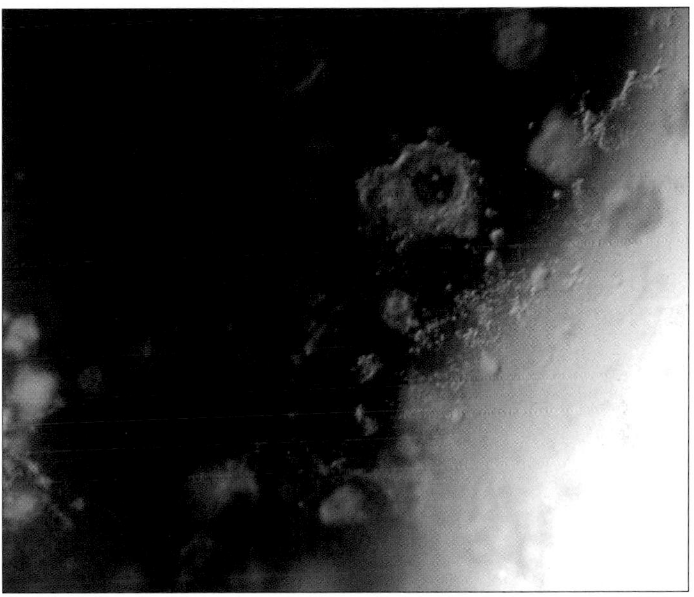

FIGURE 198.1. Granular corneal dystrophy. Note the grayish-white, sharply demarcated opacities mostly in the anterior corneal stroma that can resemble breadcrumb, snowflake or popcorn shapes. Characteristic clear intervening spaces are noted between these corneal deposits.

TABLE 198.1 – **Granular corneal dystrophy**

GCD type	Pseudonyms	Mutation in TGF beta-I
I	Classic GCD, Groenouw Type I	R555W, R124S
II	Avellino dystrohy, combined lattice/granular	R124H
III	Superficial GCD, Reis-Bücklers' corneal dystrophy, corneal dystrophy of Bowman's layer type I	R124L, R555Q, G623N Exon12 del F540
IV	French varient similar to GCD III	R124L plus del T125 and E126

- Photophobia is a common symptom.
- Corneal erosions, especially with superficial subtypes (GCD type III), occur less commonly than in patients with lattice dystrophy.
- As opacities increase in size and number, the clear intervening areas become cloudy and visual acuity is compromised. Generally, this does not occur until the 5th decade.
- The epithelium, basement membrane and far peripheral corneal stroma are typically spared.
- The prognosis with penetrating keratoplasty is excellent.
- Recurrences are common and typically have an epithelial-like whirl pattern.

DIAGNOSIS

- Observation of distinct central, anterior and mid stromal opacities with clear intervening spaces not extending to the limbus.
- Autosomal dominant inheritance.
- Mason's trichrome stain of eosinophilic hyaline deposits.
- EM findings of rod-shape bodies.

TREATMENT

- For mild cases, observation and recurrent erosion therapy.
- Soft contact lenses can be helpful.
- When reduced vision, photophobia and recurrent corneal erosions combine to sufficiently reduce the quality of life, penetrating keratoplasty is recommended.
- Graft recurrences are treated by superficial keratectomy, phototherapeutic keratectomy, or repeat penetrating keratoplasty.

SUMMARY

Granular dystrophy is an autosomal dominant stromal dystrophy which starts in the first decade of life in the anterior central corneal stroma and spreads to more posterior and peripheral areas. Later in life, as the clear intervening stromal areas become overwhelmed by the increasing number of enlarging opacities, visual acuity can be compromised. Penetrating keratoplasty is effective but often followed by recurrence in the donor tissue.

REFERENCES

Dinh R, Rapuano CJ, Cohen EJ, Laibson PR: Recurrence of corneal dystrophy after excimer laser phototherapeutic keratectomy. Ophthalmology 106(8):1490–1497, 1999.

Klintworth GK: The molecular genetics of the corneal dystrophies-current status. Front in Bioscience 8:678–713, 2003.

Krachmer JH, Mannis MJ, Holland EJ: Cornea. 2nd edn: Philadelphia, Elsevier Mosby, 2005:907–909.

Lyons CJ, McCartney AC, Kirkness CM, et al: Granular corneal dystrophy. Visual results and pattern of recurrence after lamellar or penetrating keratoplasty. Ophthalmology 101(11):1812–1817, 1994.

Rodrigues MM, Streeten BW, Krachmer JH, et al: Microfibrillar protein and phospholipid in granular corneal dystrophy. Arch Ophthalmol 101(5):802–810, 1983.

199 JUVENILE CORNEAL EPITHELIAL DYSTROPHY 371.51

(Meesmann's Corneal Dystrophy)

Peter R. Kastl, MD, PhD
New Orleans, Louisiana

ETIOLOGY/INCIDENCE

Meesmann's corneal dystrophy has autosomal dominant inheritance, as do most corneal dystrophies. This rare disease infrequently causes discomfort and minimal (if any) visual loss.

COURSE/PROGNOSIS

Mild discomfort and slightly decreased vision may occur in later life.

DIAGNOSIS

Clinical signs and symptoms

- Corneal findings include epithelial cysts, irregular astigmatism, superficial haze.
- Other clinical findings include decreased vision, ocular irritation.

Laboratory findings

Slit-lamp examination findings include epithelial bleb-like lesions that appear to direct illumination as whitish-gray, small punctate opacities but that on retroillumination appear as clear, spherical vesicles. The overlying epithelium is clear. Histopathologically, small cysts are found throughout the epithelium, which are the vesicles seen on retroillumination. These contain debris and are most numerous in the anterior one-third of the epithelium. Electron microscopy demonstrates a 'peculiar substance' in the cytoplasm that is seen more often in the basal cells. This substance appears to be fibrillogranular material, probably derived from degenerated cytoplasmic filaments.

TREATMENT

Treatment is not usually required. The use of bandage soft contact lenses can reduce any symptoms. If the vision is markedly decreased, debridement or even lamellar keratoplasty can be performed.

COMPLICATIONS

Corneal debridement can cause scarring and infection. The prolonged wearing of soft contact lenses can result in infection. Patients wearing soft lenses on a long-term basis should be examined periodically for lens wear side effects.

REFERENCES

Alkemade PP, Balen AV: Hereditary epithelial dystrophy of the cornea: Meesmann type. Br J Ophthalmol 50:603–605, 1966.

Fine BS, Yanoff M, Pitts E, Slaughter FD: Meesmann's epithelial dystrophy of the cornea. Am J Ophthalmol 83:633–642, 1977.

Irvine AD, Corden LD, Swensson O, et al: Mutations in cornea-specific keratin K3 or K12 genes cause Meesmann's corneal dystrophy. Nat Genet 16:184–187, 1997.

Meesmann A: Über eine bisher nicht beschreibene dominant vererbte Dystrophia epithelialis corneae. Ber Dtsch Ophthalmol Ges 52:154, 1938.

Pameijer JK: Über eine fremdartige familiare oberflächliche Hornhaut-veränderung. Klin Monatsbl Augenheilkd 95:516, 1935.

Roca PD: Meesmann's hereditary epithelial dystrophy (differential diagnosis). Eye Ear Nose Throat Mon 48:424 425, 1969.

Swensson O, Swensson B, Nolle B, et al: [Mutations in the keratin gene as a cause of Meesman-Wilke corneal dystrophy and autosomal dominant skin cornification disorders]. Klinische Monatsblatter für Augenheilkunde 217(1):43–51, 2000.

Thiel HJ, Behnke H: [On the extent of variation of hereditary epithelial corneal dystrophy (Meesmann-Wilke type)]. Ophthalmologica 155:81–86, 1968.

Thiel HJ, Caesar R: [Histologic and electron microscopic studies of hereditary corneal epithelial dystrophy (Meesmann-Wilke)]. Albrecht Von Graefes Arch Klin Exp Ophthalmol 174:134–142, 1967.

Tremblay M, Dube I: Meesmann's corneal dystrophy: ultrastructural features. Can J Ophthalmol 17:24–28, 1982.

200 KERATOCONJUNCTIVITIS SICCA AND SJÖGREN'S SYNDROME 370.33

James V. Aquavella, MD
Rochester, NY

ETIOLOGY/INCIDENCE

Sjögren syndrome is an autoimmune disease consisting of xerostomia (dry mouth), keratoconjunctivitis sicca, often associated with dryness of the nasal and genital mucosa. Primary Sjögren's is seen in individuals with the systemic immune dysfunction in the absence of connective tissue disease as well as in individuals lacking both systemic dysfunction and connective tissue disease. Secondary Sjögren's includes patients with defined connective tissue disease (rheumatoid arthritis, lupus).

The exact incidence is unknown; one Swedish study suggests 0.4% prevalence. Estimates for the United States are between 1 and 2%. There is a nine to one prevalence for females, and the condition is most often seen in postmenopausal women although there are a number of reports of women afflicted in their 20 s and 30 s.

One of the prime findings is lymphocyte infiltration of secretory glands. While the lachrymal and salivary glands are most frequently effected a more widespread involvement of secretory glands is not unusual.

COURSE/PROGNOSIS

While the prognosis is good, severe dry eyes can result in infection, ulceration, perforation and diffuse corneal scarring and vascularization leading to a much more guarded visual prognosis.

DIAGNOSIS

Clinical signs and symptoms

Ocular signs and symptoms are similar to those of other dry eye conditions. Burning, itching, foreign body (sandy) sensation, mucous discharge, photophobia and blurred vision may be present. The condition usually is more comfortable in the early AM with exacerbating symptomatology as the day progresses. Desiccating environmental factors may be implicated with symptom fluctuation.

While there have been European and American diagnostic criteria promulgated, in general dry mouth, dry eye and autoimmune disease constitute the diagnostic triad. The most comprehensive factors are decreased salivary flow, decreased lachrymal flow, lymphocyte glandular infiltration, the absence of nasal stimulated reflex tearing and the presence of serum antibodies.

Laboratory findings

Positive lip and lachrymal grand biopsy in conjunction with positive antinuclear antibody (ANA), rheumatoid factor (RF), anti-Ro (Sjögern specific A), and anti-La (Sjögern specific B) assist in establishing the diagnosis. Helper T cells are the predominant lymphocyte infiltrator along with B and CD4 lymphocytes. Epstein–Barr virus may play a role. An elevated IgG level has been shown to have a high specificity and positive predication value in predicting positive biopsy results.

TREATMENT

Systemic

Immunosuppressive agents such as cyclosporin A, trenonin, and corticosteroids have been utilized in severe cases. Oral bromhexine or pilocarpine has been advocate to improve lachrymal function.

Topical

The mainstay continues to be frequent application of tear substitutes (often non-preserved to avoid secondary irritation). For recurrent inflammation judicious use of topical steroids may be indicated. Existing tears may be conserved with punctual occlusion and the use of moist chamber goggles.

Cyclosporin A may have a role in increasing lachrymal function. Antibiotics may be necessary in secondary infection.

Other adjuncts

Hydrophilic bandage lenses, partial tarsorrhaphy, amniotic membranes have all been utilized with varying success. Controlling environmental humidification and airflow is helpful.

COMPLICATIONS

Secondary bacterial infection/ulceration and perforation can occur. The incidence of lymphoma in Sjögren's is elevated.

COMMENTS

This is a condition which is often managed well with minimal lifestyle modifications but which has the potential for debilitating corneal blindness. Aggressive management, involvement of other disciplines (rheumatology, immunology, oral biology, dentistry, OBGYN) can create the comprehensive approach, which will produce the best results over the long term.

REFERENCES

Daniels TE, Whitcher JP: Assocaiton of patterns of labial salivary gland inflammation with keratoconjunctivitis sicca. Arthrtis Rheum 37:869–877, 1994.

Pepose JS, Akata RF, Pflugfelder SC, Vopight W: Mononuclear cell phenotypes and immunoglobulin gene rearrangements in lacrimal gland biopsies from patients with Sjörgren's syndrome. Ophthalmology 97(12):1599–605, 1990.

Pflugfelder SC: Lacrimal gland epithelial and immunopathology of Sjögren's syndrome. In: Homma M, ed: Proceedings of the IV International Sjögren's Syndrome Syposium, Kugler. Am Steleveen, 1994.

201 KERATOCONUS 371.60

Brandon D. Ayres, MD
Philadelphia, PA
Christopher J. Rapuano, MD
Philadelphia, PA

ETIOLOGY/INCIDENCE

Keratoconus is a noninflammatory corneal disorder that involves abnormal thinning of the corneal stroma; thinning usually occurs in either the central or inferior cornea. It is most often bilateral, although severity can be very asymmetric. True unilateral keratoconus is infrequent. Keratoconus affects approximately 1 in 2000 and is the second most common cause of primary corneal transplants. In approximately 10% of cases, there is a familial history with an autosomal dominant inheritance pattern. It also can be associated with systemic conditions such as osteogenesis imperfecta, Down syndrome and atopic disease.

The biochemical cause of the corneal thinning in keratoconus is not fully understood. Altered proteoglycan synthesis has been implicated as has alteration in the nitric oxide pathway allowing activation of proteolytic enzymes that weaken and thin the cornea and decreased activity of corneal enzyme inhibitors. Contact lens wear and eye rubbing have also been implicated as primary causes of keratoconus.

COURSE/PROGNOSIS

The first symptom of keratoconus often appears between the ages of 15 and 30 years and is a slow progressive decrease in vision in one or both eyes. In the early stages, keratoconus is painless, and the eyes appear quiet; the condition may progress slowly for 10 to 20 years, often becoming stationary. As the condition progresses, the corneal mires become increasingly irregular, and thinning may extend to the limbus in advanced cases. Rarely, a rupture occurs in Descemet's membrane, resulting in:

- Acute hydrops (profound local corneal edema);
- Pain;
- Sudden deterioration of vision.

The hydrops usually resolves spontaneously over 3 to 6 months. In the acute phase, patching the eye relieves the discomfort in most cases. Interestingly, the episode often results in scarring and flattening of the cone and occasionally the return of functional visual acuity; however, if resolution is not apparent after 6 months, penetrating keratoplasty may be required.

DIAGNOSIS

Examination and laboratory findings

The distinctive patterns of keratoconus revealed with computerized corneal topography usually show inferior steepening with central irregularities. Rigid contact lens wear (especially of long duration) can confuse the diagnosis by inducing irregular astigmatism that may be permanent. This condition, corneal warpage, is classically associated with PMMA hard contact lenses. Diagnosis may require corneal mapping at intervals with the lenses not being worn over an extended period (several months). Other diagnostic signs of keratoconus include:

- Irregularity and doubling of keratometer mires (early sign);
- Scissors reflex on retinoscopy (early sign);
- Fleischer's ring (a partial or complete ring of hemosiderin pigment in deep epithelium, at the cone base);
- Vogt's striae (stress lines in the steep axis in posterior cornea);
- Corneal scarring at the apex of the cone;
- Prominent corneal nerves (uncommon);
- Annulus of the cone on retroillumination (moderate and advanced keratoconus);
- Munson's sign on downgaze (protrusion of lower eyelid) in severe cases.

Differential diagnosis

- Pellucid marginal degeneration: inferior thinning with flat central cornea.
- Keratoglobus: entire peripheral cornea steep and thinned; can be extremely thin in the periphery.
- Posterior keratoconus: accentuated posterior corneal steeping and thinning.
- Terrien's marginal degeneration: peripheral corneal thinning with lipid deposition which can cause irregular astigmatism.

All of these possible alternative diagnoses are relatively rare.

TREATMENT

Local

In early keratoconus, spectacle correction may be sufficient. As the disease advances, corrective spectacle lenses become increasingly heavy and objectionable to many patients, who then require contact lens correction. Hard contact lenses such as rigid gas-permeable lenses are usually required for good visual acuity in patients with keratoconus. Ninty percent of patients do well with contact lenses.

During progression of the condition, the patient may require frequent changes in lenses, with each successive pair requiring careful fitting, to permit the lens to move but also to resist ejection by normal blinking. Contact lenses themselves have been implicated in the exacerbation of corneal thinning, subepithelial scarring, and recurrent corneal erosion. Eye rubbing is thought by many physicians to aggravate keratoconus. All patients should be told not to rub their eyes.

Hydrops treatment involves the following:

- Discontinue contact lens wear;
- NaCl 5% drops and ointment;
- Patching;
- Some advocate short course of topical steroids;
- Cycloplegia for pain;
- Conservative follow up;
- Penetrating keratoplasty if edema does not resolve (uncommon) or visually significant scarring occurs (common).

For episodes of allergic reactions/atopy, the patient should be discouraged from rubbing the eyes; additional symptomatic treatment includes:

- Cold compresses;
- Antihistamine eyedrops or pills;
- Mast cell stabilizer eyedrops;
- Nonsteroidal anti-inflammatory drops.

Surgical

Penetrating keratoplasty is performed when the patient's vision or tolerance of contact lenses deteriorates; there is a greater than 95% success rate. Corneal scarring and high keratometric values have been implicated as risk factors in progression of disease ultimately leading to corneal transplant. Postoperatively, many patients will still require contact lenses for best visual acuity, but the correction will usually be milder and well tolerated.

Lamellar keratectomy, either with a blade or excimer laser, can be used to remove raised superficial scars at the apex of the cone, which may improve contact lens tolerance. Lamellar keratoplasty is advantageous in that it avoids the problem of endothelial rejection, however, is technically very difficult and the final vision may be suboptimal.

Alternatives such as:

- Thermokeratoplasty;
- Epikeratoplasty;
- Intrastromal corneal ring segment implantation (Intacs) are used in special circumstances but rarely achieve as good a visual outcome as a full-thickness graft.

SUPPORT GROUP

National Keratoconus Foundation
733 Beverly Blvd., Suite 201
Los Angeles, CA 90048
www.nkcf.org
FAX (310) 360-9712
E-mail: info@nkcf.org

REFERENCES

Bron AJ: Keratoconus. Cornea 7:163–169, 1988.

Ihalainen A: Clinical and epidemiological features of keratoconus genetic and external factors in the pathogenesis of the disease. Acta Ophthalmol Suppl 178:1–64, 1986.

Kenney MC, Nesburn AB, Burgeson RE, et al: Abnormalities of the extracellular matrix in keratoconus corneas. Cornea 16:345–351, 1997.

Krachmer JH, Feder RS, Belin MW: Keratoconus and related noninflammatory corneal thinning disorders. Surv Ophthalmol 28:293–322, 1984.

Rabinowitz YS: Keratoconus. Surv Ophthalmol 42:297–319, 1998.

Sray WA, Cohen EJ, Rapuano CJ, et al: Factors associated with the need for penetrating keratoplasty in keratoconus. Cornea 21:784–786, 2002.

202 LATTICE CORNEAL DYSTROPHY 371.54 *(Lattice Dystrophy Type I, Lattice Dystrophy Type II, Lattice Dystrophy Type III, LCD-I, LCD-II, LCD-III, Meretoja's Syndrome, Biber-Haab-Dimmer Dystrophy, Familial Amyloid Polyneuropathy Type IV)* AND AVELLINO DYSTROPHY 371.54

Douglas L. Meier, MD
Portland, Oregon

Lattice corneal dystrophy type I

ETIOLOGY

Lattice corneal dystrophy type I (LCD-I) is an autosomal dominant dystrophy that usually affects both eyes symmetrically. It is characterized by a localized corneal deposition of amyloid that is unrelated to systemic disease.

COURSE/PROGNOSIS

It appears in the first or second decade of life as characteristic refractile anterior stromal branching filamentous lines, focal white dots or dashes, or faint central stromal opacities. The deposits are prominent centrally and spare the peripheral 2 to 3 mm of cornea. The dystrophy is slowly progressive, with the lesions involving the deeper cornea and the opacity becoming denser and visually disabling, usually by the third or fourth decade. Occasionally, the first symptoms of the disease are noted in childhood or in the sixth or seventh decade; there is a considerable variation among affected family members in the age at which symptoms appear.

DIAGNOSIS

Clinical signs and symptoms

Symptoms of photophobia, foreign body sensation, and pain from recurrent corneal epithelial erosions may be prominent in some patients. As corneal sensation decreases, the recurrent erosions become less painful. Irregular surface corneal astigmatism further decreases functional vision.

Laboratory findings

The characteristic histologic finding in the stroma is a fusiform deposit of amyloid that pushes aside the collagen lamellae, probably corresponding to the lattice lines and dots seen clinically. A degenerative pannus is seen with portions of Bowman's membrane replaced by the deposits and irregular connective tissue. Clinically, these changes are associated with recurrent erosions. The stromal deposits stain orange-red with Congo red and demonstrate apple-green birefringence when viewed with polarized light. Red-green dichroism is seen with a green filter and a polarizing filter. Metachromasia can be demonstrated after staining with crystal violet. The deposits also stain with periodic acid-Schiff, Masson's trichrome, and fluorochrome thioflavin T. Electron microscopy of the lesions shows a felt-like mass of fine (8 to 10 nm in diameter), nonbranching short fibrils without periodicity that are approximately half the size of adjacent collagen. The fibrils are sometimes associated with an amorphous electron-dense elastoid material. The source of the amyloid is not certain but probably is from abnormally functioning keratocytes. The keratocytes often have a prominent endoplasmic reticulum; they are decreased in number and show degeneration. Descemet's membrane and the endothelium are normal.

Lattice corneal dystrophy type II

ETIOLOGY

Lattice corneal dystrophy type II (LCD-II, Meretoja's syndrome, familial amyloid polyneuropathy type IV) is an autosomal dominant form of LCD with an onset of clinical signs in the third decade. It is most common in Scandinavia.

DIAGNOSIS

LCD-II is associated with systemic amyloidosis, including signs of progressive cranial and peripheral nerve palsies, dry skin, blepharochalasis, protruding lips, mask-like facies, and bundle-branch block-all of which usually develop after the age of 40. The vision is not usually as reduced as it is in LCD-I. Recurrent erosions are uncommon. The lattice lines are fewer in number and are most dense in the midperiphery extending to the limbus with relative axial sparing. Glaucoma and pseudoexfoliation (with or without glaucoma) are common. Histologically, the corneal deposits are similar to those in LCD-I, but Bowman's membrane is intact. Systemically, amyloid deposits are found in skin, nerves, arteries, and other tissues.

Lattice corneal dystrophy type III

ETIOLOGY

Lattice corneal dystrophy type III (LCD-III) has a later onset and an autosomal recessive inheritance. It was first described in Japan.

DIAGNOSIS

The lattice lines are thicker and ropy, extending from limbus to limbus. Recurrent epithelial erosions are not seen. Histologically, the amyloid deposits are in the midstroma, and Bowman's membrane is only minimally disrupted. LCD-IIIA may be a variant of type III. It occurs in whites, is associated with corneal erosions, and has an autosomal dominant pattern of inheritance.

GENETICS

In the last decade advances in genetic analyses have documented several DNA mutations which are associated with the various types of lattice corneal dystrophy. Most of the autosomal dominant corneal dystrophies are caused by the irregularities of the *βIGH3* (or *TGFβI*) gene, which is located on chromosome 5q31. The gene is responsible for the production of the protein, keratoepithelin.

Keratoepithelin is produced by the corneal epithelium but is predominantly present in the corneal stroma, especially Bowman's layer. Keratoepithelin appears to be involved in cell adhesion or corneal wound healing by blocking epithelial cell proliferation. Keratoepithelin accumulates in the corneal stroma with those dystrophies associated with mutations of the 5q31 gene.

Type I lattice dystrophy results from a mutation at codon 124, leading to a substitution of cysteine for arginine. Gelsolin is an actin filament-binding protein. The gelsolin gene appears to be affected in type II, with the *Asp187Asn* mutation causing the findings in systemic amyloidosis. Different mutations have been implicated in several other presentations of lattice dystrophy. Given this, our current classification of lattice corneal dystrophy by phenotype and histology (i.e. LCD-I, LCD-II, etc.) as reliable as once thought.

Differential diagnosis

- Reis–Bückler dystrophy.
- Herpes simplex or zoster.
- Avellino dystrophy.
- Polymorphic amyloid degeneration.

TREATMENT

- Nonsurgical: artificial tears, lubricating ointments, soft contact lenses, pressure patching.
- Phototherapeutic keratectomy: useful for superficial lesions and recurrent erosions.
- Penetrating keratoplasty: highly successful (90%), recurrent disease not uncommon but mild and occasionally requires regrafting after 10 to 15 years.

Avellino dystrophy

ETIOLOGY/INCIDENCE

Avellino dystrophy is a condition with clinical and histologic features of both lattice and granular corneal dystrophies. It was initially described in four patients from three families, all of whom trace their ancestry to Avellino, Italy. It is inherited as an autosomal dominant trait.

COURSE

Clinically, the lesions demonstrate three characteristics: anterior stromal discrete, gray-white granular deposits; mid to posterior stromal lattice lesions; and anterior stromal haze. The granular deposits are seen first, followed by the lattice lesions. In a series of 27 patients, none developed lattice lesions without first demonstrating granular lesions. The last of these three signs to appear is the stromal haze, which develops after the fifth decade. All three of these lesions become more pronounced with age.

DIAGNOSIS

The symptoms of Avellino dystrophy include foreign body sensation, photophobia, and pain, most likely from recurrent corneal epithelial erosions. In this respect, Avellino dystrophy is more like LCD-I (in which erosions are common) than granular corneal dystrophy (in which erosions are uncommon). There has been recurrence of the granular lesion in two of three patients who have had a penetrating keratoplasty for this condition.

REFERENCES

Chau HM, Ha NT, Cung LX, et al: H626R and R124C mutations of the *TGFβI* (*βIGH3*) gene caused lattice corneal dystrophy in Vietnamese people. Br J Ophthalmol 87:686–689, 2003.

Folberg R, Stone EM, Sheffield VC, et al: The relationship between granular, lattice type 1, and Avellino corneal dystrophies: a histopathologic study. Arch Ophthalmol 112:1080–1085, 1994.

Hayashida-Hibino S, Watanabe H, Nishida K, et al: The effect of *TGF-B1* on differential gene expression profiles in human corneal epithelium studied by cDNA expression array. Invest Ophthalmol Vis Sc 42:1691–1697, 2001.

Hida T, Tsubota K, Kigasawa K, et al: Clinical features of a newly recognized lattice corneal dystrophy. Am J Ophthalmol 104:241–248, 1987.

Hirano K, Hotta Y, Nakamura M, et al: Late-onset form of lattice corneal dystrophy caused by leu527Arg mutation of the *TGFβI* gene. Cornea 20:525–529, 2001.

Holland EJ, Daya SM, Stone EM, et al: Avellino corneal dystrophy: clinical manifestations and natural history. Ophthalmology 99:1564–1568, 1992.

Meisler DM, Fine M: Recurrence of the clinical signs of lattice corneal dystrophy (type I) in corneal transplants. Am J Ophthalmol 97:210–214, 1984.

Meretoja J: Lattice corneal dystrophy-Two different types. Ophthalmologica 165:15–37, 1972.

Nassaralla BA, Garbus J, McDonnell PJ: Phototherapeutic keratectomy for granular and lattice corneal dystrophies at 1.5 to 4 years. J Refract Surg 12:795–800, 1996.

Rodrigues MM, Krachmer JH: Recent advances in corneal stromal dystrophies. Cornea 7:19–29, 1988.

Stock EL, Feder RS, O'Grady RB, et al: Lattice corneal dystrophy type IIIA: clinical and histopathologic correlations. Arch Ophthalmol 109:354–358, 1991.

203 MACULAR CORNEAL DYSTROPHY 371.55
(Groenouw's Dystrophy Type II)

Alexandre S. Marcon, MD
Porto Alegre, Brazil
Italo M. Marcon, MD, PhD
Porto Alegre, Brazil
Edward J. Holland, MD
Cincinnati, Ohio

ETIOLOGY

Of the three classic stromal dystrophies (the other two are granular and lattice), macular dystrophy is the only autosomal recessive and the most severe.

COURSE/PROGNOSIS

Corneal changes are noted in the first decade of life as a diffuse clouding in central superficial stroma. With time these grayish-white spots with blurry edges extend peripherally up to the limbus and into deeper stroma. Later, opacities become denser and can result in irregularity of the epithelium and in guttate appearance of Descemet's membrane. Visual loss progresses to legal blindness by age 40 to 50.

DIAGNOSIS

Clinical signs and symptoms

- Corneal findings include small, multiple, gray-white, pleomorphic opacities with irregular borders.
- The stroma is thinner than normal.
- Other clinical findings include loss of vision and photophobia.
- Endothelial decompensation and subsequent corneal edema can also occur.

Laboratory findings

- The gene for macular corneal dystrophy is a carbohydrate sulfotransferase gene (*CHST6*) on chromossome 16 (16q22).
- Histologically macular dsystrophy is characterized by the accumulation of glycosaminoglycans.
- Lesions stain with Alcian blue, colloidal iron and PAS.
- Serum or immunohistochemical evaluation of keratan sulfate (KS) can divide the dystrophy in type 1 (KS negative) or type 2 (KS positive).

TREATMENT

Ocular

- A contact lens may slightly improve vision by 'smoothing' the corneal surface.

Surgical

- Phototherapeutic keratectomy may help in early stages.
- Penetrating corneal transplantation is the treatment of choice (lamellar can be tried in selected cases).

COMPLICATIONS

- Graft rejection.
- Disease recurrence (with any form of treatment).

REFERENCES

Akova YA, Kirkness CM, McCartney ACE, et al: Recurrent macular corneal dystrophy following penetrating keratoplasty. Eye 4:698–705, 1990.

Aldave AJ, Yellore VS, Thonar EJ, et al: Novel mutations in the carbohydrate sulfotransferase gene (*CHST6*) in american patients with macular corneal dystrophy. Am J Ophthalmol 137(3):465–473, 2004.

Klintworth GK, Vogel FS: Macular corneal dystrophy: an inherited acid mucopolysaccharide storage disease of the corneal fibroblast. Am J Pathol 45:565–586, 1964.

Marcon AS, Cohen EJ, Rapuano CJ, et al: Recurrence of corneal stromal dystrophies after penetrating keratoplasty. Cornea 22(1):19–21, 2003.

Morgan G: Macular dystrophy of the cornea. Brit J Ophthal 50:57–67, 1966.

204 MOOREN'S ULCER 370.07
(Chronic Serpiginous Ulcer of the Cornea, Ulcus Rodens)

Steven E. Wilson, MD
Cleveland, Ohio
Marcelo V. Netto, MD
Cleveland Ohio

ETIOLOGY/INCIDENCE

Mooren's ulcer is a chronic, painful, and progressive disorder of the cornea, which often is bilateral and commonly leads to severe vision loss or even loss of the eye. Ulceration and tissue destruction are initially confined to the periphery of the cornea, but may progress in some patients to involve the entire cornea. There is usually undermining and infiltration of the leading edge of the circumferential peri-limbal ulceration. The cornea often becomes thinned and opacified by vascularization as the disease progresses. Although various forms of treatment have been proposed, some cases are refractory to all forms of therapy.

The etiology of this disease remains uncertain in the majority of cases, although autoimmunity has been suggested to play a role in the pathophysiology of the disease based on reports of cell-mediated and humoral responses to Bowman's membrane, stromal and epithelial antigens, or even molecular mimicry responses against foreign antigens that resemble those in the cornea. Importantly, some patients have been identified who have an underlying chronic hepatitis due to hepatitis C virus infection and this should be excluded in every patient because it alters therapy and the potential outcome of treatment (Figure 204.1). The majority of cases, however, appear to be idiopathic. In these patients the disorder is a diagnosis of exclusion. Some other conditions that have been associated with Mooren's ulcer include trauma, alkali burns, herpes zoster, herpes simplex, parasitic infections, and cataract and corneal surgery.

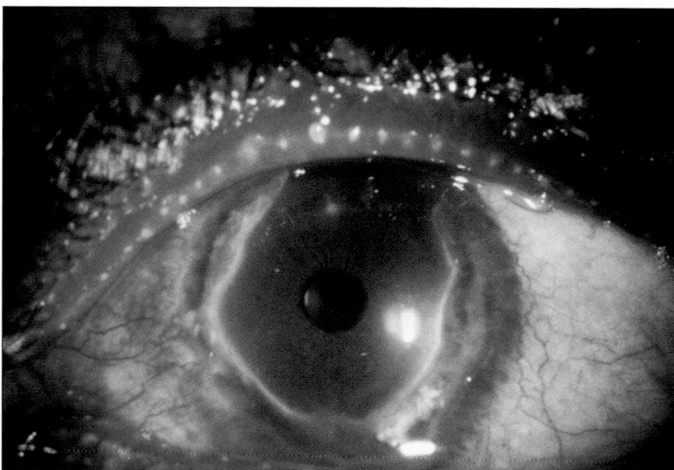

FIGURE 204.1. Hepatitis C virus-associated Mooren's like ulcer prior to treatment. The contralateral eye had similar marginal ulceration with undermining of the leading edge. (Reprinted by permission from Wilson SE, Lee WM, Murakami C, et al: Mooren's-type hepatitis C virus (HCV)-associated corneal ulceration. Ophthalmology 101:736–745, 1994.)

COURSE/PROGNOSIS

Mooren's ulcer typically begins with patchy stromal infiltrates in the periphery of the cornea. Most patients have moderate to severe pain associated with the infiltration and epithelial defects that may occur. As the disease progresses, the infiltrates usually coalesce and stromal tissue breakdown results in the formation of peri-limbal marginal ulceration. Over time the ulceration may extend for 360 degrees and progress centrally to involve the mid-peripheral and central cornea. Other ocular conditions such as episcleritis, scleritis, and iritis may be associated with the corneal ulcers in some patients.

DIAGNOSIS

The diagnosis is one of exclusion that requires an extensive search for an occult and potentially lethal connective tissue disease. A thorough review of systems and a medical examination are mandatory. Laboratory investigation includes a complete blood cell count with differential, erythrocyte sedimentation rate, rheumatoid factor, complement fixation, antinuclear antibodies, antineutrophil cytoplasmic antibody, circulating immune complexes, liver function tests, treponemal antibody absorption test, blood urea nitrogen and creatinine, serum electrophoresis, urinalysis, and chest radiograph. In addition, testing for chronic hepatitis C infection should be done. HCV antibodies are detected using EIA test and if these are present, supplemental testing with Western blotting or HCV-RNA detection can positively confirm infection. Many of these patients are asymptomatic from a systemic point of view and have minimal or no increases in blood liver enzymes. If there is a high index of suspicion, then a liver specialist should be consulted for possible biopsy to rule out chronic hepatitis

Differential diagnosis

- Infectious peripheral corneal ulcerations (*Staphylococcus aureus*, *Haemophilus influenzae*, *Moraxella* spp., herpetic, fungal).
- Peripheral corneal degenerations (Terrien's marginal degeneration, pellucid degeneration).
- Immune peripheral corneal infiltrates (staphylococcal marginal keratitis, acne rosacea, tuberculosis).
- Systemic autoimmune diseases (Wegener's granulomatosis, polyarteritis nodosa rheumatoid arthritis, systemic lupus erythematosus, relapsing polychondritis, Sjögren's syndrome, inflammatory bowel disease, a_1-antitrypsin deficiency). Some of these conditions are life-threatening and must be excluded by consultation with other specialists.

TREATMENT

The treatment of Mooren's ulcer is often unsatisfactory, especially the bilateral aggressive form. The goal of therapy is to arrest the progression of the ulcerative keratitis and to re-epithelialize the cornea.

Systemic

In cases in which underlying chronic hepatitis C virus (HCV) infection is confirmed, systemic treatment with interferon alpha, marketed as Intron A by Schering Corp. and Roferon-A by Roche Laboratories, Inc. should be instituted. Amgen Inc. also has an approved drug derived from interferon alpha called Infergen. The drug is injected subcutaneously three times a week. The authors have noted marked responses of Mooren's-like ulcers to interferon alpha in patients with confirmed HCV infection. Many of these patients had been unresponsive to other forms of treatment. A newer treatment option is Rebetron, a Schering product that combines interferon with the antiviral drug ribavirin. A liver specialist should be consulted and participate in treatment, but the ophthalmologist should be prepared to impress on other specialists the severity of the Mooren's ulcers if there is resistance to treatment because liver or other manifestations of the disease are minimal.

If chronic HCV infection is ruled out, then systemic immunosuppressive treatment can be considered, if local treatment measures are ineffective. Obviously, systemic immunosupression would likely be contraindicated in a patient with chronic HCV infection, so it is important to exclude this first. Systemic steroids should be administered first because immunosupression with chemotherapeutic agents does not take effect for several weeks. All systemic treatments should be performed in consultation with specialists knowledgeable in immunosupression.

- Initial treatment methylprednisolone 1 g/day IV in four divided doses; switch to 1 mg/kg/day prednisone PO with one of the following chemotherapeutic agents:
  - Cyclosporin A 3 to 5 mg/kg/day;
  - mMethotrexate 7.5 to 10 mg PO once a week administered with 1 mg/day folic acid;
  - Azathioprine 2 mg/kg/day;
  - Cyclophosphamide 2 mg/kg/day.

After several weeks of treatment the oral prednisone can be tapered. Frequent monitoring is needed to monitor the local response and systemic side effects of systemic immunosupression.

Local

- Cycloplegic agents (e.g. 0.5% scopolamine t.i.d.).
- Topical steroids (e.g. 1% prednisolone acetate or 1% pred nisolone phosphate every hour).
- Topical cyclosporin A 0.05% twice a day.
- Prophylactic broad-spectrum topical antibiotics (e.g. 0.3% gatifloxacin q.i.d.).
- Bandage contact lens.
- Cyanoacrylate glue over small perforations may allow healing.
- Treatment of any concomitant eye disease (e.g. meibomianitis, blepharitis, dry eyes).

Surgical

- Conjunctival recession/resection.
- Conjunctival excision may be considered if the ulcer progresses despite local and systemic medical treatment. With the patient under topical or subconjunctival anesthesia, the conjunctiva is excised extending 2 clock-hours to either side of the ulcer and 3 to 4 mm posteriorly, leaving bare sclera. The use of topical antibiotics and steroids should be continued. Tissue adhesives and a therapeutic contact lens may be beneficial.
- Superficial lamellar keratectomy.
- A central island of anterior corneal stroma can be excised to arrest the inflammatory process and to promote re-epithelialization. A lamellar corneal graft may be required.

REHABILITATION

A large tectonic graft and then a central therapeutic graft may be attempted if all other systemic and local treatment measures fail. Lamellar tectonic grafts may add structural integrity to the thinned cornea. Conjunctival flaps may be necessary for severely thinned corneas. The use of contact lenses can correct irregular astigmatism in quiescent cases.

COMMENTS

Any later surgical interventions should be performed with concurrent immunosuppression, even in apparently burnt-out diseases because of a risk of recurrence. Corneal transplantation success is typically limited by vascularization of the cornea leading to a high-risk of transplant rejection.

REFERENCES

Brown SI, Mondino BJ: Penetrating keratoplasty in Mooren's ulcer. Am J Ophthalmol 89:255–258, 1980.

Foster CS: Systemic immunosuppressive therapy of progressive bilateral Mooren's ulcer. Ophthalmology 92:1436–1439, 1985.

Moazami G, Auran JD, Florakis GJ, et al: Interferon treatment of Mooren's ulcers associated with hepatitis C. Am J Ophthalmol 119:365–366, 1995.

Wilson SE, Lee WM, Murakami C, et al: Mooren's corneal ulcers and hepatitis C virus infection: A New Association. N Engl J Med 329:62, 1993.

Wilson SE, Lee WM, Murakami C, et al: Mooren's type hepatitis C virus (HCV)-associated corneal ulceration. Ophthalmology 1994;101:736–745, 1994.

205 NEUROPARALYTIC KERATITIS

370.35

(Neurotrophic Keratitis, Trigeminal Neuropathic Keratopathy)

Ian A. Mackie, MBChB, DO, FRCS, FRCOphth
London, England

Neuroparalytic keratitis is a disease that is the potential sequela to anesthesia administration in the region of the trigeminal nerve.

ETIOLOGY

The three most common reasons for administering trigeminal anesthesia are surgery of the trigeminal neuralgias, surgery of acoustic neuromata, and herpes zoster ophthalmicus. In the course of treatment for the latter disease, about 8% of patients develop neuroparalytic keratitis. Other infrequent causes are trauma, tumors, multiple sclerosis, toxic chemical reactions, leprosy, and brain stem strokes and hemorrhages. Congenital forms, occurring notably in familial dysautonomia, (the Riley–Day syndrome) which occurs as a recessive disease in Ashkenazi Jews, may also be found. An idiopathic form has been described.

There is a notion that the disease is caused by dust and foreign matter lodging in an anesthetic eye, and protective spectacles are often fitted. These contribute very little to the management of the disease.

COURSE/PROGNOSIS

A number of studies have shown that about 15% of patients with anesthetic eyes develop serious complications. These complications may develop soon or many years after the initiation of trigeminal insensitivity. The potential for neuroparalytic keratitis associated with trigeminal insensitivity can wax and wane. This is an important concept in the long-term management of these patients.

DIAGNOSIS

To develop a true neuroparalytic keratitis, one probably must have an insensitive eye in an insensitive environment. In other words, one must have an insensitive conjunctiva as well as an insensitive cornea for the typical pathologic process to present.

Sensation in either the cornea or the conjunctiva, which may occur after trigeminal nerve or gasserian ganglion destruction and which is often present after herpes zoster infection, spares the patient from the disease.

Conjunctival sensation should be tested by gently applying the tip of a hypodermic needle to the palpebral conjunctiva above and below. This test, together with the assessment of corneal sensitivity with a wisp of cotton wool or the corner of a folded paper tissue, has important practical considerations in diagnosis and prognosis. It is, for example, sometimes difficult to differentiate the viral epitheliopathy of herpes zoster from that of neuroparalytic keratitis. In this case, the demonstration of sensation in either the cornea or the conjunctiva implies a viral etiology. Furthermore, the prognosis for the cornea after an attack of herpes zoster or after a neurosurgical procedure can be established.

All patients with anesthesia of the eye and its environment produce excess mucus. The discharge often clings to the lashes. It is important to recognize this mucus as a feature of the anesthetic condition of the eye. It does not imply infection and it does not seem to be related to the presence or absence of keratopathy. The mucus comes from conjunctival subsurface vesicles, which are greatly increased in number in this condition.

The entire palpebral conjunctiva may stain with rose bengal after gasserian ganglion destruction. This staining is probably an index of increased conjunctival cell death. It does not mean that the eye is dry and it does not seem to be related to the development of keratopathy.

About 50% of patients with trigeminal anesthesia have abnormalities of the tear film and cornea. With fluorescein, geographic drying areas are often seen in the cornea, and transient blurring of vision is common at this level of the disease. Punctate erosive corneal epitheliopathy is also common. It may have a geographic distribution and may be extensive enough to lead to a drop in visual acuity. These signs so far described can be considered stage I of the disease.

Stage II develops as an acute episode and is characterized by epithelial detachment. The patient is usually first aware of a drop in visual acuity, and the eye may be somewhat hyperemic.

Discomfort or pain, of course, is not a feature at this stage. For this reason patients should be instructed to test their vision in the affected eye frequently. Such epithelial detachments can appear in an area of cornea covered by the top lid. A gap is seen in the epithelium that is surrounded by an area of undermined epithelium extending some distance beyond the gap, and folds rapidly appear in Descemet's membrane. An aqueous flare and cells may be present.

Stage III develops when stromal lysis occurs. This may or may not be associated with infection, an early indication of which is a halo of cells in the stroma surrounding the stromal gap.

TREATMENT

Stage I

When severe, the punctate epitheliopathy is best treated with intermittent patching of the eye with tape, such as Blenderm (3M Health Care Ltd., Loughborough, LE11 1AP, England.) For a start, the eye may be patched for the whole of the wakeful day, but not during the night for fear of the tape coming in contact with the cornea. When the corneal epitheliopathy has been seen to disappear, the patching can be discontinued for one third of the wakeful day. The patient can pick the time for this uncovering to fit his or her social schedule. When again the cornea is seen to be clear, the patching can be discontinued for two-thirds of the wakeful day. As has been said before, the potential for having keratopathy waxes and wanes, and many patients will be able to proceed to uncovering the eye for the whole of the wakeful day. The tape used should be 2.5 cm wide and 6.25 cm long. The eye is shut by closing it with the top lid only, avoiding the tendency to squeeze the eye shut. The tape is held along the forefinger with about 1 cm in length being in front and unsupported by the finger. It is applied horizontally at first, to gain anchorage on the side of the nose, and then across the closed lids so that one third of the width of the tape adheres to the upper lid and two-thirds to the lower lid. Cutting the upper lid lashes greatly facilitates the application and retention of the tape. Smearing the scissors blades with petroleum jelly ensures that the cut lashes adhere to the blades and do not fall into the eye. Patients should be told to carry a mirror for periodic inspection of the closure. In the opinion of the author, mucomimetic drops do not have any influence on the punctate keratopathy of the insensitive cornea, but they seem to have some action in preventing the onset of the acute stage II of the disease.

The administration of oral tetracycline 250 mg twice daily or, better for compliance, doxycycline 100 mg on alternate days seems to diminish the amount of mucus produced by these insensitive eyes and may be continued for long periods.

Contact lenses have been advocated to control the keratopathy at this stage. However, they have several disadvantages; patients often lose their lenses during sleep, the keratopathy is difficult to assess under a contact lens, and fluorescein cannot be used without removing the lens and subsequently flushing the eye out with saline, for fear of staining the lens. The overwhelming disadvantage is the relatively frequent incidence of suppurative keratopathy. The patient is given no warning by way of pain, and the abscess is frequently well developed before a doctor is consulted. Even then, the wrong antibiotics may be prescribed by a doctor who is not familiar with the treatment of suppurative keratopathy in anesthetic, contact lens-wearing eyes. Admittedly, it is often difficult to grow organisms from these anesthetic eyes, but a broad-spectrum antibiotic, or antibiotics, against *Pseudomonas aeruginosa* infection should be chosen. This organism is known to have an affinity for contact lenses and especially those worn on an extended basis.

The ideal treatment for this developing suppurative keratopathy in neuroparalytic keratitis is first removal of the contact lens and then ofloxacin (0.3%) every 15 minutes for six hours, then every 30 minutes for the next 18 hours. On day two this is reduced to two drops hourly. On day three the frequency can be reduced to four hourly. Ceftazidime 5%, should also be used every two hours, in addition. The latter antibiotic is a third-generation cephalosporin that is highly effective against *Pseudomonas*. The incorporation of this second medication is advisable, if at all possible, because a number of *Pseudomonas* organisms (figures of 20% have been quoted) are resistant to ciprofloxacin.

Untreated, stage I of the disease can become chronic and lead to epithelial hyperplasia and underlying stromal nebulae that may be vascularized. Band keratopathy can develop.

Considerable resolution of epithelial hyperplasia can be brought about by total daily closure with Blenderm tape over a number of weeks, and this should always be tried before a corneal transplant is contemplated.

Stage II

This stage can be reached on the same day as a destructive procedure on the trigeminal nerve or its ganglion. It is an indication for urgent treatment. Atropine 1% should be instilled and the eye should be closed immediately with Blenderm or a temporary tarsorrhaphy. The injection of botulinum toxin into the levator palpebrae superioris may be indicated, but this takes about 3 days to take effect. The use of botulinum toxin to close the eye can be done in all three stages of the disease. The dose of toxin differs according to the toxin used. Botox, manufactured by Allergan and measured in mouse units, is approximately three times more powerful than Dysport, manufactured by Ipsen Ltd., also measured in mouse units. The dose for Dysport, which has been used by the author, is 10 to 20 mouse units. If a vial contains 500 units and is made up to a solution with 2.5 mL normal saline, 0.05 mL to 0.10 mL of this solution would be injected. In the case of Botox, 3 to 6 mouse units should perhaps be injected. This entails adding 2 mL of normal saline to a 100-mouse unit vial and injecting 0.06 mL to 0.12 mL.

The levator palpebrae superioris is reached by passing a 25-gauge, 2.5-mm-long needle through the skin of the upper lid, midway and just under the superior orbital rim. The needle is tracked along the roof of the orbit to avoid perforating the globe. The needle is introduced as far as it will go before the toxin is injected. This procedure produces a profound ptosis in 3 days that lasts up to 6 weeks.

On no account should a therapeutic soft contact lens be inserted at this stage. If it is, within 12 hours a very red eye, a massive hypopyon, and thick aqueous flare will surely be present. This happens in the absence of manifest corneal infection.

Stage III

The principal treatment is closure. This may be done with Blenderm tape, a temporary tarsorrhaphy, or botulinum toxin, as detailed above. Atropine should be instilled, and an appropriate antibiotic, such as ofloxacin, used topically. There is a case for a systemic antibiotic, and this should probably be ciprofloxacin 500 mg, twice daily in tablet form. This antibiotic is secreted by the lacrimal gland and penetrates the eye. Topical corticosteroids are contraindicated because they potentiate collagenase activity.

Permanent tarsorrhaphy, or repeated botulinum toxin injections into the levator palpebra are sometimes necessary for economic reasons in chronic relapsing disease. Lateral tarsorrhaphy has, in the opinion of the author, no place here. It inhibits natural blinking, and the disease process marches steadily on, concentrating on the exposed area of eye. Instead, a thin, central pillar tarsorrhaphy should be done. This can be thinned even further later on so that an 'elastic band' tarsorrhaphy remains. In this way the eye can still see when looking to either side and may have some acuity looking straight ahead.

COMMENTS

Neuroparalytic keratitis is probably a disease of abnormal corneal epithelial cell turnover. Epithelial thinning, but not stromal thinning, has been shown in monkeys after destruction of the nerve or its ganglion. This did not occur with tarsorrhaphy alone. The thinned epithelium had fewer cells. Scanning electron microscopy of the conjunctiva has shown irregularity of epithelial cells and abnormalities of epithelial microvilli.

Trophic changes in the corneal epithelium have been shown after controlled thermocoagulation of the trigeminal ganglion in rabbits. This denervation was found to markedly affect the proliferative activity of the epithelium, and mitosis was sparse.

The cyclic nucleotides, the 'second messengers' of hormone action, are involved in the regulation of corneal epithelial cell turnover. There is an imbalance in the anesthetic eye, leading to a decreased cellular turnover. Cyclic AMP has been shown to produce quiescence in cells. Cyclic GMP has been shown to initiate mitosis. Cholinergic stimulation has been shown to be associated with rapid accumulation of cellular cyclic GMP. The normal corneal epithelium is rich in acetylcholine, but the anesthetic corneal epithelium has been shown to have depleted acetylcholine. This raises exciting possibilities for topical treatment with drugs that influence the cyclic nucleotide imbalance. Blockage at the level of adenylate cyclase, which catalyses the formation of cyclic AMP, is a possibility. Beta-adrenergic-blocking drugs are obvious choices for investigation. The β receptor blocking agent pindolol has been reported to accelerate the healing of corneal epithelial defects in rabbits. This drug has been used in several corneal conditions (including neuroparalytic keratitis) with claimed success. Antiprostaglandins may also work at this level.

Unfortunately, the search for topical drugs to treat neuroparalytic keratitis does not make much economic sense. It is a relatively rare condition. Existing drugs must be tried.

Another avenue of approach may be via the cyclic nucleotide phosphodiesterases. This may be a more fertile approach owing to the apparent sensitivity of the phosphodiesterases to a wider selection of chemical structures. Dipyridamole is a phosphodiesterase inhibitor used in cardiac stress testing and as an adjunct to oral anticoagulants. Sildenafil (Viagra; Pfizer) is a type 5 selective inhibitor of cyclic GMP-specific phosphodiesterase. It also happens to be a type 6 selective inhibitor and is involved in the phototransduction of the visual cascade.

REFERENCES

Kahan A, Hammer H: Pindolol in the treatment of corneal disorders. In: The cornea in health and disease (VI Congress of the European Society of Ophthalmology), Royal Society of Medicine, International Congress and Symposium Series No. 40, London, Academic Press, 1981: 1073–1075.

Mackie IA: Neuroparalytic (neurotrophic) keratitis. In: Black CI, et al, eds: Symposium on contact lenses. St Louis, CV Mosby, 1973: 125–142.

Mackie IA: The role of the corneal nerves in destructive diseases of the cornea. Trans Ophthalmol Soc UK 98:343–347, 1978.

Schimmelpfennig B, Beuerman RW: Trophic changes in corneal epithelium after controlled thermocoagulation of the trigeminal ganglion. In: The cornea in health and disease (VI Congress of the European Society of Ophthalmology), Royal Society of Medicine, International Congress and Symposium Series No. 40, London, Academic Press, 1981: 840–843.

206 PELLUCID MARGINAL DEGENERATION 371.48

Karim Rasheed, MD, MSc, MRCOphth
Templeton, California
Yaron S. Rabinowitz, MD
Los Angeles, California

ETIOLOGY/INCIDENCE

The term *pellucid marginal degeneration* was first coined by Schalaeppi in 1957 to describe a progressive, noninflammatory peripheral corneal thinning disorder characterized by a peripheral band of thinning of the inferior cornea from the 4 o'clock to the 8 o'clock position. This thinning is accompanied by 1 to 2 mm of normal corneal tissue between the limbus and the area of thinning. The corneal ectasia is most marked centripetal to the band of thinning. The central cornea is usually of normal thickness, and the epithelium overlying the area of thinning is intact. Usually both eyes are affected, but the degree of involvement may be asymmetric. The cause of this disorder has not been clearly established, but collagen abnormalities such as occur in keratoconus have been reported.

Patients are usually 20 to 40 years old at the time of clinical presentation, and there appears to be a greater incidence in males. The condition is rare, but there may be a considerable underestimation of the incidence because patients with this condition are often misdiagnosed as having keratoconus, and 'early' cases may be diagnosed only with videokeratography.

COURSE/PROGNOSIS

As in keratoconus, this disorder is progressive. Eyes with severe disease exhibit marked corneal protrusion, which makes differentiation from keratoconus difficult in advanced cases. The area of thinning is typically epithelialized, clear, avascular and lacking lipid deposits. On careful slit-lamp examination, prominent lymphatic vessels are often detected at the inferior limbus parallel to the area of thinning. Vertical striations at the level of Descemet's membrane (similar to Vogt's striae) also may be seen in rare instances. Acute hydrops, similar to that noted in keratoconus, has been reported, but as in keratoconus, spontaneous perforation of the cornea is extremely rare.

DIAGNOSIS

Laboratory findings

Videokeratography is extremely useful in making the diagnosis and for detecting early disease that might not readily be detectable on slit-lamp examination. Videokeratography shows low corneal power along the central vertical axis, increased power as the inferior cornea is approached, and high corneal power along the inferior oblique meridians, giving the videokeratographic pattern a classic butterfly appearance (Figure 206.1). Keratometry demonstrates marked against-the-rule astigmatism. The disease is usually asymptomatic except for the progressive deterioration in vision caused by irregular astigmatism induced by the corneal ectasia.

Histological examination shows a normal endothelium and Descemet's membrane. The stroma is thinned, and Bowman's layer may have breaks or be completely absent in the affected area. Diagnosis is made by finding typical features on slit-lamp examination and confirmed by finding a classic videokeratographic pattern.

Differential diagnosis

- Pellucid marginal degeneration may be differentiated from keratoconus in most cases by the inferior band-like location of the thinning on slit-lamp examination and by the classic butterfly pattern on videokeratography.
- Keratoglobus causes generalized thinning of the cornea, with the thinning more marked at the limbus circumferentially for 360 degrees, and the entire cornea protrudes compared with regional thinning that occurs in keratoconus and inferior paralimbal thinning in pellucid marginal degeneration.
- Terrien's marginal degeneration affects a similar age group and can be bilateral. Although it also can be associated with large amounts of astigmatism, it can be differentiated from pellucid marginal degeneration because the superior cornea is predominantly affected and the area of thinning often is associated with vascularization and lipid deposition.
- Furrow degeneration has some of the features of pellucid marginal degeneration in that there is an intact epithelium and the area of corneal thinning is not vascularized, at least not in the acute phase. The differentiating feature is that the area of thinning is much closer to the limbus with virtually no intervening zone of normal cornea. Furrow degeneration may on occasion involve the superior cornea, and there may be an associated adjacent area of scleritis. The edges of the furrow are steeper than the gradual attenuation seen in pellucid marginal degeneration, and there may be a corneal infiltrate adjacent to the area of thinning. In addition, there appears to be a strong association with rheumatoid arthritis.
- Peripheral corneal melting disorders such as Mooren's ulcer or peripheral melting secondary to rheumatologic disorders are characterized by pain, which may be severe in Mooren's ulcer, and are accompanied by an epithelial defect over the area of thinning, as well as corneal vascularization adjacent to the area of thinning in the acute phase.

Reports in the medical literature suggest that keratoconus and pellucid marginal degeneration may exist in the same eye and in different eyes of the same patient.

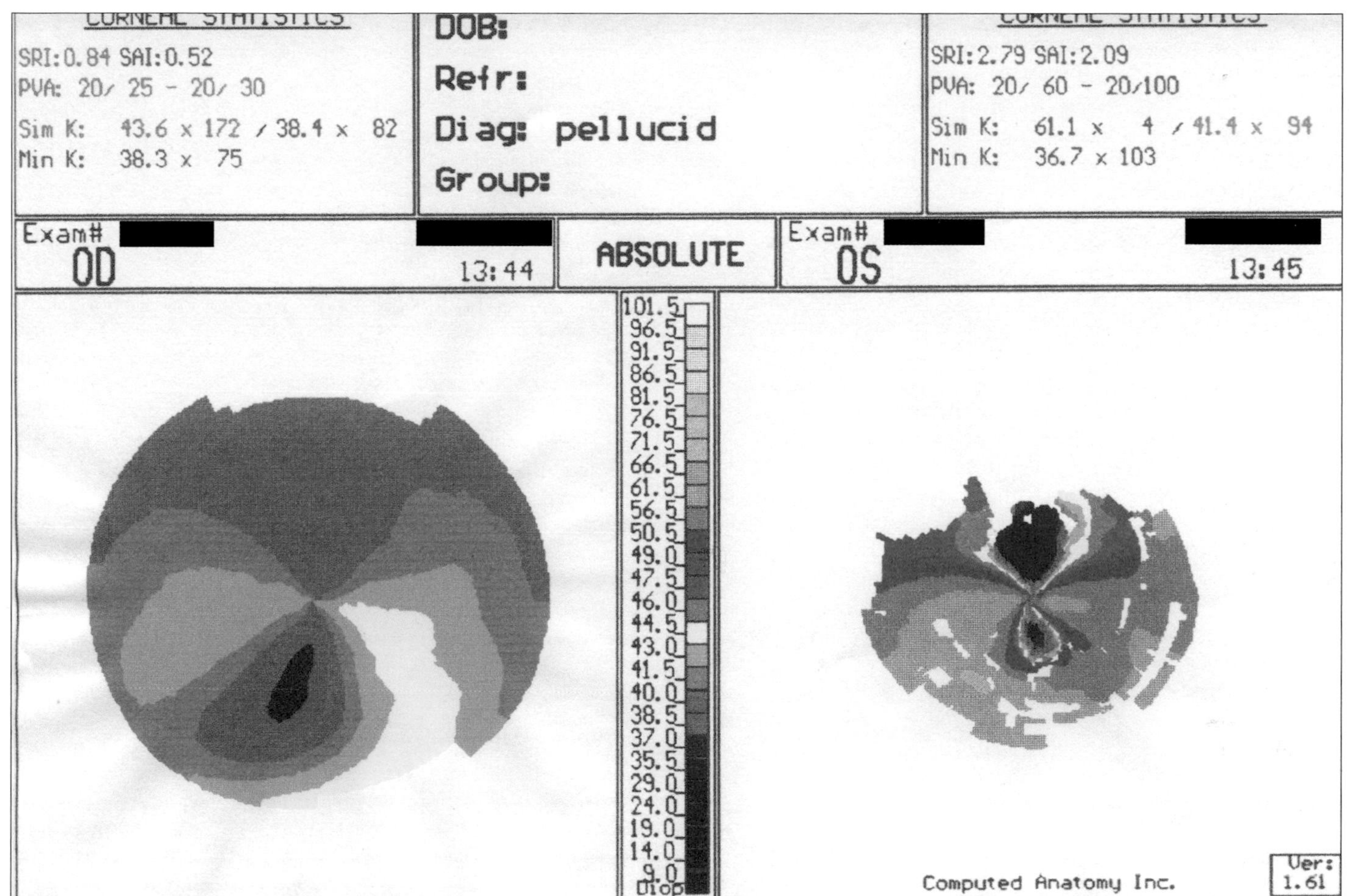

FIGURE 206.1. Corneal topography of early pellucid marginal degeneration (right eye) and advance pellucid marginal degeneration (left eye).

TREATMENT

Spectacle correction usually fails very early in the course of this disease as the degree of irregular astigmatism increases. In early to moderate cases, contact lenses are beneficial in providing visual rehabilitation. Rigid gas-permeable contact lenses are often hard to fit in patients with pellucid marginal degeneration. The problems in fitting result from the flattening of the superior cornea and the high degree of against-the-rule astigmatism that often causes the lens to dislocate inferiorly. Large diameter rigid gas permeable lenses which extend almost up to the limbus and scleral lenses made from gas permeable materials are making resurgence. A recent study found that 88.2% of eyes were successfully managed without having to resort to surgery. Of the 11.8% of patients undergoing corneal transplantation, all were able to maintain clear grafts after an average follow-up period of 9 years. These impressive results were achieved at a tertiary referral center and probably represent the best results that can currently be achieved for patients with this condition.

In patients who cannot tolerate contact lenses or in whom the ectasia is of such a degree that rigid contact lenses do not provide adequate visual acuity, surgery may be considered. A number of surgical procedures have been performed in an attempt to provide visual rehabilitation. Standard-sized penetrating keratoplasty may result in poor results because the inferior edge of the transplant must be sutured to abnormally thin cornea; this results in a high degree of postkeratoplasty astigmatism in the short term, and continued thinning of the host cornea inferiorly in the long term, which produces a situation similar to that which first necessitated surgery.

Large-diameter grafts have been tried in an attempt to remove as much of the affected cornea as possible; however, because of the proximity to the limbus and its blood vessels, these grafts are more prone to rejection. Grafts that are deliberately decentered inferiorly also work poorly because decentering causes a large degree of astigmatism and because of a higher incidence of rejection, again due to proximity to the limbus. Thermokeratoplasty and epikeratophakia are of historical interest only because the results obtained with these techniques are extremely poor.

Excision of a crescentic wedge of corneal tissue from the inferior cornea followed by tight suturing also has been reported to reduce the corneal ectasia. The procedure is usually well tolerated, but in our experience, the effect has been short lived and the thinning and ectasia recur. In addition, this procedure may be hazardous in inexperienced hands; we have noted several instances of wound dehiscence and resulting flat anterior chambers with their attendant problems when this procedure has been attempted. Crescentic lamellar keratoplasty in which a crescentic transplant is performed to reinforce the area of thinning also has been reported, but this may result in a high degree of astigmatism that necessitates a subsequent central penetrating keratoplasty.

The performance of peripheral lamellar crescentic keratoplasty followed after a few months by a central penetrating keratoplasty is the favored surgical treatment. The lamellar transplant restores normal thickness to the inferior cornea and enables good edge-to-edge apposition at the time of penetrating keratoplasty, which reduces the possibility of high postkeratoplasty astigmatism. Furthermore, the central graft that is sutured to a normal-thickness host can be treated with videokeratography-guided selective removal of sutures and astigmatic keratotomy in the usual way to reduce any residual astigmatism.

Although they are technically difficult, we have performed the two operations in the same sitting with encouraging results. Performing two keratoplasty procedures at different times necessitates the use of two separate corneas. By performing these procedures at the same time, we have been able to use tissue from the same donor, potentially reducing the antigenic load. This technique also significantly decreases the time needed to attain best-corrected acuity, which is important in these patients, who often are young and in the active working phase of their lives. The trend for progressive increase in the 'against the rule astigmatism,' which is a hallmark of this disease, appears to be abolished. Long-term follow-up will determine whether this is the optimal surgery for advanced disease.

Recently, the use of intra-corneal ring segments has been reported in patients with early to moderate disease. The early results appear encouraging.

With the increase in refractive surgery, it is extremely important to detect these patients early, because very poor results, with central corneal scarring and irregular astigmatism, have been reported for photorefractive keratectomy in undetected early cases. Incisional techniques such as astigmatic keratotomy also are contraindicated because they are highly unlikely to correct the irregular astigmatism and might result in corneal perforation in unsuspected cases.

REFERENCES

Krachmer JH: Pellucid marginal corneal degeneration. Arch Ophthalmol 96:1217–1221, 1978.

Kremer I, Sperber LT, Laibson PR: Pellucid marginal degeneration treated by lamellar and penetrating keratoplasty (Letter). Arch Ophthalmol 111:169–170, 1993.

Maguire LJ, Klyce SD, McDonald MB, Kaufman HE: Corneal topography of pellucid marginal degeneration. Ophthalmology 94:519–524, 1987.

Rabinowitz YS: Keratoconus. Surv Ophthalmol 42:297–319, 1998.

Tzelikis PF, Cohen EJ, Rapuano CJ, et al: Management of pellucid marginal corneal degeneration. Cornea 24(5):555–560, 2005.

Varley GA, Macsai MS, Krachmer JH: The results of penetrating keratoplasty for pellucid marginal corneal degeneration. Am J Ophthalmol 110:149–152, 1990.

207 PHLYCTENULOSIS 370.3

Khalid F. Tabbara, MD, ABO, FRCOphth

Riyadh, Saudi Arabia

ETIOLOGY/INCIDENCE

Phlyctenulosis is an inflammation of the cornea and conjunctiva that is induced by microbial antigens. The term *phlyctena* is a Greek word that means 'blister.' A cell-mediated immunity (delayed hypersensitivity) response occurs to microbial antigens.

- Bacteria:
  - *Staphylococcus aureus*;
  - *Mycobacterium tuberculosis.*
- Fungi:
  - *Candida albicans*;
  - *Coccidioides immitis*;
- Chlamydia:
  - *Chlamydia lymphogranulomatis.*
- Parasites:
  - *Leishmania* spp.;
  - *Ascaris lumbricoides*;
  - *Ancylostoma duodenale*;
  - *Hymenolepis nana.*
- Other.

Phlyctenulosis has a worldwide distribution. It is more common in areas in which tuberculosis is endemic. The disease occurs most frequently in children or young adults. There is a higher prevalence among females than males. Phlyctenulosis occurs more frequently in spring and summer than in autumn or winter.

COURSE/PROGNOSIS

Patients with phlyctenulosis present with photophobia, redness of the eye, irritation, and tearing. The conjunctival phlyctenule leaves no scarring, whereas corneal phlyctenule may develop localized gray infiltrates with subsequent scarring. Phlyctenulosis associated with staphylococcal antigens is triggered by active blepharitis. The most frequent site of phlyctenulosis is the limbus, and it usually occurs in the inferior quadrants of the cornea. Phlyctenulosis may result in minimal or extensive multiple nummular scars of the cornea. Salzmann's nodular degeneration may occur after healing of phlyctenulosis. When the center of the cornea is involved, corneal scarring may lead to a decrease in vision. In severe cases, corneal involvement may result in ulceration, scarring and, rarely, perforation.

DIAGNOSIS

Clinical signs and symptoms

Conjunctival phlyctenulosis

Conjunctival phlyctenulosis begins as single or multiple lesions of 0.5 to 3 mm in diameter. They appear as small, elevated, hard, pinkish lesions surrounded by a zone of conjunctival hyperemia. The lesion occurs over the bulbar conjunctiva and most frequently near the limbus. Over a few days, the nodule appears gray and soft and may develop a central necrotic lesion that may ulcerate. The lesion heals rapidly over 10 to 12 days, leaving no scar in the conjunctiva.

Corneal phlyctenulosis

Phlyctenules appear as unilateral or bilateral localized infiltrates measuring 0.5 to 2 mm. The lesion occurs at the limbus or the corneal periphery and over a period of a few days may lead to ulceration in the center. The corneal phlyctenules attract a leech of new blood vessels. Some phlyctenules show a tendency to migrate and wander in the cornea.

In severe cases, multiple phlyctenules may be seen in the cornea and may affect the visual axis, leading to scarring and a decrease in vision. Stromal involvement is typically superficial; deeper involvement may occur in staphylococcal phlyctenulosis and may rarely lead to corneal perforation.

Most nodules of phlyctenulosis start in the limbus with dilated conjunctival vessels. The infiltration may travel toward the center of the cornea, with progressive necrosis and grayish infiltrates with superficial ulceration. Scarring of the phlyctenules may take the form of a spade at the limbus with a triangular scar. In severe cases, multiple phlyctenules are seen in the cornea, and Salzmann's nodular degeneration may occur subsequently.

Laboratory findings

In patients with staphylococcal blepharitis, culture of the lids reveals *Staphylococcus* spp. In patients with tuberculosis, the tuberculin skin test is positive.

Conjunctival and corneal scrapings of phlyctenules initially may show evidence of mononuclear cells; in the late course of the disease, patients have polymorphonuclear cells. The epithelium shows degenerative epithelial cells. Usually, no eosinophils are seen in the scrapings.

Biopsy specimens of limbal phlyctenules show mononuclear cellular infiltration and polymorphonuclear cells in the epithelium and stroma. The mononuclear cells are predominantly T lymphocytes, monocytes/macrophages and dendritic cells. The T lymphocytes are mostly T helper/inducer cells. B lymphocytes and plasma cells are uncommon. The basal cell layers express HLA-DR antigens. The findings in phlyctenules are comparable to those observed in the human skin tuberculin reaction, which are considered to be classic examples of the delayed-type hypersensitivity response in humans.

Differential diagnosis

- Pingueculitis (inflamed pinguecula).
- Sterile peripheral corneal infiltrates.
- Marginal ulcers.
- Acne rosacea.
- Trachomatous pustule.
- Vernal keratoconjunctivitis.
- Infected peripheral ulcer.

The differential diagnosis of phlyctenulosis is important so as to initiate appropriate therapy. The corneal lesions of acne rosacea may closely resemble phlyctenulosis but have associated skin findings.

Pingueculitis shows no microinfiltrates. An increase in the amount of collagen in the substantia propria is seen after the pingueculitis subsides. There usually is a single lesion, there is no tendency to migrate into the cornea and there is no ulceration.

In cases of infected corneal ulcers, there is a demarcating margin with a tendency to infiltrate the center of the cornea.

In cases of peripheral corneal infiltrates, secondary to contact lenses, there is a history of contact lens use. The lesion shows no ulceration and does not migrate into the cornea.

In patients with vernal keratoconjunctivitis, the lesions are multiple with limbal hypertrophy and gelatinous infiltration of the limbus. The typical giant papillae are seen over the palpebral conjunctiva, and conjunctival scrapings show the presence of eosinophils. Patients have marked itching and may develop superficial punctate keratitis.

TREATMENT

Systemic

In staphylococcal blepharitis, patients older than 7 years can receive 100 mg doxycycline qd for 1 month.

Patients with tuberculosis should be given the appropriate systemic therapy for tuberculosis.

Local

The lids should be carefully evaluated in cases of chronic staphylococcal blepharitis. Patients should receive a vigorous regimen of lid scrubs with an antibiotic/steroid ointment to be placed twice daily for a period of 2 to 4 weeks. This may be by cleaning of the lid margin with effective baby shampoo during showers. Baby shampoo may be used to scrub the lid margin, and eyelash scales should be removed with an effective antidandruff preparation. In young children, erythromycin ophthalmic ointment may be applied twice daily at the lid margin. In addition, 0.1% topical fluorometholone eyedrops or rimexolone (Vexol) eyedrops three times daily may be given for the corneal and conjunctival phlyctenules. The treatment of corneal and conjunctival phlyctenulosis may consist of 0.1% topical fluorometholone eyedrops or rimexolone eyedrops to be given every 6 hours for a period of 10 days. The topical treatment may be tapered to once daily over a period of 4 weeks. The intraocular pressure (IOP) should be monitored for steroid-induced glaucoma. A cycloplegic agent in the form of 1% tropicamide eyedrops may be given to patients with severe corneal involvement.

COMPLICATIONS

- Peripheral corneal scarring with vascularization.
- Central scarring in central corneal phlyctenules.
- Rarely corneal perforation.
- Loss of vision.

In patients with severe corneal scarring, penetrating keratoplasty may be required for visual rehabilitation.

REFERENCES

Abu El-Asrar AM, Van Den Oord JJ, Geboes K, et al: Phenotypic characterization of inflammatory cells in phlyctenular eye disease. Doc Ophthalmol 70:352–362, 1988.

Culbertson WW, Huang AJW, Mandelbaum SH, et al: Effective treatment of phlyctenular keratoconjunctivitis with oral tetracycline. Ophthalmology 100:1358–1366, 1993.

Helm CJ, Holland GN: Ocular tuberculosis. Surv Ophthalmol 38(3):229–256, 1993.

Mondino BJ, Kowalski RP: Phlyctenulae and catarrhal infiltrates. Occurrences in rabbits immunized with staphylococcol cell walls. Arch Ophthalmol 100:1968–1971, 1982.

Ostler HB: Corneal perforation in nontuberculous (staphylococcal) phlyctenular keratoconjunctivitis. Am J Ophthalmol 79:446–448, 1975.

208 POSTERIOR POLYMORPHOUS DYSTROPHY 371.58

Nicole J. Anderson, MD
Flowood, Mississippi
R. Doyle Stulting, MD, PhD
Atlanta, Georgia

ETIOLOGY/INCIDENCE

Posterior polymorphous dystrophy (PPD) is a rare bilateral corneal disorder of Descemet's membrane and the corneal endothelium. It is typically non-progressive and often noted as an incidental finding on ophthalmic examination. It can rarely cause reduced vision from corneal edema and glaucoma.

- Inheritance is autosomal dominant with variable expression. Some cases of autosomal recessive inheritance have been reported.
- The gene locus has been identified on the long arm of chromosome 20 (20q11) and is the same locus as that involved in autosomal dominant congenital hereditary endothelial dystrophy (CHED).
- Associations have been reported with Alport's syndrome and keratoconus.
- The pathogenesis is believed to be a local metaplasia of endothelial cells to abnormal epithelial-like cells.

COURSE/PROGNOSIS

- Typical corneal findings are present from an early age, but diagnosis is not usually made until the second or third decade.
- Most cases are asymptomatic and non-progressive.
- Corneal edema may develop in mid-life, or rarely at birth.
- Glaucoma, either open-angle or closed-angle, may occur. Glaucoma can result from overgrowth and contraction of the abnormal endothelium and basement membrane over the anterior chamber angle.

DIAGNOSIS

Clinical signs and symptoms

- Slit-lamp examination shows one of three forms of the disorder. In the vesicular variant, small, round, vesicular lesions surrounded by a ring opacity are seen at the level of Descemet's membrane. Band PPD is characterized by elongated bands of roughened Descemet's membrane, with narrow, opaque, irregular ridges. In diffuse PPD, a large portion of the posterior corneal surface is invaded with a swirled pattern of thickened and opacified Descemet's membrane.
- Peripheral anterior synechia, glaucoma, iris atrophy, or corectopia may be present.

Laboratory findings

- Histologic study of the endothelium reveals multi-layered epithelial-like cells with abundant microvilli, tonofilaments and desmosomes. These cytokeratin-expressing cells arise when normal endothelial cells lose their characteristic phenotype and become epithelioid.
- Histologic study of Descemet's membrane shows a normal anterior banded zone in cases presenting after birth. The posterior non-banded zone is diminished or absent and is replaced by an abnormal posterior collagenous layer.
- Specular microscopy in vesicular PPD shows circular dark rings with scalloped edges around a light center. Band lesions appear as broad, mottled strips delineated by narrow, dark scalloped borders.

Differential diagnosis

- Iridocorneal endothelial (ICE) syndrome usually is unilateral and acquired. Endothelial cells are large and pleomorphic in ICE, rather than epithelial-like. There can be an overlap between ICE and posterior polymorphous dystrophy, causing speculation as to whether they represent different clinical entities or a spectrum of the same disease.
- Posterior corneal vesicle syndrome shows vesicles and band lesions similar to those of posterior polymorphous dystrophy, but it is unilateral and nonfamilial.
- Haab's striae resemble band lesions but have scrolled, thickened edges with smooth areas within and do not have associated vesicles.
- In children born with cloudy corneas caused by posterior polymorphous dystrophy, the differential diagnosis includes congenital hereditary endothelial dystrophy, congenital hereditary stromal dystrophy, congenital glaucoma, birth trauma, congenital infection, metabolic disorders and sclerocornea.

TREATMENT

In most cases, no treatment is necessary, as the disorder is usually non-progressive.

Ocular

- In mild corneal decompensation, topical sodium chloride drops or ointment can be administered.
- Elevated intraocular pressure should be treated medically or surgically.

Surgical

- In patients with corneal edema, penetrating keratoplasty may be necessary. Eyes with peripheral anterior synechia, elevated intraocular pressure, or both have a poor visual prognosis after penetrating keratoplasty.
- Posterior polymorphous dystrophy may recur in the graft after penetrating keratoplasty.

REFERENCES

Anderson NJ, Badawi DY, Grossniklaus HE, et al: Posterior polymorphous membranous dystrophy with overlapping features of iridocorneal endothelial syndrome. Arch Ophthalmol 119:624–625, 2001.

Háon E, Greenberg A, Kopp KK, et al: *VSX1*: a gene for posterior polymorphous dystrophy and keratoconus. Hum Mol Genet 11:1029–1036, 2002.

Krachmer JH: Posterior polymorphous corneal dystrophy: a disease characterized by epithelial-like endothelial cells which influence management and prognosis. Trans Am Ophthalmol Soc 83:413–475, 1985.

Laganowski HC, Sherrard ES, Muir MG: The posterior corneal surface in posterior polymorphous dystrophy: a specular microscopical study. Cornea 10:224–232, 1991.

209 REIS–BÜCKLERS CORNEAL DYSTROPHY 371.52

(Corneal Dystrophy of Bowman's Layer Type 1, CDB-I, Superficial Variant of Granular Dystrophy, Granular Corneal Dystrophy Type III)

David Matthew Bushley, MD
Durham, North Carolina
Natalie A. Afshari, MD
Durham, North Carolina

ETIOLOGY/INCIDENCE

Reis–Bücklers dystrophy is a bilateral, progressive, autosomal dominant corneal dystrophy with early onset affecting Bowman's layer, epithelium, basement membrane and anterior stroma. It is linked in some cases with R124L and G623D mutations in the transforming growth factor beta-induced (*TGFβI*) gene on chromosome 5q31. Reis–Bücklers dystrophy is relatively rare, though the incidence is unknown.

COURSE/PROGNOSIS

Reis–Bücklers manifests in early childhood, usually within the first and second decade of life. The initial symptom is typically recurrent corneal epithelial erosions; over time, corneal scarring and opacification occurs at the level of Bowman's layer and superficial stroma. Marked loss of vision usually occurs during the second and third decades of life.

DIAGNOSIS

Clinical signs and symptoms

The young patient usually presents with symptoms of pain, foreign body sensation and photophobia associated with recurrent corneal epithelial erosions. Clinical exam typically reveals a rough and irregular corneal surface with fine granular opacities forming a geographic pattern (rings and disc-shaped opacities) at the level of Bowman's layer. The central cornea tends to be preferentially affected, and the lesions may extend into the superficial stroma. Whereas Reis–Bücklers (CDB-I) is phenotypically similar to Thiel–Behnke honeycomb corneal dystrophy (CDB-II), electron microscopy is needed to differentiate the two clinical entities. Compared to Thiel–Behnke honeycomb corneal dystrophy, Reis–Bücklers occurs at a younger age, causes more corneal scarring, more visual impairment and exhibits a higher frequency of recurrence.

Laboratory findings

Genetically, CDB-I has mapped to a R124L mutation in *TGFβI* gene on chromosome 5q31 in many cases. Less common is a G623D mutation in the same gene. CDB-II has mapped to a R555Q mutation in *TGFβI* gene on chromosome 5q31 though another locus has been mapped to chromosome 10q23-q24.

Histopathology and light microscopy in CDB-I show band-shaped granular, Masson-positive, subepithelial deposits at the level of Bowman's layer, causing epithelial irregularity, destruction of Bowman's layer, and intermittently absent or thickened basement membrane. Transmission electron microscopy in both CDB-I and CDB-II reveals fibrocellular scar tissue ('saw-tooth' configuration) which replaces Bowman's layer, epithelial basement membrane and hemidesmosomal complexes. The two entities are differentiated by the findings in CDB-I of ultrastructural deposits of rod-like bodies whereas in CDB-II, arcuate or rounded 'curly fibers' appear in the region of Bowman's layer.

DIFFERENTIAL DIAGNOSIS

The differential diagnosis includes the corneal epithelial dystrophies, Thiel–Behnke honeycomb dystrophy (CDB-II), and superficial corneal scarring.

PROPHYLAXIS

Prophylaxis aims at reducing the frequency of recurrent corneal erosion and includes artificial tears, lubricating ointment and hypertonic agents (e.g. sodium chloride 5%).

TREATMENT

Systemic

There are no known systemic treatments for Reis–Bücklers dystrophy.

Ocular

Treatment is supportive and consists of artificial tears, lubricating ointment and hyperosmotic agents. For patients with corneal erosions, topical antibiotics and a cycloplegic agent should be added. Consideration for debridement of loose epithelium, the use of a therapeutic soft contact lens, and possible anterior stromal micropuncture are appropriate. Surgical intervention should be considered for recurrent corneal erosions or reduced visual acuity. Excimer laser phototherapeutic keratectomy (PTK) is the treatment of choice as it allows for restoration of a smooth corneal surface although some corneal opacities may remain. Unfortunately, recurrences are common. Alternatively, superficial keratectomy with a blade and peeling can be considered. Lamellar keratoplasty can be considered for deeper scarring and opacities. Options include manual (freehand) and microkeratome-assisted anterior lamellar keratoplasty (ALK). Penetrating keratoplasty (PKP) can be considered as a last resort, and recurrences in the graft are common.

COMPLICATIONS

Recurrent corneal erosions can be refractory to treatment and patients are at risk for infectious keratitis. Scarring and corneal opacification resulting from recurrent episodes may lead to reduced visual acuity and irregular astigmatism. Risks associated with PTK and other surgical interventions include loss of best-corrected visual acuity, infection, scarring, irregular astigmatism, recurrence, and, in PKP, graft rejection. Recurrence of disease is common following any of the surgical treatments.

COMMENTS

Reis–Bücklers(CDB-I) and Thiel–Behnke honeycomb dystrophy (CDB-II) are dystrophies of Bowman's layer that appear similar clinically. In the past, our understanding of these two entities was significantly impaired and confused by a lack of histologic and electron microscopic descriptions in the literature. Over the past decade, in large part due to advances in molecular genetics and the work of researchers in Europe and the United States, these dystrophies of Bowman's layer have been redefined as two distinct entities.

REFERENCES

Afshari NA, Mullally JE, Afshari MA, et al: Survey of patients with granular, lattice, avellino, and Reis-Bücklers corneal dystrophies for mutations in the *βIGH3* and gelsolin genes. Arch Ophthalmol 119(1):16–22, 2001.

Dighiero P, Valleix S, D'Hermies F, et al: Clinical, histologic, and ultrastructural features of the corneal dystrophy caused by the R124L mutation of the *βIGH3* gene. Ophthalmology 107(7):1353–1357, 2000.

Klintworth GK: Advance in the molecular genetics of corneal dystrophies. Am J Ophthalmol 128(6):747–754, 1999.

Krachmer JH, Mannis MJ, Holland EJ: Cornea. 2nd edn: Philadelphia, Elsevier Mosby, 2005.

Küchle M, Green WR, Völcker HE, Barraquer J: Re-evaluation of corneal dystrophies of Bowman's layer and the anterior stroma (Reis-Bücklers' and Thiel-Behnke types): a light and electron microscopic study of eight corneas and a review of the literature. Cornea 14:333–354, 1995.

Mashima Y, Nakamura Y, Noda K, et al: A novel mutation at codon 124 (R124L) in the *βIGH3* gene is associated with a superficial variant of granular corneal dystrophy. Arch Ophthalmol 117(1):90–93, 1999.

210 SCHNYDER'S CRYSTALLINE CORNEAL DYSTROPHY 371.56

Kristin M. Hammersmith, MD
Philadelphia, Pennsylvania
Peter R. Laibson, MD
Philadelphia, Pennsylvania

ETIOLOGY/INCIDENCE

Schnyder's crystalline dystrophy is a rare autosomal dominant disorder in which there is an abnormal bilateral deposition of cholesterol and lipid in the cornea.

There are no reports on the incidence of this dystrophy in the general population; the world's largest pedigree of patients with Schnyder's crystalline dystrophy has a Swede–Finn heritage and has been traced to the southwest coast of Finland.

The pathogenesis of the corneal changes is unknown, but it is thought to result from a localized defect of lipid metabolism. Abnormal elevations of serum lipid levels have been found in both affected and unaffected members of Schnyder's pedigrees, but some affected members may also have normal serum lipid and cholesterol measurements. Abnormal lipid storage has been reported in the skin fibroblasts of affected patients, implying a more diffuse systemic abnormality. The gene for the dystrophy has been mapped to human chromosome 1p36.2-36.3.

COURSE/PROGNOSIS

The corneal dystrophy progresses with age. Patients in their twenties demonstrate only a central corneal opacity, which may involve the entire stroma, central subepithelial cholesterol crystals, or both. These patients have excellent visual acuity with normal corneal sensation.

By age thirty, affected patients develop arcus lipoides. They may begin to note slight visual acuity reduction. Visual acuity is often considerably better than one would estimate based on slit-lamp appearance. The examination may detect the loss of Snellen visual acuity only if measured under daylight conditions. Corneal sensation also begins to decrease. Usually by age forty, patients develop a midperipheral panstromal corneal haze that fills in the donut-shaped area between the central opacity and the peripheral arcus. There will usually be some further reduction in visual acuity and corneal sensation. Often, arcus lipoides is so dense that it can be noted without the use of slit-lamp examination. By their fifties, patients may require corneal transplantation because of the increased glare and decreased vision in the daylight.

Despite the name, only 51% of affected patients have crystalline deposits. This subset of patients without corneal crystalline deposition has been identified as having Schnyder's crystalline dystrophy sine crystals. However, patients have been reported to have crystalline deposition in only one eye. Schnyder's crystalline dystrophy may be detected as early as the first decade, but the diagnosis of Schnyder's crystalline dystrophy sine crystals is more challenging and has been reported to be delayed up to the fourth decade.

DIAGNOSIS

Clinical signs and symptoms

The clinical signs of the dystrophy may include a central corneal haze, subepithelial cholesterol crystal deposition, midperipheral panstromal haze and arcus lipoides. Systemic findings may include genu valgum and hypercholesterolemia.

Laboratory findings

- Although rare sporadic cases have been reported, the vast majority of patients demonstrate a clear autosomal dominant inheritance.
- The corneal findings are predictable on the basis of patient age.
- The diagnosis may be more difficult in patients who do not demonstrate cholesterol crystals.
- Affected and unaffected patients should have serum lipid analysis because hyperlipidemias are frequent and should be treated.
- Thc loss of corneal sensation may be profound in more advanced cases.

Confocal microscopy has demonstrated loss of corneal nerves, large extracellular deposits and accumulation of highly reflective extracellular matrix.

- Histopathologic examination of corneal transplant specimens demonstrates panstromal deposition of unesterified and esterified cholesterol and lipids.
- Abnormal lipid deposition has rarely been found in basal epithelium and endothelial cells.
- Compared with normal corneas, cholesterol and phospholipid contents in affected corneas are increased more than 10- and 5-fold.
- Apolipoproteins accumulate in the affected corneas, indicating preferential deposition of high-density lipoprotein.

Differential diagnosis

- The differential diagnosis is made up of systemic abnormalities affecting lipid metabolism and resulting in central corneal clouding including lecithin-cholesterol acyltransferase deficiency, fish eye disease and Tangier disease. These diseases are differentiated because they are of autosomal recessive inheritance, they do not demonstrate anterior stromal crystalline deposits, and they have low levels of serum high-density lipoprotein.
- Other diseases with corneal crystals include cystinosis, dysproteinemias, multiple myeloma, porphyria, hyperuricemia, primary or secondary lipid keratopathy and other metabolic defects.

TREATMENT

- There is no local or systemic medical treatment that halts the progression of the corneal lipid deposition in this dystrophy.
- An alteration in serum cholesterol level has not been found to alter progression of the ocular disease.
- Penetrating keratoplasty surgery can be performed successfully in more advanced cases.
- The dystrophy can recur in the transplant; however, unlike lattice and granular dystrophy, it usually recurs many years after transplantation.
- Phototherapeutic keratectomy can be used to treat subepithelial crystals if they are causing decreased vision.

REFERENCES

Garner A, Tripathi RC: Hereditary crystalline stromal dystrophy of Schnyder. II. Histopathy and ultrastructure. Br J Ophthalmol 56:400–408, 1972.

Theendakara V, Tromp G, Kuivaniemi H, et al: Fine mapping of the Schnyder's crystalline corneal dystrophy locus. Human Genetics 114:594–600, 2004.

Weiss JS, Rodrigues MN, Kruth HS, et al: Panstromal Schnyder's corneal dystrophy: Ultrastructural and histochemical studies. Ophthalmology 99:1072–1081, 1992.

Weiss JS: Schnyder's crystalline dystrophy sine crystals: recommendation for a revision of nomenclature. Ophthalmology 103:465–473, 1996.

Weiss JS: Schnyder's dystrophy of the cornea: a Swede-Finn connection. Cornea 11:93–101, 1992.

211 SUPERIOR LIMBIC KERATOCONJUNCTIVITIS 370.32
(Theodore's Superior Limbic Keratoconjunctivitis; SLK)

Timothy Y. Chou, MD
Rockville Centre, New York
Henry D. Perry, MD, FACS
Rockville Centre, New York
Eric D. Donnenfeld, MD, FACS
Rockville Centre, New York

Superior limbic keratoconjunctivitis (SLK) was first described by Theodore and Thygeson in the early 1960s. The disease is characterized by hyperemia and thickening of the upper bulbar conjunctiva in a 'corridor'-like distribution, a fine papillary inflammation of the superior palpebral conjunctiva, punctuate erosions over the superior and perilimbal cornea, and frequently superior filamentary keratopathy.

ETIOLOGY/INCIDENCE

The cause of SLK is unknown. A viral etiology was suggested early on, but no viral particles have ever been identified histologically. There is an associated increase in incidence of thyroid dysfunction, but no other evidence that this is an autoimmune process. An allergic process is unlikely, as itching is not a typical symptom, topical corticosteroids have little benefit, and conjunctival scrapings reveal no eosinophils. Darrell described identical twins with SLK, proposing a possible genetic basis. Many seem to prefer an anatomical and mechanical explanation of the disease. Cher has attributed the development of SLK to 'blink-related microtrauma' of the eyelid against the bulbar conjunctiva. Along the same lines, Wilson and Ostler have theorized that SLK results from tight apposition of the upper eyelid, due to thyroid disease or inflammation, against a lax superior bulbar conjunctiva. The latter might be either age-related or congenital. The resulting chronic rubbing and abnormal movement of the conjunctiva would then result in characteristic findings of SLK.

The condition is usually bilateral, but it may be unilateral and is often asymmetrical. This disease is most commonly seen in patients between the ages of 20 and 67, with a mean age of 49 years. It occurs more frequently in women than men by a 3 : 1 ratio. There is no seasonal, geographic, or racial predilection. Thyroid dysfunction is found in one-quarter to one-half of patients, most often hypothyroidism or else severe Graves ophthalmopathy. One case of SLK was reported in a patient with hyperparathyroidism due to a parathyroid adenoma, with resolution of the condition following resection of the tumor. Dry eye (keratoconjunctivitis sicca) is commonly encountered, in up to half of patients.

COURSE/PROGNOSIS

SLK is a chronic condition that may last from 1–10 years or more, with a characteristic course of remissions and exacerbations. Individual attacks may last from days to months, and involve one eye or both. In most cases, periods of remission gradually lengthen until the condition eventually resolves spontaneously. Vision is not usually affected. A superior limbal pannus may develop, and scarring of the superior tarsal conjunctiva is occasionally observed, but in general there are no other serious ocular sequelae.

DIAGNOSIS

Clinical signs and symptoms

Patients with SLK usually complain of burning, irritation, tearing, foreign body sensation, pain, photophobia, mucus discharge, blepharospasm and ptosis. Subjective discomfort often seems greater than the actual clinical findings. When filaments are present, symptoms tend to be exacerbated even more (Figure 211.1).

An important initial step to properly diagnosing SLK is to have the patient look downward while the examiner elevates the upper eyelids. In this way, the characteristic superior bulbar injection is observed (Figure 211.2). It is centered at 12 o'clock, and typically arcs around the limbus for about 10 mm in the shape of an inverted trapezoid. On biomicroscopy, eversion of the upper eyelid reveals a nearly pathognomonic velvety papillary reaction along the tarsal conjunctiva. The superior bulbar conjunctiva is thickened and lusterless. Its tissue may be redundant and hypermobile. Superior limbal tissue is likewise thickened. The superior and paralimbal corneal epithelium demonstrates a fine punctate keratopathy and pannus. Filaments occur at the superior limbus and cornea in about one-third of cases. The abnormal superior conjunctival, as well as limbal and corneal surfaces stain intensively with rose bengal, and to a lesser degree with fluorescein. Corneal sensation and tear secretion, as measured by Schirmer testing, may be decreased.

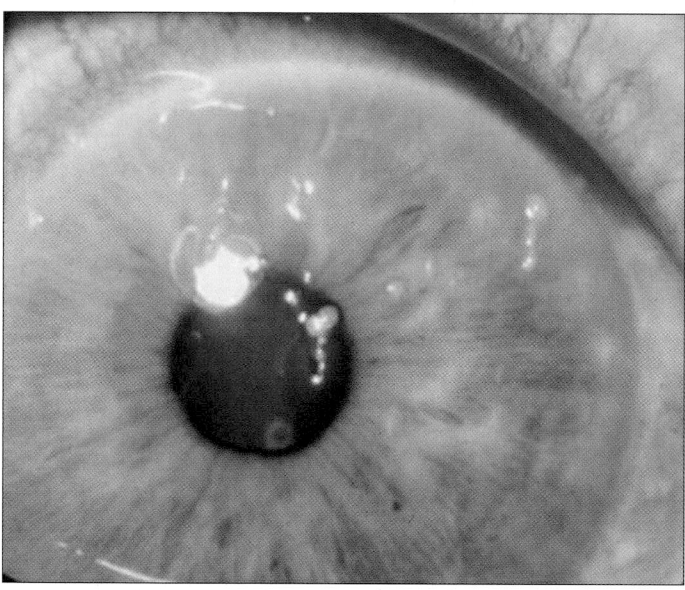

FIGURE 211.1. SLK with associated filamentary keratitis.

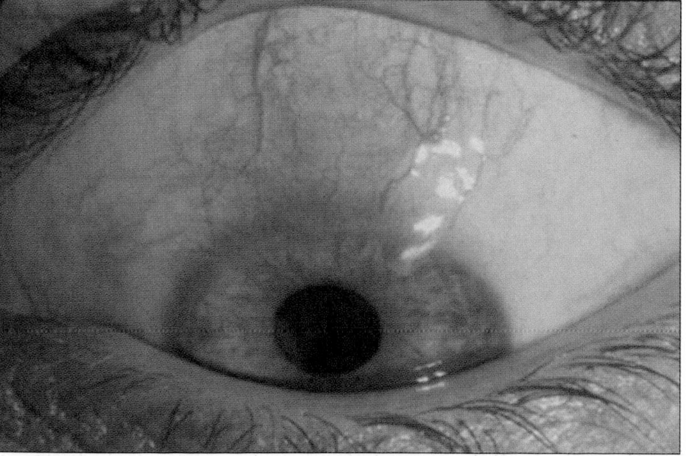

FIGURE 211.2. Classical injection pattern of the superior bulbar conjunctiva.

Laboratory findings

Diagnosis is made based on history and characteristic clinical findings. Examination of scrapings of the involved bulbar conjunctiva may be helpful. Theodore and Ferry verified Thygeson's observation that Giemsa-stained scrapings demonstrate keratinized epithelial cells. Scrapings of the upper palpebral conjunctiva show polymorphonuclear leukocytes. Biopsy of the involved bulbar conjunctiva reveals epithelial keratinization, dyskeratosis, acanthosis, balloon degeneration of the nuclei, intracellular accumulation of glycogen and hyalinized cytoplasm. There is stromal edema, as well as infiltration with polymorphonuclear leukocytes, lymphocytes and plasma cells. Goblet cells are markedly decreased. Electron microscopic examination shows a variety of nonspecific (degenerative) abnormalities within the nuclei of epithelial cells.

Patients should be advised to consult with their internists about thyroid function testing.

Differential diagnosis

The differential diagnosis is composed of conditions affecting the upper bulbar conjunctiva and cornea, and the upper palpebral conjunctiva, including the following:

- Contact lens-induced keratoconjunctivitis (CLK);
- Herpes simplex virus keratoconjunctivitis;
- Trachoma;
- Staphylococcal limbal keratoconjunctivitis;
- Floppy eyelid syndrome;
- Giant papillary conjunctivitis;
- Phlyctenular keratoconjunctivitis;
- Rosacea keratoconjunctivitis;
- Limbal vernal keratoconjunctivitis;
- Dysplasia;
- Neoplasm (case reported of sebaceous cell carcinoma misdiagnosed as SLK);
- Keratoconjunctivitis sicca;
- Retained superior perilimbal sutures.

Contact lenses can cause a keratoconjunctivitis that is clinically similar to SLK. There may be hyperemia of the superior bulbar conjunctiva, as well as irregular staining of and subepithelial infiltrates in the superior cornea. This masquerade syndrome may be related at least in part to thimerosal sensitivity and toxicity, and is not associated with thyroid dysfunction. In contrast to SLK, discontinuation of the contact lens in CLK is usually curative.

TREATMENT

Treatment remains a significant problem because there may be recurrences after the successful application of any of the following therapies.

Ocular

In patients with dry eye, initial treatment can include nonpreserved artificial tears, gels and ointments. Punctal occlusion has also been found to be useful.

Silver nitrate 0.25% to 1.0% solution is applied with a cotton-tipped applicator to the upper tarsal conjunctiva and upper bulbar conjunctiva after the instillation of a topical anesthetic agent. Irrigating solution may be used 1 minute after application. This can be repeated after 5 to 7 days and at 2- to 6-week intervals.

Scraping the superior bulbar conjunctiva with a platinum spatula may relieve symptoms for several weeks to a few months, presumably by debriding the keratinized tissue.

The worse eye may be pressure patched daily for a full week. The next week, the nonpatched eye may be patched for 1 week, with the patch changed every day. This *alternate patching technique* has also been used successfully in conjunction with the use of a bandage contact lens in the nonpatched eye.

Mast cell stabilizers such as cromolyn sodium 4%, lodoxamide tromethamine 0.1%, and ketotifen fumarate drops applied to the involved eye or eyes 4 times daily have been reported to be beneficial for some patients with SLK. When treatment is successful, it must be continued on a long-term basis because there may be recurrences upon discontinuation of the medication. The actual mechanism of how these mast cell stabilizers improve SLK is unclear.

Perry and colleagues showed improvement of symptoms and findings in 5 out of 5 patients with SLK for whom treatment with prednisolone acetate 1% and silver nitrate $^1/_2$% was ineffective, utilizing cyclosporin A 0.5% 4 times a day instead. This dose was also effective in maintaining clinical improvement when used long-term twice daily.

Vitamin A can reverse ocular keratinization. With this in mind, Ohashi and co-workers found vitamin A eye drops to be helpful in 10 of 12 patients with SLK. Vitamin A 1,500 IU/mL was more effective than 500 IU/mL.

N-acetylcysteine 10% or 20% 3–5 times a day can be used to treat the excess mucus that is related to filament formation. It may help decrease the symptoms when mucus and filaments are prominent.

Bandage contact lenses may also be used when the filaments predominate.

Surgical

Patients not responding to more conservative measures may be candidates for more aggressive treatment approaches. The superior bulbar conjunctiva may be treated with 30–50 brief focal applications of thermal cautery, after instilling topical anesthetic. Enough thermal energy should be used to burn the conjunctival epithelium and shrink the stroma, but not so much as to damage the sclera. Udell and colleagues reported success in the treatment of 8 of 11 patients (73%) with this method.

Recession or resection of the involved superior bulbar conjunctiva has been recommended for more severe cases. An arcuate 2- to 8-mm segment of conjunctiva and Tenon's tissue is removed from the 10 to 2 o'clock meridian superiorly after a peritomy incision. The remaining superior edge of the conjunctiva may be sutured to the episclera with interrupted sutures or left alone.

An alternative surgical approach was described by Yokoi et al. They resected the redundant conjunctival tissue adjacent to the area of conjunctival abnormality as defined by rose bengal staining, and successfully treated 2 of 2 eyes.

Cryotherapy for the involved superior bulbar conjunctiva has been advocated for the relief of symptoms. As with the use of silver nitrate and surgical resection, however, the symptoms may recur in days to months after treatment.

OTHER

Associated conditions such as chronic blepharitis and dry eye may aggravate symptoms; these conditions should be treated.

Dry eye

- Preservative-free artificial tears and ointments.
- Punctal occlusion.
- Avoidance of contributing environmental factors such as wind, smoke and pollution.
- Restasis used twice daily in patients with associated keratoconjunctivitis sicca.

Blepharitis

- Eyelid scrubs.
- Topical antibiotics to eyelid margins.
- Systemic tetracycline or tetracycline derivatives or systemic erythromycin.

COMPLICATONS

Because this condition is chronic, the use of corticosteroids, which have little effect, should be avoided or at least minimized. The condition does not respond to antibiotics or antiviral agents; these also should be avoided because of their potential toxicity. Caution should be taken when evaluating ptosis in patients with SLK, to ensure that they do not actually have a pseudoptosis secondary to SLK. Ptosis surgery in such patients may cause a significant increase in symptoms.

Extra precautions must be taken when treating patients who have associated decreased tear production. Close follow-up is necessary when bandage contact lenses are used, because complications from these contact lenses are more likely in patients with dry eyes. In addition, conjunctival recession or resection may not be as successful in patients who have significantly reduced tearing. Scleral melting may occur in the exposed section of the sclera after conjunctival resection in patients with severe dry eye. Management of patients with SLK who also have dry eyes should generally be more conservative.

COMMENTS

As the cause of the condition is unknown and the characteristic natural history of the disease includes periods of exacerbation and remission, care must be taken in implementing the numerous therapies recommended for this condition. This is especially true because the condition can disappear without treatment. For these reasons long-term therapy with corticosteroids should be avoided in favor of less toxic approaches including lubrication, punctual occlusion and topical ciclosporin.

REFERENCES

Confino J, Brown SI: Treatment of superior limbic keratoconjunctivitis with topical cromolyn sodium. Ann Ophthalmol 19:129–131, 1987.

Donshik PC, Collin HB, Foster CS, et al: Conjunctival resection treatment and ultrastructural histopathology of superior limbic keratoconjunctivitis. Am J Ophthalmol 85:101–110, 1978.

Grutzmacher RD, Foster RS, Feiler LS: Lodoxamide tromethamine treatment for superior limbic keratoconjunctivitis. Am J Ophthalmol 120:400–402, 1995.

Mondino BJ, Zaidman GW, Salamon SW: Use of pressure patching and soft contact lenses in superior limbic keratoconjunctivitis. Arch Ophthalmol 100:1932–1934, 1982.

Ohashi Y, Watanabe H, Kinoshita S, et al: Vitamin A eyedrops for superior limbic keratoconjunctivitis. Am J Ophthalmol 105:523–527, 1988.

Passons GA, Wood TO: Conjunctival resection for superior limbic keratoconjunctivitis. Ophthalmology 91:966–968, 1984.

Perry HD, Doshi-Carnevale S, Donnenfeld ED, et al: Topical cyclosporin A 0.5% as a possible new treatment for superior limbic keratoconjunctivitis. Ophthalmology 110:1578–1581, 2003.

Udell IJ, Kenyon KR, Sawa M, et al: Treatment of superior limbic keratoconjunctivitis by thermocauterization of the superior bulbar conjunctiva. Ophthalmology 93:162–166, 1986.

212 TERRIEN'S MARGINAL DEGENERATION 371.48

(Furrow Dystrophy, Marginal Extasia, Peripheral Furrow Keratitis)

Thomas L. Steinemann, MD
Cleveland, Ohio

ETIOLOGY/INCIDENCE

Terrien's marginal degeneration is an uncommon, slowly progressive thinning of the peripheral cornea. First described by Terrien in 1881 as a noninflammatory degeneration, its cause is still unknown. Subsequent reports have described a less common 'inflammatory' type of Terrien's degeneration that may occur in as many as one-third of affected (usually younger) individuals. The disease is commonly bilateral, but it may be asymmetric. It occurs more often in males. Patients may become symptomatic at any age, but earlier literature has described more cases occurring in middle-aged and older patients. More recent series suggest that the disease is more common in the 20- to 40-year-old age group. It has even been described in children younger than 10 years. It is usually asymptomatic unless astigmatism develops.

COURSE/PROGNOSIS

Progression of the marginal ectasia usually occurs gradually over many years. Initially, the disease process is noted superonasally, heralded by fine peripheral superficial vessels and punctate stromal opacities that coalesce gradually. At this stage, usually no thinning is noted, and the disease may resemble arcus senilis. An atypical pterygium occurring in an unusual oblique axis (pseudopterygium) has also been described as an early clinical sign.

Gradually, the stroma starts to thin in a clear zone of cornea between the marginal opacities and the limbus, forming a gutter-like furrow. The furrow remains covered with epithelium and has a sloping peripheral edge and a steel central edge. Yellow-white deposits, which appear to be lipid, are seen at the edge of the deepening furrow. The paralimbal thinning often progresses across the superior cornea. It may extend into the inferior cornea or even circumferentially, but usually the interpalpebral cornea is spared. The epithelium remains intact throughout the progression of the thinning, and patients do not typically complain of pain. Patients become symptomatic as the ectasia results in against-the-rule astigmatism. In 10% to 15% of cases, severely thinned areas may perforate, either spontaneously or with minor trauma. Occasionally, patients experience pain associated with episodic inflammation that resemble conjunctivitis, episcleritis, or scleritis. This may be treated with topical steroids.

DIAGNOSIS

The typical slit lamp appearance includes peripheral corneal thinning, sparing the limbus and most often occurring superonasally and progressing circumferentially; corneal vascularization with lipid deposits at the leading edge of the gutter; and an intact epithelium (compare with Mooren's ulcer) (Figure 212.1). There is severe against-the-rule astigmatism. Histopathology demonstrates intact epithelium with Bowman's layer fragmentation and fibrillar degeneration of stromal collagen. Descemet breaks are seen in areas of thinning.

Clinical signs and symptoms

Ocular or periocular

- Cornea: flattening of the corneal curvature in the vertical meridian, perforation (usually after minor trauma), peripheral thinning and ectasia with an overlying epithelium, peripheral vascularization and lipid deposition, corneal hydrops, intralamellar cyst, pseudopterygium.
- Other: episodic inflammation resembling conjunctivitis, episcleritis, or scleritis; high astigmatism and blurred vision.

Differential diagnosis

- Mooren's ulcer.

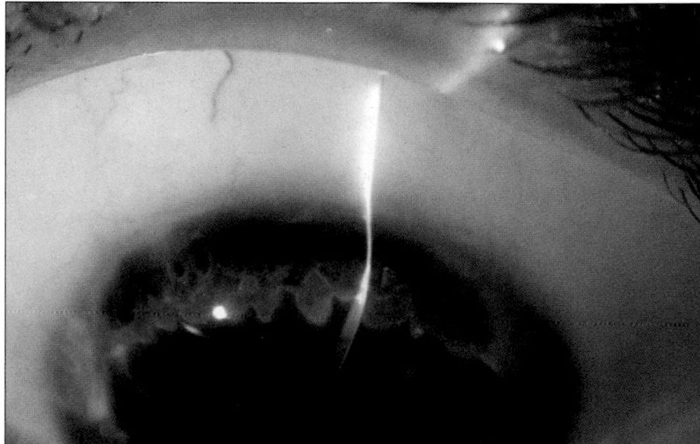

FIGURE 212.1. Terrien's marginal degeneration.

TREATMENT

Supportive

No medical therapy is effective in preventing the progression of corneal thinning. In the early stages, supportive therapy consists of spectacle correction of astigmatic refractive errors. With the progression of astigmatism, rigid contact lenses or 'piggyback' soft/rigid lens systems may be necessary.

Surgical

In advanced cases of Terrien's marginal degeneration, contact lens fitting may no longer be possible. In addition, ectatic areas may become dangerously thin. At this stage, surgical repair may be indicated both to decrease visually handicapping astigmatism and to prevent the rupture of ectatic areas through tectonic reinforcement.

Various surgical techniques have been suggested. One approach involves the excision of ectatic tissue, followed by suturing of the freshened edges of normal-thickness stroma. In another technique, a large eccentric penetrating keratoplasty is placed, although the increased possibility of graft rejection in such large transplants increases the chance of graft failure. An annular peripheral penetrating keratoplasty technique has also been described.

Inlay lamellar crescent keratoplasty has been used to treat severe thinning or perforation. With this technique, donor lamellar tissue-stroma, Bowman's layer, and, in some cases, epithelium-may be obtained by hand dissection from a whole eye.

An alternative method involves the use of a trephine that conforms to the size and curvature of the leading edge of corneal thinning. A central donor corneal button is punched using the same size of trephine; only the peripheral cornea is retained to fill the crescent-shaped defect in the host corneal bed. A lamellar graft is anchored to one edge of the keratectomy bed and alternately, cut freehand and sutured in a stepwise fashion to fill the defect.

COMPLICATIONS

In the majority of cases, conservative management is indicated. Because of the thinning and ectasia in more advanced cases, mild trauma can result in rupture of the cornea. Patients should therefore be instructed to avoid situations in which the eye might be traumatized. The use of protective eyewear may be warranted. Patients should be cautioned to seek attention for any abrupt change in visual status or for the development of pain in the eye. Because of the high risk of corneal perforation, surgeons should avoid excising a pseudopterygium in patients with Terrien's degeneration. In addition, surgery for corneal ectasia should be restricted to patients in whom astigmatism is severe and disabling or if perforation occurs or is imminent.

COMMENTS

Although Terrien's degeneration is a rare disorder, it typically presents either when the patient becomes visually symptomatic because of progressive astigmatism or after recurrent episodes of ocular irritation.

Recently a technique of collagen cross-linking with riboflavin and UVA light has been described in a rabbit model. This technique causes the collagen to thicken, increasing the cornea's stiffness and resistance to distortion and perhaps enzymatic digestion. Although the technique was described for treatment of keratoconus, itmay be applicable to Terrien's degeneration as well. This slowly progressive, generally noninflammatory disease can usually be managed conservatively, but patients must be followed periodically for progression of thinning, which can threaten the integrity of the globe.

REFERENCES

Caldwell DR, Insler MS, Boutros G, et al: Primary surgical repair of severe marginal ectasia in Terrien's degeneration. Am J Ophthalmol 97:332–336, 1984.

Goldman KN, Kaufman HE: Atypical pterygium: a clinical feature of Terrien's marginal degeneration. Arch Ophthalmol 96:1027–1029, 1978.

Kaufman HE, McDonald MB, Barron BA, Wilson SE: Color atlas of ophthalmic surgery: corneal and refractive surgery. Philadelphia, JB Lippincott, 1992:147–166.

Robin JB, Sclanzlin DJ, Verity SM, et al: Peripheral corneal disorder. Surv Ophthalmol 31:1–36, 1986.

Wollensak G, Spoerl E, Seiler T: Riboflavin/ultraviolet A-induced collagen cross-linking for the treatment of keratoconus. AmJ Ophthalmol. 135:620–627, 2003.

213 THYGESON'S SUPERFICIAL PUNCTATE KERATOPATHY 370.21

(Thygeson's Superficial Punctate Keratitis)

Parveen K. Nagra, MD

Philadelphia, Pennsylvania

Thygeson's superficial punctate keratopathy (TSPK) is a distinct clinical entity characterized by episodes of bilateral, coarse, granular, punctate epithelial opacities occurring without any ocular inflammation. Symptoms include a variable degree of ocular pain or discomfort, foreign body sensation, photophobia, and blurred vision.

ETIOLOGY/INCIDENCE

The cause is unknown. Association with viral infections has been suggested, although no definitive causation has been found. The prolonged disease course with steroid treatment may represent an altered immune response to a slow virus infection. A dyskeratosis has been postulated because of the steroidal response and the lack of inflammation in the eye. TSPK has been associated with HLA-DR3.

This keratopathy is very uncommon, affecting all races worldwide. Patients of both genders and all ages, including children, are affected.

COURSE/PROGNOSIS

TSPK is a chronic disease characterized by exacerbations and remissions. The lesions are transient, and the rate of recurrences is variable, although they often occur at weekly to monthly intervals. The natural history may be of eventual resolution within 4 years. However, in patients treated with steroids, the morbidity may last decades. There are no corneal abnormalities between attacks. While the vision may be minimally affected during episodes, the long-term visual prognosis is excellent.

DIAGNOSIS

Clinical signs and symptoms

- Punctate, scattered, epithelial lesions, with normal epithelium between lesions.
- No inflammation in the conjunctiva or anterior chamber; mild corneal stromal inflammation underlying the lesions may be present.
- Normal corneal sensation.
- Bilateral or unilateral.

Laboratory findings

- Lesions have elevated clusters of tiny gray dots, usually staining with rose bengal and fluorescein. May have a stellate appearance.
- Mucous filaments are not seen.
- No lab tests indicated.

Differential diagnosis

- Herpes simplex keratitis.
- Adenoviral keratitis.
- Staphylococcal keratoconjunctivitis.
- Keratoconjunctivitis sicca.
- Rosacea keratitis.

TREATMENT

Medical

Lubricants and topical steroids are the mainstay of treatment. Other treatments include topical cyclosporin A and therapeutic soft contact lenses. Following initiation of topical steroids, the lesions and symptoms improve rapidly.

- Fluorometholone 0.1% four times a day with slow taper over months.
- Alternatives include loteprednol 0.2%, loteprednol 0.5%, rimexolone 1%, or in advanced cases, prednisone acetate 1%.
- Patients should have regular evaluations to assess for improvement, evaluate for complications of treatment, and taper steroids.
- Cyclosporin A and therapeutic soft contact lens are effective therapies to be considered initially, when difficulty arises in tapering steroids, or steroid-related complications are noted.

Surgical

Epithelial debridement results in a rapid recurrence of lesions. Resolution has been reported following photorefractive keratectomy but not laser in situ keratomileusis.

COMPLICATIONS

The potential complications of steroid therapy and extended-wear contact lenses must always be borne in mind. The use of idoxuridine eyedrops in TSPK may result in subepithelial opacities.

COMMENTS

TSPK is not a common or communicable condition. Because it is frequently misdiagnosed and is a periodically remitting disorder, numerous ocular drugs have been used with unmerited successes and not unexpected failures. Fortunately, there is usually no residual scarring and patients have an excellent long-term visual prognosis.

REFERENCES

Darrell RW: Thygeson's superficial punctate keratitis: Natural history and association with HLA DR3. Trans Am Ophthalmol Soc 79:486–516, 1981.

Fite SW, Chodosh J: Photorefractive keratectomy for myopia in the setting of Thygeson's superficial punctuate keratitis. Cornea 20:425–426, 2001.

Goldberg DB, Schanzlin DJ, Brown SI: Management of Thygeson's superficial punctate keratitis. Am J Ophthalmol 89:22–24, 1980.

Thygeson P: Clinical and laboratory observations on superficial punctate keratitis. Am J Ophthalmol 61:1344–1349, 1966.

Nagra PK, Rapuano CJ, Cohen EJ, et al. Thygeson's superficial punctate keratitis: ten years' experience. Ophthalmology. 111:34–37, 2004.

SECTION

20 Extraocular Muscles

214 A-PATTERN STRABISMUS 378.02, 378.06, 378.12, 378.16

Ann U. Stout, MD
Portland, Oregon

A-pattern strabismus refers to a vertically incomitant horizontal strabismus in which the horizontal separation of the visual axes becomes progressively greater as gaze shifts from up to down. The A-pattern can be associated with esotropia, where the deviation is greatest in upgaze, or with exotropia, where the deviation is greatest in downgaze.

Patients with A-pattern esotropia may adopt a chin-up head posture to facilitate fusion. Patients with A-pattern exotropia may use a chin-down posture if fusion can be obtained only in upgaze.

ETIOLOGY

The numerous possible causes proposed for A-pattern strabismus include dysfunction of any of the six extraocular muscles (oblique, horizontal and vertical recti), orbital rotation or globe rotation, connective tissue (pulley) anomalies and muscle insertion anomalies.

DIAGNOSIS

There are standard prism-cover measurements in the primary position, upgaze and downgaze. Upgaze and downgaze are measured 25 to 30 degrees from the primary position. A difference between upgaze and downgaze of more than 10 prism diopters is significant. A-pattern esotropia is more common in patients with upslanting fissures, while A-pattern exotropia is more common in patients with downslanting fissures.

TREATMENT

For the clinician, determination of whether the A-pattern is due to significant superior oblique muscle overaction is imperative. In general, if a large A-pattern is present in association with superior oblique overaction, the superior oblique must be weakened to correct the pattern. Conversely, if no superior oblique overaction is present in the setting of an A-pattern, the superior oblique should not be operated on, especially if inferior oblique overaction exists.

A-pattern esotropia without oblique dysfunction

- Recess the medial rectus muscle (MR) bilaterally with upshift.
- If unilateral surgery, recess the MR with upshift and resect the lateral rectus muscle (LR) with downshift.

A-pattern esotropia with significant superior oblique overaction

- Recess the MR bilaterally (or recess the MR and resect the LR unilaterally) for esotropia in the primary position.
- Weaken the superior oblique bilaterally (see Complications).
- Weakening can be by spacer placement, tenotomy, or tenectomy.
- A-pattern should be 25 prism diopters or more if superior oblique weakening is done to avoid overcorrection.

A-pattern exotropia without oblique dysfunction

- Recess the LR bilaterally with downshift.
- If unilateral surgery, recess the LR with downshift, and resect the MR with upshift.

A-pattern exotropia with superior oblique overaction

- Recess the LR bilaterally (or recess the LR and resect the MR unilaterally) for exotropia in the primary position.
- Weaken the superior oblique bilaterally (see Complications).
- Weakening can be by spacer, tenotomy, or tenectomy.
- A-pattern should be 25 prism diopters or more if superior oblique weakening is done.

A-pattern exotropia with superior oblique overaction and dissociated vertical deviation

- This classic triad can occur as a primary strabismus entity or secondary to previous strabismus surgery, such as after MR recession for esotropia.
- Treat as A-pattern exotropia with superior oblique overaction, but superior rectus recession bilaterally can be added for dissociated vertical deviation.

A-pattern with craniofacial syndromes

- Craniofacial syndromes such as Crouzon's syndrome are frequently associated with A-pattern (or V-pattern) strabismus.
- The probable cause is orbital and/or muscle insertion rotation.

- These syndromes frequently fail to respond to oblique weakening alone.
- Oblique weakening and horizontal rectus shifts may be required.

COMPLICATIONS

- A-pattern can be converted to V-pattern.
- Conversion of A-pattern to V-pattern after superior oblique weakening is less likely if inferior oblique underaction was present before surgery.
- Torsional diplopia can occur after superior oblique weakening.
- The risk is significant if the patient has high-grade fusion before surgery.
- Superior oblique weakening should be done judiciously if patient has measurable stereopsis before surgery.
- Superior oblique weakening should not be done if patient has normal stereopsis (e.g. 40 seconds arc stereo or better) because torsional diplopia may occur.
- Graded superior oblique weakening with spacers may reduce the risk of this compared to tenotomies or tenectomies.

REFERENCES

Helveston EM: A-exotropia, alternating sursumduction and superior oblique overaction. Am J Ophthalmol 67:377–380, 1969.

Urist MJ: The etiology of the so-called A and V patterns. Am J Ophthalmol 46:825, 1958.

von Noorden GK: Binocular vision and ocular motility. 5th edn. St Louis, CV Mosby, 1996.

Wright K: Superior oblique silicon expander for Brown syndrome and superior oblique overaction. J Pediatr Ophthalmol Strabismus 28:101–107, 1991.

215 ABDUCENS (SIXTH NERVE) PARALYSIS 378.54

Raghu Mudumbai, MD
Seattle, Washington

Sixth nerve palsy is a common neuro-ophthalmic disorder. Because of the long intracranial course of the sixth nerve, abducens function may be compromised by multiple etiologies. Palsies may be unilateral or bilateral. They may be treated both medically, for example with prisms or injections of botulinum toxin, and surgically, for example by recess/resect and transposition procedures.

ETIOLOGY/INCIDENCE

In childhood, several etiologies – congenital, neoplasm, raised intracranial pressure, trauma, and post-infection – are common. Etiologies are similar in adult patients, but vasculopathies such as hypertension and diabetes are also significant causes. Sixth nerve palsy is a rare initial presentation of multiple sclerosis.

COURSE/PROGNOSIS

Prognosis varies with etiology. Cases with a vascular etiology usually resolve completely, while sixth nerve palsies arising from other causes have a more guarded prognosis. A minimum of six months is given for spontaneous resolution.

DIAGNOSIS

Clinical signs and symptoms

Symptoms include diplopia, worse in the field of the palsy and better on the opposite side except in bilateral cases. Esotropia is maximum in the field of the palsy and decreases at near. If mild, diplopia may be resolved when the patient looks towards the side opposite the palsy. Diplopia may not be present if the eye is directed towards the nose, which can block binocularity.

Differential diagnosis

Thyroid-related ophthalmopathy commonly involves the medial rectus muscle to produce a restrictive esotropia. Forced ductions or differential intraocular pressure measurements may be helpful signs. Myasthenia gravis is produced by acetylcholine receptor antibodies leading to any combination of ptosis, orbicularis weakness and extraocular muscle weakness, including isolated lateral rectus involvement. Forced generation testing reveals the weakness. Edrophonium chloride testing, the ice test and laboratory testing for acetylcholine receptor antibodies are helpful in the diagnosis. Blow-out fracture of the medial wall of the orbit can lead to entrapment of the medial rectus muscle and a restrictive esotropia. Forced ductions reveal a restriction. Duane's syndrome (Type 1), due to malformation of the sixth nerve nucleus and abnormal innervation of the lateral rectus by the third nerve, leads to unilateral or bilateral esotropia, limited abduction, enophthalmos, and narrowing of the lid fissure on abduction. Multiple sclerosis commonly produces internuclear ophthalmoplegia, which is a lesion of the medial longitudinal fasiculus and not a sixth nerve palsy. It is distinguished by contralateral abduction nystagmus and ipsilateral adduction deficit.

Sixth nerve palsy can occur in combination with other deficits leading to definable syndromes. Bilateral congenital sixth and and seventh nerve palsies occur in Mobius syndrome. In Gradenigo's syndrome, inflammation of the petrous bone, most commonly from an otitis media, leads to a sixth and seventh nerve palsies. Cavernous sinus syndrome includes third, fourth, oculosympathetic, and first division trigeminal palsies. Orbital apex syndrome adds vision loss. One and a half syndrome, resulting from a lesion of the sixth nerve nucleus and the medial longitudinal fasciculus, is recognized by an ipsilateral horizontal gaze palsy and a contralateral internuclear ophthalmoplegia. Sixth nerve palsy may be the first sign of a cavernous sinus syndrome, as the nerve travels within the substance of the sinus and thus may be the first nerve affected. Other nerves affected can include the III, IV, V_1, V_2 and the sympathetics. Orbital apex syndrome is similar, except that it does not involve V_2 and includes optic neuropathy.

TREATMENT

Ocular

Patients with mild palsies may compensate with a head turn toward the palsied side in order to maintain fusion. Large palsies or bilateral involvement may lead to voluntary closing of one eye to prevent diplopia. In cases where there is a high likelihood of improvement, occlusion by fogging one lens with tape or the use of a patch is highly useful to prevent diplopia as the amount of esotropia decreases with time. In patients unlikely to improve or who have reached maximal improvement with small residual deviation, base out prism may benefit to help patients maintain fusion. It can also be placed over the non-involved eye to decrease contracture of the medial rectus on the involved side. Permanent ground in prism is limited by the weight of the glasses and optical aberrations induced by the prism.

Botulinum toxin type A has been used in acute cases of sixth nerve palsy. Its effect lasts from weeks to several months. Two and a half to 5 units are injected into the antagonist medial rectus muscle (treatment is localized with the aid of an electromyographic electrode). This treatment may prevent long term contracture and aid in resolution of the deviation. It is more useful with smaller deviations of less than 30–40 prism diopters.

Surgical

Once it is clear that no more improvement will occur (6 to 12 months), surgical options can be employed. With time, the incomitant deviation becomes more comitant, a phenomenon known as spread of comitance. When there is some residual forced generation found in the lateral rectus, a horizontal recess/resect of the medial and lateral recti can be attempted. In complete sixth nerve palsies, a medial rectus recession can be combined with transposition of the superior and inferior recti to the lateral rectus muscle. Use of the adjustable suture technique can help improve outcomes.

An appropriate preoperative evaluation should be carried out prior to surgery. Necessary components include measurement of the deviation and evaluation of the relative strength of the lateral and medial recti. The deviation should be measured in primary, left and right gaze. Upgaze and downgaze measurements are helpful in determining if a V or A pattern is present. Muscle tone can be measured by comparing the active forced generation of the medial and lateral recti. Estimating saccadic velocity by observation or with electro-oculography may also be beneficial to gauge the amount of sixth nerve paresis. Abduction past the midline is also helpful in judging lateral rectus function. Forced duction can provide information as to whether contracture of the medial rectus is present.

In patients found to have medial rectus contraction, recession of the medial rectus should be part of the surgical plan. Maximum recession is 12 millimeters from the limbus, and additional effect can be achieved by recessing the overlying conjunctiva and Tenon's to the original insertion. The medial rectus can be placed on an adjustable suture and its resection can be combined with a resection of the lateral rectus up to 9 millimeters.

When there is minimal lateral rectus function, a transposition procedure of the vertical recti to the lateral rectus will probably be required. Transposition can either be total or by the Jensen procedure. In this procedure, the vertical recti are split and joined to adjacent halves of the lateral rectus but without disinsertion. This has the theoretical advantage of preserving anterior ciliary artery circulation to the anterior segment. There can be simultaneous medial rectus recession on an adjustable suture.

Single binocular vision in primary gaze with a limited range of fusion is a reasonable goal. Patients adapt by learning to maintain fixation in primary gaze by head rotation, a partially successful strategy. Patients, especially those with traumatic sixth nerve palsy from head trauma, should be warned that central disruption of fusion is a possibility even with good alignment.

COMMENTS

Sixth nerve palsy can result from numerous etiologies due to the long intracranial course of the nerve. Careful history taking and clinical examination supplemented by appropriate neuroimaging and laboratory testing usually leads to the correct diagnosis. While waiting for resolution, patients can be managed in the short term by patching, prism or selective use of botulinum toxin. In cases of non-resolving sixth nerve palsy, surgical improvement may be obtained with recess/resect procedures or a transposition procedure. Adjustable suture technique may also be of benefit, given the variability of recovery of lateral rectus function.

REFERENCES

Ellis FD, Helveston EM: Special considerations and techniques in strabismus surgery. Int Ophthalmol Clin 16:247–254, 1976.

Hotchkiss MG, Miller NR, Clark AW, et al: Bilateral Duane's retraction syndrome: a clinical-pathologic case report. Arch Ophthalmol 98:870–874, 1980.

Lee MS, Galetta SL, Volpe NJ, et al: Sixth nerve palsies in children. Pediatr Neurol 20:49–52, 1999

Miller NR, Newman NJ, eds: Walsh and Hoyt's clinical neuro-ophthalmology. 6th edn. Maryland, Lippincott, Williams and Wilkins, 2004.

Sanders SK, Kawasaki A, Purvin VA: Long-term prognosis in patients with vasculopathic sixth nerve palsy. Am J Ophthalmol 134:81–84, 2002.

216 ACCOMMODATIVE ESOTROPIA 378.35

Henry S. O'Halloran, MD, DOphth, FRCSI
San Diego, California
William Barry Lee, MD
Atlanta, Georgia

INTRODUCTION

Accommodative esotropia is one of the most common types of strabismus occurring in childhood. The incidence of this disorder is estimated at 0.67% to 2% in the population; however, the deviation has been found to occur as infrequently as 1 in 373 cases in some studied populations. Accommodative esotropia represents an acquired esodeviation with variable severity and intermittent onset with potential progression to a constant deviation. The disorder is most commonly hereditary in nature with some studies finding nearly 80% of affected first-or second-degree relatives, yet no pattern of inheritance or genetic locus have been identified. Less commonly, trauma or illness may be a precipitating factor. The typical age of onset is between 6 months and 5 years, with an average age of onset at 2.5 years and reports of this disease in children as young as 3 months old.

COURSE/PROGNOSIS

The natural history of accommodative esotropia with regard to spontaneous improvement or progression to nonaccommodative esotropia remains unknown. The esodeviation usually begins as an intermittent crossing of the eyes but often progresses to a constant deviation. The consequences of this deviation can result in amblyopia. Diplopia can occur but may disappear with development of a suppression scotoma in the deviating eye. Several series have quoted a high rate of monofixation (peripheral fusion with absence of central binocular fixation).

CLINICAL DIAGNOSIS

The diagnosis of refractive accommodative esotropia consists of uncorrected hyperopia in association with insufficient fusional divergence. The hyperopia averages 5 diopters with a range from 3 to 10 diopters and the angle of esotropia is approximately equal at near and distant fixation. The accommodative convergence-to accommodation (AC/A) ratio is normal. Nonrefractive accommodative esotropia consists of a high AC/A ratio. The refractive error is generally low hyperopia with an average of 2 diopters, but it can range from myopia to high hyperopia. The esotropia is greater at near fixation where greater accommodation is needed in comparison to distance fixation targets. Partially accommodative or decompensated esotropia represents an esotropia that is partially corrected with spectacle correction or an esotropia that develops from decompensation following an initially fully corrected deviation with spectacles. This form of accommodative esotropia often occurs with delayed correction.

TREATMENT

Treatment of accommodative esotropia includes prevention of amblyopia with preservation of normal visual acuity, restoration of normal ocular alignment, maintenance of binocular vision and stereopsis, and striving for an emmetropic state for both eyes. Treatment with spectacle correction is often successful in maintenance of appropriate ocular alignment, but surgical correction remains necessary in an estimated 30% of cases.

Medical

Spectacle correction

Spectacle correction is considered the initial treatment of choice for accommodative esotropia. The amount of correction is derived from a cycloplegic refraction with an appropriate cycloplegic agent such as cyclopentolate or atropine, and the full hyperopic correction is prescribed if a constant or intermittent esotropia is present. The ultimate aim is to provide the minimum correction that will maintain orthophoria under binocular conditions to encourage and expand the degree of fusional divergence. The correction is usually gradually decreased to an amount of correction that maintains orthophoria with a follow-up visit scheduled no more than 2 months after each reduction.

Single vision spectacles are used for the majority of cases; however, patients with a high AC/A ratio who have esotropia at near of 10 or more diopters should use bifocal correction. Bifocal spectacle correction should use the smallest amount of add that will restore normal ocular alignment at near with a maximum strength of up to 3.5 diopters of add. Bifocals are ordered in an executive style or large flat-top segment, with the top of the bifocal set high near the midpupil level. Progressive add bifocals commonly have the bifocal segment too low for a desirable effect. The authors use a rough rule of thumb that if the esotropia for near exceeds that for distance by 25 prism diopters, bifocals may be needed. Deviations of less than this amount may require a second office visit and assessment of esotropia for near using trial lenses.

The timing of the reduction in hyperopic correction is somewhat controversial and varies among practitioners. The authors attempt reduction of spectacle correction on a yearly basis provided that the patient is orthophoric for near and distant fixation, and each reduction is followed by a repeat examination at 6 weeks to ensure stable alignment with the weaker spectacle correction.

Contact lenses

Contact lenses may be used for treatment of accommodative esotropia in certain conditions.

- Contact lenses can include regular or toric soft contacts, rigid gas permeable contacts, and bifocal contacts.
- Advantages include reduction of accommodative effort at near and eradication of ring scotomas and prismatic effect associated with spectacle correction.
- Disadvantages include contact lens intolerance, corneal complications such as infection, and the need for strict compliance with contact lens wear and cleaning regimens.
- All lenses should be removed on a daily basis to limit risk of infection and corneal complications.

Pharmacologic agents

- Pharmacologic agents can be used alone or in combination with glasses.
- Miotics work by inducing ciliary muscle contraction and reducing accommodative effort and the need for convergence.
- Agents used include echothiophate iodide (most frequent) and demecarium bromide, both long-acting cholinesterase inhibitors.
- Commonly used to replace spectacles in the summer when swimming and other activities tend to reduce the amount of time for spectacle wear.
- Potential side effects exist including iris cysts, conjunctival hyperemia, myopia, and prolonged anesthesia with depolarizing muscle relaxants.

Surgical

Despite maximal optical and pharmacologic support, some patients develop a nonrefractive component to the esotropia. Studies estimate this occurs in 13% to 48% of patients. The goal of strabismus surgery is to correct the non-accommodative component of the esotropia.

Strabismus surgery

- Optimal correction of amblyopia before surgical correction is recommended.
- Surgical correction is recommended only when, despite full refractive correction, there is a constant esotropia of more than 10 prism diopters, precluding binocular vision and stereopsis
- Surgical results can be improved by the use of prism adaptation in which Fresnel prisms are worn in the preoperative

period and the strength of the prisms increased as the esotropia increases or until fusion is demonstrated. Surgical correction is then performed for the fully adapted esotropia angle. The surgical option of choice is bilateral medical rectus recessions, with monocular recess-resect procedures performed only when severe amblyopia is present.

- Several studies have shown a high degree of binocularity after surgery in up to 70% of patients.
- The amount of surgery to perform is controversial. Some surgeons recommend correcting the residual esotropia at distance while others use an augmented approach, correcting the average of the near deviation with and without correction.

Refractive surgery

- A method to restore ocular alignment without spectacle correction in purely refractive accommodative esotropia.
- Surgical treatment in older children and adults to correct hyperopia and hyperopic astigmatism using an excimer laser.
- Treatment can include up to 6 diopters of hyperopia and up to 6 diopters of astigmatism.
- Remains controversial in children.

AMBLYOPIA MANAGEMENT

Amblyopia associated with accommodative esotropia is usually mild and is more common when the deviation becomes constant or when anisometropia exists, particularly astigmatic anisometropia. The prognosis for vision is usually good because these children frequently have some degree of fusion before the onset of their esotropia. A standard patching regimen (i.e. 1 week of full-time patching per year of age) can be an effective means of treatment in patients that do develop amblyopia. Alternatively, part-time patching or atropine penalization therapy is used to encourage the development of fusion and stereopsis. Frequent follow-up is imperative to ensure occlusion amblyopia does not develop. Part-time patching may be indicated until 10 years of age in cases where full-time patching may pose a risk of occlusion amblyopia.

COMMENTS

The optimal agent for cycloplegia is the subject of perennial controversy. For children, we use a mixture of 1% cyclopentolate and phenylephrine 2.5%. Atropine is used when repeat refractions differ greatly or when repeated instillation of cyclopentolate is ineffective. We advise against the use of atropine before sleep because the signs and symptoms of atropine toxicity would not be noticed. Atropine penalization is an excellent alternative to patching for amblyopia therapy. One study has shown that success with amblyopia treatment is linked to a higher socioeconomic status of the parents or caregivers, and this should be considered before embarking on a complicated amblyopia regimen.

REFERENCES

Lambert SR: Accommodative esotropia. Ophth Clin North Am 14:425–432, 2001.

Ludwig IH, Imberman SP, Thompson HW, Parks MM: Long-term study of accommodative esotropia. Trans Am Ophthalmol Soc 101:155–161, 2003.

Prism Adaptation Study Research Group: Efficacy of prism adaptation in the surgical management of acquired esotropia. Arch Ophthalmol 108:1248–1256, 1990.

Weakley DR, Holand DR: Effect on ongoing treatment of amblyopia on surgical outcome in esotropia. J Pediatr Ophthalmol Strabismus 34:275–278, 1997.

Wilson ME, Bluestein EC, Parks MM: Binocularity in accommodative esotropia. J Pediatr Ophthalmol Strabismus 30:233–236, 1993.

217 ACQUIRED NONACCOMMODATIVE ESOTROPIA 378.00

F. Hampton Roy, MD, FACS
Little Rock, Arkansas

ETIOLOGY/INCIDENCE

Acquired nonaccommodative esotropia is a convergent deviation with onset after the age of 6 months. This deviation is approximately the same in all directions of gaze. It is not significantly affected by accommodation. Because normal binocular vision often exists before the onset of this disease, the prognosis for binocular function in patients with acquired nonaccommodative esotropia is better than that for those with congenital esotropia. One eye may prefer fixation in this condition. Amblyopia will develop if the deviation is unilateral and the onset occurs in childhood.

The cause of nonaccommodative acquired esodeviation is believed to be both neurogenic and anatomic. The neurogenic or innervational cause may be excessive tonic convergence or deficient tonic divergence. Anatomic factors may be anomalous medial recti insertions. Other causes of acquired nonaccommodative esotropia include stress, organic lesions, and anisometropia. Stress-induced acquired esodeviation may be precipitated by illness and emotional factors that cause a breakdown of preciously adequate fusional divergence. Patients under stress may also undergo a spasm of the near synkinetic reflex, resulting in sustained convergence with accommodative spasm and miosis. Any monocular organic lesion, such as cataract, optic atrophy, or corneal scarring, may result in an esodeviation, especially if the onset occurs before the age of 4 years. Amblyopia secondary to an asymmetric refractive error (anisometropia) may result in a secondary esodeviation. An acutely acquired esodeviation that is worse at distance should be suspected for divergence paralysis and may indicate an early lateral rectus palsy secondary to underlying neurologic disease, such as pontine tumor or head trauma. Acquired esotropia may rarely be cyclic in pattern, such as occurring every other day.

TREATMENT

Ocular

- Occlusion therapy is accomplished best at an early age (younger than 7 years). As a general rule, the schedule for rechecking patients after patching should be 1 week per year of life to ensure that amblyopia does not develop in the patched eye.
- Eyeglasses should be prescribed for significant refractive errors that may disrupt fusion. Asymmetric refractive errors

are treated with eyeglasses or contact lenses to reduce image disparity. Organic lesions that occlude vision, such as congenital cataracts, are treated as early as possible, followed by aggressive amblyopia therapy.

- Orthoptics may be indicated to eliminate sensory adaptations, such as suppression or abnormal retinal correspondence, that may have developed secondary to the esodeviation.

Surgical

- Strabismus surgery is indicated for any significant esodeviation that is still present after the completion of amblyopia therapy, refractive lens correction, and orthoptics. The surgery may be unilateral or bilateral depending on the surgeon's preference and whether the eyes freely alternate.
- Unilateral surgery consists of weakening (recession) of the medial rectus muscle and strengthening (resection) of the lateral rectus muscle. Some surgeons prefer performing unilateral surgery on patients who have a strong preference for fixation in one eye. In these cases, surgery is usually performed on the nonfixating eye.
- Bilateral medial rectus recessions are performed depending on the surgeon's preference or if the eyes are freely alternating.
- Small deviations (less than 15 prism diopters) may require a recession of only one medial rectus muscle. Deviations between 15 and 45 prism diopters usually require surgery on two muscles (recession-resection on one eye or bilateral recessions). Deviations of more than 45 prism diopters may require surgery on three or four muscles depending on the severity of the angle; however, some surgeons prefer to operate on only two muscles during the initial operation regardless of the size of the deviation.
- The use of adjustable sutures in strabismus surgery in older children and adults has significantly improved the postoperative result; this can be done with topical anesthesia at the time of surgery or within 1 day after the surgical procedure.
- Botulinum toxin type A (Oculinum) injection into an ocular muscle creates an intentional temporary paralysis that may result in improved alignment in carefully selected cases.
- Prism adaptation therapy, in which prisms are used before surgery, has been found to improve the results of surgery for acquired esotropia. Fresnel prisms are placed on eyeglasses until the angle of deviation is neutralized or fusion is obtained. This 'adapted' angle becomes the goal for a surgical correction and may reduce the reoperation rate.
- No surgery should be attempted unless preoperative measurements are accurate and consistent. At least three sets of measurements should be taken before strabismus surgery is undertaken.

Early detection

- Early detection of strabismus and amblyopia is vitally important. Children treated at an early age for amblyopia respond better to occlusion therapy than do older children. If amblyopia cannot be reversed, the prognosis for alignment of the eyes and fusion is significantly worsened.
- In patients requiring surgery, fusional results are significantly better in children who underwent surgery at an early age. In addition, obvious psychologic sequelae have been noted in children with late surgical treatment of a longstanding and cosmetically displeasing esodeviation.

COMMENTS

The treatment of acquired nonaccommodative esotropia requires a specific management plan to achieve the best possible fusional results. This plan should include a thorough ophthalmologic and strabismic evaluation, early amblyopia detection and therapy, orthoptics, and, if necessary, strabismus surgery.

REFERENCES

Abel LA, Troost BT: Acquired cyclic esotropia in an adult eye. Am J Ophthalmol 91:805–806, 1981.

Biglan AW, Burnstine RA, Rogers GL, Saunders RA: Management of strabismus with botulinum A toxin. Ophthalmology 96:935–943, 1989.

Dankner SR, Mash AJ, Jampolsky A: Intentional surgical overcorrection of acquired esotropia. Arch Ophthalmol 96:1848–1852, 1978.

Delisle P, Strasfeld M, Pelletier D: The prism adaptation test in the preoperative evaluation of esodeviations. Can J Ophthalmol 23:208–212, 1988.

Eino D, Kraft SP: Postoperative drifts after adjustable suture strabismus surgery. Can J Ophthalmol 32:163–169, 1997.

Helveston EM: Atlas of strabismus surgery. 4th edn. St Louis, CV Mosby, 1992.

Jampolsky A: Current techniques of adjustable strabismus surgery. Am J Ophthalmol 88:406–418, 1979.

Kani K: Magnetic resonance imaging measurements of extraocular muscle-path shift and posterior eyeball prolapse from the muscle cone in acquired estropia with high myopia. Am J Ophthalmol 136:482–489, 2003.

Kitzmann AS, Mohney BG, Diehl NN: Short-term motor and sensory outcomes in acquired nonaccommodative estropia of childhood. Strabismus. 13:109–114, 2005.

Kraft SP, Enzenauer RW, Weston B: Stability of the postoperative alignment in adjustable-suture strabismus surgery. J Pediatr Ophthalmol 28:206–211, 1991.

Metz HS: Acquired cyclic esotropia in an adult eye. Am J Ophthalmol 91:804–805, 1981.

Parks MM, Mitchel PR, Wheeler MB: Ocular motility and strabismus. In: Duane TD, ed: Clinical ophthalmology. Philadelphia, JB Lippincott, 1990.

Prism Adaptation Study Research Group: Efficacy of prism adaptation in the surgical management of acquired esotropia. Arch Ophthalmol 108:148–156, 1990.

Repka MX, Wentworth D: Predictors of prism response during prism adaptation. J Pediatr Ophthalmol Strabismus 28:202–205, 1991.

Rosenbaum AL: The current use of botulinum toxin therapy in strabismus. Arch Ophthalmol 114:213–214, 1996.

Scott AB: Botulinum toxin injection into extraocular muscle as an alternative to strabismus surgery. J Pediatr Ophthalmol Strabismus 17:21–25, 1980.

von Noorden GK: Binocular vision and ocular motility: theory and management of strabismus. 5th edn. St Louis, CV Mosby, 1995.

Ward JB, Niffenegger AS, Lavin CW, et al: The use of propofol and mivacurium anesthetic technique for the immediate postoperative adjustment of sutures in strabismus surgery. Ophthalmology 102:122–128, 1998.

218 BASIC AND INTERMITTENT EXOTROPIA 378.10, 378.23

Michael P. Clarke, FRCS, FRCOphth
Newcastle Upon Tyne, England
Sarah R. Richardson, DBO
Newcastle Upon Tyne, England

ETIOLOGY/INCIDENCE

Exotropia describes a divergent misalignment of the visual axes. Exotropia is less common than esotropia and is more common in the middle east, subequatorial Africa and other places with high levels of sunlight. The overall prevalence of exo deviations has been reported to be 0.4%. Exotropias are associated with ophthalmic and neuro-ophthalmic disease, particularly when these cause visual field defects, and with craniofacial syndromes.

Classification of exotropias is hampered by a lack of understanding of the biological basis of the condition, but it has proved useful to subdivide primary exotropias based on a proposed etiology of convergence and divergence mechanisms (Box 218.1).

Constant exotropias include those of infantile onset, decompensated exophorias and decompensated intermittent exotropias. Intermittent Exotropia, X(T) for short, describes an intermittent divergent misalignment of the visual axes which is initially observed when fixation is at distance rather than near, and during periods of fatigue and inattention. In intermittent distance exotropia (the so called divergence excess type) the distance deviation is 15 or more prism dioptres greater than the near deviation. In some apparent intermittent distance exotropias (the so called simulated divergence excess pattern) the near deviation increases to within 15 dioptres of the distance deviation when accommodative or convergence mechanisms are suspended. When the near deviation is within 15 dioptres of the distance deviation without the use of special tests, it is called basic, or non specific, exotropia. Intermittent exotropia can evolve into basic exotropia if the near deviation increases as the condition deteriorates. This chapter is concerned with basic and intermittent exotropia excluding convergence insufficiency.

BOX 218.1 – Classification of exotropia

1. **Primary**
   Constant
   a. Infantile
   b. Decompensated Intermittent
   c. Decompensated Exophoria
   Intermittent
   a. Convergence Insufficiency
      (i) Primary
      (ii) Undercorrected myopia
   b. Distance
      (i) True
      (ii) Simulated
      High AC/A
      Normal AC/A
   c. Basic
2. **Secondary (Sensory)**
3. **Consecutive**
   Spontaneous
   Postoperative

COURSE/PROGNOSIS

X(T) has traditionally been held to be a progressive condition, with increasing frequency of the observed distance deviation leading to an intermittent and ultimately constant deviation at near. This may then lead to loss of binocular function and stereopsis at near. This view has recently been challenged, and it now seems evident that many if not most cases of X(T) are non progressive.

DIAGNOSIS

Clinical signs and symptoms

Onset is usually before the age of 5 years, and may occur as early as the first year of life. Children with X(T) usually present to medical attention because of the observed deviation. An alternative manifestation of the condition is monocular eye closure which occurs in bright illumination. Why this occurs is unknown; it is not thought to be a means of avoiding diplopia.

Children with X(T) do not generally complain of diplopia, although they sometimes notice panoramic vision. How diplopia is avoided is unclear, as the size of the misalignment varies constantly as the viewing distance changes. The prevailing theory is that suppression of the whole of the temporal hemifield of one eye occurs under binocular conditions, when the deviation is present. Despite the presence of suppression, amblyopia is rare, as the eyes typically remain aligned fixing at near, usually with good binocular functions and stereopsis at this viewing distance.

The significance of the functional disability associated with a distance divergent deviation is also obscure. The physiological value of ocular alignment, binocular functions and stereopsis when viewing distant targets is not known. Defects of stereopsis at distance have been described in association with X(T) but it is not known if these are associated with visual disability or if they are a useful indication for treatment. Binocular visual acuity may be reduced at distance if accommodation is exerted to control the distance deviation, inducing myopia. Convergence and motor fusional amplitudes may also be affected.

Differential diagnosis

The differential diagnosis includes infantile exotropia, decompensated exophoria, near exotropia (convergence insufficiency), sensory and consecutive exotropia. Patients with infantile, sensory and consecutive exotropia generally have poor binocular functions, except in the case of sensory exotropia caused by visual field loss. Infantile exotropias may cause dissociated strabismus complex. Near exotropia has a larger angle at near fixation and good binocular functions can be demonstrated for distance fixation. It is characterized by equal vision, poor binocular convergence, normal sensory fusion and poor positive motor fusion. Patients who have decompensated exophoria present with symptoms of blurred vision, diplopia and asthenopia. Normal binocular single vision is demonstrable but often with a reduced positive fusion amplitude and reduced convergence.

TREATMENT/COMPLICATIONS

The clinical management of X(T) presents a dilemma. Conservative treatments are often ineffective and surgery may be required. However, surgical overcorrection is common, especially in younger patients, and while there may be a good cosmetic outcome despite a small overcorrection, this will be at the expense of impaired near binocular functions.

Treatment is usually requested because of the cosmetic appearance of the observed deviation. The treating physician may be concerned about the possibility of deteriorating binocular function if the strabismus is not treated. Usually the child has straight eyes and good binocular vision for near fixation, for example when reading. As the fixation distance increases, there is an increasing tendency for the eyes to diverge.

Ocular

Conservative treatments for X(T) include minus lenses, prisms, orthoptic exercises and occlusion. They may be used in isolation, or as a temporising measure in young children vulnerable to the effects of surgical overcorrection. Significant refractive errors, even hyperopic ones, should be corrected in intermittent exotropia as this will sharpen the retinal images and improve fusion. Minus lenses are sometimes used to stimulate accommodative convergence. They may be particularly helpful in patients with high AC/A ratios. Small angle X(T) (measuring <20 prism dioptres) is usually non progressive and treated conservatively, either by observation, orthoptic exercises or occlusion.

Surgical

Larger angle deviations (measuring >20 prism dioptres) are usually treated, especially if there is evidence of deterioration. Traditionally, surgical treatment has been recommended for such squints if they are observed by carers to be present at least 50% of waking hours and are poorly controlled on clinical examination. Measurements of home and clinic control of the strabismus can be combined into a score which can be used to monitor progression and as a guide to surgery (Table 218.1). While there are clear functional indications for surgery in those children who have deteriorating control of the deviation for near fixation, accompanied by deteriorating near stereoacuity, for most children with X(T) measuring >20 prism dioptres at distance fixation, the criteria for, and the benefits of, surgical intervention are poorly defined.

Most interventions, however, particularly surgery, affect the alignment of the visual axes at near almost as much as at distance. This leads to the common postoperative problem of overcorrection of the deviation at near, with potential loss of stereopsis and amblyopia, especially in younger children. Surgical conservatism, however, leads to undercorrection with a recurrence of the deviation, thought to be because of persistence of suppression mechanisms. The desired result is said to be a small initial postoperative overcorrection in order that the suppression mechanisms are disrupted, followed by a drift to alignment of the eyes over days to weeks. It is well recognized that achieving such results is difficult and unpredictable, partly because of the influence of convergence mechanisms.

Surgical tables for exotropia tend not to distinguish between different types of exotropia. The figures used by the authors, who aim at a small initial postoperative overcorrection, are shown in Table 218.2. These should be used as a guide and individual surgeons should audit their results and alter practice accordingly.

The surgical procedure should probably be bilateral lateral rectus recessions for true divergence excess exotropias, but for simulated divergence excess and basic intermittent exotropias, recess resect procedures have been demonstrated to be equally effective. Bilateral lateral rectus recessions allow easy access to the inferior oblique muscles, should there be significant oblique overaction. While many cases of intermittent exotropia have a small V pattern, oblique surgery is usually not necessary unless there is significant oblique overaction.

TABLE 218.1 – **The Newcastle control score for intermittent exotropia**

HOME CONTROL	
0 score	Squint/monocular eye closure never noticed
1	Squint/monocular eye closure seen occasionally for distance
2	Squint/monocular eye closure seen frequently for distance
3	Squint/monocular eye closure seen for distance & also near
CLINIC CONTROL NEAR	
0	Manifest only after cover test and resumes fusion without need for blink or refixation
1	Blink or refixate to control after CT
2	Manifest spontaneously or with any form of fusion disruption without recovery
CLINIC CONTROL DISTANCE	
0	Manifest only after cover test and resumes fusion without need for blink or refixation
1	Blink or refixate to control after CT
2	Manifest spontaneously or with any form of fusion disruption without recovery
NCS TOTAL (HOME + CLINIC NEAR + CLINIC DISTANCE) =	

TABLE 218.2 – **Suggested surgical numbers for intermittent exotropia**

Angle	LR Recession	MR Resection	Bilat LR Recession
20	4	3	4.5
25	5	4	5
30	5.5	4	6
35	6.5	4.5	6.5
40	7	4.5	7
50	8	4.5	8

Ideally, X(T) surgery should result in a reduction or a complete correction of the tendency for the eyes to diverge however reported cure rates are poor, averaging 51%, with one report quoting a figure as low as 31%. There is some evidence of long term loss of effect following surgery, leading to recurrent exotropia. Although successful surgery improves binocular alignment and distance stereoacuity, permanent overcorrection with total loss of BSV for distance and near is a possible complication, particularly for children operated on under the age of 5. This may lead to amblyopia in vulnerable age groups, which is not usually a feature of X(T). Reported rates of this complication vary from 0 to 40%. Patients with high AC/A ratios may be particularly susceptible to this complication.

The optimal timing of surgery is controversial: early surgery (on patients 4 years of age or younger) is advocated by some authors who believe that it produces a higher cure rate. However it is associated with a higher rate of complications, including permanent surgical over-correction with loss of BSV. Advocates of late surgery argue that better functional results are obtainable and the risk of permanent over-correction and amblyopia is greatly reduced.

If overcorrection does occur, then unless there is gross mechanical limitation a period of observation is usually appropriate. Prisms or hypermetropic correction may be of benefit. Botulinum injection into the medial rectus muscle is often effective but further surgery is necessary in some cases.

REFERENCES

Abroms A, Mohney B, Rush D, et al: Timely surgery in intermittent and constant exotropia for superior sensory outcome. Am J Ophthalmol 131.111–116, 2001.

Campos E, Cipolli C: Binocularity and photophobia in intermittent exotropia. Percept Mot Skills 74:1168–1170, 1992.

Cooper EL, Layman IA: The management of intermittent exotropia: a comparison of the results of surgical and nonsurgical treatment. American Orthoptic Journal 27:61–67, 1977.

Graham P: Epidemiology of strabismus. Brit J Ophthalmol 58:224 231, 1974.

Haggerty H, Richardson S, Clarke M, et al: The Newcastle Control Score: a new method of grading the severity of intermittent exotropia. Brit J Ophthalmol 88(2):233–235, 2004.

219 BROWN'S SYNDROME 378.61

Raghu Mudumbai, MD
Seattle, Washington
Christopher N. Singh, MD
Seattle, Washington
Peter Youssef, MD
Seattle, Washington

ETIOLOGY

Brown's syndrome results from a mechanical restriction of the superior oblique tendon that may be congenital or acquired. Symptoms may include head tilt or diplopia. It may be transitory or permanent.

DIAGNOSIS

Clinical signs and symptoms

Brown's syndrome is characterized by limitation of elevation in adduction. Limited elevation may also be present to a lesser degree in abduction. Other common clinical signs include V pattern exotropia and widening of the palpebral fissure width on attempted elevation in adduction. Most patients will be orthophoric in primary gaze. However, some patients have a hypotropia with a compensatory chin-up position or face turn. Amblyopia may be present.

Congenital

Brown's original description postulated the defect to be congenital shortening of the sheath around the reflected tendon of the superior oblique muscle. Further investigation indicates that a congenitally tight superior oblique tendon is usually responsible.

Acquired

Brown's syndrome is a secondary effect of many disorders. Iatrogenic surgical causes include procedures performed on or near the superior oblique tendon, including tuck and scleral buckling procedures and placement of glaucoma drainage devices in the superonasal quadrant. Patients with juvenile or adult rheumatoid arthritis may present with a trochleitis leading to an acquired Brown's syndrome that may be painful. Trauma with damage to the trochlea, hemorrhage into the superior oblique sheath, or entrapment of the inferior oblique muscle may also be responsible.

TREATMENT

Patients who are asymptomatic and maintain fusion in primary gaze without head turn can be managed without surgery. These patients often learn to avoid the adduction in upgaze in the involved eye that leads to diplopia.

Surgical

The goals of surgery in Brown's syndrome must be clearly identified in order to ensure reasonable expectations. When a horizontal deviation is also present or when binocular vision is absent, successful realignment may be more difficult. Intervention is reasonable if there is a hypotropia in primary gaze, if there is abnormal head position, or if diplopia is present. It is also important to note whether the Brown's syndrome is congenital and stable, or acquired and may change.

Surgical options include superior oblique tenotomy and tenectomy, simultaneous surgery on the superior and inferior oblique muscles, and the use of silicon expanders.

The goal of surgery is to establish binocular function when there is hypotropia in primary gaze. Both tenotomy and tenonectomy of the superior oblique are effective in releasing the restriction to elevation. However, both procedures lead to superior oblique palsy in the majority of cases. Therefore, concomitant weakening of the ipsilateral inferior oblique muscle has also been recommended.

A newer approach relieves the restriction of the superior oblique tendon by means of an expander. Techniques have included a suture bridge between the cut ends of the tendon after a tenotomy, but Wright introduced the use of a no. 240 silicone retinal band as a more ideal spacer. With these procedures, great care must be taken to preserve the floor of the tendon capsule. If the floor is compromised, scarring between the sclera and the silicone may result, leading to a recurrence of the restriction of the superior oblique tendon. The benefits of tissue expanders include less surgery, greater range of movement and reversibility.

COMPLICATIONS

Possible complications from surgery should always be kept in mind. These include overaction of the inferior oblique muscle from superior oblique tenotomy, which may require addition surgery on the inferior oblique muscle. The superior oblique must be completely isolated in order to prevent inadequate surgery from missed fibers. Ptosis of the upper lid may ensue. Careful dissection that stays close to the superior rectus muscle must be performed to prevent orbital fat from herniating and scarring which can lead to ocular restriction.

COMMENTS

Brown's syndrome is defined by limitation, both actively and passively, of upgaze in adduction. The congenital form is secondary to a tight superior oblique tendon. Acquired Brown's syndrome may occur in after an operation that disrupts the function of the superior oblique, as well as from inflammation of the superior oblique tendon as in rheumatoid arthritis. If the patient is asymptomatic, observation is appropriate. If diplopia, hypotropia in primary position, or a head turn is present, multiple surgical options are available. They include superior oblique weakening procedures with or without concomitant ipsilateral inferior oblique weakening procedures and the use of spacers to increase the length of the superior oblique tendon.

REFERENCES

Moore AT, Morin JD: Bilateral acquired inflammatory Brown's syndrome. J Pediatr Ophthalmol Strabismus 22:26, 1985.

Sprunger DT, von Noorden GK, Helveston EM: Surgical results in Brown syndrome. J Pediatr Ophthalmol Strabismus 28:164–167, 1991.

von Noorden GK, Oliver P: Superior oblique tenectomy in Brown's syndrome. Ophthalmology 89:303, 1982.

Wilson ME, Eustis HS Jr, Parks MM: Brown's syndrome. Surv Ophthalmol 34:153–72, 1989

Wright KW: Results of the superior oblique elongation procedure for severe Brown's syndrome. Trans Am Ophthalmol Soc 98:41–48, 2000

220 CONGENITAL ESOTROPIA 743.69
(Infantile Esotropia)

Laura B. Enyedi, MD
Durham, North Carolina
Edward G. Buckley, MD
Durham, North Carolina

ETIOLOGY/INCIDENCE

Congenital esotropia is the most common childhood strabismus, occurring in approximately 1% of children. The cause of congenital esotropia is unknown and is thought to be multifactorial. Controversy exists as to whether the primary abnormality is in the motor control system or the binocular sensory system.

COURSE/PROGNOSIS

These children are at a significant risk for developing amblyopia, although some patients maintain equal vision by alternating fixation between the two eyes (cross-fixation). Early diagnosis and treatment can result in the restoration of normal function and a delay in treatment beyond 2 years of age is associated with poor binocularity, absent fusion and no stereopsis.

DIAGNOSIS

Clinical signs and symptoms

The crossing is rarely present at birth, but usually develops by the end of the third month and is present, by definition, by age 6 months. The esotropia is large angle (30 to 70 prism diopters), constant and does not resolve with hyperopic correction. Although most patients are otherwise healthy, some have associated ocular or neurologic abnormalities that require further evaluation. There is no clear inheritance pattern, but congenital esotropia can be familial and infants with a strong family history should be observed closely for the development of strabismus. Prematurity and perinatal hypoxia are also risk factors for congenital esotropia.

Laboratory findings

The opththalmologic examination includes visual function testing by fixation preference, fix and follow response and/or preferential looking tests. The deviation is measured using prisms and alternate cover testing if possible. Krimsky or Hirschberg testing may also be used to estimate the angle of esotropia. Duction testing may reveal mild limitations of abduction and versions are examined for A- or V- patterns, indicating overaction of superior or inferior oblique muscles, respectively. Dissociated vertical deviation is commonly associated with congenital esotropia, but is not often seen on presentation. Cycloplegic refraction may reveal significant refractive errors, especially hyperopia, which may need to be corrected with spectacles prior to surgical alignment. Complete anterior segment and fundus examinations are critical to rule out structural abnormalities (e.g. cataract, coloboma, optic nerve hypoplasia, or retinoblastoma) which may cause sensory esotropia.

Differential diagnosis

The differential diagnosis of congenital esotropia includes common disorders such as psedoesotropia and accommodative esotropia as well as less common disorders such as Duane's syndrome, nystagmus blockage syndrome, sixth nerve palsy and Mobius syndrome. Sensory esotropia secondary to loss of vision from ocular or optic nerve disease must always be considered. Pseudoesotropia in which epicanthal folds and a wide nasal bridge create the false appearance of esotropia is frequently mistaken for true esotropia. Accommodative esotropia in which there is high hyperopia and / or a high ratio of accommodative convergence to accommodation usually presents in toddlers, but may also be seen in infants. The distinguishing

TABLE 220.1 – Amounts of surgical correction				
Deviation (Prism Diopters)	Bimedial Rectus Muscle Recessions (mm)	Medial Rectus Muscle Recession (mm)	and	Lateral Rectus Muscle Resection* (mm)
20	4.0	4.0		4.5
25	4.5	5.0		5.0
30	5.0	5.0		6.0
35	5.5	6.0		6.5
40	6.0	6.0		7.0
50	6.5	6.0		8.0
>50	Three-muscle surgery			

For bilateral lateral rectus resection, perform the unilateral amount listed for each eye.

features of Duane's syndrome include decreased abduction and palpebral fissure narrowing on attempted adduction. Esotropia in nystagmus blockage syndrome occurs because nystagmus is dampened by keeping the fixating eye in adduction and worsens on attempted abduction. Sixth nerve palsies present with incomitant esotropia, decreased or absent abduction and possibly other neurologic findings. Möbius syndrome is the combination of sixth nerve palsy with facial weakness, tongue abnormalities and mental retardation.

TREATMENT

Initial treatment focuses on correcting significant refractive errors and treating amblyopia. Hyperopia greater than 3 diopters should be corrected to rule out any accommodative component to the esotropia. Phospholine iodide drops may be helpful for variable deviations or deviations which are much greater at near than at distance. Definitive treatment is generally surgical and may include medial rectus recession and/or lateral rectus resection on one or both eyes. A- or V-patterns and dissociated vertical deviations, if present, may be surgically addressed simultaneously with horizontal muscle surgery. The sooner the eyes are restored to proper alignment, the better the chance for a stable long-term result (Table 220.1).

COMPLICATIONS

The most common complications from strabismus surgery are under or over corrections. A marked under or over correction, especially with a duction lag, may indicate a slipped or lost muscle. Overcorrection may be treated with prisms if the exotropia is less than 10 prism diopters. If the patient has 12 or more prism diopters of exotropia 6 to 8 weeks postoperatively, surgical repair may be necessary. Residual esotropia may be treated with spectacles if there are 2 or more diopters of hyperopia. Ten or less prism diopters of residual esotropia may be amenable to prism therapy. If the patient has 12 or more prism diopters of esotropia 6 to 8 weeks postoperatively, additional strabismus surgery may be necessary. An inadvertent ocular perforation can occur as the muscle is reattached to the globe and can rarely cause retinal detachment or endopthalmitis. Ocular perforations may benefit from intraoperative retinal cryotherapy or laser to prevent rhegmatogenous retinal detachment. Postoperative infection of the surgical site is heralded by increased redness, chemosis and purulent discharge while increased pain and decreased vision signal may indicate a more serious intraocular infection (endopthalmitis). Careful conjunctival closure is critical to avoid conjunctival cysts, conjunctival scarring and dellen formation.

COMMENTS

Close follow-up of patients after surgery is crucial because these children are still at a high risk for amblyopia and often develop other motility abnormalities such as dissociated vertical deviation and overacting inferior oblique muscles. Approximately 30% will eventually require additional surgery. Treatment results are influenced by the age at surgery, the duration of misalignment and the development of associated motility disturbances, but the majority of patients have cosmetically aligned eyes, peripheral fusion and good visual function.

REFERENCES

Helveston EM: The 19th Annual Frank Costenbader Lecture: the origins of congenital esotropia. J Pediatr Ophthalmol Strabismus 30:215, 1993.

Ing MR: The timing of surgical alignment for congenital (infantile) esotropia. J Pediatr Ophthalmol Strabismus 36:61–68, 1999.

Kushner BJ, Morton GV: A randomized comparison of surgical procedures for infantile esotropia. Am J Ophthalmol 98:50, 1984.

Parks MM: The monofixation syndrome. Trans Am Ophthalmol Soc 67:609, 1969.

Pediatric Eye Disease Investigator Group. The clinical spectrum of early-onset esotropia: experience of the congenital esotropia observational study. Am J Ophthalmol 133:102–108, 2002.

von Noorden GK: The XLIV Edward Jackson Memorial Lecture: A reassessment of infantile esotropia. Am J Ophthalmol 105:1–10, 1988.

221 CONGENITAL FIBROSIS OF THE EXTRAOCULAR MUSCLES 378.62

Forrest James Ellis, MD
Cleveland, Ohio

ETIOLOGY/INCIDENCE

Congenital fibrosis of the extraocular muscles (CFEOM) is a rare condition characterized by hypoplasia and fibrosis of the extraocular muscles. CFEOM falls in the group of syndromes characterized by congenital limitation of eye and eyelid movements (congenital cranial nerve dysinnervation syndromes). Primary neurodevelopmental abnormalities of cranial nerve nuclei occur in CFEOM type 2, while genetic defects affecting axonal transport of molecules necessary for normal extraocular muscle function and development occur in CFEOM type 1. Possible prenatal orbital penetration has been reported in isolated unilateral cases.

Three genetic subtypes of CFEOM have been identified.

- *CFEOM 1* is characterized by congenital bilateral ptosis with the eyes fixed in a position of 20 to 30 degrees infraduction. Affected individuals often adopt a chin-lift posture. Passive movement of the globes is significantly limited with forced ductions. Volitional eye movements are often limited, and convergent or divergent movements may occur with attempted vertical or horizontal gaze. Amblyopia and refractive errors are common. Penetrance appears to be complete with striking phenotypic homogeneity. The CFEOM 1 genetic locus is in the centromeric region of human chromosome 12. There is a missense mutation in an axonal transport kinesin motor protein encoded by KIF21A. The absence of the superior division of the oculomotor nerve and its corresponding midbrain a motor neurons have been described at necropsy.
- *CFEOM 2* is an autosomal recessive disorder. Affected individuals have bilateral congenital ptosis and restricted extraocular movements with the eyes positioned in abduction. The locus for CFEOM 2 has been mapped to chromosome 11q13 and involves the *ARIX* gene. This is believed to result in hypoplasia of the III and IV cranial nerve nuclei.
- *CFEOM 3* is an autosomal dominant disorder with incomplete penetrance and variable expressivity. Affected individuals demonstrate ptosis with the eyes fixed in abduction and infraduction. This disorder is clinically and genetically distinct from CFEOM 1 and CFEOM 2. The gene maps to markers on chromosome 16q.

COURSE/PROGNOSIS

- Nonprogressive.
- No spontaneous improvement.
- Vision affected by amblyopia.

DIAGNOSIS

Clinical signs and symptoms

Clinical findings vary from bilateral generalized fibrosis to fibrosis of only a single extraocular muscle. The ophthalmic findings are present at birth and are typically nonprogressive. During examination at the time of a surgical intervention, the extraocular muscles are typically thin and inelastic. Histopathologic examination of the affected extraocular muscles has demonstrated a reduced number of muscle fibers and increased fibrous tissue. CFEOM is typically an isolated phenomenon, although cases in association with other systemic disorders have been reported. Whereas most other myopathies are progressive, CFEOM is congenital and non-progressive.

- Congenital nonprogressive condition.
- Typically bilateral, but may be unilateral.
- Limitation of ocular motility, typically with ptosis of the eyelid.
- Positive forced duction.
- Synkinetic eye movements in some cases.
- A reduced number of muscle fibers and increased fibrous tissue on histopathologic examination of the affected extraocular muscles.
- Examination of family members for similar abnormalities of ocular motility.
- Family history for autosomal dominant inheritance common.
- Radiologic imaging possibly helpful in the evaluation of selected patients.

Differential diagnosis

- Duane's syndrome.
- Double elevator palsy.
- Brown's syndrome.
- Progressive external ophthalmoplegia.
- Progressive dystrophic ophthalmoplegia.
- Möbius syndrome.
- Myasthenia gravis.
- Congenital or acquired paralysis of the extraocular muscles.
- Congenital or acquired ptosis.
- Extraocular muscle entrapment (orbital fracture).
- Thyroid-related strabismus.

TREATMENT

Systemic

- Genetic counseling.
- Physical and neurologic examinations.

Ocular

- Correction of refractive error.
- Occlusion or penalization therapy for amblyopia.
- Lubrication for exposure keratopathy.

Surgical

- Goal of achieving a functional position of the eyes and eyelids; horizontal and vertical binocular alignment with the eyes in a position of slight infraduction.
- Large rectus muscle recessions typically required and preferred to rectus muscle resections.
- Conjunctival recessions augment rectus muscle surgery.
- Frontalis suspension procedures typically required for ptosis repair.

REFERENCES

Crawford JS: Congenital fibrosis syndrome. Can J Ophthalmol 5:331–336, 1970.

Engle EC, Goumnerov BC, McKeown CA, et al: Oculomotor nerve and muscle abnormalities in congenital fibrosis of the extraocular muscles. Ann Neurol 41:314–325, 1997.

Engle EC, Kunkel LM, Sprecht LA, Beggs AH: Mapping a gene for congenital fibrosis of the extraocular muscles to the centromeric region of chromosome 12. Nat Genet 7:69–73, 1994.

Hertle RW, Katowitz JA, Young TL, et al: Congenital unilateral fibrosis, blepharoptosis, and enophthalmos syndrome. Ophthalmology 99:347–355, 1992.

Traboulsi EI, Jaafar M, Kattan HM, Parks MM: Congenital fibrosis of the extraocular muscles: Report of 24 cases illustrating the clinical spectrum and surgical management. Am Orthop J 43:45–53, 1993.

222 CONVERGENCE INSUFFICIENCY 378.83

Stephen P. Christiansen, MD
Minneapolis, Minnesota

ETIOLOGY/INCIDENCE

Convergence insufficiency is a common ocular motility disturbance characterized by an exophoria or intermittent exotropia that is greatest at near fixation. It is one of the most common ocular motility causes of asthenopia. Convergence insufficiency is caused by poor fusional convergence at near fixation.

COURSE/PROGNOSIS

Patients typically present in their teens or early adulthood and complain of gradually worsening eyestrain, periocular headache, blurred vision after brief periods of reading, and sometimes crossed diplopia with near work. It is not unusual for the patient to squint one eye while reading to relieve the blurring or diplopia. Few, if any, symptoms are present at distance fixation. Symptoms are aggravated by illness, fatigue, anxiety, and prolonged near work. Untreated, the exophoria at near may break down to a poorly controlled intermittent exotropia. In most cases, convergence insufficiency is very amenable to orthoptic treatment.

DIAGNOSIS

Clinical signs and symptoms

- Remote near point of convergence. Patients are unable to maintain fixation on a fusional target as it is brought up to the tip of their nose.
- Significant exophoria or intermittent exotropia at near. More rarely, patients will be orthophoric or even exhibit a small degree of esophoria at near. However, all will have a remote near point of convergence.
- Small to non-existent exophoria at distance.
- May have reduced stereo-acuity at near.
- Normal near point of accommodation.

Differential diagnosis

- Uncorrected high hypermetropia or myopia.
- Early presbyopia. When bifocals are worn for the first time, the decrease in accommodative convergence afforded by the bifocal may be sufficient to make the patient symptomatic.
- Convergence insufficiency associated with accommodative insufficiency. Patients with combined convergence and accommodative insufficiency are usually more symptomatic than those with convergence insufficiency alone. However, symptoms alone are not sufficient to distinguish between these two entities, and all patients who present with convergence insufficiency should have accommodative amplitudes checked since satisfactory treatment will depend on a correct diagnosis. Anticholinergic drugs, closed head trauma, and viral encephalopathies should be considered in the pathogenesis of this disorder. In addition to treating the convergence weakness, plus lenses should be prescribed for reading in these patients.
- Convergence paralysis. In this condition, the patient is able to adduct the eyes, but cannot converge, and has constant diplopia at near. This is usually a result of significant closed head trauma, but can also result from a lesion in the midbrain, toxic encephalopathy, or from encephalitis. It may or may not be associated with accommodative insufficiency. Base-in Fresnel prisms in the reading add of the bifocals or ground-in prisms in a separate pair of reading glasses may be useful in restoring binocularity at near in these patients.

TREATMENT

Medical/orthoptics

- Near point of convergence exercises. An accommodative target such as the point of a pencil (hence, pencil push-ups) is placed remote to the patient's near point of convergence and gradually brought toward the tip of the nose with the patient converging to avoid diplopia. Just before there is a break in fusion, the patient holds fixation on the target for ten seconds. The 'push-up' is repeated ten times, two to four times a day until he is able to hold fixation to the tip of the nose. The exercises can be tapered and then used on an as-needed basis when the patient notices a recurrence of symptoms.
- Other forms of convergence training. Base-out prism reading, and stereogram cards may also be used by the orthoptist to improve fusional convergence.
- Base-in prisms for near only. These prisms can be ground into a separate pair of reading glasses or Fresnel membrane prisms can be fitted over the reading segment of the patient's bifocals.

Surgical

- The decision to proceed with surgery should be made with caution, and only after all orthoptic efforts have failed. Bilateral medial rectus resections are usually the most effective operation for this condition. However, the patient should be warned about the possibility of uncrossed diplopia at distance fixation after surgery. This typically resolves within one to three months post-operatively. The exophoria at near usually recurs after several years although most patients remain asymptomatic.

REFERENCES

Brown B: The convergence insufficiency masquerade. Am Orthoptic J 40:94–97, 1990.

Hermann JS: Surgical therapy for convergence insufficiency. J Ped Ophthalmol 18:28, 1981.

Nemet P, Stolovitch C: Biased resection of the medial recti: a new surgical approach to convergence insufficiency. Binoc Vis 5:213, 1990.

Phillips PH, Fray KJ, Brodsky MC: Intermittent exotropia increasing with near fixation: a 'soft' sign of neurological disease. Br J Ophthalmol 89:1120–1122, 2005.

Von Noorden GK, Campos EC: Binocular vision and ocular motility — theory and management of strabismus. 6th edn. St Louis, Mosby, 2002.

223 DISSOCIATED VERTICAL DEVIATION 378.9

(Dissociated Strabismus Complex, Alternating Sursumduction, Dissociated Vertical Divergence, Double-Dissociated Hypertropia, Occlusion Hypertropia, Dissociated Torsional Deviation, Dissociated Horizontal Deviation)

Richard J. Olson, MD
Iowa City, Iowa
Ronald V. Keech, MD
Iowa City, Iowa

ETIOLOGY/INCIDENCE

Dissociated vertical deviation (DVD) is an ocular misalignment characterized by elevation, abduction, and excyclotorsion. In most cases, the vertical deviation is the primary manifestation. Rarely, a dissociated horizontal deviation (DHD) is the predominant or only apparent feature.

DVD is usually comitant and bilateral but asymmetric. It may present as an intermittent or constant tropia or as a phoria that occurs only when fixation is disrupted. The ocular movements associated with DVD are slow and variable compared with nondissociated horizontal or vertical deviations. Most patients with DVD have sensory suppression and do not have diplopia or visual confusion.

DVD is almost always associated with infantile strabismus. The incidence of DVD in infantile esotropia is as high as 90%, though it is usually not apparent during the first year. DVD is often accompanied by a head tilt, which can be either toward or away from the eye with DVD. Inferior oblique overaction and latent nystagmus are also common.

Innervational, muscular and sensory abnormalities have all been considered, but the cause is unknown. Recent theories include Guyton's proposal that DVD is the result of damping a cyclovertical latent nystagmus, Brodsky's proposal that it is the result of a usually unexpressed dorsal light reflex, and van Rijn's proposal that it is related to asymmetry of vertical phorias also found in normals.

DVD is closely linked to subnormal fusion. It is not clear whether the lack of fusion causes the deviation or whether both conditions occur as a result of another abnormality.

DIAGNOSIS

Clinical signs and symptoms

- The detection and measurement of DVD can be difficult because it is often superimposed on a nondissociated horizontal or vertical deviation. Dissociated deviations should be considered when the deviation is slow to develop or variable with cover testing, especially when associated with the onset of strabismus in infancy.
- DVD may be distinguished from other vertical strabismus by the lack of a corresponding hypodeviation of the contralateral eye on alternate-cover testing.
- DHD may be distinguished from other horizontal strabismus by the lack of a corresponding exodeviation of the contralateral eye on alternate-cover testing.
- Determining the size of the DVD can aid surgical planning. If an eye has dense amblyopia, a prism light reflex test (Krimsky's test) may be used. If the visual acuity in the affected eye is good, the DVD can be measured by a modification of the prism cover test. Increasing amounts of base-down prism are placed in front of the DVD eye until no further downward movement of that eye is seen with alternate cover testing. A hypodeviation will be induced in the contralateral eye by the test and can be ignored.
- To assess a horizontal dissociated deviation, the same procedure is performed with base-in prism over the DHD eye until no further inward movement of that eye is seen. Movement of the contralateral eye with this test can be ignored.
- For a combined dissociated and nondissociated vertical deviation, measure the nondissociated component by adding base-up prism over the non-DVD eye until the hypodeviation is neutralized during the alternate-cover test. The next step is to measure the vertical deviation as previously described for a dissociated deviation. The actual dissociated deviation measurement is the difference between the two steps.

Differential diagnosis

- Inferior oblique overaction associated with infantile esotropia is commonly confused with DVD. The V-pattern strabismus and incomitant vertical deviation found on lateral gazes are not usually present with a pure DVD.
- Depending on the underlying strabismus condition, DHD can be confused with an intermittent exotropia, a variable angle esodeviation, or a secondary deviation after strabismus surgery.

TREATMENT

Ocular

- The correction of any ocular abnormalities that limit binocular vision may improve a coexisting DVD. This may include occlusion for amblyopia, glasses or surgery for horizontal strabismus, or orthoptics for heterophorias.
- If the vision in each eye is nearly equal and the DVD is smallest in the fixing eye, then causing a fixation switch can be helpful, either by patching or by overcorrecting or undercorrecting a refractive error with glasses or contact lenses.

Surgical

- The most commonly used procedure for DVD is a superior rectus muscle recession of 5 to 16 mm from the insertion.
- Recession and anterior displacement of the inferior oblique muscle near the temporal pole of inferior rectus muscle is another common procedure for DVD. Some surgeons recommend this surgery for isolated DVD, however, most experts prefer this approach when the DVD is associated with concomitant inferior oblique muscle overaction.

Residual DVD after large superior rectus recession may benefit from a small (5 mm or less) resection of the inferior rectus muscle. Recently, nasal myectomy of the inferior oblique muscle has been advocated if the inferior oblique muscle has previously been recessed and anteriorized.

Other surgical approaches reported in the literature include posterior fixation of the superior rectus muscle with or without recession, botulinum toxin type A injection into the superior rectus muscle, weakening of both the superior rectus and inferior oblique muscles, graded resection with anteriorization of the inferior oblique and weakening of all four oblique muscles

- DHD may be treated with lateral rectus muscle recession of 3 to 8 mm on the affected side (or ipsilateral side).

COMPLICATIONS

Although uncommon, complications from surgery for DVD include limitation of elevation (especially with the inferior oblique muscle recession with anteriorization technique) overcorrection, abnormal torsion, changes in eyelid position, and secondary overaction of the contralateral inferior oblique muscle.

COMMENTS

- Anteriorization of the inferior oblique muscle changes the muscle action from elevation to depression. Its neurovascular bundle may tether the globe causing the anti-elevation syndrome with a larger hypertropia in the contralateral eye. Many surgeons avoid unilateral inferior oblique anteriorization in part because of this complication.

It can be difficult to determine whether surgery should be performed on one or both eyes. Limiting surgery to the worst eye is effective when the patient rarely fixates with that eye. However, should the operated eye take up fixation after unilateral surgery, a large vertical deviation will result in the opposite eye. Under these circumstances, bilateral surgery may be a better choice.

- When bilateral DVDs are very asymmetric, even if bilateral surgery is performed asymmetrically, the eye with the larger DVD may be significantly undercorrected.

DVD is a common companion of early-onset strabismus, and involves elevation, abduction and excyclotorsion. Its cause is still debated. Most dissociated deviations are latent or of small magnitude and do not require treatment. Treatment is indicated when the appearance of the ocular misalignment or the resulting visual symptoms are unacceptable to the patient. Complete elimination of the deviation is difficult, especially when there is bilateral involvement.

REFERENCES

Brodsky MC: Dissociated vertical divergence: a righting reflex gone wrong. Arch Ophthalmol 117:1216, 1999.

Burke JP, Scott WE, Kutschke PJ: Anterior transposition of the inferior oblique muscle for dissociated vertical deviation. Ophthalmology 100:245, 1993.

Guyton DL: Dissociated vertical deviation: etiology, mechanism, and associated phenomena. Costenbader Lecture. J Aapos 4:131, 2000.

Schwartz T, Scott WE: Unilateral superior rectus recession for the treatment of dissociated vertical deviation. J Pediatr Ophthalmol Strabismus 28:219, 1991.

224 DUANE'S RETRACTION SYNDROME 378.71

(Stilling–Turk–Duane Syndrome, or Duane's Syndrome)

Shawn Goodman, MD

Lake Oswego, Oregon

ETIOLOGY/INCIDENCE

Duane's retraction syndrome (DRS) is a congenital, incomitant ocular motility disorder characterized by abnormal function of the lateral rectus muscle in the affected eye, together with retraction of the globe and narrowing of the palpebral fissure on attempted adduction. Generally, the lateral rectus does not abduct the eye, but instead contracts at the same time as the medial rectus on adduction. It is this simultaneous cocontraction of the medial and lateral rectus muscles on attempted adduction that causes the retraction of the globe and narrowing of the palpebral fissure when the eye is adducted.

In the primary position the ocular alignment is most commonly esotropic, but the syndrome can be present with no ocular deviation in the primary position and a minority of patients with DRS may be exotropic in primary position. EMG testing finds reduced electrical activity of the lateral rectus muscle on abduction and simultaneous electrical activity of the medial and lateral recti on adduction. Head turns to maintain binocularity are common. Marked upward or downward deviations of the eye in adduction may be seen.

DRS is most commonly unilateral, but can be bilateral. For unknown reasons, it affects the left eye more frequently (approximately 60% incidence), and approximately 60% of patients with DRS are female. There is occasionally familial inheritance, but most cases are sporadic.

DRS is believed to be due to maldevelopment or congenital absence of the sixth nerve nucleus, so that the lateral rectus muscle is instead abnormally innervated by branches of the third nerve. In the minority of patients with DRS and good abduction, it may be that the sixth nerve arrives in the orbit to innervate the lateral rectus only after branches of the third nerve have already done so. The maldevelopment or injury to developing structures probably occurs between the 4th and 8th weeks of embryogenesis, when the cranial nerves and extraocular muscles are forming. This timing also coincides with other defects in embryogenesis that can be associated with the occurrence of Duane syndrome in a minority of patients. The clinical result of this maldevelopment of the abducens nerve is a spectrum of innervational abnormalities, with varying degrees of lateral rectus muscle paresis and aberrant innervation by the oculomotor nerve.

Secondary fibrosis of non-innervated portions of the lateral rectus muscle may develop, further limiting adduction, as well as contributing to the upshoots and downshoots in adduction that are frequently seen. This has been referred to as a 'leash effect' of the tight lateral rectus muscle. A less common explanation for upshoots and downshoots is the suggestion that oculomotor branches that innervate the superior or inferior rectus muscle are contributing innervation to the lateral rectus muscle, while the oculomotor subnucleus to the medial rectus is then also contributing to vertical rectus innervation. Thus, when the eye is adducting, a vertical rectus is stimulated to contract as well, leading to an upshoot or downshoot of the eye in adduction. This latter explanation does not account for the fact that vertical rectus recessions do not successfully treat upshoots or downshoots.

Rarely the medial rectus may have subnormally-developed innervation, resulting in non-innervated and fibrotic areas in the medial rectus muscle also. The medial rectus is frequently described at surgery as being tight or fibrotic, though this may also be a secondary change due to the lack of opposing normal lateral rectus function.

DRS is present in 1–4% of strabismus patients. There are a variety of clinical findings in patients with DRS, generally divided into 3 types. The clinical spectrum across these types results from the variability of innervation of the affected lateral rectus muscle. That is, the balance of subnormal sixth nerve innervation, abnormal third nerve innervation and fibrosis in noninnervated portions of the lateral rectus muscle determines the abnormalities in ocular movements seen.

COURSE/PROGNOSIS

Many patients with DRS are able to adopt a head turn to maintain binocularity, and do so. In esotropic Type I DRS, the head turn is usually towards the affected eye, to utilize the affected eye in adduction. In exotropic Type II DRS, the head turn is usually toward the normal side, to use the affected eye in abduction.

For the most part, the deviation is stable, but one study documented a progression of the findings in many patients with DRS during the first 6 years of life. Limitation of abduction and narrowing of the palpebral fissure were seen first, with upshoot and downshoot on adduction appearing later. Marked retraction associated with enopthalmos in the primary position has been observed to be more common in adults than in children, suggesting that this finding can also be progressive over time.

DIAGNOSIS

Even though the abnormal innervations in the orbit that cause DRS occur early in embryonic life, DRS can be difficult to diagnose in a very young child. The child with binocularity will often avoid gazing in the direction of ocular misalignment, and parents will often report the abnormality as being present in the normal eye, since there is an appearance of marked overaction of the normally functioning eye if the child does look in the direction of the limitation in the affected eye.

The diagnosis of DRS can usually be made on the testing of versions. The examiner must look for limited abduction or adduction together with narrowing of the palpebral fissure on adduction.

The following classification system is commonly used:

Type I

Type I represents 70–85% of patients with DRS. It is characterized by marked to moderate limitation of abduction of the affected eye (Figure 224.3) and relatively normal adduction (Figure 224.1). There is retraction of the globe and narrowing of the palpebral fissure in adduction, due to simultaneous contraction of the medial and lateral recti (both innervated by the third cranial nerve). On attempted abduction, impulses coming from the third cranial nerve subnucleus that normally subserves the medial rectus are inhibited, and the medial rectus and lateral rectus muscles of the Duane's eye relax. This allows the globe to move forward and the palpebral fissure to widen on attempted abduction. A generally small angle of esotropia is present in the primary position (Figure 224.2). Larger angles of esotropia are occasionally seen, and exotropia occurs in about 5% of patients with type I DRS. Upshoot or downshoot of the eye in adduction may be present.

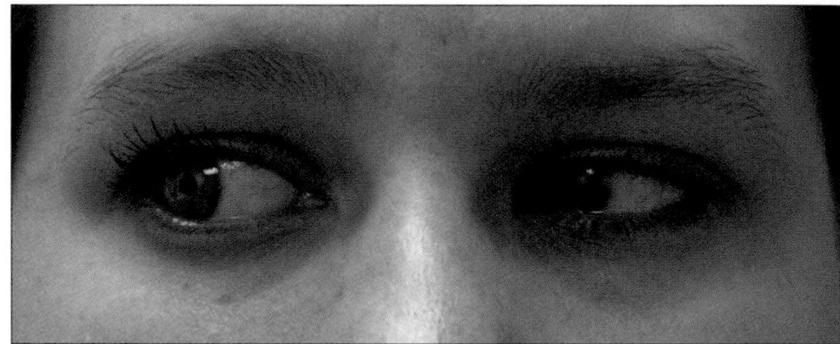

FIGURE 224.1. Type I Duane's, left eye, in adduction. Note narrowed palpebral fissure on the left.

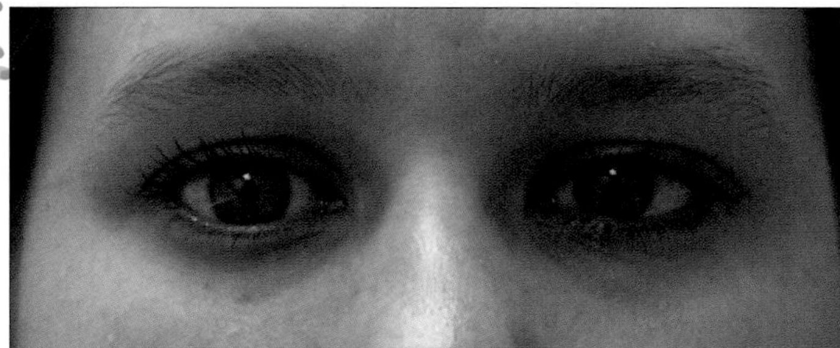

FIGURE 224.2. Type I Duane's, left eye, esotropia in primary position.

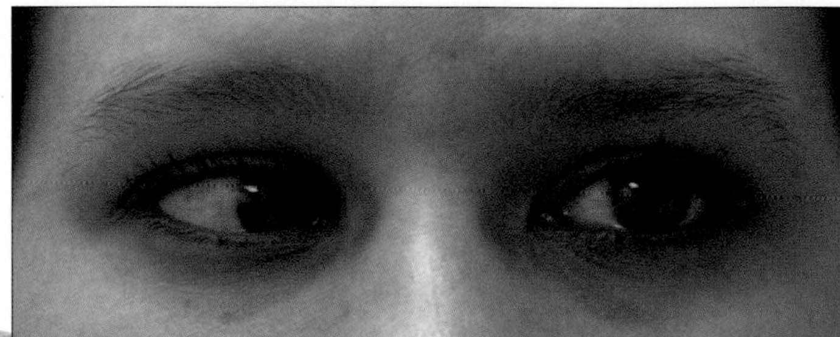

FIGURE 224.3. Type I Duane's, left eye, limited abduction.

Type II

Type II DRS comprises approximately 7% of patients. Adduction is severely limited, and there is narrowing of the palpebral fissure on adduction. Abduction is good. Exotropia usually exists in the primary position. In patients with the rare type II DRS, the sixth cranial nerve is normal and is present, but presumably it arrived at the orbit so late in embryogenesis that the anatomic adaptations (incorrect innervations) associated with type I DRS already occurred by the time the sixth cranial nerve penetrated and began to innervate the lateral rectus muscle. Thus, even though the medial rectus is normally innervated, the co-contraction of the lateral rectus markedly limits adduction.

Type III

One to fifteen percent of patients with DRS have type III. This type has been defined as limitation of both adduction and abduction, but type III is electrophysiologically identical to a type I with severe cocontraction. Retraction of the globe on attempted adduction is present. There may be little deviation in the primary position.

The above classification system is simplistic, and in approaching an individual patient the clinician must make detailed observations regarding anomalous head position, deviation in primary position, evidence of severity of co-contraction including globe retraction and overshoots, and possible bilaterality.

Further motility evaluation of the patient with DRS includes the following:

The degree of face turn can be measured by having the patient fixate on a distant target (letters or a movie) and by holding a pocket laser pointer above the patient's head, aligning the pointer with the center of the forehead anteriorly and the vertex of the posterior surface of the head posteriorly. Trigonometry reveals that at 20 feet, 21 inches to the side of fixation equals 5 degrees, 42 inches equals 10 degrees, and so on.

Assessing the location and size of the patient's single binocular field helps in defining the need for treatment in patients with DRS. Watching the child with DRS as he or she is reading or looking at pictures in the book can be a valuable diagnostic test. For instance, a child with a large exotropia in downgaze may have little face turn in the primary position, but will hold the book up directly in front of the eyes instead of down in the usual reading position.

The severity of cocontraction can be estimated by examining the degree of slowing of adduction saccadic velocities and, more practically, by recording the following parameters:

- Exodeviation in gaze opposite the eye with DRS (DRS eye in adduction) more than 3 prism diopters;
- Palpebral fissure width narrowing of 1.5 mm or more as the eye with DRS moves from the primary position (straight ahead) to full adduction;
- Near point of convergence remote beyond 6 cm;
- Upshoot or downshoot of the eye with DRS moving into adduction as the normal eye is directed into abduction and elevation or depression.

Differential diagnosis

In the majority patients with DRS, there is no other abnormality. Perhaps as many as 30% of patients with the sporadic form of DRS may have other congenital abnormalities, which can include skeletal, auricular, ocular and neural findings. Ocular anomalies, such as iris dysplasia, heterochromia, crocodile tears and morning-glory syndrome have been reported with DRS. Systemic abnormalities such as Goldenhar syndrome, Klippel–Feil syndrome, cleft palate, spina bifida, radial dysplasia, renal dysplasia, Okihiro syndrome, and deafness have all been associated with DRS.

As in DRS, an abduction deficit is also seen in sixth nerve palsy, but this only rarely occurs on a congenital basis. In complete sixth nerve palsy the resulting esotropia in primary position is large. In contrast, the esotropia in DRS, when present, is usually a small angle. Additionally, DRS has the characteristic narrowing of the palpebral fissure in adduction, a finding which is not present in sixth nerve palsy.

Although unnecessary in most cases to establish the diagnosis of DRS, saccadic velocities may be measured as a definitive diagnostic test. In DRS, both the adduction and the abduction saccadic velocities are slowed; in sixth cranial nerve palsies, only the abduction saccadic velocities are slower than normal.

Moebius syndrome has bilateral abducens palsy, but includes facial diplegia, a feature not present in DRS. It is also extremely rare.

TREATMENT

Patients with DRS need to be evaluated for refractive errors, particularly anisometropia and hyperopia. These can contribute to amblyopia and occasionally to accommodative esotropia and need to be treated prior to any surgical intervention.

The majority of DRS patients have unilateral Type 1, and these children generally maintain good binocular function and stereopsis, possibly with a head turn. For these patients any contemplated surgery is best delayed until age 5–6 or older, to avoid disrupting normal binocular development.

Indications for surgery may include anomalous head posture, strabismus in primary gaze, significant upshoot or downshoot in adduction, and cosmetically significant palpebral fissure narrowing in adduction. Surgeon and patient need to be aware of the necessarily limited goals of strabismus surgery in DRS, and that no surgery will normalize absent abduction, for instance.

In planning surgery, the lateral rectus function must be carefully analyzed, looking at the degree of anomalous innervation, and also carefully looking for the presence of any normal abducens function. Forceps force testing can be helpful to further distinguish the active, anomalous and restrictive forces in the affected eye. In a cooperative awake patient, active force generation (the examiner observes or palpates that the eye can actively abduct) and forced augmentation testing (the examiner determines whether the eye can be brought further into abduction with forceps than the patient can voluntarily move it, distinguishing restriction from paralysis), assist in determining the best surgical procedure for the patient. Under topical surgical anesthesia in a difficult management case, a patient can be asked to look in certain directions after selected muscles have been detached, to assist in predicting the results.

Surgical

Resection of the involved lateral rectus is generally not recommended, as resection intensifies the anomalous actions of the lateral rectus such as worsening globe retraction, while not improving abduction.

For Type 1 DRS (absent abduction, esotropia in primary position, and a head turn towards the affected side to fuse with the affected eye in adduction):

- The most commonly performed surgery is a medial rectus muscle recession of the affected eye. This usually reduces the head turn, but will not improve abduction beyond the midline. A large recession may reduce the binocular field by limiting adduction in the affected eye, particularly if there is significant lateral rectus co-contraction on adduction.

- A better alternative may be asymmetric medial rectus recessions, recessing the medial rectus of the unaffected eye more than that of the eye with DRS. This will better correct the esotropia in primary, and produce a 'fixation duress' in the unaffected fellow eye. This latter reduces the likelihood of recurrent contracture of the medial rectus in the involved eye.
- Caveat: if the lateral rectus has some normal abduction function, a large recession of the unaffected medial rectus may cause a large exotropia in the DRS eye, due to Hering's law.
- Transposition of all or of the lateral $^1/_2$ of the superior and inferior recti temporally, with or without posterior fixation sutures (Foster modification) has also been advocated. Transposition of the lateral half of the vertical muscles is done to preserve anterior segment circulation if the medial rectus muscle has been or will also be recessed.

For DRS with exotropia:

- Recession of the lateral rectus on the involved side may be performed for a small exotropia (less than 25 diopters).
- With a large exotropia, a large lateral rectus recession must be performed in the involved eye. Often a lateral rectus recession in the uninvolved eye is also recommended.
- Caveat: recessing the normal lateral rectus may, by Hering's law, increase stimulation to the medial rectus in the affected eye, and thus to the anomalously-acting lateral rectus in the DRS eye, increasing co-contraction not only in adduction but in primary position.
- Adding a resection of the medial rectus (i.e. a recess/resect procedure) in the affected eye for exotropic DRS is controversial. It will improve alignment but make the abduction deficit more noticeable. Medial rectus resection can also exacerbate retraction of the globe in cases with significant co-contraction.

For retraction of the globe:

- Recessing both the medial and lateral rectus muscles in the affected eye is helpful. This may need to be combined with a medial rectus recession in the uninvolved eye if esotropia is present pre-operatively.

For upshoots and downshoots seen in the DRS eye in adduction:

- Recessing the lateral rectus muscle 7–12 mm is effective in reducing this feature of co-contraction of the lateral rectus muscle (less recession is required in a more fibrotic muscle, more recession is required in a non-fibrotic muscle).
- Alternatively, a posterior fixation suture on the lateral rectus muscle can be used to reduce upshoots and downshoots.
- Y-splitting of the lateral rectus muscle (longitudinally splitting the muscle and vertically transposing the superior half superiorly and the inferior half inferiorly so that they are spread wider apart than the width of the original insertion), usually with a small recession, also improves upshoots and downshoots, and can be combined with a medial rectus recession for esotropic DRS.
- Surgery on the vertical rectus muscles is not effective in treating upshoots or downshoots.

For A and V patterns:

- The lateral rectus muscles may be transposed downward with the recession for an exotropia with an A pattern.
- The medial rectus muscles may be transposed downward together with recession for a V pattern esotropia.

COMPLICATIONS

- Large medial rectus muscle recession in the involved DRS eye, especially in the face of preoperative limitation of adduction, can markedly compromise adduction and produce a postoperative exotropia.
- New vertical deviations may be induced by lateral transposition of the vertical rectus muscles.
- Transposing the vertical rectus muscles laterally can exacerbate the unwanted actions of a severely anomalous lateral rectus such as worsening the signs of co-contraction.
- Anterior segment ischemia may occur when the vertical rectus muscles are transposed laterally at the same time as the medial rectus muscle is recessed. The risk of this may be reduced by transposing only the lateral halves of the vertical muscles (preserving the medial vessel in the unoperated medial half of each vertical muscle), or by performing the medial rectus recession as a separate procedure 4–6 months after the transposition.
- Misdiagnosis of DRS as a sixth cranial nerve palsy and subsequent large recession/resection of the horizontal rectus muscles of the eye with DRS can result in a disastrous overcorrection with exotropia in the primary position, newly induced hypertropias, intractable diplopia, and, in some cases, abduction of the eye with DRS on attempted adduction ('the splits').

REFERENCES

Barbe ME, Scott WE, Kutschke PJ: A simplified approach to the treatment of Duane's syndrome. Br J Ophthalmol 88:131–138, 2004.

Hotchkiss MG, Muller NR, Clark AW, et al: Bilateral Duane's syndrome: a clinicopathologic case report. Arch Ophthalmol 98:870–874, 1980.

Huber A: Electrophysiology of the retraction syndromes. Br J Ophthalmol 98:870–874, 1980.

Isenberg S, Urist MJ: Clinical observations in 101 consecutive patients with Duane's retraction syndrome. Am J Ophthalmol 84:419–425, 1977.

Jampolsky A: Duane Syndrome. In: Rosenbaum A, Santiago AP, eds: Clinical strabismus management. Philadelphia, WB Saunders, 1999: 325–346.

MacDonald AL, Crawford JS, Smith DR: Duane's retraction syndrome: an evaluation of the sensory status. Can J Ophthalmol 9:458–462, 1974.

Metz HS, Scott AB, Scott WE: Horizontal saccadic velocities in Duane's syndrome. Am J Ophthalmol 80:901–906, 1975.

Mims JL III: Duane's retraction syndrome in Fraunfelder and Roy (Eds), Current Ocular Therapy 5th edn, 1999.

Mims JL III: Choice of surgery for Duane's retraction syndrome. In: van Heuren WAJ, Zwaan JT, eds: Decision making in ophthalmology. St Louis, CV Mosby, 1998:112.

O'Malley ER, Helveston EM, Ellis FD: Duane's retraction syndrome-plus. J Pediatr Ophthalmol Strabismus 19:161–165, 1982.

Rosenbaum AL: The efficacy of rectus muscle transposition surgery in esotropic Duane syndrome and VI nerve palsy. Costenbader Lecture. J AAPOS 8:409–419, 2004.

Saunders RA, Wilson ME, Bluestein EC, Sinatra RB: Surgery on the normal eye in Duane retraction syndrome. J Pediatr Ophthalmol Strabismus 31:162–169, 1994.

225 ESOTROPIA: HIGH ACCOMMODATIVE CONVERGENCE-TO-ACCOMMODATION RATIO 378.35

Alvina Pauline Dy Santiago, MD
Metro-Manila, Philippines
Arthur L. Rosenbaum, MD
Los Angeles, California

The ratio of accommodative convergence (AC) to accommodation (A) [AC/A] is a measure of responsiveness of convergence for each diopter of accommodation.

ETIOLOGY/INCIDENCE

A high AC/A ratio is characterized by excessive accommodative convergence for the amount of accommodation required to focus clearly at a certain distance. Depending on available fusional divergence mechanisms, the excessive accommodative convergence results in esophoria or intermittent or constant esotropia. A high AC/A ratio occurs in as many as 50% of childhood esotropes.

COURSE/PROGNOSIS

The risk of deterioration of esotropia after successful alignment with glasses is greater in patients with a high AC/A ratio than is the risk of esotropia associated with high hyperopia alone.

DIAGNOSIS

Clinical signs and symptoms

A high AC/A ratio may develop at any age, but it usually occurs between the ages of 1 and 7 years, when the reading demand increases. It is especially common in students. Asthenopic symptoms, which are common, include eyestrain and headache. Diplopia at near is reported occasionally. Clinically, the esodeviation at near exceeds distance deviation. A high AC/A ratio may develop in hyperopic, myopic, and emmetropic patients. Amblyopia is usually not severe, unless there is concomitant anisometropic hyperopia.

Laboratory findings

In evaluating the patient with the high AC/A, perform cover-uncover testing with the full refractive error corrected. Use an accommodative target with sufficient detail to eliminate the variability of accommodation. Near measurements should be taken in primary position. Be careful not to confuse high AC/A with an increased esotropia in downgaze or the reading position that may be due to a V-pattern.

The methods of determining the AC/A ratio include the heterophoria method, the gradient method, and the fixation disparity method. The details of computations are discussed more thoroughly elsewhere. In most clinical citations, esodeviation at near that exceeds distance deviation by at least 10PD may be considered to have a high AC/A ratio. Caution should be exercised, however, in labeling patients with a high AC/A when no actual computation has been performed.

Differential diagnosis

Nonaccommodative convergence excess refers to a condition in which patients are orthotropic or have a small-angle esotropia at distance and in whom esotropia at near exceeds distance deviation by at least 15 prism diopters. The esodeviation at near does not respond to additional spherical plus lenses, which contrasts with patients with a true high AC/A ratio. The AC/A ratio is low or normal when measured using the gradient method. In these patients, tonic convergence is suspected to cause increased esotropia at near.

Undercorrected hyperopia in patients who did not receive adequate cycloplegia prior to determination of refractive error may present clinically with esotropia at near that exceeds distance deviation despite wearing the correction. Repeat cycloplegic refraction is warranted and may uncover more hyperopia than previously discovered. The best agent for cycloplegic refraction in patients with esotropia is atropine. Prolonged discomfort with atropine has prompted some ophthalmologists to use intermediate agents such as cyclopentolate that may not uncover full hyperopia.

TREATMENT

The goal of treatment is to achieve alignment at both distance and near, to less than 8 PD of esotropia. This allows peripheral fusion, and expansion of fusional amplitudes.

Ocular

Single-vision lens

The full cycloplegic correction must be tried if the patient is young enough to tolerate the full prescription (usually younger than 5–7 years); otherwise, the maximum tolerated manifest hyperopic refraction is prescribed initially. This plus correction is pushed higher, to as close to cycloplegic refraction as possible, to control residual esodeviation before prescribing bifocals. When moderate hyperopia is corrected, both distance and near deviations are decreased. This may reduce the near deviation to esophoria or infrequent intermittent esotropia with few or no symptoms.

In patients older than 10 years who have nonrefractive esotropia with high AC/A, monovision contact lenses may be effective in reducing near-angle esodeviation. This method compromises stereoacuity and may be accompanied by asthenopia.

If there is little or no hyperopia or if single-vision correction is unsuccessful, bifocals, miotics, or both may be required.

Bifocals

Prescribe bifocals only when evidence of fusion at distance (less than 10PD) can be demonstrated; the goal of bifocals is to create the same fusional situation at near. Ensure that the full cycloplegic refraction is worn and has remained unchanged before considering the use of bifocals in these situations. This has to be verified with repeat determination of cycloplegic refraction, preferably using atropine. Use only the amount of bifocal power that is required to control the near deviation (abolish the esotropia at near or convert it to a small esophoria). Bifocal power varies between +1.50 and +3.00 diopters. In children younger than 7 years, prescribe executive or D-type lenses with a segment height that bisects the pupil to ensure the use of the bifocals at near. In adults and older children, the bifocal height may be lowered to the level of the lower lid. Fresnel membrane (add-on) prisms may be used as bifocal trials to determine effectivity and power requirements; a few days may be required to judge the effect. Periodically reduce the strength of the bifocals gradually (increments of +0.75 to +1.00D) if possible, especially in patients older than 12, with the ultimate goal of eliminating the segment. There is a risk of dependency on bifocals and of prolonged hypoaccommodation. In some cases, the use of bifocals may not improve sensory fusion.

Orthoptics should be used to build fusional divergence amplitudes, especially if the correction with glasses is only partially successful.

Experience with rigid gas permeable bifocal lenses has shown conflicting results in controlling both the distance and near esodeviations. At best, these provide an alternative for patients who prefer not to use bifocals Progressive-type lenses or no-line bifocals may not achieve the desired result.

Medical

Miotics are infrequently used because of their variable efficacy and limited indications. The ideal patient is an infant or a young child who does not have significant hyperopia but has esotropia at near only and resists wearing bifocal glasses. They are used only when there is a possibility of fusion if the near deviation is improved. These are best tolerated by young esotropic patients with a high AC/A ratio.

Commonly, an anticholinesterase is administered at bedtime to reduce accommodative spasm. Echothiophate iodide (phospholine iodide) 0.03% to 0.125% daily and isofluorophate (Floropyl) ointment 0.025% every other day are some of the agents used. The need for innervationally-produced cholinesterase in the ciliary body is reduced by these agents, thereby decreasing the required accommodative effort, and lowering accommodative convergence. Side effects include pupillary constriction and accommodative spasm that limit the clinical usefulness in older children and adults. Iris tags or cysts may develop with prolonged use, although they are rarely large enough to warrant discontinuing the medication. They are minimized by the concomitant use of 2.5% phenylephrine eyedrops and are reversible with cessation of treatment.

Lenticular changes, retinal detachment, and precipitation of angle closure attack occur rarely, and are observed more often in adults than in children. Systemic side effects include nausea, vomiting, abdominal cramps, micturition, and diarrhea. There is a known drug interaction with succinylcholine and other agents used as muscle relaxants in patients undergoing general anesthesia. See Complications for information on the use of succinylcholine and other agents.

Surgical

Surgery may be required when optical means, miotics, and orthoptics fail to relieve the symptoms. An improved outcome may be achieved with prism adaptation. The application of neutralizing membrane prisms to glasses allows rudimentary fusion to develop and improves outcome Indications for surgery include restoration of fusion at near (fusion at distance should be demonstrated), motor alignment, and the possibility of increasing binocular visual field at near.

Surgical procedures for near esodeviation of more than 10 PD and distance deviation that is orthotropic or within monofixational esotropic range (fewer than 8 PD) include bilateral medial rectus muscle recession. This procedure yields the most predictable resultsDespite surgery for near deviation, the distance deviation remains controlled by (at least peripheral) fusional mechanisms. Other procedures described include a medial rectus recession up to 8 mm; and posterior fixation suture (*fadenoperation*) performed alone or combined with recession of both medial rectus muscles. There is a higher risk of overcorrection if the fadenoperation is combined with a recession. The posterior fixation suture placed on the medial rectus pulley may be as effective as a posterior fixation suture placed on the sclera.

For distance esodeviation of more than 15 PD and near esodeviation that exceeds distance deviation by at least 15 prism diopters, we perform prism adaptation, operating on the (larger) prism-adapted angle of deviation. In patients who did not demonstrate fusion before prism adaptation, prism adaptation improves sensory and motor outcome without increasing the risk for overcorrection.

Other enhanced medial rectus muscle recession procedures based on the near deviation and the distance deviationwith and without correction have also been advocated.

Despite excellent bifoveal fixation at distance, only 16% of patients achieved bifoveal fusion at near after surgery.

COMPLICATIONS

Succinylcholine, a common anesthetic agent, may result in prolonged respiratory paralysis and should not be used in patients also treated with echothiophate iodide or isofluorophate. Anticholinesterase inhibitors inactivate or deplete levels in the body of cholinesterase, an enzyme that is required to degrade cholinergic compounds such as succinylcholine. Alternative muscle relaxants that are not dependent on cholinesterase should be used. Parents should be clearly warned about this problem in case the child requires emergency surgery.

REFERENCES

Breinin GM: Accommodative strabismus and the AC-A ratio. Am J Ophthalmol 1:303–311, 1971.

Clark RA, Ariyasu R, Demer JL: Medial rectus pulley posterior fixation is as effective as scleral posterior fixation for acquired esotropia with a high AC/A ratio. Am J Ophthalmol 137:1026–1033, 2004.

Eustis HS, Mungan NK: Monovision for treatment of accommodative esotropia with a high AC/A ratio. J AAPOS 3:87–90, 1999.

Jotterand VH, Isenberg SJ: Enhancing surgery for acquired esotropia. Ophthalmic Surg 19:263–266, 1988.

Kushner BJ, Preslan MW, Morton GV: Treatment of partly accommodative esotropia with a high accommodative convergence-accommodation ratio. Arch Ophthalmol 105:815–818, 1987.

Kushner BJ: Fifteen-year outcome of surgery for the near angle in patients with accommodative esotropia and a high accommodative convergence to accommodation ratio. Arch Ophthalmol 119:1150–1153, 2001.

Leitch RJ, Burke JP, Strachan IM: Convergence excess esotropia treated surgically with fadenoperation and medical rectus muscle recessions. Br J Ophthalmol 74:278–279, 1990.

Parks MM: Abnormal accommodative convergence in squint. Arch Ophthalmol 59:364–380, 1958.

Parks MM: The monofixation syndrome. Trans Am Ophthalmol Soc 67:609–657, 1969.

Pratt-Johnson JA, Tillson G: The management of esotropia with high AC/A ratio (convergence excess). J Pediatr Ophthalmol Strabismus 22:238–242, 1985.

Prism Adaptation Study Research Group: Efficacy of prism adaptation in the surgical management of acquired esotropia. Arch Ophthalmol 108:1248–1256, 1990.

Procianoy E, Justo DM: Results of unilateral medial rectus recession in high AC/A ratio esotropia. J Pediatr Ophthalmol Strabismus 28:212–214, 1991.

Repka MX, Connett JE, Baker JD, Rosenbaum AL: Surgery in the prism adaptation study: accuracy and dose response. Prism Adaptation Study Research Group. J Pediatr Ophthalmol Strabismus 29:150–156, 1992.

Rosenbaum AL, Bateman JB, Bremer DL, Liu PY: Cycloplegic refraction in esotropic children. Cyclopentolate versus atropine. Ophthalmology 88:1031–1034, 1981.

Rosenbaum AL, Jampolsky A, Scott AB: Bimedial recession in high AC/A esotropia. A long-term follow-up. Arch Ophthalmol 91:251–253, 1974.

von Noorden GK, Avilla CW: Nonaccommodative convergence excess. Am J Ophthalmol 101:70–73, 1986.

226 EXTRAOCULAR MUSCLE LACERATIONS 871.4

Krista A. Hunter, MD
Portland, Oregon
David T. Wheeler, MD
Portland, Oregon

ETIOLOGY/INCIDENCE

Lacerations of extraocular muscles or their tendons without damage to the globe, eyelid and adjacent structures are extremely rare. Laceration of rectus muscles occurs more frequently as the oblique muscles insert on the posterior sclera and enjoy greater protection. The inferior rectus and medial rectus are the most frequently injured due to the fact that when the eye is threatened, forced closure of the eyelid is accompanied by Bell's phenomenon with upward and outward movement of the eye. This places these muscles more anteriorly and renders them more susceptible to injury. If ocular trauma involves an upper lid avulsion or penetration of the superomedial orbit, the superior oblique tendon may be lacerated. In addition to ocular trauma, there have been reports of damage to the medial rectus during endoscopic sinus surgery due to the close proximity of this muscle to the ethmoid sinus and the relatively thin medial orbital wall.

DIAGNOSIS

A lacerated extraocular muscle can be difficult to diagnose but should be suspected when profound motility disturbance is found in the setting of ocular trauma. Additional causes of trauma-related motility disturbance should be considered: orbital fracture leading to muscle entrapment, damage to a cranial nerve, and mechanical restriction from edema or hemorrhage associated with the injury. Forced ductions should be performed and would generally be free in cases of laceration although significant edema or hemorrhage could cause restriction. If the examination is delayed significantly from the time of injury, fibrosis and scarring can also lead to restriction.

Imaging studies can occasionally be a helpful adjunct but definitive diagnosis may not be possible without surgical exploration.

TREATMENT

Ideally, reattachment of the lacerated ends of the muscle or tendon should occur promptly after the acute injury. If repair is delayed, scarring and fibrosis can lead to increased difficulty finding and repairing the muscle. However, in selected cases repair may be attempted even if significant time has passed.

When a muscle is lacerated at or near its insertion, the muscle sheath and attachment to posterior Tenon's capsule prevent the muscle from retracting deeply into the orbit. In this case, the free end of the muscle or tendon may be located by following the empty sheath 'hand over hand' into the orbit. It is helpful to recall that the normal course of rectus muscles parallels the orbital wall, rather than the sclera. Painstaking effort at identifying muscle tissue is warranted. Retropulsing the globe may occasionally bring the lacerated muscle into view.

Alternative approaches for recovering a lost muscle deeper in the orbit include an anterior orbitotomy through a fornix-based transconjunctival incision and, in the case of medial rectus or superior oblique muscles, endoscopic surgery through the ethmoid sinus. The assistance of an orbital surgeon may be particularly helpful in these scenarios.

If no muscle tissue can be found for reattachment, a transposition procedure may be indicated. Full or partial tendon transfer of the two adjacent rectus muscles, with or without posterior fixation (the 'Foster modification'), may be done with retention of the anterior ciliary artery in the remaining rectus muscle. If significant concern exists about anterior segment ischemia, a muscle splitting or vessel-sparing muscle transfer technique may be used. If there is restriction of the antagonist, a subsequent recession or injection of botulinum toxin can be done.

COMMMENTS

In any case in which extraocular muscle laceration is suspected, a full and meticulous eye exam should be performed to determine the extent of the injury and rule out globe damage, fractures, or the presence of foreign bodies. Surgical exploration is frequently required.

REFERENCES

Foster RS: Vertical muscle transpositions augmented with lateral fixation. J Am Assoc Pediatric Ophthalmol Strabismus 1:20, 1997.

Helveston EM, Grossman RD: Extraocular muscle lacerations. Am J Ophthalmol 81:754–760, 1976.

McKeown CA: Anterior ciliary vessel sparing procedure. In: Rosenbaum AL, Santiago AP, eds: Clinical strabismus management: principles and surgical techniques. Philadelphia, WB Saunders, 1999:39:516–528.

Santiago AP, Rosenbaum AL: Selected transposition procedures. In: Rosenbaum AL, Santiago AP, eds: Clinical strabismus management: principles and surgical techniques. Philadelphia, WB Saunders, 1999:36: 476–489.

Thacker NM, Velez FG, Demer JL, Rosenbaum AL: Strabismic complications following endoscopic sinus surgery: diagnosis and surgical management. J Am Assoc Pediatric Ophthalmol Strabismus 8:488–494, 2004.

227 INFERIOR RECTUS MUSCLE PALSY 378.81

Richard A. Saunders, MD
Charleston, South Carolina
Richard L. Golub, MD
Phoenix, Arizona

Inferior rectus muscle palsy is an uncommon clinical entity that is almost always associated with abnormalities of one or more additional extraocular muscles. When presenting as an isolated condition, it is characterized by hypertropia of the involved eye in primary gaze position. The deviation is incomitant and becomes greater in the field of action of the involved inferior rectus muscle (i.e. when the globe is abducted and depressed). Adult patients are usually symptomatic and complain of vertical diplopia, especially in down gaze.

ETIOLOGY

- Congenital/idiopathic: long-standing condition of undetermined onset, usually diagnosed in early childhood.
- Neurogenic: oculomotor (third cranial nerve) lesions, rarely fascicular (multiple sclerosis and midbrain metastasis), nuclear or supranuclear, but may be seen in skew deviation.
- Post viral:
  - Myasthenia gravis: typically will have a fluctuating course with a history of other extraocular muscle weakness; the orbicularis oculi are usually involved.
- Orbital trauma:
  - Blowout fracture (typically posterior) with muscle entrapment or injury to the oculomotor nerve;
  - Inferior rectus muscle laceration (penetrating object, dog bite) (Figure 227.1);
  - Inadvertent orbital entry during endoscopic sinus surgery.
- Ocular surgery:
  - Extraocular muscle surgery involving:
  - Excessive recession of the inferior rectus muscle;
  - Lost or slipped muscle;
  - Muscle belly rupture in elderly patients (pulled-in-two syndrome, or 'PITS');
  - Inadvertent inferior rectus muscle injury during inferior oblique muscle myectomy.
- Retrobulbar anesthetic agents injected directly into the inferior rectus muscle (may initially result in paresis with ipsilateral hypertropia followed by muscle contracture and a permanent hypotropia).
- Placement of traction suture.
- Scleral buckle.
- Orbital surgery, such as fat pad removal.
- Miscellaneous orbital processes potentially causing rectus muscle paresis:
  - Chronic progressive external ophthalmoplegia;
  - Orbital neoplasm;
  - Rectus muscle myositis;
  - Thyroid-related immune orbitopathy: usually causes restriction but may have paretic component or association with myasthenia gravis.

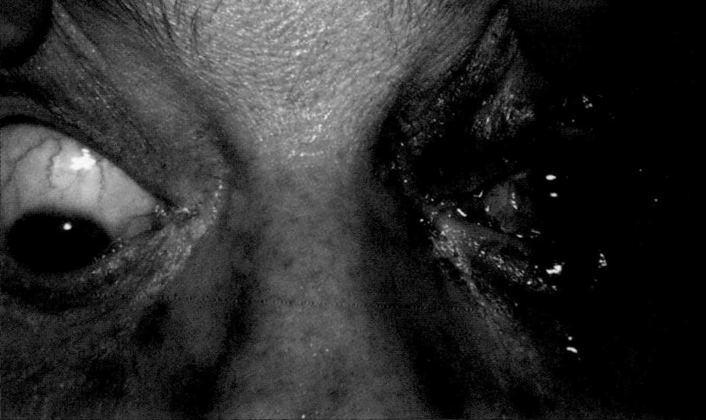

FIGURE 227.1. Traumatic rupture of left inferior rectus muscle from dog bite with absent depression of the left eye.

DIAGNOSIS

Like other cyclovertical muscle disorders, isolated inferior rectus palsy is diagnosed after a thorough history and a careful ocular motility examination. Prism and cover or Maddox rod measurements in the diagnostic gaze positions, as well as an evaluation of ocular torsion and sensory status, are essential.

Clinical signs and symptoms

- Hypertropia typically greatest in the field of action of the involved inferior rectus muscle.
- Duction limitation (not due to a restrictive process).
- Possibly a compensatory chin-down head posture with face turn toward the involved eye.
- Mild incyclotropia may be seen on sensory testing, but is rarely symptomatic.
- Bielschowsky's head-tilt test: positive, negative, or paradoxic results.
- Forced duction testing typically negative in cases of true inferior rectus muscle palsy, although paresis and restriction can coexist.
- Active force-generation testing demonstrating decreased muscle force necessary to confirm the diagnosis.

Differential diagnosis

Other ocular pathology may present a clinical picture similar to inferior rectus palsy.

For instance, superior rectus muscle restriction (e.g. Graves disease or myositis) may cause a hypertropia with down gaze limitation. The orbital floor adherence syndrome may also present with hypertropia, most pronounced or exclusively present in down gaze. It is most often seen after orbital floor fracture and represents a pseudoparesis of the inferior rectus muscle. The reduced infraduction is caused by mechanical limitation of the muscle excursion posteriorly along the orbital floor, simulating muscle 'weakness.' Patients with chronic hypertropia (e.g. longstanding superior oblique muscle palsy or skew deviation) may have limited infraduction on version testing. This problem is distinguished from inferior rectus muscle palsy by the clinical context. Duction testing can differentiate an inferior rectus paresis from a contralateral superior oblique muscle over action; ductions will shows a difference in the ability to depress the involved eye when the fellow eye is covered. Saccadic velocity elicited by optokinetic testing also can be helpful, showing a slowed saccade with inferior rectus paresis, but a normal saccade with skew deviation.

TREATMENT

Therapy for inferior rectus muscle palsy may be optical, surgical or chemical.

Ocular

For those patients with long-standing, small angle hypertropia, prisms may be beneficial. Monocular occlusion or temporary prisms may be used for patients in whom spontaneous recovery is anticipated.

Medical

Chemodenervation (botulinum toxin) of the ipsilateral superior rectus muscle is rarely indicated because of the nearly universal and often severe postinjection ptosis.

Surgical

The surgical management of inferior rectus muscle palsy should be guided by measurements in diagnostic gaze positions and results of passive duction and generated muscle force testing. Surgical options include ipsilateral superior rectus muscle recession with or without inferior rectus muscle resection, and recession or posterior fixation of the contralateral inferior rectus muscle. Weakening of the contralateral superior oblique muscle with free tenotomy is rarely indicated due to the potential for postoperative torsional diplopia and symptomatic superior oblique muscle palsy.

When ductions deficits are −3 or greater, a transposition of the horizontal rectus muscles (modified Jensen or Hummelsheim procedure) may be employed. This can be especially helpful in patients with a lost inferior rectus muscle. More recently, success with anterior transposition of the inferior oblique muscle has been described for traumatic injury or lost inferior rectus muscle.

COMMENTS

The treatment of inferior rectus muscle palsy depends on its clinical context and associated symptoms and, most importantly, on whether it presents as an isolated finding. Surgical intervention is guided by measurements in diagnostic gaze positions, the presence or absence of down gaze restriction, and the degree of rectus muscle weakness. Satisfactory outcome usually requires ocular alignment in the primary gaze and reading positions.

REFERENCES

Brodsky MC, Fritz KJ, Carney SH: Iatrogenic inferior rectus palsy. J Pediatr Ophthalmol Strabismus 29:113–115, 1992.

Greenwald MJ, Ticho BH, Engel JM: Extraocular muscle surgery. In: Krupin T, Kolker AE, eds. Atlas of complications in strabismus surgery. London, Mosby; 1993:9:10–9.11.

Olitsky SE, Notaro S: Anterior transposition of the inferior oblique for the treatment of a lost inferior rectus muscle. J of Pediatr Ophthalmol Strabismus 37:50–51, 2000.

Van Dalen JTW, Van Mourik-Noodernbos AM: Isolated inferior rectus palsy: a report of six cases. Neuro-ophthalmology 4:89–94, 1984.

von Noorden GK, Hansell R: Clinical characteristics and treatment of isolated inferior rectus paralysis. Ophthalmology 98:253–257, 1991.

228 MONOFIXATION SYNDROME

378.34

(Microtropia, Microstrabismus, Subnormal Binocular Vision, Parks' Syndrome)

M. Edward Wilson, MD
Charleston, South Carolina

It is clinically useful to divide binocular vision into central and peripheral components. Central, or macular, binocular vision involves the conscious processing of the central 3 to 5 degrees of the visual field, the 'object of regard,' by the two eyes simultaneously. Peripheral, or extramacular, binocular vision involves the processing of the remainder of the visual field beyond the central 3 to 5 degrees. Patients with monofixation syndrome can be conceptualized as having peripheral binocular vision but no central binocular vision.

The term *bifixation* has often been used to connote simultaneous fixation with both foveae. When a facultative scotoma prevents a patient from fixating with both eyes simultaneously, the term *monofixation* has been applied. When monofixation (absent central binocular vision) is combined with evidence of intact peripheral binocular vision, the patient is said to have monofixation syndrome. As the term implies, only one fovea is fixating at a time even though the extramacular portions of the retinas are functioning simultaneously and cooperatively. Unlike patients with bifixation, these individuals often have a small angle esotropia of up to 8 or 10 prism diopters. Peripheral binocular vision does not have rigid requirements for orthotropia secondary to large receptive fields serving the peripheral retina. In contrast to the looser 'point-to-area' retinal correspondence in the periphery, the small size and large number of cortical receptive fields serving macular vision require a tighter 'point-to-point' retinal correspondence centrally. Therefore, a small angle tropia is compatible with intact peripheral fusion but incompatible with intact central fusion. For this reason, microtropia or microstrabismus has been used at times interchangeably with monofixation syndrome.

ETIOLOGY

- This syndrome may represent a congenital absence of central binocular vision.
- Alternatively, infants with normal binocular vision potential at birth may lose bifixation due to prolonged strabismus (>60 days in an infant, >90 days in an older child), retaining (after the eyes are straightened by surgery or glasses) only peripheral binocular vision.
- Monofixation syndrome is seen and diagnosed most commonly after surgical realignment in childhood strabismus.
- This syndrome can also be secondary to anisometropic amblyopia.
- An idiopathic 'primary' form of monofixation syndrome can be seen, often in relatives of patients with congenital esotropia.

COURSE/PROGNOSIS

- Monofixation syndrome, once established, is permanent.
- Congenital absence of central binocular vision (primary monofixation syndrome) may predispose to strabismus just as strabismus may predispose to monofixation syndrome.
- Children with congenital esotropia most commonly develop monofixation syndrome (peripheral fusion without central fusion) when they are operated early in life. Newer studies suggest that post-operative stereopsis is better when the duration of esotropia is reduced. Bifixation (central binocular vision) may be achievable in some of these infants if the eyes are straightened within 60 days of the onset of constant esotropia.
- Monofixation syndrome promotes better stability of alignment (orthotropia or microtropia) compared with no binocular vision, but manifest strabismus of more than 8 prism diopters may recur with time.
- Central binocular vision, even when normal at birth, is tenous and easily lost if the two foveae are not stimulated simultaneously.
- Constant strabismus lasting a few months or longer may result in the permanent loss of bifixation, even in older children and adults. Peripheral fusion, in contrast, is more durable and usually returns postoperatively even after years of constant strabismus, resulting in monofixation syndrome as the postoperative sensory state of the eyes.

DIAGNOSIS

- Small angle tropia is usually present, measuring up to 8 to 10 prism diopters; however, as many as one third of patients with monofixation syndrome are orthotropic.
- Amblyopia often (but not always) coexists with monofixation syndrome.
- A history of prior surgery for infantile/congenital or childhood-onset strabismus often is present.
- This syndrome can occur without any prior history of strabismus, often in relatives of patients with congenital esotropia.
- For a definitive diagnosis, both the presence of peripheral fusion and the absence of central fusion must be established.
- The presence of peripheral fusion is indicated by the following:
  - There is subnormal (gross) stereopsis;
  - A fusion response to the Worth-four-dot at 0.33 m occurs;
  - There is tropia by simultaneous prism and cover test with overlying phoria by alternate-cover test;
  - Fusional vergence amplitudes are measurable.
- The absence of central fusion is indicated by the following:
  - Microtropia is a manifest tropia on the cover test or simultaneous prism and cover test of 1 to 10 prism diopters; larger tropias are not considered microtropias and are incompatible with monofixation syndrome -the examiner should not be misled by phorias that may overlie a microtropia;
  - Facultative macular scotoma is shown on the Worth-four-dot (patient sees two or three dots at distance despite seeing four dots at near) or Bagolini glasses (patient sees two oblique lines that form an X but with a central gap in the line from the lens over the nonfixating eye);
  - Facultative macular scotoma is shown by the deletion of letters viewed by the nonfixating eye via vectographic projection of Snellen letters (BVAT II BVS, Mentor O and O or vectographic projector chart slide, American Optical Company);
  - There is a positive 4-prism diopter base-out test (no vergence movement); this is the least reliable method and is not recommended.

Differential diagnosis

- Strabismus with pathologic cortical suppression and abnormal retinal correspondence (ARC) is characterized by the following:
  - There is no stereopsis;
  - Patients see two or three lights when viewing Worth-four-dot test at 0.33 m, rather than four as in monofixation syndrome, but may give a four-light response at 6 inches or closer (suppression scotoma in large angle esotropia is often about 6 degrees as opposed to 3 degrees with monofixation syndrome; therefore, lights must be much closer to the patient to project onto the peripheral retina outside of the larger scotoma);
  - The deviation is more than 8 to 10 prism diopters;
  - There is no phoria overlying the tropia;
  - There are no measurable fusional vergence amplitudes.
- Intermittent strabismus with bifixation is characterized by the following:
  - Patients with intermittent deviations may show suppression and ARC when deviated but retain central binocular vision when orthotropic. Perform sensory testing early in the examination, when alignment control is better;
  - Some sensory tests require glasses or goggles, which may disrupt strabismus control and fail to show bifixation.

PROPHYLAXIS

- When normal binocular vision is present in infancy, the loss of central binocular vision, and thus the development of monofixation syndrome, can be prevented by promptly correcting any acquired constant eye misalignment (with the use of glasses, surgery, prisms).
- Surgical overcorrections in the treatment of intermittent exotropia are usually constant and can result in the loss of central binocular vision if not corrected within a few months. Use glasses or prisms to promote fusion temporarily if spontaneous resolution does not occur in the first few weeks after surgery and the decision for repeat operation will be delayed.
- Infants with classic congenital/infantile esotropia have been thought to have a congenital absence of central binocular vision. For this reason, monofixation syndrome has been the desired outcome. Monofixation syndrome can be achieved with surgery within 18–24 months. Some patients, however, may retain the potential for central binocular vision. For this reason, the duration of esotropia has taken on increased significance. Monofixation syndrome may be avoided if the duration of infantile esotropia does not exceed 60 days.

TREATMENT

- Monofixation syndrome, once established, cannot be cured with orthoptic exercises or surgery.
- In hopes of preserving bifixation, infantile esotropia patients should be operated (if possible) within 60 days of the onset of constant large-angle esotropia. The onset of congenital/infantile esotropia is usually between 2 to 6 months of age.
- Treatment of amblyopia may improve the stability of alignment over time in patients with monofixation syndrome.
- When possible, monofixation syndrome should be prevented by preserving bifixation. If not, monofixation syndrome (peripheral fusion) should be the goal of strabismus treatment.
- Peripheral binocular vision, once established, is durable and can be restored even after many years of misalignment. Monofixation syndrome is an achievable functional goal of strabismus surgery even in adults whose eyes have been misaligned since childhood.

REFERENCES

Arthur BW, Smith JT, Scott WE: Long-term stability of alignment in the monofixation syndrome. J Pediatr Ophthalmol Strabismus 26:224–231, 1989.

Eustis HS, Parks MM: Acquired monofixation syndrome. J Pediatr Ophthalmol Strabismus 26:169–172, 1989.

Ing MR: Early surgical alignment for congenital esotropia. Trans Am Ophthalmol Soc 74:625–659, 1981.

Ing MR, Okino LM: Outcome of stereopsis in relation to duration of misalignment in congenital esotropia. J AAPOS, 6:3–8, 2002.

Parks MM: Monofixation syndrome. Trans Am Ophthalmol Soc 67:609–657, 1969.

Parks MM: Monofixation syndrome. In: Tasman W, Jeager EA, eds: Duane's clinical ophthalmology. Philadelphia, JB Lippincott, 1998:I:1–14.

Tychsen L: Can ophthalmologists repair the brain in infantile esotropia? Early surgery, stereopsis, monofixation syndrome, and the legacy of Marshall Parks. J AAPOS 9, 2006.

Wilson ME: Monofixation syndrome. In: Margo CE, Hamed LM, Mames RN, eds: Diagnostic problems in clinical ophthalmology. Philadelphia, WB Saunders, 1994:763–768.

229 NYSTAGMUS 379.50

Theodore H. Curtis, MD
Portland, Oregon
David T. Wheeler, MD
Portland, Oregon

Nystagmus and related ocular oscillations are repetitive involuntary eye movements that often indicate an underlying ocular or neurologic disorder. Movement can be in any direction (or more than one direction simultaneously) and may be congenital or acquired at any age. It is important to remember that nystagmus is a clinical sign that may take many different forms and about which much has been written but little is understood. This chapter will confine itself to a discussion of the more common and clinically relevant forms of nystagmus.

ETIOLOGY/INCIDENCE

The evaluation of nystagmus requires descriptive nomenclature. Most forms involve two *phases:* the first (slow drift) causes the image to move away from the fovea, and the second attempts to return gaze to the target. There are two classic *types:* pendular, in which these phases are of equal velocity, and jerk, in which the second phase is a more rapid saccadic movement. *Direction* (when present) always refers to this fast phase, although it should be recognized that the slow phase reflects the abnormality. Movement can be in any *plane* (horizontal, vertical, oblique or rotary) and has a relative *amplitude* and *frequency.* Nystagmus may be *conjugate* or *dissociated* and may vary with the direction of gaze; the field in which its intensity is minimal is referred to as the *null zone*. Alexander's Law states that jerk nystagmus increases as the eyes move in the direction of the fast component.

Asking an older child or adult if they perceive movement of the environment (oscillopsia) helps to determine age of onset; oscillopsia is absent in congenital and early acquired forms. Associated signs and symptoms may aid in localizing the lesion in acquired nystagmus to the vestibular apparatus, brainstem or cerebellum. These include hearing loss, tinnitus, vertigo, ear pain, weakness or poor coordination, numbness or paresthesias, or imbalance. Eye movement recordings and other testing as noted below may be helpful. Several types of nystagmus are presented.

Physiologic nystagmus

There are several forms of nystagmus associated with normal functioning of the ocular motor system. *End-position nystagmus* can be seen in normal individuals after prolonged gaze in extreme deviation. *Optokinetic nystagmus* (OKN) is a compensatory mechanism that functions to keep images of stationary objects on the retina during prolonged rotation of the head. The first phase (smooth pursuit) follows the target and the fast phase (saccade) resets fixation to the next image. The presence or absence of OKN is useful in assessing visual function of non-verbal and malingering patients. *Caloric nystagmus* is used in comatose patients to evaluate the vestibular system; one or both auditory canals are irrigated with either hot or cold water. *Rotational nystagmus* is useful in evaluating the ocular motor system in infants; while holding the infant in outstretched arms, the examiner pivots in place. During rotation, the fast phase is in the direction of rotation; upon stopping rotation, the fast phase reverses. Since this maneuver depends on an intact vestibular apparatus, it is an impure test of extraocular movements. Lastly, many patients can elicit *voluntary nystagmus*, which are rapid, back-to-back horizontal saccades that cannot be sustained for over 30 seconds. This ability is found in 5–8% of the population and may be familial.

Congenital (infantile) nystagmus

Few patients have onset of nystagmus precisely at birth; the term infantile is more accurate and includes nystagmus present within the first few months of life. This category is broadly divided into afferent nystagmus (due to poor vision) and efferent nystagmus (due to ocular motor disturbance); at least 90% of cases are afferent. Eye movement recordings have conclusively shown that waveform alone is not a reliable method of distinguishing between these two types; therefore, it is imperative that all infants with nystagmus undergo thorough evaluation for a primary sensory cause. Conditions known to be associated with afferent infantile nystagmus include, among others, early (usually bilateral) visual deprivation (congenital cataracts, severe glaucoma, Peter's anomaly), foveal hypoplasia (albinism, aniridia), retinal disease (Leber's congenital amaurosis, achromatopsia, macular toxoplasmosis), retinal detachment (severe retinopathy of prematurity, persistent fetal vasculature, familial exudative vitreoretinopathy) and congenital optic nerve abnormalities (coloboma, atrophy, hypoplasia). It can also accompany cortical visual impairment from a perinatal insult.

The nystagmus is typically binocular and conjugate, dampened by convergence, increased with fixation effort, and abolished in sleep. Improved visual function with convergence often translates to better near acuity, and is the basis for treating with base-out prism glasses, which sometimes improve distance acuity. Patients with high refractive errors usually benefit from contact lens correction to minimize the aberration from constant ocular movement behind thick spectacles. Attempts to reduce the amplitude and/or frequency of the nystagmus and increase foveation time have involved medication (e.g. baclofen), recession of multiple rectus muscles simultaneously, and injection of botulinum toxin (Botox) into the muscle cone. All have had limited success.

Patients with efferent nystagmus (historically known as *congenital motor nystagmus* but recently termed *idiopathic infantile nystagmus*) often have a null point in an eccentric position of gaze and manifest an anomalous head position to maximize visual acuity. Strabismus surgery, specifically an Anderson or Kestenbaum procedure, may place this null zone in primary position, thereby reducing or eliminating the head position. Variations of this technique are employed if there is accompanying strabismus or if the head position has a vertical or torsional component.

Latent nystagmus is a benign condition that appears only when one eye is covered, or when light stimulus to one eye is diminished, but can coexist with manifest nystagmus (in which case the nystagmus amplitude increases with occlusion). This is a jerk nystagmus with the fast phase toward the side of the fixing eye; it is often seen following surgery for infantile esotropia and probably results from subnormal binocular interaction. Visual acuity measurement should be performed using the polarized vectograph or blurring one eye with a high plus lens to avoid iatrogenic reduction of acuity with occlusion. So-called *manifest latent nystagmus* can occur if monocular visual loss occurs in this setting.

Acquired nystagmus

Spasmus nutans classically presents as a triad of nystagmus, head nodding and torticollis between 4 months and 3 years of age, and usually resolves within a year. The nystagmus is usually very fine, rapid and pendular, but may be vertical or rotary. It is usually asymmetric, may appear monocular, and varies over time and with position of gaze. Head nodding is inconstant and irregular, and tilting or turning of the head occurs less frequently. Pathogenesis is unknown and no treatment exists, but the condition appears to be self-limited. It is associated with strabismus and refractive error. Chiasmal glioma can present in a manner identical to spasmus nutans, prior to visibly affecting the anterior visual pathways. Some authors recommend that all patients with this condition undergo neuro-imaging; this is particularly important in the setting of visual loss, afferent pupillary defect, papilledema or optic atrophy.

Vestibular nystagmus can be divided into peripheral and central types. The etiology of peripheral disease includes labyrinthitis, acoustic neuronitis, ischemia, trauma and toxicity; the nystagmus is frequently associated with vertigo, tinnitus or deafness. It is invariably a jerk nystagmus, usually with a horizontal and rotary component, and the fast phase is toward the normal side. Central vestibular nystagmus is due to bilateral brainstem dysfunction from tumor, stroke, trauma or demyelination. This nystagmus may be purely horizontal, vertical or rotary and may change with the direction of gaze. Treatment is primarily aimed at reducing the vertigo and may include anticholinergics, monoaminergics, antihistamines, phenothiazines, benzodiazepines and butyrophenones. The sheer number of drugs involved reflects the lack of effective treatment.

Seesaw nystagmus is a dissociated pendular nystagmus in which one eye elevates while the other depresses. In the acquired form, the rising eye intorts while the falling eye extorts. In the less common congenital form, these torsional movements are reversed. Etiologies include parasellar tumors, trauma, and vertebrobasilar insufficiency; it has been reported in septo-optic dysplasia and even with severe visual loss from progressive cone-rod retinal dystrophy. Visual field results are helpful in considering neoplastic or vascular etiologies. The use of baclofen, a GABA analog, may be beneficial.

In *upbeat nystagmus*, the upgoing fast phase may be of large or small amplitude but is always present in primary position. Most patients have intrinsic brainstem or cerebellar disease. Associated conditions include multiple sclerosis, cerebellar degeneration, tumors or infarction of the medulla or midbrain, and infection or toxicity of the brainstem, such as Wernicke's encephalopathy. Treatment is directed at identification and resolution of the underlying cause.

Downbeat nystagmus is commonly seen with disease affecting the cerebellum or craniocervical junction such as cerebellar degeneration, Arnold–Chiari malformation, multiple sclerosis, trauma, tumor, infarction and many toxic-metabolic entities. The use of clonazepam, a GABA agonist, may decrease amplitude and oscillopsia. MRI may indicate a surgically correctable lesion.

Periodic alternating nystagmus (PAN) is a continuous, horizontal nystagmus in which the fast component spontaneously reverses direction approximately every two minutes. It may be congenital or indicate vestibulo-cerebellar dysfunction from stroke, tumor, multiple sclerosis, trauma, infection, drug intoxication or degenerative disease. It has also occurred with severe, acquired bilateral visual loss from cataract, vitreous hemorrhage, or optic atrophy. Correction of the visual loss may abolish the nystagmus. Other patients have responded to treatment with baclofen.

The hallmark of *gaze-evoked nystagmus* is its absence in primary position. The fast component is in the direction of gaze but its presence does not signify location or etiology. It is commonly drug-induced by anticonvulsants, sedatives, ethanol and other recreational drugs. It can also be seen with posterior fossa disease (tumor, trauma, infarct, demyelination) and is called *Bruns' nystagmus* in the setting of cerebellopontine tumors; in this case, the nystagmus is slow and coarse when looking toward the side of the lesion and fast and fine in the opposite field of gaze. Gaze-evoked nystagmus can also be seen with cranial nerve palsies, myasthenia gravis, and restrictive muscle disease such as thyroid ophthalmopathy.

Gaze-paretic nystagmus is a type of gaze-evoked nystagmus seen in patients recovering from a gaze palsy and is characterized by slow frequency and large amplitude. As with all types of gaze-evoked nystagmus, it is due to dysfunction of the neural network that integrates pursuit, saccade and vestibular signals. When this mechanism fails, the eyes drift back toward midline from an eccentric position of gaze; displacement of the image from the fovea triggers a saccadic movement to regain fixation. Two other types of gaze-evoked nystagmus are rebound nystagmus and the dissociated nystagmus seen in internuclear ophthalmoplegia. *Rebound nystagmus* can occur after prolonged eccentric gaze, with reversal of the fast phase (toward primary position), or can be seen transiently when the eyes return to primary position following sustained eccentric gaze. Both types are associated with ataxia and cerebellar disease.

Related ocular oscillations

Superior oblique myokymia is caused by rapid, torsional, monocular movements due to isolated, intermittent contraction of the superior oblique muscle. Patients report brief episodes of vertical or torsional diplopia and oscillopsia. It is best appreciated at the slit lamp or during fundoscopy and may be exacerbated with gaze into the field of action of the affected muscle. It is generally benign but may follow trochlear palsy or head trauma, and has been reported in multiple sclerosis and occasionally with cerebellar tumor. Treatment with carbamazepine may be beneficial; surgical weakening of the affected muscle is sometimes required.

Convergence retraction 'nystagmus' is seen in Parinaud's (dorsal midbrain) syndrome and is due to co-contraction of the extraocular muscles with attempted convergence or upgaze. It is a saccadic disorder, rather than a form of nystagmus, and is best seen with fixation on down-going OKN targets. Other findings in the dorsal midbrain syndrome are impaired vertical gaze, pupillary light-near dissociation, lid retraction, abnormal convergence and accommodation, and skew deviation. J. Lawton Smith has given the following age-differential: in infancy, congenital aqueductal stenosis; 10 years old, pinealoma; 20 years old, head trauma; 30 years old, brainstem vascular malformation; 40 years old, long-standing multiple sclerosis; and 50 years old, basilar artery stroke.

Several fixation instabilities are frequently seen in patients with cerebellar disease. *Square wave jerks* are back-to-back macrosaccades that first interrupt fixation and then bring about refoveation. *Ocular dysmetria* is the ocular equivalent of 'past-pointing' seen with an intention tremor: as the eyes return to primary position, they overshoot the target and oscillate about the new fixation point before coming to rest. *Ocular flutter* is a spontaneous intermittent burst of several conjugate micro-oscillations while maintaining fixation in primary position.

Opsoclonus refers to rapid, involuntary, chaotic, conjugate eye movements known as 'saccadomania' that may signal an occult neuroblastoma in children. It has also been seen in infants with an autoimmune disorder that responds to ACTH, and as a paraneoplastic manifestation in adults with visceral carcinoma. Other causes include multiple sclerosis and head trauma; it may be a benign, self-limited finding after viral encephalopathy. It is believed due to impairment of function in the pontine pause cells that normally inhibit saccadic burst cells.

Ocular myoclonus is a vertical pendular oscillation that persists during sleep and is often associated with synchronous contraction of the face, palate, pharynx and diaphragm. This is due to a lesion in the 'myoclonic triangle' which connects the red nucleus with the ipsilateral inferior olive and the contralateral dentate nucleus. GABA agonists such as valproate have been reported to decrease the movement.

Two final ocular oscillations are usually observed in comatose patients. *Ocular bobbing* is characterized by a fast, conjugate, downward movement followed by a slow drift back up to primary position, usually in the absence of any horizontal eye movement. Patients typically have a massive pontine lesion, or metabolic encephalopathy. *Ping-pong gaze* is periodic, horizontal deviation of the eyes with the direction alternating every few seconds. It is seen with bilateral infarction of the cerebral hemispheres, but the etiology is unknown.

DIAGNOSIS

- Thorough understanding of the normal mechanisms for gaze stability and the difference between physiologic and pathologic nystagmus is required.
- Meticulous history and careful clinical observation, along with a consistent method of recording the nystagmus, is essential. Clinical maneuvers – such as caloric, positional, and optokinetic stimulation – can be used to induce nystagmus for diagnostic purposes.
- If an eye movement recording laboratory is available, more accurate categorization of the abnormal eye movement can be obtained.
- Use of MRI search coil technique with a calibrated contact lens has moved from the research arena into clinical application.

Differential diagnosis

- Many forms of nystagmus indicate underlying neurologic disease. The role of the ophthalmologist is to identify the nystagmus and its localizing value so that appropriate diagnostic steps (neuro-imaging, etc.) may be undertaken. The concept of differential diagnosis is only meaningful following initial examination.
- The differential diagnosis of afferent infantile nystagmus is broad and often requires additional steps such as examination under anesthesia, ocular echography, electroretinography, visual evoked response and MRI.
- MRI should be considered in patients presenting with spasmus nutans in order to rule out glioma, especially if there is any evidence of anterior visual pathway or hypothalamic disease.
- Previously well children with opsoclonus should undergo measurement of urine vanillylmandelic acid and abdominal CT to rule out neuroblastoma.

TREATMENT

Our limited knowledge of the pathogenesis of nystagmus hinders optimal treatment. Except for the use of baclofen in PAN, few controlled clinical trials have been performed for any intervention. Careful evaluation before and during therapy, particularly noting distance and near visual acuity, is warranted. Eye movement recordings with video and/or magnetic search coils are of value.

Systemic

- Pharmacologic agents are primarily GABA agonists and potentiate the inhibitory effect of this neurotransmitter on ocular motor pathways. These drugs include baclofen, gabapentin, clonazepam, valproate and carbamazepine, among others.

- Alternative measures such as biofeedback, acupuncture, or cutaneous head and neck stimulation have been reported to decrease nystagmus in select patients.

Ocular

- Refraction with full correction should be done, as seemingly mild refractive correction can significantly improve vision in these patients.
- Optical therapies utilize prisms to place the eyes in a position of least nystagmus and thereby maximize foveation time and visual acuity. Another approach has been retinal image stabilization, which consists of high-plus spectacle lenses worn in combination with high-minus contact lenses; this is useful for monocular viewing when the patient is stationary. Contact lens wear alone has been noted to diminish congenital nystagmus, presumably by a trigeminal efferent pathway.

Medical

- Retrobulbar or intramuscular injection of botulinum toxin (Botox) has been demonstrated to abolish nystagmus temporarily, but patient satisfaction has been poor due to side effects such as ptosis or diplopia, and the need for re-injection.

Surgical

- Strabismus surgery has been utilized in certain forms of nystagmus with varying degrees of success. Anderson or Kestenbaum procedures are used to move the eyes into the 'null zone' to diminish an anomalous head position. Recessions of all four horizontal recti have been performed with mixed preliminary results. Four-muscle tenotomy has been suggested, but some studies show clinical improvement, while others show no statistically significant effect. Surgery is occasionally needed in superior oblique myokymia. In secondary nystagmus, removal of the offending lesion can improve symptoms.

COMPLICATIONS

Medical treatment should be administered by persons familiar with potential adverse drug effects. Carbamazepine can cause bone marrow suppression, baclofen is not approved for children, and clonazepam may be teratogenic; these agents should probably not be given to children or pregnant females. Surgery carries the risk of anesthesia, as well as potential loss of vision; this consideration becomes more important when potential benefits are less certain. Alternative therapy is probably harmless at worst, but should not delay diagnosis or treatment of an underlying disorder.

REFERENCES

Arnoldi KA, Tychsen L: Prevalence of intracranial lesions in children initially diagnosed with disconjugate nystagmus (spasmus nutans). J Pediatr Ophthalmol Strabismus 32:296–301, 1995.

Averbuch-Heller L, Leigh RJ: Medical treatments for abnormal eye movements: pharmacological, optical and immunological strategies. Aust New Zealand J Ophthalmol 25:7–13, 1997.

Breen LA: Nystagmus and related ocular oscillations. In: Walsh TJ: Neuro-ophthalmology: Clinical signs and symptoms. 4th edn. Baltimore, Williams & Wilkins, 1997:504–520.

Burde RM, Savino PJ, Trobe JD: Clinical decisions in neuro-ophthalmology. 2nd edn. St Louis, Mosby — Year Book, 1992:289–320.

Helveston AM, Ellis FD, Plager DA: Large recession of the horizontal recti for treatment of nystagmus. Ophthalmology 98:1302–1305, 1991.

Hertel RW, Dell'osso LF, Fitzgibbon EJ, et al: Horizontal rectus muscle tenotomy in children with infantile nystagmus syndrome: a pilot study. J AAPOS 8:539–48, 2004.

Leigh RJ, Averbuch-Heller L: Nystagmus and related ocular motility disorders. In: Miller NR, Newman NJ, eds: Walsh & Hoyt's clinical neuro-ophthalmology. 5th edn. Baltimore, Williams & Wilkins, 1998: 1461–1505.

Pratt-Johnson JA: Results of surgery to modify the null-zone position in congenital nystagmus. Can J Ophthalmol 26:219–223, 1991.

Reinecke RD: Idiopathic infantile nystagmus: Diagnosis and treatment. J AAPOS 1:67–82, 1997.

Tychsen L: Pediatric ocular motility disorders of neuro-ophthalmic significance. Ophthalmol Clin North America 4:615–643, 1991.

230 OCULOMOTOR (THIRD NERVE) PARALYSIS 378.51

Ann U. Stout, MD

Portland, Oregon

ETIOLOGY/INCIDENCE

Paralysis of the oculomotor nerve may be congenital or acquired. An oculomotor palsy may occur in association with atrochlear nerve palsy. This is significant both diagnostically and in the choice of surgical procedure.

DIAGNOSIS

Clinical signs and symptoms

Patients with this disorder typically present with symptoms of crossed diplopia with or without blurred vision. The patient may assume a head position to enable fusion. The findings are primarily ipsilateral to the lesion.

A complete paralysis includes four of the six extraocular muscles (superior, medial, and inferior rectus, as well as inferior oblique) with exotropia, hypotropia, and incyclotropia of the involved eye; paralysis of the ciliary muscle and iris sphincter, resulting in absent accommodation and a dilated pupil; and paralysis of the levator, resulting in blepharoptosis. A partial form, or paresis, produces an intermediate degree of weakness of these muscles. The upper division can be involved alone, producing a double elevator paresis with true or pseudoptosis. The lower division may be selectively involved, sparing the superior rectus and levator.

A diabetic oculomotor paresis frequently involves partial pupillary function. A sufficiently discrete nuclear lesion may involve the contralateral instead of the ipsilateral superior rectus muscle and may produce bilateral partial ptosis, although these findings are exceedingly rare.

TREATMENT

Ocular

If there is a field of single vision, bifocal correction for near vision may be needed if accommodation is impaired. If the patient is in the amblyopic age range, patching and refractive correction are required. Surgical realignment is best deferred until after amblyopia therapy is completed. Prism correction may help if the vertical deviation is small. Deformity resulting from anisocoria is particularly troubling to blue-eyed patients, and may be treated with a cosmetic contact lens painted with a pupil and an iris.

Surgical

The goal of surgery is to realign the eyes at or close to primary position. The choice of procedure depends on which muscles are involved and the completeness of the paralysis. Paresis of the vertical rectus muscles may cancel out, leaving a minimal vertical deviation, which is readily controlled with a mild head position or with prisms. In partial paralysis, there may be sufficient medial rectus function to respond well to a resection of the medial rectus muscle and recession of the ipsilateral lateral rectus muscle. Single vision across a maximum range of horizontal gaze directions is achieved by including recession of both horizontal rectus muscles on the other eye, with adjustable sutures being placed on selected or all four muscles. With very poor to no medial rectus function, if there is significant vertical rectus muscle function, the vertical rectus muscles can be transposed to the medial rectus muscle, combined with a resection and recession of these muscles for any vertical deviation. Adjustable sutures are useful here as well.

In complete paralysis of the third nerve, medial rectus function can be replaced to some extent by the transposition of a sound superior oblique muscle. The superior oblique must be weakened to alleviate the incyclotropia. The superior oblique does not respond to horizontal gaze innervation but will provide an adducting force that opposes the abducting action of the recessed lateral rectus and improves ocular alignment. The tendon can be released from the trochlea by cutting the trochlea with scissors (technically difficult). Care must be taken to avoid crushing the tendon. If the tendon is severed, then the surgeon proceeds as though the superior oblique were also paralyzed. The free tendon is resected until it is snug and sutured to the insertion of the medial rectus muscle. The new superior oblique insertion is optimally placed under the medial rectus muscle at the axis of vertical rotation (to avoid an inadvertent hypertropia).

An alternative approach to transposition of the superior oblique is to leave the trochlea intact and relocate the superior oblique tendon 2 to 3 mm anterior to the medial end of the superior rectus insertion, accompanied by the right amount of resection.

To optimize results, the lateral conjunctiva and Tenon's capsule can be recessed all the way to the orbital margin and the lateral rectus muscle should be recessed as far as practically possible. The eye can also be anchored in an adducted position for 2 weeks with orbital fixation sutures. This is especially important if the superior oblique tendon has been lost and cannot provide an adducting force. There is no value in resecting the medial rectus muscle unless it has some residual function.

Surgical elevation of the lid may be required if the ptosis is sufficiently severe. This should be deferred until after the eye is aligned. A maximal levator resection with a transcutaneous approach can suspend the upper lid; however, a frontalis sling is preferable for setting the correct lid height. Since the protective Bell's reflex is usually impaired, the ptosis should be corrected to cover only half of the cornea with the brow relaxed. Frequent blinking and moisturizing drops must be relied on to prevent corneal drying. Children tolerate corneal exposure better than adults.

In double elevator paresis without resistance to passive elevation, a full tendon transposition of the medial and lateral rectus to the insertion of the superior rectus is the operation of choice (Knapp procedure). The ptosis may be a pseudoptosis caused by the hypotropia and should not be corrected until after the strabismus repair. If it is a real ptosis, elevation of the eye will aggravate the ptosis and the patient or family should be forewarned.

A paralysis of the lower division of the third nerve (affecting the medial rectus, inferior rectus, and inferior oblique muscles) is treated by transferring the functioning superior rectus to the medial rectus muscle, the lateral rectus to the inferior rectus muscle, and tenectomizing the superior oblique muscle.

Supportive

Accurate diagnosis and appropriate medical treatment are necessary. Prism therapy is generally of limited benefit because of marked incomitance. The involved eye is occluded, if necessary, for relief of diplopia. urgery should be deferred for as long as 6 to 9 months because spontaneous recovery may occur. If so, it must be followed to its end; surgery should be considered only for the remaining deviation.

COMPLICATIONS

Because of the severe loss of function of extraocular muscles in third nerve paralysis, the only attainable goal is realignment of the eye in primary position. In patients with incomplete paralysis, a small horizontal and vertical range of fusion may be obtained, but care must be taken that the lid is not elevated too far and corneal function is not compromised. Children learn to suppress the double image; however, adults frequently require an occlusive lens because of the absence of fusion anywhere except in one direction of gaze.

COMMENTS

Total third nerve paralysis is devastating to oculomotor function, and even the limited goal of repositioning the eye near primary position is a considerable achievement. Useful function of the eye in a binocular context can be obtained only in some cases of partial paralysis. Accurate diagnosis and the ruling out of other neurological involvement are essential before any consideration can be given to surgical repair.

REFERENCES

Buckley EG, Townshend LM: A simple transposition procedure for complicated strabismus. Am J Ophthalmol 111:302–306, 1991.

Glaser JS: Infranuclear disorders of eye movements. In: Duane TD, ed: Clinical ophthalmology. Hagerstown, Harper & Row, 1982:12:1–38.

Gottlob I, Catalano RA, Reinecke RD: Surgical management of oculomotor nerve palsy. Am J Ophthalmol 111:71–76, 1991.

Peter LC: The use of the superior oblique as an internal rotator in third-nerve paralysis. Trans Am Ophthalmol Soc 31:232–237, 1933.

Scott AB: Transposition of the superior oblique. Am Orthoptics J 5:11–14, 1977.

231 SUPERIOR OBLIQUE MYOKYMIA 358.8

Andrea C. Tongue, MD
Lake Oswego, Oregon

ETIOLOGY

Superior oblique myokymia is a rare disorder reported almost exclusively in adults. Although Duane first described this condition in 1906, Hoyt and Keane, in 1970, were the first to refer to it as superior oblique myokymia, based on the clinical findings in five patients and EMG studies in one. The signs and symptoms include bouts of oscillopsia (microtremor, twitching), and vertical and/or torsional diplopia due to unilateral superior oblique muscle contractions. The disorder is often chronic and is rarely associated with any life-threatening intracranial mischief. It was considered a benign, although aggravating, disorder of unknown etiology until MRI showed that vascular compression of the fourth nerve at the root exit zone (REZ) may be one etiologic factor. Other extremely rare associated factors or potential etiologies cited are preceding superior oblique paralysis, tumors, AV fistula, demyelinating disease, adrenoleukodystrophy, lead poisoning, and stroke. All of these disorders can cause injury to the trochlear nerve and it has been postulated that the myokymia is caused by discharge of regenerating or regenerated motor neurons of the fourth cranial nerved.

COURSE/PROGNOSIS

The course appears to be chronic, with spontaneous remissions and recurrences which may be years apart. In recent years MRI studies in multiple cases have shown compression at the root exit zone of the fourth cranial nerve by a blood vessel. It appears that the right side is more frequently affected than the left in these cases

DIAGNOSIS

Clinical signs and symptoms

The clinical sign of oscillopsia is subtle and may be best detected by slit lamp examination or video photography. Symptoms include intermittent or episodic vertical jumping, shimmering, twitching, or blurring of images. Diplopia may also be present. The symptoms are usually unilateral but have been reported to be perceived as bilateral. Signs are unilateral in that no case of bilateral superior oblique myokymia has been described. Usually individual bursts of superior oblique contraction last seconds but may recur continuously for hours or days at a time. In some patients the symptoms may be provoked by down gaze and may be most easily recognized on slit lamp examination.

Laboratory findings

MRI is essential in identifying vascular compression. It should be noted that vascular contact with the trochlear nerve at the REZ was found in 14% of 30 normal volunteer subjects. Magnetic search coil technique can be used to measure the rotations of the eye during periods of superior oblique contraction. In the past, EMG studies have also shown superior oblique contraction.

TREATMENT

Systemic

Pharmacologic agents used in the treatment of this disorder include oral carbamazepine (tegretol), gabapentin, propanolol, phenytoin and baclofen. It is difficult to assess the effect of these medications because of the variable course of this disease in any individual and between individuals. The drugs may also be associated with serious and significant side effects and require ongoing and frequent laboratory and medical monitoring. Anyone prescribing these drugs should be familiar with the reported adverse effects, contraindications, and required monitoring of the patients.

Topical

Use of topical betoxalol has also been reported with varying success.

Surgical

Surgery is reserved for patients who are unable to tolerate their symptoms and do not respond or have adverse effects to medical therapy. Extra-ocular surgical procedures are directed at weakening the affected superior oblique and ipsilateral inferior oblique. Post-operative superior oblique paralysis may occur, leading to diplopia, which in some cases spontaneously resolves and in some requires further surgery. Recently the newest surgical intervention for SOM reported in the literature is intracranial micro-vascular decompression. This is a neurosurgical procedure involving a craniectomy. However, it is a procedure that attempts to correct the cause of the disease in cases where micro-vascular compression at the REZ is identified by special MRI studies. Temporary as well as lasting superior oblique paralysis (one year follow-up) has been reported in cases after micro-vascular decompression.

REFERENCES

Hashimoto M, Ohtsuka K, Suzuki Y, et al: Superior oblique myokymia caused by vascular compression. J Neuro-Ophthalmol 24:3327, 2004.

Katz SE, Anderson DP: Superior oblique myokymia as a bilateral subjective phenomenon. Can J Ophthalmol 32:256, 1997.

Palmer EA, Shults TW: Superior oblique myokymia: preliminary results of surgical treatment. J Pediatr Ophthalmol Strabismus 21:96, 1984.

Scharwey, K, Krzizok T, Sarnii M, et al: Remission of superior oblique myokymia after vascular decompression. Ophthalmologica 214:425, 2000.

Yousry I, Dieterich M, Naidich TP, et al: Superior oblique myokymia: magnetic resonance imaging support for the neurovascular compression hypothesis. Ann Neurol 51:361, 2002.

232 SUPERIOR OBLIQUE (FOURTH NERVE) PALSY 378.53

Ann U. Stout, MD
Portland, Oregon

ETIOLOGY

Superior oblique palsy is the most commonly occurring cranial nerve palsy encountered by the strabismologist. The length and pathway of the trochlear nerve across the edge of the dura (tentorium) makes it highly susceptible to minor head trauma.

Other causes of superior oblique palsy are less common and include:

- Tumor;
- Vascular abnormality;
- Diabetes;
- Iatrogenic (after sinus or orbital surgery).

Superior oblique palsy may be unilateral or bilateral and congenital or acquired.

The superior oblique tendon is also the tendon most frequently noted to be anomalous or absent.

COURSE/PROGNOSIS

As with other cranial nerve palsies, acquired superior oblique palsy (bilateral or unilateral) may resolve weeks to months after the onset; however, any deviation that persists after 6 months may be considered permanent.

DIAGNOSIS

Evaluation of the patient suspected of having superior oblique palsy should begin with a careful history, and especially with inquiry about any prior head trauma. Questions should be directed toward the presence or absence of abnormal head posture, vertical diplopia, and torsional diplopia.

Clinical signs and symptoms

Superior oblique palsy manifests in children as:

- Abnormal head posture (head tilt);
- Facial asymmetry;
- V-pattern esotropia with vertical component;
- In congenital absence of the superior oblique tendon, symptoms may include significant horizontal deviation, amblyopia, ptosis, and asymmetry of the orbits or face.

In adults, there may be additional features:

- Intermittent diplopia, which may be horizontal and vertical;
- A chin depression to avoid diplopia in bilateral cases;
- Spontaneous torsional diplopia with horizontal displacement of the tilted images in most bilateral acquired cases;
- A head tilt and turn to the side opposite the affected eye in unilateral cases.

Three-step test

An initial qualitative evaluation is carried out using a simple two-step test (Parks). A third step (Bielschowsky) includes noting whether the hyperdeviation is greater on right or left head tilt. Together these tests make up the three-step test to help in diagnosing a paresis of any of the vertically acting muscles.

Step 1

Determine which eye is hypertropic; this narrows the paretic muscle choices to four:

- The depressors on the hypertropic eye (inferior rectus, superior obique); or
- The elevators on the hypotropic eye (superior rectus, inferior oblique).

Step 2

Determine if the vertical deviation is greatest in right or left gaze:

- Right gaze involves the right vertical recti as well as the left obliques;
- Left gaze involves the left vertical recti and the right obliques;
- The gaze direction with the larger deviation will further narrow the paretic muscle choice to two, a vertical rectus and an oblique, after factoring in the results of step 1.

Step 3 (Bielschowsky head-tilt test)

The head is tilted to one side and then the other while the deviation is measured. (Bielschowsky head-tilt test). If the vertical deviation increases when the head is tilted toward the *higher* eye, the oblique muscle arrived at in step 2 is considered paretic. If the vertical deviation increases when the head is tilted toward the side of the *lower* eye, the rectus muscle identified in step 2 is considered paretic.

In general, a unilateral superior oblique palsy will create an ipsilateral hypertropia that is worse on lateral gaze away from the affected side and on head tilt towards the affected side.

Prism and cover testing should next be carried out in the nine diagnostic positions to provide a quantified evaluation.

Maddox double rod test

An essential part of evaluating the patient with suspected superior oblique palsy is the Maddox double rod test for torsion. A red Maddox rod, with the cylinders vertically oriented, is placed in front of the patient's right eye, and a similarly oriented white Maddox rod is placed in front of the left eye. The patient is asked to view a point source of light in a darkened room. The Maddox rods are then adjusted if necessary so that red and white lines appear to be parallel to the patient. The ocular torsion expressed in degrees is read directly from the trial frame holding the Maddox rods.

- *Congenital or early acquired* superior oblique palsy: no measurable torsion and no spontaneous complaint of torsional diplopia; facial asymmetry is commonly seen in the congenital form of the condition, with the fuller side of the face on the affected side. Asymmetry is secondary to head posture. Anomalies of the superior oblique tendon may be found.
- *Acquired unilateral* superior oblique palsy: measurable torsion less than 15 degrees but no spontaneous complaint of torsional diplopia; the tendon may be normal, and its condition can be assessed accurately in most cases with the use of the superior oblique traction test done at the time of surgery.
- *Bilateral* superior oblique palsy: the patient complains of torsional diplopia with horizontally separated images or has cyclotropia of more than 15 degrees, right hypertropia in left gaze, left hypertropia in right gaze, and V-pattern.

TREATMENT

Surgical

The prism and cover measurements obtained in the nine diagnostic positions in a patient with superior oblique palsy may be recorded and interpreted according to a scheme devised by Knapp:

Classes

- *Class I* has the greatest vertical deviation in the field of action of the antagonist inferior oblique muscle; it is treated with inferior oblique weakening.
- *Class II* has the greatest vertical deviation in the field of action of the underacting paretic superior oblique; it is treated with superior oblique strengthening (if the tendon is lax).
- *Class III* is an equal vertical deviation in the field of action of the antagonist inferior oblique and the paretic superior oblique; deviations of less than 20 prism diopters are treated with inferior oblique weakening and those of more than 20 prism diopters are treated with inferior oblique weakening combined with either superior oblique strengthening (if the tendon is lax), or recession of the contralateral inferior rectus.
- *Class IV* is characterized by an L-shaped pattern, with a vertical deviation in the field of action of the paretic superior oblique, the antagonist inferior oblique, and the ipsilateral inferior rectus muscles. It is treated by superior oblique strengthening (if the tendon is lax), inferior oblique weakening, and weakening of the ipsilateral superior rectus.
- *Class V* superior oblique palsy shows a greater vertical deviation in all fields of downgaze. The ipsilateral superior rectus is recessed, and with more than 20 prism diopters of hypertropia, the superior oblique is tucked (if lax) or the contralateral inferior rectus is recessed.
- *Class VI* is bilateral superior oblique palsy, characterized by a V-pattern, chin depression, bilaterally positive Bielschowsky test, right hypertropia in left gaze, left hypertropia in right gaze, and complaints of torsional diplopia with the tilted images separated horizontally. Measured cyclotropia is often more than 15 degrees. This is treated with bilateral inferior rectus recession, bimedial rectus downshift, bilateral superior oblique tucks, or a combination.
- *Class VII* is termed 'canine tooth syndrome' and displays underaction of the superior oblique muscle *and* of the inferior oblique muscle on the same side. Its origin can be trochlear trauma (resulting in a 'double Brown syndrome'), iatrogenic (e.g. an acquired Brown syndrome secondary to strengthening the superior oblique along with a residual superior oblique palsy), or local trochlear trauma complicated by closed head trauma producing a fourth nerve palsy.

Class VII is extremely difficult to treat. If the patient is able to fuse in primary gaze and has some range of fusion above and below, probably no treatment is indicated. If Brown syndrome is the most severe problem, surgical relief of the trochlear restriction may be tried with or without recession of the ipsilateral inferior rectus muscle. Iatrogenic Brown syndrome may require takedown of the tuck or recession of the resected superior oblique tendon, along with recession of the contralateral inferior rectus muscle.

- Certain types of superior oblique palsy are characterized by fairly severe torsional defects with very little vertical tropia; they may occur unilaterally or bilaterally. In such cases, the patient may benefit from anterior transposition of the superior oblique tendon by shifting the whole tendon or just the anterior fibers; an adjustable suture may be used in the procedure (Harada–Ito technique).
- *Absent or anomalous superior oblique tendon* may be treated by recession of the antagonist inferior oblique and of the ipsilateral superior rectus muscle, and by appropriate treatment of any coexisting horizontal deviation.

COMPLICATIONS

Surgery to strengthen the superior oblique tendon frequently produces an iatrogenic mechanical limitation of elevation in adduction (Brown syndrome). For this reason, tucking of the superior oblique tendon should be done in fairly small increments, graded according to the laxity of the tendon noted at surgery. In acquired superior oblique palsy, alternatives to superior oblique strengthening should be considered.

In cases of superior oblique palsy after closed head trauma, it is prudent to suspect that the condition is bilateral unless this can be definitely ruled out; this will permit the treatment of both eyes (if both are involved) without subjecting the patient to a second operation.

Prism therapy may be effective for small vertical deviations, though this is often limited by incomitance and torsion.

Surgical treatment of superior oblique myokymia may necessitate creating a superior oblique palsy. Patients with myokymia present with intermittent symptomatic oscillopsia and careful evaluation may reveal rhythmic intorsion of one eye accompanied by cyclodiplopia. This superior oblique myokymia may be transient, or it may persist and be extremely troublesome. Although superior oblique tenectomy has been suggested as a suitable treatment, this procedure may in turn result in superior oblique underaction. In this case, inferior oblique weakening may be done at the time of superior oblique myectomy or during a second procedure.

COMMENTS

Significant systemic disease is rarely associated with this condition, and extensive workup is not indicated unless other neurologic complaints warrant it. Surgical treatment can be very successful, and the assessment scheme devised by Knapp has been very useful.

REFERENCES

Ellis FD, Helveston EM: Superior oblique palsy: diagnosis and classification. Int Ophthalmol Clin 16:127–135, 1976.

Helveston EM, Giangiacomo JG, Ellis FD: Congenital absence of the superior oblique tendon. Trans Am Ophthalmol Soc 79:123–135, 1981.

Helveston EM, Krach D, Plager DA, Ellis FD: A new classification of superior oblique palsy based on congenital variations in the tendon. Ophthalmology 99:1609–1615, 1992.

Metz HS, Lerner H: The adjustable Harada-Ito procedure. Arch Ophthalmol 99:624–626, 1981.

Plager DA: Traction testing in superior oblique palsy. J Pediatr Ophthalmol Strabismus 27:136–140, 1990.

233 V-PATTERN STRABISMUS 378.03, 378.12

Jorge Alberto F. Caldeira, MD
São Paulo, Brazil

ETIOLOGY/INCIDENCE

Patients with a horizontal strabismus that becomes incomitant in vertical gaze, with more divergence of at least 15 prism diopters in the upward position as compared to the downward, are considered to have a significant V-pattern strabismus (Figure 233.1).

Horizontal, vertical and oblique muscle dysfunctions, orbital factors, and anomalies of muscle insertions (followed or preceded by cyclotorsion of the globes) can cause this incomitance. Loss of fusion may also predispose to cyclodeviations which, in turn, can produce a V-pattern. Heterotopia of extraocular muscle pulleys may be responsible for elevation or depression in adduction and a V- or A-pattern.

It is of paramount importance that a significant V-pattern is identified, properly characterized, and adequately corrected to obtain a good result, whether or not in conjunction with horizontal surgery. V-pattern is the most common anomaly among the alphabetical strabismus patterns. The relation of V-pattern : A-pattern is approximately 2 : 1.

COURSE/PROGNOSIS

Anomalous head posture is not rare in patients with a V-pattern. V esotropia with fusion in upward gaze can cause a chin depression; conversely, a patient with V exotropia and fusion in downward gaze may hold the chin in an elevated position. If the reward of fusion is not attained in any position of gaze the head posture is normal, unless there is a vertical imbalance in primary position.

A V-pattern is frequently found in association with Brown syndrome. The same holds true for bilateral paralysis of the trochlear nerve, although in some cases of unilateral paralysis the V-pattern can also be observed. In both instances, excyclotropia is a common sign, detected with the Maddox double-rod test and fundus examination.

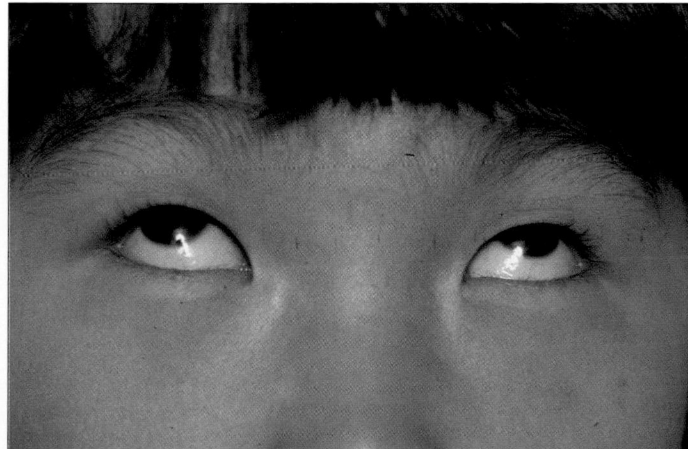

FIGURE 233.1. V-pattern strabismus.

DIAGNOSIS

If fusion is present in one postion of gaze, the effort to maintain it for a long time may cause asthenopia and/or diplopia. The deviation should be measured in the nine diagnostic positions of gaze, with the patient wearing the full refractive correction. Accommodation should be controlled with appropriate targets during the measurements. The above requirements are mandatory to avoid the appearance of a pseudo V-pattern or the concealment of a true V-pattern.

Measurements should be made at distance (6 meters) in primary position and with the eyes in position of 25 degrees elevation and 35 degrees depression, while fixating an accommodative target. The head is tilted backward or forward to obtain depression or elevation of the eyes. In very young patients an accurate prism-and-cover test in the diagnostic positions of gaze may be impossible. In this situation the examiner can move the head passively up and down, while the patient fixates a distant accommodative target. The deviation for near is measured at 33 centimeters.

In examining the binocular rotations the patient is encouraged to make extreme effort in the secondary and tertiary positions. Possible elevation in adduction, overaction of each inferior oblique and underaction of each superior oblique should be carefully registered.

The triad of bilateral elevation in adduction, bilateral overaction of the inferior oblique, and bilateral underaction of the superior oblique is more consistent in V-esotropia than in V-exotropia. Overaction of the superior oblique, bilateral or unilateral, is very seldom seen in V-esotropia, but is not rare in V-exotropia.

The significance of a V-pattern depends not only on its amount but also on whether it is functionally significant, interfering or not in the important primary and downward positions.

TREATMENT

Surgical. In most patients, an oblique muscle dysfunction is apparent and horizontal surgery should be combined with procedures on the inferior oblique muscles. Weakening surgeries on the inferior obliques have no significant effect on the deviation in primary position.

Graded recession of the overacting inferior oblique muscles is the weakening procedure of choice. Underacting superior oblique muscles frequently return to normal function after recession of the inferior obliques. Disinsertion, myotomy, or myectomy offer less predictable results than recession. The recession can be enhanced by anteriorization of the new insertion, but keeping it parallel to the temporal border of the inferior rectus. Recession and transposition (with the new insertion parallel to the insertion of the inferior rectus) usually causes some limitation of elevation. A denervation of the inferior oblique or its extirpation is very seldom indicated.

If the inferior obliques are not overacting they should not be touched. In case of a V esotropia, if both medial rectus muscles are to be recessed a downward one-half width or full tendon width transposition is indicated. If an uniocular recession-resection is planned, downward transposition of the medial rectus and upward transposition of the lateral rectus are indicated.

V exotropia without overacting inferior obliques is uncommon. Faced with a basic type of exodeviation requiring recession of the lateral rectus and resection of the medial rectus, the former is transposed upward and the latter, downward.

COMMENTS

V-pattern incomitance is a common finding in horizontal deviations. It requires a painstaking measurement of the deviation and investigation of overacting and underacting oblique muscles. A neglected significant V-pattern may transform a potentially good functional case into a disastrous one.

REFERENCES

Caldeira JAF: Some clinical characteristics of V-pattern exotropia and surgical outcome after bilateral recession of the inferior oblique muscle: A retrospective study of 22 consecutive patients and a comparison with V-pattern esotropia. Binocul Vis Strabismus Q 19:139–149, 2004.

Caldeira JAF: V-pattern esotropia: A review; and a study of the outcome after bilateral recession of the inferior oblique muscle: A retrospective study of 78 consecutive patients. Binocul Vis Strabismus Q 18:35–48, 2003.

Elliot RL, Nankin SJ: Anterior transposition of the inferior oblique. J Pediatr Ophthalmol Strabismus 18:35–38, 1981.

Goldstein JH: Monocular vertical displacement of the horizontal rectus muscles in the A and V patterns. Am J Ophthalmol 64:265–267, 1967.

Parks MM: The weakening surgical procedures for eliminating overaction of the inferior oblique muscle. Am J Ophthalmol 73:107–122, 1972.

SECTION

21 Eyelids

234 BLEPHAROCHALASIS 374.34

John H. Sullivan, MD
San Jose, California

ETIOLOGY

Blepharochalasis, a term coined by Fuchs a century ago, is a rare condition characterized by recurrent, episodic, painless periorbital edema, either unilateral or bilateral, which in its acute phase resembles angioedema. Evidence suggests an immunopathogenic mechanism, but the cause remains unknown. After repeated attacks, the eyelid skin loses elasticity and develops a characteristic thin, discolored appearance that resembles wrinkled cigarette paper or parchment. The upper eyelid fat pads may eventually atrophy, causing a typical skin concavity and psuedoepicanthal fold. The term *blepharochalasis* is frequently misused to indicate redundant skin of the aging eyelid, a common condition more accurately termed *dermatochalasis*.

- The pathogenesis is uncertain, but this condition may be immunogenic. Abundant IgA deposits are found around elastin fibers.
- Infrequently, occurrence is familial.
- There is an equal sex distribution.
- Sometimes blepharochalasis is associated with systemic illness, such as amyloidosis, dermatomyositis, or leukemia.
- There is an association with edema of the lips and thyroid enlargement in Laffer-Ascher syndrome.

COURSE/PROGNOSIS

The initial onset is usually before the age of 20 with unilateral or bilateral swelling of the eyelids and conjunctiva which can last hours to several days.

Proptosis indicates orbital involvement and the frequency and severity of repeated episodes tend to lessen with age. Occasionally, attacks are aggravated by a triggering event, such as fever, upper respiratory infection, menstruation, or weeping. Lacrimal gland prolapse is common and in the early phase, atrophy of the skin and orbital septum exposes the fat pads. There are perivascular inflammatory infiltrates during the acute stage and loss of elastin fibers in the quiescent stage. Fat atrophy eventually results in deep superior sulcus and a thin atrophic bronze-colored eyelid skin which resembles parchment. Multiple fine telangiectatic subcutaneous vessels are present and blepharoptosis results from thinning and atrophy of levator aponeurosis. Dehiscence of lateral canthal tendon causes horizontal phimosis and rounding of the lateral canthus.

DIAGNOSIS

The diagnosis is established by history and clinical features. There are no characteristic laboratory findings.

Differential diagnosis

- Angioedema: usually older age of onset; edema is seldom limited to the upper eyelids. There is an association with complement 1-esterase inhibitor deficiency and autoantibodies.
- Idiopathic lymphedema: unremitting brawny edema, usually in older patients.
- Dermatochalasis: a common aging process with redundant skin and fat prolapse.
- Tumor: progressively enlarging mass; the diagnosis is confirmed by biopsy results.
- Floppy lid syndrome: typically found in older, obese men; there is an association with papillary conjunctivitis.

TREATMENT

Active/acute phase: supportive

- Cold compresses can be used.
- Topical and systemic steroids are of limited value.

Quiescent/late stage: surgical

- Excise the redundant skin.
- Reposition the ectopic lacrimal gland.
- Reconstruct the lateral canthal tendon.
- The repair of blepharoptosis is often challenging.

COMMENTS

Little can be done to ameliorate the acute phase of blepharochalasis. The avoidance of triggering mechanisms, when present, may diminish the frequency of attacks. Immunopathologic studies are of interest, but as yet have not elucidated the cause or provided a rational form of treatment. Although not always possible, it is preferred to delay surgical reconstruction until the active phase is in complete remission. An episode of recurrent edema may spoil a satisfactory result.

REFERENCES

Bartley GB, Gibson L: Blepharochalasis associated with dermatomyositis and acute lymphocytic leukemia (Letter). Am J Ophthalmol 113:727–728, 1992.

Bergin DJ, McCord CD, Berger T, et al: Blepharochalasis. Br J Ophthalmol 72:863–867, 1988.

Custer PL, Tenzel RR, Kowalczyk AP: Blepharochalasis syndrome. Am J Ophthalmol 15;99:424–428, 1985.

Ghose S, Kalra BR, Dayal Y: Blepharochalasis with multiple system involvement. Br J Ophthalmol 68:529–532, 1984.

Held JL, Schneiderman P: A review of blepharochalasis and other causes of the lax, wrinkled eyelid. Cutis 45:91–94, 1990.

235 BLEPHAROCONJUNCTIVITIS 372.20

R. Doyle Stulting MD, PhD
Atlanta, Georgia
Evan S. Loft, MD
Atlanta, Georgia

ETIOLOGY

Blepharoconjunctivitis is one of the most commonly encountered diseases in ophthalmology. In 1982, a classification of chronic blepharitis was introduced that has served as a useful framework on which to build an understanding of this disease. This classification scheme of six clinically distinguishable groups was based on careful ophthalmologic and dermatologic examinations, cultures of the lids and conjunctiva, and lipid studies. The categories are:

1. Staphylococcal;
2. Seborrheic;
3. Mixed seborrheic/staphylococcal;
4. Seborrheic with meibomian seborrhea;
5. Seborrheic with secondary meibomianitis; and
6. Meibomian keratoconjunctivitis.

Any combination of the aforementioned entities may occur in any one patient. The latter three subtypes are commonly grouped together into one category referred to as meibomian gland dysfunction.

COURSE

Staphylococcal blepharoconjunctivitis

The symptoms of chronic staphylococcal blepharoconjunctivitis typically wax and wane, and they are usually of shorter duration than those of other types of blepharoconjunctivitis. Patients with staphylococcal blepharitis are younger (mean age, 42 years), compared to a mean age of 51 years for other types of blepharitis. Eighty percent of cases occur in women. This condition is treatable and curable, in contrast to other forms of the disease that can only be controlled.

Mixed seborrheic/staphylococcal conjunctivitis

Characteristically, these patients have a chronic history due to the seborrheic component, with periods of increased symptoms when the bacterial component becomes active.

Meibomian gland dysfunction

It is important for patients to understand that this chronic condition will require long-term lid hygiene and more aggressive treatment during exacerbations.

DIAGNOSIS

Clinical signs and symptoms

Chronic staphylococcal blepharoconjunctivitis

Clinical features of staphylococcal blepharoconjunctivitis include eyelid inflammation, erythema, possibly edema along the anterior ciliary portion of the lid, and, rarely, madarosis. The eyelid margin is frequently involved. There may be telangiectatic blood vessels along the lid margin.

Crusting of the lashes occurs with collarettes surrounding individual cilia. Anterior or posterior hordeola occur intermittently. Fifteen percent of patients develop bulbar and tarsal conjunctival changes, including injection and, when chronic, papillary hypertrophy of the tarsal conjunctiva. With acute exacerbation, a follicular response may develop over the inferior tarsal plate. A keratitis characterized by punctate epithelial erosions involving the inferior third of the cornea may occur, and may be secondary to staphylococcal exotoxin. Other possible causes of this keratitis include an abnormal blink mechanism and destabilization of the tear film. Marginal corneal infiltrates, phlyctenules, and corneal ulcers can also occur. Fifty percent of patients with staphylococcal blepharoconjunctivitis also have keratoconjunctivitis sicca that may have an associated corneal punctate epitheliopathy.

Mixed seborrheic/staphylococcal conjunctivitis

Mixed seborrheic/staphylococcal blepharoconjunctivitis exhibits signs of both types of blepharitis and an equal male/female distribution. The debris is characteristically an oily, greasy crusting on the anterior lid and collarettes on the lashes. Patients typically have more inflammation than those with seborrheic blepharoconjunctivitis alone.

Approximately 35% of patients with mixed seborrheic/staphylococcal blepharoconjunctivitis have associated keratoconjunctivitis sicca, and most patients also have seborrheic dermatitis. Keratoconjunctivitis is common in mixed seborrheic/staphylococcal blepharoconjunctivitis with mild inferior tarsal conjunctival papillary hypertrophy, bulbar conjunctival injection, punctate epithelial erosions over the inferior third of the cornea, and, rarely, follicular hypertrophy over the inferior tarsal conjunctiva.

Meibomian gland dysfunction

Meibomian gland dysfunction is most common in fair-skinned individuals, and there is an equal male/female ratio. The incidence of this disease increases with age. Keratoconjunctivitis sicca, seborrheic dermatitis and acne rosacea are frequently observed along with meibomian dysfunction. Chalazion incidence is higher in these patients. Tear break-up time is usually reduced.

Various lid margin findings may be observed on examination, including erythema, architectural irregularity, thickening, injection and telangiectasia. Meibomian gland apertures may be displaced, irregular, decreased in numbers, pouting with secretions, or plugged with yellow concretions. In meibomian dysfunction, pressure applied to the lid margins may not expulse Meibomian secretions or it can produce large amounts of cloudy or foamy secretions.

Laboratory findings

Currently, specific diagnostic tests for blepharoconjunctivitis are not available.

Eyelid and conjunctival cultures may be performed in cases of suspected staphylococcal blepharitis, especially if the condition is chronic or worsening with treatment. Antibiotics should be discontinued before culture. Of eyelid cultures from patients with chronic blepharitis, 96% were positive for *S. epidermidis*, 93% were positive for *Propionibacterium acnes*, 77% were positive for *Corynebacterium* sp., 11% were positive for *Acinetobacter* sp., and 10.5% were positive for *S. aureus*. Results of aerobic and anaerobic cultures from lids and conjunctiva showed that the only group of patients with blepharitis who had a significant percentage of positive cultures for *S. aureus* were those with clinically defined staphylococcal and mixed staphylococcal/seborrheic blepharitis. More than 80% of patients in the mixed group have positive eyelid cultures for *S. aureus*, and 50% have positive conjunctival cultures.

TREATMENT

Systemic

- Systemic antibiotics (occasionally for severe cases), such as tetracycline.

Ocular

- Warm compresses to eyelids for 5 to 10 minutes b.i.d.
- Eyelid scrubs using baby shampoo or a commercial lid scrub b.i.d.
- Bacitracin (first choice) or erythromycin ointment to the lid margins after lid scrubs and to the cul-de-sac at bedtime.
- Rarely, short-term topical steroids for hypersensitivity corneal infiltrates.
- Preservative-free artificial tears and other dry eye treatments.
- Dermatologic consultation for seborrheic dermatitis.

PRECAUTIONS

Conjunctivitis medicamentosa may occur, especially in patients with associated keratoconjunctivitis sicca. Eyelid scrubs, soaps, and artificial tear preservatives may also cause hypersensitivity and allergic reactions. The use of preservative-free tears is recommended. Discontinuation of all potentially toxic medication should result in significant improvement of keratitis medicamentosa. Alternative medical treatments must be considered in patients with specific known drug allergies or intolerance to drug-induced side effects. Use of tetracyclines during pregnancy is contraindicated.

Occasionally, more severe keratitis, phlyctenules, and corneal ulceration may require more intensive therapy.

COMMENTS

Blepharoconjunctivitis is commonly encountered by the ophthalmologist. Close observation of the specific eyelid, conjunctival, and corneal changes will help determine the type of blepharoconjunctivitis present and thus determine the type of treatment regimen best suited for the individual patient. Eyelid hygiene and topical antibiotics will cure or control staphylococcal or mixed seborrheic/staphylococcal blepharoconjunctivitis. When these therapies fail, attention should be given to other possible diagnoses or additional underlying problems. Discontinuation of all therapy and culturing or reculturing of the eyelids and conjunctiva may be indicated.

REFERENCES

Bowman RW, Dougherty JM, McCulley JP: Chronic blepharitis and dry eyes. Int Ophthalmol Clin 27:27–35, 1987.

Bowman RW, Miller K, McCulley JP: Diagnosis and treatment of chronic blepharitis. In: Focal points: clinical modules for ophthalmologists. San Francisco, American Academy of Ophthalmology, 1988.

Driver PJ, Lemp MA: Meibomian gland dysfunction. Surv Ophthalmol 40:343–367, 1996.

Groden LR, Murphy B, Rodnite J, et al: Lid flora in blepharitis. Cornea 10:50–53, 1991.

McCulley JP: Blepharoconjunctivitis. Int Ophthalmol Clin 24:65–77, 1984.

McCulley JP, Dougherty J, Deneau DG: Classification of chronic blepharitis. Ophthalmology 89:1173–1180, 1982.

Smolin G, Okumoto MA: Staphylococcal blepharitis. Arch Ophthalmol 95:812–816, 1977.

236 DISTICHIASIS 743.63

Phillip Hyunchul Choo, MD
Sacramento, California
Sumaira A. Arain, MD
Sacramento, California

Distichiasis is a condition in which lashes grow posterior to the normal row of lashes. It can be either congenital or acquired and may present as only a few isolated eyelashes, or as a complete accessory row of lashes. These lashes often rub directly on or become matted against the cornea, causing persistent eye pain and corneal damage.

ETIOLOGY/INCIDENCE

Congenital distichiasis

This is a rare condition, which may occur sporadically or as an autosomal dominant trait with variable expressivity and high penetrance. It is a developmental anomaly in which embryonic pilosebaceous units differentiate into hair follicles rather than into meibomian glands.

Congenital distichiasis can be isolated or occur in association with some forms of familial lymphedema, especially the 4th type of late-onset hereditary lymphedema that presents during adolescence. Other associated abnormalities include entropion, ptosis, congenital corneal hypesthesia, cleft lip and palate, vertebral anomalies, extradural cysts, webbed neck, yellow nails, peripheral vascular anomalies, trisomy 18, congenital heart defects, blepharocheilodontic syndrome and other systemic anomalies.

Acquired distichiasis

This is a more common form, and is often seen secondary to certain stimuli that provoke a metaplastic change within or near the meibomian gland. This metaplastic change can occur with diseases that affect both the eyelid margin and the conjunctiva, such as chronic blepharitis, staphylococcal hypersensitivity, meibomian gland dysfunction and meibomianitis, Stevens-Johnson syndrome, ocular cicatricial pemphigoid and chemical ocular injuries.

COURSE/PROGNOSIS

Distichiasis, if left untreated, may lead to corneal thinning, scarring, or even ulceration.

DIAGNOSIS

On slit-lamp examination, abnormal lashes are noted arising from or near the meibomian gland orifices. The cornea should be evaluated for any epithelial defects or signs of permanent scarring.

Clinical signs and symptoms

Symptoms may include decrease in vision, eye pain and irritation, foreign body sensation and tearing.

A penlight or slit lamp examination should reveal eyelashes growing posteriorly (along where one would expect the orifices of the meibomian glands to be) to the normal row of lashes. There may be secondary signs such as epithelial breakdown of the cornea, corneal scarring or pannus formation, and conjunctival injection and chemosis.

Differential diagnosis

Distichiasis should be differentiated from trichiasis and entropion. Trichiasis is a condition in which eyelashes grow from the normal anterior portion of the eyelid margin but are turned in or misdirected towards the eye. Entropion is a condition in which the entire eyelid margin turns inward.

PROPHYLAXIS

Proper and chronic treatment of diseases such as blepharitis and ocular cicatricial pemphigoid will decrease the stimuli to create the formation of acquired distichiatic eyelashes.

TREATMENT

Medical

No treatment may be necessary if the patient is asymptomatic and without keratopathy. For temporary symptomatic relief of epithelial breakdown of the cornea, lubricating drops and ointment are useful. Therapeutic soft contact lenses may also be helpful to protect the cornea in cases of corneal epithelial breakdown, as well as to provide symptomatic relief.

Surgical

Various surgical procedures have been described for the treatment of distichiasis. Epilation with electrolysis is useful in treating small numbers or a focal area of distichiatic lashes. This procedure is often done in the office with a local infiltrative block, while general anesthesia is required in treating infants and young children. With the aid of a slit-lamp or an operating microscope, the distichiatic eyelashes are identified and electrolysized. Various instruments such as the Ellman Surgitron (Ellman International Inc., Oceanside, NY) are commercially available for performing electrolysis of eyelashes. While performing electrolysis, it is important to treat the entire hair follicle. The eyelash should pull out effortlessly from the eyelid margin after treatment. If it does not, the follicle should be retreated. The success rate for trichiatic eyelashes is approximately 60–70%, and thus repeat treatment may be necessary, especially when treating multiple eyelashes.

Cryosurgery is an option for the treatment of a wider area of distichiasis. A double freeze-thaw treatment down to –20°C is recommended for permanent destruction of the lash follicles. Since temperatures of –30°C and lower may cause tissue necrosis and subsequent scarring, the use of a thermocouple to monitor actual tissue temperature is recommended. Furthermore, this approach is non-selective. The normal, more anterior eyelashes may also be permanently damaged by cryotherapy, leading to complete madarosis. For this reason, eyelid splitting approaches are more commonly used to treat wide areas of distichiatic eyelashes.

Lid splitting procedures involve an incision made in the eyelid margin immediately anterior to the row of distichiatic eyelashes. The use of a chalazion clamp and an ocular surgery blade are helpful. The incision is continued to about 3 mm in depth to expose the entire distichiatic eyelash follicle. Depending on the surgeon's preference, the distichiatic lash follicles can then be treated either with direct application of electrolysis, direct excision, or cryotherapy applied to the conjunctival side of the eyelid margin. Later, the incision may be closed directly with sutures, or the anterior lamella can be recessed approximately 2 mm in relation to the posterior lamella and fixated to the tarsal plate.

In 1993, O'Donnell and Collin reviewed a series of 24 patients with distichiasis who underwent treatment with epilation, cryotherapy, or a lid splitting procedure followed by cryotherapy to the posterior lamella. They found that lid splitting with cryotherapy relieved symptoms without retreatment in 87% of patients. In 1997, Vaughn and others reported the results of an eyelid splitting procedure in 17 eyelids of 5 patients with distichiasis. After the lid was split, each aberrant eyelash follicle was individually excised or microhyphrecated and subsequently removed. This approach yielded excellent functional and cosmetic results. Furthermore, White in 1975 described a surgery in which the posterior portion of the eyelid margin containing the distichiatic eyelashes was directly excised. A mucous membrane graft was then sutured in place to cover the defect.

COMPLICATIONS

All of the above treatments could result in recurrence of distichiasis, formation of trichiasis, lid notching and cicatricial entropion.

Cryotherapy may result in significant post-operative swelling of the lid and the conjunctiva. Furthermore, cryotherapy applied to the conjunctiva may aggravate an underlying conjunctival disorder, as well as cause conjunctival scarring and shortening. In addition, lid necrosis can occur if the treatment temperature is –30°C or less.

Eyelid splitting procedures may also lead to some potential complications. These include prolonged eyelid edema, keratinization of the posterior eyelid margin, and recurrence of the distichiatic eyelashes. Lastly, one should avoid damage to the normal eyelash follicles to avoid permanent madarosis.

Supported by an unrestricted grant from Research to Prevent Blindness, Inc., New York, New York.

REFERENCES

Anderson RL, Harvey JT: Lid splitting and posterior lamella cryosurgery for congenital and acquired distichiasis. Arch Ophthalmol 99:631–634, 1981.

Choo PH: Distichiasis, trichiasis, and entropion: advances in management. Int Opthalmol Clin 42(2):75–87, 2002.

Frueh BR: Treatment of distichiasis with cryotherapy. Surg Ophthalmol 12:100–103, 1981.

O'Donnell BA, Collin JR: Distichiasis: management with cryotherapy to the posterior lamella. Br J Ophthalmol 77:289–292, 1993.

White JH: Correction of distichiasis by tarsal resection and mucous membrane grafting. Am J Ophthalmol 80:507–508, 1975.

237 ECTROPION 374.10

Kostas G. Boboridis, MD, PhD
Thessaloniki, Greece

Ectropion is an eyelid malposition presenting from simple horizontal laxity to an outward turning of the lid margin away from its normal apposition to the globe. It may involve either eyelid but it mainly affects the lower.

ETIOLOGY/INCIDENCE

Ectropion is classified as both congenital and acquired. Acquired ectropion is further classified into four categories according to the underlying etiology, as involutional, paralytic, cictricial, or mechanical (Figure 237.1).

Congenital ectropion is caused by vertical shortage of the anterior lamella on the lateral third of the lower eyelid often combined with canthal tendon laxity. It is frequently associated with additional facial abnormalities as in Down syndrome, blepharophimosis and Möbius syndrome or lamellar ichthyosis. Isolated ectropion due to horizontal lid laxity is very rare congenital condition called euryblepharon.

Involutional, or *senile, ectropion* is the most common type encountered in the aging population. Senile stretching or weakening of the medial and more frequently the lateral canthal tendon, dehiscence of the lower lid retractors, atrophy of the orbicularis muscle, and hypertrophy of the tarsus with fragmentation of its elastic and collagen fibers result in an outward turning of the lid. Involutional enophthalmos may exacerbate the condition. Although the upper eyelid can be affected in a condition called floppy eyelid syndrome, involutional ectropion usually is described for the lower eyelid.

Paralytic ectropion is caused by facial nerve palsy and is often unilateral. Bell's palsy, trauma, cerebrovascular accidents, and damage to the peripheral seventh nerve during tumor removal are the most frequent causes. Loss of orbicularis muscle tone and decreased support to gravitational pull by stretching of the canthal tendons results in ectropion which becomes more pronounced with time.

Cicatricial ectropion is the result of scarring or contracture of the skin and/or orbicularis muscle causing vertical shortening of the eyelid due to trauma, inflammatory processes or skin disorders. Overzealous blepharoplasty of the lower lid can result in a cicatricial ectropion or lid retraction.

Mechanical ectropion is caused by the weight of a mass on the anterior lamella or mid-face ptosis, pulling the lid down. A tumor of the lower eyelid, fluid accumulation secondary to sinusitis, thyroid disease, lupus, or other medical problems can result in mechanical ectropion. Patients with mid-face ptosis can have sagging of the cheek and face, resulting in a mechanical ectropion.

COURSE/PROGNOSIS

All forms of ectropion, especially involutional and paralytic, worsen with time if untreated, resulting in conjunctival hypertrophy and keratinization. The increased exposure of the ocular surface may result in poor lubrication of the corneal epithelium with an increased risk of exposure keratopathy and infection. Punctum eversion, sagging of the lid and lacrimal pump failure usually result in chronic epiphora.

DIAGNOSIS

Clinical signs and symptoms

The main symptoms are chronic epiphora and recurrent conjunctivitis. Examination of the eyelid position and contour, punctum position and size, orbicularis function, Bell's phenomenon, tear film stability and patency of the lacrimal system as well as recognition of cicatricial components are all necessary in evaluating ectropion. The degree of horizontal laxity is assessed with the *distraction test,* by drawing the center of the eyelid away from the globe and measuring the distance. More than 8–10 mm is considered abnormal. The eyelid elasticity and orbicularis tone are assessed with the *snap back test* by pulling the lid from the globe and releasing it. An eyelid that snaps back only after the patient has blinked is considered abnormal. A lateral pull on the lid reveals medial canthal tendon laxity when the punctum is drawn to or beyond the medial limbus. Medial pull reveals lateral canthal tendon laxity when the palpebral angle is pulled for more than 10 mm from the lateral orbital rim.

TREATMENT

There is no systemic treatment.

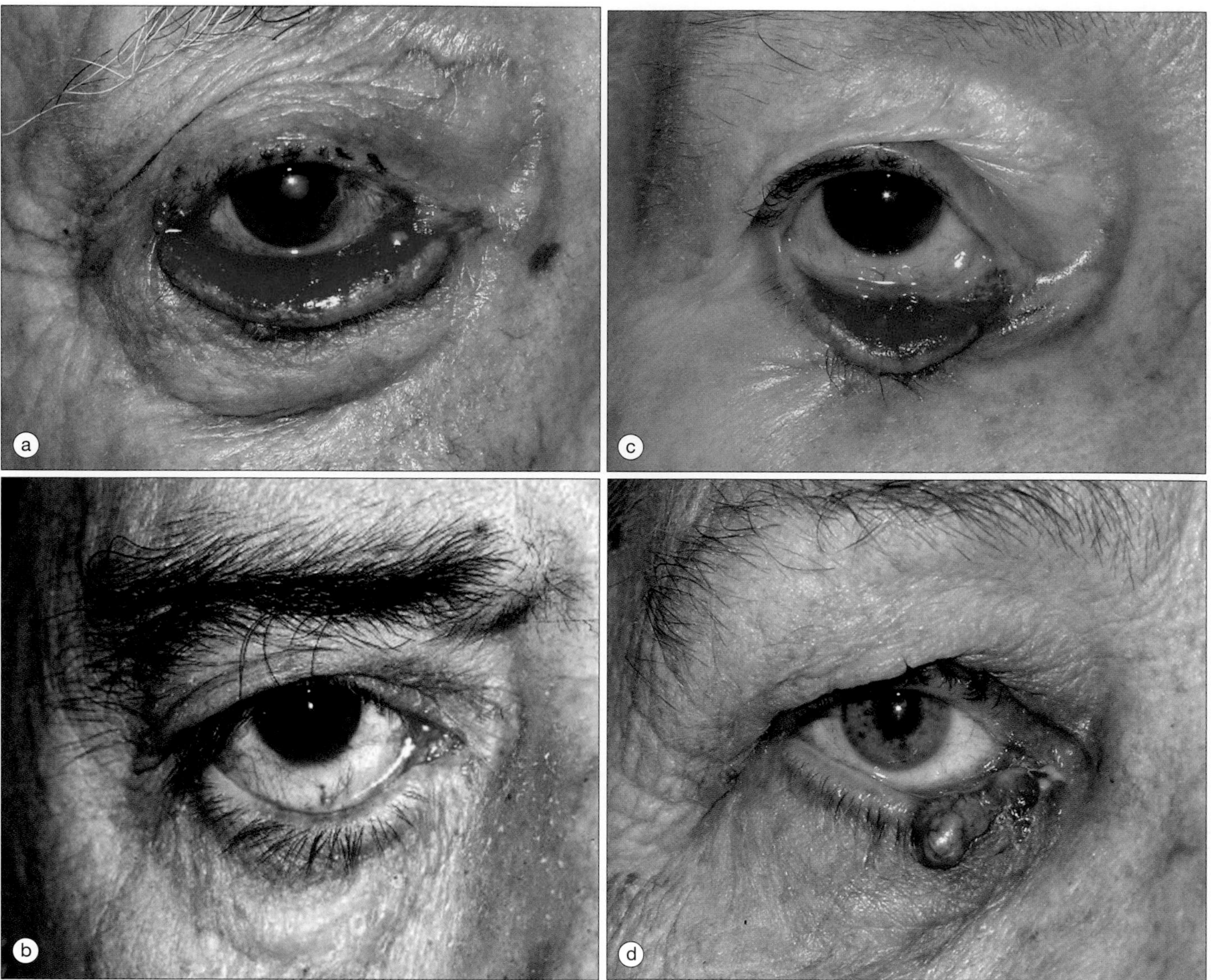

FIGURE 237.1. a) Involutional. b) Paralytic. c) Cicatricial. d) Mechanical.

Ocular

Asymptomatic or mild cases require only topical artificial tear drops. Intense lubrication and antibiotic ointment are indicated for symptomatic patients with chronic conjunctivitis. The eyelids may need to be taped closed at bedtime, especially in paralytic cases. Softening of the skin and lid margin with topical steroid ointment is beneficial in advanced cases. Intralesional steroid injection may soften the scar in cicatricial ectropion. Surgical intervention is reserved for chronic symptomatic cases that require permanent solution.

Surgical

Congenital

Severe and symptomatic cases require a full-thickness skin graft for vertical lengthening of anterior lamella combined with canthal tendon tightening.

Involutional

For mild cases, the inverting suture technique can shorten the posterior lamella and provide temporary relief. Three double-armed sutures are passed in mattress fashion through the lid, from the palpebral conjunctiva at the inferior border of the tarsus out cutaneously at the level of the orbital rim.

For generalized horizontal laxity, tightening of the lid can be performed by resecting a full-thickness wedge of the eyelid at the lateral canthal angle, as described by Bick. However, this does not address and rather exacerbates canthal tendon laxity resulting in rounding of the fissure.

For punctum eversion a medial spindle procedure is performed, in which a diamond-shaped excision of tarsoconjunctiva is performed in the posterior lamella bellow the punctum. A double armed absorbable suture engaging the retractors closes the defect and exits through the skin below the level of incision, effectively acting as an inverting and posterior lamella shortening suture.

When there is punctum eversion with horizontal laxity, the 'lazy T' procedure is indicated in which the medial spindle is combined with a medial full thickness wedge excision. If medial tendon laxity is present a canthal ligament (anterior or posterior limp) plication is also performed.

The method of choice to correct involutional ectropion and any form of horizontal laxity is the lateral tarsal strip or canthal sling procedure. This addresses the most common cause of ectropion, which is laxity of the lateral canthal tendon. A lateral canthotomy and an inferior cantholysis are performed with separation of the anterior and posterior lamellae. A tarsal strip is fashioned from the lateral tarsus by removal of skin, orbicularis and conjunctival epithelium. The lid is shortened horizontally, and the shortened tarsal strip is reattached anatomically with a nonabsorbable suture to the periosteum of Whitnall's tubercle 2 mm inside of the lateral orbital rim. The canthal angle and the skin incision are reconstructed with suture.

In addition to the tarsal strip procedure and in combination to any of the above, some surgeons believe the lower eyelid retractors must be reattached to the inferior border of the tarsus for vertical shortening of the eyelid similar to entropion repair.

Paralytic

Paralytic horizontal laxity may be transient and should be observed with conservative treatment for 3 to 6 months if the ocular surface is stable and not at risk for exposure and infection. Surgical repair is similar to that for involutional ectropion. A medial cantholpasty with the Otis Lee procedure and/or lateral tarsorrhaphy may be necessary to correct corneal exposure due to lagophthalmos and ectropion. A fascia lata sling can be used to support the eyelid in advanced cases.The fascia strip is sutured to the medial canthal tendon, placed between the orbicularis muscle and the lower lid tarsus and then attached to the lateral canthal tendon and orbital rim. Synthetic material may also used. Temporalis muscle transfer can be performed along with other reconstructive facial surgery to reanimate the lids with better functional and cosmetic results.

Cicatricial

Cicatricial ectropion is corrected by lengthening the contracted anterior lamella. Z-plasty can address an isolated scar in a particular direction. Full-thickness skin grafts or flaps from the lateral upper eyelid are necessary to relieve generalized tension and also lengthen the lid vertically.

Mechanical

Removal of the lesion causing increased weight is the treatment of choice. Tumor excision and horizontal tightening of the reconstructed lid is indicated in other cases. Occasionally, a suborbicularis oculi fat (SOOF) lift is indicated in patients with mid-face ptosis with sagging of the cheek and face causing vertical shortage of the lid.

COMPLICATIONS

Possible complications of an untreated ectropion include the following:

- Epiphora and chronic conjunctivitis;
- Conjunctival hyperemia and hypertrophy with keratinization;
- Exposure keratopathy and epithelial breakdown;
- Corneal infection with ulceration.

COMMENTS

Many procedures have been described for the treatment of ectropion. Before the appropriate treatment can be instituted, the surgeon must accurately diagnose the causative factor and type of ectropion as well as the specific anatomical structure that requires surgical intervention. In all cases of ectropion, the eye is at an increased risk for exposure keratopathy and epithelial breakdown, which may result in infection, ulceration, scarring and permanent visual loss. Patients with ectropion must be observed and correctly treated when indicated to prevent potential complications from ocular surface exposure.

REFERENCES

Anderson RL, Gordy DD: The tarsal strip procedure. Arch Ophthalmol 97:2192–2196, 1979.

Bick MW: Surgical management of orbital tarsal disparity. Arch Ophthalmol 75:386–389, 1966.

Collin JRO: Ectropion. A manual of systematic eyelid surgery. London, Churchill Livingstone, 1995: 27–40.

Leatherbarrow B: Lower eyelid ectropion. Oculoplastic surgery. London, Martin Dunitz, 2002:69–83.

Smith B: The 'Lazy-T' correction of entropion of the lower punctum. Arch Ophthalmol 94:171–2, 1976.

238 ENTROPION 370.00

Roger A. Dailey, MD
Portland, Oregon
Robert N. Tower, MD
Seattle, Washington

INTRODUCTION

Entropion of the eyelids is defined as an inversion of the eyelid margin so that the margin itself, the cilia, and sometimes the external keratinizing squamous epithelium of the eyelid are brought into contact with the surface of the eye, producing irritation and abrasion. This discussion is directed toward involutional entropion of the lower eyelid unless otherwise specified. The references provide more specific information regarding upper lid and cicatricial entropion.

ETIOLOGY

- The lower lid retractors lose control of the inferior margin of the tarsus, allowing it to rotate anteriorly and superiorly.
- The preseptal muscle tends to override the pretarsal muscle.
- Horizontal lid laxity increases the ability of the eyelid to turn in.
- Enophthalmos as occurs in aging was once thought to be a factor in this process, but this has been shown to be incorrect.

COURSE/PROGNOSIS

Entropion can occur in either the upper or lower eyelid. This condition is irritating and potentially sight-threatening in that the skin and lashes can mechanically abrade the corneal epithelium, causing pain, photophobia, and increased susceptibility to infectious corneal infiltration that could lead to scarring or progress to endophthalmitis.

Patients typically present with complaints of eye irritation, photophobia, and foreign body sensation. Occasionally, patients have noticed the in-turning of the lid and lashes; they may be using tape to keep the lid everted. With appropriate surgical management, the prognosis for full recovery is excellent with rare recurrence after surgery. Cicatricial variants (e.g. cicatricial pemphigoid) progress, and treatment tends to be more aggressive and have a lower long-term success rate. Associated corneal abnormalities usually require topical antibiotics and tear substitutes.

DIAGNOSIS

- A broad classification scheme includes congenital, cicatricial, spastic and involutional.
- The differential diagnosis includes epiblepharon, epicanthal folds, trichiasis and distichiasis.
- The history includes pain, irritation, chronic allergies, chronic glaucoma medication use, eyelid observed turning in, and associated systemic disease.
- The physical examination reveals lower eyelid laxity, conjunctival scarring with or without keratinization, eyelid observed turning in, trichiasis and superficial punctate keratitis.
- If actual lower eyelid turning-in is not see, the clinician should have the patient look up and the grasp the patient's preseptal muscle as in a 'snap test.' Then, the patient should look down, squeezing orbicularis, as the clinician lets go. This will demonstrate the entropion.

TREATMENT

Medical

Be sure to manage any associated ocular surface problems with the appropriate topical antibiotics and/or lubricants. Temporary taping of the eyelid into a better position will help avoid further keratitis until a more definitive procedure can be performed.

Surgical

Quickert sutures can be placed with the use of local anesthesia. This is a quick method to relieve the entropion and can be done in the examination lane or at the bedside. It should not be considered definitive but can last for weeks to months. One needle of double-armed suture of 5-0 chromic catgut or 5-0 Vicryl suture is placed deep in the conjunctival fornix and brought anteriorly and superiorly through the lid tissues so it exits the skin near the lid margin, beneath the lash line. The second needle is then passed in a similar fashion 3 to 4 mm lateral. Two additional double-armed sutures are placed: one medially and one laterally. The sutures are tied, causing an eversion of the lid margin.

A definitive approach to involutional entropion involves a lateral cantholysis followed by transconjunctival incision just inferior to the tarsus. The inferior retractors are then isolated and reattached to the anterior/inferior portion of the tarsus with multiple interrupted sutures. The lid then can be shortened using a tarsal strip procedure. The lateral canthus is reformed with tarsus-to-lateral rim periosteal sutures, ensuring that the tarsus is slightly posterior to the rim. Closure of the skin is completed. An alternative would be to use a subciliary incision to accomplish the same thing, particularly if there is no significant horizontal lid laxity and horizontal shortening is not necessary.

Correction of cicatricial entropion generally involves the placement of a spacer in the posterior aspect of the lower lid after transconjunctival incision. Acellular dermis or hard palate mucosa is an excellent choice; others include sclera, fascia, autogenous tarsus, nasal septal mucosa, and buccal mucosa.

COMMENTS

Involutional and cicatricial entropion requires definitive surgical treatment to avoid sight-threatening secondary corneal complications. The success rate of this surgery when performed by experienced physicians is extremely high.

REFERENCES

Anderson RL: The tarsal strip. In: Transactions of the New Orleans Academy of Ophthalmology. St Louis, CV Mosby, 1982:352–363.

D'Ostroph AO, Dailey RA: Cicatricial entropion associated with chronic dipivefrin application. Ophthalmic Plast Reconstr Surg 17(5):328–31, 2001.

Jones LT, Reeh MJ, Wobig JL: Senile entropion. A new concept for correction. Am J Ophthalmol 74:321–329, 1972.

Quickert MH, Wilkes DI, Dryden RM: Non-incisional correction of epiblepharon and congenital entropion. Arch Ophthalmol 101:778–781, 1981.

Weiss FA: Surgical treatment of entropion. J Int Coll Surg 21:758–760, 1954.

239 EPICANTHUS 743.63

Roger A. Dailey, MD
Portland, Oregon
John D. Ng, MD, MS, FACS
Portland, Oregon

The term *epicanthus* refers to a vertical fold of skin that is located between the medial canthus and the nose and may cover part or all of the inner canthus of the eye.

ETIOLOGY/INCIDENCE

- Epicanthal folds are common in infants and children of all races but are a characteristic finding in persons of all ages with Asian ancestry.
- Fetal alcohol syndrome often exhibits epicanthus.
- Rarely, the blepharophimosis tetrad can occur as a developmental anomaly, but more commonly it is transmitted as an autosomal dominant trait, linked to the *3q21-24* gene, with 100% penetrance.
- Structurally, the folds appear to be related to tension in underlying excessive orbicularis muscle, with a relative lack of attachment of the skin to the underlying structures. Differential growth rates of skin in the medial canthal area and tension placed on the skin by the underlying orbicularis also may play roles.

COURSE/PROGNOSIS

- The majority of children of Asian ancestry will lose these folds during and after puberty, but the folds persist in 2% to 5% of whites.
- Surgical management relieves the condition in as many as 90% of cases.
- Surgical complications include visible scars, asymmetry, recurrence, and, rarely, infection.

DIAGNOSIS

- The diagnosis of epicanthus is easily made on external examination.
- Amblyopia is rare in association with epicanthus and is usually associated with other problems, such as anisometropia and astigmatism.
- No spinal abnormalities have been reported from patients who have had compensatory head tilt from blepharoptosis for many years.

Types of epicanthus

Epicanthus supraciliaris is a vertical fold of skin that extends from just below the brow to an area just over the infraorbital rim, usually obscuring the caruncle.

In *epicanthus palpebralis*, the skin fold extends from the medial aspect of the upper lid to the medial aspect of the lower lid in a nearly symmetric fashion and often obscures the caruncle. This is the most common configuration.

Epicanthus tarsalis refers to a condition in which a fold begins laterally and extends over the entire eyelid, ending in the medial canthus. This is the typical Asian upper lid configuration. Epiblepharon of the upper lids is distinguished from epicanthus tarsalis by its lack of true superior palpebral fold and the presence of a fold of skin that overlaps the eyelid margin and presses the lashes against the cornea.

Epicanthus inversus is similar to epicanthus tarsalis but involves the lower lid. It usually occurs as a part of Komoto's tetrad of blepharoptosis, blepharophimosis, telecanthus, and epicanthus inversus; *blepharophimosis* refers to narrowing of the palpebral aperture in its horizontal dimension.

TREATMENT

Surgical

In general, epicanthus tarsalis, palpebralis, and supraciliaris will diminish with age as the child's nasal dorsum becomes more prominent. If ptosis repair must be performed and significantly worsens the fold, the fold can be repaired simultaneously. Often, consideration is given to surgery before the child is of school age or soon after starting school to avoid or at least minimize some of the psychologic problems regarding body image and self-esteem that can arise. Older children can be operated on with mild sedation, and the results are more predictable.

- Skin resection should be avoided in the surgical management of epicanthus tarsalis, palpebralis, and supraciliaris because it can actually accentuate the anomaly. A preferred approach is to incise the skin directly over the fold, remove the orbicularis muscle in this area, and close the skin with deep attachments to maintain a crease and remove the fold. The crease will soften with time, but the fold should not recur.
- Epicanthus inversus typically shows little improvement with age. In these children, the skin tends to be very stiff at an early age and difficult to work with surgically but becomes more amenable to intervention at a later age. This condition generally responds best to Verwey's Y-to-V operation, double Z-plasty, Mustard's technique, or the five-flap procedure. Spaeth's technique, which involves excision of a portion of the fold of skin, is generally reserved for mild cases of epicanthus inversus.
- In 1989, Anderson and Nowinski described the five-flap technique, which they consider to be the best application for epicanthus inversus. This is a modified Y-to-V procedure combined with a double Z-plasty. It has the advantage of being simple to mark out on the lid, and the flaps are small and relatively easy to transpose.
- In cases in which there is associated telecanthus, it should be repaired at the same time with medial canthal tendon resection or transnasal wiring. It is important to avoid injuring the canaliculus or lacrimal sac. A lateral canthoplasty can be performed at the same time in cases of blepharophimosis.

COMMENTS

Epicanthus supraciliaris, palpebralis, and tarsalis tend to regress spontaneously with maturity and only occasionally require surgery. Typically, this requires only resection of underlying muscle and then deep skin fixation. Epicanthus inversus rarely improves with age and generally responds to surgical managements such as a Y-to-V procedure, Z-plasties, or the five-flap technique. Amblyopia can occur in these patients and should be checked for at regular examinations in the early years of the patient's life.

REFERENCES

Callahan A: Surgical correction of the blepharophimosis syndromes. Trans Am Acad Ophthalmol Otolaryngol 77:687–695, 1973.

Hughes WL: Surgical treatment of congenital palpebral phimosis: the Y-V operation. Arch Ophthalmol 54:586–590, 1955.

Johnson CC: Epicanthus and epiblepharon. Arch Ophthalmol 96:1030–1033, 1978.

Jordan DR, Anderson RL: Epicanthal folds: a deep tissue approach. Arch Ophthalmol 107:1532–1535, 1989.

Stromland K: Visual impairment and ocular abnormalities in children with fetal alcohol syndrome. Addict Biol 9:153–7, 2004.

240 EYELID CONTUSIONS 921.1, LACERATIONS 870.8, AND AVULSIONS 871.3

Robert C. Della Rocca, MD, FACS
New York, New York
David A. Della Rocca, MD
New York, New York
John Nassif, MD
Clearwater, Florida
John Koh, MD
Southfield, Michigan

Eyelid contusions, lacerations, and canthal avulsions may result in severe functional or structural abnormalities. Complete ocular evaluation and prompt determination of the extent of adnexal injury and the absence or presence of canalicular laceration allows for appropriate and timely repair of the injury. This will promote optimum functional and cosmetic results while limiting the possibility of early and late complications.

DIAGNOSIS

Clinical signs and symptoms

On inspection of the eyelids and periorbital region, ecchymosis and edema can be very significant, obscuring the location and extent of lacerations. It is important to rule out direct or indirect ocular injury. A careful history will help in raising suspicion that systemic, ocular or orbital injury may have occurred. Visual assessment, including visual acuity testing and pupil and ocular motility evaluation should be done, in addition to slit lamp microscopy, tonometry and ophthalmoscopy. This assessment, which should include adnexal evaluation, may be limited by significant periorbital and eyelid edema. Supportive measures including the use of cool compresses can be helpful prior to detailed ocular and adnexal examination. In some cases, thorough evaluation must be delayed until anesthesia is available in the operating room. Canalicular involvement and canthal displacement must be recognized to allow for appropriate surgical planning. Ptosis is common with upper eyelid lacerations and may be due to edema or direct injury to the levator complex.

Laboratory findings

Computed tomography scanning is advised if an orbital fracture is suspected. Orbital fractures are suggested by the presence of extraocular motility dysfunction, infraorbital anesthesia, globe displacement, marked periorbital edema or signs of orbital emphysema. Magnetic resonance imaging (MRI) gives excellent soft tissue contrast, but is less effective in defining orbital fractures. B-scan ultrasonography or the other scanning modalities listed above are helpful in evaluation of the globe and optic nerve if the eyelids can not be opened secondary to edema.

TREATMENT

Severe pain is uncommon with injury to adnexal tissue. If pain control is needed we recommend acetaminophen or acetaminophen in combination with codeine. Tetanus immunization may be necessary if the patient has not had a tetanus booster within the last 5 years. Broad-spectrum antibiotics are recommended, especially in the context of animal or human bites.

If a wound is older than 2 days, we consider debridement of the granulation tissue from the wound edges at the start of the case. We recommend primary repair of the tissues unless there is significant bacterial contamination or extensive tissue loss.

Simple partial lacerations of the skin can be repaired with 6-0 nylon or silk sutures in an interrupted fashion. Full thickness lacerations are repaired in a stepwise fashion. First, the lid margin is closed using 6-0 silk sutures in 3 interrupted passes through the meibomian gland orifices, lash line and at the grey line sequentially. It is important to make sure that the placement of the first silk suture approximates the tarsal plate neatly. These three sutures are tied and left long for later tying to the skin closing sutures (away from the cornea). Next, the tarsal plate, distal to the lid margin, is closed with 5-0 absorbable suture. Last, the skin is closed with interrupted 6-0 silk sutures.

Full thickness tissue loss is uncommon and can be mimicked by edema and wound contracture. Minimal tissue loss characterized by loss of up to one-quarter of the eyelid may be managed by a full thickness closure combined with a lateral canthotomy and cantholysis. Moderate tissue loss (one quarter to one half of the eyelid) might necessitate a skin advancement flap of Tenzel to extend the length of the eyelid prior to closure. Severe tissue loss of greater than half of the eyelid length would usually necessitate an eyelid sharing procedure such as the Hughes procedure for inferior eyelid loss or the Cutler–Beard flap for upper eyelid loss.

Avulsions or lacerations of the canthus indicate the reattachment of the tissues to the appropriate level of periostium. Injury to the lateral canthus can be repaired by the creation of a lateral tarsal strip with or without a periostial flap. A medial avulsion requires the reattachment of the posterior limb of the medial canthal tendon to the posterior lacrimal crest periorbita. The use of transnasal wiring may be necessary if there is severe tissue or bone destruction.

COMPLICATIONS

- Ptosis: due to levator complex injury, severe traumatic edema (levator aponeurosis stretching and dehiscence), or on a neurogenic basis.
- Epiphora: due to canalicular laceration, lacrimal sac injury, or punctal eversion.
- Corneal exposure: due to post-repair eyelid malpositions or lagophthalmos.
- Eyelid malpositions: ectropion, entropion, eyelid retraction.
- Scar hypertrophy or depigmentation.

COMMENTS

On an emergent basis, concurrent with adnexal and canthal injuries, the presence of symptomatic and compressive orbital hemorrhage must be treated promptly with a lateral canthotomy and cantholysis. Following the cantholysis, the periorbita is opened to evacuate the hemorrhage and clots.

When possible, avoid discarding apparently devitalized tissue, whether partially or completely avulsed. Periorbital tissue has extensive vascularity and may survive trauma otherwise deemed unsurvivable. This tissue may be reattached at the site of the defect.

REFERENCES

Collin JR, Tyers AG: Colour atlas of ophthalmic plastic surgery. Churchill Livingstone, 1998:9–16:11–26.

Della Rocca RC, Bedrossian EH, Arthurs BP: Ophthalmic plastic surgery: decisions making and techniques. New York, McGraw-Hill, 2002:25–41:153–161:181–187.

Lemke BN, Della Rocca RC: Surgery of the eyelid and orbit an anatomical approach. Norwalk, Appleton and Lange, 1990:199–212.

Smith BC, Della Rocca RC, Nesi FA, Lisman RD: Ophthalmic plastic and reconstructive surgery. St Louis, CV Mosby, 1976:8–17:39–78:129–140.

241 FACIAL MOVEMENT DISORDERS
(Benign Essential Blepharospasm 333.81, Hemifacial Spasm 351.8)

John R. Samples, MD
Portland, Oregon

ETIOLOGY/INCIDENCE

Benign essential blepharospasm and hemifacial spasm are facial movement disorders that primarily affect older individuals. Benign essential blepharospasm is virtually always bilateral, but hemifacial spasm is usually unilateral. Hemifacial spasm begins with twitches in a single region of the orbicularis muscle that lasts from seconds to minutes; typically, the twitches are rather irregular and tonic in pattern. The spasm rarely recruits or extends over seconds or minutes. In contrast, benign essential blepharospasm is characterized by involuntary, tonic, sometimes-forceful closure of the eyelids that can be either intermittent or continuous. It is often associated with orofacial dyskinesia and may be associated with other movement disorders involving the trunk and the neck. These disorders are almost always axial. It is helpful to differentiate these disorders from other causes of facial spasm. Some individuals have a psychogenic cause for their blepharospasm and other individuals have dry eye conditions and other types of keratitis that stimulate a blepharospasm, particularly in response to light.

Benign essential blepharospasm is related to a central nervous system disorder that remains poorly understood.

It is sometimes part of, or found in conjunction with, Parkinson's disease and it is assumed that a common cause is shared with Parkinson's disease in these cases.

Hemifacial spasm is attributed to compression of the facial nerve by an aberrant blood vessel. It may also be caused by lesions that compress the facial nerve extra-axially, by an aneurysm or an arteriovenous malformation, or by a neoplasm that involves the cerebellopontine angle.

COURSE/PROGNOSIS

All of these conditions are usually slowly progressive but may occasionally spontaneously remit. Waxing and waning over months is not unheard of.

When a patient has hemifacial spasm, serious central nervous conditions must be ruled out. Synkinesis is observed with hemifacial spasm but not with facial myokymia. Facial myokymia is almost always a benign condition that involves a single muscle. Some patients with multiple sclerosis or brain stem tumors may have facial myokymia as a presenting sign; in this case, it usually persists indefinitely. More benign myokymias are always intermittent.

DIAGNOSIS

The hallmark of benign essential blepharospasm is the involuntary, tonic, and forceful closure of the eyelids. Often, this occurs to such a degree that it interferes with the patient's lifestyle or vision. Symptoms are typically made worse by stress, fatigue, bright lights, and driving, and symptoms are usually relieved by sleep and relaxation. Patients may have idiosyncratic factors that precipitate or alleviate their symptoms.

Hemifacial spasm tends to be more idiosyncratic in terms of its onset. Spasms are often precipitated or made worse by fatigue and stress.

TREATMENT

Systemic

Anticholinergic agents, such as trihexyphenidyl hydrochloride (Artane), may be useful in treating many patients with benign essential blepharospasm. Typically, this drug is used at a dosage of 2 mg PO b.i.d., which is slowly increased. Many patients who titrate the medicine appropriately will be able to tolerate the blepharospasm and find the medicine useful; however, side effects, including dry mouth, dry eye and drowsiness, limit the usefulness of this drug.

After anticholinergic therapy, a trial with other drugs, such as clonazepam, is sometimes warranted, but many patients are happier proceeding to botulinum toxin.

No medication has been identified as specifically curative for this condition, although medical failures are often due more to failures to attempt medical titration than to failure of the medicine to work.

For hemifacial spasm, there is virtually no successful systemic therapy, although carbamazepine has been estimated to benefit as many as 30 patients with this disorder.

Local

Injections with botulinum toxin type A provide relief for most patients with benign essential blepharospasm and hemifacial spasm. The toxin works by interfering with acetylcholine release from nerve terminals. It may provide relief from spasm for 3 months or longer. It is generally well tolerated, although some patients develop ptosis or diplopia, especially if doses are given centrally or along the midline. A typical pattern of injection places 5 units SC at each of the two sites over the brow, 5 units at each of two sites well off the midline in the upper lid, and 5 units at each of two sites in the lower lid, for a total of six injections on a side. Injections can be tailored to the individual patient's spasm.

Complications of botulinum toxin type A include ptosis, ectropion, corneal exposure, and tearing. It appears that a tolerance to toxin does not develop. Antibodies to botulinum toxin type A do not develop with the dose commonly used for these conditions.

Surgical

In benign essential blepharospasm, surgery should be reserved for individuals for whom trials with medication and botulinum toxin type A were not successful. Also, patients need to be cautioned that they may not obtain complete relief.

The most effective technique is to resect the orbicularis oculi muscles. This was initially popularized by Gillum and Anderson in 1981. The technique involves the meticulous extirpation of all of the accessible orbicularis oculi, procerus, corrugator, superciliaris, and facial nerves in post orbicular fascia. Numerous refinements have been discussed.

Decompression of the facial nerve in symptomatic cases is effective for hemifacial spasm. Surgery for cryptogenic cases and decompression of the facial nerve from aberrant blood vessels have been recommended.

The surgical approach for hemifacial spasm requires a retromastoid craniectomy and microneurosurgical techniques and should not be undertaken unless symptoms warrant. Although some patients are extremely grateful to have had this surgery, the potential risks cannot be overlooked.

Supportive

Most patients are helped by support groups, although a few patients have been adversely affected by participation when they have been exposed to patients with disease that was far more severe than their own.

Because there is substantial variability in the severity of blepharospasm, the referral of patients should be individualized so as not to increase patient anxiety.

COMMENTS

The treatment of benign essential blepharospasm has three phases: a medical phase, the trial of botulinum toxin type A, and the surgical phase. Hemifacial spasm responds best to botulinum toxin type A and, if this fails, to surgical decompression. There is no role for medication. Individuals show a substantial variation in their symptoms and their responses to medication. Both doses of medication and toxin injections require careful titration. Often several trials of toxin are required to find the dose and pattern that suits the patient best.

SUPPORT GROUP

Benign Essential Blepharospasm Research Foundation
755 Howell Street
Beaumont, TX 77706

REFERENCES

Frueh BR, Felt DP, Wojno TH, et al: Treatment of blepharospasm with botulinum toxin: a preliminary report. Arch Ophthalmol 102:1464–1468, 1984.

Gillum WN, Anderson RL: Blepharospasm surgery: An anatomical approach. Arch Ophthalmol 99:1056–1062, 1981.

Jankovic J: Clinical features, differential diagnosis and pathogenesis of blepharospasm and cranial cervical dystonia. In: Bosniak SL, Smith BC, eds: Advances in ophthalmic plastic and reconstructive surgery-blepharospasm. New York, Pergamon, 1985:4.

Jones FTW, Samples JR, Waller RR: The treatment of essential blepharospasm. Mayo Clin Proc 60:663–666, 1985.

Lingua RW: Sequelae of botulinum toxin injection. Am J Ophthalmol 100:305–307, 1985.

242 FLOPPY EYELID SYNDROME
374.9

Lee K. Schwartz, MD
San Francisco, California
Gary L. Aguilar, MD
San Francisco, California

ETIOLOGY/INCIDENCE

The floppy eyelid syndrome (FES) is an uncommon and frequently unrecognized cause of noninfectious, chronic unilateral or bilateral papillary conjunctivitis. The condition is characterized by loose, 'floppy' eyelids associated with punctate epithelial keratopathy (PEK), ptosis of lateral eyelashes and the typical conjunctival changes.

The diagnosis has been made in patients of both sexes ranging in age from 2 to 80, but the disorder most commonly affects the middle-aged, and in particular middle-aged, obese males. The floppiness of the eyelids is due to laxity of the tarsus, which is a consequence of a decrease in tarsal elastin.

There may be several pathways that lead to FES. The primary cause of the tarsal laxity has been explained by the frequent observation that the affected side in unilateral cases corresponds to the side the patient preferentially sleeps on. Pressure on the dependent eyelid during sleep may result in local ischemia and lid eversion, and may provoke the patient to rub the eyelid, exacerbating the ischemia while stretching the tarsal plate. Patients with bilateral disease commonly alternate sides while asleep or sleep face down.

Studies have shown a significant decrease in the amount of elastin within the tarsal plate and eyelid skin as compared to normal controls. It is thought that the up regulation of elastolytic enzymes, most probably induced by repeated mechanical stress, associated with eye rubbing or by sleeping habits, participates in elastic fiber degradation and subsequent tarsal laxity and eyelash ptosis in FES.

Also poor contact of the lax eyelid with the globe in conjunction with meibomian gland and tear film abnormalities may contribute further to the syndrome. Patients with more severe symptoms tend to have floppier eyelids.

A contributing factor to the syndrome appears to be an abnormality in tear film dynamics. Tear film abnormalities have been shown to be prevalent in patients with FES and are characterized by a lipid deficiency, with a consequent rapid rate of tear evaporation. The eyelid skin of FES patients is remarkable for its high temperature, high water evaporation rate, and a tendency toward hyperpigmentation.

In addition obstructive sleep apnea (OSA) may contribute to the development of FES. The physician should inquire about the presence of symptoms of nocturnal breathing disorder. OSA may contribute to local eyelid ischemia that may play an important role in the development of FES. This ischemia may be exacerbated by the hypoventilation of OSA. In addition the pressure that is placed on the dependent eyelid during sleep and/or the act of rubbing the eyelid may also contribute to the syndrome.

COURSE/PROGNOSIS

While excessive eyelid laxity has been reported in virtually all age groups, the typical FES patient is an obese middle-aged male

(37% of patients are females) who presents with a chronic red eye with a mucoid discharge. By the time the diagnosis is finally made, the patient has usually received multiple ocular medications. The duration of symptoms before diagnosis has ranged from 8 months to 14 years.

DIAGNOSIS

Clinical signs and symptoms

The syndrome is characterized by a triad of diffuse papillary conjunctivitis, a loose upper eyelid that readily everts by pulling it upward (positive lid eversion sign), and a soft rubbery tarsus that can be easily folded on itself. The lower eyelids may also be involved. Lash ptosis is common, usually involving the lateral lashes of the upper eyelid.

The consequences of untreated FES can be serious. *Staphylococcus aureus* corneal ulceration has been described, as has bilateral corneal neovascularization. Corneal scarring may occur necessitating a penetrating keratoplasty in rare cases. A case has been reported of a patient with FES and rheumatoid arthritis who had dry eyes and who developed a corneal melt with perforation; ultimately requiring evisceration after endophthalmitis supervened. This highlights the fact that comorbities may complicate FES with severe clinical consequences.

The diagnosis is often missed because patients usually present complaining of nonspecific ocular irritation and so can be confused with patients suffering from dry eyes. Typically, patients complain of a red eye(s), a foreign body sensation, eyelid swelling, dryness and a mucoid discharge. Symptoms are usually worse on waking. Patients often come in with multiple ocular medications that have been prescribed by previous physicians without success. The syndrome may be masked or complicated by a toxic medicamentosa from the numerous eye medications.

The lids may appear swollen with mucus discharge. A diffuse, velvety, papillary conjunctivitis is present in the tarsus of one or both eyelids. The upper lid may be thickened and is easily everted, (positive lid eversion sign). The eyelashes may be nonparallel and ptotic, especially laterally, tending to curl toward the globe. The cornea may show punctate epithelial keratopathy, corneal neovascularization, even ulceration.

Associated ocular findings not present in all patients

- PEK (41% to 45%).
- Keratoconus (10% to 16%).
- Blepharitis.
- Blepharochalasis.
- Blepharoptosis.
- Corneal ulcers and neovascularization.
- Dermatochalasis.
- Eyelash ptosis (loss of parallelism of cilia).
- Endotheliopathy (Chandler's syndrome, non-guttate endothelial dystrophy).
- Filamentary keratitis.
- Infectious keratitis.
- Keratotorus.
- Lower lid laxity and ectropion.
- Meibomian gland dysfunction.
- Pseudo-ptyrigium.
- Recurrent corneal erosion.
- Tear dysfunction.
- Trichiasis.

Associated systemic disorders not present in all patients

- Arteriosclerotic heart disease.
- Corneal perforation associated with rheumatoid arthritis.
- Chronic bronchitis.
- Diabetes mellitus.
- Epibulbar fasciitis.
- Gout.
- Hay fever.
- Hyperextensibility and hypermobility of joints.
- Hyperglycinemia.
- Hyperlipidemia.
- Hypertension.
- Interstitial pneumonitis.
- Mental retardation.
- Nephrolithiasis.
- Obesity.
- Obstructive sleep apnea.
- Psoriasis.

Nocturnal ectropion of the upper eyelid is probably responsible for the clinical manifestations in most patients.

It is not clear that all cases of FES represent the same syndrome. It is possible that a clinical picture similar to FES occurs in patients with lax upper eyelids of any cause.

Laboratory findings

Conjunctival scrapings reveal keratinized epithelial cells. Bacterial cultures of the conjunctiva should be obtained, and treatment should be instituted if appropriate.

Histopathologic investigations have revealed chronic conjunctival inflammation and fibrosis and scarring. Meibomian gland cystic degeneration and squamous metaplasia have been noted, along with abnormal keratinization and granuloma formation. There is no definite association with systemic diseases of collagen or elastic tissue. Various associations have been reported with keratoconus, hyperglycinemia, and other disorders.

Consider FES patients for sleep studies if OSA is suspected. Symptoms may include snoring, daytime somnolence, waking up feeling un-refreshed, apnea during sleep observed by others, waking gasping for air during the night and morning headache.

Differential diagnosis

A study of 58 patients with chronic conjunctivitis of more than 2 weeks' duration revealed that FES was the cause of chronic conjunctivitis in 2% of patients. In 31% of patients with chronic conjunctivitis, no specific cause was detected.

Because these patients often present with multiple eye medications, a toxic medicamentosa conjunctivitis and keratitis may also be present, and the underlying disorder may be missed.

Laxity of the eyelid, in general, can occur from a variety of processes, including natural ageing, hyper-elasticity syndromes, blepharochalasis and as a post-inflammatory response. Common to all these syndromes are symptoms and signs of chronic non-specific ocular surface irritation, which resolves with surgical correction of the eyelid laxity. Other conditions to consider are lax eyelid syndrome, cutis laxa, blepharochalasis syndrome, and eyelid imbrication syndrome.

TREATMENT

Ocular

- Prevention of the probable nocturnal eyelid eversion.
- Eye shield while sleeping.
- Lids taped closed at night.
- Ocular medications tapered or discontinued.
- Ocular lubricants.

Surgical

Not all symptoms are relieved by local treatment. Because the cause is simply one of excessive eyelid laxity, a surgical cure via an eyelid-tightening procedure is often necessary. An upper and a lower pentagonal eyelid resection is simple and effective. The tarsal strip or Bick procedure may also be used.

Full-thickness upper and lower eyelid resection

When performing a standard full-thickness eyelid resection on a patient with FES, it is best to treat both the upper and lower eyelids because both are affected. The principal caveat is to avoid injury to the lacrimal secretory ductules, which lie approximately 5 mm above the lateral extreme of the upper tarsus. When performing full thickness eyelid resections, the vertical excision must extend through the top of the tarsus to avoid an unsightly buckling in the upper eyelid. Back-tapering both the tarsal wedge resection posteriorly and the resection of the anterior lamella anteriorly can further enhance cosmesis.

In most cases, the wedge should be taken laterally, that is, from the area of the lateral third and medial two thirds of the eyelid. However, there are cases in which the greatest laxity occurs medially. For these cases, a new technique has been described in which a tapered, full thickness resection of 10-mm to 12-mm of eyelid is performed medially, a procedure that addresses both the laxity and cosmetic concerns.

Tarsal strip and bick procedures

The tarsal strip procedure, as described by Anderson and Gordy, also is effective. After a lateral canthotomy and lysis of both the upper and lower tendons, the upper and lower lateral eyelids are shortened. 'Tarsal strips' are fashioned from surgically thinned lateral tarsus tissue after a determination is made on the table of how much tarsus must be excised to achieve the desired tightening. The tarsal strips – cleaned of skin anteriorly, the lid margin superiorly and mucosa posteriorly – are sutured to the inner, lateral orbital periosteum, just above the lateral orbital tubercle.

The Bick procedure is much like the tarsal strip procedure and is equally efficacious. After lateral canthotomy and upper and lower cantholysis, the amount of eyelid laxity is determined. The redundant full-thickness eyelid is excised without creating tarsal strips. The tarsal edges are then affixed to the periosteum in the customary fashion.

Systemic

Treatment for OSA may improve the symptoms of FES. If obesity is present weight loss may be helpful. A change in sleep habits to avoid mechanical trauma may further support the treatment success of surgical correction.

COMPLICATIONS

The severe complications of the syndrome have included corneal neovascularization, corneal ulcer, scarring, perforation and endophthalmitis.

SUMMARY

The accurate diagnosis of FES is often initially overlooked. Ocular medicamentosa may mask the correct diagnosis. During surgical correction, the ductules of the lacrimal glands must be avoided. Early recognition will spare the patient corneal complications and unnecessary diagnostic procedures and treatment. Consider sleep studies if obstructive sleep apnea is suspected, and evaluate the patient for keratoconus.

REFERENCES

Anderson R, Gordy DD: The tarsal strip procedure. Arch Ophthalmol 97:2192–2196, 1979.

Bick MW: Surgical management of orbital tarsal disparity. Arch Ophthalmol 75:386, 1966.

Culbertson WW, Ostler HB: The floppy eyelid syndrome. Am J Ophthalmol 92:568–575, 1981.

Culbertson WW, Tseng SC: Corneal disorders in floppy eyelid syndrome. Cornea 13:33–42, 1994.

Dutton JJ: Surgical management of floppy eyelid syndrome. Am J Ophthalmol 99:557–560, 1985.

Netland PA, Sugrue SP, Albert DM, Shore JW: Histopathologic features of the floppy eyelid syndrome: Involvement of tarsal elastin. Ophthalmology 101:174–181, 1994.

243 HORDEOLUM 373.1

(Internal Hordeolum [Acute Meibomitis], External Hordeolum [Stye], Acute Infection of the Glands of Zeis or Moll's Glands)

Kevin S. Michels, MD
Portland, Oregon

ETIOLOGY/INCIDENCE

Hordeolum is usually an acute staphylococcal infection of the sebaceous glands of the eyelids. External hordeolum (stye) is caused by stasis with subsequent bacterial infection of the glands of Zeis' or Moll's glands. Internal hordeolum usually results from a secondary staphylococcal infection of a meibomian gland in the tarsal plate. Both internal and external hordeola are common sequelae of infectious blepharitis, and the most common infectious agent is *Staphylococcus aureus*. Rare cases of *Pseudomonas aeruginosa* may occur. Hordeola are more common in patients with chronic lid or skin disease or with systemic diseases such as diabetes mellitus.

COURSE/PROGNOSIS

Hordeola usually begin with painful swelling and edema of the eyelid, which becomes localized. The purulent exudate of external hordeola often breaks through the skin near the eyelash line; the suppuration of the internal hordeolum occurs on the conjunctival side of the eyelid. The prognosis is excellent unless an orbital cellulitis develops or the preauricular or submandibular nodes are involved. Hordeolum can often spontaneously improve over a 1–2 week period.

DIAGNOSIS

The diagnosis is made clinically by a localized area of tenderness in the region of obvious inflammation, but may require confirmation based on culture or biopsy results if complications occur.

Differential diagnosis

When the lesion does not resolve with appropriate therapy then preseptal cellulitis, sebaceous cell carcinoma, and pyogenic granuloma should be considered.

PROPHYLAXIS

Prophylaxis is based on lid hygiene, control of associated skin or systemic disease, and improved overall general health.

TREATMENT

Systemic

- If multiple hordeola, recurrent hordeola, or adenopathy occur, consider systemic antibiotics: 250 mg erythromycin q.i.d., 125 to 250 mg dicloxacillin, or 500 mg cloxacillan q.i.d. for as long as 2 weeks
- In chronic cases, administer prophylactic 250 mg tetracycline q.i.d. or 50 to 100 mg doxycycline qd.

Periocular

- Hot moist compresses for 5 to 15 minutes hourly or q.i.d.
- Removal of eyelashes in area to enhance suppuration.
- Once drainage occurs, topical ocular antibiotic solutions or ointments: bacitracin, erythromycin, gentamicin, tobramycin, ciloxin, and others applied q.i.d. during the acute phase.
- Topical steroids not indicated except when there is a fear of structural changes to the lid.
- Steroid injection can be considered for rare cases when excision of the lesion could lead to damage of the lacrimal apparatus, but steroids can lead to permanent skin discoloration.
- Lid hygiene.

Surgical

- The gland usually drains spontaneously.
- Stab incision, from either skin or palpebral conjunctiva depending on where the lesion is pointing, may spread infection if the incision is made before the eyelid skin or palpebral conjunctiva appears white or cream colored.
- Multiple pockets may be present; all must be incised.
- Occasionally, a firm central abscess core occurs and must be removed or the lesion will not easily heal.

If a local anesthetic is used, the injection is not administered directly in the area of inflammation but either above the upper border of the upper tarsus or below the lower border of the lower tarsus. A chalazion clamp is applied, and a horizontal incision is made over the pointing area if it is on the skin, or a vertical incision is made if the lesion is conjunctival. The lash margins should be avoided so as not to cause a lid margin defect or injury to the lash roots. The wound edges are not sutured, and postoperative warm compresses and antibiotic ointment are used until closure occurs spontaneously.

REFERENCES

Briner AM: Surgical treatment of a chalazion or hordeolum internum. Aust Fam Phys 16:834–835, 1987.

Briner AM: Treatment of common eyelid cyst. Aust Fam Phys 16:828–830, 1987.

Diegel JT: Eyelid problems: Blepharitis, hordeola, and chalazia. Postgrad Med 80:271–272, 1986.

Wilson LA: Bacterial conjunctivitis. In: Duane TD, ed: Clinical ophthalmology. Philadelphia, Harper & Row, 1979:IV:12–16.

244 LAGOPHTHALMOS 374.2

Eric A. Steele, MD
Portland, Oregon
Roger A. Dailey, MD
Portland, Oregon

ETIOLOGY

Lagophthalmos, which is the inability to fully close the eyelids, can occur for a number of reasons, including excessive projection of the eye in the orbit, inadequate vertical dimensions of either lid, contraction of the eyelid retractors or malfunction of the orbicularis oculi.

COURSE/PROGNOSIS

The presence of lagophthalmos often requires prompt efforts to protect the eye. Neglect of lagophthalmos can result in decreased vision, painful dryness, keratoconjunctivitis, corneal erosion, ulceration, and even endophthalmitis and loss of the eye.

DIAGNOSIS

Clinical signs and symptoms

The patient often presents with foreign body sensation and tearing, but may be asymptomatic if corneal hypoesthesia is present. On examination, there is incomplete closure of the eyelids. There may be associated corneal epithelial irregularities, or even ulceration with frank perforation.

TREATMENT

Appropriate therapy is dependent on an accurate diagnosis. Proptosis may be caused by congenital deformity, tumor, trauma, or thyroid related immune orbitopathy. Lid retraction can result from traumatic loss of eyelid tissue or cicatrization from many causes. Paralytic lagophthalmos secondary to decreased orbicularis oculi muscle tone commonly occurs with Bell's palsy.

Ocular

The maintenance of a moist surface on the eye is critical to the management of lagophthalmos. Treatment begins with artificial tears. Lubricating ointments protect the ocular surface longer, but cause bothersome blurring of vision, and may be best tolerated at bedtime. Punctal plugs or thermal occlusion of the puncta may be helpful, and moisture chambers or specially designed spectacles can prevent evaporative drying. A bandage contact lens can occasionally be useful in chronic irritative conditions caused by mild or partially corrected lagophthalmos, or a patch can be used for short periods of time. Long term patching has been associated with fungal infections, and even short term patching can be dangerous if corneal hypoesthesia is present.

Surgical

When the condition is severe, and protection is needed quickly prior to definitive repair, a tarsorrhaphy can be considered. A simple, effective method is to anesthetize the temporal aspect of the upper and lower eyelids with 2% lidocaine with epinephrine and use 5-0 fast absorbing gut suture (Ethicon, Somerville, NJ) to approximate the lid margins. Suture is placed beginning approximately 5 mm above the upper lid margin and passed out of the lid at the gray line and then into the opposite lid at the gray line and out through the skin approximately 5 mm below the margin. It then returns approximately 1 cm from the first pass by the opposite identical route through both lids and the ends are tied together. This provides effective corneal protection and lasts approximately one week. A similar technique using 5-0 nylon suture (Sherwood Medical, St Louis, MO) and bolsters to protect from skin breakdown can be used for a few weeks. The best permanent tarsorrhaphy (used if the other options listed below are not indicated or effective) involves creating pedicle flaps at the temporal and nasal limbus from the superior tarsus down to the inferior tarsus. This provides excellent closure while still allowing the eye to be opened for examination or administration of eye drops.

An accurate diagnosis and thorough understanding of the responsible pathology is critical for planning more definitive surgical corrections for the management of lagophthalmos. Treatment usually involves various combinations of lowering the upper eyelid, raising the lower eyelid, and providing better eyelid movement. When exophthalmos is the culprit, treatment is directed at the orbit.

The upper eyelid retraction of TRIO responds well to upper lid levator recession and graded muellerectomy. Upper or lower lid retraction from loss of tissue or cicatrisation requires pedicle flaps or anterior/posterior lamellae grafting techniques. Posterior lamellae can be reconstructed from hard palate mucosal grafting (in the lower eyelid only) or acellular dermal allograft.

Patients with facial nerve palsies can be difficult to treat. Often these patients require a gold weight implant to help with upper eyelid closure. Placement of an orbital gold weight provides excellent function and low morbidity compared to pretarsal placement. Many patients need ectropion repair via a lid shortening procedure along with midface lifting and or placement of a full thickness skin graft to the anterior lamella to allow the lower lid to maintain an acceptable position. Suborbicularis oculi fat (SOOF) lifts can be accomplished in the preperiosteal or subperiosteal plane depending on the extent of elevation needed.

Conditions that cause exposure from exophthalmos are treated by efforts to reduce tumor mass or enlarge the space available in the orbit. Systemic or local injection of steroids can help with inflammatory diseases, and chemotherapy or radiation can be effective in treating certain tumors and inflammatory conditions. The proptosis of thyroid related immune orbitopathy (TRIO) can be treated by radiation, but generally excellent outcomes are achieved with orbital decompression.

COMPLICATIONS

Although successful attempts at improving lid closure by attaching springs have been reported, problems with these devices exist. Difficulties in the adjustment and tension maintenance of the stainless-steel spring may develop, and the likelihood that the spring will eventually migrate, extrude, or break necessitates the patient's continuous proximity to a surgeon familiar with the technique. Likewise, the elastic force of a silicon rubber loop may ultimately stretch the tissue through which it passes and cause loss of some tension. While nerve anastomosis, muscle transfers, static suspension and other more exotic and definitive measures for the correction of facial paralysis can be successful, these techniques often confer some degree of facial deformity and do not always achieve sufficient ocular protection to preclude the measures outlined here.

COMMENTS

The treatment of lagophthalmos requires a logical, stepwise approach. Application of the techniques discussed in this chapter can prevent the serious complications that result from chronic ocular exposure.

REFERENCES

Bailey KL, Tower RN, Dailey RA: Customized, single-incision, three wall orbital decompression. Ophthal Plast Reconstr Surg 21 (1):1–9, 2005.

Tower RN, Dailey RA: Gold weight implantation: a better way? Ophthal Plast Reconstr Surg 20(3):202–206, 2004.

Wobig JL, Dailey RA: Oculofacial plastic surgery. New York, Thieme, 2004.

245 LID MYOKYMIA 333.2

Byron L. Lam, MD

Miami, Florida

ETIOLOGY/INCIDENCE

Myokymia is the spontaneous fine fascicular contraction of muscle without muscular atrophy or weakness. Eyelid myokymia typically involves the orbicularis oculi of one of the lower eyelids, although occasionally the upper eyelids can also be affected. These irregular contractions are usually unilateral and intermittent, and they may persist for weeks to months. Eyelid myokymia is generally benign, self-limited, and not associated with any disease. Possible precipitating factors include stress, fatigue, and excessive caffeine or alcohol intake. Rarely, eyelid myokymia may occur as a precursor or as part of facial myokymia that is characterized by continuous, involuntary movements of the facial muscles associated with multiple sclerosis and brain stem tumors.

DIAGNOSIS

Patients typically report eyelid jumping or twitching. These symptoms often improve when the eyelid is pulled manually.

Fine contractions of the eyelid are visible but are usually more apparent to the patient than to the observer. Rarely, the contractions may be vigorous enough to cause movement of the globe, producing oscillopsia and pseudonystagmus. The focus of irritation is most likely the nerve fibers within the muscle.

TREATMENT

- Reassurance and reduction in precipitating factors, if identifiable, are appropriate for most patients.
- Subcutaneous injections of botulinum toxin type A consisting of local injections of 2.5 to 5.0 units each to the affected eyelid region usually provide adequate relief lasting 12 to 16 weeks. Adverse effects include temporary lid laxity, which may produce lagophthalmos and exposure keratopathy.
- Oral quinine, antihistamines, clonazepam, or baclofen may be tried in the unlikely event that botulinum toxin type A is unsuccessful, but the efficacy of these agents has not been proved. In addition, quinine has numerous side effects and is contraindicated in pregnancy.

REFERENCES

Givner I, Jaffe NS: Myokymia of the eyelids: a suggestion as to therapy: preliminary report. Am J Ophthalmol 32:51–55, 1949.

Lowe R: Facial twitching. Trans Ophthalmol Soc Aust 11:129–133, 1951.

Reinecke RD: Translated myokymia of the lower eyelid causing uniocular vertical pseudonystagmus. Am J Ophthalmol 75:150–151, 1973.

Scott AB: Botulinum toxin for blepharospasm. In: Spaeth G, Katz LJ, Parker KW, eds: Current therapy in ophthalmic surgery. Toronto, Decker, 1989:322–324.

Sogg RL, Hoyt WF, Boldrey E: Spastic paretic facial contracture: a rare sign of brain stem tumor. Neurology 13:607–612, 1963.

246 LID RETRACTION 374.41

Dale R. Meyer, MD, FACS
Albany, New York

Lid retraction is a disorder of eyelid position that can affect the upper eyelid, lower eyelid, or both, and may be unilateral or bilateral.

ETIOLOGY/INCIDENCE

Eyelid retraction can result from an increase in retractor force, as well as from scarring or other mechanical forces. The most common cause of eyelid retraction is Graves' disease (Graves' ophthalmopathy). Eyelid retraction due to Graves' ophthalmopathy may be unilateral or bilateral, affecting the upper eyelids, lower eyelids, or both. An uncommon but important cause of upper eyelid retraction is dorsal midbrain disease. Upper eyelid retraction tends to be bilateral with midbrain conditions and when present is referred to as *Collier's sign*; often, there is associated conjugate upgaze and convergence paralysis, as well as light-near pupillary dissociation and retraction-nystagmus on attempted upgaze, the *Parinaud's syndrome*.

DIAGNOSIS

Clinical signs and symptoms

The normal resting upper eyelid position is approximately 4.0 to 4.5 mm above the central corneal light reflex, and the normal lower eyelid position is approximately 5.5 mm below the central corneal light reflex. Normally, eyelid position is symmetric (within 1 mm of the contralateral eyelid). Significant deviation of the eyelid from normal may be considered eyelid retraction.

When the upper eyelid is affected, the resting position of the upper eyelid is at a higher-than-normal level, and when the lower eyelid is affected, it is at a lower-than-normal level. Typically, *inferior scleral show* occurs when the lower eyelid is affected, and *superior scleral show* occurs with more advanced upper eyelid retraction. Upper eyelid retraction makes the person appear as if he or she is staring and can produce the illusion of exophthalmos (Figure 246.1).

Eyelid position can be affected by both vertical and horizontal gaze. In downgaze, the upper eyelid normally drops slightly or stays at the same level relative to the mid cornea or visual axis. The term *lid lag* describes the situation in which the upper eyelid assumes a higher position when the eyes are in downgaze. Lid lag is not to be confused with von Graefe's sign, which is a dynamic sign describing the pause or retarded descent of the eyelid when the eye moves from primary position to downgaze. Stellwag's sign describes retraction of the upper eyelid or eyelids associated with infrequent or incomplete blinking. Dalrymple's sign describes an abnormal vertical wideness of the palpebral fissure.

Resting eyelid position is determined by a balance of the eyelid protractors and retractors. The primary protractor of the eyelids is the orbicularis oculi muscle, which is responsible for eyelid closure and blinking. In the resting position, the orbicularis oculi muscle exhibits low-grade tonic activity only. The retractors of the upper eyelid are the levator palpebrae superioris muscle innervated by the third cranial (oculomotor) nerve and Müller's muscle, which is smooth muscle innervated by sympathetics. The lower eyelid retractors are more rudimentary and include the capsulopalpebral fascia (an extension of the capsulopalpebral head from the inferior rectus muscle) and the inferior tarsal muscle, which is also smooth muscle innervated by sympathetics.

Determination of the underlying cause of eyelid retraction is usually straightforward. History regarding previous surgery or

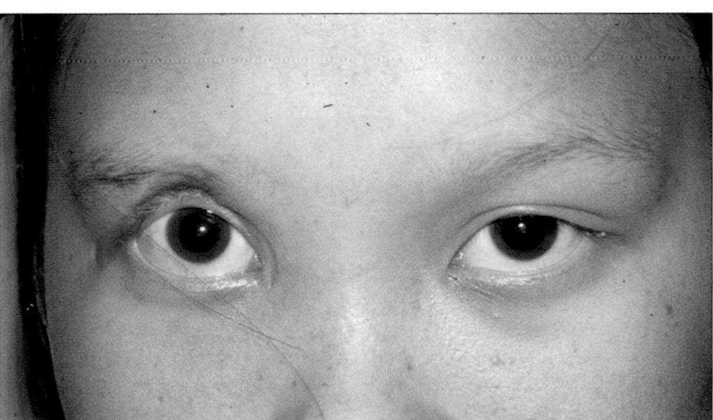

FIGURE 246.1. Congenital right upper eyelid retraction.

trauma, concomitant systemic diseases, and familial disorders should be elicited.

Laboratory findings

If the diagnosis of Graves' disease is suspected, serologic testing for total thyroxine, thyroid-stimulating hormone, and thyroid-stimulating immunoglobulins should be obtained. Orbital and head neuroimaging is not usually necessary unless the clinical and laboratory investigations do not establish the diagnosis.

Differential diagnosis

The broader differential diagnosis of eyelid retraction is diverse but can be generally classified under three categories: neurogenic, myogenic, and mechanical.

Neurogenic

- Dorsal midbrain lesions (e.g. pinealoma).
- Hydrocephalus.
- Encephalitis.
- Bulbar poliomyelitis.
- Multiple sclerosis.
- Closed head injury.
- Coma ('coma vigil').
- Epilepsy.
- Marcus Gunn (jaw-winking syndrome) trigemino-oculomotor synkinesis.
- Aberrant innervation/regeneration cranial nerve III (oculomotor nerve).
- Pseudoretraction associated with contralateral blepharoptosis.
- Weakness of orbicularis oculi (e.g. facial nerve palsy).
- Orbital floor fracture (globe hypotropia, increased innervation to superior rectus/levator).
- Sympathomimetic eyedrops (phenylephrine, apraclonidine).
- Volitional.

Myogenic

- Graves' ophthalmopathy.
- Congenital upper or lower eyelid retraction.
- Congenital hyperthyroidism.
- Congenital myotonia, myotonic dystrophy.
- Hyperkalemic.
- Periodic paralysis.
- Myasthenia gravis.
- Postsurgical.
- Inferior rectus recession (lower eyelid).
- Superior rectus recession (upper eyelid).
- Overcorrection blepharoptosis.
- Enucleation.

Mechanical

- Graves' ophthalmopathy.
- Exophthalmos (proptosis).
- Buphthalmos.
- High myopia.
- Craniosynostosis.
- Eyelid neoplasms.
- Herpes zoster ophthalmicus.
- Smallpox.
- Atopic dermatitis.
- Burns (thermal or chemical).
- After irradiation.
- Contact lens wear (or imbedded contact lens).
- Postsurgical.
- Blepharoplasty.
- Orbicularis myectomy.
- Scleral buckle.
- Osteoplastic frontal sinusotomy.
- Glaucoma filtering procedure.
- Extracapsular cataract extraction.
- Orbital floor exploration.
- Maxillectomy.
- Cheek flap.

PROPHYLAXIS

Prophylaxis of eyelid retraction is possible in some surgical procedures that may induce eyelid retraction.

- Blepharoplasty: avoidance of excessive skin excision is recommended. For lower eyelid blepharoplasty, a transconjunctival approach carries less risk of eyelid retraction than a transcutaneous approach.
- Orbitotomy: an infraciliary incision is frequently used to approach the inferior portion of the orbit for procedures such as orbital fracture repair, orbital decompression or orbital exploration, and tumor excision. Meticulous closure of the wound with avoidance of 'catching' the lower eyelid retractors or septum in the more anterior closure is recommended. It is acknowledged that even with meticulous closure, eyelid retraction of a mild nature may still occur. For this reason, whenever possible, a transconjunctival approach is recommended.
- Inferior rectus recession: lower eyelid retraction after inferior rectus recession may occur and is more likely to occur with recessions of more than 3 mm. Several surgical techniques to minimize or prevent lower eyelid retraction after inferior rectus muscle recession have been described, including extensive dissection of the inferior rectus muscle with lysis of surrounding check ligaments. Because simple wide dissection may not be adequate, more recent techniques have suggested application of countertraction at the level of the capsulopalpebral head (by advancement or suspension) at the time of the inferior rectus recession. Alternatively, primary lysis of the lower eyelid retractors 3 to 4 mm beneath the tarsus can also be performed. This procedure has the advantage of being technically simpler and is not compromised by large inferior rectus muscle recessions.

TREATMENT

The treatment of eyelid retraction will vary depending on the cause and severity. Aside from the disfigurement caused by eyelid retraction, corneal exposure is the most common complication that should be addressed.

Systemic

Systemic abnormalities contributing to eyelid retraction should be sought and corrected. For patients with Graves' disease, thyroid function should be stabilized and eyelid position should be stable for at least 6 months before elective eyelid surgery is considered.

Local

- Topical ocular lubrication (artificial tears or ointments) is used when exposure keratopathy is present.

- Guanethidine eyedrops are not usually recommended due to variable effectiveness.
- Botulinum type A (2.5–10.0 units) injected transconjunctivally just above the superior tarsal border can temporarily reduce lid retraction. The individual response to treatment is variable. Effects generally last 3–4 months. Diplopia and overcorrection (ptosis) are potential side-effects.

Surgical

- Approaches vary for upper eyelid, lower eyelid, and severity of lid retraction.
- The upper eyelid usually requires recession of Müller's muscle, levator aponeurosis, or both.
- The lower eyelid usually requires recession of lower eyelid retractors; advanced cases also require spacer graft (hard palate, ear cartilage, eye bank sclera, or other). A cheek suspension procedure may also be considered.

Upper eyelid retraction surgery

- Posterior (internal) approach.

A 4-0 silk suture is placed through the eyelid margin, and the lid is everted over a Desmarres retractor. Local anesthetic (2% xylocaine with 1 : 100,000 epinephrine) is infiltrated in the subconjunctival space above the superior tarsal border. The conjunctiva is grasped 2 to 3 mm above the superior tarsal border, and a small 'buttonhole' incision is made with Stevens scissors through the conjunctiva and Müller's muscle. The surgical plane between Müller's muscle and the levator aponeurosis is undermined with Stevens scissors, and the conjunctiva and Müller's muscle are then incised medially and laterally. The extent of the medial dissection is somewhat less than later ally to avoid overcorrection. Müller's muscle can be excised directly with Stevens scissors The patient is placed in the sitting position, and the lid position is assessed. Usually, simple recession/extirpation of Müller's muscle, as described, will produce approximately 2-mm lowering of the eyelid margin. If further lowering of the eyelid is required, the levator aponeurosis itself can be disinserted from the tarsus via the posterior approach and recessed. The patient is placed in the sitting position, and further recession of the levator aponeurosis usually can be performed through additional blunt dissection to achieve the desired eyelid position. Some surgeons suture back together the conjunctiva at the end of the procedure, but this author has not found this to be necessary or desirable. The conjunctiva usually reepithelializes in approximately 1 week. The silk suture at the lid margin can be taped down to the cheek for several days, but for less advanced cases of upper eyelid retraction, this is not necessary. Although spacer grafts have also been used to treat upper eyelid retraction, they usually are not necessary. Postoperative eyelid position can vary somewhat (either upward or downward) but usually approximates the position noted at the end of surgery.

- Anterior (external) approach.

The levator aponeurosis and Müller's muscle also can be approached from an anterior eyelid crease incision. The advantage of the anterior approach is that blepharoplasty, if desired, can be performed with further debulking of excess orbital fat. The procedure is performed after the eyelid crease is marked with a skin-marking pen, and if blepharoplasty is planned, a skin pinch technique is used to assess the amount of redundant tissue. Caution should be taken not to excise too much skin because the amount of apparent redundancy may be less when the lid is returned to a normal position. Dissection is carried down to the orbital septum, which is opened to reveal the preaponeurotic fat, which is then excised if desired. The levator aponeurosis then is disinserted from the tarsus, with less dissection performed medially than laterally to avoid overcorrection. The patient is placed in the sitting position, and the lid position is assessed. If further lowering of the eyelid is desired, Müller's muscle can be recessed/extirpated. The plane between Müller's muscle and conjunctiva is infiltrated with 2% xylocaine with 1 : 100,000 epinephrine; then, Müller's muscle is undermined and excised. With the anterior approach, the conjunctiva is usually preserved. The patient is again placed in the sitting position, and the eyelid position is checked. Further recession of the levator aponeurosis and Müller's muscle can be performed with blunt dissection. The levator aponeurosis can be secured in its recessed position with an absorbable suture. The skin is closed in the usual fashion, and the lid crease can be sutured to the superior portion of the tarsus with deeper bites to re-establish the eyelid crease.

Lower eyelid retraction surgery

Surgical correction of lower eyelid retraction can be divided into three approaches:

1. Lower eyelid retractor lysis/recession (extirpation).
2. Recession with spacers (e.g. hard palate mucosa, cartilage, sclera, acellular dermis).
3. Orbicularis/prezygomatic cheek flap advancement and fixation.

Eyelid retraction procedures are frequently coupled with horizontal eyelid tightening (e.g. tarsal strip procedure or 'lateral canthoplasty'). These techniques generally involve a conjunctival incision, with identification of the lower eyelid retractors. The eyelid retractors can be dissected from the conjunctiva, followed by recession or extirpation; alternatively, the conjunctiva and retractors can be recessed together, which is this author's favored approach. In virtually all techniques for the correction of lower eyelid retraction, some type of upward traction (usually via a Frost suture) is applied postoperatively to the lower eyelid for several days. Because gravity 'works against' lower eyelid surgery, it may be necessary to place a spacer between the recessed conjunctiva/retractors and the tarsus, particularly if the lower retraction is more than 2 mm. Hard palate mucosa grafts and auricular cartilage, as well as commercially prepared acellular dermis are useful for this purpose. Eye bank sclera can also be used, but results may be less predictable because of reabsorption and fibrosis. Finally, if lower eyelid retraction is due to a deficiency of skin such as occurs after lower eyelid blepharoplasty or burns, consideration must be given to advancement of the remaining eyelid and cheek skin, usually via dissection and mobilization of a composite cheek flap (e.g. 'SOOF lift'). In cases of extreme vertical skin deficiency, a full-thickness skin graft, usually obtained from behind the ear, may be required to adequately reposition the lower eyelid.

COMPLICATIONS

- The main complication of eyelid retraction is corneal exposure.
- Failure of eyelid retraction surgery to adequately correct eyelid retraction requires more aggressive secondary surgery, including further recession of the eyelid retractors,

consideration of spacer graft (or larger spacer), wider mobilization of skin and adjacent tissues or placement of a full-thickness skin graft, or a combination, depending on what tissue layer or layers remain 'tight.'

- Occasionally, 'overcorrection' of eyelid retraction occurs, involving the entire eyelid or segment (upper eyelid is too low or lower eyelid is too high). In the case of the upper eyelid, this can be treated with the techniques described for ptosis repair. In the case of the lower eyelid, resection/plication of the conjunctiva and underlying retractors is usually sufficient to lower the eyelid.

COMMENTS

Usually, the cause of eyelid retraction is fairly obvious based on the clinical setting and history. Graves' ophthalmopathy is the most common cause, and surgical management is aimed at weakening the eyelid retractors. Midbrain disease is an important but less common cause of upper eyelid retraction; typically, the patient has other neurologic findings that point to this cause of eyelid retraction. Postsurgical scarring and deficiency of the eyelid skin or orbital septum also may produce eyelid retraction, requiring that the shortage of these tissues be addressed. The goal of therapy is to maintain the health of the ocular surface and reduce the disfigurement associated with eyelid retraction.

REFERENCES

Bartley GB: The differential diagnosis and classification of eyelid retraction. Ophthalmology 103:168–176, 1996.

Harvey JT, Anderson RL: The aponeurotic approach to eyelid retraction. Ophthalmology 88:513–524, 1981.

Morgenstern KE, Evanchan J, Foster JA, et al: Botulinum toxin type a for dysthyroid upper eyelid retraction. Ophthal Plast Reconstr Surg; 20:181–185, 2004.

Small RG, Scott M: The tight retracted lower eyelid. Arch Ophthalmol 108:438–444, 1990.

247 MADAROSIS 374.55
(Loss of Eyelashes)

Allen M. Putterman, MD
Chicago, Illinois

ETIOLOGY/INCIDENCE

Madarosis, the loss of eyelashes, can be an undesirable cosmetic deformity. It can be caused by systemic or topical infections and inflammations, eyelid tumors, the hysteric plucking of hairs, surgery, and trauma. The hair loss may involve the entire lid but frequently involves only a segment.

DIAGNOSIS

Systemic causes of madarosis include generalized disorders, such as alopecia areata (characterized by an area or areas of sharply defined baldness) and alopecia artefacta (baldness due to the neurotic plucking of hairs or cilia). Other systemic causes of madarosis are lupus erythematosus, psoriasis, and seborrhea in which loss of eyelashes follows inflammation of the lids, as well as leprosy, syphilis, tuberculosis, sickle cell anemia, and endocrine disorders. Topical infections and inflammations, such as ulcerative and allergic blepharitis, frequently lead to the loss of cilia that is usually segmental.

Madarosis also is a complication of eyelid surgery. Absent lashes frequently occur when full-thickness segments of the lids are excised in the treatment of eyelid carcinoma. In other eyelid surgery, especially that related to the treatment of ptosis and benign tumors, lashes can be lost because of the undermining of skin from orbicularis within 2 mm of the lid margin. Traumatic lid lacerations and avulsions also are causes of madarosis.

TREATMENT

Systemic

Therapy for madarosis is aimed at treating the underlying etiologies. Medical management of systemic problems, including the emotional problems involved in alopecia artefacta, frequently leads to regrowth of the cilia. In general, lid hygiene, lid scrubs with baby shampoo, and the application of topical antibiotics (e.g. erythromycin) to the lid margins will control seborrheic blepharitis and prevent further loss of lashes. Allergic blepharitis is treated through the elimination of the offending antigens and the application of topical steroids.

Medical

The treatment of absent cilia after surgery or trauma and the control of systemic and topical infections and inflammation are difficult. Certainly, the need for treatment varies because many patients have a cosmetically acceptable appearance without lashes, especially if madarosis involves a small segment of the lid or even the entire lower lid. The easiest treatment is achieved with makeup. Eyelid liner, mascara, and false eyelashes can camouflage the defect and frequently produce a better cosmetic appearance than that achieved surgically. False eyelashes can be applied to a segment of the lid. In addition, makeup experts can attach false lashes to surrounding normal cilia through a weaving process.

Surgical

The most pleasing surgical results are achieved in patients who have had a segmental loss of lashes. The treatment consists of an eyelid excision of a full-thickness pentagon segment in the area without lashes. The surrounding normal lid segments are then connected. Three 6-0 black-silk double-armed sutures are placed through the lid margins. One suture is placed through the squared corners where the conjunctiva meets the tarsus, entering through the posterior aspect of the tarsus. The second suture is placed through the gray line. The third suture is placed through the most posterior row of cilia. The suture enters and exits from similar areas on each edge of the wound to avoid lid notching after surgery. Sutures are triple-tied, and the ends of the posterior two sutures are tied over the cilia suture, so when all six ends are cut, they point away from the cornea to avoid suture keratopathy. Two or three 6-0 Vicryl double-armed sutures are then passed through the pretarsal fascia and the anterior aspect of the tarsus on each side of the wound below the lid margin. The skin is closed with a continuous 6-0 black-silk suture.

If the normal lid segments connect with too much tension, a lateral canthotomy and cantholysis with or without a semicircular temporal flap may be needed. This is especially important in the upper eyelid, where a tight eyelid can cause ptosis. Also, it is possible to attach a segment of the lid with normal cilia to the lid segment that has a few absent cilia. Doing so decreases the area of madarosis, and a small area of absent lashes is usually acceptable. The lateral canthotomy and cantholysis and semicircular flap will leave the temporal lid segment without lashes. This also is more cosmetically acceptable than absent central lashes.

Transplantation of hairs from the eyebrow to the eyelid is another treatment of madarosis. An incision is made at the junction of the skin-lid margin over the absent lash area. The direction of the brow hairs is studied, and the hairs pointing in the desired direction are chosen. A portion of the eyebrow that is equivalent in length and width to the lid with absent cilia and consisting of four rows of hairs is excised from the eyebrow. The correct depth of the graft is critical; it must include the hair follicles while avoiding too much subcutaneous tissue. The graft is sutured to surrounding skin and lid margin so the hairs are pointing away from the cornea and correspond to the direction of the adjacent normal cilia. Usually, the outer two rows of hairs eventually slough off. This procedure commonly leads to the loss of hairs over parts of the graft and usually unsatisfactory cosmetic results.

Another alternative to lash transplantation is the removal of a segment of the normal temporal lashes and placement of them, as described, into the area of madarosis. Naugle advocated this approach and claims good results. Again, the loss of temporal lashes to create central lashes is a cosmetically desirable tradeoff. Good results have also been achieved with the placement of individual lash grafts into areas of madarosis.

Blepharopigmentation is a technique in which pigment is tattooed into the eyelids. It is chiefly advocated to simulate eyeliner or to enhance the eyelashes. However, it can also be used to simulate eyelashes and is especially effective if the eyelashes are sparse rather than totally absent. Equipment and pigment are available through Dioptics (Irvine, CA) and Alcon Surgical (Irvine, CA). Pigment is applied beneath the skin in the desired density with a rapidly pulsating needle that is covered with pigment.

COMPLICATIONS

The transplantation of eyebrow hairs into the eyelid must not be considered a cure for madarosis. The relatively high incidence of postoperative loss of transplanted brow hairs and the frequently conspicuous appearance of the brow hairs that remain should alert the surgeon to surgical failure. Blepharopigmentation initially was a popular technique but presently is used only occasionally. One of the main problems has been the difficulty of removing pigment in patients who do not like the density or the areas to which it was applied.

SUMMARY

Madarosis (loss of eyelashes) has systemic, local, hysteric, traumatic, and surgical causes. The first three categories can be treated medically. Makeup, horizontal lid shortening, and brow and lid grafts can be used to treat traumatic and surgical causes.

REFERENCES

Levine M: Blepharopigmentation. In: Putterman A, ed: Cosmetic oculoplastic surgery. 2nd edn. Philadelphia, WB Saunders, 1993:324–333.

Naugle T: Cited by Caldwell D: Eyelash loss corrected by ciliary transplantation. Ophthalmol Times 7:52–53, 1982.

Putterman AM: Basic oculoplastic surgery. In: Peyman GA, Sanders DR, Goldberg MF, eds: Principles and practice of ophthalmology. Philadelphia, WB Saunders, 1980:2292–2295.

Putterman AM: Simplified reconstruction of the eyelids. In: Tandy ME, Jr, ed: Head and neck surgery. Face, nose and facial skull, part 1. Thierre, ER Kastenbauer, 1995:1:228–237.

Putterman AM, Migliori ME: Elective excision of permanent eyeliner. Arch Ophthalmol 106:1034, 1988.

248 MARCUS GUNN SYNDROME
742.8

Roger A. Dailey, MD
Portland, Oregon
John D. Ng, MD, MS, FACS
Portland, Oregon

ETIOLOGY/INCIDENCE

The jaw-winking syndrome, described by Marcus Gunn in 1883, is one type of congenital ptosis of a synkinetic nature that classically consists of ptosis of the upper eyelid associated with involuntary retraction of the lid during contraction of the ipsilateral pterygoid muscle. This syndrome accounts for 4% to 6% of all cases of congenital ptosis.

- The condition is usually sporadic, but familial cases have been reported.
- It is almost always unilateral and more severe in downgaze.
- The often-bizarre manifestations of this syndrome are due to a congenital misdirection of part of the fifth cranial nerve that aberrantly supplies the levator muscle; therefore, stimulation to the jaw sends impulses to the variably innervated levator.
- Electromyographic studies demonstrate a synkinetic relationship between the external pterygoid muscle and the levator muscle. The lid elevates with the jaw thrusting to the opposite side (ipsilateral external pterygoid) or with the jaw projecting forward or mouth opening (bilateral external pterygoid).
- A less common type is the internal pterygoid levator synkinetic group in which the lid elevates with the muscle closing or teeth clenching. The ptosis, as well as the retraction ('winking'), varies in severity from minimal to cosmetically unacceptable, and either component may dominate the clinical picture.

COURSE/PROGNOSIS

The Marcus Gunn syndrome is persistent throughout life, although it is may become less conspicuous with time as patients learn to control or mask its features. Surgical correction can provide significant improvement in the ptosis, but the synkinetic movement persists unless the levator muscle is completely removed from the lid and attached to the superior orbital rim at the arcus marginalis or extirpated.

DIAGNOSIS

- The initial presentation typically occurs soon after birth, when the infant begins to nurse. The ptotic lid is noted to rhythmically jerk upward.
- The retraction is most commonly demonstrated by opening and closing the mouth or by moving the jaw from side to side.
- It is rarely demonstrated by coughing, smiling, the Valsalva maneuver, swallowing, inspiration, or contraction of the platysma muscle.
- Several series have reported significant associations with other ocular problems, including strabismus, anisometropia, amblyopia, and Duane's syndrome. The frequency of strabismus has been reported to be as high as 58% and includes superior rectus palsies, double elevator palsies, and horizontal deviations. Trigeminal-Abducens synkinesis has been reported.

TREATMENT

If amblyopia is present, it must be treated vigorously, and anisometropia must be corrected if it is significant.

Because the patient with Marcus Gunn syndrome brings to the clinician two separate problems (ptosis and jaw winking), the satisfactory elimination of both often is a challenging endeavor. In the evaluation of a patient, one must decide which component is more cosmetically intolerable-only then can the surgical plan be tailored accordingly and the best results obtained. A discussion with the patient or parents is important to ensure that they have realistic expectations and are aware that a compromise may be necessary.

In patients with very mild ptosis (less than 2 mm) and mild jaw wink (3 to 4 mm), one can perform a Müller's muscle conjunctival resection as described by Putterman or a levator resection; even no treatment may be acceptable. If the ptosis is moderate and the jaw winking is minimal, a levator resection is the treatment of choice. Undercorrection of the ptosis has been a complication of this approach, and it is recommended that the resection be greater (4 to 5 mm more) than in the usual case of congenital ptosis. More predictable elevation may be achieved with a combined levator resection, Muellerectomy and conjunctivotarsectomy from an anterior approach. Unfortunately, an exacerbation of the jaw wink may occur because this procedure strengthens the levator muscle and the eyelid excursion then begins at a higher level.

When the jaw-winking component is severe, a levator resection exacerbates the wink. In this case, the jaw wink must be obliterated through release of the levator aponeurosis followed by a frontalis suspension. Dryden and coworkers described a reversible technique of suturing the levator aponeurosis to the arcus marginalis of the upper orbital rim to ensure its deactivation. Bilateral levator release with fascia lata suspension of both eyelids is the procedure of choice because the often-marked asymmetry of unilateral surgery is avoided. Bilateral frontalis suspension combined with only unilateral levator excision of the affected eye also is advocated ('chicken-beard' operation). If the patient or parents refuse bilateral surgery, the frontalis suspension may be performed on the affected eye with or without prior levator release.

To effect a levator release, a skin crease incision is made, and a small amount of preseptal orbicularis is resected. The underlying septum is identified, and nearly its entire length is incised horizontally. This allows identification of the levator aponeurosis, which is released from the tarsus and attached to the arcus marginalis with multiple 5-0 Dacron sutures. Care should be taken to avoid the supraorbital neurovascular bundle. A frontalis sling of the surgeon's choice can then be performed. A double rhomboid as described by Beard is an excellent choice in this setting.

In cases in which the wink is not prominent and the levator does not have to be released, a transconjunctival frontalis suspension is an excellent option. Before the age of 3, the use of a synthetic sling is suggested, such as silicone rods or tubing. Banked fascia can be used, but in the authors' experience, this material has not been satisfactory. After the age of 3, the child's fascia lata has developed sufficiently to enable harvesting from either the midthigh or the hip area.

A stab incision is made at the upper edge of the brow where elevation of the eyelid by the surgeon's finger gives the most pleasing cosmetic appearance. This incision need not be carried down to the periosteum. A small amount of skin undermining will ensure good closure over the fascia or silicone knot later. The eyelid is then everted over a Desmarres retractor and held in place with a forceps. A fascia lata strip measuring approximately 3 mm in width and 12 to 15 cm in length is loaded on a half-circle, reverse-cutting needle (Richard Allen no. 2164-4) and passed horizontally through the lid just anterior to the superior tarsal border. This horizontal limb should measure approximately 6 to 10 mm depending on the patient's size. An attempt is made to incorporate the tarsal plate. The needle is then placed back in the lid, where it has just exited, and driven in a slightly posterior direction to an area immediately behind the superior orbital rim, 'walked' anteriorly over the rim, and brought out through the brow incision. Before this vertical fascia limb is pulled through, a small piece of 4-0 silk is placed as a marker suture at the junction of the horizontal and vertical limbs to facilitate removal of the vertical portion should repositioning of the fascia be necessary. The needle is reloaded with the opposite end of the fascia, brought through the entry site of the horizontal limb, and then directed superiorly to the brow incision in the same fashion. The result is a triangle-shaped sling with its base at the anterosuperior tarsal margin. The two vertical limbs can now be elevated to check lid margin height, contour, and symmetry. Any adjustments are made, and then the fascia is secured in the frontalis with a square knot. A 5-0 Dacron is sewn through the knot to ensure it will not slip. At this point, a good lid crease should be present, and the lid margin should be 1 to 2 mm above the desired postoperative level and in apposition with the globe.

Several modifications of the frontalis suspension have been advocated. The author favors the transconjunctival suspension in cases in which the levator has not been released. The advantages of this approach include a lesser chance of infection because it avoids low anterior skin incisions near the lash line, avoidance of visible traction lines below the skin, and facilitation of crease formation because the fascia is placed posteriorly to the orbital septum. In addition, normal attachments of the levator to the tarsus and skin are preserved so that when the frontalis muscle elevates the brow, the lid is indirectly raised and normal lid margin contour and apposition to the globe are maintained. This procedure is also inherently safer because the needle used to pass the fascia lata is never directed toward the eyeball, therefore minimizing the chance of ocular penetration.

In cases of unilateral ptosis in which the levator is released, a promising technique involving the advancement of a flap of frontalis muscle to the superior tarsus has been successful. The long-term results have not been published, but it appears to be far more successful than the corrugator muscle transpositions used in the 1960s. When an anterior approach is performed, the sling material is sutured to the tarsal surface. The Richard Allen needle is used to pass the free ends in a post-septal plane and out the suprabrow incision in the same manner as the transconjunctival approach. Fixation sutures may be used to evert the eyelashes prior to skin closure to avoid lash ptosis that can occur with frontalis suspensions.

COMMENTS

The jaw-winking syndrome is one type of congenital ptosis of a synkinetic nature that classically consists of ptosis of the upper eyelid associated with involuntary retraction of the lid during contraction of the ipsilateral pterygoid muscle. In general, the wink tends to become less noticeable with age, so if it is minimal and the patient has more than 4 mm of levator function, a standard levator resection should be highly successful. In cases of poor levator function, a frontalis suspension of some type should be used; if the wink is severe, the levator should be released from the tarsus and tacked to the arcus marginalis, followed by frontalis suspension.

REFERENCES

Beyer-Machule CK, Johnson CC, Pratt SG, Smith BR: The Marcus Gunn phenomenon. Orbit 4:15, 1985.

Bullock JD: Marcus Gunn jaw-winking ptosis: classification and surgical management. J Pediatric Ophthalmol Strabismus 17:375, 1980.

Dailey RA, Wilson DJ, Wobig JL: Transconjunctival frontalis suspension (TCFS). Ophthalmol Plast Reconstr Surg 7, 1991.

Darcet TW, Crawford JS: The quantification, natural course, and surgical results in 57 eyes with Marcus Gunn (jaw-winking) syndrome. Am J Ophthalmol 92:702–707, 1981.

Dryden RM, Fleuringer JL, Quickert MH: Levator transposition and frontalis sling procedure in severe unilateral ptosis and paradoxically innervated levator. Arch Ophthalmol 100:462, 1982.

Kodsi S: Marcus Gunn jaw winking with trigemino-abducens synkinesis. J AAPOS 4:316–7, 2000.

249 MELANOCYTIC LESIONS OF THE EYELIDS 172.1

(Ephelis, Lentigo, Nevocellular Nevus, Dermal Melanocytosis, Malignant Melanoma)

Steven A. McCormick, MD, FACP
New York, New York
Tatyana Milman, MD, FAAO
New York, New York

ETIOLOGY

Benign melanocytic lesions of the eyelids are a diverse group of congenital and acquired lesions derived from neural crest melanocytes. Three distinct cells of origin-epidermal melanocytes, nevocellular nevus cells, and dermal melanocytes-result in a variety of clinically distinct pigmented lesions of the skin. Classification schemes should distinguish among these three cell types and the location of origin. All of these cells have the capacity to synthesize and excrete melanin, the primary cutaneous pigment.

CLINICAL DIAGNOSIS

Examination should be performed in good light; the wide beam of the slit lamp is ideal. Size, location, and description of the lesion (height, surface and border characteristics, color, and so on) should be carefully recorded. The goal of the examination is to determine whether the lesion is likely to be a benign or malignant melanocytic lesion or another pigmented lesion of nonmelanocytic origin, such as seborrheic keratosis or pigmented basal or squamous cell carcinoma. Photographs of suspicious lesions are helpful in documenting the growth or changes in coloration that may signal malignancy.

The clinicopathologic features of these entities are discussed to assist the examiner in establishing the correct clinical diagnosis and in affecting appropriate management.

BENIGN LESIONS

Benign lesions derived from the epidermal melanocytes include the ephelis (common freckle), lentigo simplex, and solar lentigo ('age spot'). All commonly affect the periocular skin, as well as skin elsewhere. Ephelides are not truly tumors, but are perhaps the most common of all skin lesions, affecting all whites to some degree, as well as pigmented races. Solar lentigines are also common in whites with excessive sun exposure.

Benign tumors composed of nevocellular nevus cells are referred to as *melanocytic nevi* (clinically, the simple term *nevus* is usually applied). Nevi are classified as junctional, intradermal, or compound based on the histologic location of the nevocellular proliferation. Most of the brown to black coloration results from melanin in the superficial skin, whereas tumefaction results from a dermal component. Location in the basal epidermis (junctional component) usually imparts a darker color (black to brown) than when the proliferation is limited to the dermis (intradermal nevus). When nevus cells are present in both locations, the term *compound nevus* is applied. Common nevi tend to evolve throughout life, beginning usually as pigmented macules or papules, increasing in height and/or pigmentation (especially under the hormonal influences of puberty or pregnancy), and finally regressing with depigmentation, fat infiltration, and fibrosis. Some larger nevi may harbor hair follicles or have a papillomatous surface.

Most nevi are noted at birth or in early childhood, and it is often difficult to determine whether a given lesion is congenital or acquired. Unlike 'typical' nevi, large congenital nevi (1 cm or more in diameter and evident at birth) are treated aggressively because of their propensity to give rise to malignant melanoma in approximately 12% of the cases. An example of congenital nevus affecting the eyelids is the 'kissing' nevus, which develops in utero before the normal development of the eyelid fissure. The nevus, thus, is located on apposed areas of the upper and lower eyelids. These, like other bulky nevi, are usually removed for cosmetic or mechanical reasons.

Another special variant is the Spitz nevus, or spindle and epithelioid cell nevus. This tumor commonly presents on the face of children and young adults as a small, sharply demarcated, symmetrical, dome-shaped papule, seated in the dermis. It may be erythematous and hyperpigmented, and may enlarge rapidly (up to 10 mm), mimicking malignant melanoma. Despite its aggressive histologic appearance, this lesion is benign and self-limited.

A controversial category is the dysplastic nevus, occurring in as many as 8% of the population. These nevi are macules that are usually larger than typical nevi (more than 4 mm) and present with less distinct borders and mottled pigmentation. Some have been compared morphologically to a 'fried egg.' Dysplastic nevi may occur in two clinical settings: in patients with a familial autosomal dominant dysplastic nevus syndrome (B-K mole syndrome), and as a sporadic condition (sporadic dysplastic nevus syndrome). In B-K mole syndrome the lifetime risk for the development of malignant melanoma approaches 100%. The lifetime risk for malignant transformation in a sporadic dysplastic nevus syndrome has been estimated between 18–20%, but the majority of experts believe that most sporadic dysplastic nevi will never transform into melanoma, and do not qualify them as precancerous lesions. The histologic parameters for these lesions are likewise debated. Caution suggests close observation and excision if change or growth is documented.

Benign lesions derived from dermal melanocytes include the blue nevus and nevus of Ota. The blue nevus results from a focal proliferation of dermal melanocytes in the deeper layers of the dermis. Pigment thus situated results in slate-gray to blue coloration through the Tyndall phenomenon. The nevus of Ota is a larger area of similar skin coloration that results from a less dense distribution of dermal melanocytes (dermal melanocytosis). Ipsilateral ocular melanocytosis usually is also present, imparting slate-gray pigmentation of the sclera and increased pigmentation in the uveal tract. These patients have no increased risk for the development of cutaneous malignant melanoma, but there is a reported increased risk of uveal, orbital, and CNS malignant melanoma; therefore, regular ophthalmic examinations should be performed.

Lesions of epidermal melanocytes

Ephelis (common freckle)

- Etiology: threshold dose of UV exposure leading to the development in genetically predisposed individuals; freckles darkening with additional sun exposure; no increase in melanocytes (only increased melanin production).
- Clinical findings: small tan to brown macules on sun-exposed skin (less than 1 to 3 mm).
- Treatment: no treatment.

Lentigo simplex

- Etiology: no predilection for sun-exposed skin; no darkening of the lesions with UV exposure; multiple lesions suggesting an association with systemic syndromes (e.g. Peutz–Jeghers, LAMB, or leopard syndromes); histologically, increase in number of epidermal melanocytes; regarded by some as a form of evolving melanocytic nevus.
- Clinical findings: small brown to black macules, darker and larger than ephelis; clinically indistinguishable from a junctional nevus
- Treatment: no treatment

Solar lentigo

- Etiology: accumulative UV exposure leading to the development on sun-exposed skin of older individuals (hence the previous term 'senile lentigo').
- Clinical findings: multiple large, evenly pigmented macules on sun-exposed skin (1 to 7 mm); may gradually enlarge and coalesce; in xeroderma pigmentosum, often appear by adolescence; histologically, no obvious (or minimal) increase in the number of epidermal melanocytes (increased melanin production).
- Treatment: both UV protection and avoidance of sun exposure.

Melanocytic (nevocellular) nevi

- Etiology: hamartia of melanoblasts arrested in their normal migration and development into epidermal melanocytes; ubiquitous and affect all races; sun exposure and hormonal factors may be operative (often enlarge at puberty and in pregnancy).
- Clinical findings: morphology and pigmentation vary from small, flat macules to elevated, dome-shaped lesions; may be pedunculated and papillomatous; pigmentation ranges from tan to black; usually evenly pigmented; may increase in size over time.
- Classification: junctional, intradermal, or compound types (histologically); *dysplastic nevus* is a controversial subtype that may possibly be a precursor for melanoma; other special types includes Spitz nevus, balloon cell nevus, and congenital melanocytic nevus.
- Treatment: excisional biopsy, if indicated, or observation.

Lesions of dermal melanocytes

- Etiology: increased numbers of dermal melanocytes, forming focal tumors (blue nevi) or diffuse distribution of melanocytes (nevus of Ota).
- Clinical findings: blue nevi with slate-gray to blue pigmentation due to the deep-seated pigmentation (Tyndall's phenomenon); common in head and neck region; may be slightly raised, but epidermis not affected; nevus of Ota not usually elevated, but displays diffuse slate-gray pigmentation in distribution of the trigeminal nerve; may be bilateral; ipsilateral scleral pigmentation usually present; increased risk of *uveal, orbital, CNS* melanoma.
- Treatment: excisional biopsy of blue nevus if tumefaction is large or cosmetically undesirable; no practical treatment available for nevus of Ota.

MALIGNANT AND PREMALIGNANT LESIONS

Primary malignant melanoma of the eyelid and periocular skin is relatively rare, representing 1% to 5% of all eyelid malignancies. The incidence of cutaneous melanoma has been increasing at an alarming rate (more than 600% increase from 1950 to 2000), and undoubtedly so will the incidence of eyelid melanoma. Most melanomas arise de novo from transformed, atypical basal melanocytes, but in 25% to 35% of cases, histologic remnants of a benign nevus may be detected. The clinician must be suspicious of the 'changing mole' or any newly recognized pigmented lesion. The practitioner's task is to recognize the surface characteristics that are harbingers of malignancy. Malignant lesions tend to display irregular or notched borders rather than the smooth, symmetric borders of nevi and other pigmented lesions. They often display variegated pigmentation, ranging from pink/red to brown/black, whereas nevi tend to be uniformly pigmented. Acquired nevi tend to be less than 5 mm in diameter; malignant lesions are usually larger. However, other pigmented, nonmelanocytic lesions (e.g. seborrheic keratosis and keratoacanthoma) may be large. Change in clinical appearance and symptoms (i.e. evolution) of the lesion are uncommon in nevi, but are frequently observed in cutaneous malignant melanoma. The 'ABCDE rule' of clinical signs is a helpful mnemonic: asymmetry, border irregularity, variation in color, diameter of more than 5 mm, and evolution.

Lentigo maligna (Hutchinson's freckle) may be considered a premalignant lesion that has a natural history unlike the other types of malignant melanoma. It is a relatively common finding on the face in elderly Caucasian individuals, and often involves the lower eyelid and lateral canthal region. Lentigo maligna begins as one or more pigmented patches with irregular borders, and enlarges slowly (over several years). As the lesion expands, the pigmentation may change as some areas regress and others proliferate. Lentigo maligna may, after this protracted *in situ* phase, progress to lentigo malignant melanoma, probably the most common melanoma type affecting the eyelid skin. The appearance of nodularity within the lesion is often an indicator of progression to the invasive stage. The risk of progression appears to be low (variable lifetime risk figures are quoted: from 5% to 50%).

Malignant melanoma of the periocular skin, arising *de novo* or within a pre-existing acquired or congenital nevus, is classified as either superficial spreading melanoma or nodular melanoma. Superficial spreading melanoma, the most common melanoma subtype of the head and neck region, begins as a brown to gray or rose-colored, minimally elevated *in situ* lesion with irregular, notched borders. Unlike with lentigo maligna, the lesion is rarely more than a few centimeters in its radial growth phase and becomes minimally invasive much earlier (typically within 1 year). It is important to recognize and excise the lesion at this stage. Induration, elevation, and mottling are early signs of invasion.

Nodular malignant melanoma begins as an elevated, often darkly pigmented tumor that increases in bulk rapidly and, unlike superficial spreading melanoma, often ulcerates and bleeds. A radial growth phase is not usually recognized; an in situ lesion is not included in the classification. Because the vertical invasion occurs early, nodular melanoma usually presents with a smaller diameter than superficial spreading melanoma (often less than 1 cm). As a result of its early and aggressive invasive growth, this type of cutaneous melanoma carries the worst prognosis.

Staging schemes separate patients with local disease only (stages I and II), with local nodal metastases (stage III), or with distant nodal or visceral metastases (stage IV). Approximately 80–90% of cases are diagnosed in stages I and II, with a 5-year survival rate of around 90%. Prognosis in localized disease is gauged on the depth of invasion as measured microscopically. Breslow found that tumors of less than 0.76 mm in thickness (measured from the granular cell layer of the epidermis to the deepest extent of invasion) did not metastasize (and therefore did not require regional node dissection). In patients with tumors of more than 1.5 mm, survival rates are doubled if regional lymphadenectomy is performed. Sentinel lymph node biopsy is currently recommended for localized lesions with tumor thickness greater than 1 mm; if positive, the biopsy is followed by regional lymph node dissection. Prognosis is poor for stages III and IV; 5-year survival rates are reported as 60% for regional (stage III) disease, and 14% for distal metastatic disease. In regional disease, the number of involved lymph nodes, tumor burden within the lymph nodes, and ulceration within the primary tumor are important predictors of survival.

Lentigo maligna and lentigo maligna melanomas

- Etiology: may occur as a result of chronic, cumulative sun exposure; atypical melanocytes proliferate in the basal regions of the epidermis in Hutchinson's freckle; invasion in 5%–50% (lenitgo maligna melanoma), but usually only after many years of evolution.
- Clinical findings: slowly enlarging irregular pigmented macule or macules with irregular borders that evolve over several years; frequently involve the lateral canthal region and lower eyelid; induration, elevation, and change in coloration possible signs of invasion.
- Treatment: excision, especially if nodularity develops within the macule.

Malignant melanoma (superficial spreading or nodular)

- Etiology: may be caused by episodic, intense sun exposure; malignant transformation of basal epidermal melanocytes (or less commonly, malignant degeneration of nevus cells); growth proceeds from an *in situ* phase (recognized in superficial spreading melanoma) to invasive growth, which proceeds more rapidly in nodular melanoma.
- Clinical findings: the ABCDE rule (asymmetry, border irregularity, variation in color, diameter of more than 5 mm, evolution) is useful; pigmented macules with these features should be considered suspicious for superficial spreading melanoma; nodular melanomas present as enlarging, elevated lesions with variable dark pigmentation; evolution may be noted in up to 80%; induration and changing pigmentation are harbingers of malignancy.
- Treatment: excisional biopsy of suspicious lesions, preferably with up to 1-cm margins of resection; incisional biopsy of large lesions if the diagnosis is in question; sentinel lymph node biopsy for lesions with tumor thickness greater than 1 mm; regional lymph node dissection if positive nodes are identified.

SUMMARY

Pigmented lesions of the eyelid and periocular skin present a challenge to the ophthalmologist, but the importance of recognizing suspicious tumors cannot be overemphasized. Lesions removed early in their course carry an extremely favorable prognosis, and surgical extirpation in the facial region is accomplished with limited cosmetic effects when lesions are small. The task of the clinician is to differentiate among benign, premalignant, and malignant lesions with the use of clinical examination and review of the patient's historical observations of the lesion. The clinician must also recognize that several nonmelanocytic lesions may present as pigmented tumors; these include pigmented basal cell carcinoma, actinic keratosis, keratoacanthoma, seborrheic keratosis, and dermatofibroma. Suspicious lesions should be biopsied.

REFERENCES

Abbasi NR, Shaw HM, Rigel DS, et al: Early diagnosis of cutaneous melanoma: revisiting the ABCD criteria. JAMA 292(22):2771–2776, 2004.

Balmaceda CM, Fetell MR, O'Brien JL, et al: Nevus of Ota and leptomeningeal melanocytic lesions. Neurology 43(2):381–386, 1993.

Clark WH, Elder DE, Guerry D, et al: A study of tumor progression: the precursor lesions of superficial spreading and nodular melanoma. Hum Pathol 15:1147–1165, 1984.

Cramer SF: The histogenesis of acquired melanocytic nevi. Based on a new concept of melanocytic differentiation. Am J Dermatopathol 6 Suppl: 289–298, 1984.

Cramer SF: The origin of epidermal melanocytes: implications for the histogenesis of nevi and melanomas. Arch Pathol Lab Med 115:115–119, 1991.

Crowson AN, Magro CM, Sanchez-Carpintero I, et al: The precursors of malignant melanoma. Recent Results Cancer Res160:75–84, 2002.

Elder DE, Murphy GF: Atlas of tumor pathology: melanocytic tumors of the skin (third series, fascicle 2). Washington, DC, Armed Forces Institute of Pathology, 1991.

Grossniklaus HE, McLean IW: Cutaneous melanoma of the eyelid: clinicopathologic features. Ophthalmology 98:1867–1873, 1991.

Kienstra MA, Padhya TA: Head and neck melanoma. Cancer Control 12(4):242–247, 2005.

Le AD, Fenske NA, Glass LF, et al: Malignant melanoma: differential diagnosis of pigmented lesions. J Fla Med Assoc 84(3):166–174, 1997.

Lever WF, Schaumberg-Lever G: Histopathology of the skin. Philadelphia, JB Lippincott, 1990, pp. 756–805.

Lopransi S, Mihm MC: Clinical and pathological correlation of malignant melanoma. J Cutan Pathol 6:180–194, 1979.

Rager EL, Bridgeford EP, Ollila DW: Cutaneous melanoma: update on prevention, screening, diagnosis, and treatment. Am Fam Physician 72(2):269–276, 2005.

Spencer WH (ed): Ophthalmic pathology: an atlas and text. Philadelphia, WB Saunders, 1996:2261–2278.

Stevenson O, Ahmed I: Lentigo maligna : prognosis and treatment options. Am J Clin Dermatol 6(3):151–164, 2005.

Vaziri M, Buffam FV, Martinka M, et al: Clinicopathologic features and behavior of cutaneous eyelid melanoma. Ophthalmology 109(5):901–908, 2002.

250 ORBITAL FAT HERNIATION 374.34

(Eyelid Fat Prolapse, Orbital Fat Prolapse, Adipose Palpebral Bags, Baggy Eyelids)

Eric A. Steele, MD
Portland, Oregon
Roger A. Dailey, MD
Portland, Oregon

ETIOLOGY

Fullness of either the upper or lower eyelid can result from the herniation of orbital fat through the orbital septum, fluid retention or accumulation in the periocular tissues, prolapse of the lacrimal gland, or excess skin (dermatochalasis). Orbital fat herniation results from atrophy and dehiscence of the orbital septum allowing for forward prolapse of the orbital fat pads. In the upper eyelid, orbital fat prolapse may contribute to mechanical ptosis, as well as pose cosmetic concerns in conjunction with dermatochalasis. In the lower eyelid, fat prolapse will result in cosmetic deformity based on underlying bony anatomy and the status of other mid facial soft tissues.

- The thin nature of the orbital septum allows hereditary or involutional herniation of orbital fat.
- Thyroid immune-related orbitopathy may increase the volume of fat and lead to prolapse in the upper and lower eyelids.
- Posterior sub-Tenon injection of triamcinolone may cause ptosis and/or orbital fat prolapse.

DIAGNOSIS

The diagnosis is made on the basis of careful general medical and ophthalmologic history and clinical examination. An examination of eyelid fullness is made by palpation and ballottement of the globe with observation of the fat pads.

Differential diagnosis

- Dermatochalasis.
- Prolapsed lacrimal gland.
- Eyelid edema or blepharochalasis.
- Thyroid immune related orbitopathy.
- Festoons or cheek bags.

All of the above may be present in conjunction with orbital fat prolapse.

TREATMENT

Local

- Make-up applied by a skilled aesthetician may slightly improve the cosmetic appearance.

Surgical

Upper eyelid

- Surgical intervention in the upper eyelid will often involve simultaneous treatment of dermatochalasis.
- Surgery is performed most commonly with the patient under local or monitored anesthesia. After infiltration with a local anesthetic agent containing epinephrine, the amount of skin to be excised is marked. The lower border of skin excision coincides with the eyelid crease.
- Incision through skin and muscle is made with a scalpel or CO_2 laser. Skin and muscle are excised either in one flap or separately. The orbital septum is identified and incised in a complete horizontal 'open sky' fashion to expose the preaponeurotic fat pads.
- After supplemental injection of fat pads with anesthetic agent if necessary, the medial and central fat pads are excised as needed to obtain the desired result. Clamping of the fat pads can be used; meticulous hemostasis is mandatory.
- Care is taken to avoid resection of the lacrimal gland or overzealous resection of fat, especially in the medial central pad, to avoid an A-frame deformity or hollowed appearance after surgery.
- The skin edges are closed with a running nylon suture (6-0 or 7-0); the septum is not sutured. Crease formation stitches through the levator aponeurosis are used as desired.

Lower eyelid: transcutaneous

- The transcutaneous approach can be used where excessive skin (dermatochalasis) accompanies orbital fat herniation. Anesthesia is performed as described for the upper eyelid.

A subciliary incision is placed 2 to 3 mm below the lashes of the lower eyelid. Skin and muscle are incised with a scalpel or CO_2 laser.
- The skin-orbicularis flap is then dissected inferiorly to expose the orbital septum.
- Stab incisions or wide incision of the septum is made over the prolapsing fat pads. The fat pads (medial, central, and temporal) are teased out of their capsules and excised as needed with any combination of clamping, cautery and CO_2 laser. Meticulous hemostasis is used.
- Options at this point include a release of the arcus marginalis and draping of excess orbital fat over the orbital rim to improve contour deformities in the midface and the tear trough deformity. The redraped orbital fat can be fixed to the suborbicularis oculi fat pad or periosteum as desired with an absorbable suture.
- The septum is not closed, and the skin-orbicularis flap is draped back over the residual fat pads; then, skin, muscle, or both are excised as necessary. Care must be taken to have the patient look up and open the mouth to determine the safe amount of skin and muscle to be excised.

Lower eyelid: transconjunctival

- Transconjunctival lower eyelid blepharoplasty is the procedure of choice for most cases of pure orbital fat prolapse without significant dermatochalasis.
- After appropriate anesthesia, the globe is protected with a Jaeger lid plate using gentle pressure to prolapse the fat pads. The lower lid is pulled down by the assistant, and an incision is made through the conjunctiva and capsulopalpebral fascia to reach the orbital fat pads. The incision is placed approximately midway between the inferior border of the lower tarsus and the inferior fornix and can be made with scissors, scalpel, cutting cautery, radiofrequency, or CO_2 laser.
- The tarsus is retracted inferiorly with a Desmarres retractor, and the capsulopalpebral fascia is retracted superiorly with a traction suture. The fat pads are identified and teased from their respective capsules. Care is taken to identify and avoid damage to the inferior oblique muscle between the central and medial fat pads. Fat is removed in a graded fashion to obtain the desired result.
- Options include release of the arcus marginalis and repositioning of orbital fat across the orbital rim to correct midfacial contour abnormalities or tear trough deformity. The repositioned fat can be fixed with buried absorbable sutures or with externalized sutures removed in the postoperative period.
- The conjunctival incision is not closed.

COMPLICATIONS

Complications can result from an incomplete preoperative workup or poor surgical planning. Failure to recognize preexisting conditions such as lid laxity, lid edema, metabolic conditions (e.g. thyroid conditions, allergy, sodium imbalance), hypertrophy of orbicularis oculi, relative prominence of the globe, blepharochalasis, or lid malpositions will compromise the surgical result and patient satisfaction.

Complications include:

- Lower lid ectropion and/or retraction;
- Rounding of the lateral canthal angle;
- Upper eyelid retraction and lagophthalmos;
- Superior sulcus deformity (excessive fat removal);
- Ptosis;
- Lacrimal gland injury;
- Blindness (orbital hemorrhage).

COMMENTS

Orbital fat prolapse is primarily a cosmetic concern; thus, care for these patients should be undertaken with a thorough knowledge of anatomy, patient expectations, and surgical technique. State-of-the-art care includes the use of CO_2 laser and attention to fat preservation and repositioning techniques.

REFERENCES

Baylis HI, Long JA, Groth MJ: Transconjunctival lower eyelid blepharoplasty: technique and complications. Ophthalmology 96:1027–1032, 1989.

Dailey RA, Wobig JL: Eyelid anatomy. J Dermatol Surg Oncol 18:1023–1027, 1992.

Del Canto AJ, Downs-Kelly E, Perry JD: Ptosis and orbital fat prolapse after posterior sub-Tenon's capsule triamcinolone injection. Ophthalmology 112:1092–1097, 2005.

Hamra ST: Arcus marginalis release and orbital fat preservation in midface rejuvenation. Plast Reconst Surg 96:354–362, 1995.

Wobig JL, Dailey RA: Oculofacial plastic surgery. New York, Thieme, 2004.

251 PTOSIS 374.30 (Blepharoptosis)

Eric A. Steele, MD
Portland, Oregon
Roger A. Dailey, MD
Portland, Oregon

The term blepharoptosis refers to an abnormally low upper eyelid. The retractors of the upper lid are the levator palpebrae superioris, innervated by the superior division of the oculomotor nerve and responsible for the majority of lid elevation, and the superior tarsal (Müller's) muscle, a smooth, sympathetically innervated muscle responsible for approximately 1 to 2 mm of lid elevation. The protractor of the eyelids is the orbicularis oculi muscle, and lid position is determined by the balance of these forces.

ETIOLOGY

Ptosis has traditionally been categorized as congenital versus acquired. A mechanistic classification may be more useful in distinguishing types of ptosis and the appropriate surgical intervention. Accordingly, ptosis may be divided into myogenic, neurogenic, aponeurotic, or mechanical causes.

Myogenic ptosis

- Myogenic causes include any disorder with reduced or absent levator palpebrae muscle function secondary to maldevelopment, dystrophy, degeneration, or injury of the levator muscle.

- Congenital ptosis is usually myogenic and thought to result from abnormal development of the levator muscle (fibrofatty replacement of the normal striated muscle fibers). It may be unilateral or bilateral and is generally characterized by reduced levator muscle function, lid lag on downgaze, poor or absent lid crease, and lagophthalmos (incomplete closure). Congenital ptosis may occasionally be inherited as an autosomal dominant trait, but it is usually an isolated congenital anomaly. Ptosis is associated with many syndromes, including the blepharophimosis syndrome (an autosomal dominant condition typified by bilateral ptosis, telecanthus, epicanthus inversus, and phimosis). In addition, congenital ptosis may be associated with superior rectus dysfunction, amblyopia, astigmatism, anisometropia, and strabismus. Amblyopia, when seen with ptosis, is usually secondary to induced astigmatism or anisometropia and only rarely results from sensory deprivation. Occlusion or other treatment modalities should be continued after ptosis repair.
- Other causes of myogenic ptosis include chronic progressive external ophthalmoplegia, congenital fibrosis syndrome, disorders of the neuromuscular junction (e.g. myasthenia gravis), and muscular dystrophies such as oculopharyngeal muscular dystrophy and myotonic dystrophy.
- Occasionally, trauma may primarily damage the levator muscle itself without affecting its aponeurosis or innervation.

Neurogenic ptosis

- Neurogenic causes of ptosis include cranial nerve III dysfunction (with partial or complete ptosis depending on the site and degree of nerve involvement), Horner's syndrome (loss of sympathetic innervation to Müller's muscle, typically resulting in 2 mm or less of ptosis), Marcus Gunn jaw-winking syndrome (unilateral ptosis with synkinesis of the ipsilateral pterygoid and levator muscles such that jaw movement may result in retraction of the ptotic lid), Guillain–Barré syndrome (especially the Miller–Fisher variant in which ptosis may occur in association with ophthalmoplegia, mydriasis, ataxia, and areflexia), botulism (characterized by dilated, sluggish pupils, dry mouth, flaccid paresis, and ptosis), multiple sclerosis, and ophthalmoplegic migraine. Of course, trauma with resultant sympathetic or cranial nerve III damage may also cause ptosis on a neurogenic basis.

Aponeurogenic ptosis

- Aponeurotic or aponeurogenic ptosis is the most common cause of acquired ptosis. Stretching of the levator aponeurosis or dehiscence of its insertion onto the tarsal plate (as occurs with aging, trauma, or hard contact lens wear or after ocular surgery with a lid speculum) causes acquired ptosis, characterized by normal levator function, a high lid crease, deep supratarsal sulcus, and increased ptosis on downgaze.

Mechanical ptosis

- Mechanical causes of ptosis include cicatricial changes, lid masses, dermatochalasis, brow ptosis, and microphthalmos or enophthalmos. Floppy eyelid syndrome, characterized by lid laxity, chronic papillary conjunctivitis, and lash ptosis, may also present with ptosis.

DIAGNOSIS

Clinical signs and symptoms

- The evaluation of ptosis requires a careful history to determine the age of onset, familial incidence, rate of progression, variability/fatigability, and association with other ocular findings.

Laboratory findings

- As part of a complete ophthalmologic evaluation, motility assessment, pupillary testing, and inspection of Bell's phenomenon should be performed.
- Palpebral fissure measurement (9 mm is considered normal), margin-reflex (from upper lid to the light reflex) distance measurement, and estimation of levator excursion while immobilizing the frontalis muscle (to evaluate levator palpebrae muscle function) will determine the type of surgical intervention best suited for the patient. It is also helpful to manually elevate the ptotic lid to eliminate the effect of Hering's law and assess the amount of ptosis in the contralateral eye.
- Should any variability or fatigability be elicited, a Tensilon test and serologic evaluation for acetylcholine receptor antibodies may be helpful in diagnosing myasthenia gravis.
- In patients with mild ptosis (2 mm or less), testing with 2.5% phenylephrine eyedrops can help determine the expected result of ptosis repair via a conjunctiva-Müller's resection (see below).
- Visual field testing with ptosis and then with manual elevation of the eyelid can be used to determine the degree of visual field loss associated with ptosis. Documentation of field loss and preoperative photographs are usually required by health insurance carriers before authorization for surgical repair.

Differential diagnosis

- True ptosis must be distinguished from pseudoptosis, in which an abnormally low upper eyelid is caused by factors other than dysfunction of the lid elevators. Conditions that mimic ptosis include vertical misalignment, as occurs in hypotropia, blepharospasm, or squinting, and contralateral lid retraction, as occurs in thyroid eye disease and dermatochalasis.
- The systemic conditions and congenital syndromes associated with ptosis should be sought, and the appropriate treatment should be instituted.

TREATMENT

Surgical

- In the majority of patients with acquired ptosis, good levator function (8 mm or more) can be demonstrated, and the preferred method of repair is an external lid crease incision with reattachment or advancement of the levator aponeurosis to the tarsal plate. The lid crease should be carefully marked before infiltration of the eyelid with a local anesthetic agent. After a skin incision at the lid crease, the dissection is carried through the orbicularis muscle and orbital septum, exposing the preaponeurotic adipose tissue anterior to the levator aponeurosis. The aponeurosis is then separated from its attachments to the overlying adipose tissue and the underlying Müller's muscle. The tarsal plate is exposed, and the aponeurosis is reattached to the tarsus with sutures. When surgery is performed under local anesthesia, the patient should be raised to a sitting position to assess the lid height and contour.

- With fair levator function (5 to 7 mm), a large external levator resection (up to Whitnall's ligament in many cases) may be necessary to achieve the desired result. The procedure is similar to the external approach for levator repair. Resection of the superior tarsus is an additional technique for maximal elevation of the eyelid.
- Ptosis with poor levator function (4 mm or less) generally requires frontalis suspension. This can be performed either transcutaneously or transconjunctivally, utilizing autogenous or banked fascia lata or synthetic materials such as silicone rods. These materials are used to suspend the eyelid directly from the frontalis muscle to allow the brow to efficiently raise the eyelid. When the ptosis is unilateral, some advocate disinsertion of the (normal) contralateral levator aponeurosis combined with bilateral frontalis suspension to further stimulate frontalis use and to achieve symmetry on downgaze. The decision to modify a normal eyelid is controversial and requires thorough preoperative discussion.
- In patients with mild ptosis, excellent levator function, and a positive phenylephrine test, a conjunctiva-Möller's resection via an internal approach is effective. The lid is everted, and a segment of conjunctiva and Müller's muscle is resected using a Putterman clamp. The cut edges of the incision are sutured with 6-0 plain suture.
- For patients in whom surgery is not an option, ptosis crutches may be attached to the upper posterior rim of eyeglasses and used to mechanically elevate the lid. The lid may not close properly, however, and the patient could develop exposure keratopathy.

COMPLICATIONS

The complications of surgical ptosis management may be divided into the categories of overcorrection, undercorrection, improper suture placement, and tissue reaction.

- In general, *overcorrection* causes exposure keratitis and therefore necessitates early adjustment. The external levator approach allows loosening or removal of the sutures in the levator aponeurosis, and this adjustment can easily be performed in the outpatient clinic under local anesthesia during the early postoperative period. Overcorrection after any method of ptosis repair may cause severe exposure keratopathy and should especially be avoided in patients with poor Bell's phenomenon and weak orbicularis function, as occurs with chronic progressive external ophthalmoplegia, dystrophies, and congenital fibrosis syndrome. Occasionally, the lid must be lowered to a less functional and cosmetically appealing height to prevent keratopathy.
- *Undercorrection* is common in congenital ptosis and may necessitate repeat surgery depending on the needs and expectations of the patient and family.
- If the *sutures* attaching the frontalis sling or levator aponeurosis to the tarsus are placed too high or too low, entropion or ectropion may result. Careful attention to incorporation of levator aponeurosis within lid crease fixation sutures may also avoid lid malpositions.
- With large levator resections, *conjunctival prolapse* may result and can be treated with patching, suturing of the palpebral conjunctiva up into the fornix, or excision of the redundant tissue.
- In patients with frontalis slings, there may be exposure of silicone rods or early reabsorption of banked fascia lata, necessitating repeat surgery.
- Patients with concomitant strabismus should have their extraocular muscle surgery first because changes in extraocular muscle placement may affect lid position. In addition, if the strabismus cannot be satisfactorily treated in adults, intractable diplopia may result from elevation of the lid to a normal height.

COMMENTS

Ptosis is a complex and challenging disorder, requiring careful evaluation of the causative mechanism and surgical options to devise the most appropriate treatment strategy for each patient.

REFERENCES

Anderson RL: Aponeurotic ptosis surgery. Arch Ophthalmol 97:1123, 1979.

Callahan M, Beard C: Ptosis. 4th edn. Birmingham, Aesculapius, 1990.

Frueh BR: The mechanistic classification of ptosis. Ophthalmology 87:1019, 1980.

Wobig JL, Dailey RA: Oculofacial plastic surgery. New York, Thieme, 2004.

252 SEBORRHEIC BLEPHARITIS 372.20

Peter B. Marsh, MD
Portland, Oregon

ETIOLOGY

Seborrheic blepharitis is a common cause of eyelid inflammation which may affect the anterior or posterior lamella of the eyelids, or both, and cause significant ocular discomfort. It is frequently seen in patients with seborrheic dermatitis. Seborrheic blepharitis alone presents with inflammation of the anterior lid margin with greasy sebum secretions near the eyelashes. Posteriorly, involvement of the meibomian glands is one cause of meibomian gland dysfunction. In contrast to seborrheic blepharitis alone, this may lead to patchy inflammation of the meibomian glands which in turn can cause blockage of the glands with inspissated secretions and significant periods of exacerbation of symptoms. The exact etiology is not known. However, an altered meibum composition may be responsible, along with increased *Staphylococcus aureus* colonization of the eyelid. Although usually a chronic condition, treatment can improve symptoms, especially during times of exacerbation.

DIAGNOSIS

Clinical signs and symptoms

Patients with seborrheic blepharitis present with symptoms of ocular irritation, including burning, itching, redness, and mildly decreased vision. Meibomian keratoconjunctivitis is distinguished from other types of seborrheic blepharitis by a shorter duration of symptoms at the time of presentation and a more pronounced inflammation of the eyelids. The anterior aspects of the lids frequently are only minimally involved with deposition of an oily scurf. The prominent feature is diffuse inflammation around the meibomian glands, which are dilated with retained meibum that is not easily expressed. The orifices of the glands are obstructed and pout with these secretions. There is a marked inflammation around the meibomian glands and the orifices. Tear breakup time is frequently shortened due to the abnormal composition of the lipid tear layer.

In addition to the lid findings, an important associated condition found in these patients is aqueous tear deficiency (ATD). The symptoms of ATD are similar to those in (and may be masked by the complaints of) patients whose predominant problems are related to blepharitis. Patients with chronic blepharitis, however, have been shown to have changes in the composition of meibum, which may lead to alterations in the tear film, thereby predisposing these patients to associated ocular surface problems related to an unstable tear film. Studies have documented concurrent ATD in a high percentage of patients with chronic blepharitis. It is important to look for an accompanying dry-eye state in these patients and to treat it when present.

Laboratory findings

Although diagnosis is usually made clinically without laboratory testing, research has shown alterations in bacterial colonization and composition of meibum in patients with this condition. Aerobic and anaerobic culturing of healthy control patients and patients with each form of chronic blepharitis has revealed a significantly greater incidence of colonization, with *Staphylococcus aureus* only in the seborrheic subgroups. There was no significant difference in the incidence of coagulase negative *Staphylococcus* (C-NS), *Propionibacterium acnes*, or any other bacteria isolated in any of the various patient subgroups compared with control patients. The cultures of meibum revealed no evidence to support its role as a reservoir for bacterial colonization in any form of chronic blepharitis.

The possible role of bacterial lipases in modifying the composition of meibum and differences in the biochemical composition of meibum in the various subgroups of chronic blepharitis have also been examined by McCulley et al. Studies have shown that there is a higher percentage of C-NS species capable of de-esterifying fatty waxes and cholesteryl esters in the types of chronic blepharitis with meibomian gland involvement.

The exact role of these various meibum components has not been fully defined, but they may provide new avenues for more definitive therapeutic intervention.

TREATMENT

Systemic

When meibomian gland dysfunction is present in patients with seborrheic blepharitis, systemic treatment with tetracycline may be indicated. Usual dosage is tetracycline 250 mg PO q.i.d., doxycycline 50 mg PO b.i.d., or minocycline 50 mg PO b.i.d. These medications may improve this condition by decreasing bacterial flora on the eyelid or by decreasing bacterial lipase activity, thereby altering the composition of meibum.

Nutritional supplementation with omega-3 fatty acids (fish oil or flax seed oil) may be helpful in decreasing the inflammatory component of blepharitis and meibomitis.

Ocular

Warm compresses to the eyelids for 5 to 10 minutes b.i.d. This may be done with a warm wet washcloth or with 1 cup of dry rice in a clean sock heated in a microwave for approximately 45 seconds.

Eyelid scrubs with dilute baby shampoo or a commercial lid scrub b.i.d.

Bacitracin or erythromycin ointment applied to the lid margins after lid scrubs and to the cul-de-sac at bedtime.

Rarely, short-term topical steroids.

Topical cyclosporin A drops have been shown to decrease objective signs of meibomitis.

Preservative-free artificial tears, and punctal occlusion for associated keratoconjunctivitis sicca.

Dermatologic consultation for manifestations of seborrheic dermatitis.

COMPLICATIONS

Tetracycline or doxycycline should not be administered to children because of the effect on dental enamel; in addition, it is contraindicated in pregnant women and lactating mothers. Tetracycline should be taken on an empty stomach, such as 1 hour before or 2 hours after meals. If associated gastrointestinal irritation presents as a side effect, 100 mg of doxycycline b.i.d., which may be taken with food, can be substituted. When tetracycline is contraindicated, erythromycin is a suitable alternative.

COMMENTS

Seborrheic blepharitis is usually a chronic disease, which may have bothersome exacerbations especially if associated with meibomian gland inflammation. However, with proper diagnosis and treatment, patients can usually experience significant improvement in their symptoms. Nevertheless, the chronic nature of the disease needs to be explained to patients initially so false expections are not created. Careful examination for coexisting conditions such as dry eye and other eyelid conditions is important so that specific treatment may be initiated.

REFERENCES

Dougherty JM, McCulley JP, Silvany RE, Meyer DR: The role of tetracycline in chronic blepharitis. Invest Ophthalmol Vis Sci 32:2970–29075, 1991.

McCulley JP, Dougherty JM: Bacterial aspects of chronic blepharitis. Trans Ophthalmol Soc UK 105:314–318, 1986.

McCulley JP, Dougherty JM, Deneau DG: Classification of chronic blepharitis. Ophthalmology 189:1173–1180, 1983.

Perry HD, Doshi-Carnevale S, Donnenfeld ED, et al: Efficacy of commercially available topical cyclosporine a 0.05% in the treatment of meibomian gland dysfunction. Cornea 25(2):171–175, 2006.

Ta CN, Shine WE, McCulley JP, et al: Effects of minocycline on the ocular flora of patients with acne rosacea or seborrheic blepharitis. Cornea 22(6):545–548, 2003.

253 TRICHIASIS 374.05

Anuja Bhandari, MD, FRCOphth
Seattle, Washington
James C. Orcutt, MD, PhD
Seattle, Washington

ETIOLOGY

Trichiasis is an acquired condition in which previously normal eyelashes are misdirected toward the globe and irritate the cornea and conjunctiva. Ectropion may be associated or trichiasis may occur in isolation.

Trichiasis can occur secondary to chronic eyelid inflammation (blepharitis) or infections, e.g. trachoma, herpes simplex or zoster, or Hansen's disease. Systemic diseases such as ocular cicatricial pemphigoid, Stevens–Johnson syndrome, and toxic epidermal necrolysis are known to cause trichiasis. Trichiasis can also be the result of treatment with medications such as travaprost, pilocarpine, epinephrine, trifluridine, idoxuridine and vidarabine. Finally, mechanical or chemical trauma to the eyelids can result in trichiasis.

COURSE/PROGNOSIS

Trichiasis may lead to corneal opacification by:

- Keratinization of the conjunctiva and cornea;
- Vascularization and scarring of the cornea;
- Corneal abrasion or ulcer; and
- Corneal thinning and perforation.

Visual loss may be concurrent with these pathologic changes if they extend into the visual axis.

DIAGNOSIS

Clinical signs and symptoms

Symptoms consist of foreign body sensation, pain, photophobia, chronic irritation and decreased vision. The diagnosis is clinical, based on recognition of misdirected eyelashes emanating from the eyelid, directed toward the globe.

Differential diagnosis

Other conditions in the differential diagnosis are entropion and distichasis. Trichiasis is differentiated from entropion by the normal position of the eyelid margin. In distichiasis, a second row of eyelashes grows posterior to the normal row of eyelashes, at or near the meibomian gland orifices.

TREATMENT

Medical

Appropriate medical management of the underlying disease process (blepharitis, ocular cicatricial pemphigoid) is important in the prevention of trichiasis in untreated areas of the lids. A bandage contact lens may be worn temporarily to provide comfort and prevent corneal abrasions.

Surgical

The mainstay of treatment is surgery, usually aimed at destroying the eyelash follicle.

Epilation

Eyelashes return as early as 2 weeks after surgery.

Argon laser ablation

The argon laser provides focused energy with minimal damage to surrounding tissue, minimizing post-treatment swelling and inflammation. Local anesthetic (1% xylocaine with 1 : 100,000 epinephrine mixed with 0.5% bupivicaine) is injected. The laser is directed parallel to the shaft of the cilia and applied to a depth of 2 to 3 mm to destroy the eyelash follicle. Treatment is performed with a spot size of 50 to 100 μm, of 0.1 to 0.5 second duration at 0.3 to 2.0 W power. Forty to 50 applications per eyelash may be needed. Success rate is reported between 55 to 89%. Complications include recurrence, dimpling, notching and hypopigmentation.

Cryosurgery

Cryosurgery is most suitable when multiple, contiguous eyelashes are involved. Local anesthetic (1% xylocaine with 1 : 100,000 epinephrine mixed with 0.5% bupivicaine) is injected. A cryoprobe (with nitrous oxide as the coolant) is used. A high-flow, large surfaced probe is preferable to the retinal cryoprobe. The affected part of the lid is frozen for 30 to 60 seconds. After a complete thaw, the procedure is repeated for a total of two freeze-thaw cycles. The tissue temperature at the level of the eyelash follicle can be monitored using a thermocouple (–15° to –30°C). Success rate is reported as greater than 90% if two freeze-thaw cycles are applied. Complications include recurrence, depigmentation, hyperpigmentation, eyelid thinning or notching, eyelid edema, symblepharon, and keratinization, with activation of cicatricial ocular pemphigoid reported in one series of patients. Patients should be warned that blistering of the eyelid may follow the cryotreatment and given a topical antibiotic ointment to apply if this occurs.

Radiosurgery

The Ellman Surgitron delivers energy at 3.8MHz. Local anesthetic (1% xylocaine with 1 : 100,000 epinephrine mixed with 0.5% bupivicaine) is injected. The needle tip of the Surgitron is either inserted into the eyelash follicle (by directing it along the eyelash base) directly or used to split the lid margin along the grey line. The cut mode is used in the former technique and the cut and coagulate mode is used in the latter technique for eyelash extirpation. Success rate is reported between 67% and 83%. Complications include recurrence, lid notching, and granuloma formation.

Hyfrecation

Electrolysis of individual eyelashes has been advocated in the past. This procedure should, however, be avoided as it can result in entropion. Moreover, hyfrecation may induce heat and lead to scarring with subsequent trichiasis of adjacent eyelashes. This form of treatment should be limited to no more than 3 eyelashes total per eyelid to avoid this complicaton.

Conventional surgical techniques

Full-thickness wedge resection can be carried out where multiple contiguous eyelashes are involved, particularly in the presence of distorted eyelid margin anatomy.

Eyelid margin rotation procedures, e.g. the Lagleyze or Weis procedures, can be considered for trichiasis associated with cicatricial entropion.

Lid-splitting procedures (at the gray line) with or without insertion of a mucus membrane or amniotic membrane graft are alternatives for trichiasis associated with cicatricial entropion.

COMMENTS

For trichiasis treatment to be effective, it is important to recognize and treat any underlying pathology. The extent of the abnormal eyelashes and the underlying cause generally dictate the treatment modality. Several abnormal eyelashes may be treated with laser ablation or cryosurgery. Cryosurgery is more effective for larger eyelashes as compared with fine lanugo hair. Larger patches of eyelashes may require cryosurgery or surgery. Extensive trichiasis, with ongoing cicatricial disease, is best treated with excision and mucous membrane grafting. Timely delivery of treatment provides the best outcome for the patient and decreases the risk of corneal vascularization, scarring, and visual loss.

REFERENCES

Bearden W, Anderson R: Trichiasis associated with prostaglandin analog use. Ophthalmic Plast Reconstr Surg 20:320–322, 2004.

Berry J: Recurrent trichiasis: treatment with laser photocoagulation. Ophthalmic Surg 10:36–38, 1979.

Gossman MD, Brightwell JR, Huntington AC, et al: Experimental comparison of laser and cryosurgical cilia destruction. Ophthalmic Surg 23:179–182, 1992.

Johnson RLC, Collin JRO: Treatment of trichiasis with a lid cryoprobe. Br J Ophthalmol 69:267–270, 1985.

Rosner M, Bourla N, Rosen N: Eyelid splitting and extirpation of hair follicles using a radiosurgical technique for treatment of trichiasis. Ophthal Lasers Imaging 35:116, 2004.

254 XANTHELASMA 374.51
(Xanthelasma Palpebrarum)

Geoffrey Gladstone, MD, FAACS
Southfield, Michigan
Shoib Myint, DO, FAACS
Royal Oak, Michigan

ETIOLOGY/INCIDENCE

Xanthelasma palpebrarum, or simply xanthelasma, is a raised, soft, yellow, plaque-like, velvety lesion most commonly occurring in the medial canthal area of the eyelid. Erasmus Wilson originally described the term *xanthelasma* 100 years ago. It is derived from the Greek *xanthos*, meaning 'yellow,' and *elasma*, meaning 'beaten metal plate.' These lesions will rarely enlarge so as to obstruct vision.

Xanthelasma was considered at one time to be a degenerative phenomenon, which involved the subcutaneous and muscular tissue. Histologic studies, however, have shown it to be a pathologic change confined to the skin. Most agree that this condition commonly occurs as an isolated disorder. It has not been associated with aging or hormonal changes. The age of onset ranges from 15 to 73 years old, with the peak in the fourth and fifth decades. One-third of patients have a family history of this condition. Xanthelasma has been known to occur as a result of hyperlipemia, hypercholesteremia, obesity, and cardiovascular changes. Approximately 33% of men and 40% of women with xanthelasma have elevated cholesterol levels. Obesity was found in 26% (in women more than in men), and vascular changes were found in 18% of adults. One study, which involved 8000 healthy men and women, found xanthelasma in 1.1% of women and 0.3% of men with hyperlipidemia. It has also been associated with familial hyperlipoproteinemia type 2 and, rarely, type 3. It may be seen with xanthoma tuberosum or eruptive xanthomatoses. Patients with normal levels of serum lipids have been known to have xanthoma disseminatum. It has also been described in histiocytosis X, most commonly the Hand-Schöller–Christian type. Association with other xanthomas elsewhere is usually less than 2%.

COURSE/PROGNOSIS

With excision, the 1-year recurrence rate is 26%. The younger patients had an earlier recurrence. If all four lids are involved, the recurrence rate with excision is approximately 70% to 80%. Once plaques are established, they will remain static or increase in size.

Patients with first-time excision should be advised of a 40% to 50% success rate. Higher recurrence rates are associated with systemic hyperlipemia, the involvement of all four eyelids, and more than one recurrence after surgery.

DIAGNOSIS

Types

- Xanthelasma with lipemia, acquired or inherited.
- Hypercholesteremia, frequent.
- Hyperneutrolipemia, rare.
- Xanthelasma with normolipemia.
- Local.
- Generalized.
- Xanthoma disseminatum.
- Histiocytosis X.
- Reticulohistiocytoma cutis.

Laboratory findings

Xanthomas are foam cells with lipid found in the superficial reticular dermis. Occasionally, multinucleated giant cells (toutan cells) and fibrosis are observed. A tumor of epidermal origin is possible.

Differential diagnosis

- Myxedema.
- Cirrhosis.
- Diabetes mellitus.
- Plasma protein abnormalities.
- Amyloidosis.

TREATMENT

- Various treatment methods include dietary, medical, dermatologic, surgical, and laser.

- Patients with xanthelasma who are best treated with diet include those whose disease is associated with obesity and increased triglyceride levels.
- Dermatologic treatment includes 75% solution trichloroacetic acid, which coagulates tissue. An advantage is that it is nonsurgical and simple. Disadvantages include ectropion in lower lids, scar formation, and a recurrence rate of 50%.
- Surgical treatment involves the use of a blepharoplasty incision. Serial staged excisions should be included unless the xanthelasma is soft or immature, in which case direct elliptical excision in toto is recommended. Problems include fold asymmetry, skin shortage, webbing, scar formation ectropion, and recurrence.
- Ablation with a CO_2 laser has been used for conditions such as basal cell carcinoma, malignant melanoma, warts, acne, condylomata, hemangioma, tattoo keratoacanthoma, seborrheic keratosis, and papilloma. It has been successful in treating xanthelasma. The advantages are superior hemostasis, no suturing, no reconstructive procedure, and a high degree of patient satisfaction with minimal to no pain. A problem is that patients can get mild hypopigmentation. Scarring can be prevented because under good surgeon control, the laser will not penetrate beyond the reticular layer. After surgery, the patients can be given Aquaphor cream for 1 week.

COMMENTS

Xanthoma palpebrarum can be a challenging condition to manage. An underlying systemic condition should be sought, although most cases are isolated. Each patient is different with different expectations; therefore, the physician should accommodate the treatment to the needs of the patient. The results can be aesthetically pleasing in the right setting if done properly. The tremendous advances in medical technology should allow more efficient means of treating disorders such as this.

REFERENCES

Gladstone GJ: CO_2 laser excision of xanthelasma promotes hemostasis. Clin Laser Monthly 4:35–45, 1986.

Gladstone GJ, Beckman H, Elson LM: CO_2 laser excision of xanthelasmic lesions. Arch Ophthalmol 103:440–442, 1985.

Mendelson BC, Masson JK: Xanthelasma: follow-up on results after surgical excision. Plast Reconstruct Surg 58:535–538, 1976.

Parkes ML, Waller TS: Xanthelasma palpebrarum. Laryngoscope 94: 1238–1240, 1984.

Pedace JF, Winkelman RK: Xanthelasma palpebrarum. JAMA 193; 121–122, 1965.

SECTION

22 Globe

255 ANOPHTHALMOS 743.00

Nick Mamalis, MD
Salt Lake City, Utah
Brian A. Hunter, MD
Salt Lake City, Utah

ETIOLOGY/INCIDENCE

True or primary anophthalmos is very rare and occurs when the neuroectoderm of the primary optic vesicle fails to develop from the anterior neural plate of the neural tube during embryologic development. The diagnosis of true anophthalmos can be made only with complete absence of ocular tissue within the orbit. Secondary anophthalmos refers to the failure of the optic vesicle to form in the presence of anatomic malformations within the ventral forebrain. More commonly, children who are born with a unilaterally small orbit and no visible eye have a very small or microphthalmic globe present within the orbital soft tissue. Microphthalmos can occur due to a problem in the development of the globe at various stages of growth of the optic vesicle. The presence of an eye is necessary in utero to stimulate growth of the orbit, lids, and ocular fornices. A child born with anophthalmia commonly has a small orbit with narrowed palpebral fissure and a shrunken fornix.

- Prevalence range 0.3 to 1.9 per 10,000 live births.
- Idiopathic/sporadic or inherited (recessive, dominant, or sex linked).
- Trisomy 9, 13 through 15.
- Gene deletions chromosome 3, 7, 14. Deletions involving SOX2 and SIX6.
- Gene rearrangements (balanced *de novo* translocations) 46 XXt(1;2)(p31.2;q23); 46 XY (t8;12)(q22;q21); 46,XX, t(3;11).
- Prenatal exposures to TORCH infections (toxoplasmosis, rubella, cytomegalovirus, herpes) as well as alcohol, thalidomide, retinoic acid, hydantoin, and lysergic acid diethylamide (LSD).
- Syndromes associated with abnormalities of the CNS, genitourinary system, and in association with limb anomalies (i.e. SOX2, anopthalmia-oesophageal-genital syndrome (AEG), oligodactyly-ophthalmo-acromelic syndrome (OAS); micropthalmia-anaopthalmia-coloboma (MAC); Waardenburg anophthalmia syndrome (WAS), Lenz syndrome XLR).
- Associated with multiple syndromes with hemifacial microsomia and other craniofacial malformations (i.e. Goldenhar's syndrome, Hallermann–Streiff syndrome).

COURSE/PROGNOSIS

- True anophthalmos is a pediatric ocular emergency.
- The growth and development of the bony orbit are correlated with the growth of the globe.
- The lack of an eye or a microphthalmic eye prevents the orbit from developing properly.
- A small bony orbital cavity results not only in a cosmetic deformity but also does not allow for proper fitting of a prosthesis.
- Anophthalmos may be unilateral or bilateral.

DIAGNOSIS

Clinical signs and symptoms

Orbital

- Reduced size of the bony orbital cavity.
- Small orbital rim.
- Small or maldeveloped optic foramen.
- Lacrimal gland and ducts may be absent.
- Extraocular muscles usually absent.

Eyelids

- Microblepharism: a foreshortening of the eyelids in all directions.
- Contraction of the orbicularis oculi muscle.
- Absent or decreased levator function and lid folds.
- Shallowing of the inferior conjunctival fornix.

Globe

- Completely absent in primary anophthalmos.
- Very small, malformed globe in microphthalmos.

Laboratory findings

- On computed tomography scanning and magnetic resonance imaging, patients with bilateral anophthalmos often have an associated absence of the optic chiasm, diminished size of the posterior optic pathways, and agenesis or dysgenesis of the corpus callosum.
- Ultrasound imaging using B-scan showing complete absence of ocular tissue in anophthalmos. A-scan shows decreased axial length in microphthalmos. Transvaginal ultrasound can detect eye malformations after 22 weeks gestation; however, the sensitivity for use in detecting anopthalmia is not known.
- Patients with unilateral anophthalmos often have severe craniofacial anomalies.

Differential diagnosis

- Primary anophthalmos versus secondary anophthalmos.
- Microphthalmos: a globe with a total axial length (TAL) at least two standard deviations below the mean for age (mean TAL neonate 17 mm, adult 23.8 mm).
- Cryptophthalmos: abnormal fusion of entire eyelid margin with maldevelopement of cornea and microphthalmia. Condition is usually bilateral and associated with multiple malformations.
- Cystic eye: the failure of invagination of the optic vesicle in utero. Imaging studies reveal the presence of intraorbital cyst and intact extraocular muscles, without an optic nerve.
- Neuroimaging or histopathology may be necessary to document the true absence of ocular tissue.

TREATMENT

Ocular/Orbital

- The current preferred method for orbital expansion is to use serial implants in the growing orbit.
- Initially a solid conformer can be placed to stimulate bony orbital growth and enlarge the orbital cavity to attempt to attain normal proportions.
- Progressively increasing the size of the conformers will help progressively increase the size of the orbit to properly fit a hydroxyapatite prosthesis.
- The increase in the size of a conformer often is limited by the shortening of the eyelids and the palpebral fissure that no longer permits passage of a larger conformer.
- The horizontal length of the palpebral fissure may be increased surgically at this point by performing a lateral canthotomy from the lateral canthus to the lateral orbital wall.
- A dermis-fat graft may be placed and has the potential for post-surgical growth.
- If conformers are not tolerated, an inflatable expander (silicone balloon, or hydrophilic polymers) may be placed.
- The expander works best if placed relatively early in life (first year).
- The inflatable silicone expander is placed deep into the orbit and accessed by a tube that is usually placed through the lateral orbital wall.
- The expander is gradually filled (usually with saline) on a weekly or biweekly basis.
- The inflatable expander may allow more rapid and extensive orbital tissue expansion than the solid orbital conformers.

Surgical

- Surgical intervention should be considered after 6 months of age to adequately assess postnatal growth of the orbit.
- If conformers and expanders are not successful, the bony orbit may need to be expanded surgically.
- Osteotomy is the current preferred method for orbital expansion in cases of late referral or insufficient orbital volume in the older child.
- It is possible to enlarge the orbit in three directions-laterally, inferiorly and superiorly.
- This surgical expansion is accomplished by dividing the bony orbital rim in three parts in a stepwise fashion.
- A bicoronal approach through the scalp is often necessary when the orbital roof has to be elevated.
- Last, the eyelids need to be lengthened; this is usually accomplished by a combination of skin, mucosal, or cartilage grafts.

COMPLICATIONS

- Significant cosmetic deformities are possible if the anophthalmic orbit is not treated early.
- Even after treatment, results often are cosmetically disappointing. However, cosmetic scleral shells may be useful in microphthalmos.
- Fitted prostheses are immobile.
- Eyelids also are often short and immobile with significant malformations.

COMMENTS

Anophthalmos may cause serious psychologic problems not only due to the lack of an eye but also secondary to disfigurement of the orbit, lids, and socket. Early treatment with conformers, as well as inflatable expanders and surgery when necessary, will help decrease severe asymmetry and other cosmetic deformities.

SUPPORT GROUPS

International Children's Anophthalmia Network (ICAN). Albert Eisntein Medical Center c/o Genetics. 5501 Old York Road Philadelphia, PA 19141. Phone 800-580-4226. Email: ican@anopthalmia.org URL: www.ioi.com/ican/

National Federation of the Blind (NFB). 1800 Johnson Street Baltimore, MD 21230. Phone 410-659-9314, Email nfb@nfb.org. URL: www.nfb.org

REFERENCES

Albernaz VS, Castillo M, Hudgins PA, et al: Imaging findings in patients with clinical anophthalmos. Am J Neuroradiol 18:555–561, 1997.

Cepela MA, Nunery WR, Martin RT, et al: Stimulation of orbital growth by the use of expandable implants in the anophthalmic cat orbit. Ophthalm Plast Reconstr Surg 8:157–169, 1992.

Krastinova D, Kelly MB, Mihaylova M: Surgical management of the anophthalmic orbit, part 1: congenital. Plast Reconstr Surg 108(4):817–826, 2001.

Marchac D, Cophignon J, Archard E, et al: Orbital expansion for anophthalmia and micro-orbitism. Plast Reconstr Surg 59:486–491, 1977.

Tucker SM, Sapp N, Collin R, et al: Orbital expansion of the congenitally anophthalmic socket. Br J Ophthalmol 79:667–671, 1995.

256 BACTERIAL ENDOPHTHALMITIS 360.0

Mohan N. Iyer, MD
Houston, Texas
Eric R. Holz, MD
Houston, Texas

Endophthalmitis is defined as intraocular inflammation, and clinically, the term has come to mean intraocular infection.

Acute bacterial endophthalmitis is a serious and vision-threatening intraocular infection that requires emergent treatment. The Endophthalmitis Vitrectomy Study (EVS) was a landmark study that evaluated the roles of immediate vitrectomy and systemic antibiotics in the treatment of acute post-cataract extraction endophthalmitis. Injection of intravitreal antibiotics is the mainstay of treatment for exogenous endophthalmitis. Systemic treatment and occasionally vitrectomy and intravitreal antibiotics are required for endogenous endophthalmitis. Prophylaxis of postoperative endophthalmitis remains a controversial issue, and current recommendations include lid scrubs, use of povidone-iodine in the conjunctival fornices, and adequate aseptic technique.

ETIOLOGY/INCIDENCE

Bacterial endophthalmitis is classified based on the route of infection as either exogenous or endogenous. *Exogenous* endophthalmitis can occur following intraocular surgery, penetrating injury, or less commonly from microbial keratitis, scleritis, or an infected scleral buckle. A recent development is the occurrence of exogenous endophthalmitis following intravitreal injections of steroids or other drugs. The incidence of postoperative endophthalmitis has been reported to be:

- 0.07% to 0.12% after routine cataract surgery;
- 0.36% after secondary intraocular lens placement;
- 0.17% after penetrating keratoplasty;
- 0.06% to 1.8% after glaucoma filtering surgery.

Incidence of bleb-related endophthalmitis is greater with the use of antifibrotics because of thinner blebs, and with inferiorly located blebs presumably because of greater exposure of the bleb to bacteria-laden tear film in this location. The causative organisms in postoperative endophthalmitis are usually part of the normal ocular bacterial flora. The incidence of endophthalmitis after penetrating trauma is approximately 7%, greater in the presence of an intraocular foreign body (9% to 11%) and can be as high as 30% in the setting of rural penetrating trauma. The incidence of intravitreal injection-related endophthalmitis after triamcinolone injections is between 0.0% and 0.87%, and after ganciclovir injections is up to 0.6%. *Endogenous* endophthalmitis, also called metastatic endophthalmitis, occurs by hematogenous spread of the organism in patients with sepsis, immunosuppression, or intravenous drug use. Endogenous endophthalmitis is less common and accounts for 2–6% of all cases of bacterial endophthalmitis.

COURSE/PROGNOSIS

The course and prognosis depend on:

- The type of endophthalmitis;
- Duration of time to presentation and treatment;
- Virulence of the organism.

The prognosis for achieving good final visual acuity has increased substantially with the introduction of intravitreal antibiotics. Prior to the introduction of intravitreal antibiotics, intravenous and topical antibiotics were administered and, in a survey of cases from the years 1944–1966, 73% had final vision of hand motions or worse. In the EVS, which evaluated cases of acute postoperative endophthalmitis, at 9 to 12 months after treatment, 53% of eyes had a visual acuity of 20/40 or better, 74% had visual acuity of 20/100 or better, 15% had visual acuity of 5/200 or worse, and 5% had no light perception (LP). The most important risk factor for poor visual outcome in the EVS was an initial visual acuity of light perception (LP) only, with only 23% of patients with LP achieving 20/40 or better vision compared with 64% of patients presenting with better than LP vision. Other factors associated with poor outcome included:

- Small pupil size after maximal dilation;
- Absence of a red reflex;
- Presence of rubeosis irides;
- Findings of an afferent papillary defect;
- Corneal infiltrate or ring ulcer;
- Abnormal intraocular pressure;
- Poor media clarity with inability to distinguish any retinal vessels;
- Type of organism grown in culture.

The leading cause of final vision less than 20/40 was an abnormality of the macula.

The prognosis for retaining good vision is generally better in cases that are culture-negative or culture-positive for coagulase-negative staphylococci, and in cases of chronic or delayed-onset endophthalmitis, i.e. those presenting 6 weeks after cataract surgery. However, the prognosis for patients with bleb-associated, post-traumatic, and endogenous endophthalmitis is generally worse than for patients with acute postoperative endophthalmitis. In bleb-associated endophthalmitis, infection with more virulent organisms is more frequent, and pre-existing glaucoma may limit final vision. Post-traumatic endophthalmitis is associated with a poor visual prognosis with approximately 30% of patients achieving visual acuity better than 20/400. Cases associated with *Bacillus cereus* or with rural trauma portend an especially poor prognosis. Trauma-induced changes may also directly affect the final outcome. Poor prognosis in endogenous endophthalmitis has been attributed to delay in diagnosis, diffuse infection (panophthalmitis), and infection with virulent and in particular,gram-negative organisms. Pooled analysis of cases reported between 1976 and 1985 showed that only 41% of patients had counting fingers (CF) or better vision, 26% had no light perception, and 29% required evisceration, a trend that has remained unchanged in analyses since 1986. In addition, a 5% mortality rate due to extraocular spread of infection has been reported.

DIAGNOSIS

The diagnosis of endophthalmitis is usually made on clinical grounds. Vitreous inflammation greater than expected is the key diagnostic finding that should lead to the suspicion of endophthalmitis.

Clinical signs and symptoms

- Acute postoperative endophthalmitis.

Presenting symptoms in the EVS

- Decreased vision.
- Pain.
- Red eye.
- Swollen lid.
- Hypopyon.

Examination findings revealed

- Visual acuity less than 5/200 (86%).
- Light perception (26%).
- Hypopyon (86%).
- No retinal vessel visible by indirect ophthalmoscopy (79%).
- Afferent pupillary defect (12%).
- Corneal wound abnormality (5%).
- Corneal infiltrate or ring ulcer (5%).

While pain is generally considered a key presenting symptom, it should be noted that nearly a quarter of the patients in the EVS presented without pain. In addition, hypopyon was absent in 14% of the patients.

- Chronic postoperative endophthalmitis usually presents as an anterior uveitis weeks to months after the intraocular procedure. It may respond transiently to corticosteroid treatment. The presence of vitreous inflammation and posterior capsular opacities or plaques are highly suggestive of chronic endophthalmitis.
- Bleb-related endophthalmitis. Patients can present with bleb-related endophthalmitis months to years after glaucoma filtering surgery with symptoms of:
  - Ocular pain;
  - Redness;
  - Decreased vision;
  - Clinical signs.
- Bleb leak.
- Conjunctival injection and chemosis.
- Inflamed bleb.
- Hypopyon.
- Anterior and vitreal inflammation.

It is important to distinguish blebitis from bleb-related endophthalmitis because treatment methods are different for the two entities. When the inflammation is localized to the bleb with the absence of a hypopyon or vitreal inflammation, it is termed 'blebitis.'

- Post-traumatic endophthalmitis. Patients with penetrating injuries and with intraocular foreign bodies may have intraocular inflammation and signs similar to acute postoperative endophthalmitis on presentation or after primary repair. Endophthalmitis is suspected mainly on clinical grounds in these cases.
- Intravitreal injection-related endophthalmitis. Patients may present with anterior and vitreal inflammation within one week of an intravitreal injection. Pseudo-endophthalmitis, presumably as a result of reaction to the concomitant vehicle or dispersion of steroid particles into the anterior chamber simulating a hypopyon, should be cautiously distinguished from endophthalmitis by the lack of significant decrease in vision, significant pain, and severe vitreal inflammation.

Laboratory findings

Microbiologic studies of vitreous and anterior chamber specimens obtained are recommended, mainly to determine the infectious organism and to direct treatment in the event of need for reinjection of intravitreal antibiotics. Bacterial endophthalmitis is a clinical diagnosis, and empiric treatment with broad-spectrum antibiotics is initiated emergently well before microbiology results become available. In addition, the rate of culture-negative vitreous samples, whether or not a vitrectomy is performed, is approximately 30%. Gram stain, aerobic and anaerobic cultures are routinely obtained. Based on findings of the EVS, gram stain results should not be used solely in determining the choice of antibiotics in the treatment of endophthalmitis, and vitrectomy does not result in a greater rate of culture-positive specimens. Cultures of conjunctiva or cornea may theoretically have a role in post-traumatic endophthalmitis cases, but are not expected to add information when aqueous and vitreal samples are obtained. Patients with endogenous endophthalmitis should have a work-up for infectious diseases to identify an extraocular focus of infection. This should include cultures of blood and urine as well as evaluation of indwelling intravenous lines, and other studies determined by history and physical findings. In reported series of endogenous endophthalmitis, blood cultures were more likely to be positive than vitreous cultures. However, in the absence of positive cultures from extraocular studies, aqueous and vitreal cultures are recommended to aid in diagnosis.

The microbial spectrum in the different types of endophthalmitis is as follows:

- Acute postoperative (EVS):
  - Gram-positive coagulase-negative micrococci (mostly *Staphylococcus epidermidis*) (70%);
  - Other gram-positive (24.2%);
  - *Staphylococcus aureus* (9.9%);
  - *Streptococcus* (9%);
  - *Enterococcus* (2.2%);
  - Miscellaneous (3.1%).
- Chronic postoperative endophthalmitis:
  - Gram-positive coagulase-negative micrococci, mostly *Staphylococcus epidermidis*;
  - Other gram-positive organisms, *Staphylococcus aureus*, *Streptococcus* spp.;
  - *Propionibacterium acnes*;
  - *Corynebacterium* spp.;
  - *Actinomyces* spp.;
  - *Nocardia*;
  - Fungi.
- Bleb-related endophthalmitis:
  - *Staphylococcus* spp., *Streptococcus* spp.;
  - *Haemophilus influenzae*;
  - *Enterococcus* spp.;
  - Fastidious gram-negative rods;
  - *Pseudomona aeruginosa*.
- Post-traumatic endophthalmitis:
  - Coagulase-negative *Staphylococci* spp.;
  - *Staphylococcus aureus*, *Streptococcus* spp.;
  - *Bacillus cereus*;
  - *Propionibacterium acnes*;
  - Fungi;
  - Others.
- Endogenous endophthalmitis: gram-positive organisms, mainly:
  - *Streptococcus pneumoniae*;
  - *Staphylococcus aureus*;
  - Group A and group B *Streptococci*;
  - *Bacillus ceres*.

Gram-negative organisms:

- *Klebsiella* spp.;
- *E. coli*;
- *Pseudomonas* spp.;
- *N. meningitides*;
- *Serratia marcescens*;
- *Listeria monocytogenes*;
- *N. asteroids*.

- Intravitreal injection-related endophthalmitis:
  - Gram-positive coagulase-negative *Staphylococcus* spp.;
  - *Streptococcus* spp.;
  - *Mycobacterium chelonae*.

Differential diagnosis

- Acute postoperative endophthalmitis:
  - Phacoanaphylactic endophthalmitis, a granulomatous inflammation with keratic precipitates as a result of immune reaction to lens proteins;
  - Aseptic endophthalmitis, a severe sterile uveitis that may present with a hypopyon and mild vitreous inflammation. Pain and progressive vision loss are not characteristic. This condition usually resolves with topical steroid treatment.
- Chronic postoperative endophthalmitis:
  - Pre-existing uveitis;
  - Sterile inflammation attributed to reaction to contaminants on the intraocular lens, such as polishing compounds;
  - Rebound inflammation related to abrupt discontinuation of steroid drops;
  - Iris or vitreous incarceration in the wound, resulting in a low-grade inflammation;
  - Uveitis-glaucoma-hyphema syndrome;
  - Fungal endophthalmitis.
- Bleb-related endophthalmitis:
  - Blebitis, presenting classically as 'white on red,' with the bleb appearing white against inflamed conjunctiva;
  - Anterior uveitis;
  - Uveitis-glaucoma-hyphema syndrome.
- Post-traumatic endophthalmitis:
  - Phacoanaphylactic endophthalmitis;
  - Sterile inflammatory reaction to uveal incarceration or intraocular foreign body;
  - Sympathetic ophthalmia with bilateral anterior uveitis with keratic precipitates, vitreous inflammation, presence of depigmented nodules (Dalen–Fuchs' nodules) at the level of the retinal pigment epithelium, and choroidal thickening on B-scan ultrasonography.
- Endogenous endophthalmitis:
  - Non-infectious anterior uveitis;
  - Fungal endophthalmitis;
  - Intraocular lymphoma;
  - Retinoblastoma in children.
- Intravitreal injection-related endophthalmitis:
  - 'Pseudo-endophthalmitis,' or non-infectious endophthalmitis, seen after intravitreal triamcinolone injection, presumably as a result of toxic or inflammatory reaction to the drug, the vehicle in which the drug is suspended, or a contaminant in the preparation. This condition is seen in the immediate post-injection period, typically within two days. The presenting signs of hypopyon, anterior and vitreal inflammation, and decreased vision make it difficult to distinguish this entity from infectious endophthalmitis. With observation, the inflammation resolves within one week.

PROPHYLAXIS

Preoperative and intraoperative preventive measures have been proposed and employed in an attempt to decrease the incidence of endophthalmitis. Since the source of organisms in postoperative endophthalmitis is most commonly the patient's ocular flora, the goal is to reduce the bacterial load and treat any external eye disease prior to operating. An evidence-based assessment of bacterial endophthalmitis prophylaxis found that several measures have been considered, including preoperative povidone-iodine, lash trimming, saline irrigation, topical antibiotics, antibiotic-containing irrigating solutions, and postoperative subconjunctival antibiotics. The use of preoperative povidone-iodine received the strongest recommendation.

Preoperative measures include:

- Treatment of blepharitis, conjunctivitis, dacryocystitis, and periocular infections;
- Use of adequate aseptic techniques with sterile preparation of eyelashes, eyelids, and periocular skin, and draping of eyelashes and lid margins;
- 5% povidone-iodine solution instilled in the conjunctival fornices;
- Topical preoperative antibiotics, which are widely used and theoretically lead to decreased bacterial load on the ocular surface. Some antibiotics, such as fluoroquinolones, may have adequate aqueous penetration. However, despite these theoretical considerations and routine use, clinical studies are yet to demonstrate their efficacy in preventing endophthalmitis.

Intraoperative measures include:

- Use of meticulous aseptic technique;
- Avoidance of placement of intraocular lens on the ocular surface prior to introduction into the eye;
- Use of heparin surface-modified intraocular lenses, based on demonstration of decreased bacterial adherence in vitro. The use of low molecular weight heparin in the irrigating fluid failed to demonstrate a statistically significant reduction in the rate of culture-positive anterior chamber aspirates;
- Placement of a 10-0 nylon suture in the incisional wound if there is capsular rupture, vitreous loss, or any concern about wound integrity. Recent evidence suggests an increased risk of postoperative endophthalmitis with sutureless corneal incisions; thus, a low threshold for placement of suture to avoid microleaks from the wound is recommended;
- Subconjunctival injection of antibiotics, which remains controversial. This method has been shown to reduce ocular flora more than topical antibiotics. However, in a retrospective 10-year review of the incidence of postoperative endophthalmitis, 23 out of 54 (42%) patients with culture-positive endophthalmitis had received prophylactic subconjunctival antibiotics at the end of their surgeries, and of these, 14 (61%) were sensitive to the antibiotics used. Subconjunctival gentamicin, in particular, should be avoided given the risk of irreversible macular infarction;
- Postoperative topical antibiotics, which are in routine use despite the lack of data proving their benefit in the prevention of endophthalmitis;
- Use of antibiotics in the irrigating fluid, not recommended by the authors. The Center for Disease Control and Prevention recommends against the routine use of vancomycin in the irrigating fluid given the risk of emerging vancomycin resistance. The use of aminoglycosides in the irrigating fluid should be avoided given the risk of macular toxicity from incorrect dilution of the antibiotic. Cases of endophthalmitis have been reported despite the use of this measure.

Other prophylactic measures recommended include avoidance of an inferior bleb in glaucoma filtering surgery, use of aseptic techniques with povidone-iodine and isolation of lashes with a lid speculum for in-office intravitreal drug injections. In trauma cases, identification and removal of intraocular foreign bodies, prophylactic intravitreal injection, and systemic prophylaxis in high risk cases, such as rural injuries or contaminated wounds, are recommended.

TREATMENT

The EVS laid the foundation for current practice in the treatment of acute post-cataract extraction endophthalmitis. The findings of the EVS cannot be strictly extrapolated to bleb-related endophthalmitis, post-traumatic endophthalmitis, or endogenous endophthalmitis. Variations in presentation and organisms in these other entities predicate the methods of treatment. The antibiotics for intravitreal injections have essentially remained unchanged for over a decade. Fourth-generation fluoroquinolones, moxifloxacin and gatifloxacin, are recently developed broad-spectrum antibiotics with effective gram-positive and gram-negative coverage. Oral gatifloxacin has been shown to achieve adequate intravitreal concentrations in humans. Studies conducted in animals have documented that intravitreal moxifloxacin appears safe in doses up to 150 micrograms/ml, and may have a role in the treatment of endophthalmitis following further study (unpublished data).

Acute postoperative endophthalmitis

The EVS showed that systemic antibiotics did not confer a benefit in the treatment of acute postoperative endophthalmitis. Furthermore, the study showed a benefit from immediate vitrectomy only in patients presenting with visual acuity of light perception (LP). For patients who presented with light perception vision, immediate vitrectomy with intravitreal antibiotics results in a three-fold increase in the rate of achieving a visual acuity of 20/40 or better, a two-fold increase in the rate of achieving a visual acuity of 20/100 or better, and a decrease by half in the rate of severe visual loss to less than 5/200. For patients presenting with hand motions or better vision at 2feet, immediate vitrectomy did not confer a benefit over vitreous tap.

Systemic

- Systemic antibiotics are not recommended based on EVS findings, but may be considered in severe cases, especially with orbital involvement.
- Prednisone 1mg/kg/day PO for 5 to 10 days with rapid taper may be considered if there are no contraindications.

Local

Topical antibiotics

- Fluoroquinolones (e.g. ciprofloxacin, ofloxacin, or the newer fluoroquinolones, gatifloxacin or moxifloxacin) q.i.d. to q1-2 hour dosing.
- Fortified drops, especially in cases with wound abscesses (e.g. 50 mg/mL vancomycin and 50 mg/mL ceftazidime) qid to q1-2 hour dosing.
- Topical steroids (e.g. 1% prednisolone acetate) qid to q1-2 hour dosing.
- Topical cycloplegics (e.g. cyclopentolate 1%, 0.25% scopolamine hydrobromide, or 1% atropine sulfate) b.i.d.

Surgical

Obtaining specimens for microbiology

- Anterior chamber tap: 0.1 to 0.2 cc of aqueous fluid aspirated with a 27–30-gauge needle attached to a tuberculin syringe and inserted through the limbus.
- Vitreous needle tap biopsy: 0.1 to 0.3 cc of vitreous fluid aspirated with a 22–27-gauge needle inserted via the pars plana. If the tap is dry, the patient will need a mechanized vitreous biopsy.
- Pars plana vitrectomy and mechanized vitreous biopsy: A 20-gauge pars plana sclerotomy is made followed by introduction of a vitreous cutter/aspirator (or a disposable 23-gauge vitrector) attached to a 1–3 cc syringe, and 0.5 cc of vitreous fluid is manually aspirated while the vitrector is cutting. Pars plana vitrectomy is then performed and the vitreous cassette is also submitted for microbiological studies.

Intravitreal injections

- Separate injections of vancomycin (1 mg in 0.1 cc) plus ceftazidime (2.25 mg in 0.1 cc). Amikacin (400 mcg in 0.1 cc) may be substituted for ceftazidime, if the patient is allergic to beta-lactam antibiotics.
- Dexamethasone 400 mcg/0.1 cc — not routinely used because of conflicting reports of its efficacy.

Subconjunctival antibiotics

- Use is controversial and generally not recommended given poor penetration into the vitreous cavity. May consider in cases of wound abscess, or other anterior segment infections.
- Vancomycin 25 mg and ceftazidime 100 mg (used in the EVS).

Additional procedures

- If no improvement or stabilization is seen by 36 to 60 hours after intravitreal antibiotic injections, repeat antibiotic injections guided by culture results are recommended. In this timeframe in the EVS, nearly 9% had an additional procedure performed. If not initially performed, a vitrectomy should be considered.
- Additional late procedures include vitrectomy for media clearance, macular pucker or retinal detachment, posterior capsulotomy, scleral buckling, and glaucoma surgery.

Chronic postoperative endophthalmitis

This condition presents as recurrent or persistent postoperative intraocular inflammation that may be partially steroid responsive. Commonly, posterior capsular opacities or plaques may be seen. A vitrectomy is almost always indicated in this situation, and the timing of the surgery may be determined based on the severity of the inflammation.

Systemic

Systemic antibiotics and steroids not usually indicated.

Local

Topical antibiotics, steroids and cycloplegics as described above for acute postoperative endophthalmitis.

Surgical

- Anterior chamber and vitreous tap with intravitreal antibiotics may be adequate if no sequestration of organisms in the capsular bag is noted.

- Cases with sequestration of infected material in the capsular bag require a partial capsulectomy and removal of any residual cortex, combined with vitrectomy and injection of vancomycin (1 mg in 0.1 cc) and ceftazidime (2.25 mg in 0.1 cc) into the capsular bag/vitreous cavity. If the infection persists despite this measure, a complete capsulectomy with intraocular lens explantation and reinjection of intravitreal antibiotics as guided by culture results is recommended.
- Antibiotic irrigation of the capsular bag, without capsulectomy or intraocular lens removal, has been reportedly successful in some cases.

Bleb-related endophthalmitis

In cases of blebitis, where the infection is limited to the bleb without intraocular involvement, topical and systemic therapy is typically curative. In early-onset bleb-associated endophthalmitis, the organisms are similar to acute post-cataract endophthalmitis and the visual prognosis is likewise favorable. In delayed-onset endophthalmitis, which is the more common situation, the organisms are more virulent, including *Streptococcus* spp. and *Haemophilus influenzae*, with resultant poor prognosis. Aggressive treatment of bleb-associated endophthalmitis is recommended, with vitrectomy irrespective of the presenting visual acuity, intravitreal antibiotics, and systemic antibiotics, despite their lack of clinical efficacy in the EVS.

Systemic

- Vancomycin 1 g every 12 hours IV, plus either 1 g of ceftazidime IV every 12 hours, or ciprofloxacin 750 mg PO every 12 hours, or gatifloxacin 400 mg qd.

Local

- Topical vancomycin (50 mg/mL) and ceftazidime (50 mg/mL).
- Topical steroids and cycloplegics as described.

Surgical

- Immediate vitrectomy, anterior chamber and vitreous biopsies, and intravitreal vancomycin (1 mg in 0.1 cc) and ceftazidime (2.25 mg in 0.1 cc).
- Subconjunctival vancomycin 25 mg and ceftazidime 100 mg.

Post-traumatic endophthalmitis

Early vitrectomy with intravitreal, subconjunctival, topical, and systemic antibiotics should be used in the doses listed above. Immediate vitrectomy in suspected cases is recommended over vitreous tap and inject even if the presenting vision is better than LP. Retained intraocular foreign bodies should be suspected and ruled out with ultrasound and computed tomography scans. Prompt removal of any retained intraocular foreign body is indicated.

Endogenous endophthalmitis

A concerted effort to identify the source of the infection must be made, if not already known. In a review of a large series of reported cases, only about half were treated with intravitreal antibiotics. Systemic intravenous antibiotics are first initiated, as this condition is caused by hematogenous spread of organisms. In patients who develop or fail to have improvement of endogenous bacterial endophthalmitis while on appropriate systemic antibiotics despite therapeutic blood levels for 24 to 36 hours, vitreous tap/inject or vitrectomy with intravitreal antibiotic injection is indicated. The choice of antibiotics may be determined by available blood culture results. Endogenous fungal endophthalmitis can usually be clinically distinguished from bacterial endophthalmitis, but in cases in which no underlying systemic infection is known and the vitreous involvement is severe, vitrectomy with intravitreal injection of antibiotics with or without amphotericin (5 micrograms in 0.1 mL) may be indicated.

Intravitreal injection-related endophthalmitis

There have been few case reports of this entity. In one study, 3 of the 8 culture-positive cases ended up with no light perception vision, and two of those eyes had undergone vitrectomy with intravitreal antibiotics. The choice of treatment methods for this condition must be based on the judgment of the clinician, with early vitrectomy, intravitreal antibiotics, and systemic antibiotics offered in clinically severe cases.

COMPLICATIONS

Complications of endophthalmitis include corneal edema or decompensation, persistent intraocular inflammation, cataract, glaucoma, hypotony, residual vitreous opacity, retinal toxicity (due to enzyme and toxin release and rarely due to antibiotic treatment), cystoid macular edema, and epiretinal membrane. Retinal detachment occurs in 5 to 21% of cases. In the EVS, a final visual acuity of no light perception was noted in 5% of cases, and phthisis occurred in 2% of the patients. Contiguous spread and development of panophthalmitis is a possible complication that may require enucleation.

COMMENTS

Bacterial endophthalmitis is a vision-threatening intraocular infection requiring prompt diagnosis and treatment. Intravitreal injection of antibiotics is the mainstay in the treatment of endophthalmitis. The EVS showed that in cases of acute post cataract extraction endophthalmitis, systemic antibiotics conferred no additional benefit, and that immediate vitrectomy was only beneficial for patients with LP vision on presentation. However, these recommendations should not be strictly extrapolated to other types of endophthalmitis. The decisions for vitrectomy and the use of systemic antibiotics should be based on the type of endophthalmitis and severity of vitreous involvement.

REFERENCES

Benz MS, Scott IU, Flynn HW, Jr, et al: Endophthalmitis isolates and antibiotic sensitivities: a 6 year review of culture proven cases. Am J Ophthalmol 137:38–42, 2004.

Ciulla TA, Starr MB, Masket S: Bacterial endophthalmitis prophylaxis for cataract surgery: an evidence-based update. Ophthalmology 109:13–24, 2002.

Endophthalmitis Vitrectomy Study Group: Results of the Endophthalmitis Vitrectomy Study: a randomized trial of immediate vitrectomy and of intravenous antibiotics for the treatment of postoperative bacterial endophthalmitis. Arch Ophthalmol 113:1479–1496, 1995.

Han DP, Wisniewski SR, Wilson LA, et al: Spectrum and susceptibilities of microbiologic isolates in the Endophthalmitis Vitrectomy Study. Am J Ophthalmol 122:1–17, 1996.

Hariprasad SM, Mieler WF, Holz ER: Vitreous and aqueous penetration of orally administered gatifloxacin in humans. Arch Ophthalmol 121:345–350, 2003.

Jackson TL, Eykyn SJ, Graham EM, et al: Endogenous bacterial endophthalmitis: a 17-year prospective series and review of 267 reported cases. Surv Ophthalmol 48:403–423, 2003.

Kresloff MS, Castellarin AA, Zarbin MA: Endophthalmitis. Surv Ophthalmol 43:193–224, 1998.

Mac I, Soltau JB: Glaucoma-filtering bleb infections. Curr Opin Ophthalmol 14:91–94, 2003.

Moshfeghi DM, Kaiser PK, Scott IU, et al: Acute endophthalmitis following intravitreal triamcinolone acetonide injection. Am J Ophthalmol 136:791–796, 2003.

Nelson ML, Tennant MTS, Sivalingam A, et al: Infectious and presumed noninfectious endophthalmitis after intravitreal triamcinolone acetonide injection. Retina 23:686–691, 2003.

Olson RJ: Reducing the risk of postoperative endophthalmitis. Surv Ophthalmol 49:S55–S61, 2004.

Reynolds DS, Flynn HW Jr: Endophthalmitis after penetrating ocular trauma. Current Opin Ophthalmol 8:32–38, 1997.

Speaker MG, Menikoff JA: Prophylaxis of endophthalmitis with topical povidone-iodine. Ophthalmology 98:1769–1775, 1991.

257 FUNGAL ENDOPHTHALMITIS 360.1

Rohit R. Lakhanpal, MD
Houston, Texas
Thomas A. Albini, MD
Houston, Texas
Eric R. Holz, MD
Houston, Texas

ETIOLOGY/INCIDENCE

Fungal endophthalmitis is classified according to its source. It is classified as *exogenous* when associated with an external source such as penetrating trauma, previous intraocular surgery (cataract extraction, penetrating keratoplasty, filtering bleb procedures or vitrectomy), or direct spread from corneal or scleral fungal infection. Exogenous fungal infections occur in immunocompetent individuals and are frequently seen in agricultural workers or in patients with organic foreign bodies, such as soil, leaves, or twigs in their eyes.

Endogenous fungal endophthalmitis results from the hematogenous spread of fungal infection to the eye from elsewhere in the body. Sources for endogenous fungal endophthalmitis include:

- Systemic opportunistic infections in immunocomprised hosts, as seen in:
  - AIDS;
  - Renal failure;
  - Severe burns;
  - Prolonged corticosteroid use;
  - Chemotherapeutics;
  - Hyperalimentation;
  - Solid organ or bone marrow transplantation.
- Endocarditis (especially after cardiac valvular surgery).
- Gastrointestinal ulceration or surgery.
- Indwelling or long-term IV catheters.
- Shunts or prostheses.
- IV drug abuse.

Often the source cannot be identified, and as many as half of patients with presumed endogenous fungal endophthalmitis have negative blood cultures and negative systemic evaluations.

Obtaining a careful history will be helpful in determining the most likely organism. For example:

- *Candida* species (yeasts) may cause endogenous or exogenous endophthalmitis and are more commonly associated with indwelling catheters, chronic antibiotic use, abdominal surgery, diabetes, immunosuppression with high dose corticosteroids or cytotoxic agents, intravenous drug abuse, and perioperative post-surgical endophthalmitis secondary to contamination of lens implants or irrigation fluids.
- *Aspergillus* species (septate filamentous fungi) may be associated with exogenous (grain farmers, poultry breeders, trauma) or endogenous endophthalmitis (intravenous drug abuse, cardiac surgery, liver transplantation, and leukopenia).
- *Fusarium* species (septate filamentous fungi) are associated with leukopenia, intravenous drug abuse, ocular surgery and predisposing keratitis.
- *Blastomycosis* species and *Cryptococcus* species may cause ocular infection through endogenous spread and may occasionally spread to the central nervous system.

The incidence of exogenous fungal endophthalmitis varies from 2–13% of all cases of exogenous endophthalmitis. The visual prognosis in exogenous fungal endophthalmitis is worse than that in endogenous disease, especially in those cases of endophthalmitis initially presenting as fungal keratitis. Organisms identified in exogenous fungal endophthalmitis associated with visual outcome 20/400 or better include *Cylinrocarpon, Tubercularia, Aspergillus, Paecilomyces,* and *Candida*; on the other hand, *Acremonium* and *Fusarium* species are associated with worse final visual acuity. *Candida* and *Aspergillus* are the most common cause of endogenous endophthalmitis, but *Cryptococcus neoformans, Pseudoallescheria boydii,* and other fungi have been reported. The incidence of endogenous fungal endophthalmitis has increased in the last few decades, correlating with the increased prevalence of the sources of endogenous infections listed above. Although the visual prognosis for patients with endogenous endophthalmitis has improved with more aggressive therapy, half of patients treated at one tertiary care center had final visual acuity of 20/50 or worse in spite of aggressive management. In multiple studies, high mortality rates, as high as 77% at two months, have been seen in patients with endogenous fungal endophthalmitis.

PATHOPHYSIOLOGY

The mechanism of exogenous fungal infections begins with the traumatic or surgical breakdown of conjunctival or corneal epithelium, providing the organism with a site of entry. Ulceration and abscess formation may follow. Localized immunosuppression, typically from topical corticosteroids, increases the likelihood of invasive fungal infections. Unlike bacterial keratitis, fungal organisms more often penetrate through the cornea into the anterior chamber causing progressive hypopyon and anterior chamber inflammatory membranes. This endophthalmitis can subsequently spread to include vitritis and chorioretinitis.

In endogenous fungal endophthalmitis, fungi gain access to the eye most often via the choroidal or retinal circulations. Patients with candidemia are at higher risk for this complication, with the rate of *Candida* endophthalmitis in these patients between 28 and 45% of cases. Infection typically begins as a chorioretinitis. On histopathology, *Candida* endophthalmitis is characterized by small foci of retinal and uveal infection and suppurative granulomatous inflammation with multiple small foci of suppurative vitritis and infection. In contrast, *Aspergillus* endophthalmitis is most often localized to the subretinal and subretinal pigment epithelial spaces, and is associated with foci of deep retinal necrosis or chorioretinitis, vascular invasion, and a single larger area of suppurative vitritis. These characteristics are consistent with the clinical findings that visual recovery is less common with *Aspergillus* and positive vitreous cultures are more often obtained with *Candida*.

DIAGNOSIS

Clinical signs and symptoms

Fungal endophthalmitis presentation varies depending upon the:

- Size of the intraocular inoculation;
- Patient's relative immunocompetency;
- Concomitant administration of corticosteroids and antifungal agents during the initial infection period.

Most often, patients present 7 to 14 days after inoculation with:

- Conjunctival injection;
- Varying levels of pain (mild or absent);
- Often only mildly decreased vision.

The presentation of fungal endophthalmitis is typically more indolent than that seen with bacterial endophthalmitis, with a slower onset and more chronic course. Anterior chamber reaction, including hypopyon, and vitritis with whitish plaques on the pars plana, lens capsule or intraocular lens may develop. Alternatively, the eye may be white and quiet. Typically, exogenous endophthalmitis excites more pronounced pain and anterior segment inflammation, while endogenous endophthalmitis produces less pain and a quieter anterior segment.

More fulminant infections may cause:

- Fibrinous membranes in the anterior chamber;
- Vitreous veils, snowballs, and/or calcific plaques in the posterior segment.

Endogenous fungal endophthalmitis may also be associated with:

- White, fluffy retinal infiltrates;
- Retinal hemorrhages.

Funduscopy of *Candida* endophthalmitis characteristically reveals focal white superficial retinal lesions associated with a fluffy white overlying vitritis. Multiple white-centered superficial retinal hemorrhages can also be seen. Subretinal infiltrates sometimes coalesce into a white subretinal nodule. In contrast, *Aspergillus* endophthalmitis produces a more severe chorioretinitis, with more rapidly progressing larger lesions, as well as vasculitis and areas of retinal necrosis and retinal hemorrhage. A large yellow macular infiltrate often develops, with preretinal or subretinal exudative layering to form a pseudohypopyon of the posterior pole. Other fungi may produce a chorioretinitis similar to that seen with *Candida*.

Often, initial examination of patients at risk for fungal endophthalmitis by an ophthalmologist may be unremarkable; however, days to weeks later, fungal endophthalmitis develops in spite of continuous systemic antifungal treatment. For this reason, some authorities recommend repeat examination of patients with candidemia two weeks after an initial negative exam.

Laboratory findings

A thorough history and ophthalmologic examination often strongly suggest the causative pathogen. Obtaining a fungal culture *prior* to the initiation of antifungal therapy is essential; this may be the only way to determine the identity of the infectious filamentous fungus or yeast while allowing for drug sensitivity testing, if necessary. Fungal culture may not be necessary in those cases where systemic cultures have already isolated the pathogen.

Acquisition of vitreous fluid either by aspiration alone (i.e. vitreous tap) or during vitrectomy provides a higher yield than aqueous fluid from the anterior chamber. In the Endophthalmitis Vitrectomy Study, there was no added benefit of vitrectomy over aspiration alone. However, diagnostic vitrectomy is preferable to vitreous tap because aspiration without vitrectomy induces traction at points of vitreoretinal adhesion and may miss a focal vitritis. Syringes containing intraocular fluids are capped and taken directly to the microbiology laboratory for smears and inoculation of culture media. The vitrectomy canister is sealed and sent for vacuum filtration or centrifugation. If only a small amount of vitreous is available, tryptic soy broth (usually used for swabs) can be drawn into the specimen syringe along with a small air bubble, and mixed.

Smears are best prepared by placing one drop of each specimen on a glass slide and using a spatula to spread in a circular area 1 cm in diameter. These are then left to dry and carried to the microbiology laboratory for fixation and staining. Gomori's methenamine silver (GMS) and calcofluor white, and Acridine Orange stains may be used to stain for organisms. Blood agar and Sabouraud's dextrose agar containing gentamicin are the preferred culture media. One drop of specimen can be placed in brain heart infusion broth warmed to room temperature. Two specimen drops are placed on a calcium alginate swab, which can then be placed in the bottom of a Thioglycolate broth warmed to room temperature. Aspirates may also be sent for PCR for fungal DNA if available to facilitate early preliminary identification.

In every case, fungal cultures should be incubated at least 4 to 6 weeks for observation. Some laboratories routinely discard cultures that have no growth after 48 hours, but some fastidious organisms may be quite slow growing; cultures for suspected fungal endophthalmitis discarded before 28 days may be falsely read as negative.

TREATMENT

Therapy for fungal endophthalmitis may be instituted medically and/or surgically. Initially, removal of infecting exogenous agents (e.g. indwelling catheter), treatment of an external fungal infection (e.g. keratitis), and/or treatment of systemic conditions that may predispose to endogenous endophthalmitis (e.g. neutropenia secondary to chemotherapeutics) is warranted.

Medical

Medical therapy may be ocular or systemic. Prior to instituting therapy, however, aqueous and vitreous cultures are sent to microbiology for sensitivities.

Ocular

Ocular therapy for fungal endophthalmitis may be:

- Topical;
- Subconjunctival;
- Intravitreal.

Topical ophthalmic antifungal agents, while effective for fungal keratitis or scleritis (e.g. natamycin 5% ophthalmic suspension), do not provide adequate intravitreal drug levels required for the treatment of endophthalmitis. Poor vitreous penetration is also seen following subconjunctival deposition of antifungal agents. In addition, this route of administration has a higher risk of local side effects, such as pain at the site of injection. Intravitreal injection is then performed. Amphotericin B (5 μg in 0.1 mL) may be effective for most forms of fungal endophthalmitis. If a patient has not undergone pars plana vitrectomy (PPV), then the half-life of intraocular amphotericin B is approximately one week, and one should not repeat injection until that time has elapsed. In contrast, if a patient has undergone PPV, the drug is cleared within 24 hours of administration.

Systemic

Systemic therapy may be:

- Parenteral;
- Oral.

Intravenous drugs currently available for fungal endophthalmitis include:

- Amphotericin B;
- Fluconazole.

Both agents are effective against a wide spectrum of fungi and act by binding to sterols in fungal cell membranes, increasing cell membrane permeability and causing leakage of cell contents leading to cell death. Amphotericin B is given intravenously in doses of 0.5 mg/kg/day or 1 mg/kg every other day in a single infusion over 4 hours. The patient also must be premedicated with ibuprofen and diphenhydramine for some of the uncomfortable side effects. Fluconazole is a third-generation imidazole that may be administered either parenterally or orally in doses ranging from 200 mg to 400 mg/day.

In the past, the most effective oral agents against fungal endophthalmitis have been:

- Flucytosine is effective against *Candida* and *Cryptococcus* species, particularly when added to amphotericin B. However, resistance has been noted in over 50% of fungal isolates tested against the drug. In addition, there have been side effects reported, the most serious of which is pancytopenia; others include elevated liver function tests and hepatomegaly;
- Fluconazole has good antifungal activity, but after several weeks the physician must be aware of clinical depression setting in, which may necessitate discontinuance of the drug;
- Ketoconazole is another effective antifungal agent, particularly against *Blastomyces* and *Histoplasma* species;
- Itraconazole, another third-generation imidazole, is effective when combined with amphotericin B against *Aspergillus, Cryptococcus, Blastomyces,* and *Histoplasma* species.

Recently, a new antifungal agent, voriconazole, has been approved by the Food and Drug Administration (FDA) for systemic fungal infection. Voriconazole is a second-generation synthetic derivative of fluconazole, differing from this drug by the addition of a methyl group to the propyl backbone and by the substitution of a triazole moiety with a fluoropyrimidine group. These structural changes result in a higher affinity for the fungal enzyme lanosterol 14-a-demethylase, thus preventing the conversion of lanosterol to ergosterol. Since ergosterol is essential to fungal cell membrane synthesis, depletion causes disruption of the membrane and cell lysis. Voriconazole has demonstrated greater activity against all *Candida* and *Aspergillus* species than all other antifungals currently available. Also, all endemic fungal pathogens, such as *Fusarium, Histoplasma, Blastomyces, Paracoccidioides,* and *Cryptococcus* species, are fully susceptible to voriconazole.

Voriconazole achieves therapeutic concentrations in both the aqueous and vitreous both after oral and intravitreal administration. Examination of the safety of intravitreal use of voriconazole showed: normal adult rats were injected with differing concentrations of voriconazole in one eye while the fellow eye was injected with saline, thus serving as a control. Serial electroretinogram (ERG) measurements of maximum scotopic b-wave, b_{max}, intensity needed for half saturation, $I_{0.5}$, and saturated a-wave amplitude were measured in all eyes. Determination was made that there was no statistically significant difference in these parameters recorded between control eyes and voriconazole-injected eyes in any concentration groups. Histologic examination with light microscopy did not reveal any retinal abnormality in the eyes with 5 to 25vμg/mL intravitreal voriconazole. No statistically significant difference was noted between eyes treated with different concentrations of voriconazole versus the fellow control eyes treated with saline in terms of ERG findings. Thus, because of its broad spectrum of coverage, low MIC_{90} levels for the organisms of concern, good tolerability, and excellent bioavailability with oral administration, voriconazole may represent a major advance in the prophylaxis or management of both exogenous and endogenous fungal endophthalmitis.

Surgical

In most cases of fungal endophthalmitis, pars plana vitrectomy may be helpful to:

- Retrieve vitreous samples for culture of the causative organisms;
- Remove the bulk of infective material;
- Sterilize the vitreous cavity;
- Improve aqueous circulation into the vitreous to circulate therapeutic drug molecules and to wash out offending fungal elements.

When there is no specific vitreous pathology, one must search for fungal elements to culture from all sites. Often, centrifugation or filtration of vitreous specimens can concentrate organisms and improve the chances of obtaining a positive culture. In cases of recurrent infection or inflammation in patients with an intraocular lens, removal and culture of the intraocular lens implant and the entire capsular bag should be considered to reduce potential scaffolding for infection. Iridectomy may also be indicated if suspicion exists. In general, the chances of obtaining a positive culture increase greatly with aspiration of white, fluffy opacities, calcific plaques, or opacified portions of residual capsule rather than the relatively low yield of obtaining clear vitreous.

In most cases, pars plana vitrectomy must be combined with intravitreal injection of antifungal agents and concomitant oral or intravenous therapy. The prevailing treatment of choice currently is PPV with intravitreal injection of amphotericin B plus oral voriconazole, thus achieving adequate vitreous concentration of two fungicidal drugs after clearing the infectious debris. Choosing an agent that has a low risk of retinal toxicity is important; this is another important reason that voriconazole is an effective choice.

COMMENTS

Generally, final outcomes after the development of fungal endophthalmitis depend upon a variety of factors:

- Timing of trauma or surgery to presentation;
- Type of matter inoculated (i.e. vegetable matter has poorer prognosis);
- Relative immunocompetency of the individual;
- Timing of administration of immunosuppressive agents and antifungals;
- Isolation of organism by culture;
- Access to medical care.

If all factors are equal, some fungi have better prognosis than others do. For example, in *exogenous* endophthalmitis, visual outcome of 20/400 or better is more likely when isolates include:

- *Cylinrocarpon*;
- *Tubercularia*;
- *Aspergillus*;
- *Paecilomyces*;
- *Candida*.

On the other hand, these species are associated with worse final visual acuity:

- *Acremonium*;
- *Aspergillus*;
- *Fusarium*.

In *endogenous* endophthalmitis:

- *Candida* and *Aspergillus* species are the most common causes;
- *Cryptococcus neoformans*, *Pseudoallescheria boydii* as well as other fungi have been reported.

Patients with *Candida* tend to have better outcomes than those with *Aspergillus* due to the fact that *Candida* infections are more accessible (i.e. in the vitreous versus in the deep retina and RPE). However, all patients with endogenous endophthalmitis are very ill. In fact, as stated earlier, high mortality rates, as high as 77% at two months, have been reported in multiple studies. Thus, mortality tends to be much higher in the *endogenous* versus the *exogenous* group.

REFERENCES

Barza M, Pavan PR, Doft BH, et al: Evaluation of microbiological diagnostic techniques in postoperative endophthalmitis in the Endophthalmitis Vitrectomy Study. Arch Ophthalmol 115:1142–1150, 1997.

Binder MI, Chua J, Kaiser PK, et al: Endogenous endophthalmitis: an 18-year review of culture-positive cases at a tertiary care center. Medicine 82:97–105, 2003.

Flynn HW, Jr: The clinical challenge of endogenous endophthalmitis. Retina 21:572–574, 2001.

Hua G, Pennesi M, Shah K, et al: Safety of intravitreal voriconazole: electroretinographic and histopathologic studies. Trans Am Ophthalmol Soc 101:183–189, 2003.

Pettit TH, Olson RJ, Foos RY, et al: Fungal endophthalmitis following intraocular lens implantation: a surgical epidemic. Arch Ophthalmol 98:1025–1039, 1980.

Pflugfelder SC, Flynn HW Jr, Zwickey TA, et al: Exogenous fungal endophthalmitis. Ophthalmology 95:19–30, 1988.

Rao NA, Hidayat AA: Endogenous mycotic endophthalmitis: variations in clinical and histopathologic changes in candidiasis compared with aspergillosis. Am J Ophthalmol 132:244–251, 2001.

Stern WH, Tamura E, Jacobs RA, et al: Epidemic postsurgical *Candida parapsilosis* endophthalmitis: clinical findings and management of 15 consecutive cases. Ophthalmology 92:1701–1709, 1985.

SECTION

23 Intraocular Pressure

258 ANGLE RECESSION GLAUCOMA 921.3

Sarwat Salim, MD, FACS
Memphis, Tennessee
Raghu Mudumbai, MD
Seattle, Washington

ETIOLOGY

Angle recession glaucoma is one of the manifestations of blunt ocular trauma. The contusion leads to shearing forces between the anterior uvea and its various attachments. Damage can occur to the iris, trabecular meshwork (TM), or ciliary body. Angle recession involves rupture of the face of the ciliary body, resulting in a tear between the longitudinal and circular fibers of the ciliary muscle. Initially, this may be masked by the concomitant presence of hyphema, a common clinical presentation that occurrs after anterior segment trauma. Although a large percentage of patients may exhibit some level of angle recession on gonioscopy, only 4%–10% of these patients will develop angle recession glaucoma. The term angle recession glaucoma is somewhat misleading because the resultant glaucoma is not secondary to angle recession, but due to the initial trauma to the trabecular meshwork. Tears in the trabecular meshwork, along with degenerative changes and scarring, can lead to obstruction of aqueous outflow.

COURSE

Acutely, patients may have elevated intraocular pressure (IOP) from associated co-morbidities, such as hyphema, iridocyclitis, or pupillary block resulting from ectopia lentis with or without vitreous prolapse. In some cases, the IOP may be low secondary to decreased production of aqueous humor from associated inflammation, transient increase in outflow facility from disruption of structures in the angle, or due to the presence of a cyclodialysis cleft.

As previously mentioned, only a small minority of these patients develop late glaucoma. The risk of glaucoma appears to be related to the extent of angle recession. Usually, angle recession greater than 180° is deemed a considerable risk. In addition to the aforementioned changes described in the TM, another mechanism leading to chronic IOP elevation is due to formation of a Descemet's-like membrane lined by endothelial cells over the drainage angle.

Spaeth et al showed that approximately 50% of patients with traumatic glaucoma developed open angle glaucoma in the unaffected, nontraumatized eye, suggesting that patients who develop angle recession glaucoma may have an underlying predisposition to developing glaucoma, which may be accelerated by the additional insult of trauma.

Since angle recession glaucoma may not occur for months or years after the original trauma, these patients need to be followed regularly.

DIAGNOSIS

Clinical signs and symptoms

Acutely, the eye may be difficult to examine because of inflammation and hyphema. Once the view has cleared, attention should be paid to anterior chamber depth. The affected eye may appear deeper. On gonioscopy, characteristic findings of angle recession include widening of the ciliary body band, torn iris processes with resultant whitening of the scleral spur, and irregular and darker pigmentation in the angle. Peripheral anterior synechiae may be present. It is prudent to compare the angle appearance between the two eyes to evaluate subtle differences. Also, different quadrants within the same eye should be inspected carefully.

Other angle abnormalities from trauma such as iridodialysis (tear of the iris root) or cyclodialysis cleft (separation of the ciliary body from the scleral spur) may be detected.

Corneal blood staining, cataract, lens subluxation or dislocation, vitreous hemorrhage, retinal commotion, and retinal dialysis may be concomitantly present and accompany glaucoma.

Differential diagnosis

Acutely, many factors may contribute to elevated intraocular pressure. The trabecular meshwork may be overwhelmed by red blood cells and their byproducts or by inflammatory cells from iridocyclitis. Later, ghost cell glaucoma may develop. Chronic treatment with steroids can lead to steroid-induced glaucoma. Other differential diagnoses for unilateral glaucoma should be entertained, including pseudoexfoliative glaucoma and neovascular glaucoma. Unrelated open angle glaucoma and uveitic glaucoma should also be considered.

TREATMENT

In the acute setting, treatment should be directed at lowering intraocular pressure and controlling inflammation.

Ocular

Topical steroids with cycloplegic agents may be helpful for both inflammation and pain control. Aqueous suppressants, including beta blockers, carbonic anhydrase inhibitors, and alpha agonist agents should be used to control IOP. Osmotic agents, by reducing vitreous volume, may provide acute but transient pressure reduction.

Medical

With chronic IOP elevation, medical therapy with aqueous suppressants should be attempted first. Miotics are usually ineffective in these cases and can actually cause paradoxical rise in pressure. Prostaglandin analogs may provide the benefit of bypassing the compromised trabecular meshwork and increase the uveoscleral outflow.

Surgical

Laser trabeculoplasty is usually not successful due to distortion of the angle anatomy and TM scarring. Filtration surgery with the use of antimetabolites is the most effective surgical procedure in these cases. Glaucoma drainage devices play a role in cases of failed filtering surgery or in patients who are not candidates for trabeculectomy due to excessive scarring from the initial trauma. In eyes with limited visual potential, a cyclodestructive procedure may be an alternative option.

COMPLICATIONS

The clinician should be mindful of complications associated with medical and surgical intervention. These include worsening of asthma and heart failure with beta blockers, allergic reactions to $alpha_2$ agonists, and paresthesias, acidosis, fatigue, renal stones, and other adverse effects of carbonic anhydrase inhibitors. Filtration surgery poses risks of late onset bleb leaks with hypotony maculopathy and infection. Drainage implants can present a different set of problems, including corneal decompensation, tube retraction and erosion, and strabismus. Proper instruction ofpatients combined with a good clinical exam and frequent follow-up visits can, we hope, detect or prevent these problems.

COMMENTS

The clinician should be cognizant of both the short-term and long-term risks of glaucoma in patients who have suffered blunt ocular trauma. Patients presenting with hyphema should be evaluated with gonioscopy at an appropriate time to check for the presence of angle recession and other abnormalities. Usually, angle involvement of greater than 180° confers approximately a 10% risk for development of angle recession glaucoma. Since glaucoma can occur at any time after injury, regular follow-up examinations are mandatory for these patients, with particular attention to tonometry, gonioscopy, and optic nerve examination.

REFERENCES

Girkin CA, McGwin G, Jr, Long C, et al: Glaucoma after ocular contusion: a cohort study of the United States Eye Injury Registry. J Glaucoma 14:470–473, 2005.

Kaufman JH, Tolpin DW: Glaucoma after traumatic angle recession: a ten-year prospective study. Am J Ophthalmol 78:648–654, 1974.

Mermoud A, Salmon JF, Barron A, et al: Surgical management of post-traumatic angle recession glaucoma. Ophthalmology 100:634, 1993.

Salmon JF, Mermoud A, Ivey A, et al: The detection of post-traumatic angle recession by gonioscopy in a population-based glaucoma survey. Ophthalmology 101:1844, 1994.

Shields MB: Textbook of glaucoma. 4th ed. Baltimore, Williams & Wilkins, 1997:339–344.

Spaeth GL: Traumatic hyphema, angle recession, dexamethasone hypertension and glaucoma. Arch Ophthalmol 78:714–721, 1967.

Tumbocon JA, Latina MA: Angle recession glaucoma. Int Ophthalmol Clin 42:69–78, 2002.

259 CORTICOSTEROID-INDUCED GLAUCOMA 365.31

John R. Samples, MD
Portland, Oregon

ETIOLOGY/INCIDENCE

Corticosteroids may cause elevated intraocular pressure (IOP) through any route of administration, including oral, inhaled, topical, and periocular. Individuals vary a great deal in sensitivity to corticosteroids. Pulmonologists are sometimes skeptical that inhaled steroids will raise pressure, and it may be best to recommend that the patient get checked two weeks after this medication is started. Approximately one-third of otherwise healthy individuals will have some type of IOP elevation in response to the use of corticosteroids. Age may be an important factor in determining this; children may be particularly susceptible. Steroid-induced glaucoma in children has been reported, and in some instances, congenital glaucoma may be corticosteroid related.

The popularity of intravitreal corticosteroid injections by retinal specialists has increased the occurrence of steroid-induced glaucoma. It may be warranted to check such patients two or three weeks after an injection. Patients with already compromised optic nerves should be followed especially closely.

In addition to the age of the patient, the magnitude and duration of IOP elevation is determined by dose, route of administration, frequency, duration of exposure, and predisposition of the individual to respond to corticosteroids. (The time of onset suggests a biochemical mechanism.) Because most individuals have normal optic nerves, patients with elevated IOP secondary to corticosteroid therapy may not have glaucomatous damage.

The elevation of IOP is related to biochemical abnormality in the trabecular meshwork. Several specific hypotheses have been put forward. Impaired outflow may be related to impaired enzymes in the trabecular meshwork.

COURSE

The course remits with discontinuation of corticosteroid and may be altered with decreased potency of drug. In some instances where the response to the intravitreal injection of steroid is aromatically effective, it may be best just to continue the injections and treat the glaucoma.

DIAGNOSIS

Clinical signs and symptoms

Ocular or periocular

- Eyelids: slight ptosis.
- Lens: cataracts, particularly posterior subcapsular cataracts.
- Other: increased intraocular pressure; visual field loss.

TREATMENT

Ocular

- Discontinue the use of corticosteroids when steroid-induced glaucoma is suspected if the underlying condition permits. Whether the IOP falls will depend on the concurrent presence of uveitis or other conditions that raise the IOP. Most pressure reductions occur two weeks after steroid is discontinued.
- Alteration in the trabecular cells and in the cellular events surrounding outflow may occur as a result of corticosteroid use. Patients with corticosteroid-induced IOP elevations respond to the usual antiglaucoma medications, including miotics, epinephrine, dipivefrin, β-adrenergic antagonists, and carbonic anhydrase inhibitors. As with ocular hypertension, there may be no need to treat mildly elevated pressure if the optic nerve is normal.
- Corticosteroid glaucoma generally does not respond to laser trabeculoplasty.
- If a topical ocular steroid is needed, it is sometimes useful to use a weaker synthetic steroid, such as fluorometholone or loteprednol etabonate, which will cause less pressure elevation for a given amount of antiinflammatory effect.
- Topical nonsteroidal anti-inflammatory drugs that are sufficiently potent to penetrate the eye and have significant anti-inflammatory action are available.
- Topical nonsteroidal anti-inflammatory drugs may have significant potency as well as a useful anti-inflammatory effect when used four times a day in lieu of a corticosteroid.
- The metabolism of steroids in systemic tissues, as well as the eye, seems to be a major determinant of steroid effects and side effects.
- A major part of the increased potency of steroids, such as dexamethasone, systemically is due to substitutions occurring on the cortisol molecule, some of which decrease degradation and others of which increase binding to steroid receptors. In direct contrast, steroids that are synthesized using progesterone rather than cortisol as the foundation molecule, such as fluorometholone and medrysone, seem to be particularly susceptible to degradation. In the eye, both medrysone and fluorometholone have a lesser tendency to raise the IOP, but they are not considered as efficacious, probably because of the inactivation due to metabolism.

Surgical

- Corticosteroid-induced glaucomas may require filtering surgery if they do not remit. Any decision to perform surgery must be based on the appearance of the visual field, as well as that of the optic nerve. Occasionally, corticosteroid-induced glaucomas are observed in the presence of a functioning filter or a Seton procedure.
- Glaucomatologists vary in their opinions on whether steroid-induced pressure elevations can be a significant problem when an outflow-enhancing procedure, such as trabeculectomy or a Seton procedure, has been performed.
- The diagnosis of steroid-induced IOP elevation after filtration should include consideration of other causes of bleb failure, such as closure of the internal aspect of the filtering fistula and subconjunctival scarring.

COMPLICATIONS

Whenever a patient undergoes corticosteroid therapy, a baseline examination and close follow-up are mandatory. Patients who are treated with oral prednisone on a long-term basis or who have recurrent intravitreal corticosteroid injections may be particularly at risk and should have an eye examination to ensure that they have not developed steroid-induced glaucoma.

In addition to the side effects of corticosteroids, steroid injections can also cause problems due to the preservatives used and due to the direct toxicity of high steroid concentration on certain cell types. Periocular methyl prednisone preparations may causesteroid-related effects for longer than is generally appreciated.

COMMENTS

Many corticosteroid-induced glaucomas result from the inappropriate use of corticosteroids for minor conditions, such as eye irritation or contact lens discomfort. Also, it is not uncommon for patients who have been treated with oral steroids to have pressure elevations. The failure of a physician to recognize corticosteroid-induced glaucoma may lead to needless visual loss and difficult medicolegal problems.

REFERENCES

Agrawal S, Agrawal J, Agrawal TP: Management of intractable glaucoma following intravitreal triamcinolone acetonide.[comment]. [Comment. Letter] Am J Ophthalmol 139(3):575–576, author reply 576, 2005.

Armaly MF: Effect of corticosteroids on intraocular pressure and fluid dynamics. I. The effect of dexamethasone in the normal eye. Arch Ophthalmol 70:482, 1963.

Armaly MF: Effect of corticosteroids on intraocular pressure and fluid dynamics. II. The effect of dexamethasone in the glaucomatous eye. Arch Ophthalmol 70:492, 1963.

Armaly MF: Statistical attributes of steroid hypertensive response in the clinically normal eye. Invest Ophthalmol Vis Sci 4:187, 1965.

Jampol LM, Yannuzzi LA, Weinreb RN. Glaucoma and intravitreal steroids. [Editorial] Ophthalmology 112(8):1325–1326, 2005.

260 EXFOLIATION SYNDROME 365.52

(Pseudoexfoliation Syndrome, Pseudoexfoliation Glaucoma, Exfoliative Glaucoma, Capsular Glaucoma)

Andrew G. Iwach, MD
San Francisco, California
Ümit Aykan, MD
Istanbul, Turkey
H. Dunbar Hoskins, Jr., MD
San Francisco, California

ETIOLOGY/INCIDENCE

The exfoliation syndrome occurs when ocular tissues synthesize an abnormal protein, which may obstruct the trabecular meshwork. Exfoliation syndrome with glaucoma appears to be a secondary glaucoma in which exfoliation material and pigment obstruct the trabecular meshwork, with an associated elevation in intraocular pressure

- Once thought to occur primarily in Scandinavia, exfoliation syndrome is now known to occur throughout the world.
- There is a higher prevalence in certain areas of the world.
- Prevalence increases with age.
- Exfoliation syndrome occurs equally in both sexes.
- This syndrome presents unilaterally in one-third to one half of cases; however, as many as 43% of cases become bilateral in 5 to 10 years.
- As many as 7% of patients with exfoliation syndrome are initially diagnosed with glaucoma, but an additional 15% are found to have only elevated IOPs without optic nerve damage.
- Causes are related to mechanical obstruction by exfoliative material of exotrabecular origin, apparent production of exfoliative material by trabecular cells, and abnormal regulation of elastin synthesis, degradation, or both in the optic nerve.
- The main risk factor for glaucoma is the degree of chamber angle pigmentation rather than the amount of exfoliation.
- Exfoliation may be a risk factor for angle-closure glaucoma.
- Exfoliation syndrome is a risk factor in the evolution and treatment of exfoliative glaucoma and cataract.
- A poorer functional outcome and an increased incidence of preoperative and postoperative complications and senile cataract should be anticipated after surgery.
- The severity of glaucoma is related to the amount of exfoliative material present in the cribriform region.

DIAGNOSIS

Clinical signs and symptoms

- Patients with exfoliation syndrome present with a pattern on the anterior lenticular surface consisting of a central translucent disk surrounded by a clear zone, which in turn is surrounded by a granular gray-white area with scalloped edges that is best seen after pupillary dilation.
- Dandruff-like flakes of exfoliative material are deposited on the conjunctiva, corneal endothelium, trabecular meshwork, iris, pupillary margin, ciliary processes, zonules, and anterior hyaloid face in aphakic eyes.
- The amount of angle pigmentation is moderate, and distribution is patchy.
- Transillumination defects of the iris and reduced response to mydriatics are associated with exfoliation syndrome.
- The amount of exfoliative material correlates with the IOP and is inversely correlated with the number of axons in the optic nerve.
- Quantification may be achieved with flare measurement and biochemical protein determination, which affect pharmacologic and surgical treatment.
- Expect greater visual field loss and more difficulty in gaining control of IOP on presentation than with primary open-angle glaucoma.
- Expect a higher mean range of IOP, a higher maximum IOP, and a higher minimum IOP.
- In eyes with exfoliation syndrome, a small optic disk does not predispose to glaucoma. The optic disk does not show pathognomonic features for exfoliation.
- Fluorescein angiography of the iris reveals a decreased number of vessels, neovascularization, and leakage from the vessels.
- The extensive blood-aqueous barrier breakdown in eyes with exfoliation syndrome after intraocular surgery is a risk factor for early or late postoperative complications. Resulting alterations in the blood-aqueous barrier should be considered in the medical and surgical treatment.

Differential diagnosis

Significant fluctuation in the diurnal curve of the IOP distinguishes exfoliative glaucoma from primary open-angle glaucoma and may be an important factor in predicting any subsequent poor response to medical therapy.

TREATMENT

The treatment of glaucoma associated with exfoliation syndrome is similar to that for primary open-angle glaucoma. More aggressive management is warranted.

- IOP is typically high in exfoliative glaucoma, so the response to medical treatment is less favorable.
- The glaucoma in exfoliation syndrome tends to be less responsive to medical therapy than in primary open-angle glaucoma, and a higher percentage of exfoliative glaucoma patients require surgical intervention.
- Laser trabeculoplasty has its highest initial success rate in exfoliative glaucoma, although the IOP may rise again within a few years.
- Filtering surgery has a high success rate.
- Expect a higher incidence of vitreous loss during cataract surgery in exfoliation syndrome.
- Patients respond well to timolol initially but then have a higher IOP and significant fluctuation in the diurnal curve.
- Latanoprost causes a marked and sustained IOP reduction in eyes also being treated with timolol.
- Although the initial response to argon laser trabeculoplasty in exfoliative patients is greater, the long-term outcome is similar to that of primary open-angle glaucoma.
- Phacoemulsification can be well tolerated if a careful preoperative protocol is followed, including pupillary dilatation, wide capsulorhexis, and total nucleus hydrodisection.
- Trabecular aspiration is a new proposed mode to treat exfoliation glaucoma.

COMPLICATIONS

- Exfoliation syndrome is a risk factor for retinal vein thrombosis.
- Exfoliative glaucoma is a risk factor for accelerated cataract progression after trabeculectomy.
- Abnormal extracellular matrix production and vascular abnormalities may cause degenerative tissue changes, and atrophy of muscle cells might potentiate the reduction in dilating properties of the iris.
- There is an increased incidence of the intraoperative and postoperative complications, including insufficient dilata-

tion of the pupil, tearing of the posterior capsule, loss of the vitreous, modifications of the corneal endothelium, increased postoperative IOP, and more frequent opacification of the posterior capsule.
- Comorbidity with acute cerebrovascular disease is more common with exfoliative glaucoma than with primary open-angle glaucoma.

SUPPORT GROUP

Glaucoma Research Foundation
490 Post Street, Suite 1427
San Francisco, CA 94102

REFERENCES

Henry JC, Krupin T, Schmitt M, et al: Long-term follow-up of pseudoexfoliation and the development of elevated intraocular pressure. Ophthalmology 94:545, 1987.

Jonas JB, Papastathopoulos KI: Optic disk appearance in pseudoexfoliation syndrome. Am J Ophthalmol 123:174–180, 1997.

Konstas AG, Stewart WC, Stroman GA, Sine CS: Clinical presentation and initial treatment patterns in patients with exfoliation glaucoma versus primary open-angle glaucoma. Ophthalmic Surg Lasers 28:111–117, 1997.

Layden WE, Shaffer RN: Exfoliation syndrome. Am J Ophthalmol 78:835, 1974.

Ritland JS, Egge K, Lydersen S, et al: Exfoliation glaucoma and primary open-angle glaucoma: associations with death causes and comorbidity. Acta Ophthalmol Scand 82(4):397–400, 2004.

261 GLAUCOMA ASSOCIATED WITH ANTERIOR UVEITIS 365.62

Leon W. Herndon, MD
Durham, North Carolina

ETIOLOGY

Increased intraocular pressure (IOP) can occur with any type of ocular inflammation, and it can be acute, transient, or chronic. Anterior uveitis influences IOP through a delicate balance between aqueous humor production and resistance to aqueous outflow. Usually, the production of aqueous is diminished in anterior uveitis; if this reduction is greater than the increase in resistance to outflow, the IOP will be low. In other cases, the increased resistance to aqueous outflow may be sufficiently greater than aqueous production, leading to pressure elevation.

The causes of glaucoma associated with anterior uveitis can be divided into two categories, depending on whether the angle is open or closed.

OPEN ANGLE

- Inflammatory cells (polymorphonuclear leukocytes and macrophages) can infiltrate the trabecular meshwork, leading to IOP elevation.
- The increased protein content of the aqueous humor with the inflammatory reaction can result in compromise of aqueous outflow.
- Damage to trabecular cells after engulfing inflammatory debris may reduce outflow.
- Corticosteroids can cause IOP elevation.

CLOSED ANGLE

- The angle can be closed by extensive peripheral anterior synechiae or neovascularization.
- Posterior synechiae can lead to pupillary-block angle closure.
- Ciliary body swelling can cause forward rotation of the iris-lens diaphragm, leading to angle closure.

DIAGNOSIS

Laboratory findings

- Signs of acute iridocyclitis include ciliary flush, slight miosis, varying degrees of aqueous flare and cell, and frequent keratic precipitates.
- Chronic anterior uveitis often produces few or no symptoms but is particularly prone to cause secondary glaucoma.
- The IOP may vary in uveitic glaucoma due to variations in aqueous secretion, amount of outflow obstruction, and dose of corticosteroids being used at the time.
- A variety of noninvasive and invasive studies can be used to determine the cause of the uveitis, including serology, skin tests, chest radiographs, conjunctival biopsy, and anterior chamber paracentesis.

TREATMENT

Systemic

- Carbonic anhydrase inhibitors can be administered orally or intravenously.
- Systemic hyperosmotic agents are used to rapidly lower IOP and include oral glycerin, oral isosorbide, and intravenous mannitol.

Ocular

- Treatment should be directed at the underlying cause of the ocular inflammation.
- Inflammation can be treated with topical and systemic nonsteroidal anti-inflammatory agents; topical, periocular, and systemic corticosteroids; and systemic immunosuppressive agents.
- Ocular hypertension and glaucoma can be treated with topical β-blockers, alpha agonists, and carbonic anhydrase inhibitors.
- Miotics should be avoided because they may lead to increased inflammation.
- Prostaglandin analogs should probably be avoided because they may have a deleterious effect on the inflammatory cascade.

Surgical

Closed-angle glaucoma

- Laser iridotomy should be performed to reestablish communication between the posterior and anterior chambers.

- The argon or Nd : YAG laser, or both, may be used.
- Transient anterior chamber inflammation is a potential complication of laser iridotomy.
- Surgical iridectomy should be performed when laser iridotomy is unsuccessful or contraindicated.

Open-angle glaucoma

- Trabeculodialysis:
  - A modified goniotomy is used in children and young adults with uncontrolled uveitic glaucoma;
  - The technique involves disinsertion of trabeculum from the scleral spur, allowing direct access into Schlemm's canal;
  - The procedure has a success rate ranging from 56% to 60% in children and young adults.
- Trabeculectomy:
  - Postoperative cellular response in uveitic glaucoma can accelerate the wound-healing process and lead to failure of the trabeculectomy;
  - Antimetabolite therapy in association with trabeculectomy has been shown to improve the outcome of trabeculectomy in uveitic glaucoma with success rates of 75% to 95%.
- Drainage implant:
  - There are different types of implant tubes for draining the aqueous from the anterior chamber to the subconjunctival space but few published reports of using drainage implants in patients with uveitic glaucoma;
  - One series reported a success rate of 95.8% at 3 months and 91.7% at 6 months, 12 months, and 24 months after Baerveldt glaucoma drainage implantation in uveitic glaucoma.

COMPLICATIONS

The use of antimetabolites in glaucoma surgery is associated with an increased risk of complications, such as hypotony, bleb leaks, and endophthalmitis.

Postoperative inflammation or reactivation of the uveitis has been reported to occur in 5.2% to 31.1% of patients with uveitic glaucoma.

Cataract progression is very common in the patient with uveitic glaucoma due to use of topical corticosteroids and after filtration surgery. If possible, the surgeon should allow the anterior chamber to be free of inflammation for at least 3 months before proceeding with elective cataract surgery.

COMMENTS

There are a number of inflammatory disorders commonly associated with secondary glaucoma, including Fuchs' heterochromic iridocyclitis, glaucomatocyclitic crisis, sarcoidosis, and juvenile rheumatoid arthritis. Management of these conditions, as well as of other uveitic glaucomas, may be difficult because of the numerous mechanisms involved in their pathogenesis. The goal of treatment is to minimize permanent alteration of aqueous outflow and to prevent damage to the optic nerve.

REFERENCES

Ceballos EM, Parrish RK, Schiffman JC: Outcome of Baerveldt glaucoma drainage implants for the treatment of uveitic glaucoma. Ophthalmology 109:2256–2260, 2002.

Moorthy RS, Mermoud A, Baerveldt G, et al: Glaucoma associated with uveitis. Surv Ophthalmol 41:361–394, 1997.

Prata JA, Neves RA, Minkler DE, et al: Trabeculectomy with mitomycin C in glaucoma associated with uveitis. Ophthalmic Surg 24:616–620, 1994.

Skuta GL, Parrish RK: Wound healing in glaucoma filtering surgery. Surv Ophthalmol 32:149–170, 1987.

Sung VC, Barton K: Management of inflammatory glaucomas. Curr Opin Ophthalmol 15:136–140, 2004.

Wright MM, McGehee RF, Pederson JE: Intraoperative mitomycin-C for glaucoma associated with ocular inflammation. Ophthalmic Surg Lasers 28:370–376, 1997.

262 GLAUCOMA ASSOCIATED WITH ELEVATED VENOUS PRESSURE 365.82

John R. Samples, MD

Portland, Oregon

ETIOLOGY

Systemic disorders that raise the episcleral venous pressure can cause glaucoma as the increased pressure creates resistance to outflow in Schlemm's canal, thus raising intraocular pressure.

- Schlemm's canal is connected to the episcleral and conjunctival veins by a complicated system of vessels. Most vessels carrying aqueous humor from Schlemm's canal are directed posteriorly, with the majority draining into episcleral veins.
- A few vessels cross the subconjunctival tissue and drain into conjunctival veins.
- Episcleral veins drain into the cavernous sinus via the anterior ciliary and superior ophthalmic veins, whereas the conjunctival veins drain into the superior ophthalmic or facial veins via the palpebral and angular veins.
- The normal episcleral venous pressure ranges between 8 and 10 mm Hg. Patients with primary open-angle glaucoma do not appear to have episcleral venous pressure elevations; in fact, there may be a negative correlation, with ocular hypertensive patients having significantly lower episcleral venous pressure.

DIAGNOSIS

Clinical signs and symptoms

Elevated venous pressure is one means by which patients with thyroid eye disease may have elevated intraocular pressure.

- Elevated venous pressure may occur in association with a carotid cavernous fistula.
- The most consistent finding in patients with an elevated episcleral venous pressure is tortuous episcleral and bulbar conjunctival vessels.
- When the meshwork is open, there may be blood reflux into Schlemm's canal. An experienced ultrasonographer may be able to detect a dilated superior ophthalmic view in some of these patients.

Categories

Venous obstruction

In patients with thyroid eye disease, contracture of extraocular muscles and infiltration of the plasma cells and lymphocytes into the orbit may lead to an elevated venous pressure.

It must be kept in mind that thyroid dysfunction may lead to an elevated venous pressure as well as abnormal scleral rigidity. Retro-orbital tumors, cavernous sinus thrombosis, and lesions that obstruct venous return from the head also may cause venous obstruction and elevated venous pressure.

Carotid cavernous fistula

The typical carotid cavernous fistula occurs as a result of severe head injury; a large fistula is created between the internal carotid artery and the surrounding cavernous sinus venous plexus. The condition is characterized by pulsating exophthalmos, a bruit over the globe, conjunctival chemosis, engorgement of episcleral venous veins, and restriction of motility with evidence of ocular ischemia. The shunting of the internal carotid cavernous fistula causes high flow and high pressure. A more recently appreciated form of carotid cavernous fistula is the 'low-flow' shunt. These small fistulas may occur without a history of trauma. In these cases, the shunt is fed by a meningeal branch of the intracavernous internal carotid artery or external carotid artery that empties directly into the cavernous sinus or adjacent dural vein that connects with the cavernous sinus. Whether the patient has a high- or low-flow shunt, elevated pressure occurs. Venous backpressure may increase the episcleral venous pressure, which is the most common cause of intraocular pressure rise with the fistula. Angle-closure glaucoma has also been reported in association with carotid cavernous fistula.

Sturge–Weber syndrome

In this syndrome, a hamartoma arises from the vascular tissue and produces a characteristic port-wine stain hemangioma of the skin in a trigeminal distribution. Several mechanisms of glaucoma are possible in these patients, but at least some patients seem to have an open anterior chamber angle with low arteriovenous pressure, usually associated with stooping over or a Valsalva maneuver.

Idiopathic

These patients are elderly with no family history of the condition. The cause of the elevated venous pressure is unknown, and the associated glaucoma may be severe.

TREATMENT

- The treatment for glaucoma associated with elevated venous pressure is the same as that for other forms of glaucoma.
- In cases in which a carotid cavernous fistula or low-flow shunt is present, pharmacologic glaucoma control should be considered before surgical intervention is contemplated when the glaucoma is the only condition prompting consideration of surgery.
- In some instances, angiography alone is sufficient to prompt low-flow fistulas to close spontaneously.

Surgical

- If surgical intervention is necessary, a filtering procedure should be used.
- There is no doubt that these patients are at substantially increased risk for uveal effusion and expulsive hemorrhage. This should be included in the consent process. It has been recommended that drainage of the suprachoroid be routinely performed at the time of surgery.
- Prophylactic sclerotomy should routinely be performed at the same time as the filtering procedure.

PRECAUTIONS

Repair of carotid cavernous fistulas may be hazardous and is a controversial area in neurosurgery. If glaucoma is the sole cause for intervention, one should be certain that it is significant and difficult to treat, and that visual field progression is present. Elevated episcleral venous pressure as a cause of glaucoma is often overlooked. Because these patients do have increased complications at the time of filtering surgery, careful consideration of episcleral and conjunctival vessels before filtration is always indicated.

The consenting process should inform the patient that there is increased risk of choroidal hemorrhage when trabeculectomy is performed. Alternative, non-penetration surgeries for glaucoma may be useful in these cases.

REFERENCES

Bellows AR, Chylach LT, Jr, Epstein DL, et al: Choroidal effusion during glaucoma surgery in patients with prominent episcleral vessels. Arch Ophthalmol 97:493–497, 1979.

Harris GJ, Rice PR: Angle closure and carotid cavernous fistula in a series of 17 cases. Am J Ophthalmol 48:585–597, 1959.

Palestine AG, Young BR, Pipegras DG: Visual prognosis and carotid cavernous fistula. Arch Ophthalmol 99:1600–1603, 1981.

Podos SM, Minas TF, MacRif J: A new instrument to measure episcleral venous pressure: Comparison of normal eyes and eyes with primary open angle glaucoma. Arch Ophthalmol 80:209–213, 1968.

Radius RL, Maumenee AE: Dilated episcleral venous vessels and open-angle glaucoma. Am J Ophthalmol 86:31–35, 1978.

263 GLAUCOMA ASSOCIATED WITH INTRAOCULAR TUMORS 365.64

(Tumor Related Glaucoma, Melanomalytic Glaucoma, Melanocytomalytic Glaucoma, Neovascular Glaucoma, Angle Closure Glaucoma)

Carol L. Shields, MD
Philadelphia, Pennsylvania
Jerry A. Shields, MD
Philadelphia, Pennsylvania

ETIOLOGY/INCIDENCE

A number of intraocular tumors can produce ipsilateral elevation of the intraocular pressure. In such instances, there may be a delay in clinical recognition of the underlying neoplasm while the patient is treated for the secondary glaucoma. In cases of malignant tumors, this delay in diagnosis can have serious consequences.

In contrast to the primary glaucomas, which are generally bilateral, tumor-induced secondary glaucomas are almost always unilateral. The mechanism of the secondary glaucomas varies with the location, size, and type of tumor. Malignant tumors in the iris and ciliary body are more likely to obstruct aqueous outflow by directly infiltrating the trabecular meshwork. More posteriorly located intraocular neoplasms can produce anterior displacement of the lens-iris diaphragm causing angle closure, they can induce iris and angle neovascularization causing neovascular glaucoma, or they can liberate tumor cells in the anterior chamber angle, blocking aqueous outflow.

Primary tumors of the uvea

Nevus

Uveal nevi are benign lesions which rarely produce secondary glaucoma. Occasionally, however, localized or diffuse uveal nevi can lead to secondary glaucoma. This most often occurs with a melanocytoma or with a diffuse nevus of the iris. Melanocytoma is a specific variant of nevus which usually occurs in the optic disc, but which can arise anywhere in the uveal tract. Those located in the optic disc or choroid rarely produce secondary glaucoma whereas those which occur in the ciliary body or iris are more likely to produce secondary glaucoma by anterior chamber angle infiltration with discohesive tumor or necrotic cells, often engulfed by macrophages (melanocytomalytic glaucoma).

Melanoma

Of all patients with uveal melanoma, secondary glaucoma is found in approximately 3%.

Iris melanoma is associated with secondary glaucoma in 7 % of cases and the most common mechanism of glaucoma is direct invasion of the trabecular meshwork by tumor tissue. Occasionally spontaneous hyphema is the cause of increased intraocular pressure. The diffuse iris melanoma produces a classic syndrome of acquired hyperchromic heterochromia and ipsilateral glaucoma. Iris melanoma invasion into the angle and secondary glaucoma are the two most important risk factors for metastases.

In contrast to iris melanoma, ciliary body melanoma tends to attain a fairly large size prior to diagnosis. Ciliary body melanomas cause secondary glaucoma in 17% of cases and the mechanisms include anterior displacement of the iris with secondary angle closure or direct invasion of the trabecular meshwork. Less commonly, hyphema, necrosis, or iris neovascularization, are found as the cause of secondary glaucoma.

Published studies show that only 2% of patients with choroidal melanoma have secondary glaucoma. When secondary glaucoma occurs due to a choroidal melanoma it is from iris and angle neovascularization (56%) or anterior displacement of the lens-iris diaphragm and secondary angle closure (44%). Large necrotic choroidal melanomas can occasionally produce intraocular inflammation or hemorrhage, which can further contribute to secondary glaucoma.

Others

Other rare uveal tumors such as neurilemomas, leiomyomas, neurofibromas can produce secondary glaucoma by the same mechanisms.

Metastatic tumors to the uvea

Malignant tumors from distant primary sites metastasize via hematogenous routes to the uveal tract and rarely to the retina or optic nerve. Choroidal metastases only produce secondary glaucoma when they attain a large size, whereas iris and ciliary body metastases frequently produce secondary glaucoma because of their tendency to be friable and also involve the angle structures. In our series of patients with uveal metastases, secondary glaucoma was found in 64% of iris metastasis, 67% of ciliary body metastasis, and 2% of choroidal metastasis.

Iris and ciliary body metastases usually produce secondary glaucoma by seeding into the anterior chamber angle and trabecular meshwork, mechanically blocking aqueous outflow. In some cases, a solid growth of tumor cells can assume a ring type infiltration of the trabecular meshwork resulting in intractable glaucoma.

Metastatic tumors to the choroid appear as single or multiple elevated or diffuse lesions often associated with a secondary nonrhegmatogenous retinal detachment. The most common mechanism of glaucoma with choroidal metastases is angle closure due to anterior displacement of the lens-iris diaphragm secondary to total retinal detachment. Neovascular glaucoma can occur in advanced cases with total retinal detachment.

Primary tumors of the retina

Tumors of the sensory retina include retinoblastoma, vascular tumors, glial tumors, and others. Retinoblastoma, the most important retinal tumor, frequently produces secondary glaucoma. In rare instances, advanced retinal capillary hemangiomas can produce secondary glaucoma in association with a total retinal detachment.

In our series of 248 patients with retinoblastoma, 17% of 303 affected eyes had secondary glaucoma. The secondary glaucoma was due to iris neovascularization in 72%, angle closure secondary to anterior displacement of the lens-iris diaphragm in 26%, and tumor seeding into the anterior chamber in 2%. In cases with iris neovascularization, secondary hyphema sometimes contributed to the mechanism of glaucoma. The presence of iris neovascularization and secondary glaucoma in an eye with retinoblastoma is a statistical risk for optic nerve invasion, choroidal invasion, and eventual metastases.

Tumors of the nonpigmented and pigmented epithelium

Tumors of the nonpigmented epithelium of the ciliary body include medulloepithelioma, adenoma, and adenocarcinoma. The medulloepithelioma (previously called diktyoma) is an embryonic ciliary body tumor which becomes clinically apparent in the first few years of life. In two large series of medulloepithelioma, secondary glaucoma occurred in approximately 50% of cases. In these cases, glaucoma occurred secondary to iris neovascularization or from direct invasion of the anterior chamber angle structures by the tumor. In some instances, hyphema or cysts in the anterior chamber also contributed to obstruction of aqueous outflow.

Acquired tumors of the nonpigmented ciliary epithelium are rare, slow growing benign or lowly malignant lesions and they rarely produce secondary glaucoma. Primary tumors of the pigmented epithelium (adenoma and adenocarcinoma) of the iris, ciliary body, and retina are rare. The mechanisms of glaucoma are the same as those of malignant melanoma.

Lymphoid tumors and leukemias

Lymphoid tumors and leukemias can produce a similar infiltration of the uveal tract and retina. The most important lymphoid tumors of the intraocular structures include benign reactive lymphoid hyperplasia (BRLH) of the uvea and malignant lymphoma, particularly large cell lymphoma (histiocytic lymphoma, reticulum cell sarcoma). Secondary glaucoma most often occurs from direct infiltration of the anterior chamber angle and thickening of the iris and ciliary body by tumor cells. This results in blockage of aqueous outflow and secondary elevation of intraocular pressure.

Systemic hamartomatoses (phakomatoses)

The classic phakomatoses include encephalofacial hemangiomatosis (Sturge–Weber syndrome) neurofibromatosis (von Recklinghausen's syndrome), retinocerebellar capillary hemangiomatosis (von Hippel–Lindau syndrome) and tuberous sclerosis (Bourneville's syndrome). The two which are more likely to be associated with either infantile or juvenile glaucoma include encephalofacial hemangiomatosis and neurofibromatosis.

COURSE/PROGNOSIS

The course and prognosis of the patient depends on the primary tumor type, location, size, and other features. Glaucoma associated with iris melanoma is associated with a worse ocular and systemic prognosis compared to iris melanoma without glaucoma. Glaucoma associated with retinoblastoma is associated with a greater risk for optic nerve and choroidal invasion of the tumor, imparting a greater risk for metastatic disease.

DIAGNOSIS/LABORATORY FINDINGS

Clinical

- Examination may show an intraocular mass.
- Slit lamp biomicroscopy may reveal neovascularization of the iris.
- Gonioscopy may reveal angle invasion by tumor or angle vessels.
- Transillumination may show a ciliary body or choroidal shadow.

Ocular tests

- Ultrasonography may demonstrate an intraocular mass.
- Ultrasound biomicroscopy can show anterior chamber angle invasion or ciliary body tumor.
- Fluorescein angiography or indocyanine green angiography may demonstrate an intraocular mass or show iris neovascularization.
- Magnetic resonance imaging or computed tomography may reveal an intraocular mass with characteristics suggestive of a specific tumor type.

Systemic tests

For patients with uveal melanoma, a complete physical examination, liver function tests, liver imaging test (ultrasound or magnetic resonance imaging), and chest x-ray is recommended and should be repeated on a six month basis by the patient's oncologist. For patients with uveal metastases, a complete oncologic evaluation by the general oncologist is warranted. Breast cancer is the most common uveal metastasis. For patients with retinoblastoma, cautious ocular and systemic care by an ocular oncologist and pediatric oncologist is warranted. For patients with leukemia and lymphoma, systemic evaluation by the oncologist is recommended. Ocular involvement with leukemia carries an extremely poor systemic prognosis. Retinovitreal lymphoma tends to be associated with central nervous system lymphoma while uveal lymphoma is associated with systemic lymphoma. For patients with phakomatoses, a multidisciplinary approach with neurologist, dermatologist, pediatrician, and ophthalmologist is recommended.

Differential diagnosis

- Uveitic glaucoma.
- Neovascular glaucoma from other causes.
- Hemolytic glaucoma.
- Iridocorneal endothelial syndrome.
- Endophthalmitis.

PROPHYLAXIS

Treatment of the tumor at an early stage is a good measure to prevent glaucoma. However, some treatments, especially charged particle radiotherapy and plaque radiotherapy, can eventually lead to glaucoma.

TREATMENT

Medical

The management of glaucoma secondary to intraocular tumors should depend upon the type of tumor. In cases of benign tumors, it is often appropriate to first treat the glaucoma medically. In cases of malignant tumors, it may be appropriate to first treat the tumor in hopes of relieving the glaucoma. In cases of uveal melanoma, melanocytoma, metastasis, and lymphoid infiltration, the glaucoma may resolve with the primary treatment of the tumor either by surgical resection, radiotherapy, or chemotherapy. If the glaucoma persists despite effective therapy, then medical management of the secondary glaucoma is warranted. Generally, antiglaucoma eyedrops and systemic carbonic anhydrase inhibitors are instituted as necessary.

Surgical

Most melanocytic iris tumors should be managed initially by periodic observation and any associated glaucoma should be managed medically. If the tumor shows evidence of growth or if the secondary glaucoma cannot be controlled, then surgical intervention should be considered. In cases of circumscribed tumors, excision of the tumor by a partial iridectomy or iridocyclectomy may improve the glaucoma but further medical treatment of the glaucoma may be necessary. Trabeculectomy should be avoided until all conservative methods, including argon laser trabeculoplasty and ciliary body destructive procedures are attempted. In the case of a diffuse iris melanoma with secondary glaucoma, enucleation is generally necessary. Fine needle aspiration biopsy is indicated to differentiate melanoma from melanocytoma or nevus. We have found that open biopsy of an iris tumor or filtering surgery to control glaucoma in cases of diffuse iris melanoma can predispose to extrascleral extension of the tumor. In the case of iris melanocytoma, the liberated pigment in the trabecular meshwork may gradually disappear following complete excision of the main tumor.

Small ciliary body melanomas can be managed by periodic observation until growth is documented before initiating treatment. Somewhat larger tumors can be managed by local resection or episcleral plaque radiotherapy. Most tumors which are large or infiltrative enough to produce secondary glaucoma are generally best managed by enucleation of the affected eye. Careful medical evaluation and follow-up is warranted because of the relatively high risk of metastatic disease in cases of ciliary body melanoma with secondary glaucoma. In our series of patients with ciliary body melanoma, 50% of patients with secondary glaucoma died from metastatic melanoma within two years of the diagnosis.

The options in management of choroidal melanomas are well outlined in the literature and include serial observation, photocoagulation, transpupillary thermotherapy, radiotherapy, local resection, enucleation and even orbital exenteration. Unfortunately, choroidal melanomas that have produced secondary glaucoma are generally so large that enucleation is necessary.

In some cases of uveal metastases associated with secondary glaucoma, the glaucoma may ultimately require laser or surgical trabeculectomy, cyclocryotherapy, retrobulbar alcohol injection, or even enucleation. Since most affected patients have a poor systemic prognosis, enucleation should be avoided if possible and the goal should be to make the patient comfortable.

The management of retinoblastoma should depend upon the overall clinical findings and can include enucleation, chemotherapy, radiotherapy, cryotherapy, thermotherapy, and photocoagulation. In cases with secondary glaucoma, the tumor is usually quite advanced and enucleation is considered the treatment of choice. In most cases of retinoblastoma associated with secondary glaucoma, the optic disc cannot be visualized ophthalmoscopically because of the large tumor within the eye. Therefore, it is particularly important in these cases to obtain a long section of optic nerve stump along with the globe at the time of enucleation, since the most important route of extraocular extension of this tumor is through the optic nerve to the central nervous system.

Management of small intraocular medulloepitheliomas consists of an attempt at local resection by a cyclectomy. Unfortunately, it is extremely difficult to completely remove such tumors and recurrence is common, eventually requiring enucleation. In cases with glaucoma, enucleation is usually necessary because of pain or suspected malignancy.

IRRADIATION AND CHEMOTHERAPY

The management of iris and ciliary body metastases should be systemic chemotherapy or other management which the patient is receiving for the systemic cancer. If the ocular tumor continues to proliferate, then external beam radiotherapy to the eye, giving 3500–4000 cGy (Rad) to the affected eye in divided doses over a four week period should be initiated. If the uveal metastasis is the patient's only active metastatic focus then local plaque radiotherapy is certainly justified. Plaque radiotherapy takes approximately 4 days and minimizes radiation to the uninvolved remainder of the eye and orbit. If any associated secondary glaucoma does not resolve following chemotherapy and radiotherapy, acetozolamide, timolol or other medications should be continued to control the intraocular pressure and to keep the patient comfortable. In many instances, the glaucoma will progress relentlessly and laser or filtering surgery can be attempted. This decision should be made in light of the patient's prognosis and enucleation should be avoided if the systemic prognosis is dismal. In some instances, enucleation is warranted for pain relief.

The appropriate management of intraocular lymphoid tumors and leukemias is ocular radiotherapy combined with the chemotherapy that the patient may be receiving for the systemic disease. In the case of BRLH, about 2000 cGy (rad) is generally sufficient, whereas in the case of malignant lymphoma about 3000–4000 cGy may be necessary to bring about good resolution of the tumor. In some cases, the glaucoma resolves with the radiotherapy or chemotherapy, but in cases with severe glaucoma, this treatment may not help and enucleation of the eye, if it is blind and painful, may be necessary.

COMPLICATIONS

A patient who presents unexplained unilateral glaucoma could be harboring an unsuspected intraocular malignant tumor. It is usually contraindicated to perform laser surgery or filtering procedures until a complete ophthalmologic examination including careful indirect ophthalmoscopy is performed to exclude the possibility of tumor. In cases where the posterior pole or ciliary body cannot be viewed because of opaque media, ultrasonography, transillumination or other procedures are necessary to rule out a tumor. It is particularly important not to perform glaucoma surgery or vitrectomy on a child with vitreous cells and unilateral glaucoma until the possibility of retinoblastoma is excluded.

COMMENTS

Management of tumor-induced glaucoma usually consists of enucleation because most cases are due to advanced uveal melanoma or retinoblastoma. In cases of benign tumors, medical therapy can be attempted first followed by laser or surgical therapy. It should be emphasized that the management of glaucoma secondary to iris tumors is a very difficult problem, because many such tumors are relatively benign histopathologically and all efforts are made to control the glaucoma by medical or laser treatment prior to surgical intervention. Trabeculectomy is controversial in the management of iris melanomas because of the possibility of tumor spread into the filtering bleb and episcleral tissues.

REFERENCES

Char DH, Quivey JM, Castro J, et al: Helium ions versus iodine 125 brachytherapy in the management of uveal melanoma: a prospective randomized dynamically balanced trial. Ophthalmology 100:1547–1554, 1993.

Girkin CA, Goldberg I, Mansberger SL, et al: Management of iris melanoma with secondary glaucoma. J Glaucoma 11:71–74, 2002.

Shields CL, Materin MA, Shields JA, et al: Factors associated with elevated intraocular pressure in eyes with iris melanoma. Br J Ophthalmol 85:666–669, 2001.

Shields CL, Shields JA, Gross N, et al: Survey of 520 eyes with uveal metastases. Ophthalmology 104:1265–1276, 1997.

Shields CL, Shields JA, Shields MB, Augsburger JJ: Prevalence and mechanisms of secondary intraocular pressure elevation in eyes with intraocular tumors. Ophthalmology 94:839–846, 1987.

Shields JA, Annesley WH, Spaeth GL: Necrotic melanocytoma of iris with secondary glaucoma. Am J Ophthalmol 84:826–829, 1977.

264 GLAUCOMATOCYCLITIC CRISIS
364.22
(Posner–Schlossman Syndrome)

Abraham Schlossman, MD, FACS
New York, New York

ETIOLOGY/INCIDENCE

Glaucomatocyclitic crisis is unilateral glaucoma characterized by recurrent attacks of glaucoma that are usually associated with signs of mild cyclitis. The condition generally occurs in patients between 20 and 50 years old, with individual attacks of ocular hypertension lasting from a few hours to 1 month but very rarely more than 2 weeks.

Multifactorial causes have been postulated for this syndrome; the condition has been reported in association with:

- Allergies;
- Herpes simplex virus infection (but not herpes zoster);
- Immunogenetic disorders;
- Stress-related disorders such as peptic ulcer;
- Primary vascular abnormality.

The mean incidence and prevalence rates of the condition reported in one study were 0.4 and 1.9, respectively, in 100,000 population.

PROGNOSIS

The prognosis is excellent with prompt treatment, with no permanent changes detectable in the visual fields after an attack.

DIAGNOSIS

- Sudden onset.
- Mildly blurred vision, diminished visual acuity (temporary).
- Colored haloes around lights.
- Mild ocular discomfort.
- Unilateral; recurrences always in same eye (very rarely bilateral).
- Slight mydriasis (pupil of affected eye larger than that in the other eye and reactive).
- Intraocular pressure of affected eye between 40 and 60 mm Hg (fluctuates).
- Anterior chamber cells and minimal flare.
- Corneal epithelial edema, keratic precipitates (few, 25 or less; unpigmented); persist as long as 1 month after intraocular pressure has returned to normal.
- Ciliary flush.
- No posterior synechiae or iris atrophy.
- Rare glaucomatous cupping of optic nerve, after many attacks.

TREATMENT

Ocular

Treatment of the ocular hypertension should be limited to the attack and should consist of the use of mild miotics such as:

- Prostaglandin analogues;
- Ophthalmic beta blockers.

Topical ocular corticosteroids (one to four times daily) are used to control inflammation and are especially helpful during the acute phase.

Occasional pupillary dilation with:

- Phenylephrine 2.5% usually permits confirmation that no synechiae are forming.

Surgery is contraindicated; iridectomy and filtering operations do not prevent recurrences.

Supportive

To control the patient's pain and apprehension during attacks, analgesics, tranquilizers, or both may be helpful. Follow-up examinations are important to monitor pressure elevation and inflammation.

COMPLICATIONS

Strong miotics, and perhaps strong mydriatics, are contraindicated in the treatment of glaucomatocyclitic crises because they tend to aggravate the symptoms by producing pain, congestion, and spasm of the ciliary muscle.

In view of the ineffectiveness of surgical measures and the benign and self-limited nature of the disease, there exists no indication for any surgical intervention in this syndrome; medical therapy between attacks is not indicated.

Topical corticosteroids give good results by allaying ciliary irritability; however, if such treatment is prolonged, steroid-induced glaucoma may occur.

COMMENTS

The value of recognizing this syndrome lies in the fact that surgical procedures not only are unnecessary but also are definitely contraindicated in this condition. Glaucomatocyclitic crises differ from acute narrow-angle glaucoma and glaucoma secondary to uveitis in that the angle of the anterior chamber is open, even at the height of an attack, and the eye is white with minimal pain during attacks. Also, facility of outflow is normal between attacks, and provocative tests give normal responses.

REFERENCES

De Roetth A, Jr: Glaucomatocyclitic crisis. Am J Ophthalmol 69:370–371, 1970.

Knox DL: Glaucomatocyclitic crises and systemic disease: Peptic ulcer, other gastrointestinal disorders, allergy and stress. Trans Am Ophthalmol Soc 86:473–495, 1988.

Posner A, Schlossman A: Syndrome of unilateral attacks of glaucoma with cyclitic symptoms. Arch Ophthalmol 39:517–535, 1948.

Posner A, Schlossman A: Further observations on the syndrome of glaucomatocyclitic crises. Trans Am Acad Ophthalmol Otolaryngol 57:531–536, 1953.

Yamamoto S, Pavan-Langston D, Tada R, et al: Possible role of herpes simplex virus in the origin of Posner-Schlossman syndrome. Am J Ophthalmol 119:796–798, 1995.

265 PRIMARY CONGENITAL GLAUCOMA 743.20
(Primary Infantile Glaucoma, Buphthalmos)

Maria Papadopoulos MBBS, FRACO
London, England
Peng Tee Khaw PhD, FRCP, FRCS, FRCOphth, FIBiol, FRCPath, FMedSci
London, England

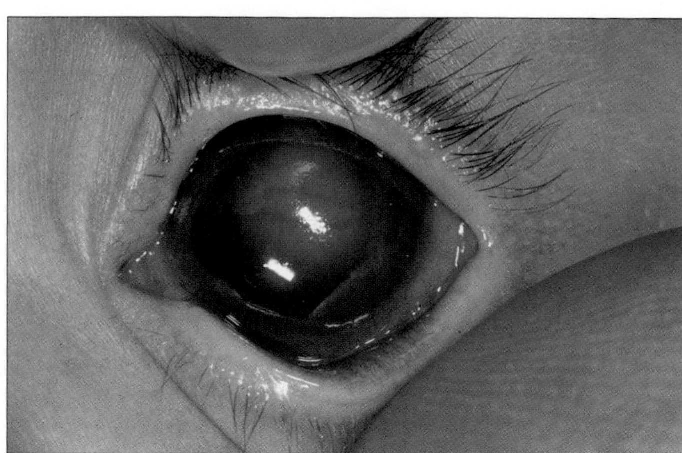

FIGURE 265.1. Corneal clouding in pediatric glaucoma.

ETIOLOGY/INCIDENCE

Primary congenital glaucoma (PCG) is a rare condition characterized by isolated trabeculodysgenesis causing aqueous outflow obstruction. Developmental arrest of tissue in the anterior chamber angle leads to the characteristic appearance of an immature angle on gonioscopy. This is the most common cause of glaucoma in infancy. Most cases are idiopathic, but autosomal recessive inheritance with variable penetrance is reported in familial cases. *GCL3A* is the major locus for PCG, accounting for 85–90% of familial and 27% of sporadic cases. Mutations of the *CYP1B1* gene, which encodes for enzyme cytochrome P4501B1, are the primary molecular defects in the majority of cases.

COURSE/PROGNOSIS

It is a blinding condition if untreated or poorly treated. Visual prognosis depends on:

- Early diagnosis;
- Prompt surgical intervention for successful intraocular pressure (IOP) control;
- Correction of ametropia;
- Rigorous amblyopia treatment.

DIAGNOSIS

This condition occurs more frequently in male children and is typically bilateral. It usually manifests in the neonatal or infantile period (<6 months). Photophobia, lacrimation and blepharospasm due to corneal epithelial or stromal oedema are common presenting features, with corneal clouding the most frequent physical sign (Figure 265.1). Buphthalmos is noticed if the eyes are particularly large or if enlargement is asymmetrical or unilateral. Optic disc cupping is reversible if not advanced.

Differential diagnosis

- Secondary glaucomas: A complete ocular and general physical examination is vital in making the correct diagnosis.
- Corneal enlargement (megalocornea, congenital high myopia): PCG is distinguishable primarily by corneal signs (Haab's striae) and elevated IOP with optic disc cupping.
- Corneal clouding (obstetric trauma, congenital corneal dystrophies, metabolic disorders, inflammatory / infectious diseases): The IOP, corneal diameters and optic disc are normal.
- Epiphora and photophobia (nasolacrimal duct obstruction): PCG is distinguishable by the absence of discharge with epiphora.

TREATMENT

Medical

- Medical therapy plays a temporizing role only.
- Preoperatively, pilocarpine 0.5–1% every 6–8 hours may lead to an improvement in symptoms, suggesting a favorable response to angle surgery.
- The beta blockers of choice are betaxolol, or timolol 0.1%.
- If necessary, oral acetazolamide should be cautiously administered in a dosage of 5–10mg/kg every six hours just prior to surgery.

Surgery

- Surgery is the principal modality of treatment.
- Angle surgery, goniotomy and trabeculotomy, is first line treatment. Both procedures have similar high rates of success in favorable cases (Figure 265.2).
- Filtration surgery, trabeculectomy with antimetabolite, is indicated following failed angle surgery or as a primary procedure when the patient is unlikely to respond sufficiently to angle surgery (e.g. if the child is older than three).
- Drainage implants offer refractory eyes the best chance of long-term success but are associated with higher complication rates.
- Cyclodestructive procedures are rarely indicated.

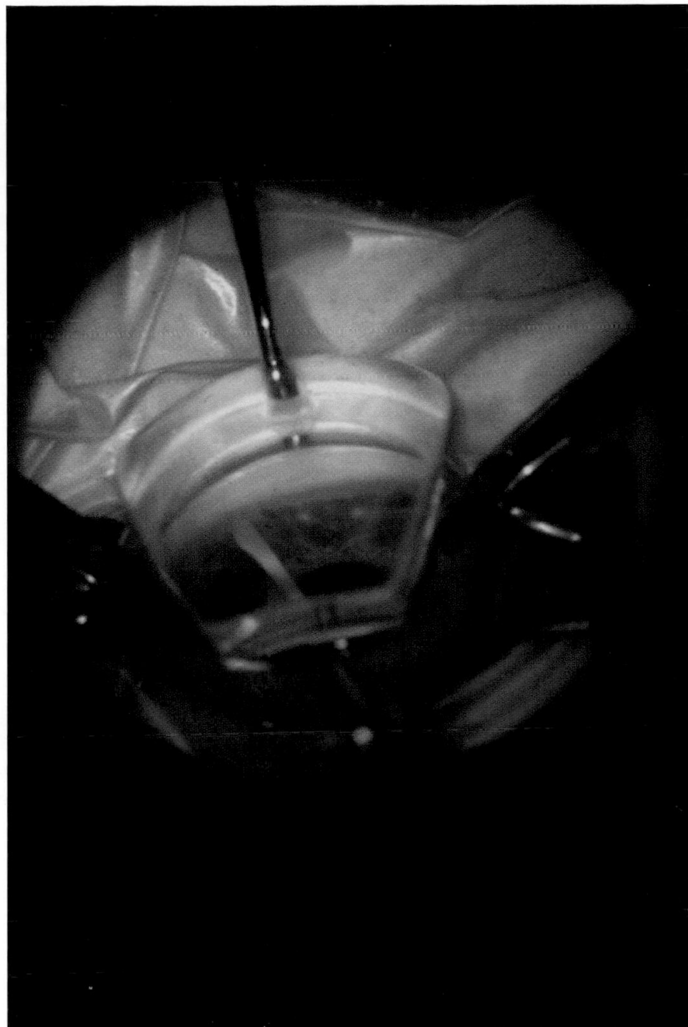

FIGURE 265.2. Goniotomy under direct visualization after stripping oedematous epithelium with alcohol.

COMMENTS

PCG is a serious condition for which early diagnosis and treatment are vital to optimize visual prognosis. The suspicion of glaucoma in a child should always be seriously treated with urgency to avoid serious visual impairment.

REFERENCES

Anderson DR: The development of the trabecular meshwork and its abnormality in primary congenital glaucoma. Trans Am Ophthalmol Soc 79:481–485, 1981.

Budenz DL, Gedde SJ, Brandt JD, et al: Baerveldt glaucoma implant in the management of refractory childhood glaucomas. Ophthalmol 111:2204–2210, 2004.

Cunliffe IA, Molteno ACB: Long-term follow-up of Molteno drains used in the treatment of glaucoma presenting in childhood. Eye 12:379–385, 1998.

Sidoti PA, Belmonte SJ, Liebmann JM, et al: Trabeculectomy with mitomycin-C in the treatment of pediatric glaucomas. Ophthalmology 107:422–429, 2000.

Stoilov I, Akarsu AN, Sarfarazi M: Identification of three different truncating mutations in cytochrome P4501B1 (CYP1B1) as the principle cause of primary congenital glaucoma (Buphthalmos) in families linked to the GLC3A locus on chromosome 2p21. Hum Mol Genet 6:641–647, 1997.

266 JUVENILE GLAUCOMA 365.14

Marianne E. Feitl, MD
Chicago, Illinois
Theodore Krupin, MD
Chicago, Illinois
Angelo P. Tanna, MD
Chicago, Illinois

The nonspecific term 'juvenile glaucoma' has traditionally been used to describe a heterogeneous group of glaucomas occurring in later childhood or early adulthood; age limits for this grouping are after the onset age of most cases of developmental (infantile) glaucoma and before the manifestation of most adult primary glaucomas.

ETIOLOGY/INCIDENCE

Juvenile-onset open-angle glaucoma, by convention, refers to chronic open-angle glaucoma diagnosed in patients between 10 and 35 years old. Unfortunately, because of a low index of suspicion on the part of the physician, the diagnosis of glaucoma in this age group is easily overlooked. In a large series of patients with glaucoma, only a small number, approximately 0.2%, were diagnosed within this age interval.

Juvenile-onset chronic open-angle glaucoma is a rare form of glaucoma that is inherited as an autosomal dominant trait with 10 to 20% of cases having mutations in the myocilin gene (*MYOC*). This gene was previously known as the trabecular meshwork-inducible glucocorticoid response (*TIGR*) gene. The 1q23-24 region of the long arm ofchromosome 1 has been identified as the location responsible for this condition (*GLC1A*). Mutations in *MYOC* are associated with only 2 to 4% of adult-onset primary-open glaucoma patients. Work is currently underway to determine the role myocilin plays in the pathogenesis of glaucoma, as well as to further delineate the roles of other genes responsible for juvenile-onset glaucoma.

COURSE/PROGNOSIS

Mild cases of developmental congenital glaucoma may go unrecognized until later in childhood; these children do not have signs of ocular discomfort and have perfectly clear corneas with only:

- Mild corneal enlargement; or
- Breaks in Descemet's membrane (Haab striae).

Intraocular pressure (IOP)-induced buphthalmos, progressive myopia, and corneal changes do not occur in children older than three years. Affected patients develop high pressure (commonly more than 50 mmHg) within the first two decades of life. The average age at diagnosis is 18 years (range, 8 to 30 years).

Juvenile open-angle glaucoma patients have a longer axial length than normal, and are more often myopic, but lack other ocular or systemic abnormalities. Visual field damage tends to be more symmetric superior-inferiorly than in adult-onset chronic open-angle glaucoma. Gonioscopy shows open iridocorneal angles without abnormal pigmentation, iris processes, or embryonic tissue. Topical medications usually are effective initially in controlling IOP, but filtration surgery may be required for long-term glaucoma control.

Primary angle-closure glaucoma is extremely rare in young persons; when present, it is usually of the plateau iris type. It may also be seen in this age group in patients with a strong family history of primary angle-closure glaucoma. Angle-closure glaucoma in children as a result of pupillary block is usually associated with other ocular disorders, including:

- Anterior uveitis;
- Iridociliary cysts;
- Microcornea;
- Microspherophakia(Weill–Marchesani syndrome);
- Dislocated lens (Marfan's syndrome or homocystinuria);
- Persistent hyperplastic primary vitreous;
- Retrolental fibroplasia;
- Nanophthalmos;
- Idiopathic lens subluxation;
- Intraocular surgery, particularly after the removal of congenital cataracts.

Following laser iridotomy, patients need to be monitored for recurrent angle closure and the need for additional medical, laser, or incisional surgical intervention.

DIAGNOSIS

Clinical signs and symptoms

Juvenile-onset glaucoma can occur in conditions associated with abnormal iridocorneal angles:

- Aniridia;
- Iridocorneal dysgenesis (Axenfeld's or Rieger's syndrome);
- Sturge–Weber syndrome;
- Neurofibromatosis;
- Lowe's syndrome.

Several of these conditions have been mapped genetically. Other conditions associated with glaucoma in the juvenile-onset age group include:

- Traumatic angle recession;
- Hyphema;
- Glaucomatocyclitic crisis;
- Rubeosis iridis;
- Retinoblastoma;
- Neoplasia,including the phakomatoses;
- Juvenile xanthogranuloma;
- Acute leukemia;
- Medulloepithelioma (also may cause secondary glaucoma).

Another important cause of secondary glaucoma is previous surgery for congenital cataract. One study demonstrated that chronic glaucoma appears to occur more often after cataract surgery performed before the age of 9 months. Another study of pediatric cataract patients without persistent hyperplastic primary vitreous showed that cataracts alone were not associated with ocular hypertension or glaucoma in the absence of surgical removal of the cataract.

Glaucoma may occur in patients with:

- Congenital rubella due to iridocyclitis;
- Angle anomalies resembling primary congenital glaucoma or mesodermal dysgenesis;
- Intumescent lens;
- Pupillary block after cataract extraction.

Although many ocular abnormalities are usually noted in the neonatal period, glaucoma may have its onset in later childhood or young adulthood. These later-onset glaucomas are most often found in eyes with microphthalmia and cataracts.

Patients with juvenile rheumatoid arthritis (JRA) havea significant incidence (8 to 24%) of uveitis that may lead to glaucoma. Female patients and patients with monoarticular or pauciarticular JRA have a higher incidence of iridocyclitis than those with the polyarticular form. Because patients are often asymptomatic, they must be examined frequently for ocular involvement. Of note, no parallel has been found between the activity of their idocyclitis and the joint disease. Iritis may first develop in patients older than 16, althogh an earlier onset is more common.

Other important causes of uveitis that may foster glaucoma include:

- Sarcoidosis;
- Ankylosing spondylitis;
- Herpes zoster;
- Syphilis;
- Tuberculosis.

Differential diagnosis

Some cases of juvenile-onset glaucoma resemble adult-onset primary open-angle glaucoma. The possibility of steroid-induced open-angle glaucoma must be eliminated by a careful history, especially in contact lens wearers.

In contrast to primary open-angle glaucoma, which characteristically occurs in patients older than 40, there is a preponderance of male patients and of myopia in juvenile-onset glaucoma.

Central corneal thickness should be measured in young patients with suspected glaucoma or elevated IOP. In adults, the relationship between pressure and central corneal thickness is approximately 2.5 mmHg for each 50 microns (i.e. 0.5 mmHg/10 microns) change from an average thickness of 540 microns. One study suggests a larger effect in children: an average of 1.5 mmHg for a 10% difference in central corneal thickness was observed in white children 5 to 15 years of age.

Pigmentaryglaucoma may have its onset during this age interval. These patients characteristically show midperipheral iris transillumination defects and pigment deposition on the corneal endothelium (Krukenberg's spindle), trabecular meshwork, iris, lens, and peripheral retina. Pigmentary glaucoma becomes less severe in some patients with advancing age. This relates to increasing axial length of the lens, causing an increased relative pupillary block that elevates the peripheral iris above the lens zonules, decreasing pigment liberation.

IOP in pigmentary glaucoma is subject to large fluctuations, which must be considered in evaluating the response to medical treatment. These patients occasionally manifest the classic symptoms of an acute IOP rise, particularly after an iris pigment 'shower' due to mydriasis or physical exercise. Pigmentary dispersion is linked to the *7q36* gene.

TREATMENT

Ocular

Most patients with juvenile open-angle glaucoma should be given a trial with medical therapy. The availability of several new classes of IOP-lowering medications has greatly increased therapeutic options. Treatment is tempered by the same considerations as with the adult glaucomas. However, there are no formal trials on the use of glaucoma medication in children. Available data is mainly based on cases series. Due to their smaller size, younger children face potentially higher serum drug levels than adults. Lid closure and nasolacrimal occlusion to minimize systemic absorption of topical medications are important. Children are less likely than adults to complain of drug side effects and thus must be watched and questioned more carefully.

The beta-adrenergic antagonists should be used with caution in children, although these agents can be effective. Nonselective beta blockers should be avoided in patients with asthma because of their bronchospastic effects. Asthma induced in children may be evidenced by nocturnal coughing, rather than wheezing as commonly seen in adults. Bradycardia and apneic spells may also occur. Beta-blockers also should be used cautiously in patients with heart problems, including congestive heart failure.

Betaxolol, a selective beta1-antagonist, may be better tolerated in patients with pulmonary disease. However, it can still trigger asthma in susceptible individuals.

The topical alpha-adrenergic agonists apraclonidine and brimonidine are effective IOP-lowering agents that decrease aqueous production and possibly increase uveoscleral outflow. Apraclonidine is less lipophilic than brimonidine, with reduced drug penetration of the blood-brain barrier. This property may reduce systemic and central nervous system side effects. Caution has been advised in the use of brimonidine in children, due to the risk of centrally mediated systemic hypotension and central nervous system depression. Fatigue and fainting attacks have been reported. A dry mouth may also occur. Serious potential systemic side effects demand particular caution when these agents are used in younger patients.

The prostaglandin-related drugs latanoprost, travaprost, and bimatoprost increase uveoscleral outflow, thereby lowering IOP. Once daily administration enhances compliance. Conjunctival injection, increased iris pigmentation and increased eyelash growth are ocular side effects. Systemic side effects are infrequent and mild. Although these agents can be excellent ocular hypotensives, their long-term safety profile is not yet known. IOP reduction is reported to be greater in older children than in very young patients. As with all of these agents, there is less clinical experience in children than in adults, so caution and a discussion of the possible risks with the patient and parents are warranted.

Topical carbonic anhydrase inhibitors such as dorzolamide and brinzolamide provide better tolerance and greatly reduced systemic side effects than are associated with the oral forms of these agents. While these agents decrease aqueous production, they are less effective than beta-blockers in lowering pressure. Dorzolamide and timolol are additive in their pressure-lowering effects, and a combined preparation (Cosopt) is available. Carbonic anhydrase inhibitors are sulfonamide derivatives, and the topical preparations may be contraindicated in patients with a documented sulfa allergy.

The oral carbonic anhydrase inhibitor acetazolamide, in total daily oral doses of 15 mg/kg, is administered to children in two to four divided doses. Side effects include loss of appetite, gastrointestinal disturbances, parasthesias, metabolic acidosis, and lethargy. Side effects may present differently in children, including bedwetting, failure to thrive, and disturbed hyperactive behavior. The risk of renal calculi should be borne in mind and indicated to the parents. Methazolamide is an alternative oral agent that may cause fewer side effects than acetazolamide.

Oral carbonic anhydrase inhibitors can be associated with bone marrow depression and aplastic anemia. This side effect, while theoretically possible with topical agents because of systemic absorption, has not been reported.

Topical miotic therapy with pilocarpine, carbachol, and pphospholineiodidedecreases IOP by increasing trabecular outflow. These drugs are effective ocular hypotensive agents, particularly in children with open iridocorneal angles. Unfortunately, they induce miosis and myopia, disabling symptoms that prevent their use. Phospholine iodide also produces cataract. Systemic side effects include nausea, vomiting, diarrhea, abdominal cramping, salivation, sweating, bradycardia, hypotension, branchospasm, muscle weakness and CNS stimulation.

Phospholine iodide is an excellent miotic drug in aphakic or pseudophakic eyes. A 1/8% solution is currently available (WyethPharmaceuticals) for twice-daily administration, with some patients responding to daily delivery.

Medical

Young patients should be examined frequently until the maintenance of a satisfactory IOP level is achieved. In the absence of credible visual fields, one must rely more heavily on correlation of IOP and stability of optic disc damage.

Aggressive treatment of iritis associated with juvenile rheumatoid arthritis, using systemic cycloplegics and steroids, should be instituted to prevent peripheral anterior syncchiae or neovascular membranes. In addition, topical cycloplegics increase uveoscleral outflow,which may reduce IOP. Glaucoma can be caused by either prolonged, inadequately treated intraocular inflammation or steroid treatment. Anti-glaucoma therapy should be instituted if necessary. Topical miotics are to be avoided because these agents can increase intraocular inflammation and decrease uveoscleraloutflow, resulting in a paradoxical rise in IOP.

Medical therapy usually is less effective in juvenile-onset than in adult-onset primary glaucoma. Long-term medical control of the glaucoma is often poor and surgery may be required.

Surgical

Surgery should be undertaken whenever medical therapy has not resulted in good control. Prolonged use of topical agents may adversely affect wound healing after glaucoma surgery.

Iridectomy is the procedure of choice in primary or secondary angle closure. Mechanical and technical incompatibilities of the slit-lamp-based laser and the need for general anesthesia may dictate a surgical iridectomy. The increasing availability of an operating microscope YAG laser delivery system allows performing a laser iridotomy.

Goniotomy or trabeculotomy is indicated as the initial surgery in eyes with congenital glaucoma. These procedures have a lower success rate after the age of three years. However, good results may still be obtained with trabeculotomy in infantile and juvenile glaucoma. One retrospective study showed a success rate for trabeculotomy of 60% in congenital glaucoma, 96% in infantile glaucoma, and 76% in juvenile glaucoma.

Retrospective studies of uveitic glaucoma in children have showed that one or two goniotomy procedures were often successful in obtaining pressures under 21 mmHg, although most patients continued to need glaucoma medication after surgery.

Surgical outcome is adversely affected by increased age, peripheral anterior synechiae, prior surgeries, and aphakia.

Filtration surgery is less likely to be successful in juvenile than in adult glaucomas. The lower success rate in young patients may relate to increased postoperative scarring and to the types of glaucomas that tend to occur in this age group. Postoperative bleb encapsulation is more common in patients with juvenile glaucoma. Trabeculectomy has a poor prognosis in eyes that have had prior surgery and eyes with secondary glaucoma, particularly neovascular and aphakic glaucoma. The use of adjunctive antifibrotic agents (e.g. 5-fluorouracil or mitomycin C) increases the trabeculectomy success (see below).

Age as an isolated factor may have its greatest influence on surgical outcome in patients younger than 30. In one series, trabeculectomy for primary glaucoma was successful in 25 of 30 (83%) of patients 30 to 49 years old, but in only 4 of 9 patients (44%) younger than 30. In youth, Tenon's tissue is more extensive, postoperative hypotony may be prolonged, wound healing may be more vigorous, and postoperative examination is often less than ideal.

Because limbal surgical landmarks can be obscure, transillumination at the time of surgery is recommended to avoid placing the sclerostomy incision too posteriorly. A lamellar scleral flap helps identify the limbal surgical anatomy, in particular the scleral spur. The scleral flap lowers the incidence of a postoperative flat anterior chamber and results in a thicker, more diffuse filtration bleb. However, the surgeon should remember that the sclera might be thinner in the juvenile glaucoma eye, making scleral flap dissection more difficult.

Corticosteroids should be used after filtration surgery to diminish postoperative inflammation and scarring of the bleb. A sub-Tenon's injection of a short-acting corticosteroid, such as dexamethasone or triamcinolone, at the completion of surgery and the use of topical corticosteroid drops or ointment after surgery are recommended. Adjunctive antifibrotic agents should be used to slow wound healing and scar formation and to increase the success rate of trabeculectomy in this patient population. Intraoperative application of 5-fluorouracil or Mitomycin C is an option in these patients. Postoperative subconjunctival injections of 5-fluorouracil may be impossible for very young patients without general anesthesia or office sedation. Both of these drugs are associated with thinner, more cystic blebs and may carry a higher rate of complications, such as wound leaks, chronic hypotony, and possibly late endophthalmitis.

Releasable scleral flap sutures may be used at the time of surgery in young patients to control postoperative bleb function and to reduce the occurrence of early postoperative hypotony. These sutures are removed at the time of examination under anesthesia. Enhanced healing responses in young patients shorten the interval when removal of these sutures must be performed to increase blebfunction.

Argon laser suture lysis may be used to titrate bleb function in older, more cooperative patients.

The risks of both early and late bleb-associated ocular infection must be carefully explained to patients and parents, and they must be advised to seek medical care immediately should any signs or symptoms occur.

Cyclodestructive treatments have several useful applications in the management of juvenile glaucoma. Diode or Nd : YAG transscleral laser procedures result in less inflammation and have a lower incidence of phthisis bulbi than cyclocryotherapy. Laser cyclodestructive procedures may be used to provide IOP control in circumstances where filtration surgery has not been successful or has a low success rate, particularly aphakic glaucoma. Conjunctival hyperemia and anterior chamber reaction are the most common side effects. Multiple treatments may be needed to achieve satisfactory lowering of pressure. Results in pediatric patients are similar to those for adults for efficacy and safety.

Endoscopic diode laser cyclophotocoagulation appears to be less effective than externally applied diode laser cyclophotocoagulation. Aphakic patients may have an increased risk of significant postoperative complications such as retinal detachment.

Cyclocryotherapyhas a higher complication rate (e.g. phthisis bulbi and loss of vision) when used to treat neovascular glaucoma.

Posterior tube drainage implants have been used to treat patients with juvenile-onset glaucoma when filtrating surgery has failed. Encouraging results have been reported with various glaucoma drainage implants. These devices place an open plastic tube into the anterior chamber that is attached to an equatorial episcleral plate, resulting in a posterior bleb over the area of the encapsulated explant. Success is related to diagnosis, number of previous glaucoma procedures, and surgeon experience.

COMPLICATIONS

Perhaps the most unfortunate error clinicians make in treating patients with juvenile-onset glaucoma is failing to recognize the condition early. The fellow eyes of patients with apparent uniocular congenital glaucoma should be followed very carefully for possible late-onset congenital glaucoma. Young patients with advancing high myopia should be regarded as potential candidates for glaucoma. Applanation tonometry is preferable to Schiotz tonometry in these patients because of their low ocular rigidity. A positive family history of glaucoma in children should suggest an examination of the patient's relatives and siblings.

COMMENTS

With the availability of hand-held portable applanation tonometers, IOP can usually be measured in the office; this should be considered part of the complete pediatric ophthalmologic examination whenever glaucoma is suspected and should be performed in all patients who can cooperate. Gonioscopy may be performed successfully in many children, often with surprising ease. Reliable visual fields are difficult to obtain in young children. Goldmann kinetic perimetry is the preferred method. This places more responsibility on the ophthalmologist for accurate assessment of stability of glaucomatous optic nerve damage.

Routine examination of the optic disc should be performed in all patients. In children on whom tonometry cannot be performed, the disc examination may reveal suspected or definite damage from elevated IOP. In those patients, further examination with the patient under anesthesia is warranted. If possible, optic disc photography or other optic nerve and retinal nerve fiber layer measurements should be done in individuals with suspected or proven juvenile-onset glaucoma. Rapid increase and reversal of disc cupping occur more frequently in children with glaucoma than in adults.

REFERENCES

Badlani VK, Quinones R, Wilenshy JT, et al: Angle-closure glaucoma in teenagers. J Glaucoma 12:198–203, 2003.

Barsoum-Homsy M, Chevrette L: Incidence and prognosisof childhood glaucoma. Ophthalmology 93:1323–1327, 1986.

Chew E, Morin JD: Glaucoma in children. Pediatr ClinNorth Am 30:1043–1061, 1983.

Ho CL, Wong EY, Walton DS: Goniosurgery for glaucomacomplicating chronic childhood uveitis. Arch Ophthalmol 122:838–844, 2004.

Mori M, Keech RV, Scott WE: Glaucoma and ocularhypertension in pediatric patients with cataracts. J AAPOS 1:98–101, 1997.

Neely DE, Plager DA: Endocyclophotocoagulation formanagement of difficult pediatric glaucomas. J AAPOS 5:221–229, 2001.

Rabiah PK: Frequency and predictors of glaucoma afterpediatric cataract surgery. Am J Ophthalmol 137:30–37, 2004.

Richards JE, Lichter PR, Boehnke M, et al: Mapping ofa gene for autosomal dominant juvenile-onset open-angle glaucoma to chromosomclq. Am J Hum Genet 54:62–70, 1994.

Richter CU, Shingleton BJ, Bellows AR, et al: Thedevelopment of encapsulated filtering blebs. Ophthalmology 95:116–118, 1988.

Ritch R, Chang BM, Liebmann JM: Angle closure inyounger patients. Ophthalmology 110:1880–1889, 2003.

Rosenberg LF, Krupin T: Implants in glaucoma surgery.In: Ritch R, Shields MB, Krupin T, eds: The glaucomas. Glaucoma therapy. 2nd edn. St Louis, Mosby-Year Book, 1996:III:1783–1807.

Ritch R: Pigmentary glaucoma: a self-limited entity. Ann Ophthalmol 15:115–116, 1983.

Sheffield VC, Stone EM, Alward WL, et al: Geneticlinkage of familial open angle glaucoma to chromosome Iq21-q31. Nat Genet 4:47–50, 1993.

Talbot AWR, Russell-Eggitt: Pharmaceutical managementof the childhood glaucomas. Exp Opin Pharmacother 1(4):697–711, 2000.

Waheed S, Ritterband DC, Greenfield DS, et al: Bleb-related ocular infection in children after trabeculectomy with mitomycinC. Ophthalmology 104:2117–2120, 1997.

Walton DS: Juvenile open-angle glaucoma. In: ChandlerPA, Grant WM, eds: Glaucoma. 3rd edn. Philadelphia, Lea &Febiger, 1986:528–529.

Weisschuh N, Schiefer U: Progress in the genetics ofglaucoma. Dev Ophthalmol 37:83–93, 2003.

Wiggs JL, Lynch S, Ynagi G, et al: A genomewide scanidentifies novel early-onset primary open-angle glaucoma loci on 9q22 and20p12. Am J Hum Genet 74:1314–1320, 2004.

Zak M, Fledelius H, Pedersen FK: Ocular complicationsand visual outcome in juvenile chronic arthritis: a 25-year follow-up study.Acta Ophthalmol Scan 81:211–215, 2003.

267 LENS-INDUCED GLAUCOMA 365.51

Rober L. Stamper, MD
San Francisco, California
Stephanie M. Po, MD
Walnut Creek, California
Michelle Nee, MD
San Francisco, California

Lens-induced glaucoma may occur as three different secondary open-angle glaucomas: phacolytic, lens-particle, and phacoantigentic glaucoma. It also can occur as a pupillary block from lens intumescence (phacomorphic glaucoma) or lens dislocation (ectopia lentis).

SECONDARY OPEN ANGLE GLAUCOMAS

Phacolytic glaucoma (lens protein glaucoma)

This type of lens-induced glaucoma arises from leakage of lens protein through an intact lens capsule in the setting of a mature or hypermature (Morgagnian) cataract. Heavy-molecular-weight proteins (greater than 150 × 106 daltons) are fourteen-fold more concentrated in mature lens cortices than in immature cataracts. In vitro experiments have demonstrated that these high molecular weight proteins can directly obstruct the aqueous outflow channels. In addition, protein-engorged macrophages, whose normal function is to phagocytose debris within the trabeculum, probably contribute to the outflow obstruction.

Clinical findings mature or hypermature cataract

- Open angle.
- Corneal edema.
- Acute rise in intraocular pressure associated with pain and redness.
- Heavy aqueous flare.
- White fluffy material on lens capsule or floating in anterior chamber.
- Diagnostic paracentesis, phase-contrast microscopy, and Milipore filter technique establish presence of macrophages (though this is not always present).

Differential diagnosis

- Uveitic glaucoma.
- Phacomorphic glaucoma.
- Pupillary block glaucoma.
- Neovascular glaucoma.
- Lens Particle glaucoma.
- Phacoanaphlactic glaucoma.

Treatment

Medical

- Topical β-adrenergic antagonist, carbonic anhydrase inhibitors, α_2 agonist, prostaglandin agonists.
- Topical steroids.
- Hyperosmotic agents.
- Oral Carbonic anhydrase inhibitors.

Surgical

- Removal of cataract usually restores normal intraocular pressure.

If intraocular pressures are still high at time of surgery, gradually entering the anterior chamber with slowly decompress the globe

Lens particle glaucoma

This type of lens-induced secondary open angle glaucoma differs from phacolytic glaucoma in that actual fragments of cortical lens material are obstructing the trabecular meshwork. These fragments have been liberated into the anterior chamber from trauma, or from iatragenic causes, such as after cataract surgery or Nd-Yag capsulotomy.

The severity of the clinical course often will vary with the amount of free cortical lens material, and the onset of glaucoma can occur months to years later.

Clinical findings

- Corneal edema.
- Heavy cellular reaction and flare, possible hypopyon.
- Lens material in the angle.

Differential diagnosis

- Phacolytic glaucoma.
- Steroid-induced glaucoma.

- Uveitic glaucoma.
- Pseudoexfoliative glaucoma.

Treatment
Medical
- Topical β-adrenergic antagonist, carbonic anhydrase inhibitors, α_2 agonist, prostaglandin agonists.
- Topical steroids.
- Topical cycloplegics.
- Hyperosmotic agents or oral carbonic anhydrase inhibitors.

Surgical
- Removal of all residual lens material.

Phacoantigenic glaucoma
This is a rare granulomatous inflammatory reaction seen after lens injury that is refractory to topical, systemic and subconjuctival corticosteroids. It may occur after extracapsular cataract extraction ,or after spontaneous, traumatic, or surgical rupture of the lens capsue, and after intraocular infection. The mechanism of this type of glaucoma is thought to be autoimmune. The natural tolerance to lens protein is lost, and a T-cell mediated immune complex reaction ensues. Histopathology shows a zonal granulomatous inflammation characterized by a core of lens material surrounded by polymorphonuclear cells, which is surrounded by a zone of epithelioid and giant cells, which in turn is bordered by nonspecific mononuclear cells.

Clinical findings
- Keratic precipitates on corneal endothelium.
- Anterior chamber reaction with residual lens material and hypopyon formation.
- Vitritis.
- Anterioar and posterior synechiae formation.
- Diagnostic paracentesis may reveal foamy macrophages.

Differential diagnosis
- Infectious endophthalmitis.
- Uveitic glaucoma.
- Phacolytic glaucoma.

Treatment
- Topical β-adrenergic antagonist, carbonic anhydrase inhibitors, α_2 agonist, prostaglandin agonists.
- Topical steroids.
- Topical cycloplegics.
- Hyperosmotic agents or oral carbonic anhydrase inhibitors.

Surgical
- Pars plana vitrectomy to remove all residual lens material and posterior capsule.
- Removal of capsule manually with forceps after injection of a-chymotrypsin beneath the iris.

Pupillary block mechanisms phacomorphic glaucoma
In this condition, an intumescent senile cataract can push the iris forward and narrow the iridocorneal angle, leading to relative pupillary block. Patients with a hyperopic refractive error and a crowded or narrow anterior segment are most at risk, and only rarely before the fifth to seventh decade of life. Factors such as dim light, emotional stress, and drugs can cause the pupil to become mid-dilated and exacerbate pupillary block.

Clinical findings
- Presence of a mature cataract.
- Shallow anterior chamber.
- Iridotrabecular apposition on Gonioscopy.
- Corneal edema.
- Markedly elevated intraocular pressure.

Differential diagnosis
- Plateau iris syndrome.
- Pupillary block from forward lens movement due to zonular weakeness.
- Phacolytic glaucoma.

Treatment
Medical
- Topical β-adrenergic antagonist, carbonic anhydrase inhibitors, α_2 agonist, prostaglandin agonists.
- Hyperosmotic agents.
- Oral Carbonic anhydrase inhibitors.

Surgical
- Argon laser iridoplasty to open angle.
- Laser iridotomy to bypass papillary block.
- Cataract extraction.

Note: Miotics may exacerbate angle closure attack by increasing iridolenticular contact and should be used with caution. In the setting of plateau iris syndrome, miotics are often useful after creation of a peripheral laser iridotomy to bypass papillary block.

Ectopia lentis
Ectopia lentis is a condtion in which the lens is displaced from its normal central position within the posterior chamber. Partial zonular weakening or breakage can lead to subluxation of the lens such that it is no longer centered within the pupillary aperture, but rather displaced to one side, or located entirely behind the iris. Complete zonular breakage leads to dislocation of the lens such that the lens may remain behind, within, or in front of the pupillary aperture. The lens may even migrate in its entirety into the anterior or posterior chambers. Ectopia lentis can be hereditary and/or associated with systemic disorders such as Weill–Marchasani, Marfans, sufite odxidase deficiency, and homocystinurea. The condition can also arise from trauma, surgical complications and ocular diseases such as exfoliation syndrome, high myopia, and uveitis.

Dislocation of the lens can result in elevated intraocular pressure from a pupillary block mechanism if the lens moves forward and becomes wedged in the pupillary sphincter.

Clinical findings
- Visual acuitiy disturbances such a refraction change, monocular diplopia, amblyopia, defective accommodation.
- Lenticular astigmatism that cannot be corrected by refraction.
- Iridodonesis.
- Phacodonesis.
- Observable alteration in lens postion with change in gaze postion.
- Disparity in anterior chamber depth between the two eyes.

- Conical shape of iris in the sphincter area on Gonioscopy.
- Observable subluxation or dislocation of the lens.

Treatment

Medical

Miotics should be used cautiously, as they can exacerbate a pupillary block. If the anterior chamber shallows after use of a miotic, it can be reversed with a cycloplegic.

If the angle opens with a miotic, complete dislocation must be suspected. The patient should be placed in a supine position to allow posterior migration of the lens, and be given an oral hyperomotic agent and topical anti-hypertensive drops.

If the lens becomes trapped in the pupillary aperture or in the anterior chamber, the patient should be placed supine and the pupil dilated. Putting pressure on the central cornea may help reposit the lens into the posterior chamber.

Surgical

- Laser iridotomy to bypass pupillary block mechanism.

Lenses that dislocate into the vitreous may float freely,settle inferiorly, or become attached to the retina. Most can be treated conservatively. Surgical removal of the lens via pars plan vitrectomy is indicated if it causes phacolytic glaucoma.

REFERENCES

Epstein DL: Diagnosis and management of lens-induced glaucoma. Opthahalmology 89:227–230, 1982.

Epstein DL, Jedziniak JA, Grant WM: Identification of heavy molecular weight soluble protein in aqueous humor in human phacolytic glaucoma. Invest Opthahalmol Vis Sci 17:398–402, 1978.

Epstein DL, Jedziniak JA, Grant WM: Obstruction of aqucious outflow by lens partricles and by heavy molecular weight soluble lens proteins. Invest Opthalmol Vis Schi 17:272–277, 1978.

Lane SS, Kopietz LA, Lindquiest TD, et al: Treatment of phacolytic glaucoma with extracapsular cataract extraction. Opthathlmology 95:749–753, 1988.

Pollard ZF: phacolytic glaucoma secondary to ectopia lentis. Ann Opthal 7:999–1001, 1975.

268 MALIGNANT GLAUCOMA 365.20 *(Ciliary Block Glaucoma, Aqueous Misdirection, Ciliolenticular/Ciliovitreal Block)*

Hau T. Nguyen, MD
Portland, Oregon
George A. Cioffi, MD
Portland, Oregon

ETIOLOGY/INCIDENCE

Malignant glaucoma is a relatively rare but serious condition originally described by von Graefe in 1869. He described a condition characterized by shallowing or flattening of the anterior chamber and elevated intraocular pressure. The descriptor 'malignant' denotes the poor response to conventional treatment. Since the original description, many theories regarding the pathophysiology of malignant glaucoma have been proposed. Investigators have based these theories upon the observation that aqueous humor outflow from the posterior chamber is obstructed. It has been suggested that aqueous obstruction by the ciliary processes in apposition to the anterior hyaloid or lens equator results in accumulation of aqueous in the vitreous cavity, and the term ciliary block glaucoma originated. Other terms used in reference to this condition include *aqueous misdirection, direct lens block glaucoma, and ciliolenticular (or ciliovitreal) block.*

Classically, malignant glaucoma presents following filtration surgery for angle-closure glaucoma, occurring in 2–4% of patients, even many years after intervention. Occurring indiscriminately in phakia, pseudophakia, or aphakia, it has been reported to occur during or after virtually every other intraocular surgery including cataract extraction, laser iridotomy, surgical iridectomy, retinal detachment surgery, placement of glaucoma drainage devices, Nd : YAG and diode laser cyclophotocoagulation, and as a complication of retinopathy of prematurity. Cessation of cycloplegics or the institution of miotics can induce or worsen the condition.

The precise mechanism of malignant glaucoma remains elusive; however, most investigators accept the hypothesis proposed in 1954 by Shaffer. He felt that a relative block to anterior movement of aqueous exists near the junction of the ciliary processes, lens equator, and anterior vitreous face leading to diversion of aqueous posteriorly into, around, and behind the vitreous body. Chandler and Grant later proposed that the additional factor of lens zonule slackness could contribute to the forward movement of the lens-iris diaphragm; therefore, mydriatic-cycloplegic therapy to tighten the zonules and force the lens posteriorly would help to break the attack. More recently, Quigley and colleagues proposed that the mechanism of malignant glaucoma involves choroidal expansion leading to increases in intraocular pressure and anterior outflow. As there is a finite ability to transmit fluid through the vitreous cavity, intraocular pressure elevates due to buildup of aqueous humor behind the vitreous, pushing it forward carrying the lens and iris with it.

COURSE/PROGNOSIS

In the treatment of malignant glaucoma, it is usually necessary to continue cycloplegia indefinitely, despite resolution. Of note, sensitization to atropine may occur at any time and alternative treatment with hyoscine may or may not be successful. Despite the available medical and surgical interventions, malignant glaucoma can recur with a frequent need for reoperation and poor visual outcome.

DIAGNOSIS

Clinical signs and symptoms

The clinical picture consists of elevated intraocular pressure (IOP) and a persistently shallow anterior chamber both peripherally and centrally, despite a patent iridotomy. Of note, in eyes that have undergone filtration surgery, the intraocular pressure may be low or normal. In this setting, malignant glaucoma is very likely if choroidal detachments and suprachoroidal hemorrhage are ruled out. β-scan ultrasonography may show aqueous pockets within the vitreous cavity.

Differential diagnosis

The differential diagnosis of malignant glaucoma includes pupillary block, choroidal detachment, and suprachoroidal hemorrhage.

- Patients with pupillary block will present with pain, elevated IOP, and a shallow peripheral anterior chamber; however, the central anterior chamber is frequently maintained. This condition is relieved by iridotomy.
- Choroidal detachment presents in hypotonous eyes with a shallow anterior chamber. Ophthalmoscopy reveals a dome-shaped serous elevation that is light brown in color, which can be confirmed by β-scan if not readily visible.
- Patients with suprachoroidal hemorrhage present with significant pain, elevated IOP, and a shallow anterior chamber in the periphery. The eye tends to be more inflamed than with serous choroidal detachments and the dome-shaped elevation is dark red by ophthalmoscopy. β-scan can also be used to confirm the diagnosis.

In addition, processes that push the lens and iris anteriorly can cause an acute or subacute IOP elevation with a shallow anterior chamber. Thus, a careful search should be made for space-occupying lesions such as tumors or cysts of the iris, ciliary body or retina, or even massive subretinal hemorrhage. Transudation of fluid after a CRVO can hydrate the vitreous, leading to anterior movement of the lens-iris diaphragm and resultant peripheral and central shallowing of the anterior chamber, mimicking malignant glaucoma.

TREATMENT

Systemic/local

For many years, miotic therapy was used to treat malignant glaucoma. It was found to be unsuccessful and in fact may worsen or precipitate the attack. The first reported success of medical therapy came in 1962 with the use of mydriatic-cycloplegic drops. Mydriatic-cycloplegic drops now form a crucial part of the medical management of malignant glaucoma, with the concurrent use of topical aqueous humor suppressants, oral carbonic anhydrase inhibitors, and hyperosmotics. This combination may be tried for 4 to 5 days and is successful in approximately 50% of cases. If medical therapy fails, then surgical intervention is indicated.

Surgical

Surgical intervention consists of argon laser treatment of ciliary processes, Nd : YAG laser hyaloidotomy, and incisional surgery. The key to surgical intervention lies in creating a channel of communication between the vitreous cavity and the anterior chamber, allowing for normalization of pressures between the two chambers.

Herschler first reported the use of argon laser to shrink ciliary processes via the peripheral iridectomy to treat malignant glaucoma. Successful treatment required shrinkage of 2 to 4 processes. Nd : YAG laser hyaloidotomy has also been described to be successful in treating pseudophakic and aphakic malignant glaucoma. The procedure involves photodisruption of the lens capsule and the anterior vitreous face.

For cases in which medical and laser therapy fail, pars plana vitrectomy is warranted. In the phakic patient, lensectomy at the time of vitrectomy may be considered when there is marked corneal edema, dense cataract, or when the anterior chamber does not deepen during vitrectomy. Primary posterior capsulectomy may also be performed at the time of vitrectomy and lensectomy for improved surgical success. In the pseudophakic patient, it is important to remove capsular and zonular material behind iridectomy sites in order to establish a free channel for aqueous flow.

COMMENTS

Ultrasound biomicroscopy (UBM)

Ultrasound biomicroscopy (UBM) is a relatively new modality in the visualization of the anterior segment. It is used to obtain real time images of anterior segment structures, allowing for identification of irido-corneal touch, appositional angle closure, anterior rotation of the ciliary body, and ciliary body-iris. The system uses 50- to 100-MHz transducers that are incorporated into a β-mode clinical scanner. Higher frequency transducers are used for fine resolution of superficial structures, whereas lower-frequency transducers are used for increased depth of penetration. Resolution ranges from 20 to 60 microns, with tissue penetration approximately to a depth of approximately 4 mm.

UBM studies have allowed identification of a subset of patients with malignant glaucoma in whom the pathologic mechanism is due to annular ciliary body detachment rather than aqueous misdirection. Liebmann and colleagues found the presence of fluid accumulation limited to the supraciliary space, which was detectable only by UBM. Drainage of the supraciliary fluid with reformation of the anterior chamber resulted in normal ocular anatomy and IOP.

REFERENCES

Chandler PA, Grant WM: Mydriatic-cycloplegic treatment in malignant glaucoma. Arch Ophthalmol 68:353, 1962.

Greenfield DS, et al: Aqueous misdirection after glaucoma drainage device implantation. Ophthalmology 106:1035–1040, 1999.

Quigley HA, Friedman DS, Congdon NG: Possible mechanisms of primary angle-closure and malignant glaucoma. J Glaucoma 12:167–180, 2003.

Ruben S, Tsai J, Hitchings R: Malignant glaucoma and its management. Br J Ophthalmol 81:163–167, 1997.

Weiss DI, Shaffer RN: Ciliary block (malignant) glaucoma. Trans Am Acad Ophthalmol Otolaryngol 76:450, 1972.

269 NORMAL-TENSION GLAUCOMA (LOW-TENSION GLAUCOMA)

365.12

Teresa C. Chen, MD
Boston, Massachusetts

Normal-tension glaucoma (NTG) is a progressive optic neuropathy characterized by retinal nerve fiber layer thinning, optic nerve head cupping, and visual field defects. Clinical signs are similar to those found in patients with chronic open angle glaucoma, but documented intraocular pressures are within the statistically normal range. In order to make a diagnosis of normal-tension glaucoma, other causes of optic neuropathy must be ruled out.

ETIOLOGY/INCIDENCE

Normal-tension glaucoma is more common than was previously recognized. Although the prevalence of NTG relies heavily on the definition of the disease, population-based studies have found that anywhere from 10% to 48% of all open angle glaucoma patients in the United States, Europe and Scandinavia have NTG, and up to 66% in the Japanese population have NTG.

This form of glaucoma is more common in the elderly. It is unusual in patients younger than 50; the mean reported age in clinical studies generally is in the 60s. Normal-tension glaucoma is more common in patients of Asian ancestry. The Baltimore Eye Study also suggests that normal-tension glaucoma may be more common in blacks than in whites; however, there are few studies that specifically study race and NTG. There appears to be a genetic component to the disease. In 1998, Sarfarazi et al reported a linkage of a normal-tension glaucoma phenotype in a large British family to a locus on chromosome 10p15-p14 (GLC1E). In 2002, Rezaie et al reported that sequence variations in the optineurin (OPTN) gene were associated with the development of familial NTG in the original GLC1E family as well as 8 other families with NTG.

Normal-tension glaucoma appears to be more common in myopic patients. Some studies have suggested that a significant majority of patients with NTG are women; however, this may reflect the fact that there are more women than men in the elderly population. Systemic hypotension, both postural and nocturnal, may be more common in patients with NTG. Migraines and other vasospastic disorders may be more common in patients with NTG; however, a few Japanese-based studies have failed to find this association.

COURSE/PROGNOSIS

Although reduction of intraocular pressure is more difficult if pressure is already in the statistically normal range, the Collaborative Normal Tension Glaucoma Study has shown that a 30% reduction of intraocular pressure can slow down visual field loss. However, since the disease continues to progress in 20% of eyes even when intraocular pressure has been reduced 30% or more from baseline, other factors besides intraocular pressure may play a role. The Collaborative Normal Tension Glaucoma Study has also shown that about half of untreated normal tension glaucoma patients do not exhibit progression over 5 to 7 years of follow-up. There is wide variation in rates of deterioration, and the urgency and aggressiveness of treatment in NTG and perhaps all chronic glaucoma should be tempered by the stage of the disease at presentation and the expected rate of natural decline. It is important to know which patients are at risk for more rapid visual field loss, especially when potentially harmful treatment is considered. Although age and untreated intraocular pressure influence NTG prevalence, the Collaborative Normal Tension Glaucoma Study showed that risk factors for more rapid visual field loss include the following: disc hemorrhage (risk ratio 2.72), migraine (risk ratio 2.58), and female gender (risk ratio 1.85). This study also suggested that Asians may have a slower rate of progression (p = 0.005). Although the smaller number of African Americans in the study may have prevented a statistically verified conclusion (p = 0.8265), the few black patients enrolled had a tendency for more rapid progression. A reported family history of glaucoma and a field defect threatening fixation did not seem to affect the rate of progression.

DIAGNOSIS

Clinical signs and symptoms

A complete ocular and systemic history should include the following: possible past documentation of elevated intraocular pressure by another physician, prior steroid use, symptoms of intermittent angle closure glaucoma, past trauma, history of blood loss, transfusion, anemia, cardiogenic shock, cardiovascular disease, migraines, and Raynaud's phenomenon.

Ocular examination should include slit-lamp examination to rule out other causes of glaucoma (pseudoexfoliation, pigment dispersion syndrome, inflammation, scarring); serial tonometry (diurnal curve); gonioscopy (trabecular meshwork pigmentation, peripheral anterior synechiae, intermittent or chronic angle closure); fundus examination, including optic nerve evaluation for cupping, hemorrhages, disc asymmetry, etc; red-free nerve fiber layer examination; retinal examination for non-glaucomatous retinal diseases that may cause visual field loss; and computerized visual field examination.

As technology improves, imaging modalities may prove useful (e.g. optical coherence tomography, scanning laser polarimetery [GDx], and confocal scanning laser ophthalmoscopy [HRT]).

Work-up should be individualized for the particular patient since not all patients require an extensive work-up. Patients should have a complete examination by a general medical practitioner. Vascular disease (hypertension and diabetes risk factors), neurological abnormalities, and blood pressure evaluations should be stressed. Carotid ultrasound and electrocardiogram should be done when indicated. Imaging studies (CT or MRI scan) may be indicated if the history or examination is atypical for NTG or if rapid progression occurs despite intraocular pressure reduction. Atypical features may include the following: younger age, optic nerve pallor disproportionate to the degree of cupping, non glaucomatous visual field defects (e.g. respecting the vertical mid-line, bi-temporal field loss, etc.), and markedly asymmetric disease.

Laboratory findings

Blood tests to rule out other causes of optic neuropathy may include the following: syphilis testing (fta-abs), ANA, CBC, ESR (erythrocyte sedimentation rate), SPEP (serum protein electrophoresis).

Differential diagnosis

- Undetected past elevations of intraocular pressure: incomplete diurnal curve measurements, intermittent angle-closure glaucoma, past steroid-induced glaucoma, previous hyphema, burnt-out pigmentary glaucoma.
- Inactive uveitic glaucomas: Fuch's heterochromic iridocyclitis, herpetic or viral trabeculitis, Posner–Schlossman glaucomatocyclitic crisis, etc.
- Non-glaucomatous ischemic optic nerve disease: anemia, cardiogenic shock, carotid occlusive disease, arteritic or nonarteritic ischemic optic neuropathy.
- Other causes of optic neuropathy resembling glaucoma: optic nerve inflammatory disease, chiasmal lesions, pits and colobomas, optic nerve compressive lesions, traumatic optic neuropathy.

TREATMENT

Until other risk factors for field progression are elucidated, the mainstay of NTG treatment is similar to that for chronic open angle glaucoma and is the lowering of intraocular pressure.

Ocular

Many neuroprotective agents are designed to help improve optic nerve blood flow and function. Some potentially useful medications include calcium channel blockers (e.g. nifedipine, nimodipine), serotonin antagonists, betaxolol, dorzolamide, brimonidine, and memantine. The specific use of these agents for optic nerve blood flow improvement or for neuroprotection should not be practiced until their benefits are more definitively shown in humans.

Medical

All of the major classes of glaucoma medications have been used to treat NTG (i.e. beta blockers, alpha adrenergic agonists, carbonic anhydrase inhibitors, prostaglandin analogues and miotics).

Surgical

Available surgical treatments include argon laser trabeculoplasty, selective laser trabeculoplasty, trabeculectomy with or without antimetabolites (i.e. mitomycin C and 5-fluorouracil), tube shunt surgery, and cyclodestructive procedures.

COMMENTS

The Collaborative Normal Tension Glaucoma Study is the first national, multi-center, prospective, randomized study to prove that lowering of intraocular pressure slows down glaucomatous progression in NTG. It also emphasized that a significant proportion of NTG patients still exhibit disease progression despite lowering of intraocular pressure. This underscores the need for further research on the pressure-independent causes of NTG, which may ultimately yield better treatment strategies in the future. As new genes associated with NTG are found, this may also provide another distant venue for treatment in these patients.

SUPPORT GROUPS

Glaucoma Support Network
Glaucoma Research Foundation
490 Post Street
Suite 830
San Francisco, CA 94102
(415) 986-3162
Toll free: 800-826-6693
Fax: 415-986-3763

Glaucoma Research Foundation: http://www.glaucoma.org/living/support_net.html

INTERNET RESOURCES

American Academy of Ophthalmology: http://www.aao.org

REFERENCES

Anderson DR, Drance SM, Schulzer M: Collaborative Normal-Tension Glaucoma Study Group. Natural history of normal-tension glaucoma. Ophthalmology 108(2):247–253, 2001.

Collaborative Normal-Tension Glaucoma Study Group. Comparison of glaucomatous progression between untreated patients with normal-tension glaucoma and patients with therapeutically reduced intraocular pressures. Am J Ophthalmol 126(4):487–497, 1998.

Collaborative Normal-Tension Glaucoma Study Group. The effectiveness of intraocular pressure reduction in the treatment of normal-tension glaucoma. Am J Ophthalmol 126(4):498–505, 1998.

Drance S, Anderson DR, Schulzer M: Risk factors for progression of visual field abnormalities in normal-tension glaucoma. Am J Ophthalmol 131:699–708, 2001.

Sarfarazi M, Child A, Stoilova D, et al: Localization of the fourth locus (GLC1E) for adult-onset primary open-angle glaucoma to the 10p15-p14 region. Am J Hum Genet 62(3):641–652, 1998.

270 OCULAR HYPERTENSION 365.04

Adam C. Reynolds, MD
Oklahoma City, Oklahoma

ETIOLOGY/INCIDENCE

Ocular hypertension is elevated intraocular pressure (IOP) without any evidence of glaucomatous optic neuropathy. It is not a disease; however, increased eye pressure is the most important risk factor in the development of open angle glaucoma. Ocular hypertension can be categorized similarly to glaucoma with various possible mechanisms of etiology associated with an open or closed (or narrow) angle and associated primary or secondary causes. This chapter will deal with primary ocular hypertension, a condition similar to primary open-angle glaucoma (POAG).

Ocular hypertension has been defined as a mean intraocular pressure greater than 21 mmHg. Based on several different population studies, two standard deviations above mean IOP of 15–17 mmHg occurs at a cutoff of approximately 22 mmHg. In populations of European descent, primary ocular hypertension has been reported in approximately 5% of persons aged 50 years and older. In the United States this translates to approximately 3.9 million individuals. However, ocular hypertension in the United States is more common in individuals of African descent. Several very well-known studies show the exponential rise in the incidence of glaucoma in individuals with IOPs in the 25 mmHg range, particularly in African Americans.

It is important to recognize, however, that ocular hypertension is only one of many factors contributing to the development of glaucomatous optic neuropathy and associated vision loss. Patients with ocular hypertension belong to the much larger group of patients at risk for glaucoma, including those with atypical or asymmetrical optic discs or strong family histories of glaucoma. The Ocular Hypertension Treatment Study (OHTS) has provided a great deal of new information on the risk of glaucoma development from ocular hypertension and the impact of treating ocular hypertension on glaucoma.

COURSE/PROGNOSIS

The majority of patients with ocular hypertension do not develop glaucoma even when followed for as long as 20 years. In the OHTS study, approximately one in ten untreated individuals went on to develop glaucoma after 5 years of observation. Although this rate will undoubtedly be higher over time, only a subset of these patients would be expected to suffer functional vision loss. Additionally, in some epidemiologic studies, more than 50% of patients diagnosed with glaucoma have IOPs under 21 mmHg at the time of diagnosis; in 20–30% of patients, untreated IOPs above 21 mmHg are never detected. In light of the fact that populations with elevated IOPs have a low incidence of glaucoma, delineating other risk factors becomes very important.

DIAGNOSIS

The OHTS study confirmed many known risk factors contributing to increased rates of glaucoma development in patients with ocular hypertension. Increasing age, increased IOP, increased myopia, increased mean deviation levels on an otherwise normal visual field, and increased cup-disc ratios were all confirmed in multivariate analysis to be independent risk factors for the development of glaucoma. One of the most interesting findings in OHTS was the importance of central corneal thickness (CCT) in delineating the risk of glaucoma development. Thinner than normal CCT correlated with increased risk, while thicker than normal CCT correlated with decreased risk. Although it was previously known that variations in CCT affect the accuracy of applanation tonometry, and some of the effect of CCT in the OHTS study is undoubtedly due to necessary adjustments of the IOP measurements, in the OHTS study central corneal thickness was found to be a risk factor independent of IOP. This has led to speculation that will need to be confirmed with further study, that a thinner central cornea may reflect other structural differences in at-risk eyes and signal a greater susceptibility to glaucoma development in ocular hypertension. It is well known that African Americans have thinner CCT measurements compared with Caucasians. In the OHTS study, decreased CCT and increased cup-disc ratios completely accounted for the increased risk of glaucoma development in African Americans compared to Caucasians in the study.

There have been many conflicting studies about the contribution of systemic diseases to the risk of glaucoma development in ocular hypertension. Neither the presence of systemic hypertension or reported diabetes was found to contribute to increased risk in the OHTS study. Other epidemiologic evidence, however, does indicate that these diseases contribute to increased risk.

TREATMENT

We now have more information about which ocular hypertensive patients should be treated and which it is more appropriate to observe. Key considerations should include patient-specific risk factors for progression to glaucoma, the potential benefit of treatment, the potential harm of treatment, the potential difference in outcomes if treatment is initiated before or after glaucoma is detectable, and the optimal degree of IOP reduction. Considerations of the patient's and physician's expectations and level of anxiety are important considerations as well.

Several additional factors were not considered in the OHTS study. These include the presence of beta type peripapillary atrophy or peripapillary hemorrhages (Drantz hemorrhages), asymmetry of the optic nerves, the presence of cerebrovascular disease, the status of the other eye, family history, new technologies to assess the nerve fiber layer, and newer visual field technologies that can possibly detect glaucoma earlier. Currently, there is insufficient evidence that technologies to measure the nerve fiber layer or different visual field strategies, such as frequency doubling technologies (FDT), are predictive of the development of glaucoma in ocular hypertension, but it is thought that in general, they can detect glaucomatous optic neuropathy earlier than has been possible. All of these factors could be considered in deciding to treat or observe a particular patient. The next few years should provide more data for assessing their value to the assessment of ocular hypertension.

Once a decision to treat has been reached, the strategies of initial treatment have traditionally been the same as the treatment of typical high IOP in POAG. Initial monotherapy with topical beta-blockers to lower the IOP by approximately 25% is the recommended practice. Other topical medications and laser trabeculoplasty may also be used, but surgery should be preserved for definite progressive glaucoma. Careful consideration of risks and benefits is important as treatment becomes more aggressive in ocular hypertension, as compared to treating progressive POAG.

Whether treatment or observation is elected, the patient should receive appropriate serial examinations to monitor IOP, visual fields, and status of the optic nerve. Patients are typically seen every 6 to 12 months. In the OHTS study, the most common end point for patients whose diagnosis was converted from ocular hypertension to glaucoma was progressive optic nerve changes consistent with glaucomatous optic neuropathy. Therefore, serial stereo disc photography, careful observation of the optic nerves, and possibly serial nerve fiber layer analysis should play an important role in ongoing assessment.

COMMENTS

In the OHTS study, approximately 9% of untreated vs. 4.5% of treated patients developed glaucoma after 5 years. Treatment reduced the incidence of glaucoma in this study population by 50%. However, it is important to realize that the number of patients needed to treat (NNT) to prevent the development of one case of glaucoma in this study was 20. Calculations from several different long-term studies of ocular hypertension and its progression to glaucoma and visual loss show that treatment reduces the risk of progression from untreated ocular hypertension to blindness by 1.2% to 8.1% over 15 years.

It is obviously not appropriate to treat all patients with ocular hypertension. In addition to the factors mentioned above, the patient's age and expected life span need to be considered in assessing the risk of a typically very slowly progressive chronic disease that usually affects visual function only in its late stages. No treatment for ocular hypertension is without risk. Although generally well tolerated, with few short-term side effects, decades of treatment with topical anti-glaucoma drops do increase the risk for cataract development (in the case of topical beta blockers). We currently do not know the 20-year or longer side effect profile of prostaglandin analogues, as they have only been in use for about 10 years.

Ocular hypertension in not a disease in itself, but its occurrence does increase the risk of developing primary open-angle glaucoma. Significant numbers of patients can probably be safely followed with observation only, but in patients with high-risk characteristics, which have now been more thoroughly defined, treatment is appropriate to prevent or delay the development of glaucoma. Treatment, if deemed appropriate, is much the same as for POAG, and has been shown to delay or avert progression to glaucoma in high-risk patients. It is imperative to carefully assess the risk-benefit relationship of therapy, taking into account possible long-term side effects and costs of treatment as well as an individual's lifestyle weighted against the benefits of IOP lowering therapy.

REFERENCES

Brandt JD, Beiser JA, Kass MA, et al: Central cornea thickness in the Ocular Hypertension Treatment Study. Ophthalmology 108:1779–1788, 2001.

Friedman DS, Wilson MR, Liebmann JM, et al: An evidence-based assessment of risk factors for the progression of ocular hypertension and glaucoma. Am J Ophthalmol 138(Suppl):S19–S31, 2004.

Gordon MO, Beiser JA, Brandt JD, et al: for the Ocular Hypertension Treatment Study Group: The ocular hypertension treatment study: baseline factors that predict the onset of primary open-angle glaucoma. Arch Ophthalmol 120:714–720, 2002.

Quigley HA, Enger C, Katz J, et al: Risk factors for the development of glaucomatous visual field loss in ocular hypertension. Arch Ophthalmol 112:644–649, 1994.

Weinreb RN: Ocular hypertension: defining risks and clinical options. Am J Ophthalmol 138(Suppl):S1–S2, 2004.

Weinreb RN, Friedman DS, Fechtner RD, et al: Risk assessment in the management of patients with ocular hypertension. Am J Opthalmol 138:458–467, 2004.

271 OCULAR HYPOTONY 360.3

Steven L. Mansberger, MD, MPH
Portland, Oregon
David J. Wilson, MD
Portland, Oregon

Ocular hypotony lacks a specific definition. However, clinicians consider an eye to be hypotonous when low intraocular pressure (IOP) results in anatomical or functional abnormalities to the eye. Therefore, hypotony is not a specific diagnosis but a constellation of clinical signs resulting from other ocular conditions. The level of IOP that creates hypotonous changes varies from individual to individual, and depends on the speed of onset and the underlying cause of the decreased IOP. Generally, no ocular effects are noted until the IOP is less than 6 mm Hg; however, hypotonous changes can occur at higher intraocular pressures.

ETIOLOGY/INCIDENCE

IOP is produced by a balance between aqueous formation, facility of aqueous outflow, and episcleral venous pressure. Ocular hypotony is usually the result of decreased aqueous formation and/or increased facility of aqueous outflow; reduced episcleral venous pressure is not a common cause.

The incidence of ocular hypotony will be different according to the etiology of the hypotony. For example, ocular hypotony may be common after glaucoma surgery.

COURSE

The course of hypotony depends on the underlying cause (see Differential diagnosis below) and the efficacy of treatment.

DIAGNOSIS

Low intraocular pressure by itself is not considered ocular hypotony unless it creates functional or anatomical abnormalities to the eye. For example, patients with surgically altered or naturally thin corneas may routinely have intraocular pressures in the single digits. Similarly, patients with myotonic dystrophy have low intraocular pressures, but they rarely have functional or anatomical abnormalities as a result of the hypotony.

Ocular hypotony may manifest by several different clinical signs. These include corneal striae, aqueous flare, choroidal folds, choroidal effusions, and macular folds. Low intraocular pressure with a difference in IOP (more than 3 mm Hg) between fellow eyes is also a common presentation.

A complete history and thorough ophthalmic examination will usually uncover the cause of ocular hypotony. To properly examine a hypotonous eye, clinicians should perform biomicroscopy of the conjunctiva, cornea, anterior chamber, iris, and posterior pole; test for a positive Seidel; and perform a careful gonioscopy. For the Seidel's test, the clinician should apply the fluorescein in a highly concentrated form; otherwise, he or she may miss small leaks. If the leak is not detected, the clinician should perform gentle digital pressure during Seidel testing to diagnose an intermittent or slow leak. Clinicians should perform gonioscopy prior to dilation because mydriatic eye drops may close a small cyclodialysis cleft. In cases of a small cyclodialysis cleft, clinicians may need to perform gonioscopy after filling the anterior chamber with a cohesive viscoelastic to allow a better view of the angle.

In some cases, clinicians will have difficulty determining the cause of hypotony. In these cases, ultrasound biomicroscopy may be helpful diagnosing an anatomical abnormality such as a supraciliary effusion or tractional ciliary body detachment.

Differential diagnosis

Ocular hypotony may arise from a number of distinct ophthalmic conditions. As well, a primary cause of hypotony may lead to a secondary cause of hypotony. For example, a wound leak after glaucoma surgery (increased aqueous outflow) may lead to ciliochoroidal detachment (decreased aqueous formation). To properly treat hypotony, the clinician must diagnose the primary cause. We list the most common causes to provide a differential diagnosis, but multiple simultaneous causes for hypotony may be present.

Decreased aqueous formation

Ciliochoroidal detachment or effusion

- Anterior proliferative vitreoretinopathy.
- Cyclodialysis cleft. This provides a conduit for fluid to collect under the ciliary body.
- Retinal cryotherapy and panretinal photocoagulation. Extensive panretinal treatment may result in ciliochoroidal edema.
- Lens capsular contraction syndrome may create centripetal tension on the zonule and ciliary body resulting in a ciliochoroidal detachment.
- Idiopathic ciliochoroidal effusion in persons with high myopia.
- Hypoproteinemia.

Ciliochoroidal dysfunction or cyclitis

- Uveitis.
- Antimetabolites for glaucoma surgery.
- Systemic medications.

- Intravenous or intravitreal cidofovir used for the treatment of cytomegalovirus retinitis.
- Oral sulfa-like medications: acetazolamide, sulfa antibiotics, topiramate, etc.
- Cyclophotocoagulation or cyclocryotherapy ablation.
- Prolonged intraocular procedures (transient hypotony).
- Ciliary body tumors.
- Postradiation treatment.
- Intraocular copper foreign bodies.

Vascular

- Carotid vascular disease or occlusion of other tributaries to the ciliary body (ophthalmic artery and long posterior ciliary arteries) resulting in ocular ischemia.
- Temporal arteritis.
- Retinal vascular occlusions (central retinal artery or vein).

Miscellaneous

- Dehydration.
- Diabetic coma.
- Uremia.
- Systemic hypertensive medications (beta-adrenergic antagonists, clonidine).
- Hemifacial atrophy.

Increased facility of outflow

Surgical

- Corneal, scleral, or conjunctival wound leak after intraocular surgery.
- Glaucoma surgery.
- Occult ocular perforation (e.g. retrobulbar needle injuries).

Traumatic

- Cyclodialysis cleft (also after complicated intraocular surgery).
- Topical cholinergic medications (pilocarpine, carbachol, echothiophate, etc.) may open a previously closed cyclodialysis cleft.
- Ruptured globe.

Uveitis may create increased uveal scleral outflow.

Retinal abnormalities

- Rhegmatogenous retinal detachment.
- Retinal tears and retinotomies.

TREATMENT

The most important factor in treating ocular hypotony is diagnosing the primary cause of the low intraocular pressure. We describe the common treatments below, but clinicians will need to employ specific treatments for each primary cause of hypotony.

Conservative treatments include the use of corticosteroids and topical cycloplegic agents, and avoiding medications that augment hypotony. Corticosteroids help improve ciliary body function by decreasing inflammation that may cause decreased aqueous production and increased uveal scleral outflow. They may be given orally, topically, or locally. Topical cycloplegic eye drops relax the lens, iris, and ciliary body, decreasing the potential space for subciliary effusions. These drops may allow small cyclodialysis clefts to close, as well as reduce inflammation by increasing the blood-brain barrier. Clinicians should limit topical and systemic medications that reduce aqueous production such as oral beta-adrenergic antagonists.

Cyclodialysis clefts are common causes of hypotony. Clinicians have reported successful treatment with topical mydriatic drops, argon laser photocoagulation, diathermy, cryotherapy, and surgical closure, among other methods. We prefer a staged approach that begins with conservative treatments (steroids, mydriatics), followed by argon laser photocoagulation of the cyclodialysis cleft, and finally surgical repair. More information, including surgical techniques, is available from previous manuscripts (see References below).

Early postoperative hypotony occurs commonly with glaucoma filtration surgery. In most cases, hypotonous changes resolve spontaneously over two to four weeks with conservative treatment. In the meantime, patience and vigilance are required by the clinician and patient. The eye does not require surgical intervention unless lens-corneal touch or 'kissing' choroidal effusions are present. In cases that do not resolve spontaneously, a ciliochoroidal effusion is commonly present and requires drainage. However, the mechanism and pathogenic role of ciliochoroidal effusions is unclear, and previous studies show that detachment of the ciliary body with silicone oil does not result in hypotony in a monkey model. In addition, the eye may develop reccurrence of ciliochoroidal effusions after surgical drainage and may require further surgery, especially when inflamed. In summary, most hypotonous eyes do not usually require treatment in the early postoperative period after glaucoma surgery, but when required, drainage of ciliochoroidal effusions is essential.

Late postoperative hypotony, 6 months or more after glaucoma surgery, is usually related to leaking or overfiltering blebs. Conservative treatments may resolve the hypotony in a minority of cases, but these eyes usually require a bleb revision. In a bleb revision, a surgeon will remove the avascular, necrotic conjunctival tissue and replace it with healthy conjunctiva. This will resolve the hypotony in the majority of cases. A recent study by Bashford has shown that the length of time of hypotony maculopathy is not related to improvement in visual acuity, and most patients will recover good visual acuity even after a long period (6 months or more) of hypotony. This suggests that the surgeon can delay bleb revision until all conservative treatments have failed.

The clinician must anticipate that successful treatment of hypotony may result in severely elevated intraocular pressure. This usually occurs with the normalization of aqueous production and a short-term decrease in trabecular outflow. The clinician should warn the patient of the symptoms of ocular hypertension and should evaluate the patient soon after treatment and at regular intervals. Clinicians should use topical aqueous suppressant glaucoma medications to treat the ocular hypertension until physiologic trabecular outflow returns.

COMMENTS

Clinicians consider an eye to be hypotonous when low intraocular pressure (IOP) results in anatomical or functional abnormalities to the eye. Treatment of hypotony requires an extensive history and complete ophthalmic examination. An accurate diagnosis is the cornerstone to treatment. While selected cases of ocular hypotony may resolve with conservative treatment, some eyes may require surgical intervention when the benefits outweigh the risks of the surgery.

REFERENCES

Barasch K, Galin MA, Baras I: Postcyclodialysis hypotony. Am J Ophthalmol 68:644–645, 1969.

Brubaker RF, Pederson JE: Ciliochoroidal detachment. Surv Ophthalmol 27:281–289, 1983.

Maumenee AE, Stark WJ: Management of persistent hypotony after planned or inadvertent cyclodialysis. Am J Ophthalmol 71:320–327, 1971.

Ormerod LD, Baerveldt G, Sunalp MA, Riekhof FT: Management of the hypotonous cyclodialysis cleft. Ophthalmology 98:1384–1393, 1991.

Pederson JE, Gaasterland DE, MacLellan HM: Experimental ciliochoroidal detachment: Effect on intraocular pressure and aqueous humor flow. Arch Ophthalmol 97:536–541, 1979.

272 OPEN-ANGLE GLAUCOMA 365.10

Emily Patterson, MD
Portland, Oregon

ETIOLOGY/INCIDENCE

Open-angle glaucoma (OAG) is a chronic bilateral ocular disease characterized by optic nerve damage manifested in morphologic and psychophysical changes. The anterior chamber angle is open, and there are no known ocular or systemic causes for the optic nerve damage. The morphologic changes include progressive loss of optic nerve fibers, optic nerve cupping, and thinning of the optic nerve rim, as noted on ophthalmic examination. The psychophysical changes include visual field (VF) defects such as nasal steps, arcuate scotomata, paracentral scotomata, and generalized depression.

The traditional triad on which the diagnosis of OAG was based included optic nerve changes, VF defects, and elevated intraocular pressure (IOP) to least 21 mmHg. However, it has become abundantly clear that a significant portion (approximately 30%) of patients with typical optic nerve or VF changes never have elevated IOP, whereas a similar proportion of patients with OAG continue to have progressive optic nerve and VF changes despite a lowering of the IOP to a 'normal' level.

The current concept of OAG is that it is a progressive optic neuropathy with elevated IOP as a major, but certainly not the only, risk factor. Furthermore, it is a multifactorial and heterogeneous disease whose diagnosis is really made by exclusion. Many cases historically been included under the rubric 'primary' OAG have been shown with advancing knowledge and diagnostic tools to be secondary glaucomas, such as pigmentary glaucoma and pseudoexfoliation glaucoma.

The cause of OAG remains unknown, but many risk factors have been identified. Elevated IOP is a major risk factor, with higher IOPs associated with greater risk and greater severity of optic nerve damage even in the normal-pressure OAG group. Other risk factors documented in various clinical trials include large optic nerve cup, thin central cornea, high myopia, older age, positive family history, African or Latino ancestry, diabetes mellitus, systemic hypertension, and history of migraine headaches.

The genes for several types of secondary OAG and subsets of juvenile- and adult-onset OAG have been identified, and it is almost certain that other genes for this heterogeneous disease will be identified soon.

In the United States, 2.2 million persons have been diagnosed with OAG, and it is estimated that at least another 2 million persons have undiagnosed OAG. Among Americans, it is the third most common cause of blindness in the United States, and in blacks of African ancestry, it is the leading cause of blindness. In the United States, with more than 3 million office visits per year related to OAG, it is not only a major ocular but also a major public health and economic problem. Worldwide, it is estimated that 65 million people have glaucoma and 5 million are blind from the disease.

COURSE/PROGNOSIS

OAG is a chronic disease for which there is no cure-only control. Until the end stages of the disease, when VF loss encroaches on visual fixation, there are no symptoms to warn the patient. Because it is considered unethical to withhold treatment from a patient with OAG, the natural history of the untreated disease is poorly documented. Not all risk factors for this disease have been identified, much less quantified. To further confound the elucidation of its natural history, there is a normal attrition of all nerve cells with age, including the nerve cells in the optic nerve.

Available studies show that 4% of white patients and 8% of black patients with OAG are legally blind due to this disease. Controlled studies of patients at high risk for glaucoma suggest that medical treatment may decrease the risk of developing glaucoma by 50%. The incidence of debilitating visual loss from OAG is low and treatment can significantly improve disease prognosis. However, because of the large number of people afflicted with this disease, the magnitude of the effect of this disease is still substantial.

DIAGNOSIS

Clinical signs

Intraocular pressure

- As many as 30% of patients have 'normal' IOP (less than 21 mmHg) at all times
- As many as 50% have 'normal' IOP at any single IOP measurement.
- IOP of at least 21 mmHg should arouse suspicion of OAG; the higher the IOP, the greater the likelihood of OAG.
- Asymmetry of IOP with difference between eyes greater than several millimeters of mercury is also suspicious.

Optic nerve

- Size of optic nerve cupping: there is a wide variation in the normal optic nerve cup size, but cups of more than 50% are suspicious. The larger the cup, the more suspicious.
- Asymmetry of optic nerve cupping: physiologic optic cups may be large, but the two eyes should be symmetric. An asymmetry of more than 10% is suspicious; the greater the asymmetry, the greater the likelihood of OAG. Asymmetric cupping associated with ipsilateral higher IOP is even more suspicious.
- Shape of optic nerve cup: physiologic cupping tends to be round with an intact, even rim of nerve tissue. Glaucomatous nerve cupping tends to be uneven with more vertical cupping toward the inferotemporal and superotemporal

regions preferentially. Notching of optic nerve rim tissue is suspicious.

- Depth of optic disk cupping: with glaucoma, there tends to be a backward bowing of the optic nerve tissue. With progression, the cup gets deeper with excavation to the level of the lamina cribosa so that the cribiform pores becomes visible.
- Atrophy of optic nerve tissue: this is manifested in the loss of the normal pink color of the optic nerve and loss of peripapillary nerve fibers. Red-free light through the ophthalmoscope makes observation of nerve fiber loss easier. Computerized instruments can be used to measure peripapillary retinal nerve fiber thickness and to compare measurements over time, allowing documentaion of progressive nerve fiber layer loss.

Disk hemorrhages

Hemorrhages on or near the disk margin occur in approximately 1% of the population older than 40. The prevalence of disk hemorrhages in patients with OAG ranges from 5% to an estimated 60% over the lifetime of someone with OAG. The presence of disk hemorrhages is strongly associated with OAG, especially the normal-pressure type.

Visual fields

The current standard instrument for detecting VF changes is the automated, computerized, threshold static perimeter. Glaucomatous VF changes include, but are not limited to, generalized depression, nasal step, paracentral scotoma, and arcuate scotoma extending to the blind spot. Newer testing strategies with short wavelength visual stimuli (SWAP) and frequency doubling techniques may prove to be better predictive screening tests.

Differential diagnosis

As noted, the diagnosis is made by exclusion of other conditions. Most important, gonioscopy of the anterior chamber angle must be performed in every eye suspected of having glaucoma. Gonioscopy not only separates the two major groups of glaucoma (OAG from angle-closure glaucoma [ACG]) but also is critical in identifying many major types of secondary OAG. Only after eliminating ACG, secondary OAG (such as pigmentary, pseudoexfoliative, and uveitic glaucoma), and glaucoma from systemic causes (such as elevated episcleral venous pressure and corticosteroid-responsive glaucoma) can the diagnosis of primary OAG be made. As our diagnostic ability improves, it is certain that more secondary causes of OAG will be identified and therefore removed from this heterogeneous category.

PROPHYLAXIS

Early identification of OAG, with appropriate observation and intervention where indicated, remains the most important element in the treatment of this disease. Unfortunately, IOP measurement as a screening method has been shown to be inadequately sensitive or specific. Evaluation of the optic nerve, a VF examination, and an IOP measurement are essential elements in a reliable screening test for OAG. The American Academy of Ophthalmology Preferred Practice Pattern guidelines for quality eye care state that a periodic comprehensive ocular examination is the best way to identify the patient at high risk of developing OAG. All asymptomatic patients older than 65 should have a comprehensive ocular examination every 1 to 2 years. All blacks older than 20 should have a comprehensive ocular examination every 3 to 5 years, and those older than 40 should have one every 2 to 4 years.

TREATMENT

The therapeutic goal in OAG is to prevent initial or progressive optic nerve damage and VF loss. Although the aim is not to treat a specific number, setting a 'target' IOP range for an individual may be appropriate and beneficial. In general, the more damage there is to an optic nerve, the lower the IOP necessary to prevent further damage. The rapidity in the development of the present damage, the extent of damage in the fellow eye, older age, positive family history, African or Hispanic ancestry, and presence of systemic risk factors all dictate a lower target IOP. As a general rule, target pressure should be 20–30% below the initital IOP, even if initial IOP is the 'normal' range. If the initial IOP is high, the target IOP should be less than 21 mmHg. The side effects of treatment must be factored into the target IOP equation, so minimal and acceptable side effects with an IOP closest to target range should be the goal. Finally, in achieving the target IOP, a 'ladder of treatment' is usually used, starting with the safest, lowest dosage and the easiest to use and least expensive treatment. If this is inadequate, the next step up the ladder in terms of increasing side effects, inconvenience in use, and increase in cost is either added or substituted until a satisfactory IOP is achieved. Periodically, the target IOP should be revisited. If optic nerve damage has progressed, a lower target IOP is indicated; if the optic nerve is stable and/or the side effects become intolerable, a higher target IOP may have to be accepted.

The traditional treatment ladder has been to start with medical therapy, followed by laser therapy, and finally surgery intervention. The discussion that follows will adhere to this format, although new treatment paradigms are evolving and are discussed.

Medical

Eyedrops

β-Blockers

- Nonselective (β_1 and β_2).
- Timolol 0.25% and 0.5% qd or b.i.d.
- Timolol gel 0.25% or 0.5% qd.
- Levobunolol 0.25% or 0.5% qd or b.i.d.
- Carteolol 1% QD or b.i.d.
- Metipranolol 0.3% QD or b.i.d.

Side effects:

- Cardiorespiratory: bradycardia, increased heart block, decreased cardiac output, exercise intolerance, congestive heart failure, difficulty breathing, asthma;
- Central nervous system: depression, mood changes, tiredness, confusion, and impotence in men.

- Selective (β_1).
- Betaxolol 0.25% suspension and 5% qd or b.i.d.

Side effects:

- Lesser incidence of pulmonary and central nervous system side effects;
- Lesser incidence of ocular hypotensive effects.

IOP is decreased by as much as 30% by decreasing aqueous production.

Ocular hypotensive effect is less in patients already on systemic β-blockers.

β-Blockers remain the first-line treatment for most patients.

Sympathomimetic agonists

Nonselective (a_1 and a_2)

- Epinephrine bitartrate 2% b.i.d. to q.i.d.
- Epinephrine borate 0.5%, 1%, or 2% b.i.d. to q.i.d.
- Epinephryl borate 0.5%, 1% b.i.d. to q.i.d.
- Epinephrine hydrochloride 0.5%, 1%, or 2% b.i.d. to q.i.d.
- Dipivefrin hydrochloride 0.1% (a prodrug of epinephrine) b.i.d. to q.i.d.

Selective a_2

- Apraclonidine 0.5%, or 1% b.i.d. or t.i.d.
- Brimonidine 0.2% b.i.d. or t.i.d.

IOP is decreased 25% by decreasing aqueous production and increasing uveoscleral outflow.

Side effects:

- Cardiovascular: systemic hypertension, tachycardia, arrhythmia with nonselective agents;
- Local allergy: most with apraclonidine, least with brimonidine, intermediate with others;
- Cystoid macular edema: in aphakic or pseudophakic eyes with open capsule with nonselective agents;
- Oral dryness with brimonidine;
- Central nervous system: fatigue, drowsiness with brimonidine.

Because of the high incidence of side effects and because they are minimally additive to the ß-blockers, most of the nonselective sympathomimetic agents are used infrequently. The addition of an epinephrine compound to a selective β-blocker is comparable in magnitude of IOP lowering to a nonselective β-blocker alone. Apraclonidine is useful in blunting the IOP spikes after laser procedures, but it is not effective in eyes already on treatment with this medication. In addition, the efficacy of apraclonidine decreases with chronic use. Brimonidine may be used as an alternative first-line medication when β-blockers are contraindicated.

Prostaglandin analogs

- Latanoprost 0.005% qd.
- Travoprost 0.004% qd.
- Bimatoprost 0.03%.
- Prostaglandin F_{2a} analogs.
- Decrease IOP 25% to 30% by increasing uveoscleral outflow.
- Totally additive to β-blockers, partially additive to cholinergic agents.

Side effects:

- Changes color of light irides to darker, increases pigmentation of periocular skin;
- Increases eyelash thickness, number, length and color;
- Anterior uveitis and cystoid macular edema reported; aphakic and pseudophakic eyes with open posterior capsules may be at greater risk with incidence of approximately 5% in these eyes;
- Recurrence of herpes simplex hepatitis has been reported.

Latanoprost has been approved for first-line treatment of glaucoma patients. Travoprost shows mean IOP reduction up to 1.8mmHg greater in black patients than white.

The combination of a β-blocker in the morning and latanoprost in the evening is a very effective treatment protocol.

Carbonic anhydrase inhibitors

Systemic

- Acetazolamide 125, 250, and 500 mg time release b.i.d. to q.i.d.
- Dichlorphenamide 50 mg b.i.d. to q.i.d.
- Methazolamide 25 and 50 mg b.i.d to t.i.d.

Side effects:

- Gastrointestinal: nausea, vomiting, anorexia, metallic taste;
- Genitourinary: urinary frequency, kidney stones, acidosis;
- Central nervous system: malaise, depression, loss of libido, numbness and parathesia of extremities;
- Hematologic: aplastic anemia, thrombocytopenia (rare);
- Allergic: because all carbonic anhydrase inhibitors are sulfonamide derivatives, they should be used with caution in persons with a history of allergy to sulfur compounds.

With multiple and sometimes severe side effects and the current availability of topical carbonic anhydrase inhibitors, chronic use is infrequent. Pressure-lowering effect is maximal with full-dose acetazolamide, with slightly less effect from systemic methazolomide and topical dorzolamide.

Topical

- Dorzolamide 2% b.i.d. to t.i.d.
- Brinzolamide 1% b.i.d. to t.i.d.
- Decreases IOP as much as 25% through a decrease in aqueous production.
- Additive to β-blockers (further 10% to 20% decrease in IOP).

Side effects:

- Stinging on instillation, greater with dorzolamide than brinzolamide because of lower pH of dorzolamide;
- Ocular allergy and sensitivity, approximately 20%.

With significantly fewer side effects than the systemic carbonic anhydrase inhibitors, dorzolamide has become a valuable second-line and, sometimes, first-line medication.

Combination β-blockers and carbonic anhydrase inhibitors

- Timolol 0.5% and dorzolamide 2% b.i.d.

The ease of use of a single eyedrop may improve compliance and reduce washout effect of two different eyedrops instilled one immediately after the other. IOP lowering is equivalent to the concomitant use of timolol b.i.d. and dorzolamide b.i.d. in carefully controlled clinical trials, but in the real world where compliance is a problem, combination therapy may have a better effect than concomitant treatment with two different medications. Ocular and systemic side effects are comparable in incidence to those of timolol and dorzolamide.

Parasympathomimetic agonists

Parasympathomimetic agents decrease IOP by 20% by increasing the facility of outflow.

Direct acting (cholinergic)

- Pilocarpine hydrochloride 0.25%, 0.5%, 1% to 6%, 8%, and 10%, (multiple brands, including generic) b.i.d. to q.i.d.
- Pilocarpine nitrate 1%, 2%, and 4% b.i.d. to q.i.d.
- Pilocarpine hydrochloride gel 4% QHS.
- Pilocarpine slow release (20 equivalent to 2% pilocarpine, 40 equivalent to 4% pilocarpine) every 5 to 7 days.
- Strengths of more than 4% usually have no greater therapeutic effects.

Direct and indirect acting

- Carbachol 0.75%, 1.5%, 2.25%, and 3% qd to t.i.d.

Indirect acting

- Echothiophate iodide 0.03%, 0.06%, 0.125%, and 0.25% qd to b.i.d.
- Demecarium bromide 0.125% and 0.25% qd to b.i.d.

Side effects:

- Cholinergic: nausea, vomiting and diarrhea, and pulmonary congestion due to increased pulmonary secretion;
- Ocular: ciliary muscle contraction resulting in pain and fluctuating myopia, miosis resulting in decreased vision, especially at nighttime; increased incidence of cataracts, detached retina, especially with stronger, indirect-acting sympathomimetic agents;
- Indirect sympathomimetic acts through inhibition of acetylcholine esterase. Because of systemic absorption, the body is depleted of acetylcholine esterase and pseudocholine esterase with chronic use; if the muscle relaxant succinylcholine is used in general anesthesia, prolonged respiratory paralysis may occur.

Parasympathomimetic agents are additive to β-blockers and carbonic anhydrase inhibitors, and partially additive to latanoprost.

Because of ocular side effects, they are relegated to a second- or third-line medication.

Laser therapy: argon laser trabeculoplasty

- Successful in decreasing IOP in 90% of adult OAG.
- Average decrease 4 to 8 mmHg.
- In general, the higher the IOP, the greater the absolute and percentage decrease in IOP
- Approximately 55% still under control after 5 years.
- Retreatment possible but success rate lower, duration of effect not as long, and post-treatment elevation of IOP more frequent.
- More effective in older patients than in younger patients.

Complications

- Post-treatment iritis, inflammation, and transient elevation of IOP common.
- Few serious complications.

Indications

- Usually tried after medical therapy is ineffective or intolerable.
- Initial treatment with argon laser possibly beneficial for some patients.

Contraindications

- Glaucoma secondary to iritis, angle recession, neovascularization of the angle, or congenital glaucoma.

Laser therapy: selective laser trabeculoplasty

Similar to ALT, but avoids thermal response in trabecular meshwork cells, instead inducing a primarily biologic response. Retreatment believed to be more successful in SLT than ALT.

Surgical

Filtration surgery

Trabeculectomy is currently the operation of choice. An opening into the eye near the limbus is made beneath the conjunctiva and a partial-thickness scleral flap. The scleral flap offers some resistance to the egress of aqueous, minimizing the chances of hypotony, and the resultant conjunctival bleb allows diffusion of the aqueous through the conjunctiva onto the surface of the eye.

In eyes without previous surgery, the success rate is approximately 75%. In eyes with previous surgery, the success rate is lower. In blacks and in younger patients, the success rate is believed to be lower as well because of more rapid healing and scarring.

Traditionally, filtration surgery has been performed only after medical and laser therapy have failed. Recent studies suggest that initial surgery may be equally beneficial and as cost effective as medical or laser therapy.

Surgical complications

Hemorrhage, infections, and wound leaks, although rare, are possible with any surgical procedure. Complications unique to the eye undergoing a filtration operation include hypotony, flat anterior chamber, choroidal effusion, and suprachoroidal hemorrhages in the perioperative period, with progression of cataract, failure of filtration, and endophthalmitis occurring as late problems.

The postoperative use of 5-fluorouracil and the intraoperative use of mitomycin C to decrease fibrosis and scarring increase the chances of successful filtration and have found wide acceptance, especially for high-risk eyes. This gain in greater filtration is offset by an increased incidence of persistent wound leak, hypotony maculopathy, and late-onset endophthalmitis.

Because the incidence of endophthalmitis in a filtered eye is at least 1% per year, proper education of the patient regarding early infection ('blebitis') is critical in preventing this blinding complication. Early treatment of blebitis with topical antibiotics and steroids is almost always effective.

Tube-shunt procedures

When excess conjunctival scarring from previous surgery limits the chances for successful trabeculectomy, various tube-shunt implants may be placed to drain aqueous from the anterior chamber to a mechanically maintained subconjunctival space posterior to the limbus.

All of the different implants share the common problems of blockage of the internal or external ostia of the drainage tube, external erosion of the implant, hypotony, insufficient IOP lowering, and fibrosis of the conjunctival space.

Generally, these procedures are reserved for eyes in which standard surgery has failed.

Cyclodestructive procedures

When all attempts at filtration surgery, with or without an implant, have failed and the IOP is still too high, a cyclodestructive procedure may be considered. By destroying the ciliary processes, the source of aqueous production, the IOP is lowered.

Initially, this was performed with a cryoprobe applied to the sclera over the ciliary processes. However, cyclocryotherapy has been supplanted by transscleral laser destruction of the ciliary processes (YAG or diode laser) or direct application of laser to the ciliary processes (transpupillary or endoscopic with argon or diode lasers).

Because this procedure results in nonreversible destruction of the ciliary processes, hypotony may result. With cyclocryotherapy, the incidence of hypotony was up to 50%. With the various laser modalities, this complication is significantly less.

Post-treatment inflammation, iritis, and pain are also less common with laser treatment than with cryotherapy.

This often is the treatment of last resort when everything else has failed and the IOP must be reduced to decrease pain and prevent corneal decompensation.

COMPLICATIONS

There are several problems unique to OAG. It is a chronic disease for which there is no cure; lifetime follow-up and treatment are necessary. Until the end stages of the disease, there are no symptoms; it is therefore understandable that one nickname for OAG is the 'silent thief.' Yet the medications to treat this disease are expensive and must be taken daily. They can cause a large number of ocular and systemic side effects which are sometimes life-threatening. Successful treatment with medications, lasers, or surgery does not result in any tangible benefit obvious to the patient. The patient has to accept on faith alone that there is control of the OAG. In accepting surgery, the patient has to subject an apparently normal eye to pain, discomfort, transient and sometimes permanent decrease in vision, and the remote possibility of losing the eye. Even if surgery is successful, the patient's vision is not improved, and the patient must suffer the cosmetically displeasing and possibly uncomfortable 'lump' under the eyelid. The only comfort to the patient is the assurance from the physician that their condition is controlled.

Compliance with any medical therapy is difficult, and it is easy to see why it is a major problem in OAG. Studies have shown that as many as 50% of patients do not take their eye medications conscientiously. Failure to achieve target IOP, or progression of disease despite IOP that is measured at target during office visits, is often due to lack of patient compliance. Education of the patient and the family therefore is of paramount importance with OAG. Prescribing the appropriate treatment is only half of the physician's responsibility to the patient. Without proper education so that the patient may appreciate the magnitude of the problem and the importance of adhering to the treatment regimen, even the most efficacious medications and surgical procedures will fail.

Some of the major complications of medications used in the treatment of glaucoma have been mentioned. It is important that patients are informed of these potential side effects and urged to call the physician with any new or unexplained symptoms after the institution of a new antiglaucoma medication. Also, it is important that patients be told to inform their primary care physicians of all new glaucoma medications. Finally, patients should be instructed either to close the lids for several minutes or to occlude the puncta after the use of eyedrops to minimize systemic absorption and side effects.

COMMENTS

The traditional approach to the treatment of OAG has been to initiate therapy with medications. When maximal tolerable medical therapy failed, argon laser was used. When that failed, surgery was the last resort. Articles have been published that question this approach. Should laser or even surgery be the initial treatment of choice in a newly diagnosed case of OAG? These are valid questions and there should be no dogma in the treatment of this difficult disease. The side effects of medical therapy are common and potentially serious, and they can drastically alter the patient's quality of life and even threaten the patient's survival. The compliance problem must be factored into the treatment equation. Furthermore, the high cost of medications and a patient's inability to keep regular follow-up appointments may justify earlier or even initial laser therapy or filtration surgery. Strong family or racial history, history of glaucomatous loss in a fellow eye, advanced optic nerve cupping and VF loss on the initial examination, and older age all justify early surgical intervention. Studies are available and other studies are under way to help guide physicians and patients in addressing these questions. The most important fact to remember is that the patient with OAG is a unique individual and requires the individualized supervision of a caring eye physician.

REFERENCES

American Academy of Ophthalmology: What's New : Primary Open-Angle Glaucoma Preferred Practice Pattern™ Limited Revision 2003. San Francisco, American Academy of Ophthalmology, 2003.

Hitchings R, Tan J: Target pressure. J Glaucoma 10(5) Supp 1:S68–S70, 2001.

Jampel MD: Laser trabeculoplasty is the treatment of choice for chronic open-angle glaucoma. Arch Ophthalmol 116:240–241, 1998.

Kass MA, Heuer DK, Higginbotham EJ, et al: The ocular hypertension treatment study: a randomized trial determines that topical ocular hypotensive medication delays or prevents the onset of primary open angle glaucoma. Arch Ophthalmol 120:701–713, 2002.

Lichter PR, Musch DC, Gillespie BW, et al: Interim clinical outcomes in the collaborative initial glaucoma treatment study (CIGTS) comparing initial treatment randomized to medications or surgery. Ophthalmology 108:1943–53, 2001.

273 PHACOANAPHYLACTIC ENDOPHTHALMITIS 360.19

(Endophthalmitis Phacoanaphylactica, Phacoanaphylactic Uveitis, Phacoantigenic Uveitis)

Matthew Giegangack MD
Portland, Oregon

ETIOLOGY/INCIDENCE

Phacoanaphylactic endophthalmitis historically has been viewed as an inflammatory disease of the eye resulting from immunologic sensitization of a patient to lens protein released from its sequestered capsular bag by a lens injury, whether surgical, traumatic, or spontaneous. The fact that the liberation of lens protein only rarely causes an immune response has led investigators to conclude that an alteration in the natural tolerance of the body to lens protein is essential for lens protein to become antigenic; this process seems to be T-cell mediated.

Phacoanaphylactic endophthalmitis may occur after penetrating ocular trauma involving the lens, 'uncomplicated' extracapsular cataract surgery, or cataract extraction complicated by posterior luxation of lens material.

COURSE

Onset of inflammation may be as early as 24 hours after a lens injury (although this is more consistent with an infectious cause) or as late as 2 weeks after a lenticular insult. The condition typically presents 3 to 5 days after injury in patients already sensitized to lens protein, whereas 10 to 14 days is more common after initial lens injury.

DIAGNOSIS

Clinical signs and symptoms

Clinically, phacoanaphylactic endophthalmitis may present with a spectrum of signs ranging from a mild anterior uveitis to a severe hypopyon uveitis resembling infectious endophthalmitis.

Ocular

- Eyelid edema.
- Anterior chamber cells and flare.
- Hypopyon.
- Corneal edema.
- Mutton-fat precipitates.
- Striae in Descemet's membrane.
- Conjunctival chemosis, hyperemia.
- Anterior and/or posterior synechiae.
- Pupillary membranes.
- Pupillary seclusion.
- Decreased vision.
- Retinal detachment.
- Secondary glaucoma.

DIAGNOSIS

Because endophthalmitis can have a toxic, mechanical, or infectious cause, a careful history (particularly with respect to recent ocular trauma and concomitant systemic infections) is vital.

Diagnostic ultrasonography is helpful to compensate for hazy media, in identifying retained intravitreal lens material, and to visualize early vitreous organization, indicating the need for prompt vitrectomy and possible intravitreal corticosteroids.

Diagnostic vitrectomy may be performed in an attempt to isolate infectious organisms, depending on the severity of the inflammation. Although intensive systemic and intravitreal antibiotics are essential to salvage an infected eye, they are of no value in the management of phacoanaphylactic endophthalmitis.

Differential diagnosis

Phacoanaphylactic endophthalmitis is readily confused with infectious endophthalmitis; in both conditions, early etiologic diagnosis is imperative to preserve visual function because prolongation of either leads to irreversible damage to ocular structures.

TREATMENT

Aggressive treatment, directed at the most likely cause, is essential; prompt suppression of inflammation to prevent the destruction of ocular tissues by the inflammatory process is the hallmark of therapy. Whenever possible, this may be facilitated by:

- Vitrectomy to remove retained lens material.

Ocular

Vigorous anti-inflammatory therapy consistent with the severity of inflammation should be initiated without delay. High-dose systemic corticosteroids such as:

- Prednisone 80 to 120 mg/day may bring rapid improvement; the dose should be tapered as rapidly as possible.

The therapeutic armamentarium also includes topical corticosteroids:

- Prednisolone acetate 1.0% every hour; and/or
- Sub-Tenon's injections* of corticosteroids (preferably aqueous, not depot).

Cycloplegic/mydriatic agents also can be beneficial.

As the inflammation subsides, the gradual dissolution of intravitreal retained lens material can be monitored with ultrasonography.

REFERENCES

Hodes BL, Stern G: Phacoanaphylactic endophthalmitis: echographic diagnosis of phacoanaphylactic endophthalmitis. Ophthalm Surg 7:60–64, 1976.

Marak G: Phacoanaphylactic endophthalmitis. Surv Ophthalmol 36:325–339, 1992.

Smith RE, Weiner P: Unusual presentation of phacoanaphylactic endophthalmitis following phacoemulsification. Ophthalm Surg 7:65–68, 1976.

274 PIGMENTARY DISPERSION SYNDROME AND PIGMENTARY GLAUCOMA 365.13

James A. Savage, MD
Henderson, Nevada

ETIOLOGY/INCIDENCE

Pigmentary glaucoma is a chronic open-angle glaucoma characterized by loss of pigment from the iris pigment epithelium and its subsequent deposition onto structures of the anterior and posterior chambers. Such pigment shedding and deposition are normal consequences of aging, but occasionally are so pronounced that they constitute *pigmentary dispersion syndrome* (PDS). In PDS, the shedding of pigment is evident as midperipheral radial iris transillumination defects (Figure 274.1). The

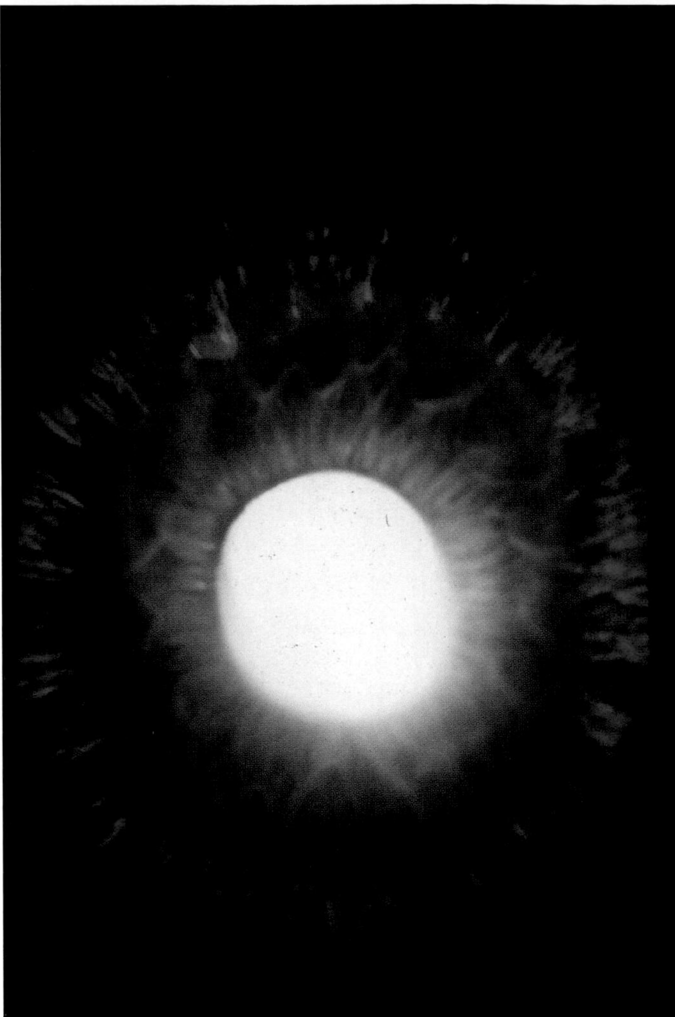

FIGURE 274.1. Iris transillumination defect.

liberated pigment is deposited on the trabecular meshwork, posterior corneal surface (Krukenberg's spindle), and other anterior segment structures. This syndrome is typically found in myopic men during early middle age and less often in women (usually women are older at onset). PDS is rare in black, Hispanic, and Oriental populations and has a male/female incidence of approximately 1 : 1. In some eyes with PDS, the trabecular deposition of pigment causes permanent damage to the aqueous outflow channels, decreases the facility of aqueous outflow, and raises the intraocular pressure, leading to glaucomatous optic nerve and visual field damage; this condition is called *pigmentary glaucoma*, and it has a male/female incidence of approximately 2 : 1.

Pigmentary dispersion syndrome

- Theories of mechanism of pigment shedding.
  - There is mechanical contact between iris pigment epithelium and underlying zonular bundles. Concave iris, elongated zonules, both, other?
  - In reverse pupillary block, some patients experience lessening of iris concavity and pigment shedding after peripheral iridectomy, glaucoma surgery with iridectomy, lens subluxation, or increased relative pupillary block due to cataract formation.
  - There is an intrinsic abnormality of the pigmented epithelium.

These theories are not mutually exclusive; for example, a defective pigment epithelium may be required for a concave iris to shed pigment.

- PDS is typically found in myopic men in early middle age (the patient tends to be older and less myopic if female).
- Most cases appear to be sporadic, although reports of familial incidence suggest an autosomal dominant multifactorial inheritance with delayed expression and variable penetrance.

Pigmentary glaucoma

- Elevated intraocular pressure and typical glaucomatous optic nerve and visual field damage occur due to decreased facility of outflow secondary to pigment-induced degeneration of trabecular structures. The exact mechanism for this pigment-induced damage to outflow pathways is unknown. Some eyes with moderate pigmentary dispersion develop severe glaucoma, whereas other eyes with severe pigment dispersion never develop glaucoma. Approximately 50% of patients with PDS can be expected to develop pigmentary glaucoma (this occurs most commonly in males).

COURSE/PROGNOSIS

Some patients with PDS may have this condition for many years without developing pigmentary glaucoma. The degree of pigment shedding and deposition does not correlate with the future development of pigmentary glaucoma. However, in patients with asymmetric pigmentary glaucoma, the glaucoma tends to be worse in the eye with the most pronounced pigment dispersion.

Pigmentary glaucoma is a chronic open-angle glaucoma that is sometimes punctuated by 'storms' of pigment released into the anterior chamber spontaneously or after pharmacologic mydriasis or exercise. These events can be confused with anterior chamber cells from active anterior segment inflammation, requiring careful examination to differentiate. Pigment storms may present as acute pressure-induced corneal edema with blurring and rainbows.

With advancing age pigment shedding, transillumination defects, and elevated intraocular pressure may abate. It has been speculated that reverse pupillary block decreases with decreasing accommodation and increased lens volume as a consequence of aging.

DIAGNOSIS

Clinical signs and symptoms

Pigmentary dispersion syndrome

- There are radial midperipheral iris transillumination defects, which may be difficult to see with dark and thick iris stroma.
- Pigment deposition on:
  - Corneal endothelium (Krukenberg's spindle);
  - Schwalbe's line (Sampoelesi's line);
  - Trabecular meshwork;
  - Anterior iris surface (sometimes heterochromia in asymmetric cases);
  - Anterior lens capsule;
  - Zonular fibers;
  - Posterior lens surface at zonular insertion (Zentmayer's ring or Scheie's line);
  - Interior of filtration blebs.

- Pigment granules are free in the anterior chamber (greatly increased during pigment 'storms').
- There is myopia.
- The anterior chamber is deep with a concave midperipheral iris, the concavity suggesting reverse pupillary block.
- There is mild iridodonesis.
- The condition is usually bilateral and symmetric; asymmetry may be due to concurrent unilateral development of exfoliative syndrome (increases pigment deposition in affected eye), cataract formation with increased relative pupillary block (decreases), or miosis (e.g. with Horner's syndrome [decreases]).

If pigment dispersion is unilateral, it is important to rule out ocular neoplasm, especially ocular melanoma.

Pigmentary glaucoma

All of the findings for PDS exist plus decreased outflow facility, elevated intraocular pressure, and typical glaucomatous optic nerve and visual field damage.

Differential diagnosis

- Normal eyes with aging (trabecular pigment less marked and less circumferential than in PDS).
- Exfoliative syndrome (older patients, more often unilateral, exfoliative material visible, iris transillumination defects at pupillary margin rather than in its midperiphery).
- Secondary pigmentary glaucoma after cataract extraction and posterior chamber intraocular lens implantation (more common if lens in sulcus than in capsular bag, iris transillumination defects correspond to the location of intraocular lens haptics and/or optic).
- Uveitis (iris transillumination defects such as with herpes zoster or other anterior uveitis, pigment dispersion with anterior uveitis, and pigment granules in anterior chamber from PDS, which may be confused with inflammatory cells).
- Ocular neoplasms (usually unilateral):
  - Iris ring melanoma;
  - Other ocular melanoma;
  - Cysts and other neoplasms of iris and ciliary body.
- Melanocytosis (usually unilateral).
- Ocular trauma:
  - Surgical and accidental;
  - Hyphema;
  - Angle recession;
  - Ghost cell glaucoma (confusion between khaki-colored erythroclasts and liberated pigment granules).
- Acute angle closure.
- Amyloidosis.
- Ocular irradiation.
- Siderosis.
- Hemosiderosis.
- Rhegmatogenous retinal detachment.
- Diabetes mellitus.
- Adie's pupil.

TREATMENT

Treatment is similar to that for primary open-angle glaucoma. Patients with PDS should be followed as glaucoma 'suspects,' with periodic evaluation of intraocular pressure, optic nerve, and visual fields. Also, the clinician should document changes in pigment shedding (iris transillumination defects) and pigment deposition.

Medical

In general, medications used to treat PDS and pigmentary glaucoma are the same as for primary open angle glaucoma. Miotics are used to lower intraocular pressure and to lessen the concavity of the midperipheral iris, iridozonular contact, and, hence, the shedding of pigment. Pilocarpine and other parasympathomimetics have the disadvantage of frequent side effects of brow ache and blurred vision, especially in young patients. In addition, there is an increased risk of retinal detachment with the use of parasympathomimetics in this typically myopic population. Pilocarpine in the form of Pilopine-HS gel or Ocuserts may offer a more gradual, steady, and better tolerated effect than pilocarpine drops every 6 hours.

Dapiprazole, a selective a-adrenergic blocker, produces miosis without cyclotonia and therefore may be much better tolerated than parasympathomimetics such as pilocarpine.

Surgical

Laser therapy

- Argon and selective laser trabeculoplasty:
  - Appear to have equivalent efficacy;
  - Longer-term success is better in younger patients (suggests an increased resistance to the beneficial effects of laser as the disease progresses over time);
  - There may be dramatic improvement in intraocular pressure, but there is some risk of a transient or lasting increase in intraocular pressure after trabeculoplasty;
  - Titrate the laser power to the minimum required to generate the desired visible effect on the trabecular meshwork.
- Laser iridectomy:
  - The contour of the midperipheral iris is changed (possibly eliminates 'reverse pupillary block');
  - Its beneficial effect might be to interrupt the process of pigment shedding/deposition/trabecular damage rather than to immediately lower the intraocular pressure.
- Argon laser iridoplasty:
  - Efforts to flatten the iris and to decrease iridozonular contact with this technique have not shown promise. In addition, inflammation and liberation of pigment from this technique may cause temporary or lasting worsening of intraocular pressure, and the iris concavity can actually be worsened. In view of these findings, the technique appears to be contraindicated in PDS and pigmentary glaucoma.

Filtration surgery

- The success of glaucoma filtration surgery for pigmentary glaucoma appears to be similar to that in primary open-angle glaucoma.

COMPLICATIONS

The side effects of glaucoma medications in general apply. The side effects of miotics, in particular, are ciliary spasm and retinal detachment in this young and myopic population. Increased intraocular pressure after laser procedures may be transient or lasting. The usual possible complications of filtration surgery also apply.

REFERENCES

Campbell DG: Pigmentary dispersion and glaucoma: A new theory. Arch Ophthalmol 97:1667–1672, 1979.

Farrar SM, Shields MB: Current concepts in pigmentary glaucoma. Surv Ophthalmol 37:233–252, 1993.

Farrar SM, Shields MB, Miller KN, et al: Risk factors for the development and severity of glaucoma in the pigment dispersion syndrome. Am J Ophthalmol 108:223–229, 1989.

Migliazzo CV, Shaffer RN, Nykin R, et al: Long-term analysis of pigmentary dispersion syndrome and pigmentary glaucoma. Ophthalmology 93:1528–1536, 1986.

Sugar HS, Barbour FA: Pigmentary glaucoma: a rare clinical entity. Am J Ophthalmol 32:90–92, 1966.

275 PLATEAU IRIS 743.8

Robert Ritch, MD
New York, New York
Clement Chee Yung Tham MD, FRCS, FCOphth(HK)
Hong Kong, China

The term 'plateau iris' was first used by Tornquist in 1958 to describe an anatomic configuration in which the iris is inserted anteriorly on the ciliary body face and the iris root angulates forward and then centrally. The result is somewhat akin to a bird's-eye view of a mesa (hence the name): the iris surface appears flat and the anterior chamber deep on slit lamp examination, but the angle is narrow on gonioscopy, with a sharp drop-off of the peripheral iris. By contrast, in pupillary block angle-closure glaucoma, the most common form of angle-closure glaucoma, the anterior chamber is shallow and the iris surface tends to be convex (iris bombé) (Figure 275.1).

Despite laser iridotomy, the angle of an eye with plateau iris can remain narrow, and the angle can be closed either spontaneously or by dilating the pupil, thus resulting in angle closure.

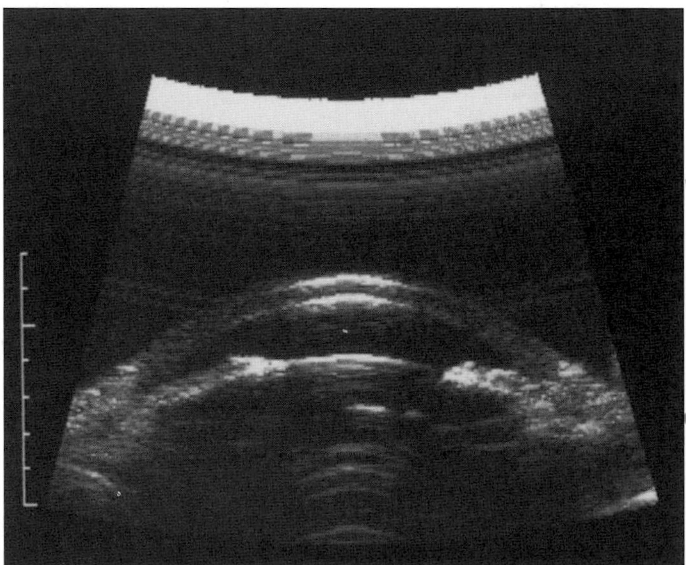

FIGURE 275.1. High frequency ultrasound image of plateau iris syndrome.

This situation is uncommon. Plateau iris syndrome refers to the development of angle closure, either spontaneously or after pupillary dilation, in an eye with plateau iris configuration despite the presence of a patent iridectomy or iridotomy. Some patients may develop elevated intraocular pressure (IOP) or even acute angle-closure glaucoma.

ETIOLOGY/INCIDENCE

Plateau iris results from large and/or anteriorly positioned ciliary processes holding up the peripheral iris and maintaining its apposition to the trabecular meshwork. Two subtypes exist, differentiated according to the level of the structures on the angle-wall occludable by the iris, or the 'height' to which the plateau rises. In the complete syndrome, which comprises the classic situation and is rare, the angle closes to the upper trabecular meshwork or Schwalbe's line, and IOP rises when the angle closes with pupillary dilation. In the incomplete syndrome, which is far more common, the angle closes partially, leaving the upper portion of the filtering meshwork open, and IOP does not change. The incomplete syndrome is clinically significant in that these patients can develop PAS months to years after a successful iridotomy produces what appears as a well-opened angle.

Patients with plateau iris tend to be female, younger (30s to 50s) and less hyperopic than those with relative pupillary block, and often have a family history of angle-closure glaucoma. The fact that iridociliary apposition in plateau iris syndrome persists after cataract extraction suggests that this is a heritable anatomic configuration and not secondary to lens size or position. The younger the patient, the greater the component of angle-crowding by the plateau configuration and the less pupillary block necessary for occludability. Most patients, however, have some element of relative pupillary block superimposed upon a plateau iris configuration, but the extent of pupillary block necessary to induce angle-closure is accordingly less in eyes with plateau iris.

COURSE/PROGNOSIS

If plateau iris syndrome is not diagnosed and treated properly, repeated episodes of angle closure can produce peripheral anterior synechiae and permanent elevation of IOP. The angle can narrow progressively with age due to enlargement of the lens, so that an angle with plateau configuration which does not close after iridotomy may do so some years later. Periodic gonioscopy is required. Argon laser peripheral iridoplasty (ALPI) is the definitive treatment for plateau iris. It is highly effective in eliminating residual appositional closure after laser iridotomy caused by plateau iris syndrome and the effect is maintained for years, although a small proportion of patients may require retreatment.

DIAGNOSIS

The diagnosis of plateau iris configuration can be made with indentation gonioscopy prior to iridotomy. A diagnosis of plateau iris syndrome, however, requires prior elimination of any component of pupillary block by iridotomy.

The anterior chamber is usually of medium depth and the iris surface slightly convex. On gonioscopy, the iris root angulates forward and then centrally. In relative pupillary block, indentation gonioscopy pushes the iris root posteriorly, opening the angle. In plateau iris, the ciliary processes prevent posterior movement of the peripheral iris, resulting in a configuration in which the slit beam follows the curvature of the iris to its deepest point at the periphery of the lens where the ciliary processes begin, then rises again over the ciliary processes before dropping peripherally (double hump sign). Greater force is needed to open the angle than in pupillary block because the ciliary processes must be displaced, and the angle does not open as widely.

Differential diagnosis

If the patient presents with elevated IOP, careful indentation gonioscopy should be performed, as in all cases of glaucoma, so that the condition is not confused with open-angle glaucoma because of the normal depth of the anterior chamber and relatively flat iris surface on direct examination. The most common cause of differential diagnostic confusion on routine examination is a prominent peripheral iris roll. With this iris picture, however, the peripheral iris does not occlude the angle on dilation, and it does not predispose to angle-closure glaucoma.

If the angle remains closed after iridotomy for pupillary block, the first step in the differential diagnosis is to determine whether the closure is appositional or synechial by indentation gonioscopy. If appositional, plateau iris can be diagnosed as above. The other two categories of angle-closure in the differential are phacomorphic glaucoma (intumescent lens) and malignant (ciliary block, aqueous misdirection) glaucoma, in which the anterior chamber is flat or extremely shallow.

Iris and ciliary body cysts can also produce acute or chronic angle-closure. These produce a plateau iris type of configuration (pseudo-plateau iris) and are usually easily diagnosed, as the angle is closed either in one quadrant only or, if there are multiple cysts, intermittently. However, when angle closure mimicking pupillary block occurs, a high index of suspicion and careful gonioscopy are needed to distinguish it from ciliary body and iris cysts.

PROPHYLAXIS

If the angle is spontaneously or pharmacologically occludable with closure above the level of the scleral spur, argon laser peripheral iridoplasty is indicated.

TREATMENT

Treatment must be targeted at the cause of angle-closure, in this case the ciliary body and iris root. If pupillary block is either not a component mechanism of the angle-closure or has been eliminated by iridotomy, it is necessary to find a way to eliminate the physical blockage of the angle. Argon laser peripheral iridoplasty compresses the iris root and creates a space where none was before. This procedure alters the configuration of the plateau iris periphery to remove the sharp angulation. Laser settings of 500 microns spot size, with an exposure time of 0.5 second, and an intensity of 200 to 300 mW achieve sustained contraction of the peripheral iris. If miotics are needed for control of IOP after iridotomy, then iridoplasty is indicated only if the angle remains spontaneously appositionally closed on miotics. If iridoplasty does not relieve all the apposition, weak miotic therapy, such as 2% pilocarpine at bedtime, may open the remaining angle.

If plateau iris configuration is diagnosed incidentally in an eye with an open angle, caution should be exercised in dilation and the patient followed gonioscopically at routine intervals for signs of progressive angle closure. If the angle continues to be narrow, it is sometimes difficult to determine if there is progressive closure of the angle. Monitoring the eye with indentation gonioscopy is valuable for showing progressive angle closure.

REFERENCES

Lowe RF: Plateau iris. Aust J Ophthalmol 9:71, 1981.

Pavlin CJ, Ritch R, Foster FS: Ultrasound biomicroscopy in plateau iris syndrome. Am J Ophthalmol 113:390–395, 1992.

Ritch R: Plateau iris is caused by abnormally positioned ciliary processes. J Glaucoma 1:23–26, 1992.

Ritch R, Tham CCY, Lam DSC: Argon laser peripheral iridoplasty in the management of plateau iris syndrome: long-term follow-up. Ophthalmology 111:104–108, 2004.

Wand M, Pavlin CJ, Foster FS: Plateau iris syndrome: ultrasound biomicroscopic and histological study. Ophthalmic Surg 24:129, 1993.

276 PRIMARY ANGLE-CLOSURE GLAUCOMA 365.20

(Primary Closed-Angle Glaucoma)

Emily Patterson, MD

Portland, Oregon

ETIOLOGY/INCIDENCE

Primary angle-closure glaucoma is caused by increased intraocular pressure due to obstruction of aqueous humor outflow from the anterior chamber, which results from closure of the angle by the peripheral root of the iris. It is a bilateral disease and affects patients with anatomically narrow angles. The trabecular meshwork is structurally and functionally normal before closure of the angle takes place.

In its early stages, closure of the angle is nothing more than contact between the trabecular meshwork and the root of the iris, and it is reversible once pupillary block is eliminated. Over time, however, the root of the iris develops adhesions to the trabecular meshwork, forming peripheral anterior synechiae that cannot be relieved by breaking the pupillary block.

Although the mechanism of the pressure rise is the same in each patient, symptoms vary markedly depending on the magnitude and speed of the intraocular pressure rise.

- Angle shallowing, and then closure, develops in eyes with an anatomically narrow anterior chamber angle.
- Relative pupillary block, which obstructs the flow of the aqueous from the posterior chamber into the anterior chamber, plays an important role in the pathogenesis of the disease.
- The condition usually occurs in those older than 40, with a predilection for women. This is because as the lens ages, it grows in its anterior-posterior diameter and crowds the anterior chamber. Women are believed more susceptible because their eyes are slightly smaller.

- Hyperopia is a strong risk factor for this condition. Hyperopic eyes are shorter and their anterior segments more crowded than emmetropic or myopic eyes.
- It is less common than primary open-angle glaucoma in whites and blacks but much more common in Inuits; the incidence in Asians is intermediate.

COURSE/PROGNOSIS

With prodromal or intermittent angle-closure glaucoma, symptoms are caused by the rapid elevations and decreases of the intraocular pressure. A steamy, hazy cornea is caused by the abrupt rise in pressure as a result of sudden angle occlusion. Symptoms classically include foggy or hazy vision with rainbow-colored haloes around lights. Ocular congestion or discomfort may occur. Symptoms spontaneously subside in a few hours if the pupillary block is relieved by miosis. The miosis may occur when the patient goes to a brighter environment or goes to sleep.

In the acute attack of primary angle-closure glaucoma, the symptoms are precipitated by pupillary dilation resulting from mydriatic drops, dim light, or emotional upset. Once angle closure is established, the symptoms of the intermittent or prodromal attack intensify and endure; they include blurred vision and haloes, conjunctival injection, and severe pain. In addition, nausea and vomiting may occur and are due to autonomic stimulation.

In chronic primary angle-closure glaucoma, the intraocular pressure rises insidiously as the closed area of the angle gradually increases, and patients may be totally free from symptoms or may experience some ocular discomfort and haloes. This variant may mimic chronic open-angle glaucoma if the gonioscopic findings are missed.

DIAGNOSIS

Clinical signs and symptoms

Ocular

Two major subtypes of primary angle-closure glaucoma-acute angle-closure glaucoma (indicated as A) and chronic angle-closure glaucoma (indicated as C) show different ocular signs:

- Anterior chamber: shallow (A and C), flare (A), clear (C);
- Chamber angle: closed (A and C) or narrow (C);
- Conjunctiva: chemosis (A), hyperemia (A);
- Cornea: epithelial edema (A), folds in Descemet's membrane (A), hypesthesia (A), pigment on the posterior surface (A);
- Iris: convex (C), forward displacement (A), peripheral anterior synechiae (A and C), posterior synechiae (A), sector atrophy, usually in the upper half (A);
- Lens: glaukomflecken (A);
- Pupil: dilation, vertical ovalization, mid-dilated, fixed position (A);
- Miscellaneous: increased intraocular pressure (A and C), visual field defects (A and C).

Differential diagnosis

- Chronic angle-closure glaucoma can be differentiated from primary open-angle glaucoma with a narrow angle by gonioscopy.
- In acute angle closure, the differential includes: secondary angle-closure glaucoma due to dislocated lens; phacolytic glaucoma; secondary angle-closure glaucoma due to an intumescent cataract; and secondary angle-closure glaucoma due to uveitis (inflammatory glaucoma).

TREATMENT

Systemic

- Hyperosmotic agents are preferred to break an acute attack: oral glycerin in a 50% solution at a dose of 2 to 3 ml/kg, oral isosorbide in doses of 1 to 2 g/kg is preferred in patients with diabetes, and isosorbide is usually tolerated better than glycerin.
- In patients with nausea or vomiting, 20% mannitol IV may be given in a dose of 1 to 2 g/kg, although 500 mg of acetazolamide IV is better.

Ocular

- Treatment is indicated to break an acute attack and control the intraocular pressure until laser iridotomy can be performed, or to manage residual glaucoma after an acute incident.
- Cholinergic agents should be used to pull the iris away from the angle in the eyes in acute attack: one or two drops of 1% to 3% pilocarpine every 5 minutes for 4 doses and then every 1 to 2 hours.
- In an acute case, β-adrenergic-blocking agents, topical carbonic anhydrase inhibitors, and prostaglandin analogs may be added to the regimen of miotics. Corticosteroids (e.g. 1% prednisolone acetate), are useful in controlling inflammation. Dipivefrin is contraindicated before iridotomy, and brimonidine may be less effective or ineffective.
- In a chronic case, medical treatment without laser iridotomy should be temporary.
- The treatment of chronic angle-closure glaucoma after laser iridotomy is similar to that of primary open-angle glaucoma.

Surgical

The treatment of primary angle-closure glaucoma consists of laser iridotomy or peripheral surgical iridectomy after the intraocular pressure has been normalized. In acute angle-closure glaucoma, the eye should be operated on promptly. Iridectomy may be done surgically, or argon or Q-switched Nd:YAG laser may be used to create an iridotomy (laser iridotomy). If the acute attack of angle closure does not respond to intensive medical therapy, filtration surgery may be considered.

In chronic primary angle-closure glaucoma, laser iridotomy is the operation of choice. It should be performed urgently, even if intraocular pressure is completely normalized with medical therapy, in order to prevent progression to synechial angle closure. Filtration surgery should not be performed unless iridotomy has failed to normalize the intraocular pressure.

Other

- The patient with acute primary angle-closure glaucoma should be hospitalized to initiate the intensive medical therapy that is usually a prelude to surgery.
- Analgesics may be used to control pain; the administration of 300 to 600 mg of aspirin every 6 to 8 hours is usually adequate.

COMPLICATIONS

Intravenous hyperosmotic agents cause headache, dizziness, nausea, and vomiting; oral glycerin particularly tends to induce nausea. Urinary retention may be brought about by intense diuresis. Pulmonary edema and congestive heart failure may be precipitated in elderly patients with borderline cardiac and renal function; this is especially true of mannitol, which greatly increases blood volume. Cellular dehydration, including cerebral dehydration, occurs more often with mannitol and may result in mental disorientation.

COMMENTS

Acute primary angle-closure glaucoma is an ophthalmic emergency and requires immediate medical therapy. All medical measures should be used simultaneously to normalize the elevated intraocular pressure. Once the pressure is brought under control, indentation gonioscopy with a Zeiss four-mirrored lens or other indirect goniolens is necessary to confirm the diagnosis and to evaluate the extent of peripheral anterior synechiae. The more extensive the peripheral anterior synechiae, the more likely that antiglaucoma medications will be needed to maintain a normal intraocular pressure after iridotomy. The fellow eye should also be treated with topical miotics to avoid an acute attack until iridotomy can be performed on it as well. Prophylactic laser iridotomy is preferable to surgical iridectomy because of its safety and convenience. Occasionally an iridotomy may fibrose and close, especially in the setting of intraocular inflammation, and may need to be repeated once or more before it remains open.

Chronic primary angle-closure glaucoma should also be treated surgically even when the intraocular pressure is normalized with medication. Because pupillary block cannot be eliminated by medical therapy, peripheral anterior synechiae will progress in the setting of chronic or intermittent angle closure, regardless of the intraocular pressure.

REFERENCES

Fleck BW, Fairley EA: A randomized prospective comparison of operative peripheral iridectomy and Nd:YAG laser iridotomy treatment of acute angle closure glaucoma: 3 year visual acuity and intraocular pressure control study. Br J Ophthalmol 81:884–888, 1997.

Sakuma T, Sawada A, Yamamoto T, et al: Appositional angle closure in eyes with narrow angles: An ultrasound biomicroscopic study. J Glaucoma 6:165–169, 1997.

Saw SM, Gazzard G, Friedman DS: Interventions for angle-closure glaucoma: an evidence-based update. Ophthalmology 110(10):1867–1868, 2003.

Sugar HS: Surgical decision, technique and complications of peripheral iridectomy for angle-closure glaucoma. Ann Ophthalmol 7:1237–1241, 1975.

Wolfs RCW, Grobbee DE, Hofman A, et al: Risk of acute angle-closure glaucoma after diagnostic mydriasis in nonselected subjects: The Rotterdam study. Invest Ophthalmol Vis Sci 38:2683–2687, 1997.

SECTION

24 Iris and Ciliary Body

277 ACCOMMODATIVE SPASM 367.53
(Spasm of the Near Reflex)

Cameron F. Parsa, MD
Baltimore, Maryland

ETIOLOGY/INCIDENCE

Accommodative spasm refers to an episodic, excessive contraction of the ciliary muscle. In some cases, it may result from the direct effects of parasympathomimetic drugs such as pilocarpine. In general, however, the term is used to describe spontaneous excess parasympathetic activity as part of the near reflex triad (e.g. accommodation, miosis, and convergence). The term is often used interchangeably with *spasm of the near reflex*, although not all components of the near reflex triad may always be apparent. Just as accommodation, convergence, and miosis may be present to different degrees, so, too, may the symptoms vary in patients with spasm of the near reflex.

Short-lived, episodic, isolated symptomatic spasm of the near reflex in nearly all cases is considered to be functional in origin (this should not be misinterpreted to indicate that it is voluntary). A high incidence of personality disorders is noted in individuals in these instances, and nonphysiologic visual loss may be an associated sign in some. Nevertheless, an examination should be performed to ensure that accompanying signs (e.g. nystagmus, papilledema, ataxia, endocrine abnormalities) are not overlooked and that associated disease is not missed.

The exact anatomic locus for episodic spasm of the near reflex remains unknown in the rare cases with underlying organic disease; presumably, it may arise from disruption at a number of sites. Any condition that may stimulate pathways of the near reflex, or supranuclear control, have been reported to cause accommodative spasm:

- Posterior fossa tumors;
- Central nervous system infections;
- Head trauma;
- Cerebrovascular injuries;
- Metabolic or toxic disorders;
- Vestibular disorders.

Morphine can provoke spasm of the near reflex via the supranuclear inhibition of parasympathetic inhibitory neurons, and *excessive alcohol intake* also may cause temporary spasm.

DIAGNOSIS

Clinical symptoms

Patients may present with one or more of the following symptoms:

- Blurred vision;
- Diplopia;
- Brow ache (bilateral), headache.

Attacks accompanied by 'discomfort' may prompt some patients to squint their eyelids, mimicking photophobia; excessive convergence effort may produce:

- Frank esotropia with diplopia;
- Unilateral or bilateral limitation of abduction.

Functional episodes of spasm are generally brief, typically lasting only seconds to minutes. When produced by head trauma, symptoms, though milder, may last for years, often without discernable miosis. Spasm can also be sustained when physiological in nature, to improve acuity when refractive error is poorly corrected.

Clinical signs

- Excessive accommodation, resulting in pseudomyopia (up to 10 diopters), easily noted when comparing manifest to cycloplegic refractions.
- Marked bilateral miosis, which may increase further on attempted abduction.
- Variable, intermittent convergence.
- Monocular occlusion of either eye (interrupting the stimulus for convergence) allows full abduction, as well as pupillary dilation.
- Oculocephalic testing (doll's head maneuver) demonstrating full range of eye movements.

In cases associated with organic disease, visual input may not be necessary to maintain spasm, and diagnostic signs present in functional cases (e.g. pupillary dilation during monocular occlusion) may be absent. An investigation for underlying disease should be initiated at this point. Rarely, occlusion of an eye can fail to 'break' an attack even in functional cases. Such so-called monocular or unilateral cases of accommodative spasm simply require the occlusion of the *dominant* eye to block the visual input, alleviating the spasm. It should be remembered that in functional cases, any attention directed to the eyes, including monocular occlusion, may precipitate an attack.

Accommodative spasm can also result from physiologic efforts. Prolonged monocular near work causing over-accommodative effort (i.e. instrument myopia or instrument accommodation) may also habituate an individual to develop accommodative spasm whenever binocularity is interrupted. Furthermore, miosis can also be invoked as part of the near-reflex triad for the purposes of improving acuity, with symptoms then related to excessive convergence.

Differential diagnosis

When excessive convergence is the presenting component of the triad, the differential diagnosis may include:

- Sixth nerve palsies;
- Thyroid eye disease (involving the medial rectus muscles);
- Simple convergent strabismus;
- Divergence insufficiency. In some cases, however, poorly corrected refractive errors or presbyopia can elicit compensatory miosis to help improve acuity via the near-reflex triad, with or without accommodative ability. Over a sustained period, the associated excessive convergence input to the medial rectus muscles may itself cause alterations producing a divergence insufficiency;
- Oculomotor apraxia or horizontal gaze palsy (congenital or acquired) with convergence substitution movements;
- Substitutive convergence movements in response to other underlying disorders (e.g. myasthenia, multiple sclerosis, stroke, etc.). Activation of the near reflex may be elicited to assist in horizontal gaze or to reduce a potential exotropia. However, in most instances, the near reflex is not invoked in primary gaze;
- Parinaud's syndrome, which can mimic some aspects of spasm of the near reflex, such as excessive accommodation and convergence; however, pupillary near-light dissociation, not miosis, is a feature of Parinaud's syndrome.

TREATMENT

Ocular

Intermittent attacks of accommodative spasm may occur over periods lasting from weeks to years. Treatment is generally based on the relief of symptoms but may take a variety of forms, often depending on whether the patient also manifests excessive convergence. Younger patients tend to present complaining of blurring of vision from the excessive accommodation; the combination of:

- Cycloplegics, such as atropine, to break the accommodative component; and
- Refractive correction for distance with reading addition will eventually provide symptomatic relief from associated problems in most cases. If cycloplegic therapy is discontinued, however, symptoms may recur. Paradoxically, minus lenses have also been used to correct some degree of pseudomyopia and provide clearer vision; over time, one may be able to reduce the power of the lenses.

Although this last approach is well accepted by some patients, particularly those with spasm consequent to head trauma, it would have no effect in reducing the convergent drive and diplopia or any other symptomatology; its success in some patients may be related to functional pathogenesis.

Patients with presbyopia who present with spasm of the near reflex may complain of excessive convergence rather than blurred vision. Approaches focused on accommodative efforts alone in this population may work in fewer instances. Aside from the correction of any refractive error to reduce the drive for acuity-enhancing miosis:

- Monocular occlusion can be used therapeutically, as well as in diagnosis; if the episodes of spasm are brief and infrequent, closing of one or both eyes during an attack may be the most practical treatment. If episodes are very frequent or long, monocular occlusion with a patch may be preferred, similarly, glasses with the medial third of each lens frosted or with semi-translucent tape placed to occlude vision while the eyes are converged may resolve excessive convergent drive.

Supportive

In patients with attacks that are *episodic*, reassurance and a careful explanation of the condition should be provided; in certain cases, psychiatric counseling may be of benefit. In several reports, barbiturate or benzodiazepine use, occasionally with hypnotic suggestion of orthotropia, provided temporary relief, underscoring the supranuclear and functional origin of this entity in the near totality of episodic cases. Particularly in patients with isolated *sustained* findings, however, an underlying physiologic need, i.e. accommodative or miotic compensation for refractive error, may be at fault. Only in rare instances, either from previous head trauma or with other pathology noted on examination is organic disease is the cause.

REFERENCES

Chan RV, Trobe JD: Spasm of accommodation associated with closed head trauma. J Neuro-Ophthalmol 22:15–17, 2002.

Cogan DG, Freese CG, Jr: Spasm of the near reflex. Arch Ophthalmol 54:752–759, 1955.

Dagi LR, Chrousos GA, Cogan DC: Spasm of the near reflex associated with organic disease. Am J Ophthalmol 103:582–585, 1987.

Guiloff RJ, Whitely A, Kelly RE: Organic convergence spasm. Acta Neurol Scand 61:252–259, 1980.

Ohashi T, Kase M, Hyodo T, et al: Long-lasting organic spasm of the near reflex. Jpn J Ophthalmol 32:466–470, 1988.

278 ANIRIDIA 743.45
(Congenital Aniridia, Hereditary Aniridia)

David Sellers Walton, MD
Boston, Massachusetts
Garyfallia Katsavounidou, MS
Boston, Massachusetts

ETIOLOGY/INCIDENCE

Aniridia is a rare (1 : 80,000), genetically determined bilateral pan-ocular disorder characterized by decreased visual acuity and abnormal development of the cornea, iris, filtration angle, retina, and optic nerve and complicated by progressive keratopathy, cataracts, glaucoma, and further visual loss. Ocular examination in infancy typically reveals near-complete but variable absence of the irides. The corneas are small, abnormally thick, and possess a zone of peripheral epithelial opacifacation. Pendular nystagmus is often (90%) present. The visual acuity is typically impaired and when tested in early childhood confirms decreased acuity between 20/200 and 20/80 related to retinal foveal hypoplasia.

Occurrence is sporadic or familial (66%), and transmission supports autosomal dominant inheritance. Haploinsufficiency secondary to a mutation of one aniridia gene (*PAX6*) or chromosomal deletion causes aniridia. *PAX6* is located in the highly conserved PAX 6 region on chromosome 11 (11p13) and encodes a highly conserved PAX protein. Penetrance is high, and its clinical expression is variable. Over 200 *PAX6* mutations have been identified. When aniridia is caused by a chromosomal deletion (11p⁻), the Wilms' tumor gene (*WT1*), located 700 kb telomeric from *PAX6*, may also be affected, putting the patient at risk (50%) for a Wilms' tumor and other abnormalities found in the WAGR syndrome (Wilms' tumor, genitourinary anomalies, developmental delay). When aniridia is associated with a chromosomal deletion, the ocular defects seem to be clinically more severe.

COURSE/PROGNOSIS

Aniridic eyes often experience progressive visual deterioration. Visual loss occurs secondary to progressive corneal opacifacation, uncontrolled glaucoma, and cataract formation. Cortical lens opacities are present by 10 years of age, associated with slow lens growth, and progress with age. Glaucoma has been described in 5–75% of reported aniridic patients with onset typically in the first decade. Keratopathy typically progresses centripetally and may become associated with dense central dense opacifacation and secondary vision loss. These dystrophic complications of aniridia develop slowly with variable expression between patients.

DIAGNOSIS

Clinical signs and symptoms

- Diagnosis is made by ophthalmologic examination with recognition of the pathonomonic corneal opacifacation, iris hypoplasia, and foveal hypoplasia. Familial occurrence provides additional diagnostic evidence.
- Aniridic glaucoma is detected on the basis of intraocular pressure measurements associated with responsible gonioscopic abnormalities.

Laboratory findings

- Chromosomal deletion (11p–) is detected by cytogenetic analysis with the use of high-resolution banding.
- Submicroscopic deletions of the Wilms' tumor gene are recognized with the FISH technique.
- PCR genotyping of halotypes across PAX6- WT1 region for homozygosity provides evidence of a chromosomal deletion.

Differential diagnosis

- Rieger syndrome with iridocorneal dysgenesis.
- Congenital coloboma of the iris.
- Hereditary iris hypoplasia.
- Traumatic iris injury.
- Surgical iris coloboma.
- Bilateral congenital mydriasis.
- Isolated internal ophthalmoplegia.
- Gillespie syndrome.
- Primary congenital newborn glaucoma.

PROPHYLAXIS

Early goniosurgery to shift the iris insertion more posteriorly away from the trabecular meshwork may decrease the incidence or delay the onset of acquired glaucoma.

TREATMENT

Medical

- Medical glaucoma therapy for increased intraocular pressure.

Surgical

- Filtration glaucoma or glaucoma drainage device surgery for glaucoma resistant to medical therapy.
- Keratolimbal allograft for corneal epithelial decompensation.
- Cataract extraction and intraocular lens implantation.
- Occlusion therapy for acute symptomatic corneal epithelial failure.

SUPPORT GROUP

USA Aniridia Network
1138 N. Germantown Pkwy-Siute 101
Cordova, Tennessee, 38016
Ph: 901-752-8835
Fax: 901-757-4022
E-mail: info@aniridia.net
Website: www.aniridia.net

REFERENCES

Chen TC, Walton DS: Goniosurgery for prevention of aniridic glaucoma. Arch Ophthalmol 117:1144–1148, 1999.

Glaser T, Walton DS, Maas RL: Genomic structure, evolutionary conservation and aniridia mutations in the human *PAX6* gene. Nat Genet 2:232–239, 1992.

Gupta KB, DeBecker I, Guernsey DL, et al: Polymerase chain reaction-based risk assessment for wilms tumor in sporatic aniridia. Am J Ophthalmol 125:687–692, 1998.

Mayer KL, Nordlund ML, Schwartz GS, et al: Keratoplasty in congenital aniridia. The Ocular Surface 1:74–79, 2003.

Nelson NB, Spaeth GL, Nowinski TS, et al: Aniridia: a review. Surv Ophthalmol 28:621–642, 1984.

Riccardi VM, Sujansky E, Smith AL, et al: Chromosomal imbalance in the aniridia-Wilms' tumor association: 11p interstitial deletion. Pediatrics 61:604–610, 1978.

279 CILIARY BODY CONCUSSIONS AND LACERATIONS 921.3

Igor Westra, MD, MSc
Wilmington, North Carolina

ETIOLOGY

Ciliary body concussions and lacerations are injuries that usually accompany damage to other structures of the eye. Mild blunt trauma may produce a transient iritis with cells and flare in the anterior chamber and anterior vitreous, as well as a relative hypotony. More severe blunt trauma may result in pupillary sphincter rupture, iridodialysis, angle recession, and cyclodialysis. Cyclodialysis is defined as separation of the ciliary body from the scleral spur and may be associated with hyphema, choroidal detachment, hypotony, and inflammation.

Ciliary body concussions and lacerations are secondary to blunt or perforating penetrating trauma. Automobile air bag and paintball injuries are modern causes of ciliary body trauma. Lacerations of the ciliary body usually result from perforations or penetrations, as of the cornea or anterior sclera; however, some objects that penetrate the skin of the lid at or even outside the orbital rim may bypass the conjunctival sac and produce scleral and uveal penetration posteriorly. Penetrating injuries caused by small projectiles may create anterior, as well as posterior, lacerations.

COURSE/PROGNOSIS

Once the choroid is separated from the sclera, aqueous may drain into the suprachoroidal space. This commonly results in profound hypotony. Prolonged hypotony may result in irreversible complications, including iris atrophy, angle-closure glaucoma, cataract, loss of retinal pigment epithelium from crests of choroidal folds, cystoid macular edema, optic atrophy, and phthisis bulbi. Decreased function of the ciliary body may also lead to difficulty with accommodation. Other late manifestations of blunt trauma include secondary glaucoma associated with major circumferential areas of angle recession. Extensive ciliary body injuries may involve necrosis of major portions of the pars plicata and lead to extensive fibrosis or atrophy. Massive fibrosis and vascularization of the vitreous may follow, with subsequent retinal detachment.

DIAGNOSIS

- There is a history of trauma.
- Slit-lamp ophthalmoscopy and gonioscopy should be performed, looking for angle recession, hyphema, shallow anterior chamber, Tyndall effect, iris atrophy, iridodialysis cellular debris, cyclodialysis cleft, sphincter rupture, and cataract.
- Eyes injured by blunt trauma require gonioscopic evaluation. When there is a hyphema, the examination is carried out after it clears. If a hypotonous cyclodialysis cleft is suspected, use of the Goldmann three-mirror lens is recommended.
- Tonometry is performed, looking for hypotony.
- Indirect ophthalmoscopy is performed, looking for detachment, exudative detachment rupture, choroidal folds, Berlin's edema, dialysis, retinal hemorrhages, vitreous hemorrhage, macular edema, papilledema, and optic nerve atrophy.
- Indirect ophthalmoscopy, orbital radiography, computed tomography scanning, and ultrasound evaluation may be used to locate a foreign body.

TREATMENT

Ocular

- Protection from further injury is provided by using a Fox shield.
- A topical cycloplegic, such as 1% atropine twice per day or 1% cyclopentolate four times per day, may be administered.
- Topical corticosteroids may be given four to six times per day to limit the inflammatory reaction. In the presence of hyphema, bed rest and the administration of 50 mg/kg aminocaproic acid orally every 4 hours for 5 days decrease the occurrence of recurrent hemorrhage. Tranexamic acid 75 mg/kg/day in three divided doses is another choice. Both these agents reduce the incidence of secondary bleeding through the inhibition of the conversion of plasminogen to plasmin. These oral agents may cause nausea, vomiting, dizziness and postural hypotension. They should not be used in pregnant patients or in patients with renal or hepatic impairment. Topical aminocaproic acid, one drop every 6 hours for 5 days, has been designated as an orphan drug and may be available soon in the United States. It has the advantage of minimal systemic side effects.
- Sedation and pain medication may be necessary for patient comfort.
- If a cyclodialysis cleft is found, medical treatment with 1% atropine twice a day for 2 to 6 weeks is used in an attempt to approximate the ciliary body and sclera. Unless there is significant uveitis, corticosteroids are avoided because they inhibit the scarring necessary for cleft closure.
- Reversal of hypotony by any means within 2 months results in the best visual acuity. A delay in treatment results in the loss of one to three Snellen lines of ultimate visual acuity. Spontaneous closure seldom occurs after 6 weeks.

Surgical

- If the ciliary body concussion has resulted in a shallow anterior chamber, a hypotonous cyclodialysis cleft is suspected. Pilocarpine 2% is administered to maximize the pupil constriction and open clefts. The chamber is deepened by making a stab incision and intracamerally infusing the sodium hyaluronate. Retrobulbar anesthesia is administered. A stab incision is made at the limbus, sodium hyaluronate is injected through the incision, and the pressure is adjusted to between 10 and 20 mm Hg by releasing aqueous humor. The stab incision is then closed with a single 10-0 nylon suture. The angle can then be examined by gonioscopy, and argon laser photocoagulation can be performed. To avoid postoperative ocular hypertension, the anterior chamber is irrigated with balanced salt solution through the reopened limbal incision, and sodium hyaluronate is aspirated out through a second stab incision. These incisions are subsequently closed with 10-0 nylon, with care taken to bury the knots. A subconjunctival injection of an antibiotic such as 125 mg of cefuroxime should be given. Atropine 1% one drop twice a day and an antibiotic drop, such as moxifloxacin or gatifloxacin one drop three times per day, are given. Corticosteroids are avoided.
- In a few cases, hidden clefts may be found by injecting fluorescein into the anterior chamber and making sclerostomies over the ciliary body in all four quadrants. Detection of fluorescein in the suprachoridal fluid confirms the presence of an occult cyclodialysis cleft. Immersion B-scan ultrasound or ultrasound biomicroscopy may also be helpful.
- If medical treatment of the hypotonous cyclodialysis cleft has failed, laser treatment is administered. After expansion of the anterior chamber with sodium hyaluronate, as

described, contiguous rows of argon laser burns causing bubble formation are delivered to the scleral surface. A Goldmann lens with 100- to 200-μm spot size, 0.1-second time setting, and high power settings of 2000 to 3000 mW is recommended. The uveal surface is also treated but with a lower power setting of 1000 mW, which causes an intense blanching. In cases in which prelaser anterior chamber deepening is not required, retrobulbar anesthesia is recommended for patient comfort. Atropine 1% drops twice a day are used for several weeks.

- Contact transscleral diode laser treatment of the cleft areas has also been effective. The anterior chamber is expanded as described. The Iris 'G' probe (Iris Medical Instruments, Mountainview, CA) is used to apply laser to the cleft using settings of 1500 mW and 1500 milliseconds. Two rows of treatment are applied 1.5 mm posterior to the limbus for the extent of the cleft. Postoperative medical management is the same as that with argon laser treatment.
- Laser treatment is usually effective, but if several laser sessions have been unsuccessful, other surgery may be necessary. Techniques include vitrectomy and intraocular gas tamponade, ciliochoroidal diathermy, cycloplexy, cryoablation, and an anterior scleral buckling procedure.
- When surgical repair of a ciliary body laceration is performed, cultures should be taken of the wound.
- Ciliary body tissue is excised only if it is necrotic, severely traumatized, or grossly contaminated. If a cyclectomy is necessary, encircling transscleral diathermy may be indicated to decrease bleeding and subsequent ciliary body detachment.
- Meticulous reconstruction of corneal and scleral lacerations by microsurgical techniques should be undertaken as soon as possible after careful evaluation. The surgical goals are to maintain the contour of the eye and obtain a liquid-tight seal.
- The loss of corneal or scleral tissue may require replacement with patch grafting.
- For corneal closure, 10-0 nylon sutures are used; 7-0 or 8-0 nonabsorbable sutures are preferred for scleral repair.
- Suturing of the ciliary body laceration is rarely indicated.
- After primary repair of the lacerations, secondary repair may be necessary for the management of associated injuries, such as disrupted lens, vitreous hemorrhage, vitreous traction, retinal breaks, and retinal detachment. Although some believe that immediate vitrectomy is preferable, a 7- to 10-day interval allows for choroidal hemorrhages to recede, decreases the risk of intraoperative hemorrhage, and allows for spontaneous separation of the posterior hyaloid, which makes the procedure safer. Safety is also enhanced by preoperative ultrasound evaluation of eyes where the view of the posterior pole is limited.
- Delay of secondary repair past 2 weeks runs the risk of severe intraocular proliferative membranes. Vitrectomy is carried out under controlled conditions with an infusion line to keep the intraocular pressure constant and instrumentation that passes through 0.88-mm sclerostomies.
- Scleral buckling may be required for retinal pathology or is placed prophylactically by some surgeons.
- Postoperative medications consist of topical antibiotics, such as moxifloxacin or gatifloxacin three times per day for 1 week, 1% prednisolone acetate four times per day for several weeks depending on inflammation, and 0.25% scopolamine twice a day for several weeks.

COMPLICATIONS

Complications include decreased accommodation, cataract, secondary glaucoma, cystoid macular edema, and phthisis bulbi.

PRECAUTIONS

When faced with a ciliary body laceration associated with a severely traumatized eye, the question of a primary enucleation may arise. Primary enucleation of traumatized eyes should be avoided, especially if there is any visual function. Patients appreciate that everything possible has been done to save their eyes. Often, traumatized eyes look better after primary and secondary repair, and occasionally remarkable recoveries occur. Sympathetic ophthalmia is a remote possibility that should be discussed with the patient. If secondary repair has failed, enucleation can still be performed within the 2-week time period that is thought to be protective from sympathetic ophthalmia.

COMMENTS

Concussions and lacerations of the ciliary body usually accompany injuries to other ocular structures; an examination that is as complete as possible should be carried out as promptly as feasible without exacerbating the injury. Delay in examination may allow hemorrhage and inflammation to obscure intraocular details. Ophthalmic ultrasound can be a valuable adjunct. Lacerations require immediate treatment, and hypotonous cyclodialysis clefts should be treated within a 2-month period. Patients with ciliary body injuries require long-term follow-up to watch for complications, such as cataract and angle recession resulting in glaucoma.

REFERENCES

Brooks AMV, Troski M, Gillies WE: Noninvasive closure of a persistent cyclodialysis cleft. Ophthalmology 103:1943–1945, 1996.

Brown SVL, Mizen T: Transscleral diode laser therapy for traumatic cyclodialysis cleft. Ophthalmic Surg Lasers 28:313–317, 1996.

Crouch ER, Crouch ER: Trauma: ruptures and bleeding. In: Tasman W, ed: Clinical ophthalmology. Philadelphia, JB Lippincott, CD-ROM, 2006:4:61.

Ormerod LD, Baerveldt G, Sunalp MA, et al: Management of the hypotonous cyclodialysis cleft. Ophthalmology 98:1384–1393, 1991.

Recchia FM, Aaberg T, Sternberg, P: Trauma: principles and techniques of treatment. In: Ryan SJ, ed: Retina. Philadelphia, Elsevier, 2006:2379–2402.

280 FUCHS' HETEROCHROMIC IRIDOCYCLITIS 364.21
(Fuchs Uveitis Syndrome)

Thomas J. Liesegang, MD
Jacksonville, Florida

Fuchs heterochromic iridocyclitis is readily recognized by its classic clinical appearance, which includes heterochromia of the irides (usually the lighter iris is present in the involved eye), the absence of conjunctival inflammation, specific atrophic changes on the iris surface, minimal cell and flare, widely scattered small nonconfluent keratic precipitates, vitreous cells, the absence of posterior synechiae, a complicated cataract, and occasional glaucoma. The expanded form of the disease has been described by several authors as having additional findings and a poorer prognosis.

ETIOLOGY/INCIDENCE

Fuchs heterochromic iridocyclitis can occur at all ages in both sexes. It may present as an asymptomatic finding early in its course with minimal ocular symptoms of floaters or in some patients only after the development of a cataract. The disease is recognized in approximately 5% of patients presenting with uveitis. In approximately 10% of cases, the disease is bilateral, and clinical astuteness is required to make the diagnosis. If the disease is unilateral at presentation, it usually remains a unilateral disease. The diagnosis is made based on clinical findings; there are no distinct laboratory findings.

- From 1.2% to 4.5% of patients with uveitis.
- No racial or sexual predilection.
- From 7.8% to 10% with bilateral disease.
- No definitive HLA or familial concurrence.
- Unknown cause: probably immune (hypersecretion of plasma cells, antibodies against corneal epithelial protein, anterior chamber immune response to antigen, possibly viral).
- Cause may be multifactorial or may be initiated by multiple single stimuli.

COURSE/PROGNOSIS

- Frequently asymptomatic or mild; fluctuates over time.
- Long insidious course.
- Occasional symptoms of discomfort, ciliary injection, increase in floaters.
- Visual loss from vitreous debris, progressive cataract, glaucoma.
- Cataract surgery generally successful.
- Variable course of glaucoma, may be progressive and refractory.
- Vitreous debris possibly requiring vitrectomy.

DIAGNOSIS

Clinical signs and symptoms

Classic features

- Quiet external eye.
- Heterochromia with involved eye lighter in color:
  - Paler hue to involved iris;
  - In brown eyes, may be very subtle.
- Unilateral disease:
  - Bilateral in 10%, frequently missed when bilateral.
- Anterior iris atrophy, especially peripupillary:
  - Atrophy of anterior and posterior layers;
  - Blunting, flattening, blurring, or washed-out appearance of iris crypts.
- Hyaline keratic precipitates with intervening filaments:
  - Small, round, nonpigmented, translucent keratic precipitates;
  - Keratic precipitates can extend up the entire back surface of the cornea;
  - Cotton-wisp filaments between precipitates.
- Minimal anterior chamber cell and flare:
  - Variable at each examination.
- Occasional iris crystals.
- Absence of posterior synechiae a distinguishing feature.
- Occasional gelatinous iris nodules:
  - Busacca nodules on the iris surface;
  - Koeppe's nodules at the pupillary margin.
- Vitreous humor cells:
  - Dust-like or may progress to heavy, stringy veils.
- Cataract beginning with posterior subcapsular changes:
  - Tendency to progress to mature white cataract.
- Occasional secondary glaucoma.
- Amsler's sign (hyphema or filiform hemorrhage after sudden reduction in intraocular pressure during surgery or with minor trauma):
  - Finding consistent with the rubeosis recognized in the expanded spectrum of disease.
- Occasional chorioretinal scars:
  - Pathophysiology unclear: probably unrelated to toxoplasmosis.
- Long insidious course.
- Prognosis good.

Expanded spectrum of Fuchs' syndrome (frequently not recognized)

- A panophthalmic disease.
- Any age affected.
- Occasionally presents with red external eye.
- Absent or reversed heterochromia (hence author's preference for term Fuchs uveitis or Fuchs uveitis syndrome) (Figure 280.1):
  - Anterior iris atrophy may allow darker posterior iris layer to dominate.
- Heterochromia may be without evident iris atrophy.
- Iris atrophy may be without evident heterochromia.
- Patchy atrophy of posterior pigmented layer of iris.
- Pupil irregular from sphincter atrophy.
- Frequent small peripheral anterior synechiae.
- Increased visibility of iris radial vessels.
- Fine iris rubeosis or gross rubeosis:
  - Vessels meandering over the iris surface in some patients;
  - Angiography to confirm ischemic vasculopathy and infarction.
- Spontaneous or induced hyphema.
- Cataract developing in all patients:
  - Iris atrophy may progress as the cataract matures.
- Prognosis variable with cataract surgery.
- Secondary glaucoma in up to 60%:
  - Initially partially inflammatory, later refractory;
  - Poor prognosis with glaucoma;
  - Multiple mechanisms, including peripheral anterior synechiae, rubeotic vessels, trabecular sclerosis, abnormal felt-like membrane in angle;
  - Intraocular pressure may go up dramatically after YAG discussion.

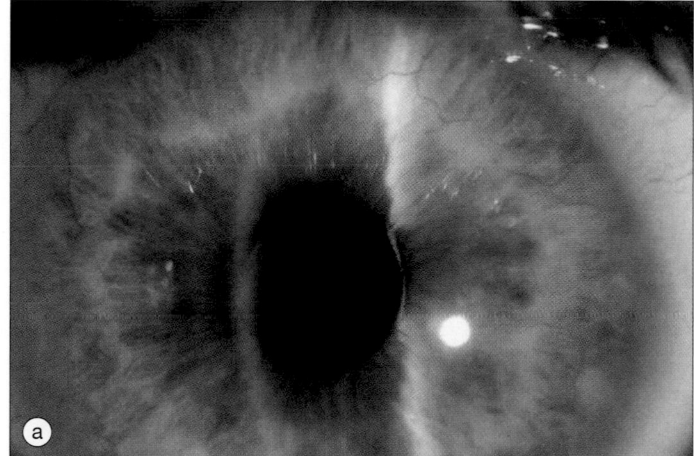

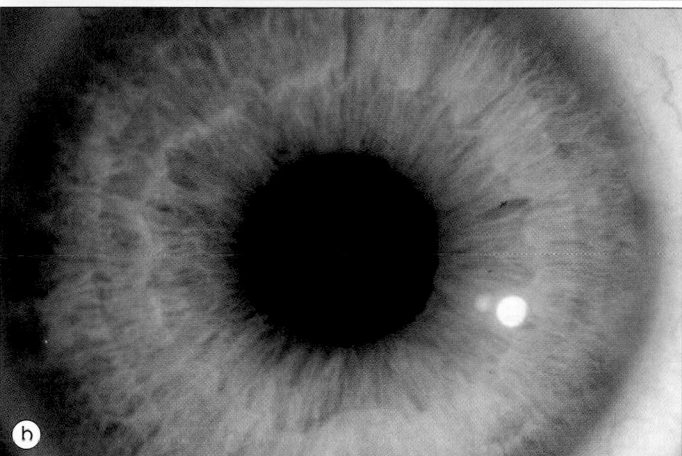

FIGURE 280.1. Fuchs uveitis in a blue eyed individual. a) Subtle iris heterochromia in left eye with iris atrophy and poor iris details, slightly irregular pupil, loss of iris ruff, and early iris neovascularization superiorly. b) Normal right iris.

- Dense vitreous veils or vitreous hemorrhage:
  - Occasionally, vitrectomy required.
- Increased incidence of central and peripheral corneal edema:
  - Abnormal endothelial pattern on specular microscopy;
  - Poor tolerance of intraocular surgery in some;
  - Occasional pattern of Brown–McLean syndrome (peripheral edema);
  - Cellular and humoral immune response to major corneal stromal antigen.

Laboratory findings

- No distinct histopathologic or electron microscopic findings.
- No distinctive laboratory features.
- Several research laboratories reporting immunologic findings: Significantly higher levels of TNF-α in the aqueous humor and sera; Predominant CD8+ T cell subset infiltrating the anterior chamber suggesting an antigen-driven process.

Clonal nature and predominantly $CD8^+$ T-lymphocyte infiltration are suggestive of a viral pathogenesis, perhaps from rubella or HSV.

Differential diagnosis

- Idiopathic or viral uveitis.
- Lens-induced glaucoma.
- Pars planitis.
- Posner–Schlossmann syndrome.

TREATMENT

- In most instances, therapy not indicated.
- Occasionally, discomfort, ciliary injection, floaters treated with topical corticosteroids.
- Cycloplegics not indicated.
- Cataract surgery usually successful but higher risk of vitreous debris or vitreous hemorrhage.
- YAG discission occasionally accompanied by very high intraocular pressure.
- Glaucoma may be difficult to control; treated with topical or systemic therapy, but a high rate of glaucoma surgery.
- Laser trabeculoplasty may be contraindicated.
- Rubeotic glaucoma may require enucleation.
- For both cataract and glaucoma surgery, poorer prognosis with the expanded form of disease compared with classic presentation.

COMPLICATIONS

- Progressive cataract.
- Refractory glaucoma.
- High intraocular pressure after YAG discussion.
- Vitreous debris or hemorrhage.
- Dilated pupil.
- Occasional peripheral or central corneal edema.

COMMENTS

This entity is easily recognized in its classic form; there is a better prognosis for cataract surgery and less severe glaucoma. It is easily missed in its expanded form (which is more frequent); there is a poorer prognosis for cataract surgery and more severe glaucoma. Patients must be monitored for cataracts and glaucoma. Minimal therapy is preferred for uveitis. Since heterochromia is frequently absent, the author prefers the term Fuchs uveitis syndrome.

REFERENCES

Jones NP: Fuchs' heterochromic uveitis: An update. Surv Ophthalmol 37:253–272, 1993.

Labalette P, Caillau D, Grutzmacher C, et al: Highly focused clonal composition of CD8(+) CD28 (neg) T-cells in aqueous humor of Fuchs' heterochromic cyclitis. Exp Eye Res 75:317–325, 2002.

La Hey E, de Jong PT, Kijlstra A: Fuchs' heterochromic cyclitis: review of the literature on the pathogenetic mechanisms. Br J Ophthalmol 78:307–312, 1994.

Liesegang TJ: Fuchs' uveitis. In: Pepose JS, Holland G, Wilhelmus K, eds: Ocular infection and immunity. St Louis, Mosby, 1996.

Quentin CD, Reiber H: Fuchs heterochromic cyclitis: rubella virus antibodies and genome in aqueous humor. Am J Ophthalmol 138:46–54, 2004.

Ram J, Kaushik S, Brar G, et al: Phacoemulsification in patients with Fuchs' heterochromic uveitis. J Cataract Refract Surg 28:1372–1378, 2002.

281 IRIDOCORNEAL-ENDOTHELIAL SYNDROME 364.51

Elisabeth J. Cohen, MD
Philadelphia, Pennsylvania

Iridocorneal-endothelial (ICE) syndrome includes clinical variations previously referred to as progressive (essential) iris atrophy, Chandler's syndrome, Cogan–Reese syndrome, and iris nevus syndrome.

ETIOLOGY/INCIDENCE

ICE is a unilateral, progressive, relatively uncommon, nonfamilial condition with onset during young adulthood associated with variable iris and endothelial abnormalities and peripheral anterior synechiae (PAS). All forms of ICE are associated with glaucoma due to obstruction of aqueous outflow that is more responsive to surgical than medical treatment.

The etiology of ICE is unknown, although there is speculation about possible causes. Herpes simplex virus DNA has been identified by polymerase chain reaction in the endothelia of some ICE patients by one group of investigators. Another theory is that ocular surface epithelial cells end up on the back of the cornea in the course of abnormal corneal development in utero.

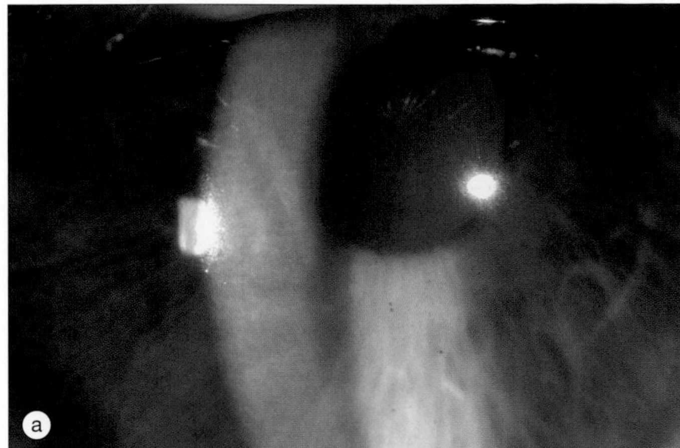

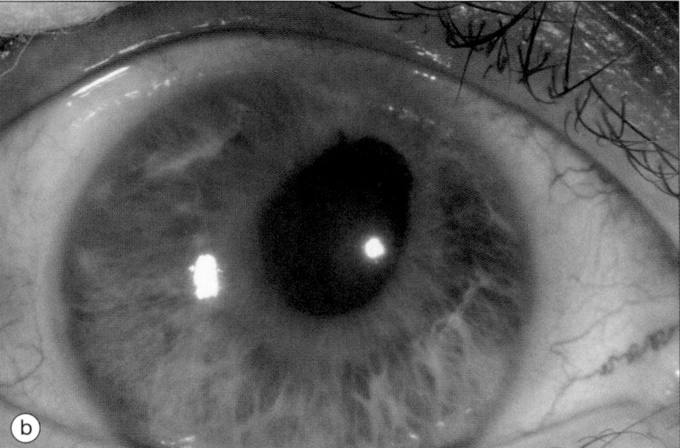

FIGURE 281.1. a) and b) Patient with ICE syndrome who has corneal edema, ectopion uveae, and localized peripheral anterior synechiae.

COURSE/PROGNOSIS

ICE usually progresses slowly. Patients with early changes should be observed regularly to monitor the IOP, cornea, and optic nerve.

DIAGNOSIS

Clinical signs and symptoms

Iris changes include atrophy, holes, nodules, ectropion uveae (Figure 281.1), and corectopia. Corneal changes by slit lamp exam include a fine hammered silver appearance of the endothelium and corneal edema.

Laboratory findings

ICE is primarily a clinical diagnosis, although specular and confocal biomicroscopy can be helpful. Abnormal corneal endothelium produces basement membrane that progressively covers the anterior chamber angle and anterior iris and contracts, pulling the pupil toward the membrane and causing iris atrophy away from the membrane and PAS near it. Specular microscopy may demonstrate 'ICE' cells, unless corneal edema prevents visualization. ICE cells are not hexagonal and there is a reversal of the normal light/dark pattern, so that the cells look dark and the cell borders appear light. ICE cells correlate with the epithelialization of endothelial cells seen in some cases on histopathology in this condition. Confocal microscopy can visualize the endothelium even in the presence of corneal edema, revealing epithelial-like endothelial cells with hyperreflective (white) nuclei.

Differential diagnosis

The differential diagnosis of ICE includes posterior polymorphic dystrophy (PPD) Axenfeld–Rieger syndrome and Fuchs' dystrophy. PPD is an inherited, autosomal dominant endothelial dystrophy associated commonly with bilateral focal vesicular changes and scalloped ridges in asymptomatic patients, and less often with diffuse corneal edema. There is epithelialization of the endothelium. Corectopia, PAS, and glaucoma can occur, but iris changes are milder and glaucoma is less common than in ICE. Axenfeld–Rieger syndrome is a congenital, bilateral, autosomal dominant condition characterized by marked iris changes including atrophy, holes and corectopia and, frequently, glaucoma. However, the endothelium is normal, and the cornea is normal except for a prominent Shwalbe's line. In Fuchs' dystrophy there are bilateral guttae which are larger than the endothelial changes in ICE.

TREATMENT

Medical

When glaucoma develops, medical treatment with aqueous suppressants can be tried initially, but usually surgery is required. Corneal edema, when present, may initially respond to lowering intraocular pressure and hypertonic saline drops during the day and ointment at bedtime. Persistent corneal edema can be caused by progressive endothelial degeneration from the disease and/or trauma from glaucoma surgery.

Surgical

Trabeculectomy with an anti-fibrotic agent is sometimes successful, but glaucoma drainage implants, subsequently or initially, tend to be more successful. Multiple glaucoma procedures are often necessary.

If corneal edema causes reduced visual acuity which interferes with normal activities, glaucoma is controlled, and recovery of vision is not limited by glaucomatous optic neuropathy, then penetrating keratoplasty can be performed in ICE patients with fair success. ICE patients have a higher than average risk of graft rejection and failure, but clear grafts can be obtained in a number of cases. If multiple graft failures occur, glaucoma is controlled after a glaucoma drainage implant procedure, and the visual acuity is limited by the cornea, a permanent keratoprosthesis may be an option to consider in these patients.

REFERENCES

Alvarado JA, Underwood JL, Green WR, et al: Detection of herpes simplex viral DNA in the iridocorneal-endothelial syndrome. Arch Ophthalmol 112:1601–1609, 1994.

Alvim PTS, Cohen EJ, Rapuano CJ, et al: Penetrating keratoplasty in iridocorneal endothelial syndrome. Cornea 20:134–140, 2001.

Doe EA, Budenz DL, Gedde SJ, et al: Long-term surgical outcomes of patients with glaucoma seconday to the iridocorneal endothelial syndrome. Ophthalmology 108:1789–1795, 2001.

Eagle RC, Font RL, Yanoff M, et al: Proliferative endotheliopathy with iris abnormalities: The iridocorneal endothelial syndrome. Arch Ophthalmol 97:2104–2111, 1979.

Garibaldi DC, Schien OD, Jun A: Features of the iridocorneal endothelial syndrome on confocal microscopy. Cornea 24:349–351, 2005.

282 IRIS BOMBÉ 364.74

Rodrigo J. Torres, MD
Portland, Oregon
George A. Cioffi, MD
Portland, Oregon

ETIOLOGY/INCIDENCE

Iris bombé refers to a specific configuration of the iris visible on clinical examination in which the peripheral iris is circumferentially bowed anteriorly towards the cornea in a convex fashion, while the central iris remains relatively deep in the anterior chamber. This configuration is most commonly seen in the setting of primary pupillary block, but can also be seen with pupillary block from seclusio pupillae, intraocular lenses (particularly anterior chamber intraocular lenses), and vitreous extension into the anterior chamber in an aphakic eye. Therefore, patients with a history of anterior uveitis and annular posterior synechiae, patients with an anterior chamber intraocular lens without a patent peripheral iridotomy, and patients at high risk of a primary angle closure attack are the patients most commonly presenting with an iris bombé configuration.

COURSE/PROGNOSIS

Left untreated, iris bombé results in irreversible scarring and closure of the anterior chamber angle, obstruction of conventional aqueous outflow, and significant elevation of the intraocular pressure. Permanent glaucomatous optic nerve damage is likely to result from recurrent attacks of acute angle closure. Furthermore, scarring of the angle can develop with sequelae of chronic angle closure glaucoma. However, iris bombé is very responsive to early treatment, with avoidance of recurrent attacks, optic nerve damage, and chronic angle closure.

DIAGNOSIS

Clinical signs and symptoms

- van Herick technique: peripheral anterior chamber <1/4 corneal thickness.
- Gonioscopy: Angles appositionally closed 360 degrees, may open slightly with compression.
- Elevated intraocular pressure.
- Pain.
- Nausea.
- Corneal edema.
- Ciliary flush.

Differential diagnosis

- Plateau iris syndrome.
- Aqueous misdirection.
- Phacomorphic glaucoma.
- Suprachoroidal effusion or hemorrhage.

High resolution ultrasound imaging can assist diagnosis in cases with severe corneal edema.

PROPHYLAXIS

- Prevention of seclusio pupillae by controlling anterior chamber inflammation with topical steroids and mydriatics.
- Prophylactic surgical or YAG laser peripheral iridotomies in aphakes and patients with anterior chamber intraocular lenses, seclusio pupillae, or narrow angles at high risk for an attack of primary angle closure.
- Lysis of adhesions for recent onset seclusio pupillae with topical atropine sulfate 1% and 10% phenylephrine. If unresponsive, consider intracameral t-PA injection (12.5 μg/0.05 cc sterile water.)
- Surgical lysis of posterior synechiae in cases of seclusio pupillae.

TREATMENT

Systemic

Hyperosmotics (IV mannitol 20%, 1–2 mg/kg over 45 minutes) and carbonic anhydrase inhibitors (acetazolamide 250–500 mg IV or PO).

Ocular

Aqueous suppressants (beta blockers, alpha agonists, topical carbonic anhydrase inhibitors).

Surgical

When cornea clears:

- YAG laser peripheral iridotomy or surgical peripheral iridotomy;
- Lysis of posterior synechiae.

COMPLICATIONS

- Acute angle closure glaucoma.
- Chronic angle closure glaucoma.

REFERENCES

Duke-Elder S, Perkins ES: System of ophthalmology. Diseases of the uveal tract. St Louis, CV Mosby, 1966:IX:177–179.

Shields MB: Textbook of glaucoma. Maryland, Williams & Wilkins, 1998:177–194.

Skolnick CA, Fiscella RG, Tessler HH, et al: Tissue plaminogen activator to treat impending pupillary block glaucoma in patients with acute fibrinous HLA-B27 positive iridocyclitis. Am J Ophthalmol 129:363–365, 2000.

Tomey KF, Traverso CE, Shammas IV: Neodynium-YAG laser iridotomy in the treatment and prevention of angle closure glaucoma: a review of 373 eyes. Arch Ophthalmol 105:476–481, 1987.

Van Buskirk EM: Pupillary block after intraocular lens implantation. Am J Ophthalmol 95:55–59, 1983.

283 IRIS CYSTS 364.6
(Intraepithelial Cysts, Epithelial Implantation Cysts, Congenital Iris Cysts)

Kenneth C. Swan, MD
Portland, Oregon

Iris cysts are intraepithelial cysts originating between the epithelial layers and stromal cysts that (1) are congenital or (2) are implanted by surgery or caused by trauma.

ETIOLOGY

- Intraepithelial cysts represent an incomplete obliteration or reestablishment of the space between the two layers of the secondary optic vessel. The outer layers composed of pigment epithelium usually present as a black globular mass behind the iris. Peripherally, the cysts may present as globular protrusions as the overlying iris stroma is pushed anteriorly. The cyst may extend through the iris into the anterior chamber. More than one cyst may be noted in the same eye or in the other eye.
- Pigmented iris nodules and cysts also may occur as a proliferative response to miotic therapy for glaucoma or accommodative esotropia.
- Epithelium-lined stromal cysts may be congenital or result from intraocular implantation of surface epithelium by surgery or trauma. Poor wound apposition and delayed healing of the stromal wound predispose to epithelial ingrowth. Accidental incarceration of lens capsule in the wound also increases the risk of implantation cyst after extracapsular cataract extraction.

COURSE/PROGNOSIS

- Intraepithelial cysts are stationary and rarely require treatment.
- Iris cysts produced by miotic therapy partially recede when myotics are discontinued. Occasional mobilization of the pupil reportedly reduces their development.
- Some implantation and embryonal epithelial cysts remain small and stationary. Most slowly enlarge, and they may fill the anterior chamber, with potential loss of vision. Enlarging cysts may distort the pupil and lead to keratopathy, iridocyclitis, and glaucoma.

DIAGNOSIS

Differential diagnosis

- Stromal cysts are semitransparent and contain opalescent fluid.
- Intraepithelial cysts are heavily pigmented and usually do not transilluminate. Dilation of the pupil reveals the characteristic smooth, rounded posterior surface.
- Echographs help to differentiate intraepithelial cysts from melanoma, as well as to determine posterior extension of stromal cysts.

TREATMENT

- Intraepithelial cysts rarely progress and do not require treatment.
- Iris cysts induced by miotics partially recede when miotics are discontinued. Occasional mobilization of the pupil reportedly decreases their rate of formation.
- Management of the implantation or embryonal epithelial cysts is in large part dependent on the growth pattern. Some small cysts may remain stationary and asymptomatic. These should be observed at regular intervals because they may increase dramatically after a dormant period. Several forms of treatment have been reported to be effective, including chemical cauterization, laser photocoagulation of the cyst walls, diathermy, cryocoagulation, and block excision with cornea sclera transplant. Irradiation has been ineffective and has been abandoned.
- For cysts that involve the corneal or limbal stroma, chemical cauterization is effective. A discission knife is used to make a track into the cyst. The knife is withdrawn, and a short, blunt-tipped 30-gauge needle attached to a 2-mL syringe containing 0.5 mL of 20% trichloroacetic acid is introduced. The cyst is aspirated, and then, without withdrawal of the needle, the mixture of cyst fluid and trichloroacetic acid is carefully injected. The clear walls of the cyst and the protein in the cyst fluid immediately turn white. The cyst contents are aspirated to collapse the cyst completely before the needle is withdrawn. Suction is maintained as the needle is withdrawn to avoid spread of the acid into the stromal tissue. Only minimal coagulation of the conjunctiva occurs at the puncture site. Iris cysts not in contact with the wall of the eye cannot be injected safely.

PRECAUTIONS

- When injecting sclerosing fluids, such as 20% trichloroacetic acid, great care must be taken to inject only into the cyst. Inadvertent injections into the anterior chamber can cause irreversible corneal iris and lens damage. Coagulation and surgical excision also require great care; disruption of the cyst wall can convert a localized epithelial cyst into a diffuse epithelial growth.

REFERENCES

Capo H, Palmer E, Nicholson DH: Congenital cysts of the iris stroma. Am J Ophthalmol 116:228–232, 1993.

Foster RK: Block excision of postoperative anterior chamber cysts. Trans Am Ophthalmal Soc 93:83–104, 1995.

New Sidoti PA, Valericia M, Chem N, et al: Echographic evaluation of primary cysts of the iris pigment epithelium. Am J Ophthalmal 120:161–167, 1995.

Rosenquist RC, Fraunfelder FT, Swan KX: Treatment of conjunctival epithelial cysts with trichloracetic acid. J Ocul Ther Surg 4:51–55, 1985.

Swan KC: Iris pigment nodules complicating miotic therapy. Am J Ophthalmol 37:886–889, 1954.

Swan KC: Epithelial cell cysts of the anterior chamber treated by acid injections. Doc Ophthalmol 18:363–370, 1979.

284 IRIS MELANOMA 190.8

R. Max Conway, MD, PhD, FRANZCO
Sydney, New South Wales

ETIOLOGY/INCIDENCE

Iris melanoma is a malignant neoplasm arising from iris melanocytes.

The annual age-adjusted incidence of uveal melanoma in predominantly Caucasian populations is approximately 4.3 per million, of which 2–5% comprise iris melanoma. Individuals with pale or blue irides are reported to be at higher risk for developing iris melanoma. The etiological role of sunlight remains inconclusive.

COURSE/PROGNOSIS

Iris melanomas usually grow locally into the anterior chamber or along the iris surface and commonly invade the anterior chamber angle and anterior ciliary body by local extension. Overall, 2.6%–11% of iris melanomas are reported to metastasise after 10 years. Increased risk for metastasis is associated with increasing age, ciliary body involvement, elevated intraocular pressure, diffuse variant, prior surgical intervention, extra-ocular extension and mixed or epithelioid cell histology.

DIAGNOSIS

Clinical signs and symptoms

Most iris melanomas are asymptomatic at presentation and are diagnosed in middle-aged patients when the lesions are small and vision excellent. Iris melanoma usually appears as a pigmented, unilateral, solitary nodule in the lower half of the iris. (Figure 284.1a) Abnormal vascularization, pigment dispersion, ectropeon uveae, compression or distorsion of surrounding tissues, sector cataract, sentinel vessels, heterochromia, spontaneous hyphema and chronic uveitis may be present. Atypical variants include amelanotic, multifocal and diffuse varieties.

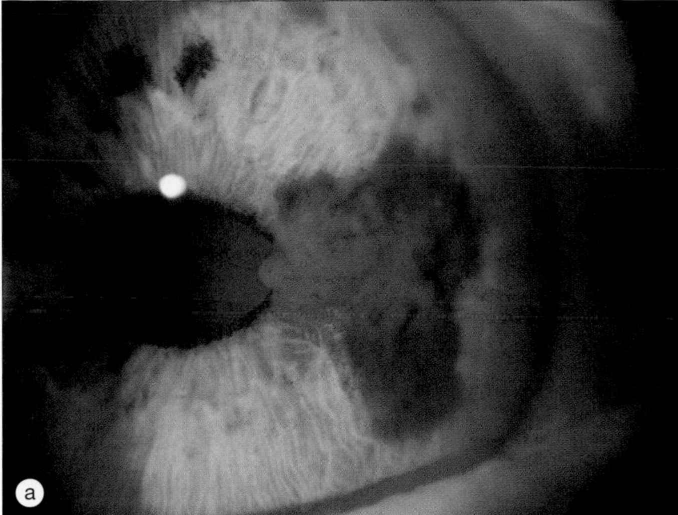

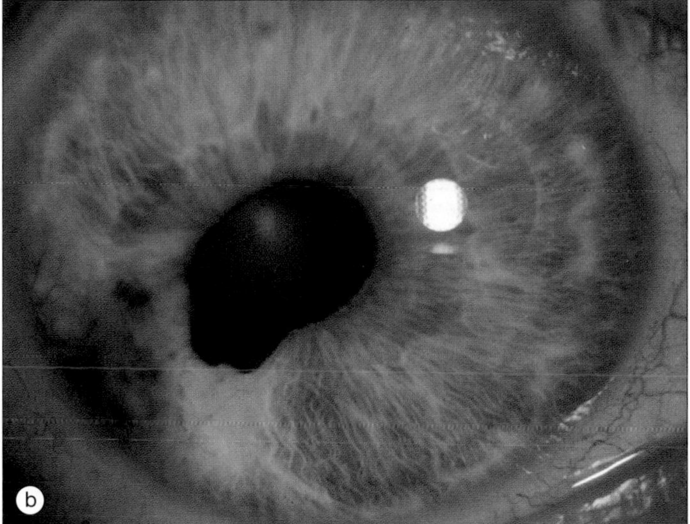

FIGURE 284.1. Clinical photograph of iris melanoma (a) and amelanotic variant (b).

(Figure 284.1b) Glaucoma may occur in association with tumour invasion into the trabecular meshwork.

As the metastasis rate is low and most patients have excellent vision, it is the practice at our institution to document growth by serial examination prior to embarking upon intervention. Serial examination includes clinical photography and ultrasound biomicroscopy to obtain objective measurements of tumor dimensions for comparison over time. Iris fluorescein angiography may have a useful adjunctive diagnostic role by demonstrating hotspots of increased fluorescein leakage due to tumor vessels with increased permeability.

Differential diagnosis

Iris nevus is the most common differential diagnostic entity. In contrast to melanomas, nevi are usually flat or mildly elevated (<1mm), <3mm in basal extent, produce minimal compression or distorsion of surrounding tissues, are not associated with pigment dispersion, do not cause glaucoma and show no or slow growth tendency. Other pigmented lesions which need to be considered include iris cysts, melanosis, melanoctyoma, foreign bodies and iris atrophy/ICE syndrome. Secondary involvement of the iris by a CB melanoma is important to recognize as it alters prognosis and therapy. These commonly appear as cresent-shaped, pigmented masses arising from the ciliary body. UBM and B-scan ultrasonography are very helpful tests for excluding a ciliary body component in association with an iris mass. Amelanotic lesions which may be confused with iris melanoma include metastases and vascular lesions.

TREATMENT

Besides growth tendency, other factors which may initiate intervention include large size, multifocal tumors, tumor-related glaucoma or extra-scleral extension. Recent years have seen a trend towards the conservative treatment of uveal melanomas, including iris melanoma. Modalities which may be used include resection with iridectomy/iridocyclectomy or various forms of radiotherapy (plaque brachytherapy or charged particle therapy). Enucleation remains the treatment of choice for tumors unsuited to conservative modalities. In all patients, long-term post-treatment follow-up is advisable for the early detection of recurrence or metastases.

COMMENT

If a suspicious lesion is circumscribed and slow growing, careful observation is recommended. Accelerated growth in the lesion is the most common sign of malignant transformation.

REFERENCES

Conway RM, Chew T, Golchet P, et al: Ultrasound biomicroscopy: role in diagnosis and management in 130 consecutive patients evaluated for anterior segment tumors. Brit J Ophthalmol (in press 2005).

Conway RM, Chua WC, Qureshi C, Billson FA: Primary iris melanoma: diagnostic features and outcome of conservative surgical treatment. Br J Ophthalmol 85:848–854, 2001.

Shields CL, Materin MA, Shields JA, et al: Factors associated with elevated intraocular pressure in eyes with iris melanoma. Br J Ophthalmol 85:666–669, 2001.

Singh AD, Shields CL, Shields JA: Prognostic factors in uveal melanoma. Melanoma Res 11:255–263, 2001.

Singh AD, Topham A: Incidence of uveal melanoma in the United States: 1973–1997. Ophthalmology 110:956–961, 2003.

Vajdic CM, Kricker A, Giblin M, et al: Sun exposure predicts risk of ocular melanoma in Australia. Int J Cancer 101:175–182, 2002.

285 IRIS PROLAPSE 364.8

David Litoff, MD
Boulder, Colorado

ETIOLOGY/INCIDENCE

Iris prolapse is an uncommon intraoperative or postoperative complication of cataract surgery. It can also occur with glaucoma surgery, corneal transplantation, or as the result of an acute degenerative process, infection, or penetrating injury. With phacoemulsification and small incision cataract surgery, iris prolapse is becoming increasingly rare. The mechanism of iris prolapse involves the pressure posterior to the iris being greater than the pressure anterior to the iris. If these conditions exist and a wound leak is present, the iris can bow anteriorly into the wound. Iris prolapse is a serious condition that can lead to significant complications if left untreated.

Etiologies for intraoperative iris prolapse include the following:

- Low height of the infusion bottle or slow infusion rate;
- Wound leak due to poor wound construction;
- Floppy iris;
- Excessive eyelid squeezing;
- Posterior misdirection of fluid;
- Excessive viscoelastic injected posterior to iris;
- Retrorbital or expulsive hemorrhage;
- Excessive volume of retrobulbar anesthetic injection.

For postoperative iris prolapse, etiologies include:

- Poor wound construction or closure;
- Trauma or increased pressure on the globe;
- Excessive coughing;
- Pupillary block;
- Poor wound healing.

Iris prolapse unrelated to surgery may be caused by:

- Corneal or scleral penetrating injury;
- Perforation due to a corneal or scleral perforating ulcer;
- Perforation due to an immunologic melting disorder.

DIAGNOSIS

Iris prolapse is a clinical diagnosis with recognition of iris tissue presenting in a corneal or scleral wound. Associated findings may include an irregular pupil, a filtering bleb, or a shallow anterior chamber.

PROPHYLAXIS

The prevention of iris prolapse requires careful attention to wound size, configuration, location, and closure. The prevention of intraoperative iris prolapse during cataract surgery requires careful attention to bottle height and flow rates. During surgery, care must be taken that excessive viscoelastic is not be placed posterior to the iris, pushing the iris anteriorly out of the wound. The prevention of postoperative iris prolapse involves the use of an eye shield to prevent inadvertent trauma in the early postoperative period.

COMPLICATIONS

Severe complications can occur as the result of iris prolapse. One of the most significant complications is endophthalmitis. The prolapsed iris can act as a scaffold for bacteria growth into the anterior chamber. Other complications include epithelial or fibrous ingrowth and cystoid macular edema.

TREATMENT

Intraoperative

Treatment of intraoperative iris prolapse involves first recognizing the etiology. If the iris prolapse is secondary to a wound leak, then the wound size should be decreased by placing a suture. If pressure from a lid speculum is causing excessive pressure on the globe, then the speculum should be repositioned or switched to a different type. If excessive eyelid squeezing is resulting in iris prolapase, then a lid block can be helpful in reducing the pressure on the globe. Recognizing posterior misdirection of fluid as the cause of posterior pressure can be much more difficult. When no other cause is found and the anterior chamber has shallowed significantly, posterior misdirection of fluid should be suspected. This can occur during the hydrodissection of the cataract, but more commonly occurs during phacoemulsification with the infusion of fluid. Other causes of intraoperative iris prolapse, such as choroidal hemorrhage, should be ruled out prior to making the diagnosis of fluid misdirection. If fluid misdirection is the cause of iris prolapse, placing some pressure on the anterior surface of the lens can sometimes slowly result in a regression of the fluid anteriorly. Intravenous mannitol can shrink the vitreous and also be beneficial in treating fluid misdirection. If this maneuver is unsuccessful then a vitreous tap should be performed to reduce the posterior pressure.

Medical

In the early postoperative period, iris prolapse can be treated with a strong miotic. The miotic will result in constriction of the iris which occasionally pulls the prolapsed portion or the iris out of the wound. The late occurrence of an iris prolapse that is small and covered with conjunctiva can often be observed without treatment.

Surgical

If medical treatment is unsuccessful in repositioning the iris, surgery is often needed. If the iris prolapse is large and more than 96 hours old, it is better to excise the prolapsed iris because it is usually necrotic. The iris should be excised if there is any evidence of epithelial or fibrous growth on the iris. Repositioning iris with epithelium can result in epithelial ingrowth with significant complications.

REFERENCES

Allan BDS: Mechanism of iris prolapse: a qualitative analysis and implication for surgical technique. J Cataract Refract Surg 21:182–186, 1995.

Francis PJ, Morris RJ: Post-operative iris prolapse following phacoemulsification and extracapsular cataract surgery. Eye 11:87–90, 1997.

Jaffe NS, Jaffe MS, Jaffe GF: Cataract surgery and its complications. 5th edn. St Louis, CV Mosby, 1990:577–58.

Naylor G: Iris prolapse: who? when? why? Eye 7:465–467, 1993.

Taguri AH, Sanders R: Iris prolapse in small incision cataract surgery. Ophthal Surg Lasers 33(1):66–70, 2002.

286 PARS PLANITIS 363.21

(Angiohyalitis, Chronic Cyclitis, Cyclitis, Peripheral Uveitis, Peripheral Uveoretinitis, Vitreitis)

Sema Oruc Dundar, MD
Aydin, Turkey

ETIOLOGY/INCIDENCE

Pars planitis is an idiopathic inflammatory condition characterized by cells and debris in the vitreous and exudates and snowbank formation along the peripheral retina and pars plana. It occurs in patients between the ages of 5 and 40 years. There is a bimodal distribution pattern with peaks between the ages of 5–15 and 25–35 years. Pars planitis is usually bilateral and frequently asymmetric in severity. It represents 4–16% of all uveitis cases seen in referral practices.

The cause of pars planitis is unknown. Histopathologic and clinical findings suggest a possible autoimmune basis. Several studies have associated HLA-DR2 with pars planitis, suggesting an immunogenetic predisposition. An association was also found with HLA-DR15, a suballele of HLA-DR2.

COURSE/PROGNOSIS

The clinical course of the disease can vary from self-limited to chronic with exacerbations. It can be divided into three categories; 10% of the patients have a self-limited course with gradual improvement, 59% suffer a prolonged course without exacerbations, and 31% show a smoldering course with exacerbations.

The visual prognosis in most patients is relatively good. The most important factor that affects the final visual outcome is the presence of macular involvement.

DIAGNOSIS

Clinical signs and symptoms

The onset is typically insidious and blurred vision and floaters are common complaints. Signs of pars planitis may include:

- Vitritis (mild, moderate, or severe);
- Mild or absent anterior chamber cellular reaction;
- Clumps of inflammatory cells visible in the vitreous;
- Exudate (snowbank) over the inferior peripheral retina and pars plana;
- Vascular sheathing, neovascularization;
- Cystoid macular edema;
- Vitreous hemorrhage;
- Cyclitic membrane formation;
- Cataract;
- Glaucoma;
- Retinal detachment;
- Retinoschisis.

Differential diagnosis

There are no specific tests that establish the diagnosis of pars planitis, which is classically made by observing a snowbank or membrane over the inferior peripheral retina and pars plana. The differential diagnosis includes sarcoidosis, multiple sclerosis, Lyme disease, toxocariasis, intraocular lymphoma and HTLV1.

TREATMENT

Systemic

The goal of therapy is to eliminate or diminish long-term visual loss. The treatment aim is not to eradicate all inflammation but to ameliorate sight-threatening complications. Some clinicians do not treat the disease until visual acuity drops to 20/40, whereas others institute treatment for visually disabling cystoid macular edema in patients with better visual acuity.

Corticosteroids are the mainstay of therapy. Patients who have bilateral disease or whose disease is recalcitrant to periocular steroids can be treated with oral corticosteroids. The dose of oral corticosteroids is usually 1 mg/kg/day for 2 to 3 weeks with a slow taper on the basis of clinical response as well as the ocular and systemic complications of such therapy. Antiulcer medications should also be prescribed. In many cases, steroids must be tapered slowly over a period of several months and alternate day therapy is essential in these patients to reduce steroid induced complications.

Other systemic immunosuppressive agents have been used to treat patients whose disease is recalcitrant to other treatment modalities. A good therapeutic response has been reported with the use of chlorambucil, azathioprine, cyclophosphamide, methotrexate and cyclosporin A. All immunosuppressive medications have significant systemic side effects.

Ocular

Periocular corticosteroids are very effective in treating many cases of pars planitis, and especially in treating unilateral asymmetric disease. They have the advantage of causing minimal systemic corticosteroid complications. Triamcinolone acetonide (40 mg/mL) or methylprednisolone acetate depot preparation (80 mg/mL) is injected.

Periocular injections may be delivered to the retroseptal space or the sub-Tenon's space. One study has shown that the superotemporal posterior sub-Tenon's approach is more effective in placing the steroid close to the macula than the inferior approach. The conjunctiva is anesthetized topically. The upper eyelid is retracted and the patient is instructed to look inferonasally. The needle is placed bevel toward the globe and advanced through the conjunctiva and Tenon's capsule using a side-to-side movement in order not to penetrate the globe accidentally. The needle is kept as close to the globe as possible. The needle is advanced to the hub of needle; and the steroid injected into the sub-Tenon's space. Injections can be repeated every 2 to 3 weeks. Two or three injections should be given over a 6 to 8 week period before concluding that injections are no effective.

Surgical

Cryotherapy of the inferior snowbank has been advocated in patients intolerant of corticosteroids. The cryotherapy is administered directly to the areas of exudates. The iceball should cover the entire area of exudate and overlap the uninvolved areas of retina and ciliary body by one probe width. A single depot injection of corticosteroids is given after the procedure. Patients are usually given at least 3 months before additional treatment is applied. Peripheral scatter photocoagulation also appears to be an effective alternative to cryotherapy in patients with neovascularization of the vitreous base.

Pars plana vitrectomy has been advocated for management of more severe complications of pars planitis, including those with persistent vitreous hemorrhage, dense vitreous debris that is not responsive to medical therapy, persistent cystoid macular edema, retinal detachment, and macular pucker.

COMPLICATIONS

Complications of corticosteroid therapy are numerous and can be seen with any mode of administration. Ocular complications from corticosteroids include the possible development of posterior subcapsular cataract and potentially elevated intraocular pressure.

All immunosuppressive drugs have significant side effects and their use should be monitored by a physician expert in their use. The major side effects of cyclosporin A are nephrotoxicity and hypertension. Therefore, kidney function and blood pressure must be checked regularly. Patients should be informed of all side effects and risks of immunosuppressive agents.

COMMENTS

Many patients with pars planitis require no treatment. As cystoid macular edema is the leading cause of significant visual loss in pars planitis, most treatment is aimed at elimination of cystoid macular edema.

Generally, treatment is not given unless there is a decrease in visual acuity. The clinician should decide the level of visual acuity to aim at treating the patients. Treatment decisions should be made on an individual basis.

REFERENCES

Henderly DE, Gentsler AJ, Rao NA, et al: Pars planitis. Trans Ophthalmol Soc UK 105:227–232, 1986.

Kaplan HJ: Intermediate uveitis (pars planitis, chronic cyclitis) — a four step approach to treatment. In: Saari KM, ed: Uveitis update. Amsterdam, Excerpta Medica, 1984:169–172.

Oruc S, Duffy BF, Mohanakumar T, et al: The association of HLA class II with pars planitis. Am J Ophthalmol 131:657–659, 2001.

Oruc S, Kaplan AD, Galen M, et al: Uveitis referral pattern in a Midwest University Eye Center. Ocular Immunol Inflamm 11:287–298, 2003.

Smith RE, Godfrey WA, Kimura SJ: Chronic cyclitis.I: course and visual prognosis. Trans Am Acad Ophthalmol Otolaryngol 77:760–768, 1973.

287 RUBEOSIS IRIDIS 364.42

Masanori Ino-ue, MD, PhD
Kobe, Japan

ETIOLOGY/INCIDENCE

Neovascularization of the iris (rubeosis iridis) is a feared complication of a variety of ischemic diseases, often resulting in a severe, usually intractable type of secondary glaucoma.

In our clinic, one-third of rubeosis iridis cases are attributable to diabetic retinopathy, 17% to retinal vein occlusion, and 13% to carotid occlusive disease. One-third are related to other causes, with post-vitrectomy and post-lensectomy procedures being the most predominant. Following central retinal artery obstruction, 1% to 2% of patients develop rubeosis iridis. These patients may have associated carotid artery obstruction. Intraocular tumors, prior retinal detachment surgery, and uveitis may also lead to rubeosis iridis.Localized anterior segment ischemia has been shown to be the cause of rubeosis iridis in Fuchs' heterochromic iridocyclitis, pseudoexfoliation syndrome, and trauma to the anterior ciliary blood vessels during retinal detachment or strabismus surgery.

The age at the time of development of rubeosis iridis is younger in patients with diabetic retinopathy compared to patients with retinal vein occlusion or carotid occlusive disease.

Sex distribution differs depending on the etiology. Due to the prevalence of other underlying diseases, more males with carotid artery disease develop rubeosis iridis.

The increasing incidence of diabetes mellitus is a major predisposing factor for development of rubeosis iridis, with diabetic retinopathy as the most common association. Bilateral rubeosis is most often seen in patients with diabetes. Patients with underlying diabetes are also prone to develop retinal vein occlusion and carotid occlusive disease.

With the availability of newer diagnostic techniques for carotid occlusive disease coupled with the decreased incidence of rubeosis iridis after retinal vein occlusion secondary to retinal photocoagulation, carotid occlusive disease is becoming a more prominent cause of rubeosis iridis.

DIAGNOSIS

Clinical signs and symptoms

There are four stages in the clinical course of rubeosis iridis, including the pre-rubeosis stage. In may be useful to consider each stage for proper management.

In the pre-rubeosis stage, new vessels on the iris or in the angle are not clinically detectable. The many conditions that may lead to rubeosis iridis have been mentioned previously. Diabetes mellitus, hypertension and arteriosclerosis are the most important systemic predisposing factors, with previous ocular surgery an additional consideration. These patients should undergo a careful fundus fluorescein angiography and slit-lamp examination. Quantitative laser photometry with iris fluorescein angiography may be helpful in detecting occult rubeosis.

The first visible sign of rubeosis iridis appears in stage 2. Tiny tufts of new vessels at the pupillary margin, which may be difficult to detect in a dark iris, can be visualized with the slit-lamp. High magnification is essential for early detection. At this stage, the angle is not yet involved and the intraocular pressure is normal.

In the third stage, the patches of new blood vessels in the iris grow and coalesce. New thin-walled vessels start to invade the iris stroma. At the angle, vessels cross the ciliary body and scleral spur and may extend to the trabecular meshwork. On gonioscopy, the anterior chamber angle will still appear open. Some patients may present with intraocular pressure elevations.

Later, new vessels become more florid and a fibrovascular membrane begins to cover the anterior surface of the iris. The iris surface becomes flat, an ectropion uvea may be present, the pupil is dilated and the iris displaces forward.

Peripheral anterior synechiae (PAS) occur randomly. As the PAS extend and coalesce, angle closure occurs. The findings in gonioscopy are critical in the management of rubeosis iridis. Glaucoma may result from the occurrence of hyphema, the presence of PAS, or from the leakage of protein and cells from the new vessels. The intraocular pressure values in neovascular glaucoma due to carotid occlusive disease may be normal or even subnormal. An eye with low perfusion may have normal intraocular pressure values but is susceptible to damage.

Spontaneous arrest or even total regression of rubeosis iridis may occur. In such cases, the iridi have a flat and scarred appearance.

PROPHYLAXIS

As prophylaxis against the development of rubeosis iridis, patients with retinal hypoxia associated with central retinal vein occlusion and proliferative diabetic retinopathy should undergo panretinal photocoagulation. To prevent development of rubeosis iridis in high-risk eyes after vitrectomy, extensive endophotocoagulation may be a valuable adjunct procedure. Controlling hypertension in diabetic patients is another form of prophylactic therapy. In carotid occlusive disease, panretinal photocoagulation is perceived as partially effective in preventing late-onset rubeosis iridis. Carotid artery surgery should be performed before the development of rubeosis iridis.

TREATMENT

Ocular

Eyes with diabetic retinopathy, or post-retinal vein occlusion cases that develop early stage rubeosis iridis, with minimal or no angle involvement may benefit from adequate panretinal photocoagulation. Rubeosis iridis may regress in such cases. Even in cases with carotid occlusive disease, panretinal photocoagulation may still reduce iris rubeosis to a certain degree.

In late-stage rubeosis, synechial angle closure may cause severe neovascular glaucoma. Although panretinal photocoagulation cannot reverse angle closure, it may cause regression of new vessels and prevent further closure of the angle. If patients have undergone prior filtration surgery, extensive photocoagulation should be performed.

If panretinal photocoagulation is not possible, retinal cryotherapy is an alternative procedure. Peripheral transscleral retinal diode photocoagulation is also effective in treating patients with rubeosis iridis.

Medical

In secondary open-angle glaucoma, anti-glaucoma medications will be effective to some degree. Topical atropine (1%) twice a day, as well as topical steroids four times per day, are effective in reducing pain and decreases ocular inflammation.

In the latter stages of the disease, any medication acting on aqueous outflow is contraindicated. Medications that reduce aqueous production may be beneficial but may not be sufficient to normalize the intraocular pressure. Hyperosmotic agents may be required for temporary control of marked elevations in intraocular pressure.

Surgical

A vitrectomy–lensectomy procedure is indicated when the lens or vitreous is hazy. However, even if the media are clear, in active early-stage rubeosis iridis, vitrectomy-lensectomy is meant to be an anti-vasoproliferative surgical procedure. This surgery involves extensive endophotocoagulation to the peripheral retina. Silicone oil tamponade also supports rapid regression of rubeosis iridis.

Goniophotocoagulation refers to the direct application of laser to the angle vessels. It is effective in the early stages of rubeosis iridis, prior to the onset of open-angle glaucoma.

Filtration surgery in eyes with active rubeosis may be complicated by intra- and post-operative hemorrhage leading to a high risk for late bleb failure. After adequate panretinal photocoagulation, administration of anti-glaucoma medications and topical atropine or steroids, and the use of hyperosmotic agents, trabecular filtration surgery with application of mitomycin C may be effective in regressing active rubeosis iridis.

To resolve the problem of bleb failure in filtration surgery, drainage implants are being employed. However, problems with stent and valve procedures remain.

In carotid artery occlusive disease, increased blood flow to the ciliary body after carotid artery surgery may result in increased aqueous humor production, resulting in a dramatic increase in intraocular pressure. If rubeosis iridis and neovascular glaucoma are present prior to carotid surgery, the indications for surgery should be carefully reconsidered.

In end-stage neovascular glaucoma, cyclo-destructive surgery may be the most reasonable therapy for pain relief. Cyclocryotherapy and transscleral cyclophotocagulation with Nd:YAG laser may be performed.

COMMENTS

Based on experimental and clinical observations regarding angiogenesis, administration of anti-angiogenic factors may inhibit the development of rubeosis iridis or may cause its regression. Intravitreal injection of crystalline cortisone may be useful in the treatment of neovascular glaucoma. Furthermore, photodynamic therapy with verteporfin is a promising new treatment option for rubeosis iridis and neovascular glaucoma in place of goniophotocoagulation.

REFERENCES

Adamis AP, Shima DT, Tolentino MJ, et al: Inhibition of vascular endothelial growth factor prevents retinal ischemia associated iris neovascularization in non-human primate. Arch Ophthalmol 114:66–71, 1996.

Bartz-Schmidt KU, Thumann G, Psichias A, et al: Pars plana vitrectomy, endolaser coagulation of retina and the ciliary body combined with silicone oil endotamponade in the treatment of uncontrolled neovascular glaucoma. Graefes Arch Clin Exp Ophthalmol 237:969–975, 1999.

Gartner S, Henkind P: Neovascularization of the iris (rubeosis iridis), Surv Ophthalmol 22:291–312, 1978.

Ino-ue M, Azumi A, Kajiura-Tsukahara Y, et al: Ocular ischemic syndrome in diabetic patients. Jpn J Ophthalmol 43:31–35, 1999.

Miller JW, Stinson WG, Gregrory WA, et al: Phthalocyanine photodynamic therapy of experimental iris neovascularization. Opthalmology 98:1711–1719, 1991.

288 UVEITIS 364.3

(Iritis, Iridocyclitis, Intermediate and Posterior Uveitis, Noninfectious Chorioretinitis)

Eric Lowell Singman, MD, PhD

Lancaster, Pennsylvania

ETIOLOGY

While most cases of uveitis (inflammation of the uveal tract) are idiopathic or posttraumatic, a growing number of infections, malignancies, autoimmune diseases and pharmaceuticals have been recognized as etiologic.

Systemic and ocular infections associated with uveitis include tuberculosis, syphilis, Lyme disease, Whipple's disease, HIV, herpesviremia, enteroviremia, toxoplasmosis, toxocariasis, cat scratch fever, chlamydiosis (either trachoma or genitourinary tract infection of patients with reactive arthritis), streptococcemia (e.g. in subacute bacterial endocarditis) and opportunistic fungal infections such as aspergillosis.

Malignancies can not only cause uveitis through opportunistic infection (e.g. lymphoma, leukemia) or autoimmune activity (e.g. carcinoma [lung or breast]-associated retinopathy and melanoma-associated retinopathy) but can also mimic uveitis (e.g. retinoblastoma, ocular melanoma, and leukemia).

Autoimmune diseases inciting uveitis include sarcoidosis, Behçet's disease, Reiter's syndrome (reactive arthritis), inflammatory bowel syndrome-associated spondylarthropathy, rheumatoid arthritis, multiple sclerosis, systemic lupus erythematosis, Crohn's disease, ankylosing spondylitis, Vogt–Koyanagi–Harada syndrome and sympathetic ophthalmia.

Pharmaceuticals reported to trigger uveitis include erythopoetin, sulfonamides, topical prostaglandin and cholinergic analogs, bisphosphonates, rifabutin, and certain vaccinations including varicella and mumps/measles/rubella.

DIAGNOSIS

Clinical signs and symptoms

Symptoms of uveitis include pain, tearing, photophobia, restricted versions and visual loss. Signs include tenderness, redness, periorbital edema, chemosis, secondary glaucoma, anterior chamber- posterior chamber- and vitreous-debris (cells and/or proteinaceous exudation, i.e. flare), retinal- and choroidal-infiltration, nerve fiber layer infarcts (i.e. cotton wool spots), papilledema, macular edema and retinal vasculitis.

Longterm sequelae of uveitis include iris synechialization, cystoid macular edema, posterior subcapsular cataract, glaucoma, band keratopathy, keratoconjunctivitis sicca, retinal detachment and neovascularization, all of which can lead to permanent visual loss.

Differential diagnosis

Underlying infections and malignancies that masquerade as uveitis must be excluded from the differential diagnosis prior to treatment. In all cases, the timing of onset and duration of symptoms are important clues toward diagnosis. A lack of response to therapy or significant recrudescence after therapy should prompt further investigation and possible reevaluation of the diagnosis.

In many cases, uveitis is treated empirically unless there is compelling information in the history or physical examination to do otherwise. Examples of patients who might be treated empirically include an otherwise healthy young person with a mild, unilateral iritis, or a patient with a known history of juvenile rheumatoid arthritis who has previously responded to a topical steroid. Conversely, if a patient has a repeat bout of iritis, bilateral iritis or a severe case, a diagnostic workup is recommended (Figure 288.1). Furthermore, if a patient with Crohn's proffers that they are an outdoors enthusiast or sexually promiscuous, a directed workup should be offered to ensure that their uveitis might not be from some other entity (e.g. Lyme disease or syphilis respectively).

Laboratory findings

When a workup is initiated, it is strongly recommended that tests for certain illnesses routinely be included in first line

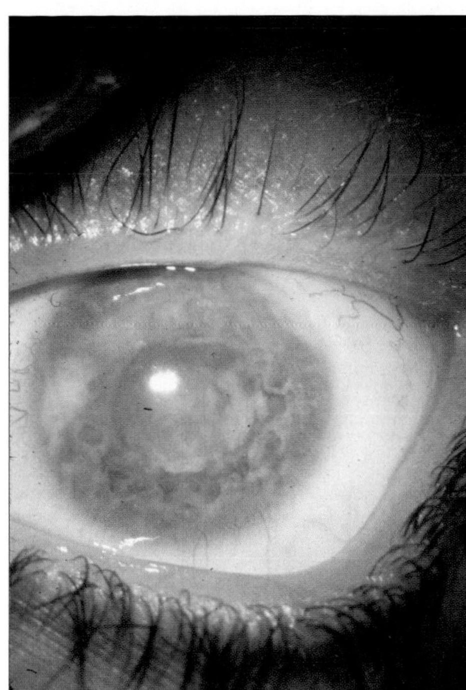

FIGURE 288.1. Iritis with pupillary membrane.

studies unless the history suggests otherwise. These include a chest radiograph, purified protein derivative (PPD) immune challenge administered subcutaneously, fluorescent treponemal antibody (FTA-ABS) and Lyme C6 peptide, to search for evidence of sarcoidosis, tuberculosis, syphilis and Lyme disease, respectively.

Patients with complaints of joint pain should be further evaluated for autoimmune and infectious arthritides, particularly lupus, rheumatoid arthritis and Lyme disease. Evaluation of the serum for the presence of antinuclear antibody (ANA), anti-double stranded DNA antibody (anti-dsDNA Ab), rheumatoid factor (RF), cyclic citrullinated peptide antibody (CCP Ab), Lyme-C6 peptide antigen and antibody, Western blot and polymerase chain reaction (PCR) could be performed.

At times, certain diagnoses will lead the differential list based upon the clinical picture, such as in a patient with hematochezia (e.g. suspected Crohn's disease) or a patient with a classic chorioretinal distribution of inflammation (e.g. birdshot chorioretinopathy); confirmation of the diagnosis is still important. In such cases, it may be useful to search for the presence of particular human leukocyte antigen (HLA) serotypes known to be associated with uveitis. Examples include HLA B27 (ankylosing spondylitis, Reiter's syndrome, psoriatic arthritis and inflammatory bowel disease-associated spondylarthropathy), HLA B5 and B51 (Behçet's disease), HLA B7 (serpiginous choroiditis) and HLA A29 (birdshot chorioretinopathy).

In some patients who do not respond to therapy, a diagnostic paracentesis of the anterior chamber or vitrectomy could be quite helpful. Often, these procedures are the only way to diagnose lymphoid malignancies masquerading as uveitis.

TREATMENT

Treatment of uveitis is dependent on the etiology, duration of disease, severity and location of inflammation, as well as the potential complications of therapy. For infectious uveitis, treatment is directed at the inciting organism; this generally leads to elimination of the inflammation. There are times when judicious use of steroids can help reduce collateral damage caused by inflammation. Treatment of immune-mediated uveitis is determined more by severity and location than by etiology.

Systemic

Oral steroids are the mainstay of systemic therapy against uveitis that has not responded to topical or periocular medication and that is not associated with infection or malignancy. The goal of therapy is to maximize anti-inflammatory efficacy while minimizing side effects. Often, the inflammation will not be eliminated but only reduced to a tolerable level. For the first four weeks, prednisone 60 mg daily is prescribed. Once the inflammation is controlled, a gradual tapering schedule is implemented. Pulse intravenous steroid therapy (1 gm/day methylprednisolone × 3 days) can be used as initial therapy in some patients.

A trial of immunosuppressant therapy is suggested by the International Uveitis Study Group for patients with bilateral disease, and/or vision loss below 20/50 and/or failure to respond to steroids. Currently used agents include cyclosporin A (2.5–5 mg/kg PO daily), hydroxychloroquine, and cytotoxic agents such as azathioprine, chlorambucil, cyclophosphamide, and methotrexate (7.5–25 mg/week). Novel agents such as anti-TNF monoclonal antibody, thalidomide, tacrolimus and interferon-alpha are currently being evaluated and have shown some promise. Nonsteroidal anti-inflammatory agents such as indomethacin and flurbiprofen are of limited value. Immunosuppressive therapy should be monitored closely by oncologists or rheumatologists.

Ocular

Topical therapy for iritis should include a steroid and cycloplegic. As a general rule, medications that cause lesser adverse effects provide a weaker therapeutic response.

Steroid preparations include prednisolone, dexamethasone, rimexolone and fluorometholone; therapy should be initiated as soon as possible. Intensive therapy, such as hourly dosing or employing medication-soaked pledgets placed in the conjunctival fornices may give more rapid relief. Thereafter, drops are prescribed every 4–6 hours. Dexamethasone is available as an ointment.

Periocular steroid injection is an excellent choice for unilateral and/or posterior uveitis. For anterior uveitis, the depot site is the subconjunctival space of the inferior fornix, while for posterior inflammation, a superotemporal depot in the sub-Tenon's space or anterior placement with a trans-septal approach is suggested. Available preparations include dexamethasone, betamethasone, triamcinolone and methylprednisolone. Shorter acting compounds such as dexamethasone may be preferred where the risk of steroid-induced glaucoma is unknown. Injections of 1mL can be repeated every 2–6 weeks and the injection site should be varied to ensure adequate delivery of drug.

Choices of cycloplegics include cyclopentolate (0.5–2% t.i.d.), homatropine (2–5% b.i.d.), and atropine (1% b.i.d.). The inflamed eye metabolizes the cycloplegic agents more rapidly so dosing may have to be increased. However, the goal of cycloplegia is to reduce pain without maintaining constant mydriasis, so as to prevent anterior and posterior synechialization.

Glaucoma secondary to 360 degree posterior synechialization is best treated with peripheral laser iridotomy.

Vitrectomy is an option for severe vitreous opacification that has failed other therapy. Cryotherapy and laser photocoagulation may be considered for localized pars plana exudates. Cataract surgery is optimally performed in a quiescent eye. In all cases, surgery on an eye that is or was inflamed has greater risks of complications.

COMPLICATIONS

Ocular toxicity from periocular or topical ocular steroids include posterior subcapsular cataract, glaucoma, central serous retinopathy and an increased risk of fungal infections or herpetic infections.

Systemic corticosteroids can not only cause all the aforementioned adverse effects associated with local steroid placement, but can also cause or worsen osteoporosis, adrenal suppression, hyperglycemia, acne, peptic ulcer disease, pseudotumor cerebri and psychosis.

Inadvertent intraocular injection of corticosteroids could result in blindness. Even well placed periocular steroid injections can cause localized ptosis, fat atrophy and more nonspecific sequelae of injection including hemorrhage, infection and allergy.

Steroid induced glaucoma can be controlled with topical eye drops, removal of the depot steroid, reduction or discontinuation of the steroid, and surgery. At times it may be difficult to determine whether the glaucoma is from the steroid, the uveitis or both. Withdrawal of steroid can cause pseudotumor cerebri and Addisonian crisis.

Immunosuppressive medications have particular toxicity, and all predispose patients to opportunistic infections. None should be administered to a woman prior to knowing her gestational status. It is recommended that a nonpregnant woman use birth control while receiving this therapy. High dose cyclosporin A is associated with nephrotoxicity, hepatoxicity, hirsuitism, hypertension, gingivitis, malaise and lymphoma. All cytotoxic agents cause hemotologic cytopenias. Methotrexate is fairly safe, although one should watch for hepatoxicity by monitoring liver function tests. Nutritional support with folate 1 mg/day should be included during methotrexate therapy.

COMMENTS

As the genetics of immunopathogenesis are explored, it is hoped that we will come to a point where the preponderance of cases will not have to be deemed idiopathic; the diagnosis of idiopathic uveitis must be one of exclusion. If the clinician feels that the list of diagnostic possibilities has been exhausted and the patient is not improving or is worsening, referral to a tertiary level treatment center is strongly advised.

The ophthalmologist is in a unique position to help the patient with uveitis. Uveitis is often a presenting sign in many diseases. Hence, it behooves the ophthalmologist to coordinate his efforts with the patient's primary care provider to ensure that the presence of an underlying pathology be considered. The ophthalmologist can help guide testing for a systemic problem. If such is discovered, the ophthalmologist can help protect the eye from the adverse effects of both illness and therapy.

REFERENCES

Antel J, Birnbaum G, Hartung H-P: Clinical neuroimmunology. Malden: Blackwell Science; 1998.

Brazis PW, Stewart M, Lee AG: The uveo-meningeal syndromes. Neurologist 10:171–184, 2004.

Durrani OM, Meads CA, Murray PI: Uveitis: a potentially blinding disease. Ophthalmologica 218:223–236, 2004.

Foster CS, Vitale AT: Diagnosis and treatment of uveitis. New York: WB Saunders; 2002.

Vavvas D, Foster CS: Immunomodulatory medications in uveitis. Int Ophthalmol Clin 44:187–203, 2004.

SECTION

25 Lacrimal System

289 CONGENITAL ANOMALIES OF THE LACRIMAL SYSTEM 743.65

(Congenital Nasolacrimal Duct Obstruction, Dacryocystitis, Dacryocystocele, Accessary [Anlage] Punctum, Punctal Stenosis, Canalicular Stenosis)

David K. Coats, MD
Houston, Texas

ETIOLOGY/INCIDENCE

The most common congenital anomaly of the lacrimal drainage system is outflow obstruction, which may be present in as many as 5–6% of infants. The most common site of obstruction is at the distal portion of the nasolacrimal duct near its entry into the inferior meatus. Here, a membrane known as Hasner's membrane, fails to regress, producing symptomatic outflow obstruction.

Less common clinical anomalies include punctal atresia or stenosis, canalicular atresia or stenosis, and accessory lacrimal puncta. A dacryocystocele is a congenital anomaly that may develop when there exists an obstruction at the valve of Hasner distally and a proximal obstruction at the valve of Rosenmuller. A dacryocystocele is typically obvious in the first few weeks of life and can be associated with dacryocystitis and/or respiratory distress as described below.

COURSE/PROGNOSIS

When the obstruction of the lacrimal drainage system is distal to the nasolacrimal sac, the symptoms are overflow tearing and recurrent mucopurulent discharge, as bacteria and debris sequestered within the lacrimal sac reflux onto the ocular surface. When the obstruction is proximal to the lacrimal sac, the symptoms are typically tearing only, with little or no mucopurulent discharge. Tearing is rarely present at birth in patients with lacrimal outflow obstruction, but usually develops in the first weeks of life. Among the most prominent symptoms are mucopurulent debris on the lashes upon awakening that may result in adhesion of the upper and lower lids together. Pressure on the nasolacrimal sac will often result in obvious reflux of tears and/or mucupurulent material from the punctum.

Nasolacrimal outflow obstruction will resolve spontaneously during the first year of life in most patients. More than half of patients will be asymptomatic by 6–8 months of age and approximately 90% will be asymptomatic by 1 year of age. Dacryocystitis occasionally develops and can be life threatening in young infants. Dacryocystitis commonly occurs in association with a dacryocystocele. Respiratory distress can occur in infants with a unilateral or bilateral dacryocystocele because of the presence of cystic dilation of the nasal mucosa at the distal end of the nasolacrimal canal, which blocks the nasal passage.

Symptoms that are notably absent in infants with lacrimal outflow obstruction include photophobia and corneal clouding. When present, a more ominous condition, such as congenital glaucoma, should be considered.

DIAGNOSIS

Clinical testing

Though children are inherently difficult to evaluate, office testing can be of value in selected cases when the clinical diagnosis is not obvious. An increased tear lake is almost always present. A dye disappearance test can be performed by placing fluorescein drops in the inferior cul-de-sac. In a child with an intact lacrimal drainage system, the dye will typically egress through the lacrimal drainage system within 3 to 5 minutes, with minimal or no overflow onto the cheeks. In a child with lacrimal outflow obstruction, in contrast, the fluorescein dye remains in the tear meniscus for a prolonged period of time and often overflows onto the cheek. Reflux of tears and/or mucopurulent material from the punctum with pressure on the nasolacrimal sac is probably the simplest confirmatory test in a young child.

DIFFERENTIAL DIAGNOSIS

The majority of children who present with persistent tearing and/or discharge, will be diagnosed with a nasolacrimal duct obstruction. The diagnosis is generally obvious. A number of more serious problems can masquerade as a nasolacrimal duct obstruction, and include congenital glaucoma, keratitis, uveitis, trichiasis, and corneal foreign body. These more serious problems can usually be readily distinguished from a simple nasolacrimal outflow obstruction by the presence of photophobia, corneal clouding, corneal enlargement, and/or persistent ocular redness, none of which occur in the child with isolated nasolacrimal duct obstruction.

TREATMENT

Nasolacrimal outflow obstruction

Because nasolacrimal outflow obstruction spontaneously resolves during the first year of life in most children, conservative therapy is typically warranted. Nasolacrimal sac massage is often recommended several times per day, both to empty the nasolacrimal sac and to potentially hasten resolution of the obstruction. Topical antibiotics are usually prescribed when mucopurulent discharge is present throughout the day. Topical antibiotics typically need not be used when discharge is present only upon awakening. Systemic antibiotics are indicated in the presence of an associated dacryocystitis and/or preseptal cellulitis.

Surgical

Probing of the nasolacrimal drainage system can be done in an office or operating room setting. Office probing is limited to smaller children, typically those less than 1 year of age. The recommended age at initial probing varies among practitioners, with some probing as early as 4 to 6 months of age, while others wait until a year or more of age. Probing in the office is done under topical anesthesia after wrapping the child in a blanket or restraining the child in a papoose board.

There are a number of surgical treatment options available for children undergoing treatment in the operating room. Many surgeons prefer probing and irrigation alone as the initial treatment for all children, reserving adjunctive therapies, such as silicone tube intubation and balloon dilation, for treatment failures. Other surgeons prefer to use adjunctive measures at the time of initial probing when treatement is performed under general anesthesia. If probing is performed alone, without adjunctive measures, irrigation of the lacrimal drainage system with fluorescein dyed saline solution and suction retrieval from the nose should be used to confirm patency of the lacrimal drainage system.

Silicone tubes can be placed in the lacrimal drainage system as a stint to reduce the tendency for the newly opened duct to close. A variety of tube delivery systems are available, including monocanalicular and bicanalicular systems. Tubes may be removed in the office weeks to months after placement, depending on the preference of the surgeon.

Balloon catheter dilation has been reported to be an effective primary surgical treatment for nasolacrimal duct obstruction. A collapsed balloon is placed through the punctum and into the nasolacrimal canal. It is then inflated to dilate the lacrimal drainage system. Because of the high cost of balloon catheters relative to other treatment options, many surgeons reserve balloon catheters for special situations, including treatment failures.

Controversy exists regarding the timing and method of treatment for children with dacryocystoceles. Certainly the child with respiratory distress should be treated urgently. For those without respiratory distress, some authors recommend massage and systemic antibiotics, with observation to allow time for spontaneous resolution. Others, citing a high incidence of dacryocystitis, recommend probing as soon as possible after the diagnosis is made. Initial probing can be performed in the office. Treatment failures are common and repeat treatment in the operating room is sometimes needed. Surgical removal of an associated intranasal mucocele, when present, may be needed to affect resolution. Identification and treatment of intranasal mucoceles can be facilitated by use of nasal endoscopy.

COMPLICATIONS

Complications of surgical treatment for lacrimal outflow obstruction are uncommon. Recurrence or persistence of symptoms may occur in a small number of patients. Damage to the mucosa lining the lacrimal outflow system, or creation of a false passage can occur and may render future treatment more difficult. Damage to the nasal mucosa and adjacent turbinates can occur, but is infrequent.

COMMENTS

Punctal stenosis can be overcome by dilation and/or a snip punctalplasty to enlarge the punctal opening. Puncture of a membranous covering over the puncta will relieve obstructions from this cause. Canalicular stenosis can be overcome by passing probes of gradually increasing diameter, followed by stenting to promote maintenance of the newly enlarged canaliculus.

Dacryocystorhinostomy and conjunctivodacryocystorhinostomy are occasionally indicated in children who fail standard treatment for lacrimal outflow obstruction. These procedures are generally deferred until children are 5 to 6 years of age, and are needed infrequently.

Ectopic (anlage) lacrimal ducts do not require treatment unless symptomatic. Tearing and/or discharge from an anlage duct may require treatment. The anomalous duct is removed intact by ligating it near the lacrimal sac followed by excision of the ectopia duct and closure of the overlying skin.

Nasolacrimal outflow obstruction tends to be more complex in patients with mid-face anomalies, including children with Down syndrome. In children with Down syndrome, abnormalities of the lacrimal drainage system proximal to the lacrimal sac predominate, including canalicular stenosis and canalicular atresia. Adjunctive therapies such as silicone tube intubation and balloon dilation are often considered during initial treatment.

Symptomatic nasolacrimal duct obstruction is common in infants, affecting up to 6% of newborn infants. Conservative treatment is typically recommended because spontaneous resolution will occur in most patients. Some surgeons recommend probing in the office as early as 4 to 6 months of age, while others wait until the child is a year or more of age. When performed in the operating room, probing and irrigation alone can be utilized as the initial treatment or probing can be combined with an adjunctive measure such as silicone tube intubation or balloon catheter dilation initially.

Complications of lacrimal outflow obstruction are uncommon and primarily involve infection of involved and surrounding tissues, and respiratory obstruction in the case of dacrycystoceles. Complications associated with treatment are also uncommon and can be minimized by proper selection of probes, adjunctive measures, and optimal technique. Failure of standard probing with or without adjunctive measures is uncommon, though repeat treatment is sometimes needed. Dacryocystorhinostomy and conjunctivodacryocystorhinostomy are rarely required.

REFERENCES

Lueder GT: Balloon catheter dilation for treatment of older children with nasolacrimal duct obstruction. Arch Ophthalmol 120:1685–1688, 2002.

Paul TO, Shepherd R: Congenital nasolacrimal duct obstruction: natural history and the timing of optimal intervention. J Pediatr Ophthalmol Strabismus 31:362–367, 1994.

Paysse EA, Coats DK, Bernstein JM, et al: Management and complications of congenital dacryocele with concurrent intranasal mucocele. J AAPOS 4:46–53, 2000.

Yuen SJA, Oley C, Sullivan TJ: Lacrimal outflow dysgenesis. Ophthalmology 111:1782–1790, 2004.

290 DACRYOADENITIS 375.00

John D. Ng, MD, MS, FACS
Portland, Oregon

Dacryoadenitis is an inflammatory enlargement of the lacrimal gland. Acute or chronic dacryoadenitis may affect the palpebral and/or orbital lobes separately.

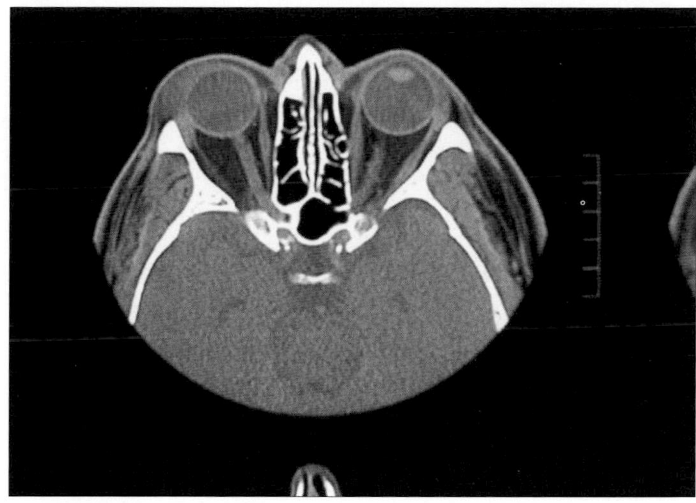

FIGURE 290.1. Computed tomography (CT) showing inflammatory enlargement of lacrimal gland in right orbit.

ETIOLOGY

Dacryoadenitis may be caused by infection, sarcoid, Sjögren syndrome, Graves disease, lupus, Wegener granulomatosis, or benign lymphoepithelial lesions.

COURSE/PROGNOSIS

- The disease may run a brief course and then resolve. Alternatively, it may progress to suppuration.
- Acute orbital is rarer than palpebral lobe involvement:
  - Acentuated symptoms include pain and adenopathy;
  - Proptosis is common;
  - Limited ocular motility with diplopia, occasional convergent squint, ptosis, edema and erythema may occur.
- Chronic dacryoadenitis:
  - There is painless swelling in the upper/outer eyelid, with ptosis;
  - A hard mass is palpable under the superolateral rim of the orbit;
  - Displacement of the globe downward and inward occurs with diplopia on looking up and out, but proptosis is rare.

DIAGNOSIS

- Patients with acute palpebral dacryoadenitis usually present with orbital pain.
- Edema and S-shaping of the upper lid occur.
- There may be a preauricular lymph node.
- Palpation of the lid shows a tender nut-shaped swelling continuous with neither the orbit nor the ciliary margin.
- The conjunctiva may be injected and chemotic, with/without mucous discharge.
- CT — enlarged gland, no bony destruction (Figure 290.1).

TREATMENT

Systemic

- Treatment is determined by the cause.
- When dacryoadenitis is a complication of systemic disease, therapy is directed toward the overall treatment of the generalized disorder.
- Dacryoadenitis from a viral disease (most commonly, mumps) should be treated symptomatically:
  - Heat or cold is applied locally;
  - Bed rest and salicylates are recommended.
- Dacryoadenitis secondary to sarcoidosis should be treated with systemic corticosteroids.
- Use appropriate antibiotic therapy if the causative agent is identified in a bacterial infection.

Ocular

- Lavage the conjunctival sac if discharge is present.
- Replacement therapy is instituted with tear substitutes.

Surgical

- Incision and drainage are indicated if suppuration occurs;
- Incise through the conjunctiva, avoiding the ductules, if the palpebral lobe is involved;
- Incise through the skin if the orbital lobe is affected.

COMMENTS

It is generally believed that lacrimal gland enlargements are caused by tumors or inflammations, with inflammations representing the more frequent cause. Among granulomatous diseases resulting in lacrimal gland inflammation, sarcoidosis and Sjögren's syndrome are the most prominent. The lacrimal gland may also undergo chronic inflammation and, ultimately, fibrosis as sequelae of radiation or loss of innervation. Lacrimal gland enlargement may be due to causes other than inflammation, such as nutritional deficiencies, alcoholism, diabetes, tumors, and the use of certain drugs. The infrequency of reported cases of dacryoadenitis reflects the fact that the lacrimal gland is housed in a bony cavity that is not regularly palpated and can conceal moderate enlargement.

REFERENCES

Kostic DA, Linberg JV: Lacrimal gland tumors. In: Tassman W, Jaeger EA, eds: Clinical ophthalmology. Philadelphia, Lippincott, Wilkins & Wilkins 2004:2:40:5–7.

Mafee MF, Edward DP, Koeller KK, Dorodi S: Lacrimal gland tumors and simulating lesions. Clinicopathologic and MR features. Radiol Clin North Am 37(1):213–239, 1999.

Jakobiec FA, Jones IS: Orbital inflammations. In: Duane TD, ed: Clinical ophthalmology. Haggerstown, Harper & Row, 1982:II:64–69.

291 DACRYOCYSTITIS AND DACRYOLITH 375.30

Robert N. Tower, MD
Seattle, Washington

ETIOLOGY/INCIDENCE

Dacryocystitis is an inflammation in the lacrimal sac resulting from stasis of tears in the lacrimal drainage system and secondary infection by bacteria or fungus. It may be present in infancy (congenital nasolacrimal duct obstruction), affecting 2% to 6% of live births, or maybe an acquired condition. It most frequently presents in middle age, but it is not restricted to any age group.

Dacryolith is a concretion of material in the canaliculi, lacrimal sac, or nasolacrimal duct. It partially or completely obstructs the drainage of tears. Dacryoliths are frequently present in fungal canaliculitis, and as a distinct entity it may be present in many patients with chronic dacryocystitis and a patent nasolacrimal duct.

Infantile dacryocystitis

Causes include incomplete canalization of the nasolacrimal duct, with an obstructing membranous remnant; nasolacrimal duct atresia; facial cleft; and dacryocele.

Acquired dacryocystitis

- Chronic or acute infection is a common denominator.
- Trauma, nasal fracture or surgery, and laceration or blunt trauma to lacrimal sac are causes.
- In functional block, the nasolacrimal duct is patent, but lacrimal excretory function is compromised.
- Dacryolith is present in 15% to 20% of patients with functional block.
- Tumor is intrinsic in the lacrimal sac or extrinsic and impinging on the sac or duct.
- Granuloma, inflammatory or infectious disease are the causes.
- Retained foreign body, including the Silastic tubing from prior lacrimal intubation, can be a cause.

Canaliculitis

- The origin is usually fungal: *Candida, Aspergillus, Nocardia,* and *Actinomyces* spp., among others.
- A bacterial origin is unusual except after trauma.

COURSE/PROGNOSIS

Infantile dacryocystitis

Congenital nasolacrimal obstruction usually presents in the first 6 weeks of life with epiphora and chronic mucopurulent discharge in one or both eyes. Most infants will have spontaneous resolution of the condition within the first 6 months of life, and more than 90% are reported to outgrow the problem by one year.

Acquired dacryocystitis

Acquired dacryocystitis may be acute or chronic. Acute dacryocystitis presents with painful, sometimes massive, enlargement of the lacrimal sac at or below the level of the medial canthal tendon and in the medial lower eyelid. If not treated, spontaneous rupture and drainage through the skin are common. A dacryocutaneous fistula may result. With proper therapy, the acute infections resolve in 7 to 14 days (Figure 291.1).

Chronic dacryocystitis, with or without dacryolith, is characterized by recurring episodes of epiphora or mucopurulent discharge, often but not always associated with a nontender fullness below the medial canthal tendon. Acute dacryocystitis may be superimposed on the chronic condition. Bloody tears may be a sign of lacrimal sac dacryolith or tumor.

Canaliculitis

Fungal canaliculitis is usually a unilateral disorder with thickening of the nasal eyelid and canthal erythema. It should be suspected in anyone with chronic unilateral nasal angle blepharoconjunctivitis that does not respond to typical antibiotic therapy. Compression of the canaliculus often will cause reflux onto the eye of a creamy pus containing 'sulfur granules.' Canaliculitis is found most commonly in the Midwest and other farming areas of the United States.

DIAGNOSIS

Infantile dacryocystitis

- Typical epiphora and discharge in the absence of conjunctival erythema are virtually pathognomonic.
- The fluorescein dye retention test will indicate poor lacrimal drainage in the involved eye.
- Digital pressure over the lacrimal sac may express mucopurulent material onto the globe.

Acquired dacryocystitis

Acute

- A typical clinical presentation is usually all that is needed for diagnosis.

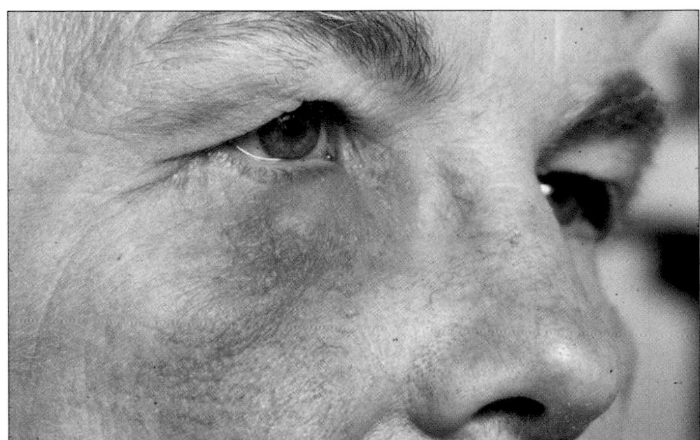

FIGURE 291.1. Dacryocystitis.

- The fluorescein dye retention test will confirm lacrimal drainage disorder and may be useful if inflammatory signs are minimal.
- Massage over the lacrimal sac often recovers a pus reflux through the canaliculus. Culture usually grows gram-positive cocci and much less often gram-negative cocci. In children, *Haemophilus* spp. is common.

Chronic

- Epiphora, with or without mucus, is almost always present.
- Tests of lacrimal excretory function, including fluorescein dye retention and primary and secondary Jones tests, should indicate reduced tear drainage.
- Palpable dilation of the lacrimal sac during irrigation is typical, and if the nasolacrimal duct is completely obstructed, irrigant will reflux out the opposite canaliculus. In some patients, however, irrigation of the lacrimal system may not indicate any obstruction.
- Culture of lacrimal sac reflux is usually not necessary for appropriate treatment.

Canaliculitis

- A clinical picture combined with expression of pus from the canaliculus and not from the lacrimal sac is diagnostic.
- Appropriate stains of slide preparations may identify a fungus.
- Culture for fungus is usually indicated, though therapy will be necessary before return of the results of such cultures. They may lead to proper alteration of therapy in resistant cases.

Differential diagnosis

Infantile dacryocystitis

- Punctal or canalicular atresia: usually, there is epiphora without mucus.
- Conjunctivitis: conjunctiva is red, and the problem resolves with topical antibiotics.
- Conjunctival foreign body: the onset is usually later, with an acute presentation and red eye.
- Nasal mucosal edema: inferior meatus is obstructed, and tearing is produced secondarily: The problem resolves with decongestants.

Acquired dacryocystitis: chronic

- Punctal or canalicular stenosis: there is epiphora without mucus; probing and irrigation will reveal upper system obstruction.
- Epiphora is secondary to a poor lacrimal pump:
  - Cranial Nerve VII palsy is present;
  - Eyelid deformity preventing lid movement occurs;
  - Senile eyelid laxity with or without ectropion is present;
  - Flaccidity.

TREATMENT

Systemic

- Chronic dacryocystitis rarely requires systemic therapy, even in infants.
- Acute dacryocystitis in childhood may be a medical emergency, requiring hospitalization and intravenous antibiotics.
- Acute dacryocystitis in adults is treated with oral broad-spectrum antibiotics: 500 mg azithromycin once, followed by 250 mg q.i.d. for 4 days, or 500/150 mg amoxicillin/clavulanate t.i.d. for 10 days. The medication is changed if the culture grows a resistant organism.

Ocular

Acquired dacryocystitis

- Acute:
  - Warm compresses and antibiotic eyedrops are applied q.i.d.;
  - If the sac is distended, decompress it by introducing a lacrimal probe or cannula through the lower canaliculus into the sac; gentle pressure will usually empty the sac contents onto the conjunctiva. Rarely, it is necessary to use percutaneous drainage with an 11 blade. Perform this in the line of the future dacryocystorhinostomy incision in case a dacryocutaneous fistula forms, after the resolution of infection, evaluate the cause of stasis and perform the appropriate surgery to prevent recurrences.
- Chronic:
  - Antibiotic drops may be applied twice daily until surgical intervention;
  - Gentle digital decompression is applied twice or three times daily until surgery.

Canaliculitis

- Topical nystatin 20,000 U/mL q.i.d. is used for most fungal agents.
- Topical penicillin 50,000 U q.i.d. is used for *Actinomyces* spp.
- Express canalicular dacryoliths and gently irrigate with the antifungal solution every 2 to 3 days.

Surgical

Congenital nasolacrimal duct obstruction

- When surgery is required, simple probing in the office or operating room is successful 90% of the time.
- Intubation of the nasolacrimal duct with Silastic tubing to act as a stent in the duct is required occasionally. Dacryocystorhinostomy is needed rarely.
- Dacryocele without infection may respond as typical nasolacrimal duct obstruction. When the infection is present, probing must be combined with intranasal examination for nasolacrimal duct cyst, and excision if one is found.

Acquired dacryocystitis

- External dacryocystorhinostomy.
- Endonasal endoscopic dacryocystorhinostomy.
- Balloon catheterization has been reported with some success.

COMPLICATIONS

Probing

- Laceration of puncta or canaliculi can occur.
- False passage formation can occur in the eyelid.

Dacryocystogram

- Dye extravasation outside the canaliculi or tear duct causes inflammation and possible necrosis of soft tissue.

Silastic tubes

- If the tube is too tight, it will cheese-wire the punctal opening.
- Incomplete removal of tubing may result in late scarring of the anastomosis.
- Leaving the tube in place for more than 6 months increases risk of late scarring.

Dacryocystorhinostomy

- Retrobulbar or preseptal hemorrhage can be severe.
- Postoperative intranasal hemorrhages may require nasal pack or, rarely, cautery of the ethmoid artery.
- Scarring of the anastomosis and late failure are most commonly a result of an osteotomy that is too small. Postoperative infection or hemorrhage also increases the risk of late failure.

COMMENTS

External dacryocystorhinostomy has a success rate of 95% when performed by experienced surgeons. Although it requires a facial incision, the cosmetic result usually is excellent. It is the only surgical approach to the lacrimal sac that allows full examination for dacryoliths, granulomas and tumors.

Intranasal endoscopic dacryocystorhinostomy has the advantage of avoiding a skin incision, but it has a significant learning curve. It can achieve rates of success near that of the external approach in experienced hands.

Balloon catheterization is a more recent innovation that appears to have some limited success in the appropriately selected patient population. It is unlikely to supplant standard dacryocystorhinostomy.

Although chronic dacryocystitis may resolve spontaneously in infants, it will usually be a recurring problem in older children and adults until surgical intervention. Acute dacryocystitis should be controlled medically, but surgery should then be performed to prevent the disabling return of the same problem.

Canaliculitis may respond to medical therapy, but if it persists uncontrolled beyond 3 to 4 weeks, it also should be treated surgically.

REFERENCES

Campolattaro BN, Luedder GT, Tychsen L: Spectrum of pediatric dacryocystitis: medical and surgical management of 54 cases. J Pediatr Ophthalmol Strabismus 34:143–153, 1997.

Lee TS, Woog JJ: Endonasal dacryocystorhinostomy in the primary treatment of acute dacryocystitis with abscess formation. Ophthal Plastic & Reconstr Surg 17(3):180–183, 2001.

Yazici B, Hammad AM, Meyer DR: Lacrimal sac dacryoliths: predictive factors and clinical characteristics. Ophthalmology 108(7):1308–1312, 2001.

Zappia RJ, Milder B: Lacrimal drainage function. 1. The Jones fluorescein test. Am J Ophthalmol 74:154–159, 1972.

292 EPIPHORA 375.20

John L. Wobig, MD
Portland, Oregon
John D. Ng, MD, MS, FACS
Portland, Oregon

ETIOLOGY

Epiphora is the result of hypersecretion or failure of the lacrimal excretory system to function. Many conditions cause epiphora. Stimulation of the fifth cranial nerve due to any pathologic condition, such as corneal foreign body, trichiasis, corneal ulcer or nasal pathology will cause a reflex hypersecretion. Aberrent facial nerve regeneration can cause crocodile tearing. Abnormalities of the tear distribution and pump systems such as entropion, ectropion or lid retraction as well as constriction or complete closure of the punctum, canaliculi, tear sac, or tear duct may also result in epiphora.

COURSE/PROGNOSIS

The course of epiphora depnds on the etiology and if treated medically or surgically, can be cured.

DIAGNOSIS

Laboratory findings

- Schirmer's test.
- Basic secretion test.
- Primary dye test (Jones test 1).
- Secondary dye test (Jones test 2).
- Lid snap-back test.
- Diagnostic probing.
- Slit lamp examination.

TREATMENT

Ocular

Local disorders of the eye that cause reflex hypersecretion are treated conservatively, with treatment directed toward the cause, e.g. lid hygeine and doxycycline for meibomianitis and epilation for trichiasis. Massage of the tear sac in conjunction with antibiotic drops is used for dacryocystitis. Injection of botulinum toxin into the main lacrimal gland has been used to treat hypersecretion from aberrant facial nerve regeneration.

Surgical

A conjunctival dacryocystorhinostomy with Jones tube placement is preferable to removal of the accessory lacrimal gland lobe if hypersecretion cannot be treated conservatively.

Surgery on the distributional system is usually done to correct entropion or ectropion.

- Punctal occlusion.
- Open strictures with Habb needle knife under the microscope or slit lamp.

- One-snip procedure: cut posterior punctum for 2 mm; follow with several dilations.
- Silicone intubation.
- Canalicular obstructions.
- Silicone intubation.
- Conjunctivodacryocystorhinostomy.
- Tear sac obstructions.
- Dacryocystorhinostomy.
- Silicone intubation.
- Nasolacrimal duct obstruction.
- Early probing for infants.
- Dacryocystorhinostomy (DCR) for adults.
- Balloon dacryoplasty with intubation may be used in selected cases such as partial obstruction although with less long-term patency compared with DCR.

PRECAUTIONS

Probing for therapeutic purposes should be confined to infants, whereas probing in adults should be limited to diagnostic testing. Dacryocystorhinostomy is the preferred treatment for most cases of epiphora, and a dacryocystectomy should be avoided except for tumors. Lacrimal surgery necessitates a thorough knowledge of the lateral wall of the nose.

COMMENTS

A lacrimal evaluation should include inspection, palpation, and the proper diagnostic test. The lacrimal distributional, secretory, and excretory systems should be evaluated to properly diagnose the underlying cause of epiphora.

REFERENCES

Tenzel RR: Canaliculo-dacryocystorhinostomy. Arch Ophthalmol 84:765, 1970.

Veirs ER: Lacrimal Disorders: Diagnosis and treatment. St Louis, CV Mosby, 1976.

Wobig JL: The office management of the lacrimal excretory system. JCE Ophthalmol December:13–24, 1978.

Wobig JL: Lacerations of the lacrimal excretory system: ocular trauma. New York, Prentice Hall, 1979.

Wobig JL: Epiphora, causes and treatment. Perspect Ophthalmol 5:177–181, 1981.

293 LACRIMAL SYSTEM CONTUSIONS AND LACERATIONS 871.4

Louise Mawn, MD
Nashville, Tennessee

ETIOLOGY

Both intentional and accidental sharp and blunt trauma can injure the lacrimal system. Full thickness laceration of the palpebral and lacrimal segments of the lid can result from objects such as coat hangers, knives, tree branches, children's toys, innocuous trauma from fingernails or blunt trauma from a fist. Dog bites to the medial canthal and lacrimal area are more common in toddlers and young children (Figure 293.1).

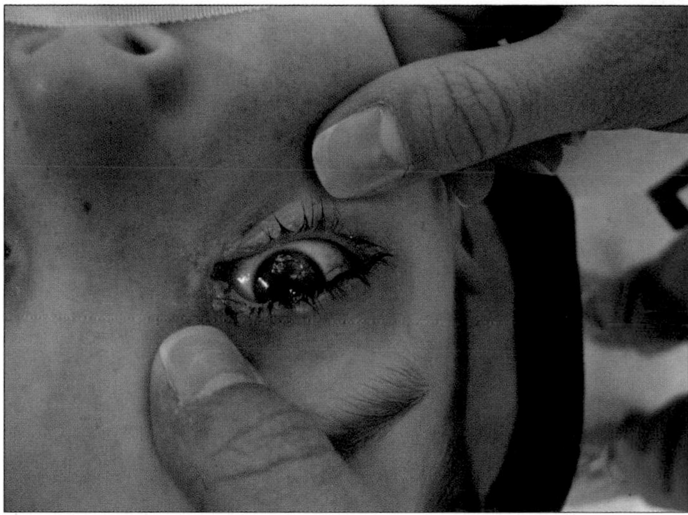

FIGURE 293.1. An 8 year old boy with a laceration of his right superior canaliculus sustained during a fall.

INCIDENCE

Facial lacerations accounted for an estimated 1.97 million Emergency Department visits in the United States in 2002. Eyelid lacerations make up a smaller percentage of those visits. An epidemiological study of 180 patients seen at the University of Munich between 1997–1999 found 16% of all eyelid injuries involved the lacrimal system. Forty four percent of the eyelid injuries were associated with injuries to the eyeball.

COURSE

Most frequently patients with a laceration of the periocular area present for emergent evaluation. Although some controversy exists in the method of repair and whether to repair an isolated laceration of a canaliculus, most ophthalmic plastic surgeons favor repair.

PROGNOSIS

Microsurgical repair of the lacerated canaliculus has been reported to achieve patency rates as high as 94%–100%. Cases with extensive medial canthal trauma have a lower success rate.

DIAGNOSIS

Any laceration involving the medial portion of the eyelid needs careful examination to exclude injury to the lacrimal drainage system. The mechanism of injury must be carefully documented. Suspicion of deeper injury must be high in medial canthal injuries with foreign bodies. Imaging with focus on extension into the anterior cranial fossa through the orbital roof should be obtained.

Clinical signs and symptoms

Epiphoria on the injured side and bleeding from the laceration site are the most common presenting signs and symptoms.

Differential diagnosis

Laceration of the periocular tissue without lacrimal system involvement.

PROPHYLAXIS

Following injury from a dog bite, the relationship of the animal to the victim and future risk should also be ascertained and appropriate steps taken to reduce the chance of subsequent injury as there is a significant risk of repeat attack.

TREATMENT

Systemic

In contaminated wounds from animal bites or vegetable matter, coverage for the most likely pathogens should be started immediately. Dogs habor a multitude of bacteria including p.multocidia and dysgenic fermenter 2. Antibiotic coverage should be broad spectrum. Frequently Keflex is used as a first choice. A tetanus booster should be given if it has been more than 5 years since the last booster in an immunized patient; tetanus immunoglobulin may be necessary in a non-immunized patient. Rabies prophylaxis is rarely needed in domestic pets but may need to be considered in wild animals and the immunization status of the animal should be noted.

Ocular

The status of the globe and visual function must first be determined. Any injury to the globe takes priority over the lacerated canaliculus or periocular tissue. Once the globe is determined to be stable, the injured eyelid tissue must be handled with delicate instruments and precision.

After carefully cleaning the tissue, the laceration should be replaced in its anatomic location. Rarely once the tissue is irrigated and replaced in its original location is there actual loss of lid tissue.

Medical

The wound should be gently irrigated with antibiotic solution such as 50,000 units Bacitracin in 500 cc normal saline. High pressures should be avoided as bacteria can be propelled further into the tissue. Depending on the degree of contamination both oral and topical antibiotics may be given for the first 10 days. An antibiotic-steroid ointment combination may help decrease both infection and inflammation. If the lacrimal drainage system has been repaired, an antibiotic-steroid drop should be given with slow taper over four weeks post-operatively.

Surgical

Numerous techniques exist to repair a lacerated canaliculus including bicanalicular stent placement through either a round eyed pigtail probe technique, or through stents placed through the nasal lacrimal duct, or a monocanalicular stent through a single disrupted canalicular system. The disrupted canaliculus can be identified by the white cuff of tissue around the lumen of the canaliculus. An advantage to the pigtail probe technique is that the angle anatomy can be casted into position be securing the relationship through the lacrimal sac and opposing canaliculus. Passing the pigtail probe requires proper instruction in this technique as the probe must be carefully passed through the lacrimal system and gently guided through the medial canthal anatomy exiting through the proximal section the proximal segment and intact portion of the system can then be intubated with a 6-0 prolene suture. The probe can then be passed through the distal segment and this segment also intubated with the 6-0 prolene suture. A 24 mm piece of Crawford stent is then passed over the 6-0 prolene suture. Pericanalicular suture of 7-0 vicryl may be required to further oppose the severed ends of the canalicular system. At most 3 interrupted sutures are passed at the inferior, anterior and superior aspect of the peri- canalicular tissue. If the medial canthal tendon is also severed, prior to securing these sutures, a 4-0 vicryl suture should be passed from the pretarsal orbicularis to the deep canthal periosteum to re-secure the posterior limb of the medial canthal tendon. The pericanalicular sutures can then be tied and the 6-0 prolene suture within the Crawford stent tied and the knot rotated into the intact segment of the lacrimal system.

COMPLICATIONS

Post-operative epiphoria or ectropion of the medial lower lid and or puncta are the most common complication encountered after these injuries.

COMMENTS

High speed or projectile injuries often allow for deep penetration of foreign bodies. Any trauma involving vegetable matter such as wood must be carefully evaluated to determine if any retained vegetable matter may be present. This will most commonly involve computed tomographic imaging and additional imaging with magnetic resonance imaging may be required. The retained wood must be removed as it will cause further soft tissue inflammation, infection and disruption of function. This type of trauma will sometimes cause fracture of the roof of the orbit as the foreign body penetrates the orbit and extends through the roof to the anterior cranial fossa. Neurosurgical consultation should be obtained.

REFERENCES

Burroughs J, Soparkar C, Patrinely J, et al: Periocular dog bite injuries and responsible care. Ophthal Plast Reconstr Surg 2002:18(6):416–419; discussion 419–420.

Herzum H, Holle P, Hintschich C. Eyelid injuries: epidemiological aspects. Ophthalmologe 98(11):1079–1082, 2001.

Jordan DR, Nerad JA, Tse DT: The pigtail probe, revisited. Ophthalmology 97(4):512–519, 1990.

Kersten RC, Kulwin DR. 'One-stitch' canalicular repair. A simplified approach for repair of canalicular laceration.Ophthalmology 103(5):785–789, 1996.

Reifler DM: Management of canalicular laceration. Surv Ophthalmol 36:113–132, 1991.

Singer AJ, Thode HC, Hollander JE: National trends in ED lacerations between 1992–2002. Am J Emerg Med 24(2):183–188, 2006.

294 LACRIMAL GLAND TUMORS 224.2

Eric A. Steele, MD
Portland, Oregon
Roger A. Dailey, MD
Portland, Oregon

ETIOLOGY

Lacrimal gland tumors can arise from cells of epithelial origin, such as acinar or ductal elements, or from nonepithelial cells, such as inflammatory, neural, vascular, or fatty elements. More than half of all lacrimal gland tumors are nonepithelial in origin.

Epithelial tumors are evenly divided into benign and malignant lesions. The most common benign lesion is the benign mixed tumor (pleomorphic adenoma), whereas adenoid cystic carcinoma, adenocarcinoma, and malignant mixed cell tumor are typical epithelial malignancies. Of these, adenoid cystic carcinoma is the most common.

Nonepithelial tumors of the lacrimal gland include inflammatory and lymphoid lesions. Idiopathic orbital inflammation, which is also known as orbital pseudotumor, is the most common inflammatory process affecting the lacrimal gland. When the inflammation is limited to the lacrimal gland, this is also referred to as inflammatory dacryoadenitis. Lymphoid lesions occur along a disease spectrum from benign reactive lymphoid hyperplasia to malignant lymphoma.

COURSE/PROGNOSIS

- *Benign mixed tumor* presents with slowly progressive painless proptosis. The globe is displaced downward and medially. Prognosis is excellent if the tumor is completely excised with an intact capsule.
- *Adenoid cystic carcinoma* and *adenocarcinoma* are often associated with pain and rapid growth. Adenoid cystic carcinoma spreads via perineural invasion, whereas adenocarcinoma metastasizes to regional and distant lymph nodes. Both conditions have a poor prognosis.
- *Malignant mixed tumor* arises from benign mixed tumor that has been neglected or incompletely excised. The prognosis is poor.
- *Idiopathic orbital inflammation* typically presents acutely with pain, erythema, and tenderness. The lacrimal gland may be involved in isolation or in conjunction with other orbital structures.
- *Lymphoid lesions* tend to occur in older patients and to have a more insidious onset than does idiopathic orbital inflammation. Both benign and malignant diseases present with a slow onset of proptosis, downward displacement of the globe, ptosis, and, diplopia. A salmon-colored patch can be seen if conjunctival involvement is present. Reactive lymphoid hyperplasia has a good prognosis, although there can be malignant degeneration. Of patients with lacrimal gland lymphoma, 35% have or will develop systemic disease.

DIAGNOSIS

Laboratory findings

In addition to the history, radiologic studies play a key role in diagnosis. Computed tomography (CT) of the orbits is usually the preferred imaging modality since it provides excellent images of any associated bony changes.

- Benign epithelial lesions typically appear as a circumscribed mass with pressure remodeling but no destruction of the bony lacrimal fossa.
- Malignant epithelial lesions are typically ill defined, with lytic destruction of bone and intralesional calcification on CT scanning.
- Idiopathic orbital inflammation shows diffuse lacrimal gland enlargement, often with poor definition of gland margins due to inflammation in surrounding tissues. If a discrete mass is present, it typically conforms to the globe.
- Benign and malignant lymphoid lesions mold to the globe and other adjacent structures, without bony changes on CT. The margins often are quite well defined.

TREATMENT

Surgical

- Care must be taken to completely excise a benign mixed tumor, since residual tissue can degenerate into a malignant mixed tumor.
- The treatment of adenoid cystic carcinoma is controversial. Surgical options include wide local excision and orbital exenteration. Postoperative radiation therapy has been used with both surgical approaches. The prognosis has been poor regardless of the treatment modality, with few long-term survivors.
- Adenocarcinoma and malignant mixed tumor are also treated with tumor excision or orbital exenteration.
- Idiopathic orbital inflammation is treated initially with oral steroids and then with radiotherapy or antimetabolites if the patient becomes steroid dependent. Rapid improvement with steroid treatment supports the diagnosis of pseudotumor, although this must be interpreted cautiously because some orbital neoplasms transiently improve with steroid treatment. Atypical cases or lesions that do not respond to steroids may require incisional biopsy for diagnosis.
- Surgical treatment for lymphoid lesions is limited to incisional biopsy for diagnostic purposes. Reactive lymphoid hyperplasia is treated with low-dose radiation. A diagnosis of lymphoma warrants a systemic evaluation for extraorbital disease. If the disease is confined to the orbit, radiation is the treatment of choice. If extraorbital disease is present, chemotherapy, radiation, or both may be used.

REFERENCES

Kennerdell JS, Flores NE, Hartsock RJ: Low-dose radiotherapy for lymphoid lesions of the orbit and ocular adnexa. Ophthal Plast Reconstr Surg 15(2):129–133, 1999.

Tse DT, Neff AG, Onofrey CB: Recent developments in the evaluation and treatment of lacrimal gland tumors. Ophth Clin North Am 13 (4):663–681, 2000.

295 LACRIMAL HYPERSECRETION
375.20

Michael A. Bearn, FRCOphth
Elgin, Scotland

Lacrimal hypersecretion is excess secretion of tears from the main or accessory lacrimal glands.

The symptom of excess tearing may be due to lacrimal hypersecretion, pseudoepiphora (commonly in dry eye states), functional epiphora (normal syringing and abnormal dye disappearance test [DDT]) outflow obstruction or eyelid malpositions.

Epiphora (overflow of tears on the cheek) is the result of imbalance between tear production and drainage.

INCIDENCE

Tearing is a very common symptom. Unpublished data of 100 consecutive adult patients attending an epiphora clinic showed approximately one third due to outflow obstruction, one third due to eyelid malposition and one third due to hypersecretion.

In several cases however epiphora was due to a combination of factors.

AETIOLOGY

The lacrimal nucleus in the pons receives an afferent input from the trigeminal nerve and a central input. The efferent pathway is in branches of the facial nerve synapsing in the sphenopalatine ganglion.

Causes of hypersecretion are divided into central, reflex trigeminal , irritation of the efferent pathway and abberent regeneration. In addition primary lacrimal gland pathology has been described as a cause.

Central: emotion or pain, hysterical.
Reflex trigeminal: corneal pathology.
Conjunctival.
Meibomian gland dysfunction (MGD).
Nasal.
Photopic, asthenopic.
Space occupying lesions irritating the efferent pathway.
Crocodile tears in abberent facial nerve regeneration.

Primary lacrimal gland. Tumours and fistulas have been reported as causing hypersecretion.

In children lacrimal hypersecretion is uncommon. Causes include albinism, buphthalmos, epiblepharon, crocodile tears, blepharitis and idiopathic.

DIAGNOSIS

Clinical signs and symptoms

- Slit lamp examination, DDT, Schirmers test, eyelids for MGD, palpate the lacrimal gland.
- Tests of tear drainage.

Differential diagnosis

- Pseudoepiphora, functional and obstructive.

TREATMENT

Ocular

- Treat the cause. Botulinum toxin injected into the lacrimal gland is effective for crocodile tears.

Medical

- Metalloproteinase inhibitors can be useful for chronic ocular surface disorders.

Surgical

- Lid malpositions and trichiasis.

COMPLICATIONS

- Discomfort, blurring, excoriation.

COMMENTS

Symptomatic tearing is a balance of tear production and excretion. When treating the patient with epiphora it is important to identify and treat all the factors.

Hypersecretion may be helped therefore by increasing the drainage or lid position and partial obstructive cases by treating any causes of hypersecretion identified.

Simple reassurance may be all that is necessary.

REFERENCES

Clark WN: Lacrimal hypersecretion in children. Paediatric Ophthalmol Strabismus 24:204, 1987.

Duke Elder S: System of ophthalmology: Neuro-Ophthalmology. Vol XII. London: Henry Kimpton, 1971.

Jones L, Linn M: The diagnosis of the causes of epiphora. American Journal of Ophthalmology 67:751–754, 1969.

Riemann R, Pfennigsdorf S, Riemann E, et al: Successful treatment of crocodile tears by injection of botulinum toxin into the lacrimal gland: a case report. Br J Plast Surg 52:230–231, 1999.

Zappia RJ, Milder B: Lacrimal drainage function 2. The fluorescein dye disappearance test. Am J Ophth 74:160, 1972.

296 LACRIMAL HYPOSECRETION
375.15

James V. Aquavella, MD
Rochester, New York

Lacrimal hyposecretion is characterized by a deficiency of aqueous tear production by the lacrimal gland. Accessory lacrimal glands located in the conjunctiva do not constitute a significant source of tears.

ETIOLOGY/INCIDENCE

Lacrimal gland hyposecretion can be congenital or more frequently acquired as the result of trauma, disease or simply aging. The incidence of reduced tear film is greater in post-menopausal women, consistent with changes in adrogenic hormonal levels. Some reports indicate that as many as 15 million individuals in the United States may experience symptoms associated with lacrimal dysfunction.

Lymphocytic infiltration of the lacrimal gland as a result of autoimmune disease has been associated with subsequent tear film inadequacy. Dry eye syndrome can be the result of tear film dysfunction, or associated with reduced tear volume, altered tear composition, increased evaporation, or inflammatory modulators.

These conditions may coexist in varying degrees, making it difficult to establishment a precise diagnosis. Sjögren's syndrome is a severe form of dry eye characterized by lacrimal hyposecretion, dry mouth, and arthritis, as well as immunologically modulated ocular surface inflammation.

COURSE/PROGNOSIS

The symptoms of this condition span a spectrum which extends from relatively annoying ocular discomfort to irreversible corneal scarring leading to legal blindness. In most individuals the surface irritation is chronic and associated with only minor visual disruption. Sjögren's syndrome, ocular cicatrical pemphigoid, and Stevens–Johnson syndrome can have devastating long-term effects.

DIAGNOSIS

Isolated lacrimal hyposecretion must be differentiated from the other causes of dry eye and from chronic blepharitis and meibomian gland dysfunction.

TREATMENT

Ocular

The mainstay of therapy is the use of ocular surface lubricants, applied frequently in liquid or ointment form. When very frequent instillation is necessary, preservative-free vehicles are indicated. Concurrent use of topical anti-inflammatory or immunosuppressant agents is often necessary. Punctal occlusion or the use of protective goggles and hydrophilic contact lenses may be necessary.

COMPLICATIONS

Corneal neovascularization and scarring may result. Increased incidence of ocular surface infection is common. Corneal ulceration and secondary perforation may occur.

COMMENTS

With attention to dissecting factors in the patient's environment, and moderate lifestyle modifications this condition can be well managed in most cases. There is no specific therapy which has been shown to consistently improve lacrimal secretion, so artificial tears are the mainstay of treatment. Severe forms need frequent involvement of a corneal subspecialist.

SUPPORT GROUP

Sjögren's Syndrome Foundation, Inc.
333 North Broadway
Jericho, NY 11753

REFERENCES

Aquavella JV, Boghani S, Sjögren syndrome. Chapter in E-Medicine, www.emedicine.com Updated May 2005.

Lemp MA: Report of the National Eye Institute/Industry workshop on clinical trials in dry eyes. CLAO J 21:221–232, 1995.

Mircheff AK: Understanding the causes of lacrimal insufficiency: implications for treatment and prevention of dry eye syndrome. In: Research to prevent blindness science writers seminar. New York, Research to Prevent Blindness, 1993:51–54.

Sullivan PA, Sato EH: Immunology of the lacrimal gland. In: Albert DM, Jakobiec FA, eds: Principles and practice of ophthalmology: basic sciences. Philadelphia, WB Saunders, 1994:479–486.

Wang J, Aquavella JV, Zhao Y, Chung S: Tear dynamics measured with real-time otpicla cohenece tomography.[Abstract], Journal of Vision 4(11):89a, 2004.

297 UVEOPAROTID FEVER 298
(Heerfordt's Syndrome, Uveoparotitis)

Frederick W. Fraunfelder, MD
Portland, Oregon

ETIOLOGY/INCIDENCE

Heerfordt syndrome (uveoparotid fever) consists of bilateral uveitis and parotid gland enlargement and is generally thought to be caused by sarcoidosis. It is often associated with systemic symptoms and cranial nerve palsy, usually the seventh nerve. Sarcoidosis is increasingly recognized as a cause of multifocal choroiditis and panuveitis. Severe dry eye is also a common occurrence with this condition.

COURSE/PROGNOSIS

Facial palsy and parotid swelling are usually transient and do not recur, but even with systemic steroid treatment, about one-fourth of patients are left with a chronic mild uveitis that requires continuing minimal systemic or local steroid treatment. There is an increased incidence of severe sarcoidosis in the African American population. When sarcoid uveitis is severe, it is particularly likely to be associated with raised intraocular pressure during the active stage. Later, broad adhesions across the drainage angle resulting from the fibrosis of iris nodules may lead to chronic closed-angle glaucoma. As in any other case of uveitis, secondary cataracts may form.

DIAGNOSIS

Clinical signs and symptoms

The signs of the syndrome may be incomplete and are usually associated with other ophthalmic and general manifestations of sarcoidosis. Posterior uveitis frequently accompanies the anterior uveitis but may appear to be present alone with 'snowball' vitreous opacities and haze and whitish fundus lesions. Retinal vasculitis affecting the veins may be a prominent feature in some cases, but fluorescein angiography reveals that it is much more frequent than would be suspected on routine ophthalmoscopy.

Only rarely are lacrimal glands clinically swollen, but they are frequently affected as revealed by evidence of tear deficiency in 65% of sarcoid patients compared with 6% of matched control patients. The eyes feel 'gritty,' especially in a dry or smoke-laden atmosphere, and are prone to recurrent infection of the conjunctivae and lid margins. The hyalinized epithelial cells of the exposed conjunctiva and cornea stain with rose bengal, and especially in uveoparotid fever, mucus filaments may be attached to the corneal epithelium, causing pain and photophobia. The tear film is thinned with an accelerated break-up time of less than 10 seconds. Schirmer's test confirms a reduction of tear flow. Conjunctival follicles with sarcoid histology are commonly present in the lower fornix and are a valuable source of biopsy material.

Both the cornea and conjunctiva may be involved in the deposition of calcium salts in exposed areas when sarcoidosis is complicated by hypercalcemia. In the cornea, this appears as a band opacity and may be associated with redness and discomfort. Some patients may become uremic from renal calcinosis. In addition to the facial palsy, in which the nerve may be involved above or below the level at which it is joined by the chorda tympani, sarcoid deposits at the base of the brain may cause other cranial nerve palsies and a variety of neurologic effects depending on the situation of the granulomas.

Diabetes insipidus and hypopituitarism from hypothalamic lesions may also occur. The optic nerve itself may be affected, with visual loss being associated with papilledema or optic atrophy. Finally, the skin of the eyelids may be disfigured by sarcoid papules.

Ocular and periocular signs include:

- Conjunctiva: follicles, hyperemia, keratoconjunctivitis sicca;
- Cornea: band keratopathy, keratoconjunctivitis sicca;
- Eyelids: sarcoid nodules in skin;
- Iris, ciliary body or choroid: sarcoid nodules, uveitis;
- Lacrimal system: decreased tear secretion, infiltration of lacrimal gland;
- Optic nerve: atrophy, papilledema, internal ophthalmoplegia;
- Retina: vasculitis, mainly affecting veins;
- Sclera: episcleral nodules, episcleritis;
- Vitreous: haze, snowball opacities;
- Other: diplopia, paralysis of seventh nerve, proptosis due to orbital sarcoid granulomas, secondary cataract, secondary glaucoma, visual loss.

Laboratory findings

- Noncaseating epithelioid cell follicles in biopsy material from the liver, skin, lymph nodes, or conjunctiva.
- Radiographic changes in the lungs.
- Low tuberculin sensitivity.
- Serum angiotensin-converting enzyme level elevated.
- Whole-body gallium isotope scans (^{67}Ga) taken up by active cells at inflammatory sites, especially sarcoid granulomas.
- Kveim–Siltzbach skin test.
- Leukemia.
- Lymphoma.
- Tuberculosis.
- Sjögren's syndrome.
- Mumps.
- Waldenström's macroglobulinemia.

TREATMENT

Systemic

Systemic corticosteroid treatment is essential for all patients with Heerfordt's syndrome. It will usually control the uveitis and retinal vasculitis, lead to resolution of the swollen parotid glands, improve the keratoconjunctivitis sicca by resolving lacrimal gland lesions, and restore a normal blood calcium level by increasing urinary excretion and decreasing intestinal absorption of calcium.

In general, the corticosteroid dose is kept as low as is possible to produce the desired response. Initially, the administration of 40 to 60 mg/day prednisone orally in conjunction with topical ophthalmic prednisolone, hydrocortisone, betamethasone, or dexamethasone may be necessary to control uveitis. This dosage may be slowly reduced over a period of months but must never be withdrawn abruptly.

Central nervous system lesions usually resist treatment and may occasionally present grave therapeutic problems, especially if a large dose is required for a long period. Skin lesions are usually resistant to corticosteroid treatment and may be disfiguring. To avoid higher corticosteroid doses, 200 mg of chloroquine may be given twice daily, although the cornea and retinal function must be reviewed regularly during treatment for signs of toxicity.

Ocular

The usual topical ophthalmic treatment for uveitis by mydriasis and cycloplegia is 1% atropine solution or ointment, 1% cyclopentolate solution, or 5% phenylephrine solutions. Corticosteroids (topical, 0.1% dexamethasone alcohol; 1.0% prednisolone acetate, or 0.5% prednisolone sodium phosphate) are used at a frequency of up to twice hourly and gradually reduced. Subconjunctival or retrobulbar injection is the initial treatment for severe uveitis, with betamethasone sodium phosphate 4 mg or a slow-release preparation of methyl prednisolone acetate 20 mg. A combined injection of corticosteroid with a mydriatic and local anesthetic may be particularly useful, for instance, Mydriacaine No. 2, a mixture containing epinephrine acid tartrate 216 µg, atropine sulphate 1 mg, procaine hydrochloride 6 mg, boric acid 5 mg, sodium metabisulphite 300 µg, sodium chloride 300 µg, and water for injection to 0.3 mL.

Keratoconjunctivitis sicca is usually treated with one of the artificial tear preparations, but in the case of filamentary keratitis, a mucolytic agent may be required at intervals, such as 5% to 10% acetylcysteine. Acute band keratopathy usually responds to reduction of the serum calcium level but may require surgical removal. EDTA (edetate disodium), chelates calcium and allows one to remove it from the surface of the cornea. The argon fluoride excimer laser, which produces an ultraviolet radiation that is readily absorbed by all tissues and penetrates by only a few micrometers, causes photoablation in which the tissues are vaporized and also can be used to remove a band opacity.

COMMENTS

The use of topical and systemic corticosteroid therapy is essential, but the possibility of corticosteroid-induced cataract or secondary glaucoma must be borne in mind and care must be taken to exclude other diseases such as diabetes, tuberculosis, or peptic ulcer because the usual regimen may require modification. Indomethacin may be considered in acute uveitis, and azathioprine may allow a 50% reduction in the steroid dose.

Uveoparotid fever must be regarded as a potentially severe form of sarcoidosis requiring prolonged energetic systemic corticosteroid therapy and close supervision. Its duration will depend on the progress of the disease. A delicate balance must be preserved between tissue damage by sarcoidosis and the complications of corticosteroid treatment.

Local therapy with mydriatics and corticosteroids alone is unlikely to control the uveitis of uveoparotid fever; however, these medications help raise intraocular concentrations even when systemic treatment is being given, and they may be used for local ocular defense over a long period when it is considered safe or desirable to withdraw systemic corticosteroids. Such patients should always be watched for signs of corticosteroid-induced glaucoma, which is more likely to be caused by local than by systemic treatment.

It is sometimes difficult to decide whether secondary glaucoma is caused by uveitis or corticosteroids. In either case, it is usually best to continue therapy and treat the raised intraocular pressure with anti-glaucoma medications.

Corticosteroid-induced cataracts are a therapeutic risk which may require surgery in some patients.

REFERENCES

Bruins Slot WJ: Besnier-Boeck's disease and uveoparotid fever (Heerfordt). Ned Tijdschr Geneeskd 80:2859–2863, 1936.

Blair MP, Rizen M: Heerfordt syndrome with internal ophthalmoplegia. Archives of Ophthalmology 123:1017, 2005.

Gartry G, Kerr Muir M, Marshall J: Excimer laser treatment of corneal surface pathology: a laboratory and clinical study. Br J Ophthalmol 75:258–269, 1991.

James DG, Anderson R, Langley D, Ainsley D: Ocular sarcoidosis. Br J Ophthalmol 48:461–470, 1964.

SECTION

26 Lens

298 ADULT CATARACTS 366.10

Kelly D. Chung, MD
Portland, Oregon

ETIOLOGY/INCIDENCE

Cataract is a disorder in which the crystalline lens becomes opacified. It is the leading cause of visual impairment in all but the most developed countries where cataract surgery represents one of the most common surgical procedures performed.

The etiology of the vast majority of cataracts is age-related though genetic factors probably account for around 50% of age-related cataract with systemic and environmental factors, the remainder. Diabetes mellitus, corticosteroid use, heavy alcohol use, smoking, and lifetime ultraviolet light exposure are amongst the many factors that are linked to cataract formation.

Cataract is classified according to the portion of the lens that is opacified. The major types include nuclear, cortical, and posterior subcapsular though it is common to have a mixture of these types of opacities in a given cataract. Although all types of cataract can be simply age-related cataract, posterior subcapsular cataract is commonly seen with toxicities such as uveitis or corticosteroid-induced cataracts.

DIAGNOSIS

Early cataract may not disturb vision. However, as the opacification of the lens increases, cataract can produce painless progressive decrease in visual acuity and contrast sensitivity. There may be symptoms of glare, monocular diplopia, and changing refractive error.

Cataract is diagnosed clinically, optimally with the patient's pupil dilated and slit lamp biomicroscopy. The red reflex is reduced or completely interrupted by the opacity and the opacities are directly visualized within the lens.

COURSE/PROGNOSIS

The course of cataract is generally slowly progressive with the patient experiencing from few or no symptoms early on to blurred vision, glare and changing refractive error. There is no proven way to prevent or slow the progression of cataract.

TREATMENT

Early on, managing a change in refractive error can sometimes improve a patient's visual function without further intervention.

When the vision is no longer adequate to meet the patient's activities of daily living then cataract surgery is indicated. Occasionally, cataract surgery is indicated for medical rather than functional reasons if it is blocking a view to monitoring or treating the retina, leaking lens proteins, or causing narrow angle glaucoma. The prognosis for improved vision after cataract surgery in an otherwise healthy eye is excellent.

REFERENCES

McCarty CA, Taylor HR: The genetics of cataract. Invest Ophthalmol Vis Sci 42:1677–1678, 2001.

Negahban K, Chern K: Cataracts associated with systemic disorders and syndromes. Curr Opin Ophthalmol 13:419–422, 2002.

Resnikoff S, Pascolini D, Etya'ale D, et al: Global data on visual impairment in the year 2002. Bulletin of the World Health Organization 82:844–851, 2004.

299 AFTER-CATARACTS 366.50

Christopher Graham Tinley, MBChB, MRCOphth
Devon, England

After-cataract is a term originally used to describe lens epithelial cell proliferation following cataract surgery. A broader definition may include any visually significant opacification of the intraocular lens/capsular bag complex.

ETIOLOGY/INCIDENCE

Posterior capsule opacification

By far the most common cause of after-cataract is posterior capsule opacification (PCO). Following cataract surgery, lens epithelial cells (LECs) not completely removed from the capsular bag can be divided into two entities: anterior LECs (A cells), which form a single layer on the back of the anterior capsule around the capsulorhexis and E cells, located in the equatorial region. The E cells comprise germinal cells, which are the primary cells of origin of PCO. Immediately after uncomplicated cataract surgery there are normally no cells on the posterior capsule. Opacification develops as retained E cells proliferate and migrate onto the posterior capsule.

PCO usually takes one, or is a combination of two morphological forms:

- Regeneratory: clusters of swollen, opacified, epithelial 'pearls' (bladder or Wedl cells);
- Fibrotic: posterior capsule fibrosis and wrinkling. A cells are implicated in this form of PCO, since their primary response to any stimulus is to proliferate and undergo fibrous metaplasia (Figure 299.1).

Lens epithelial cells express cytokines interleukin-1 (IL-1), IL-6, IL-8, basic fibroblast growth factor and transforming growth factor beta, which may act in an autocrine and paracrine fashion, influencing the postoperative proliferation of LECs and collagen synthesis.

PCO is still the most frequent complication of cataract surgery. It can lead to clinically significant reduction in visual acuity, impaired contrast sensitivity, glare and monocular diplopia. It also limits advances in the development of intraocular lenses (IOLs), particularly accommodative IOLs. The onset of PCO ranges from 3 months to 4 years after surgery and its incidence increases with time. With newer generation IOLs, the PCO rate is now less than 10%, 3 years after surgery. For older generation IOLs it can be as high as 40%. Underlying diseases related to changes in the blood-aqueous barrier, such as uveitis, are associated with higher rates of PCO. However, there is conflicting evidence regarding PCO rates in patients with diabetes mellitus. Pseudoexfoliation and retinitis pigmentosa are also risk factors for PCO, but the most important systemic factor is patient's youth. In pediatric eyes, the PCO rate can be greater than 80%.

Anterior capsule contraction syndrome

Anterior capsule contraction syndrome, or anterior capsule phimosis, is a rare complication after uneventful phacoemulsification surgery, where progressive shrinkage of the anterior capsule opening occurs. 'A cells' undergoing fibrous metaplasia are its cells of origin. The anterior capsule opening usually shrinks rapidly during the first postoperative month, followed by a slower contraction in the subsequent 6 months. However, progressive shrinkage is thought to be due to an imbalance between the centrifugal zonular forces and the centripetal force induced by capsular fibrosis at the capsulorhexis margin. It has been associated with several conditions, such as pseudoexfoliation syndrome, high myopia, advanced age, retinitis pigmentosa, myotonic dystrophy and diseases in which the blood-aqueous barrier is compromised (e.g. diabetes mellitus, uveitis). It is more prevalent with silicone IOLs, particularly those with plate haptics.

Contraction of the anterior capsule opening can result in a clinically significant reduction in vision secondary to IOL decentration, tilt or anterior capsule opacification. It can also interfere with visualization of the peripheral retina, retinal photocoagulation and vitreous surgery. In extreme cases, complete occlusion of the central opening may occur and excessive zonular traction can result in IOL dislocation, ciliary body detachment and retinal detachment.

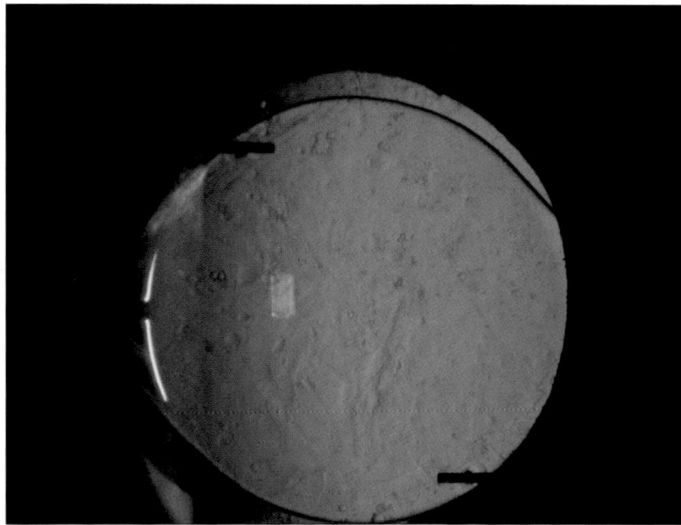

FIGURE 299.1. Posterior capsular opacity.

IOL opacification

IOL opacification is a new form of after-cataract which has emerged recently. The loss of lens transparency can alter patients' visual function according to its severity. Its incidence varies from 0% to 14%, depending on the IOL material. The most frequently affected IOLs are the hydrophilic acrylic, or hydrogel lenses. Late opacification of the lens can occur, usually 1 to 2 years after surgery, due to calcium deposition on the optic surface as well as intralenticularly. On slitlamp examination the IOL has a 'frosty' or very reflective appearance, due to multiple, fine, granular deposits. The cause of this delayed dystrophic calcification appears to be multifactorial. In addition to patient-related factors, such as systemic disease (e.g. diabetes mellitus) and ocular inflammation, factors relating to IOL manufacturing and packaging have also been implicated. Opacification has been reported in other IOL types, but occurs much less frequently.

Delayed endophthalmitis

Propionibacterium acnes is an anaerobic, gram positive bacillus of low virulence that is present in the normal flora of the eyelid margin and conjunctiva. If sequestered between the IOL optic and posterior capsule during cataract surgery, it is one of several organisms that can cause delayed endophthalmitis. It is usually diagnosed more than 6 weeks after surgery with a white plaque on the posterior capsule and persistent, low-grade intraocular inflammation. Vitritis is present in most cases, but the presence of a hypopyon and granulomatous-appearing keratic precipitates can be variable. Typically there is a transient response to topical corticosteroids and endophthalmitis may first manifest or worsen after Nd:YAG laser capsulotomy.

IOL deposits

Pigment deposits on the IOL are usually derived from contact with the posterior iris surface, but can also be inflammatory. They are particularly prevalent with posterior chamber, phakic IOLs. Chronic uveitis can lead to inflammatory precipitates on the IOL with fibrin deposition, sometimes resulting in a pupillary membrane.

DIAGNOSIS

Differential diagnosis

- Posterior capsule opacification.
- Anterior capsule contraction syndrome.

- IOL opacification.
- Delayed endophthalmitis.
- IOL deposits.

PROPHYLAXIS

Several factors contribute to the prevention of PCO. These can be divided into two groups:
- IOL factors:
- IOL optic barrier effect.

Square, truncated posterior-edged optics form a sharp capsular bend that mechanically inhibits migration of LECs over the posterior capsule.
- Maximal IOL optic-posterior capsule contact.

This enhances the barrier effect and is achieved by posterior angulation of the IOL haptics and a posterior convexity of the optic.
- Biocompatible IOLs reducing the stimulus for cellular proliferation.

Hydrophobic materials, both acrylic and silicone, have better capsular biocompatibility than hydrophilic acrylic materials. Bioadhesive optic materials create firm optic-posterior capsule contact, with more rapid formation of the capsular bend.
- Surgery-related factors:
- Hydrodissection-enhanced cortical clean-up.

Cortex and cell removal is more thorough and the number of retained LECs in the capsular bag is minimized.
- Complete 360° anterior capsule-optic overlap.

Placement of the capsulorhexis edge on the anterior surface of the optic pushes the lens posteriorly, leading to greater apposition between the IOL and the posterior capsule.
- In-the-bag fixation of the IOL.

This sequesters the IOL from the adjacent, pro-inflammatory uveal tissues and maximizes capsular contact.

In pediatric cataract surgery, a primary posterior capsulotomy, with or without anterior vitrectomy, reduces the incidence of PCO. Due to advances in pharmacology, immunology and molecular genetics, other strategies to prevent PCO have been proposed, most specifically targeting lens epithelial cells. Sealed-capsule irrigation is a promising new surgical technique that permits irrigation of the capsular bag with distilled water, while maintaining mechanical isolation from the rest of the eye. LEC lysis is induced by osmotic hydration.

TREATMENT

Posterior capsule opacification

PCO in adults is most commonly treated by means of neodynium:yttrium-aluminium-garnet (Nd:YAG) laser posterior capsulotomy. The pressure shockwave which disrupts the capsule is created when infrared light (1064 nm) is amplified and focused forming an energy plasma — a process known as optical breakdown. Commonly used Nd:YAG lasers are Q-switched or mode-locked, or both, which allows for greater efficiency, lower power settings and hence fewer side-effects.

The indications for treatment are:
- Visual symptoms due to the presence of PCO;
- To improve visualization of the fundus for diagnostic or therapeutic purposes.

Surgical technique

- The pupil is dilated prior to treatment.
- Topical anesthesia is applied and an anterior segment contact lens is placed on the eye, which decreases light reflections, helps with stabilization of the patient's globe and results in a smaller focal spot.
- The laser beam is aimed or defocused slightly posteriorly and treatment started away from the central visual axis, to keep IOL damage to a minimum.
- Approximately 1.0 mJ (single pulse) is usually adequate, but the power can be titrated according to the response. Energy settings should be kept to a minimum and should generally not exceed 2.5 mJ per pulse.
- Typically a central, cruciate pattern of punctures is performed. The procedure may be facilitated if the laser is fixed along stress lines, as the capsule retracts after it is disrupted.
- The capsulotomy opening should be at least 2.5 mm, but larger openings may be needed to alleviate symptoms of glare and allow for better visualization of the peripheral fundus. The capsular opening tends to increase in size during the first month after laser and becomes more circular, with smoothing of the edge contour from capsular tag retraction.
- If a total energy greater than 100 mJ is required, consider prescribing a short course of topical steroids. Clinicians may opt to postpone further treatment to a capsule if a small opening has already been created and they wish to avoid potentially increased risks by applying more energy.
- If post-laser IOP elevation is a concern to the clinician, 1% apraclonidine may be administered pre- and postoperatively to help prevent this.
- Dense, fibrotic PCO, as seen after pediatric cataract surgery, may require surgical discission via a pars plana approach.

Anterior capsule contraction

Radial, anterior, Nd:YAG capsulotomies can be performed to create four equally spaced radial cuts, about 1 mm in length, using an average power of 1.5 mJ. However, dense, central, fibrous plaques may not be amenable to laser treatment. In these cases, a vitrector can be used to clear the fibrotic tissue, or alternatively mechanical peeling of the membrane can be performed.

IOL opacification

Explantation and exchange of the IOL is the only available treatment.

Propionibacter endophthalmitis

Although sensitive to vancomycin, injection of intravitreal antibiotics alone is associated with a very high recurrence rate. The best result involves complete removal of the capsular plaque. If this is centrally located, it is reasonable to perform a pars plana vitrectomy with a partial capsulectomy. If the plaque extends into the periphery or the inflammation recurs, vitrectomy with total capsulectomy and IOL removal or exchange may be preferred. Overall, the visual outcome is good and patients without co-existing ocular pathology achieve an average visual acuity of 20/40 or better.

IOL deposits

The Nd : YAG laser focused anteriorly, with low energy settings (0.5–1 mJ), can be used to disrupt IOL deposits.

COMPLICATIONS

IOP elevation

The pressure rise is maximum 3 to 4 hours after laser treatment and returns to within 5 mmHg of pre-laser values by 24 hours. The exact mechanism of the IOP rise has not been fully elucidated, although several theories exist. In the majority of cases, there is no long-term effect on IOP, but a persistent IOP rise to 30 mmHg lasting longer than 1 week occurs in about 1% of patients. A late onset IOP rise of, on average 1 mmHg, has been reported in 4.5% of patients. This may not be clinically important in healthy eyes, but can potentially damage the optic nerve in eyes with glaucoma. There is no evidence of any functional permanent visual deficit as a result of these pressure rises however. High total laser energy has been shown to be related to greater increases in IOP, particularly when the energy per pulse is 2.5 mJ or greater. Patient-dependant risk factors include aphakia, glaucoma, a pre-existing IOP of more than 20 mmHg, high myopia and vitreoretinal disease.

Retinal detachment

It has been estimated that the risk of retinal detachment is four times greater after Nd : YAG capsulotomy and its incidence ranges from 0.5%–3.5%. Laser shockwaves and loss of an intact posterior capsule may initiate vitreous changes such as liquefaction and posterior vitreous detachment. These are known to cause both new tears and allow existing tears to progress to retinal detachment. Risk factors for retinal detachment post-laser include high myopia, lattice degeneration with associated holes, greater use of laser energy and larger capsulotomy size. Patients should be warned of the symptoms of retinal detachment and advised to report promptly should they occur.

Cystoid macular edema

An increased rate of cystoid macular edema (CME) is proposed to be associated with a rupture of the anterior hyaloid face. It is a rare complication (less than 1%) and is self-limiting in nature. In the event of concurrent contributing factors, such as complicated surgery, history of previous CME and retinovascular disease, the risk of CME may be more significant. Postponing capsulotomy until 6 months after surgery may reduce this risk.

Intraocular lens damage

IOL damage during Nd:YAG capsulotomy is well-documented in the form of lens pitting. Silicone lenses are most easily damaged, followed by acrylic lenses, while PMMA are the most resilient. There is a reduced rate of IOL damage as the user gains experience. Sometimes however, there may be little margin for error. By keeping energy output low and using a converging contact lens to focus the laser energy just behind the capsule, damage can be kept to a minimum. Although most lens strikes cause no significant clinical effect on visual function, even if the damage is directly within the visual axis, multiple lens strikes may potentially cause problems with glare.

IOL dislocation

IOLs may become displaced after laser treatment with reports of dislocation into the vitreous. Fortunately however, these remain rare.

Uveitis

Although transient anterior chamber flare may be seen post-laser treatment, persistent iritis or vitritis is rare. Use of topical steroids is recommended only for those patients with a history of uveitis or who have received a large amount of treatment energy.

Other

There are isolated cases of re-proliferation of lens epithelial remnants after laser capsulotomy with clinically significant reduction of vision requiring further laser treatment. Single cases of pupillary block glaucoma, aqueous misdirection, macular hole, retinal hemorrhage, uveoscleritis and spreading of endocapsular low-grade endophthalmitis have been reported.

REFERENCES

Aslam TM, Devlin H, Dhillon B: Use of Nd : YAG laser capsulotomy. Surv Ophthalmology 48:594–612, 2003.

Apple DJ, Peng Q, Visessook N, et al: Eradication of posterior capsule opacification. Documentation of a marked decrease in Nd : YAG laser posterior capsulotomy rates noted in an analysis of 5416 pseudophakic eyes obtained post-mortem. Ophthalmology 108:505–518, 2001.

Auffarth GU, Brezin A, Caporossi A, et al: Comparison of Nd : YAG capsulotomy rates following phacoemulsification with implantation of PMMA, silicone, or acrylic intra-ocular lenses in four European countries. Ophthalmic Epidemiol 11:319–329, 2004.

Bertelmann E, Kojetinsky C: Posterior capsule opacification and anterior capsule opacification. Curr Opin Ophthalmol 12:35–40, 2001.

Crowston JG, Healey PR, Hopley C, et al: Water-mediated lysis of lens epithelial cells attached to lens capsule. J Cataract Refract Surg 30:1102–1106, 2004.

Deramo VA, Ting TD: Treatment of *Propionibacterium acnes* endophthalmitis. Curr Opin Ophthalmol 12:225–229, 2001.

Findl O, Menapace R, Sacu S, et al: Effect of optic material on posterior capsule opacification in intraocular lenses with sharp-edge optics: randomized clinical trial. Ophthalmology 112:67–72, 2005.

Neuhann IM, Werner L, Izak AM, et al: Late postoperative opacification of hydrophilic acrylic (Hydrogel) intraocular lens. A clinicopathological analysis of 106 explants. Ophthalmology 111:2094–2101, 2004.

Nishi O, Nishi K, Osakabe Y: Effect of intraocular lenses on preventing posterior capsule opacification: design versus material. J Cataract Refract Surg 30:2170–2176, 2004.

Park TK, Chung SK, Baek NH: Changes in the area of the anterior capsule opening after intraocular lens implantation. J Cataract Refract Surg 28:1613–1617, 2002.

Reyntjens B, Tassignon M-J, Van Marck E: Capsular peeling in anterior capsule contraction syndrome: Surgical approach and histopathological aspects. J Cataract Refract Surg 30:908–912, 2004.

Trivedi RH, Werner L, Apple DJ, et al: Post cataract-intraocular lens (IOL) surgery opacification. Eye 16:217–241, 2002.

300 CONGENITAL AND INFANTILE CATARACTS 743.20

Krista A. Hunter, MD
Portland, Oregon
David T. Wheeler, MD
Portland, Oregon

ETIOLOGY/INCIDENCE

A cataract can be defined as any light-scattering opacity of the lens. It is estimated that congenital cataracts are responsible for 5% to 20% of blindness in children worldwide. Incidence varies from country to country. One newborn out of every 250 is estimated to have some form of cataract. One retrospective study of the prevalence of infantile cataracts in the United States showed a rate of 3–4 visually significant cataracts per 10,000 live births. This is a similar rate to a UK study which showed 3.18 per 10,000. These numbers underestimate the total number, however, since they do not take into consideration visually insignificant cataracts.

Cataracts may be unilateral or bilateral and can vary widely in size, morphology and degree of opacification from a small white dot on the anterior capsule to total opacification of the lens. Consequently, the effect on vision, course of treatment and prognosis may also be widely variable.

The causes of infantile cataracts have been the source of much speculation and research. Making a distinction between unilateral and bilateral cataracts may be useful when considering etiology.

Approximately two-thirds of bilateral congenital or infantile cataracts have an identifiable cause or are hereditary. Many genes involved in cataract formation have been identified, and inheritance is most often autosomal dominant although it can be X-linked or autosomal recessive. Within the same pedigree, there can be considerable morphologic variation. Galactosemia is an important example of an autosomal recessive condition while Lowe syndrome is the most common X-linked condition associated with cataracts.

Systemic associations with congenital cataracts include metabolic disorders such as galactosemia, Wilson disease, hypocalcemia and diabetes. Cataracts may be a part of a number of syndromes, the most common being trisomy 21. Intrauterine infections including rubella, herpes simplex, toxoplasmosis, varicella and syphilis are another cause.

In contrast, most unilateral cataracts are not inherited or associated with a systemic disease and are of unknown etiology although they do not rule out the possibility of an associated systemic disease. They are usually the result of local dysgenesis and may be associated with other ocular dysgenesis such as persistent fetal vasculature (PFV), posterior lenticonus, or lentiglobus.

Trauma is a known cause of pediatric cataracts. If there is no known history of trauma to explain an acquired cataract in this age group, investigation must be considered in children who present with other signs suggestive of child abuse.

Regardless of the etiology, prompt treatment of visually significant cataracts is necessary to allow proper development of vision.

COURSE/PROGNOSIS

The course and prognosis of pediatric cataracts is highly variable. The likelihood and rate of progression is very difficult to predict. In addition, the presence of other ocular or systemic abnormalities also contributes to the variable outcome.

The most serious complication of congenital cataracts is permanent visual impairment. When the visual axis is blocked by lens opacity during the sensitive period of visual development, irreversible amblyopia and permanent nystagmus may result. The first two months of life are the most critical for visual development; amblyopia resulting from visual deprivation after the age of 2 to 3 months can often be reversible to some degree. Visual development continues until at least 6 to 7 years of age.

Unilateral cataracts carry a less favorable prognosis than bilateral cataracts. Even a minimal opacity can create significant amblyopia. A child with a unilateral cataract is also at greater risk for anisometropia, which can complicate the picture.

In addition to clearing the visual axis by appropriate surgical technique, proper optical correction in the form of aphakic glasses, contact lenses or intraocular lens implants is essential for good visual development. This requires an ongoing commitment from both the ophthalmologist and family of the infant.

DIAGNOSIS

Clinical signs and symptoms

Cataracts present as opacities in the lens which span a spectrum from easily visible in the undilated state, and apparent to the parents or pediatrician, to much more subtle changes requiring pupillary dilation and careful examination with a slit lamp. The red reflex is an extremely useful part of the exam, as it allows the examiner to estimate the cataract's size and location within the visual axis, even in an uncooperative child.

Cataracts are classified according to their morphological appearance and location; however, making the diagnosis of a specific type of cataract can be difficult if it spreads to involve multiple layers, obscuring the original opacity.

Cataracts may be a part of another disease or syndrome, and are sometimes the initial finding that leads to the disease diagnosis. A cataract may be accompanied by other noticeable ocular abnormalities such as microcornea, megalocornea, coloboma of the iris, aniridia, or zonular dehiscence.

Often an infant with mild cataracts appears asymptomatic, which may delay the diagnosis for years. At other times, lack of reaction to light, strabismus, a failure to notice toys and faces or an apparent delay in development becomes the cause of concern. Mild cataracts may cause photophobia only in bright lights. Dense cataracts also may be discovered if they lead to the development of sensory nystagmus.

For unilateral cataracts in an otherwise healthy child, an extensive workup is not necessary. The most critical part of the workup is a thorough ophthalmologic exam including slit lamp examination of both eyes, intraocular pressure testing, and ultrasound examination of the posterior pole if it is not visible. If the exam reveals the classic appearance of a specific diagnosis such as PFV or posterior lenticonus, no further evaluation is necessary.

The first step in the diagnosis of a patient with bilateral cataracts should be a family history, including examination of family members. If there is a clear autosomal dominant pattern and the child is healthy, further evaluation is not necessary. In cases without clear family history, a thorough pediatric and developmental exam should be performed. Recommended lab workup includes TORCH titers, VDRL, serum calcium and phosphorus levels and urine for reducing substance. Additional systemic workup should be done in coordination with the pediatrician. Dysmorphic features may suggest the need for consultation with a geneticist.

Differential diagnosis

The differential diagnosis for leukocoria or "white pupil" includes retinoblastoma, persistent hyperplastic primary vitreous PFV, retinopathy of prematurity, chorioretinal colobomas, toxocariasis, Coats disease, vitreous hemorrhage and other retinal tumors. These can be distinguished by complete examinations of the anterior and posterior segment, often including ultrasound examination.

TREATMENT

Ocular

Not all pediatric cataracts require surgery. A small, partial or paracentral cataract can be managed by observation. Pharmacologic pupillary dilation with phenylephrine or tropicamide can be helpful. Dilation with atropine should be avoided. Part-time occlusion may be necessary in unilateral or asymmetric cases that develop or are at risk for amblyopia. These techniques may at least delay the need for surgery until a point when eye growth has stabilized and an IOL can be implanted with less refractive uncertainty. Because of the unpredictability in the progression of partial cataracts, these patients should be carefully monitored and if significant amblyopia develops and is unresponsive to treatment, surgical intervention should be performed.

Surgical

If the cataract(s) are felt to be visually significant, surgical intervention is the only option. The timing of surgery is critical for visual development. Most investigators recommend surgery within the first two months of life. There has been evidence to suggest that before one month of age, the risk of aphakic glaucoma is increased. In cases of bilateral cataracts, it may be advantageous to perform surgery on both eyes in the same intervention to allow for simultaneous initiation of visual rehabilitation as well as reducing exposure to general anesthesia. In this setting, treating each eye as a separate sterile procedure may reduce infection risk.

Removal of the lens can be approached through the limbus or the pars plana. The limbal approach has the advantage of maintaining the posterior capsule to facilitate posterior chamber intraocular lens (IOL) implantation if desired.

Several options exist for opening the anterior capsule in pediatric cataracts. The ideal anterior capsulectomy technique is one that results in low incidence of radial tears and is easily performed. In cases of dense cataract, dye can be used to stain the anterior capsule, making this step easier and safer. A manual continuous curvilinear capsulorhexis (CCC), which is the preferred method in adult eyes, can be difficult in pediatric cases due to the elasticity of the pediatric capsule. However, when it can be controlled and completed, it creates an edge which has a low incidence of radial tears.

A mechanized circular anterior capsulectomy, known as vitrectorhexis, has been proven to be a very good, safe alternative if the CCC is not possible. The vitrector tip is placed through a stab incision at the limbus and irrigation is provided though a sleeve around the vitrector or though a separate limbal incision. A cut rate of 150 cycles per minute is recommended. The vitrector port is oriented posteriorly, and held in the center of the capsule to create an initial opening. The opening is enlarged in a circular fashion, holding the cutter just anterior to the capsule to aspirate the capsule up into the cutter. A smooth, round capsulectomy that is also resistant to radial tears can be produced. This procedure is facilitated by using a vitrector supported by a venturi pump.

Pediatric cataracts are soft, and therefore phacoemusification is generally not needed. The lens cortex and nucleus can be removed with an irrigation-aspiration or vitrector hand piece.

To reduce the risk of posterior capsule opacification, which occurs in approximately 80% of pediatric eyes, most surgeons perform a posterior capsulorhexis at the time of surgery. The lens capsule can be filled with viscoelastic and a posterior continuous capsulorhexis made slightly smaller than the anterior one. If an IOL is to be implanted, it can be placed in the capsular bag at this time and some advocate the technique of optic capture where the optic is pressed through the posterior capsulorhexis and the haptics remain in the bag.

It is controversial whether an anterior vitrectomy should be performed at the primary surgery. It can be performed either though the limbal incisions, after making the posterior capsulotomy with the vitrector hand piece, or through the pars plana. The anterior vitreous is removed and the lens epithelial cells therefore cannot grow in the vitreous face.

IOL implantation in children is felt to be safe and acceptable in children as young as one year. In those younger than one year, the decision is more controversial and research is ongoing. The refractive goal of surgery is also controversial. Most surgeons will choose to make the child hyperopic but there is currently no agreed-upon standard. These children will need bifocal glasses for the rest of their lives.

A pars plana approach can be used when no IOL implantation is intended. An attempt is made to remove the whole cataract and the adjacent vitreous with a vitreous cutter.

Care should be taken to remove the viscoelastic entirely to prevent elevated intraocular pressure following surgery and the anterior chamber should be checked carefully for vitreous. The sclera in children is soft and elastic and it is difficult to achieve a self-sealing incision; thus the incision should be closed using 10-0 nylon or Vicryl suture.

COMPLICATIONS

Opacification of the visual axis is the most common complication of cataract surgery in children. This is a serious complication because it can lead to amblyopia. A posterior capsulorhexis and anterior vitrectomy, as previously discussed, is one way to avoid this. An IOL can prevent the formation of a Sommering 's ring, but it is also easier for the lens epithelial cells to migrate to the center of the pupil. Others have suggested that capturing the optic by placing the haptics in the bag and pushing the optic through the posterior capsularhexis may prevent opacification. If opacification occurs, a Nd:YAG laser capsulotomy can be attempted. In this age group, general anesthesia is necessary and a surgical membranectomy may be indicated if Nd:YAG laser treatment is not effective.

Secondary glaucoma is the most sight-threatening complication of pediatric cataract surgery. Open-angle glaucoma can develop months to years after the surgery. The highest incidence is found when surgery is performed on patients younger than 2 months and especially within the first month of life. An IOL may inhibit the development of secondary glaucoma. Glaucoma may also result from inflammation. Angle-closure glaucoma can result from anterior synechiae leading to pupillary block, which can be treated with a peripheral iridectomy. In some eyes, secondary glaucoma can be controlled with topical medication, but many patients will require additional surgical intervention.

Fibrinous or exudative postoperative uveitis is common due to increased tissue reactivity of these eyes. Inflammation can be treated with topical steroids. The visual axis may require clearing with the Nd:YAG laser. Tissue plasminogen activator has been recommended in cases of severe fibrin deposition on the IOL surface, threatening visual rehabilitation.

Endophalmitis is a rare but serious complication. In children, it occurs with approximately the same frequency as in adult cataract patients. Common organisms are *Staphylococcus aureus*, *Staphylococcus epidermidis* and *Staphylococcus viridans*.

The lifetime incidence of retinal detachment after cataract surgery in pediatric patients is reported to be 1–1.5%. Risk factors for retinal detachment are high myopia and repeated surgeries.

Careful surgical technique can reduce early postoperative complications such as wound leak, iris to the wound and vitreous to the wound. Retinal hemorrhages can occur, probably as a result of leaving the intraocular pressure low at the end of surgery. Iris capture of the IOL optic can cause discomfort and disfigure the pupil. This is caused by iris scarring to the posterior capsule. Risk can be reduced by careful placement of the lens at the time of surgery.

Amblyopia, strabismus and nystagmus which may have developed prior to cataract surgery may continue despite removal of the cataract(s) and must also be addressed.

In the postoperative period, it is important to prevent and keep in check any significant inflammatory reaction. The prolonged use of local steroids, nonsteroidal anti-inflammatory agents, and atropine are recommended for this purpose. Systemic steroids have not been shown to be beneficial. The eye must be monitored regularly for the development of a secondary cataract or any other early or delayed problem.

Unlike adult cataract, the management of a pediatric patient is not complete when the post-operative period is over. In some ways, the more difficult and important part of management is still ahead. Neglecting the treatment or and prevention of amblyopia or not giving proper refractive correction is leaving the work half done. Lifelong careful follow-up is essential for all patients treated for pediatric cataract.

Management of pediatric aphakia depends on the age and development of the child, the family situation,and whether there are abnormalities of other ocular structures such as the cornea. For infants, aphakic contact lenses are the treatment

TABLE 300.1 – Etiology of cataracts in children

Idiopathic	Chromosomal Cri du chat syndrome Trisomy 13 Trisomy 18 Trisomy 21 Turner syndrome
Intrauterine infection Cytomegalovirus Herpes simplex Rubella Syphilis Toxoplasmosis Varicella	Renal disease Alport syndrome Hallermann-Streiff-Francois Lowe syndrome
Other ocular diseases Aniridia Anterior segment dysgenesis Microphthalmia Persistent fetal vasculature Retinitis pigmentosa Retinopathy of prematurity	Craniofacial syndromes
Inherited Autosomal dominant Autosomal recessive X-linked	Skeletal disease Bardet-Biedl syndrome Conradi syndrome Smith-Lemli-Optiz Stickler syndrome Weil-Marchesani syndrome
Metabolic disorders Diabetes mellitus Fabry syndrome Galactosemia Galactokinase deficiency Hyperferritinemia Hypocalcemia Hypoglycemia Infantile neuronal ceroid lipofuscinosis Mannosidosis Meckel-Gruber syndrome Refsum syndrome Zellweger syndrome	Muscular disease Myotonic dystrophy
	Dermatological disease Atopic dermatitis Cockayne syndrome Incontinentia pigmenti Rothmund-Thomson
	Trauma
	Uveitis or acquired infection
	Drug induced
	Radiation induced

of choice. Contact lenses should be fitted within the first 7 days after cataract surgery. It is generally recommended to overcorrect infants (children younger than 1 year) by +2.00 to +3.00 diopters, and children between 1 and 2 years by +1.00 to +1.50 diopters. Bifocal glasses may be worn over the contact lenses. Three types of contact lenses are used in pediatric patients: silicone elastomer, rigid gas permeable, and Hydrogel.

Although not the first choice for postoperative vision correction, aphakic spectacles are an option for children who are contact lens intolerant or as a backup to contact lenses in children with bilateral aphakia. Spectacles should not be used for patients with unilateral aphakia because they disrupt binocular fusion. However, for a child without binocular potential or strabismus, unilateral aphakic spectacles in combination with patching can be used. A high refractive index lens can diminish the weight and size of aphakic spectacles, making them easier for patients to tolerate.

Amblyopia treatment must be initiated as soon as possible. For amblyopia treatment to be effective, the amblyopic eye must have not only a clear visual axis, but also the proper corrective lenses to provide the retina with a clear image. In cases of unilateral amblyopia, the amount of patching required depends on the age at which the visual axis was cleared. Generally, patching is not advised for more than half the waking hours during the first 6 months of life to allow the possibility of binocular vision development. A high percentage of children with unilateral aphakia will show a loss of visual acuity after 2 years of age; therefore, continued part-time occlusion until 7 or 8 years of age may be required. Patient and family education about amblyopia and treatment strategies is essential.

COMMENTS

Congenital and infantile cataract surgery and management is more complex than adult cataract surgery and offers different challenges. Every patient needs personalized, appropriate management regarding the timing of cataract surgery, the decision to place an IOL and its selection. Early and late postoperative follow-up and management of various expected and unexpected problems and, in particular, the steps taken to prevent or treat amblyopia are critical. Despite the additional challenges, the results can be extremely gratifying (Table 300.1).

REFERENCES

Holmes JM, Leske DA, Burke JP, Hodge DO: Birth prevalence of visually significant infantile cataract in a defined U.S. population. Ophthalmic Epidemiol 10:67–74, 2003.

Lambert SR: Cataract and persistent hyperplastic primary vitreous. In: Taylor D and Hoyt CS, eds: Pediatric ophthalmology and strabismus. 3rd edn. Philadelphia: Elsevier Saunders: 2005:47:441–457.

Pandey SK, Wilson ME, Trivedi RH, et al: Pediatric cataract surgery and intraocular lens implantation: current techniques, complications and management. Int Ophthalmol Clin 41(3):175–196, 2001.

Vishwanath M, Cheong-Leen R, Taylor D, et al: Is early surgery for congenital cataract a risk factor for glaucoma? Br J Ophthalmol 88;905–910, 2004.

Zetterstrom C, Lundvall A and Kugelberg M: Cataracts in children. J Cataract Refract Surg 31;824–840, 2005.

301 DISLOCATION OF THE LENS
379.32
(Ectopia Lentis, Luxation of the Lens, Subluxation of the Lens)

Devin M. Gattey, MD
Portland, Oregon

The crystalline lens is held in position by the zonules, small fibers arranged in a 360-degree array arising from the ciliary body and connecting to the lens capsule at the equator. They are composed of fibrillin, a protein that is defective in people with Marfan syndrome. The lens is normally suspended behind the iris and in front of the vitreous. A dislocated lens, or ectopia lentis, occurs when the lens is not in its normal position (Figure 301.1). When a lens is decentered but remains in the pupillary area, it is subluxated. A luxated lens is completely displaced from the pupillary aperture, implying complete disruption of zonular fibers. The lens may be luxated forward into the anterior chamber or posteriorly into the vitreous cavity.

ETIOLOGY/INCIDENCE

- Trauma is the most common cause of a phakic lens dislocation.
- Systemic disorders and inherited syndromes can be causes.
- In Marfan syndrome, lens dislocation is usually superior and temporal; patients may have dilation or dissection of the aorta and cardiac valvular disease.
- In homocystinuria, the lens dislocation is usually inferior and nasal. These patients may have a tendency to develop thromboembolism; it is important that the diagnosis be established before any surgical maneuvers are made that could precipitate vascular complications.
- In Weill–Marchesani syndrome, microspherophakia is typically seen and the lens is more likely to dislocate anteriorly.
- Sulfite oxidase deficiency, hyperlysinemia, focal dermal hypoplasia, Ehlers–Danlos syndrome, and mandibulofacial dysostosis are rare causes.

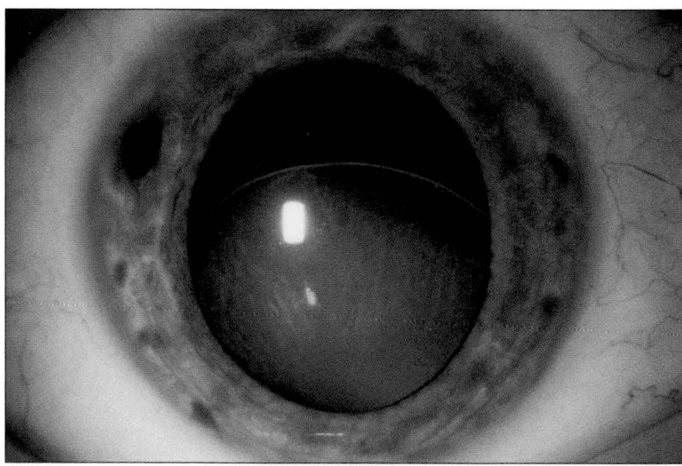

FIGURE 301.1. Simple ectopia lentis.

- Isolated ocular disorders are associated with dislocation of the lens.
- Simple ectopia lentis is usually an autosomal dominant entity that may be expressed in the first few years of life in one form and during adulthood in another form (genetic spontaneous late subluxation of the lens). Dislocation is often superotemporal and symmetric.
- Ectopia lentis et pupillae is an autosomal recessive condition that is associated with corectopia. The pupil and the lens are commonly dislocated in opposite directions.
- Other ocular disorders associated with ectopia lentis include retinitis pigmentosa, uveitis, aniridia, and pseudoexfoliation syndrome.
- Dislocation of the entire lens nucleus or of lens fragments can occur during cataract surgery.

COURSE/PROGNOSIS

- Dislocated lenses with intact capsules can be well tolerated for long periods of time without surgical intervention. Resultant refractive errors, glaucoma, and lenses luxated into the anterior chamber may cause the dislocation to become intolerable.
- Dislocated lenses in children can lead to amblyopia.
- In cases of dislocated lens material after cataract surgery, timely pars plana vitrectomy and lensectomy for the removal of the residual lens material to reduce the postoperative complications of inflammation and glaucoma can result in a favorable outcome.

DIAGNOSIS

Clinical signs and symptoms

- Besides decreased vision, patients may complain of monocular diplopia because of the decentered lens. In addition, there may be pain associated with inflammation, photophobia, and elevated intraocular pressure.
- Examination may show progressive myopia or marked astigmatism, iridodonesis, phakodonesis, vitreous in the anterior chamber, pupillary block, iritis, elevated intraocular pressure, as well as obvious dislocation of the lens or lens implant.

PROPHYLAXIS

- Patients should be advised to avoid participation in contact sports as further dislocation of the lens may occur and they are at higher risk for retinal detachments. In children, amblyopia prevention is paramount.

TREATMENT

Systemic

- Patients with spontaneous dislocation of the lens need evaluation for associated systemic disease. Genetic counseling may be appropriate for specific conditions.

Ocular

- If the subluxated lens is clear, refraction usually can be accomplished satisfactorily.
- If the lens is luxated into the vitreous cavity, an aphakic correction may be used.
- Dilation of the pupil or pupilloplasty may be useful in some phakic cases.
- Topical corticosteroids are used to control ocular inflammation in lens dislocation after cataract surgery or trauma. Typically, cycloplegics and anti-glaucoma medications are used in conjunction with the corticosteroids.
- Pupillary block glaucoma from lens dislocation may respond to mydriatics. If this is not successful, laser or surgical peripheral iridectomy should be attempted before lens removal.
- Dislocation of the lens into the anterior chamber often causes corneal edema and pupillary block with elevated intraocular pressure. Dilation of the pupil and digital pressure on the cornea through the lid with the patient in a supine position may relieve the situation by pushing the lens into the vitreous cavity.

Surgical

Indications for surgical intervention

- Visual function is decreased, either due to a cataractous lens or to a clear lens with the edge in the pupillary axis, precluding suitable phakic or aphakic correction.
- A dislocated lens leaks lens protein, leading to a lens-induced uveitis or glaucoma.
- There is irreversible luxation of the lens into the anterior chamber with pupillary block.

Techniques

- Lenses that are only slightly decentered may be approached with careful phacoemulsification. Capsular tension rings may assist implant stability. Some surgeons advocate iris or capsule retractors to decrease lens movement during extraction.
- If the lens is further dislocated with vitreous prolapsed into the anterior chamber, a pars plana approach with vitreoretinal instrumentation for lensectomy and vitrectomy is recommended. Either a sewn-in posterior chamber lens implant or an anterior chamber implant may be used.
- Lens fragments that have fallen posteriorly in the course of cataract extraction should be removed using standard three-port vitrectomy techniques, not via anterior segment approaches. A sub-total anterior vitrectomy with removal of residual anterior lens material and placement of an acrylic intraocular lens implant in the sulcus position should be attempted before the vitreoretinal portion of the surgery. The cataract wound should be closed with suturing.
- If immediate access to a vitreoretinal specialist is not possible, the dropped nucleus or retained fragments may be removed up to 2 weeks later or longer depending on the overall clinical situation.

COMPLICATIONS

- Retinal detachment may be associated with the dislocated lens after trauma, cataract surgery, or pars plana vitrectomy and lensectomy for retained lens material.
- After cataract surgery, the dislocated lens material can be associated with uveitis, leading to cystoid macular edema and glaucoma. In addition, there is the increased risk of endophthalmitis when there is vitreous loss.

- Amblyopia is the most common reason for permanently decreased vision in patients with congenital causes of lens dislocation.

COMMENTS

Congenital dislocation of the crystalline lens is often associated with serious systemic disease. Marfan syndrome is the most common of these, affecting about 5 in 100,00 people. Those afflicted with this genetic condition are prone to excessive height, scoliosis, aortic dilation, and dissecting aortic aneurysm. Ectopia lentis occurs in the majority of patients with Marfan syndrome. Homocystinuria is another genetic disorder associated with dislocation of the lens. These patients may have developmental delay, excessive height, and thrombotic vascular occlusions. This makes surgery extremely risky for these patients. Patients with congenital dislocation of the lens need to be carefully screened for these and other conditions. They also need to be evaluated carefully for amblyopia as this is the principal cause for permanently decreased vision.

Phacoemulsification is the dominant method of cataract extraction in the developed world. Dropped nucleus and retained lens fragments are not rare complications of this procedure, occurring in approximately 0.3% of cases. When this occurs, initial management by the cataract surgeon should focus on prevention of retinal detachment, not on retrieval of posteriorly located lens material. In general, it is best to clean up the anterior segment of vitreous and residual cortex and place an acrylic lens implant in the ciliary sulcus. An experienced vitreoretinal surgeon should attempt retrieval of the retained lens material. Research indicates that leaving the lens material in the vitreous cavity for up to 2 weeks does not lead to a worse visual outcome.

SUPPORT GROUPS

There are several on-line support groups for people with Marfan syndrome including:
http://www.livejournal.com/community/marfangroup/
http://health.groups.yahoo.com/group/marfans_support_and_chat/
http://www.marfan-list.org/

REFERENCES

Chandler PA: Choice of treatment in dislocation of the lens. Arch Ophthalmol 71:765–786, 1964.

Fishkind WJ: Complications in phacoemulsification — avoidance, recognition, and management. New York, Thieme Medical, 2002.

Monshizadeh R, Nasrollah S, Haimovici R: Management of retained intravitreal lens fragments after cataract surgery. Surv Ophthalmol 43:397–404, 1999.

Nelson LB, Maumenee IH: Ectopia lentis. Surv Ophthalmol 27:143–160, 1982.

Roy FH, Arzabe CW: Master techniques in cataract and refractive surgery. New Jersey, SLACK Incorporated, 2004.

302 LENTICONUS AND LENTIGLOBUS 743.36

David Lawlor, MD
Newport, Vermont

ETIOLOGY/INCIDENCE

Lenticonus is a circumscribed conical bulge of the anterior or, more commonly, posterior lens capsule and cortex. It is usually restricted to the 2- to 7-mm axial area. The conical lens surface bows forward into the anterior chamber in *anterior lenticonus* or posteriorly into the vitreous in *posterior lenticonus*. The cone is usually axial in location but may be eccentrically or, rarely, in the periphery of the lens. In *lentiglobus*, the entire posterior capsule has a globular shape. The majority of cases are of the posterior lentiglobus variety. Anterior lenticonus is rare, usually bilateral, and commonly associated with Alport's syndrome. It has also rarely occurred in patients with Waardenburg's syndrome and in patients with spina bifida. Strabismus is commonly found in patients with posterior lenticonus. Duane's syndrome, persistent hyperplasia of the primary vitreous, retinoblastoma, microphthalmia, coloboma, and anterior lenticonus have been reported uncommonly with posterior bowing of the lens capsule.

- The incidence of this anomaly is 1 to 4 in every 100,000 children. There is no sex predilection.
- The true etiology of posterior lenticonus remains unknown but many theories have been proposed:
  - Inherited weakness of a circumscribed portion of the posterior lens capsule; normal intralenticular pressure displaces the cortex posteriorly within the area of the weakened capsule;
  - Localized hypertrophy of the posterior lens cortex;
  - Traction on the posterior capsule by remnants of the hyaloid arterial system;
  - Disturbance in the tunica vasculosa lentis.
- Histopathologically, the posterior capsule is markedly thin, in contrast to the relatively thick preequatorial capsule. At the summit of the posterior cone the posterior capsule is half the thickness of a normal posterior capsule.

Most cases of posterior lenticonus are unilateral and sporadic, but many bilateral familial cases have been reported.

COURSE/PROGNOSIS

In posterior lenticonus, the bulge of the capsule increases with age, and cataractous changes progressively occur in the lens cortex inside and around the cone. Early in the course of this abnormality, there is an 'oil droplet' appearance on slit-lamp examination and in the ophthalmoscopic reflex. The axial refraction in the cone and center of the lens is myopic, whereas the peripheral reflex is hyperopic. This produces a scissoring reflex at retinoscopy, which is described as pathognomonic of the condition. Posterior lenticonus is usually detected in early infancy and progresses throughout childhood.

The progressive nature of the condition is demonstrated by the gradual opacification of the posterior cortical fibers overlying the posterior lenticonus. These cataractous changes may occur during the amblyogenic age. Amblyopia can be due to optical distortion induced by the double-lens system of the lenticonus and by visual deprivation due to cataractous changes. Occlusion therapy must be instituted before or after cataract extraction when amblyopia is present.

Patients with posterior lenticonus have a relatively good visual prognosis because the condition is rarely significant at birth, thus allowing the foveal fixation reflex to develop during the first months of life. In a series of 39 patients, Cheng and colleagues found that 19 patients (49%) achieved postoperative visual acuity of 20/40 or better. In another series by Crouch and Parks, 12 of 21 patients (63%) showed a postoperative visual acuity of 20/50 or better.

Posterior lenticonus is the most prevalent unilateral cataract in a normal-sized eye. Anterior polar cataract, congenital nuclear cataract, and persistent hyperplasia of the primary vitreous occur in microphthalmic eyes with a corneal diameter of 10 mm or less.

DIAGNOSIS

The retinoscopic 'oil droplet' appearance and scissoring reflex in the early phase of the disease and the biomicroscopic appearance of the posterior capsular bulge into the vitreous with posterior cortical cataractous changes are characteristic.

TREATMENT

Patients without significant cataractous changes can be followed or treated with dilating eyedrops, correction with glasses, or patching.

Surgical

Common indications for surgical treatment include the following:

- A decrease in visual acuity to a level of 20/70 or less after occlusion therapy;
- The loss of central fixation reflex;
- The onset of 'sensory' strabismus.

In these cases, lens extraction via a limbal incision with irrigation-aspiration or irrigation-aspiration-cutting instruments is the treatment of choice. A pars plana approach for cataract extraction has also been reported. Intraocular lens implantation is a standard procedure in patients at least 2 years old. Younger patients can be optically corrected with contact lenses. During surgery, the posterior weakened capsule bows anteriorly toward the cornea when the infusion is lowered.

COMMENTS

Posterior lenticonus or lentiglobus must be suspected in patients with unilateral progressive cataracts in normal-sized eyes with cataractous changes in the posterior cortical layer. This disease has a progressive course; it does not usually interfere with the fixation reflex during the first months of life. Surgery must be considered when visual acuity is moderately reduced from optical distortion or cataractous changes.

REFERENCES

Bleik JH,Traboulsi EI, Maumenee IH: Familial posterior lenticonus and microcornea. Arch Ophthalmol 110:1028, 1992.

Butler TH: Lenticonus posterior. Arch Ophthalmol 3:425–436, 1930.

Cheng KP, Hiles DA, Biglan AW, et al: Management of posterior lenticonus. J Pediatr Ophthalmol Strabismus 28:143–149, 1991.

Crouch ER, Parks MM: Management of posterior lenticonus complicated by unilateral cataract. Am J Ophthalmol 85:503–508, 1978.

Gibbs ML, Jacobs M, Wilkie AOM, et al: Posterior lenticonus: clinical pattern and genetics. J Pediatr Ophthalmol Strabismus 30:171–175, 1993.

Khalil M, Saheb N: Posterior lenticonus. Ophthalmology 91:1429–1430, 1984.

Mohney BG, Parks MM: Acquired posterior lentiglobus. Am J Ophthalmol 120:123–124, 1995.

Pollard ZF: Familial bilateral posterior lenticonus. Arch Ophthalmol 101:1238–1240, 1983.

Simons BD, Flynn HW: A pars plana approach for cataract surgery in posterior lenticonus. Am Ophthalmol 124:695–696, 1997.

303 MICROSPHEROPHAKIA 743.36

Adolfo Güemes, MD

Buenos Aires, Argentina

ETIOLOGY/INCIDENCE

Microspherophakia is the presence of a small and spheric lens. The lens is larger in the anteroposterior diameter, whereas the equatorial diameter is smaller than normal. The decreased equatorial diameter of a microspherophakic lens measures an average of 6.75 to 7 mm (normal, 9.0 mm), and the anteroposterior diameter is larger than normal (>5.0 mm, normal: 3.4 to 4.5 mm). The overall lenticular mass is reduced by approximately 25%. The entire lens can be visualized when the pupil is dilated. The lens curvature is increased, resulting in lenticular myopia. Microspherophakia is commonly associated with subluxed lenses. The zonules in microspherophakia are long and irregular, and some can be seen in a retracted state on the lens surface.

Microspherophakia has been attributed to an arrest of development of the lens in the fifth to sixth month of embryonic life, a time at which the lens is spheric. Anomalies in development of the ciliary body and the zonules and nutritional deficiency from the tunica vasculosa lentis have all been implicated in this arrest of development. A zonular defect with loss of the normal zonular traction on the lens could allow the lens to remain spheric instead of gradually converting to the normal biconvex shape.

Microspherophakia can be inherited as an isolated autosomal dominant or autosomal recessive disorder. A gene for the autosomal recessive form for Weill–Marchesani syndrome has been mapped to chromosome 19p 13.3-p13.2. On a survey of 396 congenital dislocated lenses, fewer than 1% were dislocated secondary to microspherophakia and Weill–Marchesani syndrome.

COURSE/PROGNOSIS

The visual prognosis in microspherophakia is poor due to the development of secondary glaucoma. Repeated episodes of elevated intraocular pressure may result in the formation of peripheral anterior synechiae.

DIAGNOSIS

Differential diagnosis

Microspherophakia is most commonly associated with the Weill–Marchesani syndrome. Patients have brachycephaly, a short body build with brachydactyly, normal or hypertrophic musculature, a broad thorax, hypoextensible joints, and microspherophakia with subluxed lenses. Less commonly, microspherophakia is associated with homocystinuria, ectopia lentis et pupillae, Marfan syndrome, Klinefelter's syndrome, chondrodysplasia punctata, mandibulofacial dysostosis, and metaphyseal dysplasia.

COMPLICATIONS

Secondary glaucoma

Secondary glaucoma is the most serious complication of microspherophakia. There are two mechanisms involved in this complication.

Pupillary block

There is a forward displacement of the lens with a greater area of iris-lens contact, which causes an increased resistance to the flow of aqueous from the posterior to the anterior chamber. Iris bombé can result from this forward lens displacement. *Inverse glaucoma* is a term used to describe an acute rise in intraocular pressure after the instillation of miotics. Miotics increase the iris-lens surface contact area, producing a pupillary block. This block can be reversed with pupillary dilation.

Angle-closure glaucoma

The loose zonules permit the lens to move forward and the peripheral iris to bow anteriorly and close an already crowded angle. Gonioscopy usually reveals normal angle structures.

Lens dislocation

Lens dislocation is a common finding. In microspherophakia associated with Weill–Marchesani syndrome, the lens dislocates downward early in life. Less commonly, the lens can dislocate into the anterior chamber after pupillary dilation. In dominant disease with microspherophakia such as Marfan syndrome, the lens moves upward in a majority of cases. Iridodonesis and phacodonesis are usually noticeable on slit-lamp examination.

Myopia

Myopia is lenticular in nature, but superimposed axial myopia has been reported in isolated autosomal dominant microspherophakia. Myopia is usually severe and progressive, beginning in early childhood. It can fluctuate according to the pupil diameter and lens position. It ranges in magnitude from −5 to −30 diopters.

PROPHYLAXIS

Topical mydriatics can be used to control pupillary block glaucoma, but mydriatics may allow the lens to dislocate anteriorly in patients with abnormal zonular attachments. A laser iridectomy can be performed before secondary glaucoma develops.

TREATMENT

Ocular

Glaucoma control is of primary concern. Standard pharmacological glaucoma treatment may not be effective. Mydriatics and cycloplegics, such as cyclopentolate and tropicamide, may be of value in preventing pupillary block glaucoma, but prolonged mydriasis may allow the lens to dislocate into the anterior chamber. In patients with microspherophakia and intact zonules or in whom the zonular integrity is unknown, miotics should never be used to break an attack of acute glaucoma. Hyperosmotic agents and carbonic anhydrase inhibitors that shrink the volume of the vitreous may permit posterior movement of the lens and relief of the pupillary block. A peripheral iridectomy is then usually necessary.

Surgical

Peripheral iridectomy

Laser iridectomy is the initial choice of treatment, after which surgical iridectomy can still be performed if the former fails. Surgical complications such as vitreous loss are more common in these patients due to the lack of vitreous face protection by lens periphery and zonules.

Lens extraction

In patients with severe lenticular myopia, lens subluxation or secondary glaucoma, lens extraction may be necessary in addition to a peripheral iridectomy. Lensectomy with anterior vitrectomy is the treatment of choice in these cases.

REFERENCES

Faivre L, Gorlin RJ, Wirtz MK, et al: In frame fibrillin-1 gene deletion in autosomal dominant Weill-Marchesani syndrome. J Med Genet 40:34–36, 2003.

Fuchs Josefine, Rosenberg Thomas: Congenital ectopia lentis. A Danish national survey. Acta Ophthalmol Scand 76:20–26, 1998.

Halpert M, BenEzra David: Surgery of the hereditary subluxated lens in children. Ophthalmology 103:681–686, 1996.

Jensen AD, Cross HE, Paton D: Ocular complications in the Weill-Marchesani syndrome. Am J Ophthalmol 77:261–269, 1974.

Johnson VP, Grayson M, Christian JC: Dominant microspherophakia. Arch Ophthalmol 85:534–542, 1971.

304 TRAUMATIC CATARACT 366.20

Dan S. Gombos, MD, FACS
Houston, Texas
George M. Gombos, MD, FACS
Brooklyn, New York

Lens opacification is a common complication after ocular trauma. It can be diagnosed at the time of injury or years later and can cause a significant decrease in vision. Distinguishing them from other cataracts (congenital, metabolic, age related) is an essential component in their management. The identification of associated ocular injuries and the anticipation of potential complications are critical to the medical and surgical approach taken by the ophthalmologist.

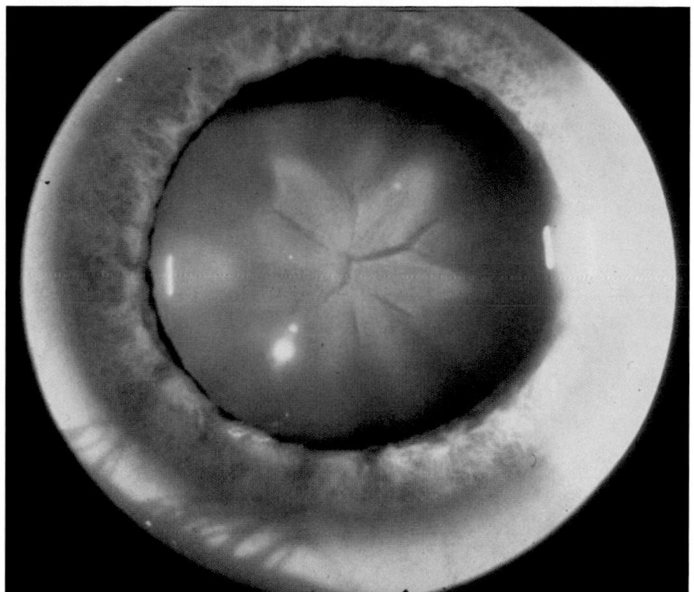

FIGURE 304.1. Acquired cataract following trauma. Photograph courtesy of Stephen Orlin, MD.

ETIOLOGY/INCIDENCE

- Lens opacification may result from perforating and nonperforating injuries to the globe. Nonperforating trauma includes contusive and concussive injuries to the orbit, head, or body.
- Traumatic cataract can occur after electric shock, radiation, or chemical injury.
- Any damage to the lens capsule can lead to cataract formation. Contusion-related injuries result in a pressure wave that may lead to dysfunction of the lens epithelium and edema of cortical lens fibers (Figure 304.1).

COURSE/PROGNOSIS

- Cataract formation (simple traumatic cataract) may be the only significant pathology after an injury. Complicated traumatic cataracts involve perforating injuries with damage to other ocular structures (cornea, iris, cilliary body, vitreous, retina).
- Opacities caused by concussive or contusive injuries may be transient, static, or progressive.
- Sharp objects (needles, pins) that cause perforating injuries can lead to focal nonprogressive lens opacities.
- When the anterior and posterior capsules are both damaged, complete lens opacification commonly occurs. This may progress rapidly, reducing vision to hand motion or light perception within hours.

DIAGNOSIS

- History of trauma.
- Lenticular opacities typical of trauma are identified.
- The form may be discrete, punctate, or rosette-shaped, or there may be scattered subepithelial changes.
- The location is commonly anterior, segmental and subcapsular.
- Late rosette opacities deep in the cortex may be found years later.
- Contusive injuries may cause a full or partial circle of iris pigment on the anterior surface of the lens capsule (Vossius' ring).
- There may be signs of trauma to other ocular structures, including the cornea, iris, zonules, and posterior pole: lens subluxation, iridodonesis, phacodonesis, shallow or deep anterior chamber, increased or decreased intraocular pressure and hyphema.

Differential diagnosis

Cataracts from other causes include age-related, metabolic, congenital, and drug-induced cataracts.

PROPHYLAXIS

- Protective shatter-resistant goggles should be worn at work.
- Childhood hazards at home and at playgrounds should be identified.
- Lead shielding should be used during radiation exposure.

TREATMENT

Medical

If the patient's visual acuity is 20/40 or better, the cataract is nonprogressive, and the eye is quiet, no specific treatment is required. Periodic reevaluation is suggested.

Surgical

Patients with traumatic cataracts should undergo surgery if the visual acuity deteriorates or there are ocular complications.

- With extensive penetrating or perforating injury, immediate surgical intervention is essential.
- Extracapsular cataract extraction or phacoemulsification is the procedure of choice. Zonular dehiscence must be anticipated.
- If the lens capsule is badly ruptured and the lens material is mixed with vitreous and blood, complete lensectomy and vitrectomy are indicated. Open-sky or pars plana techniques can be used.
- Intraocular lens implantation can be performed as part of the initial repair or as a secondary procedure if significant trauma has occurred. In patients with loss of the posterior capsule and zonular dehiscence a sutured intraocular lens may be indicated.

COMPLICATIONS

- Complications include uveitis, hemorrhage, elevated intraocular pressure (e.g. pupillary block, phacolytic glaucoma), and endophthalmitis.
- In order to avoid a fibrinous uveitis an intensive course of topical corticosteroids may be necessary.

COMMENTS

The pediatric patient

To prevent amblyopia and achieve rapid visual rehabilitation, primary intraocular lens implantation is preferred in the pediatric patient.

- Acrylic and PMMA posterior chamber lens are generally implanted. Anterior chamber lenses should be avoided. Posterior capsulotomy, if necessary, can be performed at the time of surgery or postoperatively with an Nd:YAG laser.
- A complete history, including details involving the trauma, must be obtained. Document the place, date, and time of injury, as well as the visual acuity at presentation.
- Always consider the possibility of an intraocular foreign body. When the ocular medium is not clear or the history suggests an intraocular foreign body, radiographic studies, ultrasonography, or both must be performed.

The management of traumatic cataracts requires a thorough history, physical examination, and appropriate documentation. Surgical intervention may be necessary at presentation or deferred indefinitely. Traumatic injuries vary. Dogmatic rules or surgical techniques should not be used indiscriminately. Carefully planned and modified management results in better visual outcomes.

REFERENCES

Asano N, Schlotzer-Schrehardt U, Dorfler S, et al: Ultrastructure of contusion cataract. Arch Ophthalmol 113:210–215, 1995.

Jacobi PC, Dietlein TS, Lueke C, Jacobi FK: Multifocal intraocular lens implantation in patients with traumatic cataract. Ophthalmology 110:531–538, 2003.

Koenig SB, Ruttum MS, Lewandowski MF, et al: Pseudophakia for traumatic cataracts in children. Ophthalmology 100:1218–1224, 1993.

Lacmanovic Loncar V, Petric I: Surgical treatment, clinical outcomes, and complications of traumatic cataract: retrospective study. Croat Med J 45(3):310–313, 2004.

Mian SI, Azar DT, Colby K: Management of traumatic cataracts. Int Ophthalmol Clin 42(3):23–31, 2002.

SECTION

27 Macula

305 AGE-RELATED MACULAR DEGENERATION 363.31
(Age-related Maculopathy) 362.51, 362.52

Thomas S. Hwang, MD
Portland, Oregon
Michael L. Klein, MD
Portland, Oregon

Age-related macular degeneration (AMD) is the leading cause of severe vision loss in developed nations. The pathologic changes of this chronic degenerative condition occur primarily in the retinal pigment epithelium (RPE), Bruch's membrane, and the choriocapillaris of the macular region.

The clinical hallmark of the disease is the presence of drusen (Figure 305.1). Vision loss usually results from one of the two forms of advanced AMD-central geographic atrophy and choroidal neovascularization.

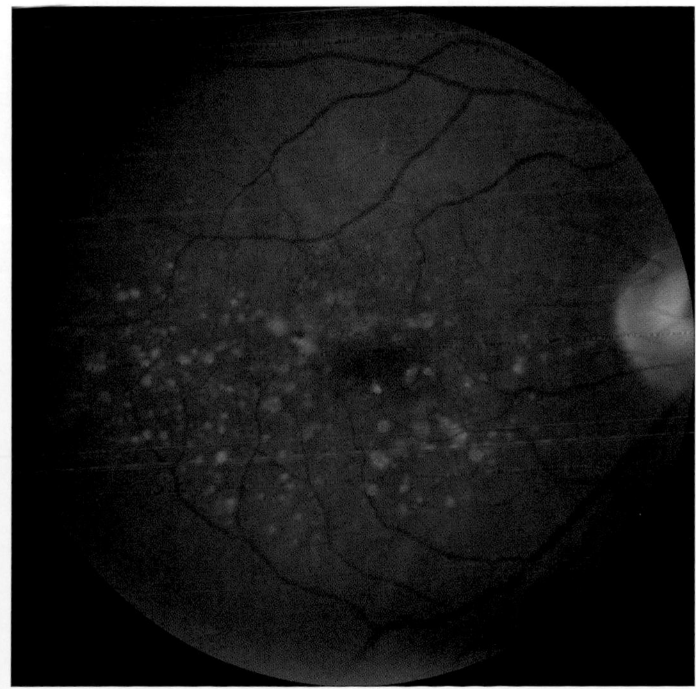

FIGURE 305.1. Age-related macular degeneration.

ETIOLOGY/INCIDENCE

The cause is unknown. Many believe that AMD represents a complex group of diseases resulting from a combination of genetic and environmental factors. Symptoms begin after the age of 50. An estimated 10% of persons older than 75 years have significant AMD with some visual loss.

Advanced AMD occurs more frequently in European-derived populations. Population-based studies have suggested that advanced AMD may be less frequent in Asian populations, and rare in African-derived populations.

Risk factors for developing advanced AMD include age, race, blue iris color, and cigarette smoking. Hypertension has been associated with an increased risk of neovascular AMD. Studies have linked serum cholesterol levels, high intake of dietary fats, and cardiovascular disease to the risk of advanced AMD, but findings to date have been inconclusive.

COURSE/PROGNOSIS

Patients without high-risk features may not develop vision loss related to advanced AMD for years. The age-related eye disease study (AREDS) showed that patients without advanced AMD but with high-risk features, defined as the presence of large drusen (>125 microns), numerous medium-sized drusen (63–125 microns), or non-central geographic atrophy had an 18% risk of developing advanced AMD in 5 years. Those patients with advanced AMD in the contralateral eye had a 46% risk of developing advanced AMD in their better eye in 5 years. Neovascular AMD is a more frequent cause of significant vision loss than is geographic atrophy. Spontaneous recovery of vision, after vision loss related to AMD, is uncommon.

DIAGNOSIS

Clinical signs and symptoms

- Most patients are asymptomatic in the early stages.
- The disease is bilateral, but often presents asymmetrically.
- Drusen and focal hyper- and hypopigmentation are common early signs.
- Patients with neovascular AMD often present with sudden vision loss or metamorphopsia.
- Ophthalmoscopic findings of choroidal neovascularization include the presence of subretinal fluid, heme, and lipid. Sometimes a subretinal membrane is visible.
- Patients with geographic atrophy may present with gradual vision loss or difficulty reading despite good central acuity.

- Geographic atrophy is characterized by a sharply demarcated area of RPE atrophy and clearly visible choroidal vasculature.
- Severe subretinal hemorrhage and breakthrough hemorrhage into vitreous cavity may occur but are uncommon.

Laboratory findings

- Fluorescein angiography is useful for defining choroidal neovascularization (CNV) and its suitability for treatment.
- Indocyanine green angiography may be useful in delineating CNV that is obscured by hemorrhage or pigment epithelial detachment, although no randomized, controlled clinical trials support their use in determination of treatment.
- Optical coherence tomography (OCT) has become a useful adjunct to fluorescein angiography in determining the amount of subretinal and intraretinal fluid leakage associated with CNV.

PROPHYLAXIS

- Smoking cessation and control of hypertension have been suggested by population-based studies as possible ways of modifying risk for advanced AMD.
- Daily nutritional supplement consisting of vitamin C, 500 mg, vitamin E, 400 IU, beta carotene, 15 mg, zinc, 80 mg, as zinc oxide and copper, 2 mg (commercially available as Preservision AREDS Formula, Bausch and Lomb one capsule twice a day), has been shown to reduce the risk of advanced AMD in patients with high risk features (large drusen, non-central geographic atrophy, or advanced AMD in contralateral eye).
- Other nutritional supplements, including lutein, zeaxanthin, and omega-3 fatty acids, show some promise but have not yet been rigorously studied.
- Clinical trials are under way to determine whether an anti-angiogenic agent could be effective in reducing the rate of advanced AMD in high-risk patients.

TREATMENT

No treatment is currently available for the non-neovascular form of AMD, other than the preventive precautions mentioned above. Several treatments are directed towards inhibiting and/or destroying choroidal neovascularization.

Systemic

No systemic treatment is available for AMD at this time, although systemically administered anti-angiogenic agents are being evaluated.

Ocular

The introduction of antiangiogenic agents has revolutionized the treatment of neovascular AMD. Ranibizumab (Lucentis, Genentech), is a humanized antibody fragment against vascular endothelial growth factor-A (VEGF-A) which has been studied in randomized clinical trials. Regardless of lesion characteristics (e.g. occult vs classic), patients treated with an intravitreal injection of ranibizumab every four weeks over a period of one to two years had a better than 90% chance of retaining their vision within 3 lines, and about 20–40% chance of improving more than three lines of vision. These results are clearly superior to previous treatments for neovascular AMD, including laser photocoagulation, photodynamic therapy, and the first anti-VEGF agent to be approved, pegaptanib sodium (Macugen, Eyetech/Pfizer/OSI).

Frequent intravitreal injections of antiangiogenic agents are associated with a small risk of serious intraocular complications, including endophthalmitis. The risk of infection is minimized by the use of a lid speculum and 5% povodine iodine solution in the conjunctival fornix prior to injection with a 30 gauge needle at the pars plana. In current clinical practice, injections are commonly delivered on a monthly basis , as had been used in most clinical trials. However, many of the treating physicians employ treatment on an 'as needed' basis. This involves close follow-up of the patient (usually at monthly intervals initially) with optical coherence tomography along with careful examination to determine if repeat injections are necessary.

Prior to the general availability of ranibizumab many physicians investigated the use of intravitreal treatment with bevacizumab (Avastin, Genentech), a humanized antibody against VEGF-A developed for treating colon cancer . Short-term observations involving many patients treated with intravitreal bevacizumab yielded favorable results which were considered by many to be comparable to those achieved with ranibizumab. While lacking the long-term evidence for efficacy and safety established for its cousin ranibizumab, the short-term favourable results and the much reduced cost of bevacizumab has resulted in its current widespread usage. A national head-to-head trial with bevacizumab and ranibizumab is planned.

Pegaptanib sodium is an aptamer specific for certain forms of VEGF. It was the first anti-angiogenic agent to be approved for the treatment of neovasular AMD. Because the newer agents have shown to be more effective, this drug has a very limited role in treatment of AMD at this time.

Photodynamic therapy (PDT) takes advantage of verteporfin (Visudyne, Novartis), light-sensitizing dye with an affinity for the neovascular tissue to selectively destroy neovascular tissue. This was the first available treatment for subfoveal choroidal neovascularization that did not result in immediate vision loss. While this treatment was superior to observation in predominantly classic lesions, and smaller occult and minimally classic lesions. PDT is seldom indicated as the first line treatment today because of the availability of antiangiogenic agents. However, its use in combination with these agents is currently being investigated, and PDT alone or in combination with intravitreal steroids continues to have a limited role in selected cases.

The Macular Photocoagulation Study (MPS) demonstrated in a randomized controlled clinical trial that laser photocoagulation for patients with neovascular AMD resulted in better visual acuity than observation alone. With the subsequent development and use of newer and more effective treatments, photocoagulation is seldom used in clinical practice today.

Surgical

The Submacular Surgery Trial examined the role of vitrectomy and submacular surgery in the treatment of CNV in AMD. In patients with hemorrhagic or subfoveal choroidal neovascularization due to AMD, vitrectomy and removal of the membrane did not result in improved outcome.

Macular translocation has been reported to be of benefit in well-selected patients, although complications leading to complete blindness can occur in both the limited and 'total 360' renditions of the surgery.

COMMENTS

Low vision aids can allow patients to read, write, and even drive. A variety of magnification devices and telescopic devices are available. A careful evaluation by a low vision specialist can significantly improve patients' functioning and their quality of life.

REFERENCES

AREDS: A randomized, placebo-controlled, clinical trial of high-dose supplementation with vitamins C and E, beta carotene, and zinc for age-related macular degeneration and vision loss. Report no. 8. Arch Ophthalmol 119:1417–1436, 2001.

Gragoudas ES, Adamis AP, Cunningham ET, Jr, et al: Pegaptanib for neovascular age-related macular degeneration. N Engl J Med 351:2805–2816, 2004.

Guidelines for using verteporfin (visudyne) in photodynamic therapy to treat choroidal neovascularization due to age-related macular degeneration and other causes. Retina 22:6–18, 2002.

Hawkins BS, Bressler NM, Miskala PH, et al: Surgery for subfoveal choroidal neovascularization in age-related macular degeneration: ophthalmic findings: SST report no. 11. Ophthalmology 111:1967–1980, 2004.

Jonas JB, Akkoyun I, Budde WM, et al: Intravitreal reinjection of triamcinolone for exudative age-related macular degeneration. Arch Ophthalmol 122:218–222, 2004.

Macular Photocoagulation Study Group: Laser photocoagulation of subfoveal neovascular lesions of age-related macular degeneration. Updated findings from two clinical trials. Arch Ophthalmol 111:1200–1209, 1993.

Toth CA, Freedman SF: Macular translocation with 360-degree peripheral retinectomy impact of technique and surgical experience on visual outcomes. Retina 21:293–303, 2001.

306 CYSTOID MACULAR EDEMA

362.53

(Cystoid Maculopathy, Irvine–Gass Syndrome)

Wayne E. Fung, MD

San Francisco, California

ETIOLOGY

Cystoid macular edema (CME) is a common cause of decreased central vision, resulting from fluid accumulation in intraretinal spaces in the macular region.

Two possible mechanisms have been postulated to explain the occurrence of CME in such a diverse array of conditions: inflammation and anoxia. The inflammatory theory may account for CME associated with cataract surgery, postscleral buckling procedures, and chronic uveitis, including pars planitis. The vascular occlusion mechanism, on the other hand, readily explains the conditions associated with obvious retinal vascular disease and retinal detachments because the outer third of the retina derives its nourishment from the choriocapillaris.

Retinitis pigmentosa and perifoveal telangiectasia also are involved with disturbances or shunts in the retinal circulation, whereas choroidal tumors have been linked either to occlusion of retinal capillaries secondary to vascular endothelial cell hypertrophy or edema, or to cyst formation through expansion of extracellular spaces by serous exudates within the inner plexiform and inner nuclear layers.

COURSE/PROGNOSIS

By far the most common situation associated with CME is cataract surgery, particularly intracapsular procedures; the surgical trauma to the anterior segment is thought to stimulate the production of prostaglandins or retard their resorption within the eye. Various investigators have found CME to occur after 40% to 60% of intracapsular cataract extractions; extracapsular surgeries result in CME in only approximately 10% of cases.

The position of an intraocular lens also can contribute to CME. Lenses suspended in the pupil have the worst prognosis, followed by anterior chamber lenses. Posterior chamber lenses implanted 'in the bag' have the lowest incidence of CME. Fortunately, the condition resolves spontaneously in 3 to 6 months in the majority of patients; however, if the anterior hyaloid face is disturbed or if formed vitreous is incarcerated in the corneoscleral wound, the condition may become chronic.

Diabetic retinopathy is the second most common condition associated with CME. It is largely seen in patients with adult-onset (after age 30) diabetes whose disease is of 10 years' duration or more. Concomitant hypertension or arteriosclerosis makes the presence of CME more likely as a complication of diabetic retinopathy.

Certain antiglaucoma medications, such as latanoprost, have been associated with an increased incidence of cystoid macular edema and anterior uveitis. Recent studies estimate that between 1% and 5% of patients taking the drug may develop anterior uveitis, CME, or both.

DIAGNOSIS

CME is considered a sign of an underlying ocular and/or systemic disease process and not an entity in itself. It is associated with many clinical situations, including the following:

- Cataract surgery;
- Diabetic retinopathy;
- Exudative age-related maculopathy (with serous macular detachment);
- Tributary or central retinal vein occlusions;
- Scleralbuckling procedures;
- Chronic uveitis, pars planitis;
- Collagen-vascular disease;
- Aphakia with topical antiglaucoma epinephrine compounds;
- Tumors of the choroid (melanoma, capillary hemangioma);
- Diabetic traction detachments;
- Retinitis pigmentosa;
- Epiretinal membranes;
- Drug reactions;
- Toxic conditions (i.e. nicotinic acid intoxication);
- Perifoveal retinal telangiectasia.

Diagnostic tests

- Slit-lamp: with Hruby lens or hand-held + 90D lens.
- Fluorescein angiogram.
- Optical coherent tomography (OCT).

TREATMENT

Systemic

Suppression of inflammation, whether it results from surgery or systemic causes, seems to reduce the incidence and duration of cystoid macular edema. Antiprostaglandin agents (nonsteroidal anti-inflammatory drugs) that have produced good results include the following:

- Fenoprofen 60 mg PO t.i.d.;
- Ibuprofen 400 mg PO t.i.d. or q.i.d.;
- Prednisone 20 mg PO t.i.d. or q.i.d. for 1 week, tapered to 40 mg/week for 2 weeks, and then to 20 mg/week for 2 to 3 weeks.

A dramatic improvement in chronic CME has been reported after treatment with:

- Hyperbaric oxygen 2 atmospheres for 1 hour twice daily.

Retinal edema largely subsided and visual acuities improved from 20/70 to 20/20 or 20/25. The beneficial effect may occur as the oxygen causes transient constriction of macular capillaries (relieving pressure on leaking vascular endothelial cell junctions) and stimulates collagen formation to seal the leaks.

Ocular

A favorable response in cystoid macular edema may occur with ocular anti-inflammatory drugs, such as the following:

- Topical 1% indomethacin in sesame oil or water, 1 drop, 3 or 4 times dail. This can be given prophylactically 1 day before cataract surgery and 3 or 4 times daily after surgery for 4 to 6 weeks;
- Topical 0.5% ketoralac trimethamine, 1 drop, 4 times daily;
- Topical 0.1% diclofenac, 1 drop, up to 4 times daily;
- Topical 1% prednisolone acetate, 1 drop, 4 times daily or 0.12%, 5 drops every 4 hours while awake;
- Sub-Tenon's or retrobulbar injection of 40 mg triamcinolone with a 27-gauge needle with the patient under topical anesthesia.

Many patients show an improvement of visual acuity within 1 to 2 weeks after the initiation of intensive corticosteroid therapy. Recent studies have shown that a single retrobulbar corticosteroid injection was as effective as three biweekly posterior sub-Tenon's injections of the same drug. Visual acuity improvements were comparable between the two groups; however, as with all steroid medications, close monitoring of the patient's intraocular pressure is required.

For topical medications, it is important to instruct the patient to keep the lids closed for 10 to 15 seconds after the instillation of drops and to apply gentle pressure over the inner canthus to trap the active medication in the ocular region and prevent its escape into the nasopharynx.

Cyclooxygenase inhibitors also have been proved to be useful adjuncts to steroid therapy, as have carbonic anhydrase inhibitors such as acetazolamide (Diamox) that facilitate the transport of water across the retinal pigment epithelium from the subretinal space to the choroid. In a recent randomized, masked, crossover trial of acetazolamide in chronic cases of uveitis, a statistically significant decrease in angiographic CME was documented, although visual acuity did not improve.

In patients with retinitis pigmentosa, oral acetazolamide has been shown to decrease CME and improve visual acuity; the question of whether a topically applied carbonic anhydrase inhibitor such as dorzolamide hydrochloride might also be effective in retinitis pigmentosa patients was recently tested. In the prospective, double-masked, crossover study, topical dorzolamide was compared with oral acetazolamide in 5 patients, and it was shown that although topical dorzolamide improved the CME angiograms of some patients, no measurable improvement in visual acuity could be documented with dorzolamide. Oral acetazolamide, however, proved to be effective in improving CME bilaterally in all subjects, whereas 3 of 5 study participants showed objective improvement in visual acuity by 7 letters or more.

Medical

Laser therapy of the retina should be considered for CME in conjunction with diabetic maculopathy, branch vein occlusion, and some cases of central retinal vein occlusion. The decision is based on the patient's visual acuity (usually 20/50 or worse) and fluorescein angiographic evidence that the CME is due to progression of intraretinal edema from vascular leakage sites to the central macula. The target or targets of treatment should be the leakage sites.

Diode (810-nm) versus argon green (514-nm) lasers were compared in a recent study of the treatment of diabetics with diffuse macular edema; the treatments involved the use of a modified grid pattern. No significant differences were found between the two laser modalities in visual improvement, visual loss, reduction in or elimination of macular edema, or the number of supplemental treatments required over the minimum 12-month follow-up. Pre-existing systemic vascular disease, however, was a limiting factor for the degree of eventual improvement, regardless of the type of laser used.

For central retinal vein occlusion, *panretinal photocoagulation* should be considered under two circumstances:

- If neovascularization is developing on the disk or on other parts of the retina;
- If there is angiographic evidence of 'nonperfusion' in the peripheral retina.

If CME is present with a central retinal vein occlusion but neovascularization of the disk and elsewhere is *absent*, a grid pattern of laser therapy across the central macula could be considered if the visual acuity has fallen to 20/50 or lower.

In this new era of anti-VEGF drugs, one wonders whether or not, drugs such as Avastin and Lucentis, have a role in treating chronic CME. The rational for their use includes their ability to reverse capillary permeability rapidly and to block intraocular VEGF. Thus far, there have been no publications on this specific subject.

In 2007, Genentech will start a prospective, randomized, multi-center study to evaluate the effectiveness of Lucentis for the treatment of Diabetic Macular Edema. The results of this study will help to answer the question just posed.

Surgical

In aphakic eyes with vitreous to the wound but without an intraocular lens, *anterior vitrectomy* through either a limbal or pars plana approach has been found to be effective in improving the patient's CME in 75% of cases. The surgical goal is to restore normal anterior segment anatomy by removing all abnormal visible vitreous connections. Because significant complications can and have occurred with this procedure, it is prudent to reserve this method until medical treatment fails.

Pars plana vitrectomy for cases of medically refractory pseudophakic cystoid macular edema was recently confirmed to be useful; 24 consecutive eyes (23 with vitreous adhesions to anterior chamber structures and 1 eye with iris capture of the intraocular lens) showed significant ($P < 0.0001$) improvement in visual acuity (mean improvement of 4.7 Snellen lines) after the vitrectomy procedure.

Pars plana vitrectomy has proved to be ineffective, however, in a handful of cases of chronic CME after uncomplicated extracapsular extraction with 'in the bag' posterior chamber lens placement. Furthermore, this vitrectomy procedure should be considered only for pars planitis or chronic uveitis after less invasive approaches have failed. Specifically, *cryotherapy* should be performed for pars planitis, whereas systemic and sub-Tenon's injection therapies for chronic uveitis should be given a thorough trial before vitrectomy is considered for either condition. This is because potential side effects of the procedure, including retinal tears, retinal detachment, and rubeosis iridis, are significant.

Finally, cystoid macular edema should be considered more a medical problem than a surgical problem. The medical armamentarium has been enlarged significantly in recent years, and it is only after medical treatment has failed and definite indications for surgery (i.e. anterior segment distortion or vitreous traction on the macula) are present that invasive procedures should be contemplated.

COMPLICATIONS

The most common adverse reactions to oral anti-inflammatory medications are the following:

- Gastrointestinal discomfort (e.g. dyspepsia, constipation, nausea, vomiting, anorexia, flatulence);
- Headache;
- Somnolence;
- Dizziness;
- Tremor;
- Pruritus;
- Tinnitus;
- Palpitations.

To minimize side effects and to facilitate absorption into the serum, these drugs should be taken 30 minutes before meals.

Oral corticosteroids should not be given to patients with a history of peptic ulcers or osteoporosis. Before sub-Tenon's injection of corticosteroids is performed, the patient should be tested for possible adverse response to steroids (e.g. elevated intraocular pressure) by topical applications because the periocular injection route most likely delivers the active ingredient to the eye for 1 month.

COMMENTS

The role of light toxicity in causing cystoid macular edema has been considered by many clinicians. Light delivered to the retina via intravitreal fiberoptic light sources during surgery has definitely been shown to be toxic to the retina; the coaxial light of an operating microscope delivered to the posterior segment of an aphakic eye is responsible for producing a pink scotoma during the first postoperative week. It is unclear what role light plays in the emergence of postoperative CME in cases of posterior vitrectomy.

REFERENCES

Fine BS, Brucker AJ: Macular edema and cystoid macular edema. Am J Ophthalmol 92:466–481, 1981.

Flach AJ: Cyclo-oxygenase inhibitors in ophthalmology. Therapeutic review. Surv Ophthalmol 36:259–284, 1992.

Fung WE, Vitrectomy-ACME Study Group: Vitrectomy for chronic aphakic cystoid macular edema: Results of a national, collaborative, prospective, randomized investigation. Ophthalmology 92:1102–1111, 1985.

Rossetti L, Bujtar E, Castoldi D, et al: Effectiveness of diclofenac eyedrops in reducing inflammation and the incidence of cystoid macular edema after cataract surgery. J Cataract Refract Surg 22(suppl 1):794–799, 1996.

Thach AB, Dugel PU, Flindall RJ, et al: A comparison of retrobulbar versus sub-Tenon's corticosteroid therapy for cystoid macular edema refractory to topical medications. Ophthalmology 104:2003–2008, 1997.

307 EPIMACULAR PROLIFERATION
362.56
(Epiretinal Fibrosis, Macular Pucker, Cellophane Maculopathy, Preretinal Macular Fibrosis)

Alexander P. Hunyor, MB, BS, FRANZCO, FRACS
Sydney, Australia
Joseph E. Robertson, Jr., MD
Portland, Oregon

Epimacular proliferation is a descriptive term for the condition in which the macular region is distorted by the contraction of a fibrocellular epiretinal membrane (ERM) that has grown across the inner retinal surface. These membranes are the result of proliferation of, and collagen formation by, one or more of the following cell types: retinal pigment epithelial (RPE) cells, macrophages, fibrocytes, and astrocytes. The presence and proportion of these cells depend on the underlying cause, which may include a precipitating event such as retinal tears, inflammation, trauma, retinal vascular disease, vitreous hemorrhage, surgery including cryotherapy and photocoagulation, and idiopathic causes. Epimacular proliferation is a common condition, although it is frequently asymptomatic and does not require surgical management. Good surgical results are achieved with vitrectomy and ERM peeling in selected cases.

ETIOLOGY/INCIDENCE

Epimacular proliferation commonly occurs without an obvious precipitating cause and then is classified as idiopathic. Posterior vitreous detachment (PVD) has been noted in 75% to 93% of eyes with idiopathic epimacular proliferation. Partial or complete PVD may cause breaks in the internal limiting membrane (ILM), allowing migration and proliferation of fibrous astrocytes. Rupture of the ILM may actually be the cause of many cases of epimacular proliferation considered to be idiopathic. PVD may also result in retinal breaks, allowing the entry of RPE cells into the vitreous cavity.

The incidence varies according to the clinical classification scheme. Autopsy studies have shown ERM in 2% to 4% of eyes. Epidemiologic studies suggest a prevalence of 7% in persons over 50 years of age. The incidence increases with advancing age, as does the incidence of PVD.

COURSE/PROGNOSIS

The majority of ERMs involving the macula are nonprogressive and require no intervention. In one study, visual acuity remained 20/30 or better in 56% and 20/50 or better in 78% of affected eyes. Patients with significant visual symptoms due to ERM may be considered for surgery. Spontaneous separation of epiretinal membranes with resolution of visual symptoms is a well-documented but rare occurrence. The prevalence of ERM increases following uncomplicated cataract surgery, but these ERMs usually have little or no impact on vision.

DIAGNOSIS

Clinical signs and symptoms

Symptoms include visual distortion (metamorphopsia) and reduced/blurred vision. The diagnosis of epimacular proliferation is established on clinical grounds. Although the semi-opaque nature of the ERM itself may contribute to visual loss, most symptoms appear to be secondary to distortion, edema, or localized detachment of the macula. The underlying cause should be sought in all cases; in apparently 'idiopathic' cases, an unrecognized retinal tear must be excluded.

- High-power biomicroscopy, preferably with a fundus contact lens, is required.
- Red-free light may facilitate the examination.

On examination, the appearance varies from thin and translucent 'cellophane' to thick opaque sheets. Retinal striae and vascular distortion are common (Figure 307.1a). PVD is usually present. Thin diaphanous ERMs are more typical of the idiopathic form. Denser ERMs are more common after retinal tear or detachment. These are probably a limited form of proliferative vitreoretinopathy. RPE cells predominate in these membranes.

Other findings include cystoid macular edema, localized traction detachment of the macula, 'pseudoholes' (round/oval openings in the ERM, usually centrally), nerve fiber layer hemorrhages, and cotton-wool spots (due to axoplasmic stasis from ERM traction). ERMs are bilateral in 20% to 30% of patients.

Several clinical features of ERMs merit specific attention when surgical intervention is considered. Vessels underlying the membrane are usually tortuous, whereas vessels peripheral to the membrane generally appear to be straight and even narrow as they are dragged toward the epicenter or the point of maximal contraction. At least one edge of the membrane is often slightly elevated, and this should be noted because it may be the best location to initiate peeling of the membrane. Failure to find such an edge does not, however, preclude the patient from being an appropriate surgical candidate.

Laboratory findings

Optical coherence tomography (OCT — Figure 307.1b) provides additional information regarding the extent of the ERM, any persistent vitreous attachments, and macular thickness. Increased vascular permeability, induced by distortion of retinal vessels, results in significant extravascular leakage on fluorescein angiography in approximately 20% of cases. Angiography may also be useful in the assessment of any underlying retinal vascular disease that may limit the final visual prognosis. Rarely, a clinically unsuspected subretinal neovascular membrane may be detected on fluorescein angiography in a patient with epimacular proliferation.

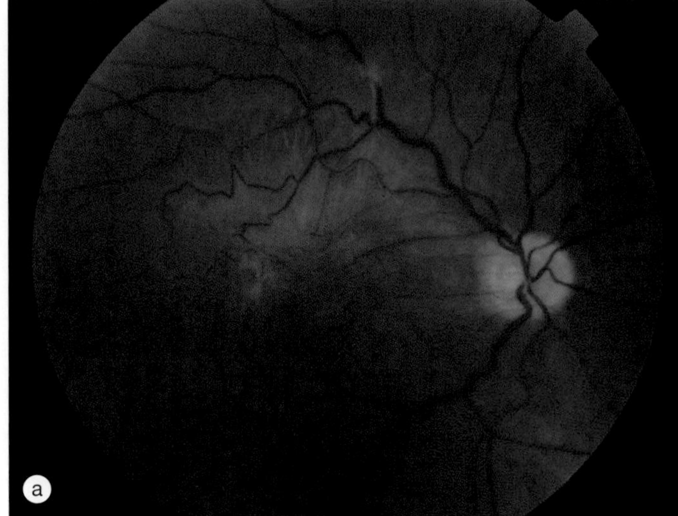

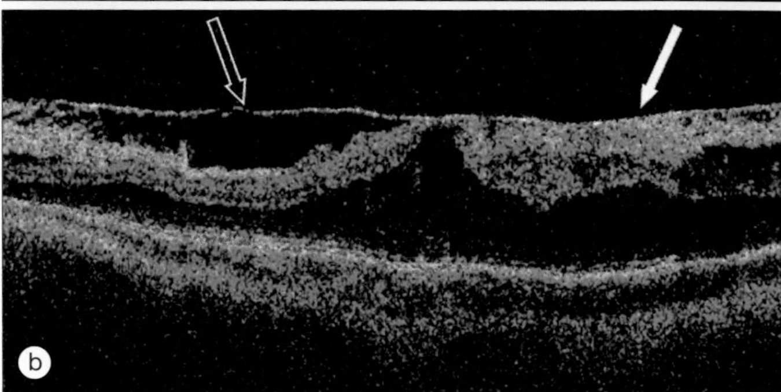

FIGURE 307.1. a) Color fundus photograph showing epiretinal membrane with vascular distortion and retinal striae. b) Optical coherence tomography (OCT) scan of epiretinal membrane with areas of separation (open arrow) and broad adherence (closed arrow) to retinal surface, with associated macular thickening.

TREATMENT

Medical

- There is no medical therapy for epimacular proliferation.
- Underlying conditions such as uveitis should be treated.
- Photocoagulation to areas of microvascular leakage due to traction from an epiretinal membrane should be avoided because it may result in further contraction of the membrane.

Surgical

Case selection

- Candidates include symptomatic patients with significant metamorphopsia or reduction in visual acuity (VA). No specific VA level is considered as a 'cutoff,' as patients with poorer VA but few/no symptoms often do not require surgery whereas patients with better VA but marked metamorphopsia may do so.
- Evaluate other causes of visual symptoms (e.g. cataract) and underlying conditions (e.g. retinal vascular disease).
- A visible 'edge' of the membrane is not a prerequisite for consideration of surgery.

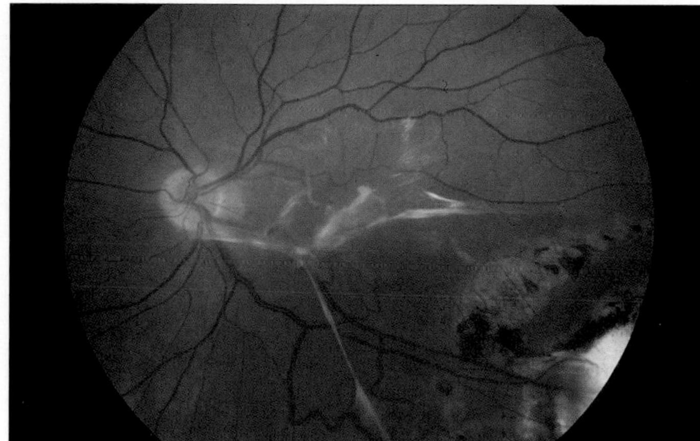

FIGURE 307.2. Epimacular proliferation adjacent to previously treated angioma.

Technique

- Various methods of ERM removal have been described.
- The common features of these techniques include the following:
  - Three-port pars plana vitrectomy approach;
  - ERM mobilization and removal with a combination of picks, microvitreoretinal blades, forceps and scissors.

Regardless of the exact technique used, the avoidance of retinal trauma with ERM manipulation and the identification and treatment of intraoperative retinal breaks (an uncommon complication) are essential. Removal of the internal limiting membrane (ILM) in addition to the ERM may reduce the rate of recurrent ERM, but its long-term effects and influence on visual outcome have not been determined. Vital stains such as indocyanine green (ICG) and trypan blue have been used to assist in visualization of ERM and ILM. The long-term effects of their use have not been established.

In large series, more than 80% of patients improve postoperatively by 2 or more Snellen lines of acuity. Five percent of patients have worse postoperative visual acuity, and 10% to 15% are unchanged. The 'average' improvement in visual acuity is 50%, although individual prediction may be difficult. Patients commonly have some residual metamorphopsia, even with much-improved visual acuity. The best postoperative vision correlates with a shorter history and better preoperative visual acuity. The macular thickness and profile on OCT rarely return to 'normal' but this does not preclude significant visual improvement.

In patients with ERM after retinal reattachment surgery, the presence of previous macular detachment confers a less favorable visual prognosis. This is not, however, a contraindication to surgery because substantial improvement in visual acuity may still result from membrane peeling. The prognostic significance of cystoid macular edema associated with epiretinal membranes is unclear because different studies have had conflicting results.

COMPLICATIONS

The most common postoperative complications are progressive nuclear sclerosis, which is visually significant in the majority of patients with long-term follow-up and is more common in older patients; and rhegmatogenous retinal detachment, which occurs in 4% to 8% of patients. Visually significant reproliferation of the ERM occurs in fewer than 5% of cases. Subretinal neovascularization is a rare complication of ERM peeling. Other complications are those common to intraocular surgery in general and vitrectomy in particular.

COMMENTS

Although epiretinal membranes are common, few patients require surgery for this condition because most membranes cause minimal or no symptoms. Most membranes remain stable over long periods of observation. The decision regarding surgery should be made based on the patient's symptoms at the time of assessment, and other causes of visual reduction such as lens opacity should be evaluated. Although the results of surgery are good, a return to completely 'normal' vision is uncommon, and patients should be made aware of this before surgery. They also should be advised of the likelihood of progressive nuclear sclerosis, which will usually require subsequent surgery, in addition to the other potential complications.

REFERENCES

DeBustros S, Thompson HR, Michels RG, et al: Vitrectomy for idiopathic epiretinal membranes causing macular pucker: Br J Ophthalmol 72:692–695, 1988.

Hillenkamp J, Saikia P, Gora F, et al: Macular function and morphology after peeling of idiopathic epiretinal membrane with and without the assistance of indocyanine green. Br J Ophthalmol 89:437–443, 2005.

Jahn CE, Minich S, Moldaschel S, et al: Epiretinal membranes after extracapsular cataract surgery. J Cataract Refract Surg 27:753–760, 2001.

Massin P, Allouch C, Haouchine B, et al: Optical Coherence Tomography of idiopathic macular epiretinal membranes before and after surgery. Am J Ophthalmol 130:732–739, 2000.

Mitchell P, Smith W, Chey T, et al: Prevalence and associations of epiretinal membranes. The Blue Mountains Eye Study, Australia. Ophthalmology 104(6):1033–1040, 1997

Wise GN: Clinical features of idiopathic preretinal macular fibrosis. Am J Ophthalmol 79:349–357, 1975.

308 MACULAR HOLE 362.54

Tina A. Scheufele, MD
Boston, Massachusetts
Jay S. Duker, MD
Boston, Massachusetts

A macular hole is a full-thickness defect in the neurosensory retina centered at the foveola resulting in a central scotoma. Vitreal traction is believed to cause centrifugal displacement of foveal retinal cells and supporting elements. With current vitreoretinal surgical techniques, successful closure and visual improvement are possible in the majority of cases.

ETIOLOGY/ INCIDENCE

Macular holes occur in 0.3% of the population over the age of 55. The incidence is 2–3 times higher in women. Approximately ten percent of patients are affected bilaterally.

Antero-posterior or oblique vitreal traction exerted on a tightly adherent prefoveolar vitreous cortex is thought to initiate hole formation. Consequently, the risk of developing a macular hole after complete posterior vitreous separation is less than 1%. In contrast, patients with full-thickness macular holes whose asymptomatic fellow eyes demonstrate vitreal-foveal traction on OCT have more than a 40% chance of developing a macular hole in the second eye.

Most macular holes are isolated, but they may occur days to weeks after blunt trauma or in patients who have high myopia with a posterior staphyloma. Additional associations include: epiretinal membranes, cystoid macular edema, rhegmatogenous retinal detachment, YAG posterior capsulotomy, hypertensive retinopathy, diabetic retinopathy, Best's disease, and adult vitelliform macular dystrophy.

COURSE/PROGNOSIS

The earliest sign of a macular hole is an abnormal vitreoretinal interface at the foveola. A stage 1A impending macular hole appears clinically as a yellow spot. Continued vitreal traction results in elevation of the foveolar retina (stage 1B impending), followed by a break in the photoreceptor layer at the umbo (stage 1B occult) with centrifugal displacement of the retinal photoreceptors, Müller cells, and xanthophyll. The clinical appearance is a small yellow ring. The patient often reports metamorphopsia, but visual acuity is usually nearly normal. Fifty percent of stage 1 holes spontaneously resolve.

A stage 2 hole is a 100–399 um full-thickness defect of the neurosensory retina. The prefoveolar vitreous cortex may separate, forming a pseudooperculum. If separation occurs at one edge of the hole, the defect appears eccentric. A true operculum is rare. Visual acuity ranges from 20/40 to 20/400.

A stage 3 hole is = 400 microns. Visual acuity is often 20/200 but (rarely) may be as good as 20/40. The vitreous cortex has separated from the central macula but remains attached to the optic nerve and often to the peripheral macula. The edges of the hole are elevated, with intraretinal cysts. A cuff of subretinal fluid may surround the hole. Nodular yellow opacities in the RPE may be found at its base.

Progression to a stage 4 hole occurs once the vitreous detaches from the optic nerve. A Weiss ring is present.

Left untreated, nearly all stage 2 holes will progress to stage 3 or 4 within 5 years. Spontaneous resolution of stage 2 or larger holes is rare. Tangential traction from epiretinal membranes may contribute to progressive enlargement.

DIAGNOSIS

The earliest visual complaint is usually metamorphopsia. Distortion may be apparent on the Amsler grid. As the hole enlarges, visual acuity declines. Untreated, vision usually stabilizes around 20/200.

Biomicroscopy has traditionally been used to diagnose and stage macular holes. Confirmatory tests may help solidify the diagnosis. While fluorescein angiography may demonstrate a hyperfluorescent window defect, the finding is non-specific. In the Watzke Allen test, most patients with a full-thickness macular hole will report a gap in a narrow vertical beam of light focused on the fovea through a condensing lens. In a similar test, a 50 micron laser aiming beam that is focused on the macular hole will not be seen if a full-thickness defect exists.

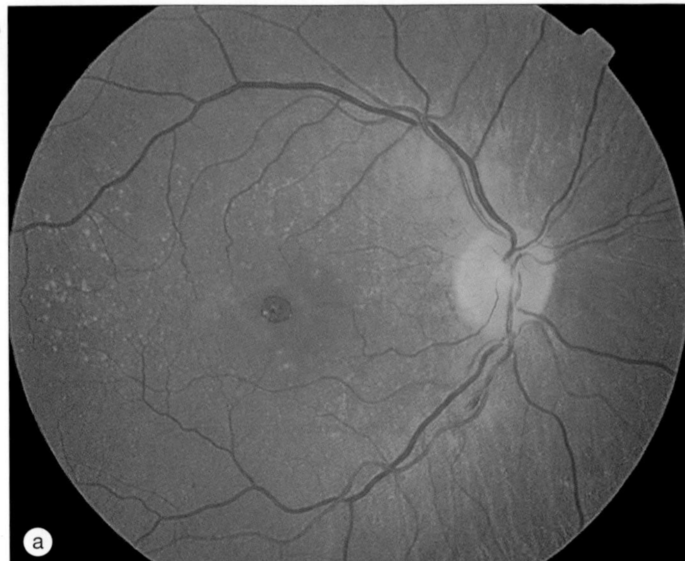

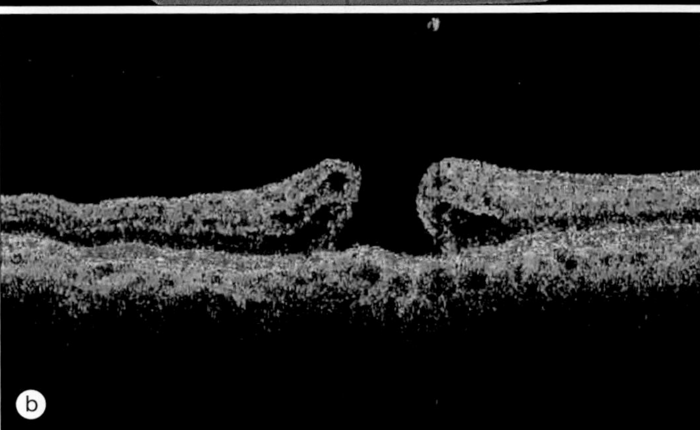

FIGURE 308.1. a) OCT of a stage 4 macular hole. Intraretinal cysts are present at the edges of the hole and a pseudooperculum is seen within the detached posterior hyaloid. Note that the hole is larger at its base than at the inner retinal surface. b) Stage 4 macular hole with a cuff of subretinal fluid and yellow deposits at its base. This patient also has macular drusen.

Optical coherence tomography (OCT) is the best ancillary test, as it can document vitreoretinal interface abnormalities not apparent biomicroscopically. It can also differentiate full-thickness macular holes from pseudoholes and lamellar holes. The basal diameter of the hole, which may correlate most with prognosis, can be measured more precisely with OCT (Figure 308.1).

Differential diagnosis

The differential diagnosis includes macular pseudoholes, lamellar holes, and cystoid macular edema.

TREATMENT

Prophylactic vitrectomy for stage 1 holes is usually not indicated. However, close observation is recommended, since 50% will progress to full-thickness defects, on average 4 months after the onset of symptoms. Occasionally traumatic macular holes, especially when small, may resolve without surgery.

Surgical management is recommended for holes graded stage 2 or higher. The overall anatomical success rate is >80% and approaches 90% for stage 2 holes. Visual acuity improves 2 or more lines in 80% of patients, and final visual acuity is 20/40 or better in 40–60% of patients. Best outcomes are associated with holes <400 um and <6 months' duration.

The surgical technique involves a standard pars-plana vitrectomy with posterior vitreous detachment; peeling of the posterior cortical hyaloid, any epiretinal membranes, and sometimes the internal limiting membrane (ILM); air-fluid exchange; and gas. Most surgeons use either 20–25% sulfur hexafluoride (SF6) or 14–16% perfluoropropane (C3F8). The patient is then positioned face down for about 7 days (range: 5–14 days).

Intravitreal adjuncts, such as indocyanine green (ICG), trypan blue, or triamcinolone acetonide, can improve visualization and peeling of the ILM and residual hyaloid. Toxicity to the retinal pigment epithelium (RPE) has been demonstrated in vitro with standard concentrations (5 mg/mL) of ICG. Newer studies show that lower concentrations (0.5 mg/mL) and shorter exposure times may be safe, but this is still being investigated.

COMPLICATIONS

Complications related to the macular hole itself are rare. In highly myopic eyes with posterior staphylomata, a macular hole can cause a rhegmatogenous retinal detachment.

Complications after vitrectomy include cataract progression (>75%), retinal detachment (3%), endophthalmitis (<1%), retinal pigment epithelial changes, cystoid macular edema, visual field defects, intraoperative enlargement of the hole and, rarely the development of choroidal neovascular membranes.

The rate of progression of nuclear sclerotic cataracts after vitrectomy is most significant in patients over age 50. Worsening of a cataract is the most common reason for decreased vision months to years after successful macular hole closure.

Temporal or inferior visual field defects may relate to mechanical damage from the air infusion; small paracentral scotomata may be caused by ILM peeling.

Late re-opening of the macular hole occurs on average 12–15 months after surgery in 2–10% of patients. Traction from epiretinal membranes (ERM) may be responsible. Cataract extraction may be associated with late re-opening, possibly due to post-operative epiretinal membrane formation or cystoid macular edema. Closure rates after a second vitrectomy are similar to that of the initial surgery, approximately 80%.

COMMENTS

OCT can help assess the success of the surgery once the gas bubble is above the macula. The edges of a closed macular hole will be apposed and the cuff of subretinal fluid gone.

Patients with poor vision may benefit from low-vision referral.

REFERENCES

Benson WE, Cruickshanks KC, Fong DS: Surgical management of macular holes: a report by the American Academy of Ophthalmology. Ophthalmology 108:1328–1335, 2001.

Casuso LA, Scott IU, Flynn HW: Long-term follow-up of unoperated macular holes. Ophthalmology 108:1150–1155, 2001.

Gass JDM: Stereoscopic atlas of macular diseases: diagnosis and treatment. 4th edn. St Louis, Mosby, 1997.

Johnson MW: Improvements in the understanding and treatment of macular hole. Curr Opin Ophthalmol 13:152–160, 2002.

Ko TH, Fugimoto JG, Duker JS: Comparison of ultrahigh- and standard-resolution optical coherence tomography for imaging macular hole pathology and repair. Ophthalmology 111:2033–2043, 2004.

309 SOLAR RETINOPATHY 363.31
(Solar Maculopathy, Solar Retinitis, Eclipse Burn, Eclipse Blindness, Eclipse Retinopathy, Foveomacular Retinitis, Photo Retinopathy, Photo Maculopathy)

Timothy L. Gard, MD
Hillsboro, Oregon

ETIOLOGY/INCIDENCE

Solar retinopathy is a well-described clinical entity, thought to be the result of a photochemical injury to the retina. This insult to the retina may be thermally enhanced as well. It is reported most often following a solar eclipse, thus accounting for its sporadic occurrence. Less common cases have occurred following direct sun gazing. Cases in which direct solar observation has been implicated in retinal damage include: military personnel assigned to survey the sky; religious or ritualistic ceremonies; hallucinogenic drug use (LSD); mental illness: and matters of secondary gain. Cases of solar retinopathy in patients sun bathing without a history of direct solar viewing have occurred in conjunction with various risk factors, including young age, emmetropia, and possibly higher than normal levels of solar radiation reaching the earth's surface have been reported.

COURSE/PROGNOSIS

Within several hours of solar exposure patients may note a central scotoma in one or both eyes, though the dominant eye is often more severely affected. Visual acuity can be normal to significantly reduced, typically from 20/30 to 20/100. Fundus examination can be unremarkable or show a small yellowish spot within the fovea. A faint gray-white border may be present as well. Over the ensuing weeks, the spot fades, becoming a reddish spot surrounded by a faintly pigmented halo and later followed by the development of a 25–200-micron lamellar defect. This small lamellar hole or depression is permanent and characteristic of solar retinopathy. Most patients recover normal or near normal vision in 3 to 9 months, though some severely affected individuals can have reduced acuity and a permanent scotoma. Factors believed to worsen the prognosis include longer exposure times, larger pupil size, younger age, clear ocular media, emmetropia, and geophysical factors favoring increased levels of solar radiation.

DIAGNOSIS

Clinical signs and symptoms

The patient's history is most helpful when considering a diagnosis of solar retinopathy. A recent eclipse in one's practice area would increase the likelihood of encountering an affected individual. Initial complaints may include a decrease in vision, central or paracentral scotoma, metamorphopsia, micropsia, chromatopsia, afterimage, and erythopsia. Both eyes may be involved but often asymmetrically, with the dominant eye more severely affected. Non-visual complaints include brow ache, headache, or both. On examination, visual acuity can vary widely, from 20/20 to 20/200. Amsler grid testing may reveal a small central or paracentral scotoma. Examination of the anterior segment is typically unremarkable, and the visual axis clear of any significant media opacity. Retinal exam can be normal or reveal varying degrees of retinal pigment epithelial (RPE) involvement. The typical presentation of acute solar retinopathy reveals a small yellow spot with a grayish border within the foveal area, though multiple spots may be evident. More subtle presentations may reveal an altered foveal light reflex or granular or punctuate irregularity to the RPE. In the more severe cases the yellow spot will change to a reddish spot that then develops into a foveal depression or 25–200-micron permanent lamellar defect.

Laboratory findings

Fluorescein angiography findings are often normal, though a small window defect may be noted. OCT findings can be normal or may show tiny hyper-reflective spots present in the inner retina. Amsler grid testing is useful in demonstrating the small central or paracentral scotoma of which patients often complain. Multifocal electroretinography has shown decreased amplitudes, with normal latencies.

Differential diagnosis

Other causes of lamellar depressions or holes include trauma and posterior vitreous detachment. Welding arc maculopathy is rare, and may require more prolonged exposure than solar retinopathy. This is in contrast to the keratitis that develops so commonly following brief exposure. The light flash or arc created by a high-voltage electrical short circuit may also produce similar retinal findings.

PROPHYLAXIS

Education is the most effective tool in helping prevent solar damage to the eye. Prior to a solar eclipse, a public awareness campaign about the risks of eclipse viewing and education about safe ways to view the event should occur. Eclipses should only be viewed indirectly using a pinhole projection system, in which a pinhole is used to form the solar image on the inside of a cardboard box or other flat, non-reflective surface. The image thus formed can then be safely observed. It is important to emphasize that sunglasses do not provide protection for solar or eclipse viewing. In our everyday practices we will encounter patients who are at relatively higher risk for sun-related ocular injury, such as aphakic patients who should be fitted with eyewear that absorbs potentially damaging ultraviolet light. Modern-day intraocular lenses are designed to provide protection, but the conjunctiva and lids can still benefit from sunglasses and a brimmed hat.

TREATMENT

No effective treatment is known.

COMPLICATIONS

Many patients with solar retinopathy have a return of normal vision and resolution of symptoms over the weeks and months that follow. Some patients have a permanent reduction in vision and persistent metamorphopsia and or scotoma.

COMMENTS

Though patients with solar retinopathy are most frequently seen after a solar eclipse, this damage also occurs in the setting of purposeful sun gazing, which can cause serious and lasting retinal damage. There appears to be significant variation in susceptibility to solar retinopathy, with numerous risk factors suggested.

REFERENCES

Gass JDM: Stereoscopic atlas of macular diseases: diagnosis and treatment. 4th edn. St Louis, Mosby-Year Book, 1997.

Mainster MA: Solar eclipse safety. Ophthalmology 105:9–10, 1998.

Sadun AC, Sadun AA, Sadun LA: Solar retinopathy a biophysical analysis. Arch Ophthalmol 102:1510–1512, 1984.

Schatz P, Eriksson U, Andreasson S, et al: Multifocal electroretinography and optical coherence tomography in two patients with solar retinopathy. Acta. Ophthalmol. Scand 82:476–480, 2004.

Yannuzzi LA, Fisher YL, Krueger A, et al: Solar retinopathy: a photobiological and geophysical analysis. Trans Am Ophthalmol Soc 85:120–158, 1987.

SECTION

28 Optic Nerve

310 ANKYLOSING SPONDYLITIS AND REITER'S DISEASE 720.0

James P. Dunn, Jr., MD
Baltimore, Maryland
Sanjay R. Kedhar, MD
Baltimore, Maryland

Ankylosing spondylitis (AS) and Reiter's disease are two of the seronegative spondyloarthropathies, disorders characterized by chronic inflammation of the peripheral and axial joints, familial occurrence, and extra-articular involvement of the skin, genitals, and eyes.

ETIOLOGY/INCIDENCE

AS usually affects young adults aged 16 to 40. Men are affected slightly more often than women and often have more severe involvement.

- Four to eight percent of the Caucasian US population is positive for HLA-B27. The prevalence is somewhat lower in other ethnic groups.
- There is a 2% cumulative lifetime incidence of uveitis in HLA-B27-positive patients. The mechanism by which HLA-B27 confers increased susceptibility to systemic and ocular disease is unclear. The HLA-B27 gene product may cross-react with foreign antigens ('molecular mimicry').
- Infection with *Chlamydia*, *Salmonella*, *Shigella*, *Yersinia*, *Ureaplasma urealyticum*, or *Campylobacter* spp. may trigger attacks of Reiter's disease.
- Uveitis develops in 20% to 40% of patients with AS and in approximately 25% of those with Reiter's disease.
- Of patients with HLA-B27-associated anterior uveitis, 24% to 69% have ankylosing spondylitis and 15% have Reiter's disease.
- In patients with systemic and ocular disease, the systemic disease is undiagnosed in more than 50% at the time of uveitis consultation; more than 80% of patients experience rheumatologic symptoms before the initial episode of uveitis.
- There is a 10-fold increased risk of AS and iridocyclitis in first-degree relatives who are positive for HLA-B27.

COURSE/PROGNOSIS

- The average attack of iridocyclitis in AS and Reiter's disease lasts about 6 weeks, with considerable variation.
- The prognosis depends on the number and severity of attacks of uveitis.
- Most clinicians believe that prompt, aggressive corticosteroid therapy for each attack reduces the risk of chronic uveitis and macular edema.

DIAGNOSIS

Clinical signs and symptoms

AS is characterized by chronic inflammation of the cartilaginous joints of the axial skeleton, including the sacroiliac joints, intervertebral spaces, and apophyseal and costovertebral articulations. Early symptoms include low back pain, which improves with activity. Fusion of the axial skeleton ('bamboo spine') can occur in untreated patients, causing marked impairment in mobility. The arthritis can also involve the shoulders, hips, knees, and feet; cervical arthropathy and heel pain (plantar fasciitis) are common symptoms. Extra-articular manifestations include cardiac conduction defects, aortic regurgitation, IgA nephropathy, amyloidosis, apical lobe fibrosis, and cauda equina syndrome. The classic ocular manifestation of AS is acute, unilateral, recurrent, nongranulomatous iridocyclitis, with attacks repeatedly affecting one eye or alternating between the eyes. Symptoms include pain, redness, and photophobia. Intervals between episodes can be months to years. After repeated attacks, chronic iridocyclitis can develop, more commonly in women. Scleritis is uncommon. Intraocular pressure at the time of an acute attack is usually normal or low (due to ciliary body dysfunction), but may increase with treatment as aqueous production normalizes and the hypertensive effects of corticosteroid therapy or peripheral anterior synechiae become manifest.

Reiter's disease consists of the triad of nongonococcal urethritis, asymmetric polyarticular arthritis of the large joints, and conjunctivitis or anterior uveitis. AS can occur in patients with Reiter's disease. Other characteristic features include keratoderma blennorrhagicum, a psoriatic skin disease, in approximately 25% of patients, and balanitis circinata. Fasciitis and tendonitis, often manifesting as heel pain, can occur. Reiter's disease is more common in men. Ocular manifestations of Reiter's disease include acute, recurrent, unilateral, nongranulomatous iridocyclitis; bilateral, mucopurulent conjunctivitis; and subepithelial or anterior stromal corneal infiltrates. As with AS-related iridocyclitis, intraocular pressure may be normal or low at the time of an acute attack but may increase with treatment.

Laboratory findings

- Laboratory values include a strong association with the histocompatibility antigen HLA-B27 and a negative rheumatoid factor and antinuclear antibody.
- AS is diagnosed with use of the modified New York criteria. Radiographic evidence of sacroiliac joint space narrowing and sclerosis is classic. Ninety percent of whites are positive for HLA-B27 compared with only 60% of blacks.
- Complete Reiter's disease is defined as the clinical triad noted above. Incomplete Reiter's disease is defined by the presence of peripheral joint disease or enthesopathy and uveitis without urethritis. Urethral culture to rule out gonorrhea or other infections is indicated in the presence of dysuria.

Differential diagnosis

- Post-traumatic uveitis.
- Herpetic iridocyclitis.
- Idiopathic acute anterior uveitis.
- HLA-B27-associated acute anterior uveitis without systemic disease.
- Syphilis.
- Sarcoidosis.
- Posner–Schlossman disease.

TREATMENT

Systemic

- Oral nonsteroidal anti-inflammatory drugs (NSAIDS) such as 25 to 50 mg indomethacin t.i.d. recommended; aspirin is usually not helpful.
- Urethritis in Reiter's disease should be treated with 250 to 500 mg tetracycline q.i.d., 100 mg doxycycline b.i.d., or 250 to 500 mg ciprofloxacin b.i.d. Children younger than 8 years should receive 40 mg/kg day erythromycin.
- Septic cases of *Salmonella*, *Shigella* and *Yersinia* spp. should be treated with 160 mg trimethoprim and 800 mg sulfamethoxazole b.i.d. or a fluoroquinolone such as 500 mg ciprofloxacin b.i.d. *Campylobacter* spp. infections should be treated with 500 mg ciprofloxacin b.i.d. or 250 to 500 mg erythromycin q.i.d. in adults or 40 mg/kg day erythromycin in children.
- Several uncontrolled studies have suggested sulfasalazine may reduce the frequency of uveitis flares in patients with AS. The initial dose of 500 mg/d should be increased by 500 mg/d at weekly intervals to a dosage of 1 g b.i.d. Up to 1.5 g b.i.d. may be used to control flares of inflammation.
- Tumor necrosis factor (TNF) antagonists such as infliximab may be effective for treatment of acute and refractory cases of HLA-B27 associated uveitis. Dosages and intervals between infusions vary between studies. Small series suggested efficacy of acute, anterior uveitis with single doses of infliximab 10 mg/kg or three doses of 3 mg/kg. Results of etanercept therapy for uveitis have been mixed.
- Successful systemic therapy does not reduce the incidence or severity of ocular disease.

Ocular

- Topical corticosteroids (e.g. 1% prednisolone acetate) are administered every 1 to 2 hours initially until the uveitis is quiet and then tapered and discontinued. A loading dose of the corticosteroid drops given every minute for five minutes at bedtime and on awakening may be helpful early in treatment.
- Cycloplegic agents (e.g. 1% atropine, 1% cyclopentolate, or 0.25% scopolamine) given b.i.d. to q.i.d. are useful in reducing pain and photophobia, as well as the risk of posterior synechiae.
- Periocular corticosteroid injections (e.g. 40 mg triamcinolone acetonide) or oral corticosteroids (e.g. 1 mg/kg prednisone) may be necessary in severe cases.
- The keratitis in Reiter's disease responds to a mild corticosteroid such as 0.1% fluorometholone q.i.d.
- Topical NSAIDS are not effective in treating uveitis.

Surgical

- Cataract surgery should be deferred until the uveitis has been quiet for at least 3 months.
- Posterior chamber intraocular lenses can usually be placed; capsular fixation is recommended.
- Surgery may precipitate an attack of uveitis. Oral corticosteroids are usually not recommended post-operatively, but a more aggressive use of topical corticosteroids can be helpful.

Other

- Physical therapy is used to maintain chest expansion, spinal mobility and range of motion.

COMPLICATIONS

- Factors affecting complications include the number of recurrences and the promptness of therapy.
- Final visual acuity can be 20/60 or less in 6% of patients and 20/200 or less in 3% of patients.
- Common complications include cataract, posterior synechiae, secondary glaucoma, and cystoid macular edema. Glaucoma and cataracts also are potential complications of corticosteroid therapy.
- Hypopyon uveitis occurs in 9% to 14% of patients with HLA-B27-positive uveitis.
- In one study, posterior segment disease (vitritis, papillitis, retinal vasculopathy, or pars plana exudates) occurred in 17% of patients with HLA-B27-associated uveitis.

REFERENCES

El-Shabrawi Y, Hermann J: Anti-tumor necrosis factor-alpha therapy with infliximab as an alternative to corticosteroids in the treatment of human leukocyte antigen B-27 associated anterior uveitis. Ophthalmology 109:2342–2346, 2002.

Jimenez-Balderas FJ, Mintz G: Ankylosing spondylitis: clinical course in women and men. J Rheumatol 20:2069–2072, 1993.

Lee DA, Barker SM, Su WP, et al: The clinical diagnosis of Reiter's syndrome. Ophthalmic and non-ophthalmic aspects. Ophthalmology 93:350–356, 1986.

Monnet D, Breban M, Hudry C, et al: Ophthalmic findings and frequency of extraocular manifestations in patients with HLA-B27 uveitis: a study of 175 patients. Ophthalmology 111:802–809, 2004.

Rodriguez A, Akova YA, Pedroza-Seres M, Foster CS: Posterior segment ocular manifestations in patients with HLA-B27-associated uveitis. Ophthalmology 101:1267–1274, 1994.

311 COMPRESSIVE OPTIC NEUROPATHIES 377.49

Julie Falardeau, MD, FRCSC
Portland, Oregon
Terry D. Wood, MD
Burlington, Vermont

Compressive optic neuropathies are diseases of the optic nerve that lead to visual loss secondary to pressure on the optic nerve, either within the orbit, inside the optic canal or intracranially.

ETIOLOGY

Compressive optic neuropathies can occur secondary to intrinsic optic nerve sheath meningioma, optic nerve glioma or masses extrinsic to the intracranial or intraorbital optic nerve. Orbital masses include cavernous hemangioma, lymphangioma, schwannoma, neurofibroma, mucocele, and malignancies such as lymphoma, metastases, multiple myeloma, sarcoma, rhabdomyosarcoma, neuroblastoma, and invasive sinus tumors. Thyroid ophthalmopathy and inflammatory disorders such as idiopathic orbital inflammatory syndrome can result in compressive optic neuropathies secondary to enlarged extraocular muscles, compromising the optic nerve at the orbital apex. Metastatic prostate carcinoma, fibrous dysplasia, Paget's disease of bone, osteopetrosis, and the hyperostoses associated with meningiomas affect the intracanalicular optic nerve. Intracranially, the optic nerve may be compressed by vascular lesions (e.g. aneurysm, dolichoectatic carotid arteries) and tumors. Intracranial tumors that affect the optic nerve include meningioma, pituitary adenoma, craniopharyngioma, metastatic tumors, and invasive sinus and nasopharyngeal carcinomas.

COURSE/PROGNOSIS

Compressive optic neuropathies usually manifest as slowly progressive visual loss. Rapid growth or acute hemorrhage into an intraorbital or intracranial tumor may present with acute visual loss and mimic an acute optic neuropathy. The prognosis is highly variable and depends on the etiology and duration of the compression.

DIAGNOSIS

Laboratory findings

Computed tomography with contrast enhancement and magnetic resonance imaging with gadolinium enhancement and fat suppression techniques are essential for diagnosis and appropriate treatment. Orbital ultrasonography can also provide useful information.

Differential diagnosis

- Ischemic optic neuropathy (arteritic or non-arteritic).
- Inflammatory optic neuropathy.
- Normal tension glaucoma.
- Demyelination.
- Traumatic optic neuropathy.
- Auto-immune optic neuropathy.
- Metabolic optic neuropathy.
- Toxic optic neuropathy.
- Congenital/hereditary optic neuropathy.

PROPHYLAXIS

- Patients with orbital inflammatory disease may require prolonged tapering of steroids to prevent relapses.

TREATMENT

Systemic corticosteroids, surgical excision, debulking, radiation therapy, and chemotherapy are used to treat compressive optic neuropathies.

Systemic

- Oral or intravenous corticosteroids can be used in thyroid-associated compressive optic neuropathy. This treatment is usually combined with an orbital decompression.
- Orbital inflammatory diseases are usually rapidly responsive to systemic corticosteroids. Steroid-sparing immunosuppressive treatment or radiation therapy should be considered for patients with significant steroid complications or in refractory cases.

Ocular

- Radiation therapy (15–20 Gy) to the extraocular muscles can be considered in cases of dysthyroid optic neuropathy; it is especially useful in refractory cases.
- Radiation therapy (50–55 Gy) is the best treatment available for patients with optic nerve sheath meningioma and documented progressive vision loss.

Surgical

- The location of a mass and its radiographic appearance are essential in determining whether the mass will be excised entirely, undergo biopsy, or be debulked.
- Encapsulated orbital masses may be removed entirely. Irregular orbital masses may undergo biopsy, be debulked, and be treated with chemotherapy or radiation therapy.
- Optic nerve sheath meningiomas are difficult to excise without visual loss. Portions of the tumor can be removed in a blind, uncomfortable eye. Intracranial extension can be approached surgically although radiation might be more beneficial.
- When there is optic canal compression by a meningioma, fibrous dysplasia, or metastatic prostate carcinomas, the optic canal can be decompressed extracranially through an external ethmoidectomy.
- The same approach can be used for dysthyroid optic neuropathy. The decompression is completed at the annulus of the optic canal because compression is occurring at the orbital apex. Combined approaches using endoscopic decompression of the medial wall and orbital apex and subciliary approaches to the orbital floor usually provide adequate decompression.
- Compressive optic neuropathies secondary to an intracranial lesion require surgical excision by a neurosurgeon via a transsphenoidal approach or through a craniotomy.

COMPLICATIONS

All orbital surgeries are fraught with the possibility of iatrogenic damage to the optic nerve. The surgical field must have complete hemostasis at the conclusion of the operation. Bleeding into the closed orbital space can also cause a compressive optic neuropathy. Significant swelling occurs after any orbital surgery. Patients routinely receive high dose systemic corticosteroids (oral or intravenous) during the perioperative period to decrease orbital swelling.

Extracranial optic canal decompression can be complicated by meningitis, cerebrospinal fluid leaks, pneumocephalus, sinusitis, esotropia, and symptomatic diplopia. The most feared complication is carotid bleeding. If attention is paid to the anatomic landmarks in the sphenoid sinus, the internal carotid artery may be avoided.

COMMENTS

Compressive optic neuropathies should be suspected in any patient with progressive vision loss associated with a relative afferent pupillary defect or with a relative afferent pupillary defect and proptosis, injection, or ophthalmoplegia. These patients require a complete evaluation including visual acuity, color vision, pupillary assessment, ocular motility evaluation, and visual field testing. Careful attention must be paid to the visual field of the contralateral eye for superotemporal quadrant field defects that are suggestive of a junctional scotoma and an anterior chiasmal mass. The optic nerve head may have a normal appearance or demonstrate atrophy, edema, shunt vessels, and large cupping. Patients may or may not have ophthalmoplegia, injection, chemosis, strabismus, proptosis, pain, resistance to retropulsion, bruits, and periorbital changes.

If patients are suspected of having a compressive optic neuropathy, they must undergo a neuroimaging study of the brain and orbits. Magnetic resonance imaging with gadolinium enhancement and fat suppression is the modality of choice.

After treatment, all patients with compressive optic neuropathy should be followed with sequential tests of visual acuity and perimetry. Afferent pupillary defects are best followed with neutral density filters.

REFERENCES

Goldberg RA, Steinsapir KD: Extracranial optic canal decompression: indications and technique. Ophthal Plast Reconstr Surg 12:163–170, 1996.

Graham SM, Brown CL, Carter KD, et al: Medial and lateral orbital wall surgery for balanced decompression in thyroid eye disease. Laryngoscope 113:1206–1209, 2003.

Li KK, Lucarelli MJ, Bilyk JR, Joseph MP, et al: Optic nerve decompression for compressive neuropathy secondary to neoplasia. Arch Otolaryngol Head Neck Surg 123:425–429, 1997.

Saeed P, Rootman J, Nugent RA, et al: Optic nerve sheath meningioma. Ophthalmology 110:2019–2030, 2003.

Schaefer SD, Soliemanzadeh P, Della Rocca DA, et al: Endoscopic and transconjunctival orbital decompression for thyroid-related orbital apex compression. Laryngoscope 113:508–513, 2003.

Turbin RE, Thompson CR, Kennerdell JS, et al: A long-term visual outcome comparison in patients with optic nerve sheath meningioma managed with observation, surgery, radiotherapy, or surgery and radiotherapy. Ophthalmology 109:890–899, discussion 899–900, 2002.

312 CONGENITAL PIT OF THE OPTIC DISC 377.4

Fion D. Bremner BSc, MBBS, PhD, FRCOphth
London, England

ETIOLOGY/INCIDENCE

Congenital pits in the optic nerve head are developmental anomalies found in 1 : 11,000 of the normal population (males = females). They are usually single, unilateral (85%) and occur most commonly in the temporal sector of larger than normal discs. Light microscopy shows herniation of dysplastic retinal tissue through a defect in the lamina cribrosa. There are no associations with other developmental anomalies, although cilioretinal arteries are present in over 50% of cases. Autosomal dominant inheritance has been described, but most cases are sporadic and the underlying genetic defect and pathogenesis are unknown.

COURSE/PROGNOSIS

Many optic pits remain asymptomatic throughout life. However, 25–75% of patients with this condition present in the third to fourth decades of life with visual loss due to serous detachment of the macula. The source of the fluid is unknown. The precipitant is probably vitreous traction, and the risk is greatest if the pit is temporal. Spontaneous anatomical reattachment occurs in 25% of cases but visual function often remains subnormal.

DIAGNOSIS

Visual acuity is usually unaffected in patients with uncomplicated optic pits, but threshold perimetry may reveal nonprogressive visual field defects, particularly arcuate scotomata. Maculopathy causes central blurring and metamorphopsia, with a drop in acuity to 6/9–6/60; there is serous elevation of the retina extending from the optic pit to the fovea, sometimes accompanied by a partial thickness macular hole (Figure 312.1). On fluorescein angiography pits show early hypofluorescence and late hyperfluorescence (staining) without leakage of dye towards the macula. Ocular coherence tomography (OCT) confirms that the fluid is mainly within a schitic cavity, accumulating under the retina only after formation of an outer leaf hole under the fovea. Rarely, an inner leaf cyst progresses to a hole and rhegmatogenous retinal detachment.

Differential diagnosis

Of pit:

- Disc coloboma;
- Glaucomatous excavation (especially normal tension glaucoma).

Of maculopathy:

- Central serous retinopathy (CSR).

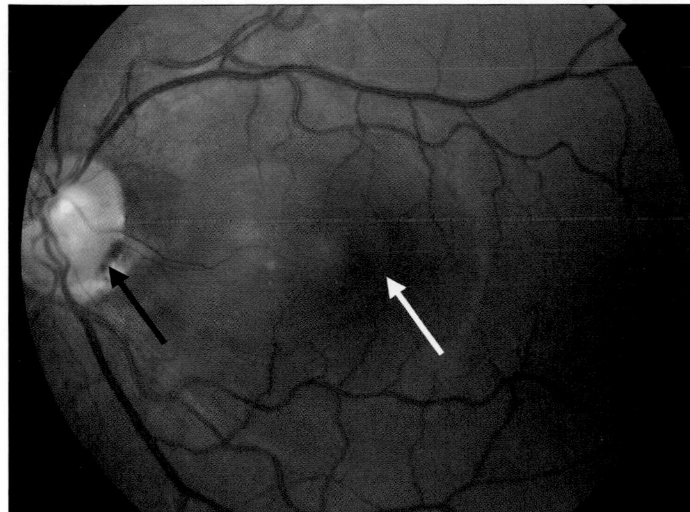

FIGURE 312.1. Congenital optic disc pit (black arrow) with serous detachment of the macula (white arrow).

TREATMENT

Uncomplicated optic pits require no treatment although prophylaxis against maculopathy has been suggested. Various measures have been tried to restore vision in patients with associated maculopathy.

Laser

Linear photocoagulation between pit and macula (to 'wall off' the subretinal fluid and prevent extension under the fovea) used to be the standard treatment but proved ineffective, probably because the fluid is mainly within a schitic cavity and not subretinal.

Surgical

Two approaches have been described, vitrectomy with gas tamponade and macular buckling. Both procedures have produced good long-term outcomes in published series.

COMPLICATIONS

Of maculopathy:

- Intraschitic haemorrhage;
- Macular cyst;
- Macular hole;
- Rhegmatogenous detachment.

Of treatments:

- Rhegmatogenous detachment;
- Cataract;
- Glaucoma.

COMMENTS

Congenital optic pits are not uncommon but are frequently overlooked. Associated serous detachment of the macula is easily misdiagnosed as CSR unless the disc is also examined carefully. The distinction is clinically important since, unlike CSR, optic pit-associated maculopathy is rarely self-limiting and without surgical treatment carries a poor prognosis for spontaneous visual recovery.

REFERENCES

Kranenburg EW: Crater-like holes in the optic disc and central serous retinopathy. Arch Ophthalmol 64:912–924, 1960.

Lincoff H, Schiff W, Krivoy D, Ritch R: Optical coherence tomography of optic pit maculopathy. Am J Ophthalmol 122:264–266, 1996.

McDonald HR, Schatz H, Johnson RN: Treatment of retinal detachment associated with optic nerve pits. Int Ophthalmol Clin 32:35–42, 1992.

Sobol WM, Blodi CF, Folk JC, Weingeist: Long-term visual outcome in patients with optic nerve pit and serous retinal detachment of the macula. Ophthalmology 97(11):1539–1542, 1990.

Stefko ST, Campochiaro P, Wang P, et al: Dominant inheritance of optic pits. Am J Ophthalmol 124(1): 112–113, 1997.

313 DRUG-INDUCED OPTIC ATROPHY 377.34

Roberto Guerra, MD
Modena, Italy
Gian Maria Cavallini, MD
Modena, Italy

Drug-induced optic atrophy is a toxic optic neuropathy ranging from partially or totally reversible forms to irreversible blindness. The condition is usually bilateral. Visual acuity may range from 20/20 to light perception, with most patients showing a visual acuity in the range of 20/200 at the time of the first examination.

ETIOLOGY/INCIDENCE

Relatively little is known about the pathogenesis of drug-induced neuropathies, but clinical signs and symptoms and the results of optic nerve conduction studies indicate that most of these neuropathies are characterized by the selective symmetric involvement of maculopapillary axons, ganglion cells, or both.

Toxic optic neuropathies seem to be directly related to the dosage and duration of treatment.

Agents that may cause optic atrophy include amiodarone, barbiturates, carmustine, chloramphenicol, chloroquine, cisplatin, corticosteroids, 2′,3′-dideoxyinosine (ddI), digoxin, disulfiram, ergotamine, ethambutol, fluoroquinolones, heavy metal compounds, halogenated 8-hydroxyquinolines, hexachlorophene, hexamethonium, iodide compounds, isoniazid, lithium carbonate, methotrexate, metronidazole, monoamine oxidase inhibitors, nitrosoureas, oral contraceptives, penicillamine, perhexiline, phenothiazines, streptomycin, tamoxifen, tryparsamide and vincristine.

Optic atrophy has been associated with vigabatrin use. Cimetidine and linezolid-associated optic neuropathies as well sildenafil-associated nonarteritic anterior ischemic neuropathy have been reported.

Optic neuropathy has been reported as a rare complication with the use of several vaccines, including rabies; smallpox; trivalent measles, mumps, and rubella; diphtheria; and bacille Calmette–Guérin.

The cocaine-exposed newborn may have optic nerve abnormalities and delayed visual maturation.

Toxic optic neuropathies are uncommon. Several reports are anecdotal, and sometimes the role of the suspected drug may have been overlooked. A higher incidence of optic neuropathy is associated with antitubercular agents, chemotherapy; or both. Ethambutol-induced optic neuropathy is rare with daily doses not exceeding 25 mg/kg. Irreversible isoniazid-induced optic atrophy has been reported with daily doses ranging from 5 to 6 mg/kg after 30 to 45 days of treatment.

RISK FACTORS

- Renal or hepatic failure, diabetes, and arteriosclerosis may enhance the neuropathic effect of the drug.
- Optic atrophy is often associated with decreased intake of vitamins B_1, B_6, and B_{12}; folic acid; amino acids; and zinc.
- Nutritional deficiency is the underlying condition of tobacco-alcohol amblyopia.
- Dietary deficiencies appear to have had a major pathogenetic role in the 1991–1993 epidemic optic neuropathy in Cuba.

COURSE/PROGNOSIS

Prodromal symptoms are unusual and may include multicolored points of light, bright lines, or fluctuating shadows in the visual field.

Central vision loss is usually progressive, bilateral, and symmetric. Loss of vision is acute when associated with poisoning from methyl alcohol and Laurocerasus berries. The optic nerve may be involved alone or in conjunction with other parts of the eye, cornea, or retina or with the peripheral nervous system. The optic nerve head appearance ranges from normal to slightly edematous, edematous, pale, or atrophic. Cecocenral scotomata are a very common finding, whereas visual field constriction (tryparsamide) and fluctuating hemianopsic defects (ethambutol) are unusual. Dyschromatopsia of the red-green axis is prominent on the blue-yellow axis. Spontaneous central vision recovery usually occurs within several weeks of drug withdrawal, although not always. Visual loss after poisoning with methyl alcohol and cyanides can be irreversible.

DIAGNOSIS

A medical history of continued drug consumption is often prominent for diagnosis. Decreased vision, visual field defects, color vision deficits, abnormal contrast sensitivity testing, and abnormal visual evoked potential recordings are diagnostic but do not sharply differentiate drug-induced neuropathies from any other retrobulbar optic neuropathy pattern.

A progressive, gradual, and symmetric central vision loss, however, is the most common clinical finding in drug-induced neuropathy.

Nonarteritic anterior ischemic optic neuropathy should be differentiated by a sudden loss of vision, unilaterality (the second optic disk may be edematous without loss of vision), patient's age, and association with hypertension, diabetes, or both. Systemic symptoms of arteritic anterior ischemic optic neuropathy include giant cell arteritis, elevated sedimentation rate, and accelerated involvement of the second eye.

TREATMENT

Discontinuation of the suspected drug at the first sign of optic nerve dysfunction remains the most efficient treatment. To treat optic neuropathy secondary to ethambutol, isoniazid, penicillamine, or quinolines, 100 to 250 mg zinc sulfate PO b.i.d. may be given. Zinc does not seem to be of value if optic atrophy is advanced. When vision does not improve in 10 to 15 weeks after ethambutol discontinuation, the only apparently successful treatment reported is the parenteral administration of 40 mg hydroxycobalamine; this should be given for 10 to 28 weeks. Most patients treated in this manner usually recover full vision. Low serum levels of vitamin B_{12} and zinc have been found in patients with tobacco-alcohol amblyopia, and 20 mg/day hydroxycobalamine In for 4 weeks may be more effective than the usual 1-mg dose. Optic neuropathy induced by a ketogenic diet can be reversed by 50 mg/day thiamine PO for 6 to 12 weeks.

COMMENTS

Drug-induced neuropathies remain a challenging problem for diagnosis and therapy. The ophthalmologist should maintain a surveillance of patients who receive high-risk drugs. Visual evoked potentials may reveal a high percentage of subclinical optic neuropathies during treatment (ethambutol).

Zinc serum levels should be checked for all patients with optic neuropathies because a close correlation exists with the clinical course of the disease. Zinc is of little value except in tobacco-alcohol amblyopia. More controlled studies are needed despite the rarity of these toxic neuropathies.

Supplemental vitamins B and folic acid are useful to restore vision in a patient with poor nutritional status.

REFERENCES

Grant WM: Toxicology of the eye. 2nd edn. Springfield, CC Thomas, 1974.

Frisén L, Malmgren K: Characterization of vigabatrin-associated optic atrophy. Acta Ophthalmol Scand 81:466–473, 2003.

Guerra R, Casu L: Hydroxycobalamin for ethambutol-induced optic neuropathy. Lancet 2:1176, 1981.

Sa'adah MA, Al Salem M, Ali AS, et al: Cimetidine-associated optic neuropathy. Eur Neurol 42:23–26, 1999.

Ten Tusscher MPM, Jacobs PJC, Busch MJWM, et al: Bilateral anterior toxic optic neuropathy and the use of infliximab. BMJ 326:579, 2003.

314 INFLAMMATORY OPTIC NEUROPATHIES 315.28

Simon J. Hickman, MA, PhD, MBBChir, MRCP
Sheffield, England

The inflammatory optic neuropathies are a diverse group of disorders defined by the presence of inflammation of the optic nerve that is not due to the demyelinating optic neuritis usually associated with multiple sclerosis. Compared with demyelinating optic neuritis the inflammatory optic neuropathies are often more painful and the visual impairment is more severe.

They present often with bilateral, simultaneous or early sequential, eye involvement.

ETIOLOGY

The inflammatory optic neuropathies are listed in Table 314.1. These conditions are rare and are often clinical syndromes without pathological confirmation. There is likely to be considerable overlap between them. The inflammation may be confined to the optic nerves or be part of a generalized multi-system disorder.

COURSE/PROGNOSIS

These conditions are important to recognize and differentiate from demyelinating optic neuritis because, in most cases, spontaneous resolution of vision does not occur. Early high-dose corticosteroid or other immunosuppressive treatment is required to restore vision and then continued maintenance immunosuppression is usually needed to maintain vision whereas in demyelinating optic neuritis corticosteroids merely speed-up recovery without affecting prognosis (Table 314.1).

TABLE 314.1 – The inflammatory optic neuropathies

Condition	Usual Clinical Features	Investigations	Treatment
Autoimmune optic neuritis	Usually bilateral, severe, progressive visual impairment Positive ANA No systemic vasculitis	Contrast-enhanced MRI orbits and brain CSF examination ANA	Corticosteroids Azathioprine Cyclophosphamide Chlorambucil
Behçet's disease	Bilateral, simultaneous or sequential, visual impairment Recurrent oral ulceration and two of: recurrent genital ulceration; uveitis; retinal vasculitis; erythema nodosum; pseudofolliculitis; papulopustular eruption; acneiform nodules or positive pathergy test	Contrast- enhanced MRI orbits and brain CSF examination Pathergy test Biopsy of ulcerated lesion	Corticosteroids Ciclosporin
Chronic relapsing inflammatory optic neuropathy (CRION)	Bilateral, simultaneous or sequential, visual impairment No evidence for sarcoidosis or vasculitis on investigation Corticosteroid responsive with relapses on withdrawal of treatment	Contrast-enhanced MRI orbits and brain CSF examination Serum + CSF ACE ANA Chest radiograph ^{67}Gallium scan	Corticosteroids Azathioprine Methotrexate
Neuromyelitis optica (NMO)—Devic's disease	Bilateral, simultaneous or sequential, visual impairment Transverse myelitis extending over several vertebral segments Monophasic or relapsing course	Contrast-enhanced MRI orbits, brain and spinal cord CSF examination Serum NMO-IgG	Corticosteroids Plasma exchange Azathioprine Rituximab
Neuroretinitis	Swollen optic disc with macular star Macular star Spontaneous recovery usual although relapsing, corticosteroid-dependent cases reported	*Bartonella*, *Borrelia*, syphilis, and Toxoplasma serology	Corticosteroids Azathioprine Appropriate antibiotics
Optic peri-neuritis	Arcuate or paracentral scotomata often with spared central vision Circumferential optic nerve sheath enhancement on MRI	Contrast-enhanced MRI orbits and brain CSF examination	Corticosteroids Azathioprine
Post-infectious Post-immunization Acute disseminated encephalomyelitis	Bilateral and simultaneous optic neuropathy Often in childhood Usually excellent prognosis	Contrast-enhanced MRI orbits and brain CSF examination	Corticosteroids
Sarcoidosis	Bilateral, simultaneous or sequential, visual impairment Isolated optic neuropathy or as part of generalized sarcoidosis More common in African, Afro-Caribbean or African-American populations	Contrast-enhanced MRI orbits and brain CSF examination Serum + CSF ACE Chest radiograph ^{67}Gallium scan Biopsy of an involved organ	Corticosteroids Methotrexate Infliximab
Systemic lupus erythematosus	Bilateral and severe simultaneous visual impairment in a patient with known SLE or with systemic features of the disease	Contrast-enhanced MRI orbits and brain CSF examination ANA	Corticosteroids Cyclophosphamide

ACE = angiotensin converting enzyme, ANA = anti-nuclear antibody, CSF = cerebrospinal fluid, MRI = magnetic resonance imaging.

DIAGNOSIS

Clinical signs and symptoms (see Table 315.1)

These conditions present as acute optic neuropathies but unlike demyelinating optic neuritis they are more often bilateral and can be more painful. Optic disc swelling, often with haemorrhage and a cellular infiltrate of the vitreous, is usually present and other signs of a systemic vasculitis or multi-system inflammatory disorder may be seen. Spontaneous improvement in vision does not occur or vision may worsen after a standard treatment course of corticosteroids.

Laboratory findings (see Table 315.1)

All patients should have gadolinium-enhanced orbital and brain magnetic resonance imaging (MRI) which will rule out a compressive lesion and may show optic nerve sheath or meningeal enhancement consistent with sarcoidosis. The brain imaging should be reviewed for asymptomatic lesions consistent with demyelination which may help to differentiate demyelinating optic neuritis from the other inflammatory optic neuropathies where lesions would not be expected. Spinal cord MRI should be performed if neuromyelitis optica is suspected. Genetic testing for Leber's mutation may be helpful in appropriate patients. Serological and other tests to investigate for the presence of sarcoidosis or a systemic vasculitis should be performed. A positive antinuclear antibody test may, however, be seen in up to 3% of patients with typical demyelinating optic neuritis.

An infectious cause, such as syphilis, Lyme disease, HIV, or tuberculosis should be excluded in appropriate patients. A cerebrospinal fluid examination is very useful in identifying infections, particularly if there is hypercellularity. The protein level is usually raised in the inflammatory optic neuropathies. There may be no oligoclonal bands or matched oligoclonal bands in both CSF and serum indicating systemic production of immunoglobulins. In demyelinating optic neuritis there may be no oligoclonal bands of immunoglobulins, or intrathecal synthesis of immunoglobulins (unmatched bands compared with serum).

Differential diagnosis

- Demyelinating optic neuritis.
- Compressive optic neuropathy.
- Infectious optic neuropathy.
- Anterior ischemic optic neuropathy.
- Leber's hereditary optic neuropathy.
- Toxic optic neuropathy.
- Nutritional optic neuropathy.

PROPHYLAXIS

Prolonged immunosuppression is usually required to prevent relapses.

TREATMENT (see Table 315.1)

These conditions are rare and in most cases randomized trials of treatment have not been performed. Treatment advice is therefore based on Class III evidence. Systemic medical treatment is required in most cases.

Treatment of a suspected inflammatory optic neuropathy should be with 1g/day intravenous methylprednisolone for 3 days followed by 1 mg/kg/day of oral prednisolone. This should be tapered at 10 mg/month after symptoms have improved and an alternate-day regimen considered. When 20 mg/day equivalent is reached then the withdrawal should be more made more slowly. If a relapse occurs on reducing the dose then high-dose prednisolone should be re-instigated, or a pulse of intravenous methylprednisolone given in severe cases, and a corticosteroid-sparing agent such as azathioprine, methotrexate or ciclosporin started before reducing the prednisolone dose again. Gastric protection and measures to try to prevent corticosteroid-induced osteoporosis need to be employed, according to local guidelines.

The specific treatment of some of the inflammatory optic neuropathies, according to the evidence that is available, is considered below.

Autoimmune and vasculitic optic neuritis

In optic neuritis associated with vasculitis (e.g. in systemic lupus eythematosus) the early addition of intravenous cyclophosphamide has been reported to be of benefit in some cases to restore vision.

Behçet's disease

Optic neuropathy is rare in Behçet's disease and is often seen in combination with retinal vasculitis. Treatment should commence with intravenous methylprednisolone followed by a tapering dose of prednisolone as described above, with the early addition of ciclosporin in treatment-resistant cases.

Neuromyelitis optica

The initial treatment of neuromyelitis optica should be as outlined above with early addition of azathioprine in most cases. Where there is a poor initial response to treatment then plasma exchange should be performed as there is evidence of humeral factors being involved in the pathogenesis of the condition and Class I trial evidence supporting this line of therapy. Rituximal may be useful for maintenance therapy in refractory cases.

Neuroretinitis

The visual loss in neuroretinitis usually recovers spontaneously and the disease does not usually recur. In a subgroup of patients, vision is not recovered without corticosteroids; long-term immunosuppression with azathioprine is required to prevent relapses. If an underlying infectious cause is found then treatment with appropriate antibiotic medication may hasten visual recovery.

Sarcoidosis

The addition of weekly methotrexate to oral prednisolone has been reported to both improve vision and reduce the corticosteroid-dose requirement in sarcoid-associated optic neuropathy. In a refractory case, infliximab may be considered.

COMPLICATIONS

Corticosteroids

In the short term, high-dose corticosteroids can cause insomnia, mild mood changes, stomach upsets, facial flushing, acne, edema and weight gain. Serious side effects reported following their use include psychosis, acute pancreatitis, avascular necrosis of the femoral head and deaths in two children from chicken pox. In the long term corticosteroids can precipitate hypertension, diabetes mellitus, cataracts and osteoporosis. Measures to try to prevent the development of osteoporosis should be undertaken according to local guidelines.

Immunosuppressant agents

By definition, use of immunosuppressant drugs can result in agranulocytosis and risk of infections, including those caused by atypical organisms. In addition: intravenous cyclophosphamide can cause nausea and vomiting, alopecia and haemorrhagic cystitis; azathioprine and methotrexate can cause liver impairment and ciclosporin is nephrotoxic. Long-term immunosuppression is associated with an increased risk of malignancies.

COMMENTS

A patient with an inflammatory optic neuropathy needs to be rapidly diagnosed because early treatment with high-dose corticosteroids and sometimes additional immunosuppressant agents are required for visual recovery, usually followed by long-term maintenance therapy to maintain vision.

SUPPORT GROUPS

National Organization for Rare Disorders, 55 Kenosia Avenue, PO Box 1968, Danbury, CT 06813-1968, USA.

www.rarediseases.org

REFERENCES

Chavis PS, Antonios SR, Tabbara KF: Cyclosporine effects on optic nerve and retinal vasculitis in Behcet's disease. Doc Ophthalmol 80:133–142, 1992.

Hickman SJ, Dalton CM, Miller DH, et al: Management of acute optic neuritis. Lancet 360:1953–1962, 2002.

Kidd D, Burton B, Plant GT, et al: Chronic relapsing inflammatory optic neuropathy (CRION): A newly recognised steroid responsive syndrome seemingly distinct from sarcoidosis. Brain 126:276–284, 2003.

Maust HA, Foroozan R, Sergott RC, et al: Use of methotrexate in sarcoid-associated optic neuropathy. Ophthalmology 110:559–563, 2003.

Myers TD, Smith JR, Wertheim MS, et al: Use of corticosteroid sparing systemic immunosuppression for treatment of corticosteroid dependent optic neuritis not associated with demyelinating disease. Br J Ophthalmol 88:673–680, 2004.

315 ISCHEMIC OPTIC NEUROPATHIES 377.41

Alfredo A. Sadun, MD, PhD
Los Angeles, California

Ischemic optic neuropathies are not rare. A variety of unusual vasculitities and other forms of vascular compromise that affect other organ systems can also produce an ischemic optic neuropathy. For example, posterior ischemic optic neuropathy is a rare result of shock usually from injury or surgery in combination with a compartment syndrome.

However, there are two causes of ischemia that have a particular predilection for the optic nerve head. Arteritic and nonarteritic anterior ischemic optic neuropathy both manifest as sudden visual loss associated with optic disc edema. Making an immediate distinction is critical to prudent management.

Arteritic anterior ischemic optic neuropathy (AAION): giant cell arteritis (GCA) or temporal arteritis

Arteritic anterior ischemic optic neuropathy is a true neuro-ophthalmic emergency and often a devastating condition. The loss of vision is very severe, often at perception of hand motions or worse and, if not treated immediately, this loss often progresses to become bilateral. Treatment is no longer effective once optic disc edema and visual loss has occurred.

Patients may be as young as 55 years, but much more commonly are past their seventh decade of life. Patients may present with loss of vision as their first symptom of GCA. However, patients may have a prodromal course of visual and systemic symptoms including amaurosis fugax, diplopia, general malaise, headache, low-grade fever, weight loss, arthralgias, and myalgias. The most specific symptom of GCA is probably jaw claudication.

Once the diagnosis is made, treatment with systemic corticosteroids is usually required for 12 to 24 months; however, some patients with GCA may require corticosteroids for many years.

AAION is the most frequent ophthalmological manifestation of GCA. However, some patients may present with central retinal artery occlusions or ophthalmoplegia that manifests as double vision from ischemia to the extraocular muscles.

ETIOLOGY/INCIDENCE

- GCA is an idiopathic autoimmune occlusive vasculitis.
- Histopathologic examination of the temporal arteries and orbital vasculature reveals a round cell (epitheliod) infiltration with destruction of the internal elastic lamina. The macrophage cellular infiltration often is accompanied by giant cell formation.
- GCA is a disease of the elderly; the youngest patient reported in the literature with an unequivocally positive temporal artery biopsy was 55 years old. The incidence of disease goes up about ten times per decade (starting at age 65, the incidence goes up ten times to 75 and 100 times to age 85).
- GCA is more common in white Americans than in black Americans and is particularly rare in Hispanics.

COURSE/PROGNOSIS

- GCA is a devastating disease, insofar as the AAION is very severe and recovery of vision extremely rare. Visual loss in the second eye is likely unless prompt therapy is instituted. This treatment is usually in the form of corticosteroids though methyltrexate and other cytotoxic therapies may be effective.

DIAGNOSIS

Laboratory findings

- The diagnosis of GCA must be suspected in all elderly patients with generalized constitutional complaints. This is particularly important if the patient complains of amaurosis fugax, diplopia, jaw claudication, or temporal headaches. Ischemic optic neuropathy with severe visual loss or a central retinal artery occlusion in a patient over 60 requires consideration of GCA.

- On presentation, blood tests to include a Westergren erythrocyte sedimentation rate (ESR) and C-reactive protein must be obtained. A CBC is also useful. The ESR is often near or above 100 in GCA. The algorithm of considering the ESR abnormal if more than half the patient's age plus 5 (for men) or 10 (for women) is only a general guideline.
- Cases of patients with GCA with normal sedimentation rates are well described, so a normal rate does not eliminate the diagnosis. The patient's clinical symptoms are the most important factor in establishing the diagnosis.
- Temporal artery biopsies are very useful to establish the diagnosis. The biopsies are best performed in the temporal region of the scalp. Even temporal artery biopsies are not completely definitive. Once again, the complete clinical picture of the patient's signs and symptoms drives the diagnosis.
- Findings of temporal artery biopsies should be interpreted by experienced pathologists.

Differential diagnosis

- The differential diagnosis of optic neuropathy due to GCA usually includes other entities that can produce optic nerve swelling and visual loss, including NAION, diabetic papillopathy, and compressive lesions of the optic nerve within the orbit.
- For central retinal artery occlusions, the differential diagnosis includes embolic events from the carotid arteries and the heart.
- Double vision from GCA often is associated with a deficit of abduction. However, in GCA, the diplopia may last only a few days, whereas in microvascular ischemic cranial mononeuropathies (often associated with diabetes or hypertension), the paralysis often persists for 8 to 12 weeks.

TREATMENT

- Once the diagnosis of GCA has been made, immediate treatment with systemic corticosteroids is essential. Some have advocated high-dose corticosteroids, especially when the visual loss has been recent, as there is a remote possibility of some recovery. After which, oral steroids are administered with a very slow taper that takes into account the serial ESR levels as well as the patient's symptoms.
- Other immunologically active medications, such as methyltrexate, cytoxan or immuran can be used to treat GCA especially in patients with diabetes or other issues that makes corticosteroid use more problematic.

COMPLICATIONS

- Patients with GCA should be followed in conjunction with an internal medicine specialist since systemic corticosteroids are associated with possible serious potentially life-threatening complications. The blindness association with GCA is permanent and hence many of the complications of corticosteroids have to be managed.
- One major advantage of obtaining a temporal artery biopsy is in anticipation of the dilemma later faced by the ophthalmologist and internist regarding the life-threatening complications of corticosteroid use.

The temporal artery biopsy is most easily read by the pathologist within 3 weeks of therapy, though more subtle histopathological changes can be determined even later. Hence, when there is a suspicion of GCA, the patient should have blood testing performed immediately, then begun on corticosteroids and then usually have the biopsy scheduled within the next week or two.

Non-arteritic ischemic optic neuropathy

Non-arteritic ischemic optic neuropathy (NAION or often just simply AION) is the second most common optic nerve disorder affecting adults, after primary chronic open-angle glaucoma. The incidence is up to 8000 new cases each year in the US. Typically the patient suffers from sudden painless severe and irreversible loss of vision in one eye. The patient is also at risk for a similar event occurring to the other eye and, given that there is no effective treatment, NAION is a devastating problem for patients and ophthalmologists alike. Most patients are in the vasculopathic age group (older than 50 years). The use of the term *non-arteritic* was adopted in large part to differentiate this condition from *arteritic ischemic optic neuropathy* (AAION), which is associated with giant cell arteritis (GCA) or temporal arteritis.

Recent studies have put into question the true natural history of the disease that was traditionally described as an abrupt loss of vision without improvement. However, the Ischemic Optic Neuropathy Decompression Trial (IONDT) has confirmed that modest improvements in vision often occur within a few months of onset.

ETIOLOGY

- NAION is hypoperfusion of the optic nerve head which is supplied by many small arterioles from the posterior artery circulation. That the etiology relates to compromised blood supply is supported by the increased incidence of NAION with vasculopathic risk factors such as diabetes and hypertension and with increasing age of the patients as well as from intravenous fluorescein angiography and orbital color Doppler imaging studies.
- Patients who present with NAION are usually 50–75 years old and have vasculopathic risk factors such as hypertension, diabetes mellitus, or atherosclerosis.
- Patients almost always have absent or very small cup-to-disc ratios (less than 0.3) in both the affected and unaffected eyes (the 'disc at risk'). The idea is that the crowded optic discs may suffer a compartment syndrome in connection with ischemia.
- There are those who believe that episodes of nocturnal hypotension may trigger NAION in susceptible patients.

PRESENTATION/COURSE/PROGNOSIS

- The patient presents with a sudden unilateral painless loss of vision often noted upon awakening. The clinical examination discloses mild to severe visual acuities, an afferent papillary defect and hyperemic optic disc edema with peripapillary hemorrhages.
- Most patients do not have any further progressive loss of vision; however, about 10% continued to deteriorate for 1 to 4 weeks.

- Patients with NAION, unlike AAION, do not have preceding episodes of amaurosis fugax or symptoms of temporal arteritis such as jaw claudication, fever, polymylagia, weight loss, or scalp tenderness.
- The natural history is classically described as non-improving and non-deteriorating. However, the IONDT report suggested a modest level of improvement in up to 40% of patients.
- Involvement of the second eye months or years later is not uncommon; studies have suggested rates up to 41%, though the IONDT suggests that 15% will go bilaterally blind.

DIAGNOSIS

NAION is diagnosed by a good clinical history of sudden and painless unilateral visual loss in the absence of the constitutional symptoms of GCA. The patient usually has some cardiovascular risk factors such as diabetes or hypertension. The examination generally reveals an unilateral optic neuropathy, an altitudinal visual field defect and unilateral disc edema with peripapillary hemorrhages. Furthermore, the contralateral asymptomatic eye will show a very small cup-to-disc ratio.

In the setting of a classic presentation of NAION, an MRI is not required; however, the patient may need evaluation for hypertension, diabetes mellitus, and anemia. In atypical presentations (or if the patient is a poor historian), neuroimaging should be performed.

TREATMENT

No effective treatment for NAION is available. The following modalities have been tried, but none have been proved beneficial:

- Anticoagulation;
- Systemic and retrobulbar corticosteroids;
- L-Dopa;
- Pentoxyfilline;
- Optic nerve sheath decompression;
- Hyperbaric oxygen.

REMARKABLE FEATURES OF NAION

- Most patients with NAION have vasculopathic risk factors such as diabetes, hypertension, or high serum cholesterol.
- Although NAION is a vasculopathic disorder, these patients do not have an increased incidence of myocardial infarction, cerebrovascular accident, or sudden death.
- The incidence of NAION peaks in the 60s. Most age related diseases (AAION, glaucoma, etc.) continue to increase in incidence with age.
- In 98% of cases, NAION occurs only once per eye.
- There is a 15–41% incidence of visual loss in the fellow eye.
- Visual loss may be preceded by posterior vitreous detachment in a small percentage of patients.
- Emboli are almost never seen, suggesting that the ischemia is usually due to watershed hypoperfusion.
- The branches of the central retinal artery just peripheral to the area of the disc edema and subsequent pallor often become focally attenuated and sheathed. Why such a response occurs in the retinal circulation is unknown, especially when the ciliary arteries are believed to be the primary site of difficulties.

DIFFERENTIATION BETWEEN AAION AND NAION

- Patients with GCA (AAION) are usually much older than patients with NAION.
- Patients with GCA generally have more severely affected visual acuity and visual field loss. NAION usually results in inferior or superior altitudinal visual field loss.
- Patients with GCA may have amaurosis fugax or double vision before a fixed visual deficit. NAION is not preceded by these symptoms.
- Patients with GCA are often systemically ill with headache, fever, malaise, weight loss, arthralgias, and myalgias. In particular, clinicians should be attentive to signs of jaw claudication. Patients with NAION are constitutionally well.
- Patients with NAION develop hyperemic optic disc edema with peripapillary hemorrhages. In contrast, in GCA there is pallid disc edema.
- Patients with NAION have a greatly increased incidence of a congenitally anomalous optic nerve in the contralateral asymptomatic eye. Detection of a contralateral optic nerve with a normal cup-to-disc ratio should raise the clinician's index of suspicion for GCA or another cause of the patient's visual loss instead of NAION.

REFERENCES

Albert DM, Searl SS, Craft L: Histologic and ultrastructural characteristics of temporal arteritis. Ophthalmology 89:1111–1126, 1982.

Arnold AC: Ischemic optic neuropathy, diabetic papillopathy, and papillophlebitis in Ophthalmology. 2nd edn. London, Yanoff & Duker 2003:1268–1274.

Hayreh SS, Podhajsky PA, Zimmerman B: Ocular manifestations of giant cell arteritis. Am J Ophthalmol 125:509–520, 1998.

Johnson LN, Arnold AC: Incidence of nonarteritic and arteritic anterior ischemic optic neuropathy: population-based study in the state of Missouri and Los Angeles County, California. J Neuroophthalmol 14:38–44, 1994.

The Ischemic Optic Neuropathy Decompression Trial Research Group: Optic nerve decompression surgery for nonarteritic anterior ischemic optic neuropathy is not effective and may be harmful. JAMA 273:625–632, 1995.

316 OPTIC NEURITIS 317.28

Simon J. Hickman, MA, PhD, MBBChir, MRCP

Sheffield, England

Optic neuritis is an inflammatory demyelinating condition of the optic nerve that usually presents as a sub-acute painful unilateral impairment of vision, although bilateral visual loss can occur.

ETIOLOGY/INCIDENCE

The incidence is 1–5 per 100,000/year. The age group principally affected is 20–49 years with females being more commonly affected. Most cases of optic neuritis are due to idiopathic inflammatory demyelination, which may occur in isolation, as a manifestation of multiple sclerosis (MS) or, rarely, as part of neuromyelitis optica. The causes of optic neuritis/MS are currently unknown. A genetic predisposition exists, as suggested by the epidemiology of the condition. Environmental factors, in particular exposure to viruses, are probably also important although, as yet, no reliable candidates have been identified. Childhood cases are seen, a higher proportion of which are bilateral with less of an association with MS.

COURSE/PROGNOSIS

The natural history of acute optic neuritis is for the pain to last for only a few days and the vision to deteriorate over a period of a few days to two weeks before spontaneously improving. Most patients show a good functional recovery. The visual acuity at one year was 20/40 or better in 95% of the placebo group of the Optic Neuritis Treatment Trial (ONTT) with a median visual acuity of 20/16. The cumulative probability of having recurrent optic neuritis after ten years' follow-up in the ONTT was 35% for either eye, although the overall visual prognosis was good with the median visual acuity being $20/16^{-2}$. The risk of MS developing at ten years in those who had clinically isolated optic neuritis on entry to the trial was 38%. The risk increased if asymptomatic brain lesions were seen on baseline magnetic resonance imaging (MRI). The risk of MS was 22% in those with no lesions and 56% when one or more lesions were present.

DIAGNOSIS

Clinical signs and symptoms

Optic neuritis usually presents as an acute unilateral impairment of vision with retro-ocular pain and pain on eye movement, although in about 10% of cases it is painless. The degree of visual loss varies from minor blurring to no perception of light in the affected eye. Decreased colour vision, a central or para-central scotoma and a relative afferent pupillary defect are also usually seen on examination. The optic disc may appear swollen but is often normal in appearance (Figure 316.1).

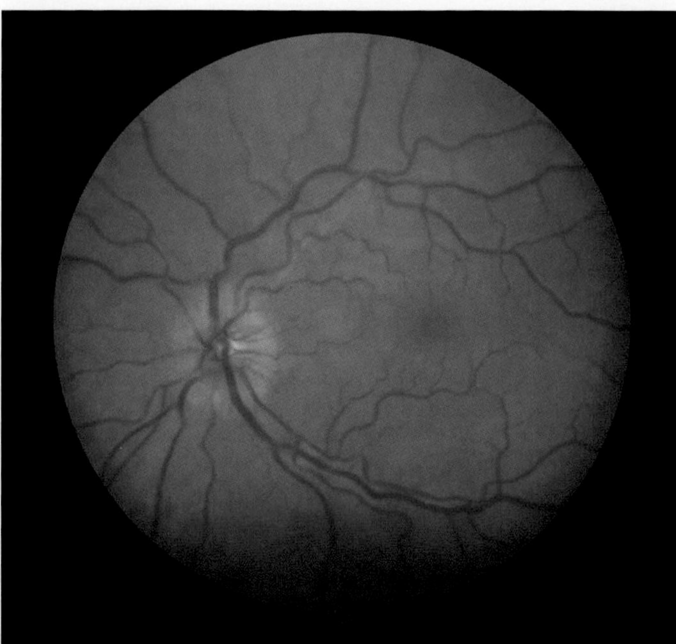

FIGURE 316.1. Typical swollen optic disc in a patient with acute optic neuritis.

Laboratory findings

In the main, optic neuritis is a clinical diagnosis and in typical cases further investigation is not essential in making the diagnosis. If any atypical features for optic neuritis lead to suspicion of an alternative diagnosis then prompt investigations are required.

Orbital MRI, particularly if gadolinium-enhanced, will usually demonstrate the symptomatic lesion. The principal use of MRI is to assess the brain for asymptomatic lesions which can help to define the risk for the future development of MS as described above. Visual evoked potentials (VEP) may not be helpful in differentiating between different causes of optic neuropathies in the acute phase, although the combination of VEP with a pattern electroretinogram may be useful in differentiating macular from optic nerve disorders. A cerebrospinal fluid (CSF) examination is useful when there is clinical doubt and an infectious or other inflammatory optic neuropathy needs to be excluded. Testing the CSF for oligoclonal bands may also help in counseling the patient about their risk for the development of MS.

Differential diagnosis

- Inflammatory corticosteroid-dependent optic neuropathy.
- Neuromyelitis optica.
- Compressive optic neuropathy.
- Infectious optic neuropathy.
- Anterior ischemic optic neuropathy.
- Leber's hereditary optic neuropathy.
- Toxic optic neuropathy.
- Nutritional optic neuropathy.
- Posterior scleritis.
- Central serous retinopathy.
- Acute zonal occult outer retinopathy (AZOOR).
- Big blind spot syndrome.

PROPHYLAXIS

The β-interferons can be used to delay the onset of MS and, thereby possibly, prevent further relapses of optic neuritis.

TREATMENT

Systemic medical treatment may be used.

Corticosteroids

High-dose parenteral corticosteroids speed up visual recovery in acute optic neuritis but do not affect long-term outcome. Intravenous methylprednisolone (IVMP) is usually administered in a dose of 1 g/day for three days, which may be followed by oral prednisolone 1 mg/kg/day for 11 days and a short dose-taper.

A meta-analysis showed that steroids reduced the number of patients without clinical improvement at 30 days (odds ratio 0.60, range 0.42–0.85) but did not cause long-term improvement in disability (odds ratio 0.96, range 0.71–1.31). The ONTT randomized patients to receive IVMP, oral prednisolone, or placebo. The benefit of IVMP in speeding up visual recovery was greatest between days four to 15 but the treatment advantage declined such that by one year no treatment benefit was seen. When the presenting visual acuity was 20/40 or better then IVMP conferred no benefit, even during the initial stages of recovery. Oral prednisolone produced no significant improvements in the rate of recovery and its use was associated with a persistent increased risk of recurrence of optic neuritis compared with IVMP or placebo.

The use of IVMP seemed to decrease the risk of the development of MS in the ONTT after two years in those patients with an abnormal brain MRI. However, the findings were based on a retrospective analysis with an open-label treatment (there was no intravenous placebo arm) with only small numbers developing MS. Also, 50 patients were lost to follow-up, which may have had a confounding effect. The apparent beneficial effect of IVMP was lost by 3 years and the use of IVMP did not affect the eventual development of neurological disability from MS.

The prognosis following childhood optic neuritis is generally excellent and in a case with mild visual impairment then the child may merely be observed. In a case with severe visual loss then three days of 15 mg/kg/day IVMP may help to improve vision, although trial data are lacking.

β-Interferons

Two recent trials have demonstrated that the β-interferons can slow down the progression to MS following an isolated demyelinating event. The CHAMPS study recruited 383 patients (192 with optic neuritis) who, in addition, had two or more clinically silent brain lesions on MRI and randomized them to receive once weekly 30 μg intramuscular interferon β-1a or placebo injections. The trial was stopped early after an interim analysis since the cumulative probability of the development of MS during the three-year follow-up period was significantly lower in the interferon group than in the placebo group (rate ratio 0.56; 95% CI 0.38–0.81; $p = 0.002$). There was also a relative reduction in new lesion activity on MRI in the interferon group ($p < 0.001$). In the ETOMS study, 309 patients (98 with optic neuritis) with four asymptomatic white matter lesions (or three if one was enhancing after administration of gadolinium) were randomized to receive once weekly subcutaneous 22 μg interferon β-1a or placebo injections. After two years the odds ratio for conversion to MS was 0.61 (95% CI 0.37–0.99; $p = 0.045$) in the treatment group compared with the placebo group, again with less new lesion formation in the treatment group ($p < 0.001$).

These results are consistent with previously reported trials of the β-interferons in relapsing-remitting MS suggesting that, in patients at high risk of developing MS, the β-interferons have reduced the relapse rate, but not necessarily the eventual occurrence of MS. Longer-term follow-up is needed to ascertain whether the development of persistent disability is delayed by early introduction of a β-interferon.

The absolute risk of developing MS after optic neuritis, even with asymptomatic brain lesions on MRI, is still relatively small and many physicians wait and re-image patients after an interval to see if new brain lesions have developed. This may then lead to a diagnosis of MS according to the McDonald criteria and a potentially greater absolute benefit of treatment with a β-interferon, although trial data to support this approach do not at present exist.

COMPLICATIONS

Corticosteroids are generally well-tolerated. Common minor adverse effects reported include insomnia, mild mood changes, stomach upsets, facial flushing, acne, edema and weight gain. However, serious side effects following their use have been reported including psychosis, acute pancreatitis, avascular necrosis of the femoral head and deaths in two children from chicken pox. The β-interferons have been particularly reported to cause influenza-like symptoms, depression and injection-site reactions, although serious adverse events are rare.

COMMENTS

Optic neuritis usually causes acute painful unilateral visual disturbance with most patients making good spontaneous recoveries. Parenteral corticosteroids can speed up the visual recovery but without affecting long-term visual prognosis; IVMP may delay the onset of MS, but this remains controversial. As significant side effects can occur with the use of high-dose corticosteroids, their use is not obligatory and an expectant approach is reasonable. The β-interferons are generally well tolerated and can delay the development of MS in patients after an isolated episode of optic neuritis if they have asymptomatic brain lesions on MRI. However, the effects on long-term development of disability are not known.

SUPPORT GROUPS

The National Multiple Sclerosis Society, 733 Third Avenue, New York, NY 10017, USA.

www.nationalmssociety.org

Multiple Sclerosis Society of Great Britain and Northern Ireland, MS National Centre, 372 Edgware Road, London, NW2 6ND, UK.

www.mssociety.org.uk

REFERENCES

Beck RW, Cleary PA, Anderson MM, Jr, et al: A randomized, controlled trial of corticosteroids in the treatment of acute optic neuritis. N Engl J Med 326,581–588, 1992.

Comi G, Filippi M, Barkhof F, et al: Effect of early interferon treatment on conversion to definite multiple sclerosis: a randomised study. Lancet 357:1576–1582, 2001.

Hickman SJ, Dalton CM, Miller DH, et al: Management of acute optic neuritis. Lancet 360:1953–1962, 2002.

Jacobs LD, Beck RW, Simon JH, et al: Intramuscular interferon beta-1a therapy initiated during a first demyelinating event in multiple sclerosis. N Engl J Med 343:898–904, 2000.

McDonald WI, Compston A, Edan G, et al: Recommended diagnostic criteria for multiple sclerosis: guidelines from the International Panel on the diagnosis of multiple sclerosis. Ann Neurol 50:121–127, 2001.

The Optic Neuritis Study Group: Visual function more than 10 years after optic neuritis: experience of the Optic Neuritis Treatment Trial. Am J Ophthalmol 137:77–83, 2004.

317 PAPILLEDEMA 377.00

Andrew W. Lawton, MD
Little Rock, Arkansas

ETIOLOGY/INCIDENCE

Papilledema is swelling of the optic discs due to increased intracranial pressure (ICP). A small percentage of patients with increased ICP in part of the subarachnoid system will have normal optic discs with spontaneous venous pulsations or a single elevated disc.

COURSE/PROGNOSIS

The early recognition of increased ICP is critical. Headaches may be the most intrusive sign of elevated ICP. Optic nerve destruction can occur, however, with devastating swiftness, even in those with few symptoms.

Causes of optic nerve damage include alteration of axoplasmic flow with interruption of the intracellular pumping process from the axon to the intraocular cell, venous stasis due to retardation of outflow through the central retinal vein, and interference with autoregulation of the central retinal artery circulation, evidenced by transient obscurations of vision. As nerve tissue is lost, the appearance of optic nerve swelling decreases until a heavily damaged optic nerve flattens out. A 4+ swollen disc may function normally while a non-edematous disc may be completely nonfunctional.

DIAGNOSIS

Clinical signs and symptoms

Patients may be unaware of visual loss despite permanent optic nerve damage. The initial visual change is enlargement of the blind spot on perimetry. In severe papilledema, encroachment of intraretinal fluid and exudates on the macula reduces central vision (Figure 317.1). The first true sign of compromise of optic nerve health is peripheral perimetric depression, particularly in the inferonasal region which may expand into arcuate bundle scotomas. Eventually, nerve fiber loss progresses until the papillomacular bundle suffers and central vision deteriorates.

Characteristic symptoms include holocranial headaches (worst on awakening) associated with neck and back pain, transient obscurations of vision, intermittent or constant diplopia, pulsatile tinnitus, and nausea with vomiting.

Initial findings on posterior segment examination include opacification of the peripapillary nerve fiber layer, venous dilation, and loss of retinal spontaneous venous pulsations. As the papilledema worsens, the optic disc develops peripheral elevation with preservation of the central cup. Hemorrhages may occur on the optic disc surface and peripapillary nerve fiber layer. The retina and choroid become distorted with the formation of Paton's lines. Chronic optic disc edema results in a haze of the anterior disc surface from gliosis, progressive optic disc pallor due to optic atrophy, and the development of pale areas (pseudo-drusen).

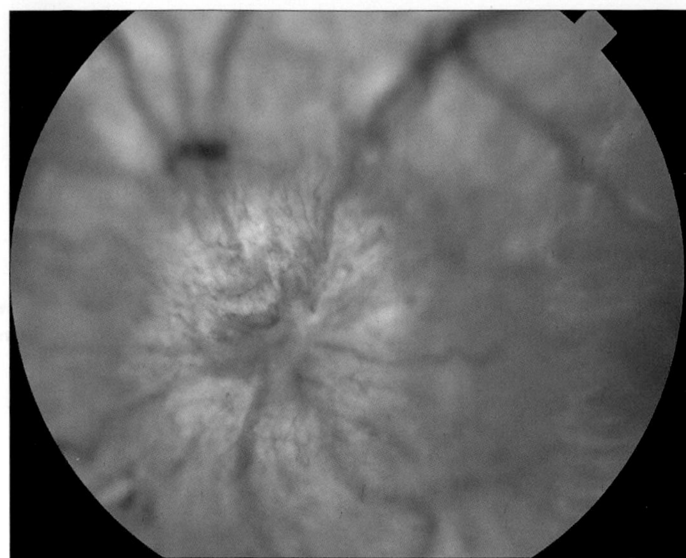

FIGURE 317.1. Papilledema.

Laboratory findings

The definition of 'elevated intracranial pressure' and the risk of injury are affected by fluctuations in ICP levels throughout the day. A pressure below 20 cm water is normal, over 25 cm abnormal, and between 20 cm water and 25 cm water potentially abnormal based on visual function. Serial lumbar punctures provide little assistance in patient care once IIH is diagnosed. In IIH, the CSF composition is normal.

Differential diagnosis

Idiopathic intracranial hypertension (IIH, pseudotumor cerebri) is elevation of intracranial pressure without a discernable etiology. Patients tend to be female, of childbearing age, and overweight. Neuro-imaging studies are normal but may show compressed ventricles. The brain shows both intracellular and extracellular edema. IIH is a diagnosis of exclusion: the MRI and the CSF composition must be normal.

Intracranial masses and hydrocephalus produce a papilledema with a higher likelihood of permanent visual loss. The mechanism underlying this process is different from that of IIH. Interruption of cerebrospinal fluid egress that can occur through infectious agents, subarachnoid hemorrhage, proteins secreted by tumors, and other intermediaries results in an extracellular accumulation of fluid. Without the counterbalancing effect of the intracellular edema present in IIH, the ventricular system and subarachnoid space expand. This imbalance puts stress on the lamina cribrosa and optic nerve vascular supply. Circadian fluctuation increases the impact by forcing the lamina cribrosa to move back and forth. External agents that may cause elevation of ICP include antibiotics (tetracycline derivatives, naladixic acid), vitamin A and its analogues, and corticosteroids. Medical conditions include severe iron deficiency anemia, sleep apnea, chronic renal disease with or without dialysis, pregnancy, arteriovenous fistulas, and dural sinus thrombosis.

TREATMENT

Systemic

The clinician should address any specific underlying cause. Discontinuation of offending medications, CPAP therapy and/

or surgery for sleep apnea, or tumor management may be successful. In the case of IIH, initiation of a supervised weight loss program may diminish the need for supportive therapy.

Patients with good central visual function, no edema in the macula, and visual field changes limited to enlargement of blind spot size can be watched. The clinician should conduct visual field tests on three visits, each 1 month apart. If function is stable or improves, future visits can be spaced further apart.

Medical

At the first evidence of optic nerve compromise, patients should receive systemic medical therapy. Acetazolamide decreases cerebrospinal fluid production and is the usual first choice. The standard initial daily dosage would be 1 gram divided in two to four doses per day. If visual function stabilizes or improves within a week, continue this dose. If optic nerve function deteriorates, one may increase the dosage by a gram daily up to 4 grams total per day. Once patients exceed a gram per day, however, the side effects of gastric upset, tingling in the hands and feet, and electrolyte imbalance result in sufficient patient discomfort to lead to poor compliance. Topiramate is a new carbonic anhydrase inhibitor that may be effective. Furosemide at 40 mg twice daily is a possible alternative to acetazolamide and topiramate with fewer systemic side effects. Both medications may result in bone marrow suppression; patients should be checked by complete blood count at regular intervals to look for anemia, leukopenia, and thrombocytopenia. Both medications may also cause problems for patients with sulfonamide allergies and may cause kidney stones.

Treatment with corticosteroids is controversial. Corticosteroids may lower ICP, but potentially dangerous rebound and further elevation of ICP may occur as corticosteroids are tapered. Corticosteroids may cause weight gain and thwart a supervised weight loss program.

Surgical

Lumboperitoneal shunting or ventriculoperitoneal shunting may result in rapid improvement in patients with both headaches and visual loss.

Optic nerve sheath decompression (ONSD) may be effective but the mechanism of its effect is unclear. It is often preferred in patients with visual loss but minimal headache complaints. Decompression of one optic nerve may relieve optic disc edema in the contralateral disc but this result is not guaranteed.

REFERENCES

Corbett JJ, Jacobson DM, Mauer RC, Thompson HS: Enlargement of the blind spot caused by papilledema. Am J Ophthalmol 105:261–265, 1988.

Friedman DI, Jacobson DM: Diagnostic criteria for idiopathic intracranial hypertension. Neurology 59:1492–1495, 2002.

Galvin JA, Van Stavern GP: Clinical characterization of idiopathic intracranial hypertension at the Detroit Medical Center. J Neurol Sci 223:157–160, 2004.

Jacobson EE, Johnston IH, McCluskey P: The effect of optic nerve sheath decompression on CSF dynamics in pseudotumor cerebri. J Clin Neurosci 6:375–377, 1999.

McGirt MJ, Woodworth G, Thomas G, et al: Cerebrospinal fluid shunt placement for pseudotumor cerebri-associated intractable headache: predictors of treatment response and an analysis of long-term outcomes. J Neurosurg 101:627–632, 2004.

318 TRAUMATIC OPTIC NEUROPATHY 377.49

Leonard A. Levin, MD, PhD

Montreal, Canada and Madison, Wisconsin

Traumatic optic neuropathy is diagnosed when there is clinical evidence of an optic neuropathy that is temporally related to head or ocular trauma in the absence of another etiology.

ETIOLOGY/INCIDENCE

Traumatic optic neuropathies are generally classified by location of injury (anterior or posterior) and type of injury (direct or indirect). Because the central retinal artery and vein enter and exit the optic nerve approximately 10 mm posterior to the globe, anterior injuries are usually associated with vascular changes in the retina. More posterior injuries do not cause acute fundus changes. Anterior direct optic nerve injuries result from penetrating ocular or orbital trauma that damages the anterior optic nerve, e.g. a knife wound that transects the optic nerve. Posterior direct optic nerve injuries result from penetrating orbital or cerebral trauma that damages the posterior optic nerve, e.g. a bullet that passes just anterior to the chiasm.

Indirect injuries are caused by forces transmitted at a distance from the optic nerve, e.g. blunt head trauma without penetration. Anterior indirect injuries are usually associated with sudden rotation of the globe from blunt trauma, such as falling and hitting the eye on the corner of a table. These commonly cause partial or total avulsion of the optic nerve, with associated bleeding and central retinal artery occlusion.

Posterior indirect optic nerve injuries result from blunt head trauma, usually transmitting a concussive force to the optic nerve and resulting in contusion or even transection. There may or may not be bone fracture(s).

The most common site of posterior indirect optic nerve injury is the optic canal; the intracranial optic nerve is the next most common site of injury. Posterior indirect injury is the most common cause of traumatic optic neuropathy. There may be little or no evidence of significant head trauma; a fall from a bicycle may suffice. In most cases there is multisystem trauma or significant brain injury.

Loss of consciousness occurs in 40 to 72% of patients with traumatic optic neuropathy. Motor vehicle and bicycle accidents are the most frequent causes of traumatic optic neuropathy, accounting for 17 to 63% of cases. Traumatic optic neuropathy may also be iatrogenic, especially after maxillofacial or endoscopic surgery, as a result of inadvertent direct injury to the optic nerve or transmitted force fracturing the optic canal.

Traumatic optic neuropathy in children is similar to that in adults.

COURSE/PROGNOSIS

The prognosis for recovery from optic nerve injuries depends in part on whether the injury is direct or indirect. Direct injuries tend to produce severe and immediate visual loss with little likelihood of recovery. Patients with indirect optic neuropathies may have spontaneous visual recovery, at variable times after injury. In some cases, visual loss only begins several hours to days after the injury. If this happens, the possibility of an intrasheath hemorrhage should be entertained, and neuroimaging repeated.

The severity of initial visual loss in patients with traumatic optic neuropathy varies dramatically from no light perception to better than 20/20 with only a visual field defect as functional evidence of disease. Patients with only light perception vision or with no light perception are less likely to improve, regardless of therapy, than are patients with vision better than light perception.

DIAGNOSIS

Clinical signs and symptoms

Injuries to the proximal portion of the optic nerve within 10 mm of the globe, anterior to where the central retinal artery enters and the central retinal vein leaves the nerve, produce a variety of disturbances that are immediately apparent in the ocular fundus, including an ophthalmoscopic picture of a central retinal or branch artery occlusion, central retinal vein occlusion, or anterior ischemic optic neuropathy. More posterior optic nerve injuries produce no immediate change in the appearance of the ocular fundus. Almost always the optic disk remains normal in appearance for at least 3 weeks and then becomes progressively paler.

Both anterior and posterior traumatic optic neuropathies are characterized by varying degrees of visual acuity loss, decreased color vision, and visual field defects. An afferent pupillary defect should be present in all cases of traumatic optic neuropathy unless there has been symmetric injury to both optic nerves. In unconscious patients, this sign is often the only clinical evidence for a posterior optic nerve injury. Occasionally there is injury to the chiasm, in which case there may be unilateral or bilateral temporal visual field defects respecting the vertical meridian. Chiasmal injury can be seen with posterior avulsion of the optic nerve, e.g. traumatic enucleation.

Laboratory findings

Neuroimaging, particularly computed tomography (CT) scanning, is important in the evaluation of a patient with traumatic optic neuropathy. CT scanning is clearly superior to magnetic resonance imaging (MRI) in delineating fractures of bone. MRI is better for imaging soft tissue, particularly the intracranial optic nerve and chiasm, and may be useful for delineating intrasheath hemorrhage or optic nerve transection within intact meninges. CT should be done with thin sections, and reconstructions performed.

From 20 to 50% of patients with posterior traumatic optic neuropathy have evidence of an optic canal fracture by neuroimaging. Even in the absence of a fracture, blood in the sphenoid sinus should raise suspicion for optic nerve injury. MRI should be performed only after a metallic intracranial, intraorbital, or intraocular foreign body has been ruled out by CT scanning or conventional radiography.

Patients with large fractures involving the optic canal are also at risk for carotid-cavernous fistulas, and may need CT angiography.

TREATMENT

Medical

Respiratory and cardiovascular resuscitation and stabilization are the first priorities in all cases of trauma, regardless of the severity of ocular injury; thus, care of the patient with a traumatic optic neuropathy often requires a team approach, involving emergency physicians, trauma surgeons, head and neck surgeons, neurosurgeons, and ophthalmologists. Medical therapy for traumatic optic neuropathy is controversial, as there is no evidence from good quality randomized trials to guide decision-making. Because visual function can spontaneously improve, observation without medical or surgical treatment is a valid option.

There is no evidence that medical treatment of anterior or direct optic nerve injuries is efficacious. For posterior indirect traumatic optic neuropathy, intravenous corticosteroids can be used. Some practioners use 'megadose' intravenous methylprednisolone, i.e., a 30 mg/kg loading dose followed by 5.4 mg/kg/hour continuous infusion for 48 to 72 hours. However, such a large dose appears to be toxic in animals, and this approach is falling into disfavor. A dose of 250 mg methylprednisolone, administered every 6 hours for 48 to 72 hours, is probably safer. Dexamethasone may be substituted for methylprednisolone, based on one trial demonstrating its equivalency in this setting.

If medical therapy produces no improvement, surgery can be considered in centers with expertise in optic canal decompression. If vision improves with treatment, the patient is placed on oral prednisone at a tapering dose. If vision deteriorates during the taper, high-dose intravenous methylprednisolone is reinstituted, diagnostic imaging is performed, and surgical decompression is considered.

Surgical

Surgical therapy for both anterior and posterior traumatic optic neuropathy is controversial, as there is no evidence from good quality randomized trials to guide decision-making. Surgery should only be considered in centers with experience with the procedures. Because of the possibility that the carotid may be iatrogenically injured, there must be informed consent regarding the risk of death or stroke.

Surgery should not be performed on an unconscious patient because of the difficulty in assessing visual function. A possible exception is when the pupil in the affected eye is amaurotic (nonreactive to light but reactive to light in the contralateral eye). The presence of a relative afferent pupillary defect indicates only that an optic neuropathy is present; it does not indicate the severity. A patient with a relative afferent pupillary defect may have 20/20 visual acuity.

An optic nerve sheath fenestration should be performed in cases of anterior traumatic optic neuropathy associated with neuroimaging evidence of an enlarged optic nerve sheath. The procedure is performed in the hopes of evacuating an intrasheath hematoma.

Decompression of the intracanalicular optic nerve via an endoscopic transnasal or transethmoidal route may be performed in cases of traumatic posterior optic neuropathy that do not respond to a 48- to 72-hour initial course of intravenous systemic corticosteroids. The procedure must include (1) removal of at least 50% of the circumference of the osseous canal, (2) removal of bone along the entire length of the canal, and (3) total longitudinal incision of the dural sheath, including the annulus of Zinn.

REFERENCES

Chuenkongkaew W, Chirapapaisan N: A prospective randomized trial of megadose methylprednisolone and high dose dexamethasone for traumatic optic neuropathy. J Med Assoc Thai 85 (5):597–603, 2002.

Goldberg RA, Steinsapir KD: Extracranial optic canal decompression: indications and technique. Ophthal Plast Reconstr Surg 12(3):163–70, 1996.

Levin LA, Baker RS: Management of traumatic optic neuropathy. J Neuroophthalmol 23(1):72–5, 2003.

Levin LA, Beck RW, Joseph MP, et al: The treatment of traumatic optic neuropathy: the International Optic Nerve Trauma Study. Ophthalmology 106(7):1268–1277, 1999.

Levin LA, Joseph MP, Rizzo JF, 3rd, Lessell S: Optic canal decompression in indirect optic nerve trauma. Ophthalmology 101(3):566–569, 1994.

319 VASCULOPATHIC OPTIC NEUROPATHIES 377.39

John G. McHenry, MD, MPH
Detroit, Michigan
Thomas C. Spoor, MD, MS, FACS
Detroit, Michigan

Vasculopathic optic neuropathies cause optic nerve damage through ischemia, leading to axonal stasis, fluid transudation into the subarachnoid space, compression of already damaged axons, neuronal death, and the further compromise of visual function.

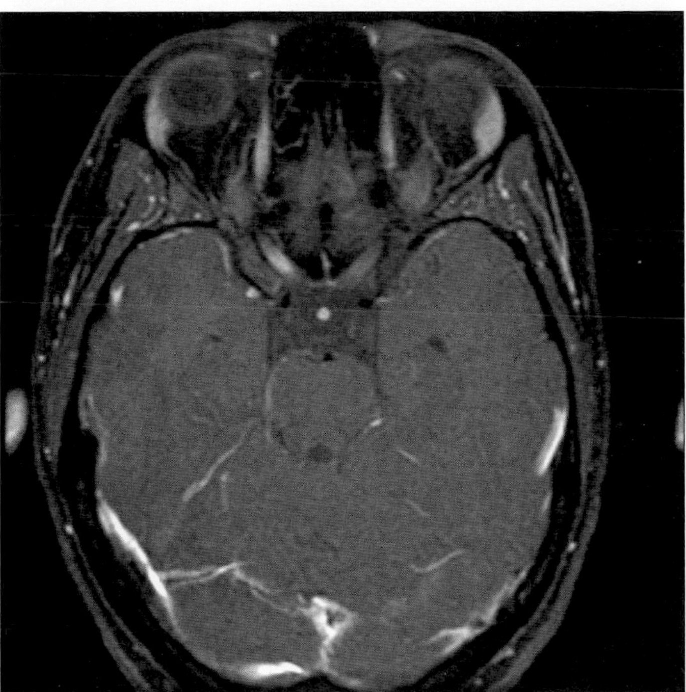

FIGURE 319.1. Vasculopathic optic neuropathies. Axial T1 with gadolinium and fat suppression displaying an enhancing right optic nerve intracranially near the chiasm. (Courtesy of Dr Robert Egan, Casey Eye Institute, Oregon Health & Science University.)

ETIOLOGY

Vasculopathic optic neuropathies include both anterior ischemic optic neuropathy (AION) and posterior ischemic optic neuropathy (PION). Patients with ischemic optic neuropathies present with sudden visual loss, often noticed on awakening. Visual function is compromised, and a relative afferent pupillary defect is present. Patients with AION develop optic disk hemorrhages, edema, and pallor, whereas patients with PION have normal to atrophic disks (Figure 319.1).

AIONs include both an arteritic form, associated with giant cell arteritis (GCA), and a more common nonarteritic form. Nonarteritic AION (NAION) occurs in a static and a progressive form, as well as a prodromal form of optic disk swelling with minimal visual loss that may resolve spontaneously. Sectoral hypoperfusion of the optic nerve may lead to static NAION. Visual acuity can range from counting fingers to 20/20. Visual loss is stable. Static NAION can also occur after severe hypoperfusion of the optic nerve, secondary to systemic hypotension or massive blood loss. In these patients, vision ranges from no light perception to counting fingers. Patients with progressive NAION have further deterioration in visual function after the initial episode of visual loss.

Progressive NAION can be seen in sleep apnea. Often, the patient with progressive NAION awakens with visual loss. In the early hours of the morning, the optic nerve is at risk: blood pressure decreases, intraocular pressure increases, ventilation decreases and oxygenation decreases. The cerebrospinal fluid becomes hypercarbic and intracranial pressure increases. These events can not only lead to optic nerve ischemia, as in NAION, but also disk swelling, as in pseudotumor cerebri. Antihypertensive medications taken at night can lead to nocturnal hypotension and potential blindness on awakening.

DIAGNOSIS

The work-up for disk swelling and hemorrhage in a patient with visual loss who is older than 45 years begins with a complete history. The review of systems focuses on visual loss, temporal pain, headaches, jaw claudication, tongue pain, and proximal muscle weakness. Questions regarding headache and sleep abnormalities and snoring are crucial. Patients are also questioned about previous malignancies. Visual acuity and the presence of a relative afferent pupillary defect or light-near dissociation are recorded. Pupillary defects are graded with neutral density filters. Computerized perimetry is performed with calculation of mean deviation and corrected-pattern standard deviation. Slit-lamp biomicroscopic examination of the optic nerve head with a 78- or 60-diopter lens is helpful and the disks are photographed stereoscopically. Finally, blood is drawn to measure the erythrocyte sedimentation rate (ESR), C reactive protein (CRP), homocystine, Protein C and S, an antiphoslipid and circulating lupus anticoagulant panel, a serum protein electrophorous (SPEP), complete blood count, rheumatoid factor and ANA, and FTA-ABS and RPR. In patients with symptoms of sleep apnea, a sleep study is performed.

The risk of GCA increases with age. It is extremely uncommon in patients younger than 50 years and increases dramatically after the age of 80. It also is more common in women than in men. Whites are more often affected than blacks or Asians. Clinical suspicions guide the evaluation. Statistically, 45- to 75-year-old patients will be more likely to have NAION than GCA. The disks will show sectoral swelling in both. Pallid edema, however, is more often seen with giant cell arteritis. Unfortunately, if not seen early, the disk may be only pale. The patient with sleep apnea may have more generalized swelling.

Young patients with diabetes mellitus, sickle cell anemia, or hypertension may present with sectoral or diffuse optic disk swelling with visual loss. There also have been reports of patients taking oral contraceptives who developed ischemic optic neuropathy. Hemoglobin electrophoresis should be performed to exclude sickle cell anemia in young black patients with disk swelling and visual loss.

PION can occur secondarily to intracranial artery or internal carotid ophthalmic artery atherosclerosis. It may also present with tumors that disrupt the blood supply to the optic nerve. Trauma can injure the pial vessels within the optic canal that supply the optic nerve, resulting in PION. The ophthalmic artery may also be disrupted by penetrating injuries or iatrogenically during paranasal sinus surgery. The fundus then will show a cherry-red spot with massive pallid edema of the optic nerve. Optic nerve vascular damage has also been implicated in radiation-induced optic neuropathy. The exact mechanism of visual loss is very complex and includes cytopathic, chromosomal, and immunologic factors, as well as vascular compromise. The common denominator of all of these PIONs is optic atrophy without antecedent disk swelling. PION is a diagnosis of exclusion.

Differential diagnosis

- Inflammatory optic neuropathies.
- Ischemic optic neuropathies.
- Metabolic optic neuropathies.
- Toxic optic neuropathies.
- Demyelination.
- Axonal degenerations.
- Traumatic optic neuropathy.
- Normal tension glaucoma.
- Sleep apnea associated optic neuropathy.
- Cross-over syndromes.

PROPHYLAXIS

Patients are counseled against smoking. They are started on a regimen of one aspirin per day. Prolonged tapering of steroids is necessary to decrease the incidence of recurrences of GCA.

TREATMENT

Systemic

The treatment for GCA is systemic corticosteroids; there are no effective treatments for NAION. The evaluation and treatment of an elderly patient with profound visual loss, pallid edema, temporal pain, and tenderness proceeds in the following manner:

- An intravenous line is started immediately, and the patient is given 500 mg methylprednisolone IV.
- The patient is next given 150 mg ranitidine or a comparable H_2 blocker or proton pump inhibitors and hospitalized. Prednisone 120 mg PO is started concurrently.
- Laboratory requests include an ESR by the Westergren method, a C reactive protein, complete blood cell count, platelets, prothrombin time, partial thromboplastin time, anticardiolipin antibodies, antinuclear antibodies, fluorescent treponemal antibody absorption test, VDRL syphilis test, electrolytes, blood urea nitrogen, and creatinine. The ESR is only one piece of information that can lead to the diagnosis of GCA; its specificity is extremely poor. Malignancies, infection, cardiovascular, and collagen-vascular diseases may raise the ESR. A rough estimate is that if the ESR is half the patient's age plus 10 for a woman, it is abnormal (just half the age for a man). The platelet count is extremely important. Giant cell arteritis is unlikely without thrombocytosis. Interleuken 6 can also be measured.
- Two hours after the first dose of methylprednisolone, the patient is started on a course of 250 mg methylprednisolone IV every 6 hours for 48 hours and is continued on 120 mg prednisone PO and 150 mg ranitidine b.i.d.
- If the temporal artery biopsy is positive, the patient is discharged on 120 mg/day prednisone plus ranitidine.
- Steroids are slowly tapered over a period of 6 months for healed arteritis and 24 months for active arteritis. This treatment is performed in conjunction with an internal medicine colleague or a rheumatologist. A systemic work-up is essential.
- Serial ESR and CRP results guide the tapering of steroids.
- If the biopsy is negative, steroids are tapered relatively quickly depending on the clinical suspicion as well as the ESR and CRP. Patients with persistent elevation of acute phase-reactants, such as platelets, will often need a biopsy of the temporal artery on the opposite side.
- Patients with a lower clinical probability of GCA are started on 80 mg prednisone with ranitidine, and a temporal artery biopsy is scheduled within the next several days.
- Patients with a higher probability of GCA are admitted to the hospital, started on a regime intravenous steroids and ranitidine, and scheduled for a temporal artery biopsy expeditiously.

COMPLICATIONS

Patients with hypertension and diabetes are at the highest risk for developing AION. There is a 15% incidence of a second event in the fellow eye. Eyes with small cup-to-disk ratios are at particular risk. Rarely, a patient will have a second event in the same eye.

Patients may awaken from major surgery bilaterally blind. It is important to differentiate blindness secondary to occipital strokes from blindness secondary to optic nerve infarcts. Initially, there may be no sign other than minimal optic disk swelling; however, if optic nerve infarction has occurred, pallid edema will ensue over the next 24 hours. The prognosis is very poor.

Some patients may have protein S or C deficiencies, antiphospholipid syndrome, an antithrombic III deficiency, factor V laden deficiencies or hyperhomocystemia. Consideration should be given in consultation with a hematologist for systemic anticoagulation with warfarin. The ciliary circulation is made up of very small vessels and may respond better to Plavix or aspirin. In patients who have progressed on aspirin, Plavix is added. There are inflammation conditions that can also lead to ischemia, such as sarcoid and lupus. These cross-over syndromes require corticosteroid therapy.

COMMENTS

A prospective randomized clinical trial that compared observation with optic nerve sheath decompression showed that decompression was not effective treatment for NAION. Current treatments are designed as prophylaxis against second events, such as nicotine patches for smokers, aspirin, Plavix, lowering intraocular pressure, increasing ocular blood flow with drozolamide, steroids for patients whose disease includes inflammatory component, warfarin in those with coagulation defects, altering the timing of antihypertensive medication in patients with elevated blood pressure and continuous positive airway pressure in patients with sleep apnea. While 40% of patients improve, 40% also worsen.

REFERENCES

Bogen DR, Glaser JS: Ischemic optic neuropathy: the clinical profile and history. Brain 98:689–708, 1975.

Borchert M, Lessell S: Progressive and recurrent nonarteritic anterior ischemic optic neuropathy. Am J Ophthalamol 106:443–449, 1988.

Clearkin L, Caballero J: Recovery of visual function in anterior ischemic optic neuropathy due to giant cell arteritis. Am J Med 92:703–704, 1992.

Costello F, Zimmerman MB, Podhajsky PA, Hayreh SS: Role of thrombocytosis in diagnosis of giant cell arteritis and differentiation of arteritic from non-arteritic anterior ischemic optic neuropathy. Eur J Ophthalmol 14(3):245–257, 2004.

Egan R: Prothrombotic and vascular risk factors in NAION. Ophthalmology 107(12):2116–2117, 2000.

Hayreh SS: Posterior ischaemic optic neuropathy: clinical features, pathogenesis, and management. Eye 18(11):1188–1206, 2004.

SECTION

29 Orbit

320 ENOPHTHALMOS 376.50

Charles N. S. Soparker, MD, PhD
Houston, Texas

ETIOLOGY

Enophthalmos is posterior displacement of the eye. This is most commonly measured in relation to the outer edge of the orbit, the orbital rim, but it may also be assessed relative to the frontal and maxillary prominences or even the contralateral eye.

The term *primary enophthalmos* indicates a congenital problem for which the cause is unknown or unproved. Some degree of facial asymmetry is common, but congenital relative enophthalmos or orbital retrusion may occur with in utero maldevelopment (e.g. plagiocephaly or microphthalmos).

Secondary enophthalmos is due to an acquired change in the volumetric relationship among the rigid bone cavity, the orbit, and its contents (predominantly the orbital fat and the eye). Expansion of the orbital cavity without change in the volume of the orbital contents (i.e. a blow-out fracture) will lead to enophthalmos. Alternatively, scarring contracture of the orbital fat and extraocular muscles may decrease soft tissue volume, making the orbital cavity less full and causing enophthalmos.

- Inadequate postnatal orbital cavity development.
- Inadequate local tissue stimulation for orbital growth.
- Intraorbital (e.g. phthisis bulbi or fat atrophy in childhood).
- Extraorbital (e.g. maxillary bone problems).
- Bone growth arrest (e.g. ionizing radiation for retinoblastoma).
- Orbital cavity expansion.
- Outward fracture of orbital bones: frequency of fracture sites: floor more than medial wall more than lateral wall more than roof.
- Surgical expansion of the orbit (as in thyroid orbitopathy).
- Silent sinus syndrome, which is spontaneous, asymptomatic collapse of the maxillary sinus and orbital floor.
- Orbital varix with presumed, slow bone erosion when the varix fills with the patient in recumbent position.
- Volumetric loss of orbital contents.
- Orbital fat atrophy.
- After concussive trauma.
- After severe inflammation or infection.
- After external beam irradiation.
- Associated with wasting disorders, such as Parry–Romberg hemifacial atrophy or linear scleroderma.
- Contraction of orbital fat.
- Scirrhous carcinomas (most commonly, metastatic breast).
- Pseudoenophthalmos.
- Pseudoenophthalmos (unilateral blepharoptosis; Horner's syndrome).
- Contralateral exophthalmos.
- Contralateral pseudoexophthalmos.
- Contralateral high myopia.
- Contralateral eyelid retraction.

COURSE/PROGNOSIS

The course varies depending on the cause. Enophthalmos due to orbit cavity expansion is generally easier to correct than that found in loss of orbital contents because the former is less frequently associated with serious systemic disease.

DIAGNOSIS

Laboratory findings

The physical examination demonstrates associated hemifacial atrophy indicates Parry–Romberg syndrome. The skin biopsy will rule out similarly appearing linear scleroderma (this is more common in children).

Associated extraocular muscle dysfunction with firm induration of the eyelids suggests scirrhous carcinoma.

Corneal computed tomography (CT) is best to evaluate blowout fractures and shows characteristic maxillary sinus hypoplasia with mucosal thickening, thinning of various antral bone walls, and increased retromaxillary fat density seen in silent sinus syndrome. Axial CT may demonstrate orbital fat atrophy. Rapid spiral CT with Valsalva may show orbital varix. Contrastenhanced CT and magnetic resonance imaging (MRI) demonstrate different features of scirrhous carcinomas. Bone scans may help to identify areas of active bone inflammation seen in osteomyelitis.

Differential diagnosis

Acquired enophthalmos must be differentiated from contralateral exophthalmos and congenital, relative enophthalmos or orbital retrusion. Many persons have some degree of facial asymmetry, and a review of old photographs is often helpful.

TREATMENT

Any related systemic or progressive disease processes should be addressed. Approximate the normal orbital bone positions before soft tissue volume loss is addressed.

The repair of orbital fractures should be as follows:

- Maintain the convexity of the posterior, medial orbital floor;
- Be certain to stabilize floor implants posteriorly on intact floor ledge;
- Release any major adhesions or scar bands to allow mobilization of soft tissues. In late post-traumatic cases, sharp rather than blunt dissection often is required;
- If using bone grafts, allow for 15% to 30% reabsorption;
- Overcorrect to obtain 1 to 2 mm of exophthalmos intraoperatively;
- Perform forced duction testing of the globe before closure.

The replacement of lost orbital soft tissue volume should be as follows:

- Perform 'forward traction' test on the globe to determine the amount of correction possible;
- Augment from the orbital walls inward with bone or synthetic materials;
- Position augmentation material beneath and behind the equator of the globe to achieve forward and upward displacement, as needed.

COMPLICATIONS

- Blindness from optic neuropathy-ischemic or compressive; either may be related to malposition of orbital implant or implants or to orbital hemorrhage.
- Orbital cellulites.
- Exacerbation of any intraocular injuries.
- Ocular motility disturbance from unreduced fractures, implant position, iatrogenic myopathy, or neuropathy.
- Damage to the infraorbital nerve.
- Implant infection, inflammatory reaction, migration, and hematic cyst formation.
- Grafted bone reabsorption.
- In cases of autologous bone or cartilage grafts, donor site complications.
- Lower eyelid retraction and immobilization.
- Facial scars (if transconjunctival approach is not used).
- Undercorrection.
- Hyperglobus due to augmentation directly beneath the globe rather than behind the equator
- Efferent pupillary defect due to damage of the ciliary ganglion or parasympathetic in the inferior division of cranial nerve III.

REFERENCES

Baujat B, Derbez R, Rossarie R, et al: Silent sinus syndrome: a mechanical theory. Orbit 25:145–148, 2006.

Cline RA, Rootman J: Enophthalmos: a clinical review. Ophthalmology 91:229–237, 1991.

Davidson JK, Soparkar CN, Williams JB, et al: Negative sinus pressure and normal predisease imaging in silent sinus syndrome. Arch Ophthalmol 117:1653–1654, 1999.

Manson PN, Clifford CM, Su OT, et al: Mechanisms of global support and posttraumatic enophthalmos: I. The anatomy of the ligament sling and its relation to intramuscular cone orbital fat. Plast Reconstr Surg 77:193–202, 1986.

Soparkar CNS, Patrinely JR, Cuaycong MJ, et al: The silent sinus syndrome: a cause of spontaneous enophthalmos. Ophthalmology 101:772–778, 1994.

321 EXTERNAL ORBITAL FRACTURES 802.8

Richard D. Lisman, MD, FACS
New York, New York
Jennifer Scruggs, MD
New York, New York

An external fracture of the orbit results in direct disjunction of any portion of the orbital rim, usually with bony orbital wall involvement. These injuries may occur in isolation or in conjunction with multisystem trauma.

ETIOLOGY/INCIDENCE

Facial bones break in predictable patterns. The superior and lateral orbital rims are the strongest rims of the orbit, and fractures are rare except at suture lines. In contrast, the medial and inferior orbital rims are weaker and more commonly sustain comminuted fractures.

Fractures of the lateral orbital wall usually occur through bony suture lines; the zygomaticofrontal suture superolaterally and the zygomatiomaxillary suture inferonasally are the weakest portions of the orbital rim. A fracture in these regions may result in a 'tripod' fracture of the zygoma (malar eminence), with the third foot of the tripod at the zygomaticotemporal suture of the zygomatic arch. Orbital floor fractures are invariably a part of this fracture complex.

Naso-orbital ethmoid fractures involve the medial wall of the orbit and often its associated lacrimal system through direct laceration or associated bony injury. These fractures may be associated with craniofacial separation (Le Fort II or III) fractures of the maxilla.

The superior orbital rim is thick and fractures are uncommon. They are usually seen in association with severe head trauma and cerebral injury.

DIAGNOSIS

Clinical signs and symptoms

The clinical diagnosis is based on observation for facial deformity as well as palpation for rim discontinuity.

- Tripod fractures of the zygoma:
  - Flattened malar eminence secondary to posterior displacement of the zygoma;
  - Palpable and painful step-offs at the zygomaticofrontal suture (lateral orbital rim) and zygomaticomaxillary suture (inferior orbital rim);
  - Lateral canthal tendon displacement and globe ptosis when the zygoma is displaced inferiorly and posteriorly;
  - Trismus, or pain and difficulty opening the mouth from irritation and contusion of the adjacent temporalis muscle or impingement of the coronoid process by displaced bone spicules;

- Hypesthesia of the infraorbital nerve with orbital floor involvement.
- Naso-orbital ethmoid fractures:
  - Flattening of the nasal bridge and possibly the forehead;
  - Telecanthus and inferior displacement of the medial canthal tendon. The ethmoid sinuses are crushed and the nasal bones and frontal process of the maxilla splayed laterally;
  - Diplopia (more common in orbital fractures with a medial component);
  - Lacrimal damage (canaliculi, lacrimal sac, or nasolacrimal duct) with tearing and/or dacryocystitis.
- Superior orbital rim fractures:
  - Neurologic manifestations with concurrent head trauma and cerebral injury;
  - Traumatic optic neuropathy: shearing injury as the force of impact at the superior orbital rim is transmitted along the orbital roof to the optic canal.

Laboratory findings
- Computed tomography:
  - Imaging with computed tomography (CT) is the gold standard to confirm the diagnosis, delineate the extent of injury, and devise a treatment plan for external orbital fractures. Plain films are inadequate. Axial and coronal CT projections should be obtained, using fine cuts (preferably 1 mm) through the orbits. Newer helical CT scanners quickly acquire these projections with no need to reposition the patient. Three-dimensional CT reconstruction, which shows dramatic presentation of the spatial relationships of the bone fragments, may offer additional benefit in complex external orbital fractures.
- Ultrasonography:
  - It has been suggested that ultrasound may play a role in visualizing fractures of the zygomatic arch and anterior wall of the frontal sinus. While ultrasound is insufficient as a diagnostic study, it has potential value intraoperatively to evaluate closed reduction of fractures where direct visualization of alignment is not possible.

TREATMENT

Systemic
A complete history and physical exam are essential to evaluate for other concurrent injures. Intracranial injuries take precedence over the management of orbital rim fractures. In addition, a full ophthalmologic examination must exclude penetrating ocular injury prior to evaluation or repair of orbital fractures.

Observation and conservative management are often preferred for up to 2 weeks before surgical intervention to allow associated hemorrhage and swelling to subside. Broad-spectrum antibiotics are commonly prescribed as communication invariably exists between the orbit and nasal cavity or sinuses. Corticosteroids may be useful to decrease edema. Minimally displaced tripod fractures of the zygoma may result in minimal or no deformity or functional disability and do not require intervention.

Surgical
Surgery is indicated when bone displacement causes cosmetic or functional defects. The surgical approach typically involves incisions to expose the bone fragments, manipulation to place them in proper anatomic position, and fixation, often with titanium microplates, to stabilize the bone.

The surgical management of a tripod fracture of the zygoma varies according to the severity of bone displacement. A depressed fracture with smooth edges may be approached through a Gillies incision posterior to the hairline at the temple. A Bristow elevator is placed between the temporalis muscle and temporalis fascia and is used to lift the zygoma into position while the other hand supports the fracture inferiorly (bimanual approach).

A displaced or comminuted fracture requires direct visualization with rigid internal fixation. Exposure of the inferior orbital rim is gained through a transcutaneous or transconjunctival lower eyelid incision with a lateral canthotomy; the transconjunctival approach is preferred and decreases the risk of lower eyelid retraction. The zygomaticomaxillary buttress is exposed through a gingivobuccal sulcus incision. A coronal approach may be necessary to visualize and plate a severely comminuted fracture of the zygomatic arch. Extremely comminuted or absent bone may be replaced with a synthetic structural device or bone graft.

Repair of naso-orbital ethmoid fractures is complex and often requires a combined coronal, transconjunctival, and oral approach in order to reconstruct the nose, lacrimal apparatus, medial canthal tendon, and frontal sinus. Proper medial canthal tendon attachment is to the posterior lacrimal crest; transnasal wiring or miniplate fixation may be used. Posttraumatic dacryostenosis is common, especially with delayed fracture repair or bone loss in the lacrimal region. Subsequent dacryocystorhinostomy is indicated for persistent tearing or dacryocystitis.

COMPLICATIONS

- Ocular: paralytic or restrictive strabismus, enophthalmos.
- Eyelids: ptosis, lid retraction, lateral canthal displacement, telecanthus, ectropion, entropion.
- Lacrimal system: obstruction, tearing, dacryocystitis.
- Surgical: hemorrhage, infection, implant extrusion.

COMMENTS

External orbital fractures occur in predictable patterns with an associated constellation of signs and symptoms. CT scanning is essential for diagnosis and surgical planning. Treatment may initially involve observation; surgery is warranted for cosmetic or functional deformities. Surgical repair may combine multiple incisions to gain access to bony fragments from different directions, with subsequent reduction and fixation of the fractures.

REFERENCES

Becelli R, Renzi G, Mannino G, et al: Posttraumatic obstruction of lacrimal pathways: a retrospective analysis of 58 consecutive naso-orbitoethmoid fractures. J Craniofac Surg 15:29–33, 2004.

Bedrossian EH, Della Rocca RC, Brazzo BG: Management of zygomaticomaxillary (tripod) fractures. In: Nesi F, Lisman R, Levine M, eds: Smith's ophthalmic plastic reconstructive surgery. St Louis, V Mosby, 1998.

Nerad, JA: Eyelid and orbital trauma. In: Nerad JA, ed: Krachmer JH (series ed.): Oculoplastic surgery: the requisites in ophthalmology. St Louis, Mosby, 2001:312–347.

Weseley R: Current techniques for the repair of complex orbital fractures: miniplate fixation and cranial bone grafts. Ophthalmology 99:1766, 1992.

Zingg M: Classification and treatment of zygomatic fractures: a review of 1,025 cases. J Oral Maxillofac Surg 50:778, 1992.

322 INTERNAL ORBITAL FRACTURES 802.8

Richard D. Lisman, MD, FACS
New York, New York
Jennifer Scruggs, MD
New York, New York

ETIOLOGY/INCIDENCE

Internal orbital fractures, commonly known as blowout fractures, involve the walls of the orbit, leaving the bony rim intact. The orbital floor is most commonly affected, followed by the medial wall; the orbital roof is rarely fractured in isolation, and the lateral wall of the orbit is fractured with involvement of the orbital rim (see External orbital fractures, discussion of tripod fracture of the zygoma).

Theories on the mechanism of injury of pure blowout fractures are twofold: the buckling theory and the hydraulic theory. The buckling theory describes direct force on the relatively thick orbital rim with transmission of that force to the thin-boned walls of the orbit. The hydraulic theory states that a blow by an object of greater diameter than the orbital entrance leads to an increase in intraorbital pressure, resulting in a fracture at the weakest portion of the orbit. Thin bones of the orbital floor (typically medial to the infraorbital canal) or medial wall are 'blown out' and orbital contents pushed into the maxillary or ethmoid sinuses.

DIAGNOSIS

Clinical signs and symptoms

Patients with orbital floor fractures may present acutely with proptosis from swelling and/or hemorrhage. Later, enophthalmos may ensue from orbital expansion associated with larger medial wall and floor fractures. Enophthalmos may also result from incarceration of orbital tissues into the maxillary antrum with resultant cicatrization. Extreme herniation of tissue may result in hypoglobus.

Diplopia is the most common complaint of patients with blowout fractures. Restrictive strabismus from entrapped orbital tissue is characteristic of smaller orbital floor fractures. Diplopia most commonly involves the vertical positions of gaze; decreased motility in upgaze is typical. The affected eye may be hypotropic (with anterior fractures) or hypertropic (with posterior fractures).

Hypesthesia in the distribution of the infraorbital nerve is very common and involves the lower eyelid, cheek, and anterior (incisor) teeth on the affected side. Subcutaneous emphysema occurs from the connection to the nasal cavity and/or sinuses.

Medial wall fractures may present acutely with epistaxis and rarely show proptosis if in isolation. Frank extraocular muscle entrapment is rare in isolated medial wall fractures, but transient horizontal diplopia may occur due to contusion of the medial rectus muscle.

A characteristic constellation of findings can be found in children with orbital floor fractures with entrapped tissue and minimally displaced bone fragments, the so-called 'trapdoor' fracture. These children may have nausea and vomiting or bradycardia (oculocardiac reflex), which are predictive of muscle entrapment. Aside from marked motility disturbance, these patients may show few additional signs of orbital trauma; thus the term 'white-eyed' blowout fracture has been used. These patients need urgent surgical repair.

Laboratory findings

Computed tomography (CT) scans of the orbit are used to confirm the diagnosis and delineate the area of the fracture. Coronal and axial views of the orbit should be obtained, using fine cuts (preferably 1 mm) through the orbits. Newer helical CT scanners quickly acquire these projections with no need to reposition the patient. Herniation of orbital tissue is thus visualized, and the position and appearance of the extraocular muscles can be noted. Occasionally, a trapdoor fracture of the orbital floor will clearly delineate an entrapped inferior rectus muscle below the floor. Orbital emphysema is frequently evident with fractures of the medial orbital wall.

TREATMENT

A complete history and physical exam are essential to evaluate for concurrent injuries. A full ophthalmologic exam must exclude penetrating ocular injury prior to repair of orbital fractures.

Medical

- Broad-spectrum antibiotics are commonly prescribed, as communication invariably exists between the orbit and nasal or sinus cavities.

Ocular

- Serial Hertel exophthalmometry and extraocular muscle measurements (with or without orthoptic documentation) are performed. Enophthalmos may develop or worsen as edema resolves. Conversely, early diplopia may improve with decreasing orbital edema.
- Forced duction testing may be performed to determine if the motility dysfunction is restrictive in nature.

Surgical

Controversy exists in the timing of the management of orbital blowout fractures. Most surgeons agree that early (before 5 days post-injury) intervention is difficult when there is excessive traumatic edema and hemorrhage; conversely, late surgery (after 14 days post-injury) may be hampered by the formation of fibrovascular scar tissue. The exception is children with a blowout fracture and restriction; in these patients scarring progresses rapidly and surgery should be performed as soon as possible.

- A conservative approach is often favored for the first 5 to 14 days after trauma to allow associated hemorrhage and swelling to subside. The patient should avoid the Valsalva maneuver, including sneezing, nose blowing, and strenuous activity (to avoid further orbital tissue incarceration or exacerbation of orbital and subcutaneous emphysema).

Indications for surgical repair of a blowout fracture include:

- Diplopia which is restrictive in etiology and is persistent or progressive, occurring in near primary or reading position;
- Enophthalmos which is cosmetically unacceptable (typically 2 mm or more). Extensive disruption of the orbital floor and/or medial wall is considered a precursor to enophthalmos and therefore a relative indication for repair.

The goal of surgery is to release entrapped orbital tissue from the fracture and to restore normal orbital volume. Multiple surgical approaches are available; some surgeons are now advocating endoscopic methods for orbital fracture repair. However, the favored approach remains as follows:

- The transconjunctival approach with a lateral canthotomy and cantholysis is preferred to expose the orbital floor; the medial wall is also accessible or may be further exposed through a transcaruncular approach. Alternatively, a cutaneous approach via an infraorbital or subciliary incision may be used.
- The preseptal plane is entered down to the inferior orbital rim.
- The periosteum is incised along the orbital rim; periorbita is elevated off the orbital floor until the fracture is reached.
- The hand-over-hand technique is used to free the orbital contents from the maxillary antrum and reduce the fracture.
- The orbital floor is typically restored with an implant (such as porous polyethelene or silastic); the implant should cover the entire floor defect with no tissue prolapsing around the implant.
- Forced duction testing of the inferior rectus muscle is used to confirm release of any entrapment before closure.

Postoperative vision assessment is important in the first several hours after surgery; corticosteroids and antibiotics are usually administered for 1 week.

COMPLICATIONS

- Nonsurgical: progressive cicatrization with worsening diplopia or enophthalmos.
- Surgical: hemorrhage, infection, implant extrusion, diplopia not improving after 6 months postoperatively, eyelid malpositions (ectropion, entropion, ptosis), pseudoptosis, lacrimal obstruction, sinus disease.

Chronic fibrosis of the inferior rectus muscle may be due to ischemic (Volkmann's) contracture of the muscle resulting from hemorrhage and edema within the muscle sheath thereby leading to a compartment syndrome. In this subgroup of patients, systemic steroids are thought to be beneficial.

REFERENCES

Converse JM, Smith B: Enophthalmos and diplopia in fractures of the orbital floor. Br J Plast Surg 9:265–274, 1957.

Chang EL, Bernardino CR: Update on orbital trauma. Curr Opin Ophthalmol 15:411–415, 2004.

Cruz AAV, Eichenberger GCD: Epidemiology and management of orbital fractures. Curr Opin Ophthalmol 15:416–421, 2004.

Kersten RC: Blowout fracture of the orbital floor with entrapment caused by isolated trauma to the orbital rim. Am J Ophthalmol 103:215–220, 1987.

Lisman RD, Smith B, Rodgers R: Volkman's ischemic contractures and blowout fractures. Adv Plastic Reconstr Surg 7:117–131, 1988.

323 ORBITAL INFLAMMATORY SYNDROMES 377.398

Peter J. Dolman, MD, FRCSC
Vancouver, British Columbia, Canada
Jack Rootman, MD, FRCSC
Vancouver, British Columbia, Canada

This chapter reviews a heterogeneous group of orbital inflammatory syndromes (OIS) defined by clinical and histologic signs of orbital soft tissue inflammation that cannot be attributed to local injury or to infection or to Graves' orbitopathy.

Traditionally, these syndromes were clumped together under the generic term 'inflammatory pseudotumor,' defined loosely as a non-neoplastic orbital inflammatory mass. Included in this broad group were lymphoid proliferations, which now are considered a separate disease spectrum ranging from benign lymphoid hyperplasia to lymphoma, (including Sjögren's disease of the lacrimal gland).

More recently, the term 'idiopathic non-specific orbital inflammatory syndromes' has been used to describe the balance of diseases, but as subsets are identified with their own characteristic clinical and pathologic patterns, this term may become obsolete. As the molecular pathways of inflammatory cascades are progressively understood, further disease subcategories will probably be described.

For now, a simple classification for OIS can be based on the primary histopathology: acute polymorphous, sclerosing, granulomatous, and vasculitic.

ETIOLOGY/INCIDENCE

OIS account for 5–10% of cases of orbital disease. The cause is unknown, but they are likely immune disorders, perhaps initiated by a preceding infection. There is no age, sex, or race predilection for most of these diseases, although acute polymorphous myositis is more common in females.

COURSE/PROGNOSIS

Acute polymorphous OIS develop over several days to weeks with pain, redness, edema, and local dysfunction. Their clinical presentation relates to the principle area of orbital involvement: anterior (globe and surrounding orbital fat), myositis (extraocular muscle), dacryoadenitis (lacrimal gland), apical (orbital apex and cavernous sinus), and diffuse (entire orbital involvement).

Sclerosing OIS develop more insidiously and lead to orbital dysfunction as a result of progressive scarring and inflammation. This disease may be linked to multifocal fibrosclerosis, including retroperitoneal fibrosis and sclerosing cholangitis.

Granulomatous OIS develop subacutely to chronically with minimal inflammatory signs around a palpable mass. Sarcoidosis is a recognized systemic syndrome with granulomata developing in the conjunctiva, uvea, skin and lungs. Xanthogranulomatoses show fat-laden histiocytes and multi-nucleated giant cells on histopathology and may have significant systemic features involving the lungs, heart or retroperitoneum.

Vasculitic OIS develop in both acute and chronic fashion, with intermittent acute relapses, and have the cardinal features of painful proptosis, possible scleritis, optic neuritis or dacryoadenitis, and occasional bilateral involvement. Diseases such as Wegener's granulomatosis or polyarteritis nodosa may have systemic, life-threatening involvement and require tissue diagnosis and evaluation and co-management by a rheumatologist.

DIAGNOSIS

Laboratory findings

Acute polymorphous OIS

- Computed tomography (CT) scans:
  - Identification of the involved areas;
  - Irregular margins surrounding the primary focus.
- Histology:
  - Tissues infiltrated with a mixed population of neutrophils, plasma cells, histiocytes, macrophages and lymphocytes.

Sclerosing OIS

- CT scans:
  - Homogeneous, dense lesions incorporating both fat and surrounding structures.
- Histology:
  - Dense collagen deposition with a relatively scant, polymorphous inflammatory infiltrate.

Granulomatous OIS

- CT scans:
  - Discrete, dense mass.
- Histology:
  - Granulomatous inflammation with epithelioid cells, histiocytes and giant cells without an identifiable local or systemic cause;
  - Xanthogranulomatous OIS have fat-laden histiocytes and multi-nucleated giant cells.

Vasculitic OIS

- CT scans:
  - Infiltrative disease focused in the lacrimal gland, diffusely through the orbit including the sclera or optic nerve sheath, and possible midline disease with opacification of the sinuses with bony destruction.
- Histology:
  - Necrotizing vasculitis with microabscess formation and variable fibrosis.

Differential diagnosis

Orbital cellulitis

- May be confused with acute anterior/diffuse OIS.
- Often opaque, contiguous sinus on CT scan.
- Biopsy sinuses for culture and sensitivities if uncertain before antibiotic or anti-inflammatory therapy.

Fungal infections

- Apical involvement with pain, vision loss and oculomotor pareses may be confused with acute polymorphous apical OIS or with apical vasculites like Wegener's granulomatosis.

Graves' orbitopathy

- May mimic acute polymorphous myositis.
- More insidious onset with less pain with ocular movements.
- Little CT evidence of inflammation involving tendons or surrounding tissue.

Malignancies

- Cicatricial neoplasms may be confused for a sclerosing OIS.
- Discrete neoplasm may mimic chronic, nongranulomatous OIS.

TREATMENT

Systemic

Oral corticosteroid

- *Acute polymorphous OIS* respond dramatically, with pain relief reported within hours.
  - *Typical acute polymorphous myositis and dacryoadenitis* controlled with lower doses of oral corticosteroids (40 to 60 mg prednisone per day) tapered over 4 to 8 weeks.
  - *Anterior, diffuse, and apical inflammations* require higher doses (60 to 100 mg/day prednisone) tapered over 8 to 12 weeks; recurrent exacerbations may occur and require a temporary increased dosage.
- *Sclerosing OIS* often become refractory to steroids requiring immunosuppressives (cyclophosphamide, methotrexate, azothioprine and cyclosporin A) for 4–6 months; initial dose of prednisone 60 to 100 mg/day for 2 weeks tapered over 8 to 12 weeks.
- *Granulomatous OIS* usually respond well to the same regimen followed for idiopathic myositis; an internist may help rule out systemic inflammatory syndromes (sarcoid, asthma) in cases of granulomatous disease and monitor side effects of long-term corticosteroids.
- *Vasculitic OIS* (Wegener's granulomatosis) may show partial response to oral corticosteroids, but typically require other immunosuppressives (cyclophosphamide) for control.

Intravenous steroids

- Methylprednisolone 1 g/day IV on alternate days for three doses; useful in acute diffuse OIS with vision loss, in sclerosing OIS, or in patients developing complications from chronic oral steroid use.
- Administered with cardiac monitor because of rare incidence of arrhythmia and sudden death.

Nonsteroidal anti-inflammatory drugs

- Ibuprofen 400 mg t.i.d. for 2 weeks tapered over 4 weeks.
- Adjunct to oral steroids to permit more rapid taper or in patients with acute OIS who are intolerant of oral steroids.
- Acute single muscle myositis may respond to non-steroidal anti-inflammatory drugs.

Cyclophosphamide

- 50–200 mg per day
- May be helpful for OIS refractory to steroids or that recur repeatedly on attempted steroid taper.
- Use in sclerosing OIS combined with steroids and cyclosporin A.

- Hematologist or oncologist should manage therapy to monitor for adverse affects (e.g. leukopenia, thrombocytopenia, hemorrhagic cystitis, sterility, and carcinogenesis).

Methotrexate

- 5–15 mg per week, requires folic acid supplement.
- May be helpful for recalcitrant cases of sclerosing OIS alone or in combination with steroids and cyclophosphamide.
- Hematologist or oncologist should supervise therapy; toxicity includes ulcerative stomatitis, leukopenia, and hepatic and renal damage.

Cyclosporin A

- Used in low doses (2 mg/kg/day) to control granulomatous OIS where steroids and cyclophosphamide are poorly tolerated.
- Used in combination with steroids and cyclophosphamide for sclerosing inflammation to prevent progression.

Ocular

Intralesional triamcinolone acetonide (20 to 40 mg) or betamethasone (6 mg) may be injected into localized OIS, including sclerotenonitis, acute polymorphous dacryoadenitis, and granulomatous inflammatory masses

Surgical

Biopsy

- Most cases of acute polymorphous OIS with characteristic clinical and radiographic features may be treated with a therapeutic trial of steroids without obtaining a biopsy.
- Lesions refractory to steroid therapy should be biopsied.
- Lacrimal gland inflammations should be biopsied because they may be confused clinically and radiologically with lymphoid proliferations (including Sjögren's), specific systemic inflammations (sarcoid, Wegener's), or epithelial neoplasia.
- Insidious or sclerosing OIS and orbital apex lesions should be biopsied to rule out cicatricial malignancy, lymphoid proliferations, and specific granulomatoses (e.g. Wegener's).

Excision

- Partial or complete removal of a granulomatous or sclerosing inflammatory mass may be helpful if the lesions are well localized and can be removed with minimal functional damage.

Exenteration

- This may be indicated for very aggressive sclerosing inflammations that cause blindness, an unsightly contracted orbit, and intractable pain despite maximal medical therapy.

COMMENTS

Acute polymorphous OIS are usually easily recognized by their characteristic clinical and radiologic features and their rapid response to corticosteroids with or without adjunctive nonsteroidal anti-inflammatory agents. A typical course of treatment is 6 to 8 weeks. Poorly responsive lesions should undergo biopsy before initiation of other anti-inflammatory treatment or radiotherapy to rule out lymphoproliferative or other specific or systemic inflammatory syndromes.

Sclerosing OIS should be biopsied early, and the patient examined systemically to rule out other sites of multifocal fibrosclerosis. Pulse-dose steroids, cyclophosphamide, azathioprine, methotrexate and/or cyclosporin A should be instituted promptly to control the disease and prevent permanent scarring and functional deficits — combination therapy of these three drugs should be seriously considered under the supervision of a rheumatologist or internist. Radiotherapy does not seem to be helpful for this disease. Local excision may help control the inflammatory mass; in relentless cases with blindness and pain, exenteration may rarely be required.

Patients identified on biopsy to have granulomatous OIS should be screened by an internist for systemic entities such as sarcoid and treated appropriately. Xanthogranulomatous OIS should be evaluated by an internist to rule out systemic involvement (including pulmonary or cardiac disease). In the absence of systemic disease, granulomatous inflammations often respond well to a brief course of systemic steroids, an intralesional steroid injection, or simple excision of the inflammatory mass.

Patients with any of the vasculitides (Wegener's necrotizing granulomatosis, polyarteritis nodosa) may present with acute or sub-acute cases of OIS, often with pain and proptosis and findings related to the part of the orbit involved (scleritis, dacryoadenitis, orbital apex). These findings may be bilateral, and involve the midline sinuses with destruction of bone. A rheumatologist should assist in the management of these patients' care, both to rule out systemic involvement and to assist in medical therapy (combined corticosteroids and cyclophosphamide).

REFERENCES

Flanders AE, Mafee MF, Rao VM, et al: CT characteristics of orbital pseudotumors and other orbital inflammatory processes. J Comput Assist Tomogr 13:40–47, 1989.

Kennerdell JS: The management of sclerosing non-specific orbital inflammation. Surv Ophthalmol 22:512–518, 1991.

Krohel GB, Carr EM, Webb RM: Intralesional corticosteroids for inflammatory lesions of the orbit. Am J Ophthalmol 101:121–123, 1986.

Mauriello JA, Flanagan JC: Pseudotumor and lymphoid tumor: Distinct clinicopathologic entities. Surv Ophthalmol 34:142–148, 1989.

Mombaerts I, Goldschmeding R, Schlingemann RO, et al: What is orbital pseudotumor? Surv Ophthalmol 41:66–78, 1996.

Rootman J, McCarthy M, White V, Harris G, Kennerdell J: Idiopathic sclerosing inflammation of the orbit: a distinct clinicopathologic entity. Ophthalmology 101:570–584, 1994.

Rootman J, Nugent F: The classification and management of acute orbital pseudotumors. Ophthalmology 89:1040–1048, 1982.

324 OPTIC FORAMEN FRACTURES 802.8

Vivian Schiedler, MD
Seattle, Washington
James C. Orcutt, MD, PhD
Seattle, Washington

Fractures of the optic foramen are usually seen in the context of a nonpenetrating blow to the head with subsequent transfer of force to the optic canal and its contents or with basilar skull fractures. The primary concern for the treating physician is the diagnosis and management of traumatic optic neuropathy. However, the benefits of medical and surgical interventions for this condition have recently been called into question.

ETIOLOGY/INCIDENCE

Traumatic optic neuropathy is most commonly seen in a young person who has had a closed head injury. Bicycle and motorcycle accidents are the most frequent causes of injury. Less frequent causes include assault and falls. Most patients are male. Loss of consciousness is common and can make the diagnosis more difficult.

- The optic nerve may be damaged directly by a displaced fracture within the foramen, but it can also be damaged in the absence of fracture by other primary mechanisms such as hematoma, crush injury, and total or partial avulsion. Pial vessels supplying the optic nerve may be severed as the result of shearing forces.
- Primary injuries, which result in permanent axonal injury, may lead to secondary mechanisms of injury such as: edema formation, ischemic necrosis, apoptosis, and reperfusion injury. Therefore, the absence of an optic foramen fracture seen on imaging studies does not rule out the diagnosis of traumatic optic neuropathy, nor does it lessen the severity of the diagnosis.

COURSE/PROGNOSIS

- In the absence of traumatic optic neuropathy, cerebrospinal fluid leak, or other localizing neurologic finding, optic canal fractures tend to heal without any significant sequelae. As with any patient who has had a closed head injury, there is a risk of developing carotid cavernous or dural cavernous sinus arteriovenous fistulas.
- If vision is lost immediately upon traumatic impact, the prognosis for visual recovery is extremely poor. If the optic nerve is transected by a bony fragment in the optic canal, visual recovery is doubtful.

However, some degree of spontaneous visual recovery, even from no light perception vision, is common in many cases of traumatic optic neuropathy. Therefore, it is difficult to ascertain whether treatment with steroids or optic canal decompression offers any significant benefit above and beyond the natural course.

DIAGNOSIS

- The diagnosis of traumatic optic neuropathy is clinical. Vision and pupillary function are abnormal in the absence of other ocular injuries. In both unconscious and conscious patients, a relative afferent pupillary defect (Marcus Gunn pupil) is necessary for the diagnosis of unilateral traumatic optic neuropathy.
- A structurally normal-appearing eye, both externally and funduscopically, is consistent with acute indirect injury to the optic nerve.

Vision loss may be delayed. It may also improve spontaneously. Therefore, careful documentation of the time interval between trauma and visual assessment is helpful.

- Once the diagnosis is suspected, a complete ophthalmologic examination should be performed to rule out other causes of visual loss and a Marcus Gunn pupil (i.e. significant retinal injury). The diagnosis of bilateral traumatic optic neuropathy requires a high level of suspicion since a relative pupillary defect may not be observed in such cases.
- A direct coronal computed tomography scan of the head and orbits using 1.5 or 2 mm cuts is the best imaging technique and may show fracture, perineural or subperiosteal hematoma, or transsection of the optic nerve. Axial cuts with coronal reconstruction are satisfactory if direct coronal views cannot be obtained.

TREATMENT

The treatment of optic foramen fractures in the setting of indirect traumatic optic neuropathy is controversial. To date, there have been no randomized controlled trials or natural history studies on optic canal fractures with or without associated traumatic optic neuropathy. There is no consensus that optic canal decompression is beneficial.

Medical

Treatment options include the use of intravenous steroids alone or in conjunction with optic canal decompression. The International Optic Nerve Trauma Study (1999) was a nonrandomized comparative interventional study of 133 patients who received either no treatment, steroids alone, or optic canal decompression with or without steroids. Treatment was no more beneficial than observation. It is estimated that 30% to 50% of patients will improve without any therapy. Thus, no standard of care currently exists regarding whether to use corticosteroids or surgery.

Recent data from animal models of optic nerve injury suggest that corticosteroids worsen axonal loss in a dose dependent manner. In addition, high doses of corticosteroids appear to contribute to apoptotic retinal ganglion cell loss. Therefore, the previously advocated megadose corticosteroid treatment of acute traumatic optic neuropathy, which was based on spinal cord injury data from the NASCIS II trial, is now falling into disfavor.

If methylprednisolone treatment is elected, a moderate dose of 250 mg every 6 hours or lower is recommended. Conscious patients should be checked for improvement in visual acuity and pupillary defect in 48 to 72 hours. If there is no improvement, the steroids should be discontinued. If there is any improvement, the steroids are continued for 5 days and then tapered rapidly. Any decline in visual acuity, visual field, or pupillary response on withdrawal of steroids warrants a repeat computed tomography scan, reinstitution of steroids, and consideration of decompression. The treatment of the unconscious patient is identical, except only the pupillary response can be followed clinically.

The choice of therapy is dependent not so much on the presence of a fracture seen on imaging studies as it is on the clinical picture. Patients who have no light perception from the time of injury have a poor prognosis, and it is unlikely that any treatment will make a difference in their clinical course. However, for patients who have delayed onset of visual loss or who lose vision upon withdrawal of steroids, especially in the setting of an obvious foramen fracture impinging the optic nerve, it is reasonable to consider more aggressive medical or surgical intervention, particularly if the patient is conscious and can understand the risks and uncertain benefits.

Surgical

Optic nerve decompression may be performed by transcranial or transethmoid routes. Transcranial decompression has been the traditional technique, but it requires a craniotomy and retraction of the frontal lobe. Transethmoid decompression, although technically more difficult, seems to be gaining popularity. It is possible to perform transethmoid decompression with the patient under local anesthesia, during which the medial wall of the optic canal is removed. Visualization of orbital structures is more difficult when this route is chosen and care must be taken to avoid iatrogenic damage to the adjacent carotid artery within the sphenoid sinus.

COMMENTS

The ideal treatment for traumatic optic neuropathy has yet to be determined. The presence or absence of an optic foramen fracture is less important in determining prognosis than is the clinical picture. Complete, immediate visual loss is a poor prognostic sign, and it is likely that any improvement seen after therapy in this setting would have occurred in the absence of treatment.

Currently, there is no standard of care for the use of corticosteroids or optic canal decompression in the treatment of traumatic optic neuropathy with or without optic foramen fracture. Recent animal data suggests that corticosteroids may be detrimental. Neither corticosteroids nor surgical decompression have proven to be definitively beneficial. Therefore, it is reasonable to withhold treatment altogether. Given the risks associated with optic nerve decompression and its uncertain benefits, patients should be directly involved in this decision. Treatment should be individualized on a case-by-case basis.

REFERENCES

Goldberg RA, Steinsapir KD, et al: Extracranial optic canal decompression: Indications and technique. Ophthalmol Plast Reconstr Surg 12:163–170, 1996.

Joseph MP, Lessel S, Rizzo J, et al: Extracranial optic nerve decompression for traumatic optic neuropathy. Arch Ophthalmol 108:1091–1093, 1990.

Levin LA, Beck RW, Joseph MP, et al: The treatment of traumatic optic neuropathy: the International Optic Nerve Trauma Study. Ophthalmol 106:1268–1077, 1999.

Steinsapir KD, Goldberg RA: Traumatic Optic Neuropathy: a critical update. Comp Ophthalmol Update 6:11–21, 2005.

Steinsapir KD, Goldberg RA, Sinha S, et al: Methylprednisolone exacerbates axonal loss following optic nerve trauma in rats. Restor Naurol Neurosci 17:157–163, 2000.

325 ORBITAL CELLULITIS AND ABSCESS 376.01

Kristi Bailey, MD
Portland, Oregon

Orbital cellulitis and abscesses are vision and potentially life threatening diseases, which require prompt evaluation and treatment of patients of all ages, particularly children and the immunosuppressed.

ETIOLOGY/INCIDENCE

- Adjacent sinus disease:
  - Accounts for >80% of cases in children.
- Skin/periocular trauma:
  - Most common cause in adults
- Dacryocystitis.
- Dental infections.
- Otitis media.
- Intracranial infection.
- Intraorbital foreign body.
- Postsurgical.
- Bacteremia.
- Endophthalmitis.
- Dacryoadenitis.

Pathogens

Bacterial

- Children:
  - *Streptococcus pneumonia*;
  - *Staphylococcus aureus*;
  - *Haemophilus influenzae*.

Incidence sharply reduced by the advent of routine vaccination. Can be highly ampicillin resistant.

- Adults:
  - Polymicrobial infections, including *S. pneumonia, S. aureus,* and gram-negative aerobes;
  - Anaerobes, including *Peptostreptococcus, Bacterioides, Clostridium,* and *Fusobacterium*.

Fungal

- Aspergillosis.
- Mucormycosis.

DIAGNOSIS

Clinical signs and symptoms

- Clincal presentation:
  - Orbital pain;
  - Proptosis;
  - Acute febrile illness;
  - Diplopia, decreased ocular motility;
  - Eyelid swelling and erythema;
  - Possible vision loss.
- Pertinent history:
  - Concurrent sinusitis or ear infection;
  - Recent trauma;
  - Recent surgery or dental work;
  - Diabetes;
  - Immunocompromised status.
- Ophthalmic examination:
  - Eyelid or periorbital edema, erythema;
  - Extraocular muscle dysfunction or pain with eye movement;
  - Conjunctival chemosis, injection;
  - Proptosis, with or without decreased visual acuity or pupillary abnormalities, color vision deficits, visual field deficits (best tested with automated static perimetry).

- Physical examination:
  - Fever;
  - Constitutional symptoms (nausea and vomiting, lethargy). More common in children.
- Laboratory:
  - Leukocytosis;
  - Positive blood cultures (more common in children).
- Computed tomography of orbits:
  - Subperiosteal abscess (direct coronal views often delineate best);
  - Adjacent sinus disease, particularly ethmoidal.
- Fungal cellulites:
  - May require tissue biopsy to confirm diagnosis (cultures often are negative).

Differential diagnosis

- Neoplasms:
  - Rhabdomyosarcoma;
  - Lymphoma;
  - Leukemia;
  - Metastastic;
  - Retinoblastoma.
- Thyroid-related ophthalmopathy.
- Orbital inflammation:
  - Orbital pseudotumor;
  - Orbital myositis;
  - Wegener's granulomatosis.
- Arteriovenous malformation.
- Carotid-cavernous sinus fistula.

TREATMENT

- Cultures:
  - Blood;
  - Conjunctiva;
  - Discharge.
- Hospitalization:
  - Intravenous antibiotics for 7 to 10 days;
  - Outpatient oral antibiotics for 5 to 7 days; if concomitant chronic sinusitis or osteomyelitis, may require 3 or more weeks of antibiotics and infectious disease or otolaryngology consultation.
- Infants:
  - Ceftriaxone 50 mg/kg IV every 12 to 24 hours (no more than 4 g/day).
- Children:
  - Nafcillin or oxacillin 12.5 mg/kg IV every 6 hours *and* cefuroxime 25 to 33 mg/kg IV every 8 hours (no more than 4.5 g/day);
  - Penicillin or cephalosporin allergy alternatives: chloramphenicol 12.5 to 25 mg/kg IV every 6 hours (hematologic monitoring).
- Adults:
  - One of the following: ampicillin/sulbactam IV 1.5 g every 6 hours; cefuroxime 1.5 g IV every 8 hours; cefoxitin 2.0 g IV every 8 hours; cefotetan 2.0 g IV every 12 hours;
  - Alternative antibiotics: ticarcillin/clavulanate 3.1 g IV every 4–6 hours; piperacillin tazobactam 3.375 g IV every 6 hours; cefotaxime 2.0 g IV every 4 hours; ceftriaxone 2.0 g IV every 24 hours.
- Sinusitis or dental abscess (upper second molar most common):
  - Oral surgery consultation;
  - May require surgical drainage.
- Fungal cellulites:
  - Aggressive surgical debridement;
  - Infectious disease and otolaryngology consultation;
  - Amphotericin B 0.8 to 1.5 mg/kg/day IV;
  - Correction of predisposing factors (e.g. metabolic acidosis, hyperglycemia).
- Orbital abscess:
  - Children younger than 9 years: often sterile or single organism; if no optic nerve compromise, may observe because these may resolve with antibiotic treatment.
- Adults:
  - Often multiple organisms;
  - Surgical drainage.
- Other treatment considerations:
  - Corneal exposure: lubricants;
  - Ocular hypertension: topical medications; systemic carbonic anhydrase inhibitors.
- Sinus disease:
  - Nasal decongestants: Children: 0.125% phenylephrine; Adults: 0.05% ocymetazoline hydrochloride;
  - Systemic antihistamines.

COMPLICATIONS

- Subperiosteal abscess (7%).
- Meningitis (2%).
- Cavernous sinus thrombosis (1%):
  - Nausea and vomiting;
  - Headache;
  - Disorientation;
  - Contralateral eyelid edema/proptosis;
  - Trigeminal nerve division I and II dysfunction;
  - Episcleral and retinal venous engorgement.
- Visual loss (1%):
  - Corneal exposure;
  - Inflammatory and neovascular glaucoma;
  - Exudative retinal detachment;
  - Optic neuritis;
  - Central retinal vein and artery occlusions.
- Intracranial abscess (1%).
- Osteomyelitis of orbital bones (1%).

REFERENCES

Ambati BK, Ambati J, Azar N, et al: Periorbital and orbital cellulitis before and after the advent of Haemophilus influenzae type B vaccination. Ophthalmology 107(8):1450–1453, 2000.

Jain A, Rubin PA: Orbital cellulitis in children. Internat Ophthalmol Clin 41(4):71–86, 2001.

Uehara F, Ohba N: Diagnostic imaging in patients with orbital cellulitis and inflammatory pseudotumor. Internat Ophthalmol Clin 42(1):133–142, 2002.

326 ORBITAL GRAVES' DISEASE 376.2
(Dysthyroid Orbitopathy, Endocrine Ophthalmopathy, Thyroid-Associated Eye Disease)

Kristi Bailey, MD
Portland, Oregon
Roger A. Dailey MD, FACS
Portland, Oregon

Thyroid-associated eye disease is the most prevalent cause of proptosis and compressive optic neuropathy in adults. Though typically a chronic form of orbital inflammation, it may have acute or subacute presentations. Associated systemic thyroid disease may or may not be present.

ETIOLOGY/INCIDENCE

Graves' disease is an autoimmune disease that affects women three or four times as often as it affects men. Typically, the patient is a woman between the ages of 25 and 50, although Graves' orbitopathy can occur at any age. A history of smoking is highly correlated with development of thyroid eye disease.

COURSE/PROGNOSIS

The spectrum of disease in Graves' orbitopathy is broad, ranging from mild symptoms to severe disfigurement and blindness.

Clinical signs and symptoms

- Dry eyes, foreign body sensation.
- Pain.
- Photophobia.
- Diplopia.
- Eyelid edema.
- Conjunctival hyperemia and chemosis.
- Decreased vision in one or both eyes.
- Eyelid retraction.
- Eyelid lag on downgaze.
- Motility disorders.
- Hyperemia over the rectus muscle insertions.
- Proptosis and exposure keratitis.
- Optic neuropathy.

Patients may present with any combination of symptoms and signs. The active phase of disease usually stabilizes within 6 months.

DIAGNOSIS

The diagnosis is made on clinical grounds that may be supported by laboratory and other noninvasive testing. The key to diagnosis is the ophthalmologic examination, including the following:

- Visual acuity, color vision;
- Pupil examination;
- Extraocular movements and motility measurements;
- Lid evaluation;
- Exophthalmometry;
- Slit-lamp examination (chemosis, keratitis, conjunctival injection);
- Intraocular pressure (looking for significant increase in upgaze relative to primary gaze);
- Fundoscopy (looking for evidence of nerve compression).

Laboratory findings

- Visual field testing.
- Forced duction testing (for restrictive myopathy).
- Computed tomography (CT) scanning or magnetic resonance imaging (MRI).
- Thyroid function testing (T_4 and thyroid-stimulating hormone).
- Thyroid-stimulating immunoglobulins.
- Endocrinology consultation.

Differential diagnosis

- Orbital myositis or pseudotumor.
- Dural or carotid cavernous fistula.
- Orbital tumors.
- Orbital vasculitis (such as Wegener's granulomatois or polyarteritis nodosa).
- Orbital cellulites.

Risk factors

There is no specific prophylactic treatment for Graves' disease to prevent the orbital sequelae. However, smoking has also been implicated as a risk factor for the development and worsening of thyroid eye disease. Patients should be counseled to stop tobacco use.

TREATMENT

Patients with Graves' orbitopathy are managed on an individualized basis according to the predominant clinical findings. Management then is directed at the specific problem or problems.

Ocular

- Ocular lubricants for burning, irritation and keratitis.
- Moisture chambers, swimmer's goggles, or humidifiers for exposure keratitis.
- Sunglasses for photophobia or tearing.
- Taping eyelids at night for lagophthalmos.
- Elevation of the head of bed at night for congestion and lid edema.
- Prisms for diplopia.
- No role for topical steroids; retrobulbar steroids of unproved effectiveness.

Systemic

- The treatment of hyperthyroidism should be performed by an internist or endocrinologist.
- Systemic corticosteroids are utilized for the treatment for congestive signs and symptoms.
- Prednisone 60 to 100 mg/day is indicated as initial, immediate treatment for vision loss from congestive optic neuropathy. If vision continues to decline or does not improve within 2–7 days, orbital decompression surgery is recommended.
- Mild diuretics such as 25 to 50 mg/day hydrochlorothiazide may reduce orbital edema.
- Systemic immunosuppressives (cyclophosphamide, azathioprine, and cyclosporine) and plasmapheresis may have benefit in carefully selected cases.

Radiation

Radiation as a steroid-sparing treatment has a controversial role in the management of the patient with Graves' disease. The primary indication is that the patient has disabling congestive symptoms, including conjunctival chemosis, prolapse, and injection, as well as rapidly progressive proptosis or optic neuropathy. External beam radiation in doses of 2000 cGy are delivered to the orbit in 10 fractions over 2 weeks. Improvement may be seen as early as 2 weeks post radiation, but may take several months for maximum benefit. Therefore, steroid therapy may be best continued for 4 to 6 weeks after completion of the radiation. An exacerbation of inflammatory and congestive symptoms lasting 2–3 weeks is not uncommon following radiation. It is sometimes necessary to increase the steroid dose temporarily during the radiation treatments. As a rule, patients who do not respond to steroids or who are in the fibrotic, non-congestive stage of the disease process will not respond to radiation. Patients at risk of retinopathy, such as diabetics, should probably not be irradiated.

Surgical

- Approximately 10% of patients with clinical Graves' disease will require surgery for myopathy, lid retraction, proptosis, or optic neuropathy.
- Orbital decompression may be performed for compressive optic neuropathy as well as for the less proptotic patient with exposure problems, orbital pain, or pressure. Coronal CT scanning and MRI can be used to identify the underlying pathology and help direct the oculofacial plastic surgeon in planning the surgical strategy.

Numerous surgical techniques for decompression of one to all four of the orbital walls have been described. The amount of proptosis reduction correlates to the number and extent of walls decompressed, as well as to the specific walls chosen.

The transantral Caldwell–Luc medial and inferior wall decompression, was the procedure of choice until the early 1980s. The use of a balanced lateral and medial decompression technique to decrease the incidence of postoperative strabismus and infraorbital parasthesias has become more prominent. The orbital floor may be added to the balanced medial and lateral wall technique for a three-wall decompression yielding further proptosis reduction. Endoscopic techniques may also be employed. The orbital roof is rarely used.

- When the restrictive myopathy of Graves' orbitopathy induces a tropia that has been stable by prism measurement for 6 months or longer (off steroids), eye muscle surgery can help restore ocular alignment. The goal is to create fusion in the primary and reading positions. Adjustable suture techniques are preferable in these patients to ensure a favorable postoperative alignment. Recessions are preferred over resections because of muscle restriction and the tendency for scar formation in the orbit of patients with Graves' disease. Overcorrection is preferred because postoperative adjustment is easier when tightening the sutures (i.e. reducing the recession).
- For patients with primarily eyelid manifestations, several eyelid surgery techniques are available. For upper eyelid retraction of up to 2 mm, excision of Müller's muscle is adequate to correct the problem. For larger amounts of upper eyelid retraction, levator surgery becomes necessary. A variety of procedures have been described, including levator stripping, levator marginal myotomy, recession of the levator aponeurosis, or placement of a spacer (e.g. sclera, dura) between the aponeurosis and the upper tarsal border. Lower eyelid retraction is approached in a similar fashion. Disinsertion or extirpation of the lower lid retractors has been used with varying success. Placement of a spacer between the disinserted capsulopalpebral fascia and the lower border of the tarsus may also be used. Sclera, cartilage, fascia, or a tarsal transplant from the upper lid have all been used successfully as spacers.
- The pathologic process of dysthyroid orbitopathy frequently leads to presenile prolapse of orbital fat in the upper and lower eyelid. This prolapse is caused by a combination of factors, including orbital congestion and inflammation, weakening of the orbital septum, and an increase in the volume of orbital fat. Cosmetic blepharoplasty should be approached with this in mind, concentrating on a more aggressive approach to fat removal while being conservative with skin excision.
- When indicated, orbital decompression should be undertaken before strabismus or eyelid surgery because the decompression may alter the ocular alignment and eyelid position. Similarly, eye muscle surgery, especially inferior rectus recession, will affect the position of the eyelids. Accordingly, when eye muscle surgery is indicated, it is usually done before any contemplated eyelid surgery. Cosmetic blepharoplasty is best reserved for last when patients with Graves' disease require more than one ophthalmic surgical procedure.

COMPLICATIONS

The side effects and complications of corticosteroid therapy are well known. Chronic steroid therapy should be managed with the assistance of an internist or endocrinologist.

Orbital radiation should be performed by a radiation specialist who is experienced with irradiation of the orbit. The retrobulbar area is treated while the globe itself is shielded. Every patient should be informed of the risk, albeit very slight, of radiation-induced cataract or retinopathy.

Complications of orbital decompression include diplopia and strabismus, globe dystopia, periorbital paresthesia and dysesthesia, CSF leak, intraparynchemal injury, lacrimal gland injury, temporalis muscle atrophy, hematoma, globe or optic nerve injury, inadequate decompression, infection, ptosis, or vision loss.

Complications of surgery for lid retraction include ptosis (usually more prominent nasally), persistent retraction (usually more prominent temporally), contour abnormalities, ocular irritation or lid thickening induced by spacers (e.g. sclera), and damage to the lacrimal gland and its ducts.

Eye muscle surgery for restrictive myopathy has the same risks as standard strabismus surgery; however, exposure is usually more difficult because of the tethering effect of the muscles. Adhesions and scarring are more of a problem because of the orbital inflammation, especially in reoperations.

REFERENCES

Bailey KL, Tower RN, Dailey RA: Customized, single-incision, three-wall orbital decompression. Ophthal Plast Reconstruct Surg 21(1):1–9; discussion 9–10, 2005.

Baldeschi L, et al: Early versus late orbital decompression in Graves' orbitopathy: a retrospective study in 125 patients. Ophthalmology. 113(5):874–878, 2006.

Bartalena L, et al: An update on medical management of Graves' ophthalmopathy. J Endocrinolog Invest 28(5):469–478, 2005.

Hatton MP, Rubin PAD: Controversies in thyroid related orbitopathy: radiation and decompression. Internat Ophthalmol Clin 45(4):1–14, 2005.

Kennerdell JS, Maroon JC, Buerger GF: Comprehensive surgical management of proptosis in dysthyroid orbitopathy. Orbit 6:153–179, 1987.

Mizen TR: Thyroid eye disease. Sem Ophthalmol 18(4):243–247, 2003.

Putterman AM: Surgical treatment of thyroid-related upper eyelid retraction. Ophthalmology 88:507–512, 1981.

Rootman J: Graves' orbitopathy. In: Rootman J, ed: Diseases of the orbit. Philadelphia, JB Lippincott, 1988:241–280.

327 ORBITAL HEMORRHAGES 376.32

Klaus D. Teichmann, MD, FRCSC, FRACO, DiplABO
Riyadh, Saudi Arabia

Orbital hemorrhage often occurs acutely. Because there is little room for expansion, any substantial hemorrhage behind the orbital septum will raise intraorbital and intraocular pressure (IOP) and may cause orbital compression or compartment syndrome. The globe is pushed forward until it reaches the limits of anatomic constraint. If bleeding continues, rising intraorbital pressure will compromise blood circulation of the optic nerve and possibly of the globe. Central retinal artery occlusion (CRAO), high IOP, choroidal ischemia, anterior or posterior ischemic optic neuropathy, and direct compressive optic neuropathy are mechanisms by which vision can be lost.

In milder cases, where there is no significant or progressive visual loss, imaging studies, laboratory tests, and a complete work-up may be performed. In severe cases with rapid or progressive visual loss, immediate orbital decompression should be considered to save visual function. Imaging can be undertaken once vision has improved (or at least stabilized). Vision-threatening acute orbital hemorrhage constitutes one of the few true ophthalmologic emergencies, and every ophthalmologist should be prepared to provide prompt and effective treatment.

ETIOLOGY/INCIDENCE

Blunt or penetrating orbital trauma frequently is associated with orbital hemorrhage. Its incidence after retrobulbar injection is reported at 1% or higher but can be significantly reduced with proper technique. Less commonly, periocular or sinus surgery is responsible: orbital hemorrhage was associated with 0.055% of cosmetic lid surgeries (1 in 2000 cases), wITH permanent visual loss in 0.0045% (1 in 20000 cases). Values are higher for orbital surgery.

Violation of the orbital fat is a common cause for postoperative orbital hemorrhage, as traction on orbital fat can tear deep orbital vessels. Local vascular disease (e.g. venous anomalies, advanced atherosclerosis, aneurysms of the ophthalmic artery, arteriovenous malformations, carotid cavernous sinus fistula, lymphangioma, hemangioma) predisposes to orbital hemorrhages, as do some systemic disorders including hypertension, anemia, leukemia, hemophilia and other clotting disorders, uremia, scurvy, sickle cell disease, and malaria. Orbital hemorrhage may occur spontaneously or be precipitated by an increase in venous pressure (e.g. Valsalva maneuvers such as coughing, straining, labor, and weight-lifting and prolonged head-down positioning).

COURSE/PROGNOSIS

Orbital hemorrhage usually takes a benign course, with spontaneous resolution or hematic cyst formation and without any visual loss. Temporary or permanent loss of vision may occur, however, due to retinal or optic nerve damage (particularly with arterial hemorrhages and optic nerve sheath hematomas). Survival time of retinal tissue after a CRAO may be less than 2 hours, whereas permanent optic nerve damage can occur in less than 3 hours. In certain cases, however, all (or some) vision may be regained even when treatment is delayed for several hours or days. Vision regained after the institution of therapeutic measures can be lost again if bleeding continues. Therefore, frequent monitoring over 24 to 48 hours is mandatory. Orbital hemorrhages tend to develop during the first 24 hours after surgery, particularly in the first 3 hours, but may occur as late as several days postoperatively.

DIAGNOSIS

Clinical signs and symptoms

The diagnosis is usually based on history (trauma, surgery, local or systemic predisposing disease) and the typical clinical findings, as follows:

- Symptoms include:
  - Ocular, orbital, and/or periorbital pain;
  - Sensation of pressure;
  - Nausea, vomiting;
  - Diplopia;
  - Dimming of vision up to total unilateral (or bilateral) loss of vision.
- Signs include:
  - Tight or swollen eyelids with or without ecchymoses, ptosis, or lid retraction;
  - Tense orbit with or without proptosis;
  - Immobile globe;
  - Hemorrhagic chemosis of the conjunctiva;
  - High IOP;
  - Cloudy cornea;
  - Afferent pupillary defect or motor anomalies of the pupil;
  - Disk pallor or hyperemia;
  - Disk edema;
  - Pulsating or collapsed retinal arteries;
  - Choroidal folds.

A cherry-red spot and cloudy swelling of the retina are rare. Features suggestive of central retinal vein occlusion indicate possible optic nerve sheath hemorrhage.

Differential diagnosis

This includes orbital compression syndromes without hemorrhage:

- Orbital cellulites;
- Emphysema of the orbit;
- Fluid exudation after thermal burns (particularly where there is facial involvement);
- Carotis-cavernous sinus fistula;

- Granulocytic sarcoma (acute myelogenous leukemia);
- Rhabdomyosarcoma;
- Metastatic neuroblastoma (in children).

PROPHYLAXIS

- Before any ocular and orbital surgery, systemic hypertension, renal disease, Graves' disease, and glaucoma should be noted as factors predisposing to orbital hemorrhage, as should the use of platelet inhibitors (aspirin, dipyridamole, ticlopidine), nonsteroidal antiinflammatory drugs or warfarin. Suspected bleeding disorders should be elucidated based on prothrombin time (PT), partial thromboplastin time (PTT), platelet count, and bleeding and clotting times.
- During surgery, meticulous hemostasis should be maintained with cautery, ligatures, hemostats and simple compression. Traction on the orbital fat should be minimized. Prolapsed fat is removed with unipolar cautery, and visible vessels are coagulated before resection. The distal stump of fat should be examined for bleeding before being released into the orbit. Moist absorbable gelatin sponge segments, soaked in thrombin solution and applied to sites where fat was excised, may help promote hemostasis.
- The use of epinephrine in local anesthesia is not without risk: it may provoke a marked rise in blood pressure, as well as causing a deceptively bloodless field during surgery. Diffuse oozing may then set in once pharmacological vasoconstriction has subsided.
- A rubber (Penrose) drain or a suction drain (Hemovac) is advisable for deep orbital surgery.
- In any orbital surgery, the wound should not be closed until bleeding has stopped completely.
- After completion of the surgery, tight bandages, if used at all, should not be left on for longer than 30 to 60 minutes. If pain is reported, they should be removed immediately and the surgical site should be most closely monitored.
- Gauze pads soaked in iced saline may decrease postoperative swelling and abort hemorrhage.
- After any lid or orbital surgery, the patient's head should be elevated 30 to 40 degrees.
- Close postoperative observation is mandatory. Patients should be asked to immediately report severe or sudden pain. In case of doubt, look for proptosis or ecchymosis; check IOP, vision and pupillary action; examine the fundus for optic disk swelling or pallor and to rule out complete or partial CRAO. Postoperatively, vomiting, coughing, strenuous physical activity and bending over should be avoided for several days.

TREATMENT

Systemic

- Most orbital hemorrhages require no treatment; patients should merely be observed.
- Imaging studies (computed tomography, magnetic resonance imaging, ultrasound) may provide valuable information about extent and location of a hemorrhage (intraconal, extraconal, within optic nerve sheath, subperiosteal, sub-Tenon, preseptal), possible associated bony injuries, intracranial injury, intraocular or intraorbital foreign bodies, and underlying disease (e.g. lymphangioma).
- Imaging studies are crucial in diagnosing optic nerve compression, which may be present even when intraorbital pressure is normal.
- Preliminary orbital decompression may be required before time-consuming imaging studies are performed. These should, however, be requested wherever possible because they are likely to provide valuable diagnostic information, as well as guidance for definitive surgical management.
- Relevant laboratory tests, if not done before surgery, should be performed if a bleeding diathesis is suspected.
- Medication is used to control blood pressure and bleeding disorders.
- Analgesics (not aspirin) and antiemetics are administered as required.
- Intravenous acetazolamide or hyperosmotic agents cannot effectively decompress the orbit, but may be tried.
- Systemic steroids (e.g. 250 mg methylprednisolone IV every 6 hours for several days) may be given to reduce orbital swelling, decrease vascular permeability, and protect the optic nerve from ischemic damage.
- Megadose steroids (e.g. methylprednisolone: initial dose of 30 mg/kg IV; followed by 5.4 mg/kg/hour IV for 48 hours) may be given in the presence of optic nerve sheath hemorrhage.
- If vision recovers, taper the steroids over one week.
- If vision fails to regenerate, discontinue the steroids after 2 days.
- Other neuroprotective agents are under investigation and may be useful in the future.

Ocular

- Lubrication to prevent exposure keratopathy.
- Topical medications to lower IOP are usually ineffective but may be tried.
- Ice-cold compresses may reduce tissue swelling, stop bleeding, and prolong survival time of neural tissue.
- Direct compression applied to the orbit may help arrest bleeding, but compromises perfusion. The same is true for compression of the ipsilateral carotid artery.

Surgical

Surgical decompression is the cornerstone of therapy for orbital hemorrhage. It can be achieved in different ways: (1) through the release of orbital tension by means of canthotomy, cantholysis, or fracturing the orbital floor, or (2) through drainage of blood from the orbit.

- Lateral canthotomy and inferior cantholysis (possibly followed by superior cantholysis) effectively lower a raised intraorbital pressure. Straight scissors are used for making a horizontal cut from the lateral canthal angle to the orbital rim. The lower eyelid is stretched anteriorly and the inferior crus of the lateral canthal tendon is severed with the scissors, at which time the lower eyelid should swing away from the globe.
- If decompression is inadequate after cantholysis, the orbital septum may need to be opened across the eyelids.
- In the absence of a surgical wound, Steven scissors can be inserted through the conjunctiva and Tenon's capsule in the inferior nasal quadrant, between the medial and the inferior rectus muscles. By inserting and spreading the scissors (but not cutting), or by inserting an 18-gauge needle, a retrobulbar hemorrhage can at times be drained.

- Where there is a surgical wound, it should be opened, any hematoma should be drained, and bleeding vessels should be cauterized or tied.
- Subperiosteal hemorrhages can be drained directly.
- If drainage fails, a small curved mosquito clamp can be inserted through an opening made in the inferior nasal fornix. The closed clamp is advanced posteriorly, with its convex side upwards, along the medial orbital floor for about 20 mm. Rotational pressure then is applied, breaking the orbital floor and the maxillary sinus mucosa. The defect is enlarged by spreading and rotating the blades of the clamp. This maneuver may be facilitated by a preceding lateral canthotomy and inferior cantholysis.
- Exploration of the orbit may become necessary if hemorrhage continues, in order to identify the source of the bleeding and permit meticulous cautery of bleeding points, drainage of fluid blood, and removal of clots. The most likely source of bleeding is the ophthalmic artery or its branches (including the anterior and posterior ethmoidal arteries). The latter can be approached by means of a semicircular incision medial to the nasal canthus, followed by wide opening of the periosteum and removal of ethmoidal cells including the lamina papyracea.
- In diffuse oozing, the local application of hemostatic agents (e.g. topical thrombin, absorbable gelatin sponge, microfibrillar collagen) and compression may achieve hemostasis. In some cases of diffuse bleeding, the increased volume of orbital tissues may require extensive decompression through removal of the orbital floor and the medial orbital wall.
- If optic nerve compression is localized to the orbital apex, the posterior ethmoid should be removed.
- For optic nerve sheath hematomas, fenestration of the optic nerve sheath and removal of blood clots is mandatory in cases where visual function fails to recover after orbital decompression.
- Intraoperatively, pupillary response to light, flash visual evoked potentials, or — provided the patient is awake — visual acuity can serve as guides for success of decompression. The wound should be closed only after all bleeding has ceased. Insertion of a drain is advisable.

COMPLICATIONS

Complications include permanent loss of vision, delayed wound healing, infection, hematic cyst formation, cholesterol granulomas, discoloration of the skin, fibrosis, enophthalmus, motility restriction, diplopia, lid retraction, ectropion, entropion, and infraorbital nerve anesthesia (which may be transient).

COMMENTS

Preseptal orbital hemorrhages do not require surgical intervention.

Direct compression of the optic nerve may be present in the absence of raised intraorbital pressure. It can be due to optic nerve sheath hematoma, subperiosteal hemorrhage near the orbital apex, or large intraconal blood clots. Surgical evacuation through a medial or lateral orbitotomy or via an ethmoidectomy (near the orbital apex) is often required if the optic nerve is compromised.

For non-vision-threatening subperiosteal hemorrhages, surgical drainage is recommended only if the blood has not spontaneously resorbed after a few weeks.

Anterior chamber paracentesis as an emergency measure in orbital hemorrhage may convert a hard globe with a formed anterior chamber into a hard globe with an absent anterior chamber. Because its effect is small and the procedure is fraught with complications, it is not recommended as treatment of high IOP in the presence of a high intraorbital pressure.

REFERENCES

Bains RA, Rubin PAD: Blunt orbital trauma. Int Ophthalmol Clin 35:37–46, 1995.

Hargaden M, Goldberg SH, Cunningham D, et al: Optic neuropathy following simulation of orbital hemorrhage in the nonhuman primate. Ophthal Plast Reconstr Surg 12:264–272, 1996.

Liu D: A simplified technique of orbital decompression for severe retrobulbar hemorrhage. Am J Ophthalmol 116:34–37, 1993.

Yung CW, Moorthy RS, Lindley D, et al: Efficacy of lateral canthotomy and cantholysis in orbital hemorrhage. Ophthal Plast Reconstr Surg 10:137–141, 1994.

SECTION

30 Retina

328 ACQUIRED RETINOSCHISIS 361.10, 361.12 *(Degenerative Retinoschisis, Senile Retinoschisis)*

M. Vaughn Emerson, MD
Portland, Oregon
J. Timothy Stout, MD, PhD
Portland, Oregon

ETIOLOGY/INCIDENCE

Acquired retinoschisis is a degenerative condition in which splitting of the peripheral retina occurs at the level of the outer plexiform layer. This results in the formation of an inner layer (closer to the vitreous) and an outer layer (closer to the retinal pigmented epithelium). The resulting schisis cavity gives the retina a cystic appearance, which in more extensive cases may appear bullous.

The condition occurs in 1% to 4% of the population; it occurs in 7% of patients older than 40 and is most frequent in patients older than 50. This distinguishes it from juvenile retinoschisis, which occurs in a much younger population. Juvenile retinoschisis is characterized by schisis at the level of the nerve fiber layer and an X-linked recessive mode of transmission, and is associated with mutations in the *XLRS-1* gene. Acquired retinoschisis is usually bilateral (77–85%) and has a predilection for the inferotemporal peripheral retina (80%). The incidence is equal in men and women.

The pathogenesis is unknown. Circulatory compromise may be a factor because the peripheral retina is in a circulatory 'watershed' zone. Chronic vitreous traction, perhaps associated with the chronic motility effects of accommodation on the peripheral retina, may also play a role.

COURSE/PROGNOSIS

- Patients are usually asymptomatic, and the condition is discovered on routine examination of the peripheral retina.
- Schisis extends posterior to the equator in 74% of eyes. Progression of posterior extent (more than two disk diameters) occurs in 3% of eyes.
- Circumferential extension (extension of more than one clock hour) is seen in 6% of eyes.
- A new area of developing retinoschisis is seen in 10% of eyes.
- Two percent of eyes will demonstrate spontaneous disappearance of retinoschisis.
- New retinal breaks occur in 6% of eyes, in either the inner or the outer layer of the retinoschisis.
- Schisis-associated retinal detachment occurs in 6% of eyes when fluid passes through an outer layer break and the outer layer comes into apposition with the inner layer.
- Of eyes with outer-layer breaks, 50% to 60% will develop schisis-associated detachments.
- Symptomatic progressive retinal detachment that extends beyond the limits of the schisis cavity occurs in 0 to 0.05% of eyes.

DIAGNOSIS

Clinical signs and symptoms

- Acquired retinoschisis is generally very slowly progressive, as a result, patients are typically asymptomatic. Rarely, posterior extension or associated retinal detachment may lead to severe visual loss.
- New onset of symptoms (photopsias, floaters, or visual field loss) may occur in conjunction with an unrelated posterior vitreous detachment and are usually not related to the schisis.
- The refraction is hyperopic in 80% of patients.
- The inner layer may be pitted in appearance, and 70% of eyes have tiny, glistening yellow-white dots.
- Degenerative retinoschisis may be associated with peripheral cystoid degeneration and pars plana cysts.
- Peripheral blood vessels may appear sclerotic.
- Inner layer breaks, which are usually tiny and difficult to detect ophthalmoscopically, occur in 2% of eyes.
- Outer layer breaks, which are often much larger and have characteristic rolled edges, are present in 4% to 5% of eyes.
- The presence of inner- and outer-layer breaks rarely occurs and may lead to retinal detachment.

Laboratory findings

- An *absolute* scotoma in the area of the retinoschisis is present on visual field testing (in contrast to a *relative* scotoma in retinal detachment).
- Ultrasonography (including B-scan and ultrasonic biomicroscopy) demonstrates a minimally mobile, thin membrane in the retinal periphery that cannot be decompressed with scleral depression (in contrast to rhegmatogenous

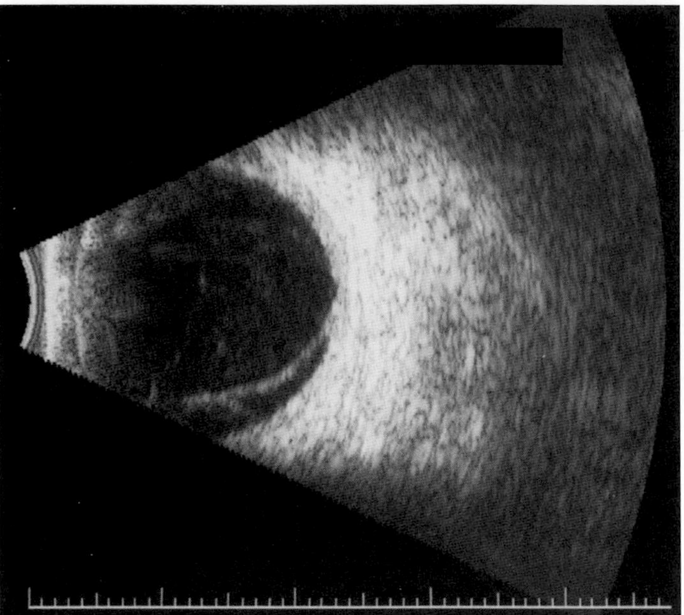

FIGURE 328.1. B-scan ultrasound of retinoschisis.

retinal detachment, in which the subretinal space can be decompressed). This may be useful in cases in which medial opacity inhibits indirect ophthalmoscopy (Figure 328.1).

- Laser photocoagulation will cause a whitening reaction in the outer layer (in contrast to a retinal detachment in which a reaction to laser photocoagulation will not be apparent).
- Optical coherence tomography (OCT) can be used to help differentiate between schisis and detachment.

Differential diagnosis

- Rhegmatogenous retinal detachment: unilateral, relative scotoma on visual field, no reaction to laser photocoagulation; progressive, elevation may be decompressed with scleral depression.
- Retinal macrocyst: associated with long-standing rhegmatogenous retinal detachment; other signs of chronicity may also be seen, including demarcation lines and retinal atrophy and thinning.
- Exudative retinal detachment: shifting fluid may be seen; signs of inflammation or tumor of the retina or choroid may be apparent.
- Tractional retinal detachment: foci of fibrovascular proliferation causing traction are seen; the retina has a concave appearance; traction can cause a secondary retinoschisis, but this is a different entity.
- Choroidal detachment: the detachment is a solid structure under the retina, associated with hypotony; detachment may be present for 360 degrees and apices may localize to the vortex veins.
- Optic nerve pit: from 30% to 40% of patients with optic nerve pit have macular detachment, which may in fact be a macular schisis cavity.
- Venous occlusive disease: patients with central or branch retinal vein occlusion may develop secondary retinoschisis in the distribution of the affected vein; this will be located in the posterior part of the retina and not the periphery, as is seen in acquired retinoschisis.
- Juvenile retinoschisis: this is associated with young males, an X-linked recessive mode of transmission, and a higher percentage of vitreous hemorrhage (21%) and retinal detachment (16%).

PROPHYLAXIS

Although prophylaxis has been recommended in the past to prevent the progression of retinoschisis or to prevent the formation of a rhegmatogenous retinal detachment, no modality (diathermy, retinal cryopexy, laser photocoagulation) has been demonstrated to be clinically beneficial and in some cases may have worsened the outcome (resulting in retinal detachment, vitreous hemorrhage, maculopathy and proliferative vitreoretinopathy). As a result, prophylactic treatment of acquired retinoschisis is not advised. Asymptomatic localized nonprogressive schisis detachments and retinoschisis with outer layer breaks are the only known precursors of symptomatic progressive retinal detachments and thus should be monitored every 6 months. Treatment should be administered only if symptomatic retinal detachment is seen.

TREATMENT

The treatment of acquired retinoschisis is limited to patients who develop symptomatic, progressive schisis-associated retinal detachments. Local or systemic nonsurgical treatment is not necessary. Bilateral patching of the eyes may be helpful in decreasing the height of the retinal detachment, making surgical intervention easier.

Surgical

- Configuration of the outer layer breaks will determine the mode of treatment.
- Larger and posterior outer layer breaks are difficult to treat with a standard scleral buckle; buckling is associated with a higher incidence of macular distortion.
- Smaller and peripheral outer layer breaks causing schisis-detachments are treated with a standard scleral buckle, retinal cryopexy, and external subretinal fluid drainage. The external drainage is attempted in the bed of the outer layer break; this may allow the drainage of subretinal fluid and collapse of the schisis cavity. Even if the retinoschisis cavity does not collapse, as long as the outer layer break is supported, the retina should remain attached.
- For schisis detachments with large and posterior outer-layer breaks, pars plana vitrectomy with internal drainage, laser photocoagulation, and gas-fluid exchange is recommended. Pars plana vitrectomy is performed; as much of the posterior hyaloid as can be removed without tearing the inner layer of the schisis cavity is removed. If an inner-layer break overlies a posterior outer-layer break, internal drainage is done through the inner-layer break to drain subretinal and schisis cavity fluid. If an inner-layer break is not present, endodiathermy is used to make an opening in the inner layer over a posterior outer-layer break. Once the retina is flattened, endolaser is used to surround the outer-layer breaks; any areas that are not sufficiently flat are treated with retinal cryopexy. Long-acting gas or silicone oil is injected into the vitreous cavity. A scleral buckle to support the vitreous base may also be placed. Reported complications of this approach include cataract, epiretinal membrane, and proliferative vitreoretinopathy requiring additional surgery.

REFERENCES

Ambler JS, Meyers SM, Zegarra H, et al: The management of retinal detachment complicating degenerative retinoschisis. Am J Ophthalmol 107:171–176, 1989.

Byer NE: Clinical study of senile retinoschisis. Arch Ophthalmol 79:36–44, 1968.

Byer NE: Long-term natural history study of senile retinoschisis with implications for management. Ophthalmology 93:1127–1137, 1986.

George NDL, Yates JRW, Moore AT: Clinical features in affected males with X-linked retinoschisis. Arch Ophthalmol 114:274–280, 1996.

Sneed SR, Bodi CF, Folk JC, et al: Pars plana vitrectomy in the management of retinal detachments associated with degenerative retinoschisis. Ophthalmology 97:470–474, 1990.

329 ACUTE RETINAL NECROSIS 362.84 *(Necrotizing Herpetic Retinopathy)*

Mark S. Blumenkranz, MD
Menlo Park, California

Acute retinal necrosis is an ocular viral syndrome predominantly affecting the retina that is associated with four cardinal features:

- Confluent peripheral retinal necrosis with discrete borders associated with rapid circumferential progression in untreated eyes;
- Occlusive vasculopathy with predominantly arteriolar involvement;
- Vitreous and anterior chamber inflammation;
- Variable optic neuropathy.

If untreated, the disease is associated with rapid progression and severe vision loss, with bilaterality common. If untreated, more than three-fourths of patients will develop complex forms of retinal detachment and severe vision loss.

ETIOLOGY/INCIDENCE

The disease is thought to be caused by recrudescence of infection in the retina and adjacent ocular tissues with members of the herpes simplex virus-most typically herpes varicella virus and less often herpes simplex viruses I and II in immunocompetent individuals. Most cases are thought to represent reactivation of dormant virus from the dorsal root ganglia followed by hematogenous or neurotransmission spread to the eye. The distribution of the disease appears to be worldwide, wit an annual approximate calculated incidence of 4.25 in 1 million population in one study. This represents approximately 2.5% of the patients with uveitis seen at a large referral center. Males are thought to be more commonly affected than females, representing approximately two-thirds of reported cases. HLA phenotypes Bw62, DR4, and HLA-DR9 have been associated with increased frequency and severity of disease.

COURSE/PROGNOSIS

The course of untreated acute retinal necrosis is usually unfavorable in most patients; if the disease is untreated, most patients develop extensive zones of confluent necrotizing retinitis, optic neuropathy, and, ultimately, retinal detachment (more than 75% of patients). Most commonly, there is a documented history of antecedent infection with herpes simplex, herpes varicella zoster, or simplex virus, although this may be remote, dating back to childhood chickenpox. A mild or limited form of acute retinal necrosis may follow acute herpes varicella zoster virus infection (chickenpox), particularly in adults, but this is exceedingly rare in children. A particularly severe form of acute retinal necrosis with distinctive features, termed *progressive outer retinal necrosis,* may occur in immunocompromised patients, particularly those with human immunodeficiency virus (HIV) infection. However, most patients with acute retinal necrosis are immunologically normal and have no immediate active preceding infection, although the necrosis occasionally follows an episode of shingles. With modern therapy, including antiviral drugs, anti-inflammatory medications, antithrombotic therapy, and laser prophylaxis, many of the most severe complications of the disease can be ameliorated or prevented.

DIAGNOSIS

Laboratory findings

The diagnosis is generally established on the basis of the characteristic slit-lamp and ophthalmoscopic findings, including:

- Acute vision loss secondary to vitreous inflammation, retinitis, and optic neuropathy, to varying degrees;
- Pain secondary to anterior uveitis or scleritis;
- Peripheral confluent zones of creamy-appearing necrotizing retinitis with dentate margins and circumferential spread;
- Obliterative vasculopathy-predominantly arteriolar sheathing and occlusion with associated peripheral retinal capillary nonperfusion.

Laboratory findings may demonstrate evidence of a previous infection with herpes varicella zoster or herpes simplex virus, although acute rises in titers of IgM to either agent are uncommon. Direct sampling of intraocular fluid by conventional viral culture techniques, and particularly polymerase chain reaction methods, may be useful although it is generally not required to establish the diagnosis.

- Suggested laboratory evaluation should exclude other treatable infectious processes and specific immunologic syndromes and should include complete blood cell count, sedimentation rate, antinuclear antibody, rheumatoid factor, VDRL syphilis test, fluorescent treponemal antibody absorption test, neurologic studies for HIV, blood urea nitrogen, creatinine, urinalysis, chest radiograph, and skin testing with purified protein derivative (PPD), in addition to serologic studies for evidence of prior infection with herpes simplex virus, herpes varicella zoster virus, and cytomegalovirus.
- In patients with severe vision loss out of proportion to ophthalmologic findings or other symptoms, including headache, change in mental status, or dermatologic manifestations of viral infection, optional tests may include computed tomography or magnetic resonance imaging of the orbit and optic nerve, aqueous tap for assessment of intraocular antibody production of herpes viruses and herpes viral DNA by polymerase chain reaction (if available), and vitrectomy in severe cases associated with atypical clinical presentation,

associated immunocompromise, or retinal detachment or in patients found to be resistant to initial therapy.

Differential diagnosis

- Syphilitic neuroretinitis.
- Cytomegalovirus retinitis.
- Toxoplasmic retinal choroiditis.
- *Candida albicans* endophthalmitis.
- Acute multifocal hemorrhagic retinal vasculitis.
- Behçet's disease.
- Sarcoidosis.
- Ocular lymphoblastic lymphoma.

PROPHYLAXIS

There is no generally accepted prophylaxis for the development of disease in the first eye, but the use of intravenous and oral aciclovir, valciclovir or famciclovir and possibly other antiviral agents, is thought to be protective against the subsequent development of viral infection of the fellow eye in patients who present initially with unilateral disease. In addition, in patients who have active necrotizing retinitis, barrier peripheral laser photocoagulation of the retina may be effective in preventing the later development of retinal detachment.

Retinal detachment prophylaxis

Ultimately, the most frequent cause of vision loss in patients with acute retinal necrosis is late retinal detachment commonly associated with proliferative vitreoretinopathy. The use of peripheral laser photocoagulation to demarcate zones of anterior necrotic retina from the remainder of the retina appears to be beneficial in reducing the likelihood of this complication. In one series, only 17% of patients receiving laser photocoagulation developed retinal detachment, compared with approximately two-thirds of patients not receiving photocoagulation. The photocoagulation is limited to the anterior periphery and demarcates zones of necrotic retina in a nonspecific, diffuse panretinal pattern. Because patients may have associated pain and media opacities, retrobulbar anesthesia and the use of longer wavelengths, particularly yellow, red, and infrared, may be helpful. Patients with more severe intraocular inflammation may not have sufficient media clarity to permit this and therefore may be at higher risk for retinal detachment. The benefits of prophylactic vitrectomy and photocoagulation for this condition have not been established, nor have the prophylactic effects of scleral buckling, although this may be of value when media opacities prevent prophylactic photocoagulation.

TREATMENT

Systemic

The mainstay of treatment for this condition is antiviral therapy directed against members of the herpes simplex virus family. The traditional drug of choice is 1500 mg/m^2/day aciclovir IV in three divided daily doses. Aciclovir is active against both herpes simplex and herpes zoster virus at dosages thought to be achieved within the eye after intravenous administration. Aciclovir may also be administered via the oral route, although the efficacy of this route of administration has not been well established relative to intravenous aciclovir. More recently, valciclovir and famciclovir have surpassed oral aciclovir because of superior bioavailability. The drug may be administered at a dosage of 1000 mg/day to 4 g/day IV and is available in either 200 or 800 mg strengths. After 7 to 10 days of intravenous administration, it is recommended that patients receive oral therapy for an additional 3 weeks because active viral particles have been identified in eyes that have received intravenous therapy for 1 week. Newer agents thought to have greater bioavailability than aciclovir via an oral route are available and may be substituted, although clinic experience remains limited with these agents; these include famciclovir, which has been found to be effective in the treatment of patients with acute herpes zoster in the prevention of postherpetic neuralgia in doses of 500 mg t.i.d. Valciclovir may also be administered at 1000 mg/day TID and is thought to be as effective as five daily doses of 800 mg of aciclovir in the treatment of cutaneous herpes zoster infection. One recent study suggested that 1000 mg/day of valciclovir (Valtrex) was as effective as intravenous aciclovir in a small series of patients.

Anti-inflammatories

The second component of therapy in this disease consists of reduction in intraocular inflammation, particularly in the vitreous cavity, to reduce the likelihood of subsequent vitreous scarring, contracture, and late retinal detachment. The administration of oral prednisone or equivalent corticosteroids in dosages of 0.5 to 1.5 mg/kg/day is recommended approximately 24 to 48 hours after the initiation of antiviral therapy, to be gradually tapered over 1 to 3 weeks. The exact duration of steroid therapy is dictated by the severity of the intraocular inflammation and any associated complications of therapy.

Antithrombotics

Because patients have visual loss associated with arteriolar occlusions in the retina and optic nerve, antiplatelet therapy with aspirin is thought to be potentially beneficial. Platelet hyperaggregation may be increased and can be treated with aspirin 500 to 650 mg/day. The use of more aggressive forms of anticoagulation, including heparin or Coumadin, does not appear to be warranted.

Ocular

Most patients have associated anterior granulomatous uveitis, including keratic precipitates and anterior chamber cell and flare, often related to fibrinoid changes in the aqueous. Topical steroids and cycloplegics are useful in reducing pain and inflammation; the use of topical antiviral agents is not considered necessary.

Surgical

In patients who develop retinal detachment, vitrectomy can be of benefit in reattaching the retina and improving vision. Previous studies suggest that although scleral buckling may be effective in some patients, vitrectomy is required to relieve vitreoretinal traction and permit optimal tamponade with either gas (preferably) or silicone oil (if necessary) in patients due to the large number, size, and posterior extent of retinal breaks. The use of a supplementary scleral buckle associated with vitrectomy may be associated with ocular complications, including ocular hypertension, fibrin syndrome, and choroidal detachment. This is not absolutely required in patients in whom adequate vitreous traction release associated with photocoagulation and long-term tamponade can be achieved, although it is not contraindicated.

COMPLICATIONS

The principal complications are complex retinal detachment associated with proliferative vitreoretinopathy, optic atrophy, cataract, macular epiretinal membrane, and hypotony. Giant tears of the retinal pigment epithelium have been described, and patients with severe intractable inflammation or irreparable retinal detachment frequently develop phthisis bulbi.

REFERENCES

Aslanides IM, de Souza S, Wong D, et al: Oral valacylovir in the treatment of acute retinal necrosis. Retina 22:352–354, 2002.

Blumenkranz MS, Clarkson J, Culbertson WW, et al: visual results in complications after retinal reattachment in the ARN syndrome: the influence of operative technique. Retina 9:170–174, 1989.

Blumenkranz MS, Culbertson WW, Clarkson JG, et al: Treatment of the ARN syndrome with intravenous acyclovir. Ophthalmology 93:296–300, 1986.

Culbertson WW, Blumenkranz MS, Haines H, et al: The ARN syndrome. Part 2: histopathology and etiology. Ophthalmology 89:1317–1325, 1982.

Duker JS, Blumenkranz MS: Diagnosis and management of the ARN syndrome. Surv Ophthalmol 35:327–343, 1991.

Engstrom RE, Holland GN, Margolis TP, et al: The progressive outer retinal necrosis syndrome (PORN): a variant of necrotizing herpetic retinopathy in patients with AIDS. Ophthalmology 101:1488–1502, 1994.

Figueroa MS, Garabito I, Guiterrez C, et al: Famciclovir for the treatment of ARN syndrome. Am J Ophthalmol 123:255–56, 1997.

330 BRANCH RETINAL VEIN OCCLUSION 362.36

Thomas Hwang, MD
Portland, Oregon
Michael Klein, MD
Portland, Oregon

ETIOLOGY/INCIDENCE

Branch retinal vein occlusion (BRVO) is a common disorder characterized by downstream effects of blocked blood flow in a branch retinal vein. The blockage most frequently occurs at an arteriovenous intersection. Rarely, an underlying inflammatory condition may cause secondary branch retinal vein occlusion in locations other than arteriovenous crossings.

It is thought that venous occlusion results in increased capillary pressure and subsequent damage of the capillaries, resulting in ischemia. The exact mechanism for this process is not clearly understood. One important response to ischemia is production of vascular endothelial growth factor (VEGF), which promotes vascular permeability and neovascularization. Capillary damage and increased hydrostatic pressure combined with factors such as VEGF result in leakage and retinal edema. Ischemia, retinal edema, and retinal neovascularization are the major causes of vision loss from BRVO.

Population based studies have found the prevalence of BRVO to be 0.6–1.0%, depending on the age distribution of the group being studied. The condition occurs more frequently in older patients, usually in the seventh decade of life. Hypertension is a consistent risk factor found across multiple studies. Other risk factors, such as glaucoma, diabetes, smoking, cardiovascular disease, and body mass index, are reported by some but not by all.

COURSE/PROGNOSIS

The natural history of a branch retinal vein occlusion varies widely. In some patients, it may be an incidental finding without any symptoms. The location and the extent of retinal involvement as well as perfusion status are important determinants of the prognosis. Vision loss usually results from macular edema, macular ischemia, or complications of neovascularization, including vitreous hemorrhage, traction detachment, and rubeosis irides. The overall prognosis is good for patients with branch retinal vein occlusion, as 50–60% will maintain visual acuity of 20/40 or better after one year.

DIAGNOSIS

Clinical signs and symptoms

Patients with branch retinal vein occlusion usually present with decreased vision. The hallmark of an acute branch retinal vein occlusion is intraretinal hemorrhages in the territory of a retinal vein branch (Figure 330.1). Nerve fiber layer infarcts, retinal edema, intraretinal lipid exudation, and venous dilation and tortuosity are also commonly seen. Branch retinal vein occlusions of the superotemporal quadrant are most frequently found, but occlusions involving the nasal quadrants probably present rarely to the ophthalmologist.

With time, the intraretinal hemorrhages resolve. Sclerosis of both arterioles and venules in the affected area, telangiectatic-appearing vessels-which may represent capillary dilation or

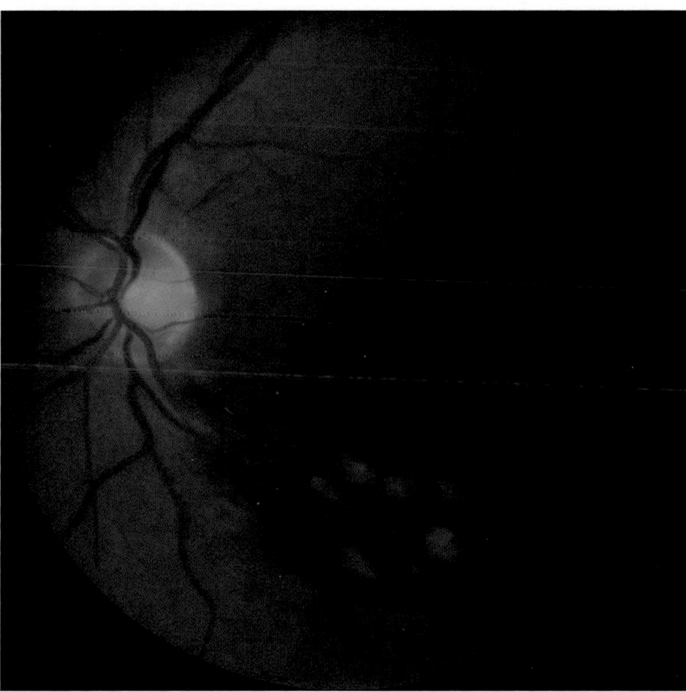

FIGURE 330.1. Branch retinal vein occlusion.

collaterals and microaneurysms are common findings in patients with chronic BRVO. Without the characteristic intraretinal hemorrhages, diagnosis of a chronic branch retinal vein occlusion can be challenging.

Vision loss in branch retinal vein occlusion is caused by macular edema, macular ischemia and neovascular complications. Macular edema may be present in both acute and chronic phases of the disease. Occasionally, distant peripheral vein occlusion can result in macular edema, supposedly mediated by factors such as VEGF.

Eyes with significant capillary non-perfusion may develop retinal neovascularization, and some of these will develop vitreous hemorrhage. Rubeosis irides is an infrequent but serious complication of branch retinal vein occlusion, occurring in about 1% of affected eyes.

Laboratory findings

When patients with branch retinal vein occlusion present with extensive retinal hemorrhages, ancillary testing such as fluorescein angiography is not useful, as the hemorrhages obscure too much of the retinal vasculature.

Once the hemorrhages have cleared sufficiently, a high-quality fluorescein angiogram should be obtained to determine the perfusion status. Non-perfused branch retinal vein occlusions, or those with five or more areas of retinal capillary non-perfusion, have a 40% chance of retinal neovascularization. Sixty percent of these patients may develop vitreous hemorrhage. Those with perfused branch retinal vein occlusion are thought to be at low risk for neovascular complications.

The angiographic appearance of the parafoveal capillaries can guide determination whether the vision is limited by perfused edema or ischemic changes. A branch retinal vein occlusion is considered to have perfused edema when the parafoveal capillary network is intact and leakage is present from the vessels. This determination is particularly important for patients being considered for grid laser photocoagulation (see below) as the Branch Vein Occlusion Study results can only be applied to those patients with perfused edema.

Fluorescein angiography could also be helpful in situations when telangiectatic vessels are present. The characteristic appearance of collateral vessels can help make a diagnosis of chronic branch retinal vein occlusion. In those situations when clinical determination of neovascularization versus telangiectatic vessels is impossible, marked, early angiographic leakage from the vessels can help make a diagnosis of neovascularization.

High-resolution optical coherence tomography (OCT) is helpful in following retinal edema in the setting of branch retinal vein occlusion. Objective and quantitative retinal thickness measurements can aid in treatment decision making, especially when newer pharmacologic agents are considered.

Differential diagnosis

Diabetic retinopathy and hypertensive retinopathy can have many of the characteristics of branch retinal vein occlusion, including intraretinal hemorrhages, nerve fiber layer infarcts, macular edema, lipid exudation and retinal neovascularization. Branch retinal vein occlusions differ from those conditions in their localization along a retinal vein territory.

Retinal vasculitides with venous involvement, such as sarcoidosis and Eales disease, may have some features of vein occlusion, such as venous sheathing and tortunosity. They may also have associated branch retinal vein occlusions. These underlying conditions should be considered, especially when branch retinal vein occlusion occurs in atypical locations, i.e. away from arteriovenous crossings.

Patients with retinal macroaneurysms may present with retinal hemorrhages and macular edema that appear to follow a vascular territory. This condition is also associated with hypertension. Fluorescein angiography may be helpful in identifying macroaneurysms. Branch retinal vein occlusion may occur concurrently as a result of a macroaneurysm.

Sclerotic arterioles of chronic branch retinal vein occlusion can be mistaken for old branch artery occlusion. Associated telangiectatic changes of the vessels are usually not present with arterial occlusion.

The telangiectatic-appearing vessels of a chronic branch retinal vein occlusion can mimic the appearance of idiopathic parafoveal retinal telangiectasis and the two can be difficult to differentiate. While many cases can be distinguished based on location, history and longitudinal follow-up may be necessary in others.

Sometimes the same telangiectatic-appearing vessels as appear in BRVO are mistaken for intraretinal microvascular abnormalities (IRMA) of diabetic retinopathy. Although the two conditions both cause dilated, tortuous intraretinal capillaries, IRMA in diabetic retinopathy is usually not concentrated in a quadrant along a vascular territory.

PROPHYLAXIS

No effective means of prophylaxis is known.

TREATMENT

Systemic

Systemic anticoagulation has not been shown to prevent or affect the clinical course of branch retinal vein occlusion and is not recommended at this time.

Ocular

Most treatments for BRVO are aimed at specific vision-threatening complications of the disease. Limited surgical options have been tried to reverse the underlying vascular occlusion and thus eliminate the inciting causes of those downstream complications. They are discussed in the following sections.

Medical

Pharmacotherapy for BRVO is aimed at treating macular edema. Although the Collaborative Branch Vein Occlusion Study (BVOS) has shown that grid laser photocoagulation is effective for increasing the chances of visual improvement with treatment for perfused macular edema (discussed below), there remained many eyes that did not respond to laser treatment or the results of the BVOS could not be applied.

There is most published experience with intravitreal corticosteroids, particularly triamcinolone acetonide. The actions of corticosteroids are multiple and non-specific, but include reduction of vascular permeability. Many have reported significant and sometimes dramatic improvement in vision and macular thickness with intravitreal triamcinolone acetonide at doses ranging from 2 to 25 mg. At least temporary improvement of vision and OCT evidence of decreased retinal thickness were seen in eyes that did not respond to BVOS-style laser or meet the criteria for grid laser.

Patients with persistent macular edema following laser photocoagulation could be considered for treatment with intravitreal triamcinolone acetonide. Eyes that are not eligible for BVOS grid laser because they have ischemic edema should first be observed, since spontaneous resolution of edema may be more frequent in these eyes than those with perfused edema.

Typically, the eye is anesthetized with subconjunctival lidocaine or with lidocaine gel. Superior anesthesia is achieved when lidocaine is left in place for several minutes. A solution of 5% povodine iodine is applied to the conjunctiva before the application of lidocaine gel, if used. With a lid speculum in place, a 27 g or 30 g needle is used to inject 0.1 cc of 40 mg/cc suspension of triamcinolone acetate into the vitreous through the pars plana. (The pars plana is measured 3.5 mm behind the limbus with calipers.) After injection, the speculum is removed and indirect ophthalmoscopy is performed to confirm perfusion of the optic nerve and alert the clinician to any immediate complications. Occasionally a paracentesis is necessary to bring the intraocular pressure to a safe level. Intraocular pressure is checked 10–20 minutes after the procedure. Many practioners routinely recommend antibiotic drops 4 times a day for 3 days, despite lack of evidence for their effectiveness in preventing endophthalmitis. Patients are discharged with instructions to return immediately if they have increased pain and decreased vision. The intraocular pressure should be checked in approximately 3 weeks, as steroid-induced pressure response is typically seen in this time frame.

Enthusiasm for intravitreal injection of triamcinolone acetonide is tempered by its many limitations. Even in cases with the most dramatic positive effect, the duration of this effect is limited. In a non-vitrectomized eye, the effect seems to last about 3 months, although the observed duration is highly variable. The effect is more abbreviated for vitrectomized eyes. Accelerated cataract formation is a frequent complication. Steroid-induced ocular hypertension occurs in about one-third of patients. While most can be treated with topical medications, a few need surgical treatment to relieve unacceptably high intraocular pressure. Multi-centered controlled clinical trials are under way to evaluate the efficacy and safety of intravitreal triamcinolone acetonide versus the current standard of care. Similar trials are being conducted for sustained-release corticosteroids.

Drugs with specific anti-VEGF activity are also being studied for treatment of macular edema caused by BRVO. Agents such as pegaptanib sodium, bevacizumab, ranibizumab, and anecortave acetate have the potential to decrease vascular permeability and reduce macular edema without the adverse effects of corticosteroid therapy. No medication, however, including triamcinolone acetonide, has been approved for use in treatment of macular edema caused by BRVO.

Surgical

Laser photocoagulation

Recommendations for laser photocoagulation are based on the Collaborative Branch Vein Occlusion Study (BVOS), a multicenter, randomized clinical trial sponsored by the National Eye Institute. The mechanism through which laser photocoagulation works is not clearly understood.

- *Grid laser photocoagulation for macular edema*: BVOS found that BRVO patients with persistent, perfused macular edema confirmed by high-quality fluorescein angiogram, vision 20/40 or worse, and vein occlusion of 3 to 18 months' duration were twice as likely (63% vs. 36%) to gain 2 or more lines of vision with grid laser photocoagulation at 3 years compared to observation. It is important to wait 3 to 6 months after the onset of disease to allow for clearing of hemorrhage, as hemorrhage can obscure adequate view for fluorescein angiogram, and laser photocoagulation through heme is theoretically more likely to result in complications. Also, as many eyes spontaneously improve in the first few months, waiting can obviate unnecessary treatment.

The protocol laser photocoagulation was performed in a grid pattern with argon blue-green laser, in the territory of the vein occlusion, between the major arcades and the foveal avascular zone. Recommended treatment parameters were duration of 0.1 second, 100 micron spot size and power setting sufficient to produce 'medium' white burn.

For patients who meet the above criteria, this treatment should certainly be considered, as its use is supported by the best evidence available for treatment of BRVO-related macular edema. Many experts warn not to extrapolate the results to patients who fall outside of the inclusion criteria for BVOS, particularly those with vision better than 20/40, non-perfused edema, and insufficiently cleared hemorrhages.

- *Scatter laser photocoagulation*: BVOS found that BRVO patients with 5 or more disc areas of non-perfusion had a 41% chance of developing retinal neovascularization, usually in the first 6 to 12 months after occlusion. Prophylactic scatter laser photocoagulation in the affected territory was found to reduce the incidence of neovascularization by 50%. However, prophylactic treatment is not routinely recommended, as many eyes (60%) would be treated unnecessarily.

Scatter laser photocoagulation is recommended when retinal neovascularization is found, as 60% of untreated eyes go on to develop vitreous hemorrhage. Treatment reduces the risk by 50%. Recommended parameters for treatment includes peripheral scatter with argon blue-green laser, spot size between 200–500 microns, duration of 0.1 second, and power setting sufficient to produce a medium white burn.

Vitrectomy with or without sheathotomy

Since BRVO occurs at arteriovenous crossings in patients with increased risk for arteriolar disease, and at such crossings the sheath is shared by the arteriole and the venule, liberating the vessels from the confining sheath may theoretically improve blood flow through the venule and reverse some of the downstream effects of a vein occlusion. This technique has been tried by a few surgeons but has not been adopted by many.

A recent report has suggested that vitrectomy without sheathotomy may be as effective in improving vision in patients with macular edema and BRVO as vitrectomy with sheathotomy. It is difficult to say whether the improvement in vision in these reports represents truly superior results from laser photocoagulation, since many patients in these series had contemporaneous cataract surgery and treatment with triamcinolone acetonide. More studies are necessary to determine whether these surgical treatments are beneficial in this setting.

COMMENTS

Treatment for macular edema caused by BRVO is evolving. Currently, laser photocoagulation is the only proven treatment available for this condition. Alternative treatments that may provide better visual outcome are being actively sought. The trials that are currently under way may better guide us in the future to incorporate new surgical and pharmacological modalities into the practice pattern.

REFERENCES

Branch Vein Occlusion Study Group: Argon laser photocoagulation for macular edema in branch vein occlusion. Am J Ophthalmol 98:271–282, 1984.

Branch Vein Occlusion Study Group: Argon laser scatter photocoagulation for prevention of neovascularization and vitreous hemorrhage in branch vein occlusion: a randomized clinical trial. Arch Ophthalmol 104:34–41, 1986.

Eye Disease Case-Control Study Group: Risk factors for branch retinal vein occlusion. Am J Ophthalmol 116:286–296, 1993.

Klein R, Klein BE, Moss SE, Meuer SM: The epidemiology of retinal vein occlusion: the Beaver Dam Eye Study. Trans Am Ophthalmol Soc 98:133–141, 2000.

Opremcak EM, Bruce RA: Surgical decompression of branch retinal vein occlusion via arteriovenous crossing sheathotomy. a prospective review of 15 cases. Retina 19:1–5, 1999.

331 CENTRAL OR BRANCH RETINAL ARTERIAL OCCLUSION 362.31

Amar Alwitry MD, MRCS, MRCOphth, FRCOphth
Derby, England
Aaron Osbourne MD, MRCOphth
Nottingham, England

Retinal arterial occlusions can be divided into two main subtypes: central retinal artery occlusion (CRAO) and branch retinal artery occlusion (BRAO). Patients with CRAO usually present with profound monocular vision loss, often down to the level of counting fingers or seeing only hand motions. In BRAO the visual loss is partial with a scotoma or visual field loss corresponding to the portion of the retina supplied by the occluded branch retinal artery. If a major macular arterial tributary is involved the visual loss may be profound Occasionally amaurosis fugax, or transient blindness in one eye, may occur hours or days before the onset of the arterial occlusion. In approximately 25% of eyes with CRAO, the presence of a cilioretinal artery results in sparing of part or all of the macula. Conversely, occlusion of a cilioretinal artery in isolation causes a corresponding scotoma. The significance of managing patients with retinal artery occlusion goes beyond attempts to restore vision. Approximately 90% of patients with CRAO have an associated underlying disease, the identification and treatment of which may reduce complications or increase longevity for the patient. Moreover, protecting vision in the fellow eye is of paramount importance as retinal arterial occlusion is often associated with a poor visual prognosis.

ETIOLOGY/INCIDENCE

The true incidence of CRAO is unknown. It occurs more frequently in older males (male: female ratio 2:1) with patients typically being early in their seventh decade of life. The disease affects both eyes in 1% to 2% of patients. Of all retinal artery occlusions 60% involve the central retinal artery, 35% involve the branch retinal artery, and 5% involve the cilioretinal artery.

Emboli are the most common cause of retinal artery occlusions, particularly in the elderly. Emboli arising from platelet-fibrin clots may originate from ulcerated atheromas in the carotid artery, from mural thrombi secondary to myocardial infarction or atrial fibrillation, or from mitral valve prolapse. Cholesterol emboli are frequent and often arise from carotid ulcerations that release plaque into the arterial circulation. Calcific emboli usually develop secondary to diseased aortic or mitral valves.

Other sources of emboli include:

- Septic endocarditis (leukoemboli);
- Tumors, e.g. atrial myxoma, a benign cardiac tumor in young patients;
- Fat emboli from long bone fractures;
- Amniotic fluid emboli;
- Talc or cornstarch coagulums in intravenous drug abusers;
- Corticosteroid boluses from facial or orbital injections may (rarely) travel retrograde into the central retinal artery;
- Materials used in cardiac procedures and contrast from angiography.

Nonembolic causes of retinal artery occlusion include:

- Direct thrombosis of the retinal arteries may occur secondary to hemorrhage into an ulcerative arteriosclerotic plaque;
- Vasculitis, including temporal arteritis and systemic lupus erythematosus;
- Posterior inflammatory conditions such as toxoplasma chorioretinitis and Behçet's disease;
- Coagulopathies such as disseminated intravascular coagulation. Antiphospholipid syndrome and sickle cell disease can also cause thrombus formation;
- Occlusion of vessels due to prolonged elevation of intraocular pressure above systolic blood pressure. This may result from vitreoretinal surgery or unrecognized pressure on the eye during general anesthesia;
- Occlusive pressure in the central retinal or ophthalmic artery may develop from intraorbital implants, tumors, edema, hemorrhage, or intraorbital injection;
- Migraine may cause retinal artery occlusion in young patients;
- Idiopathic; Susac's syndrome is a rare microangiopathy characterized by the clinical triad of encephalopathy, hearing loss and multiple BRAOs. This has been reported in patients aged between 16 and 58. The cause remains unknown but an autoimmune basis is thought to be likely.

COURSE/PROGNOSIS

Transient or partial obstruction of the central retinal artery may lead to recovery of some or all visual function in minutes or hours, but permanent visual loss is usually a prominent feature of complete arterial occlusion.

By definition visual loss which resolves fully within 24 hours is a transient ischemic attack of the retinal circulation, or amaurosis fugax. There is evidence, however, that more than 90 minutes of ischemia will result in permanent retinal damage and concomitant visual loss.

Intuitively, both presenting and final visual acuity are likely to be far worse with CRAO than BRAO. The gradient of the partial pressure of oxygen from the patent choroidal circulation to the retina after CRAO is adequate for prolonged survival but not for sustained physiological viability of the inner two-thirds of the retina. Experimental complete occlusion of the central retinal artery in rhesus monkeys for longer than 97 minutes resulted in irreversible retinal damage which became massive by 240 minutes.

Clinically, the patient's CRAO may not be complete, in which case recovery of partial vision may occur hours or days after the onset of symptoms. The prognosis for visual recovery varies with the site of occlusion, being worse with more proximal occlusions such as those in CRAO and better with the distal occlusions seen in BRAO.

In CRAO, 70% of eyes have a final vision of 20/400 or worse. In contrast, 90% of eyes with BRAO retain vision of 20/40 or better.

DIAGNOSIS

Clinical signs

- In CRAO a relative afferent pupillary defect is almost invariably present. Retinal whitening and edema are visible, with maximal whiteness occurring approximately 70 minutes after deprivation of blood flow through the central retinal artery. Intracellular edema does not occur at the fovea which is devoid of ganglion cells. The characteristic cherry-red or brown spot occurs because the light reflex from the intact choroidal vessels remains visible at the fovea (Figure 331.1). The affected retinal arteries may appear thin and empty or have pulsatile or stationary blood segments that look like 'boxcars' or 'cattle trucking.' The veins are darker than normal due to stagnation of blood and poor oxygenation. Approximately one-third of patients have incomplete occlusion of the central retinal artery with some oxygenated blood flow to the retina; the presenting visual acuity in these patients may range from 20/30 to hand motion. When occlusion is incomplete, final visual acuity correlates positively with visual acuity at presentation and negatively with duration of visual impairment.
- In BRAO the retinal whitening is in the distribution of the affected artery (Figure 331.2). The site of the obstruction is most often at the bifurcation of the arteries where emboli are likely to become lodged. Arterial abnormalities similar to those in CRAO may be observed and emboli are visible in more than half of all eyes with BRAO.

Cholesterol emboli, also known as Hollenhorst plaques, are bright-yellow refractile crystals (Figure 331.3). Platelet-fibrin emboli are barely visible, grayish, nonrefractile plugs that tend to be mobile. Calcific emboli are large, white, oval, moderately refractile bodies at or near the optic disk.

Laboratory findings

- As one of the most dramatic sights in ophthalmology, the diagnosis is usually made clinically and, in the case of acute

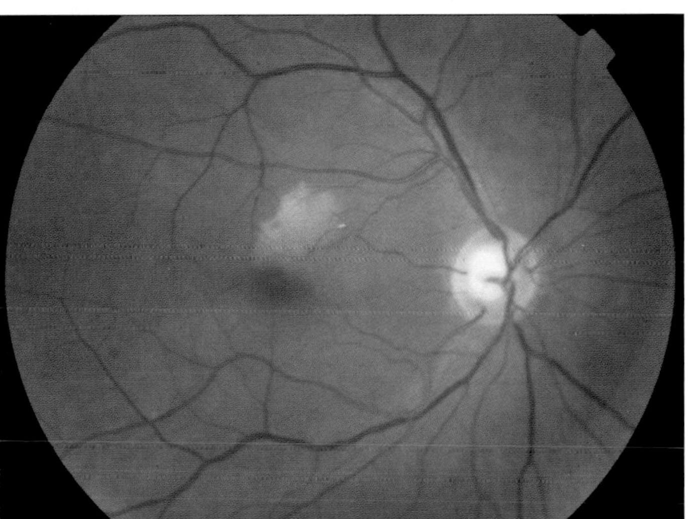

FIGURE 331.2. A color fundus photograph of a patients right eye showing the area of retinal whitening corresponding to the area of retina affected by the branch retinal artery occlusion. An embolus is clearly visible within the vessel.

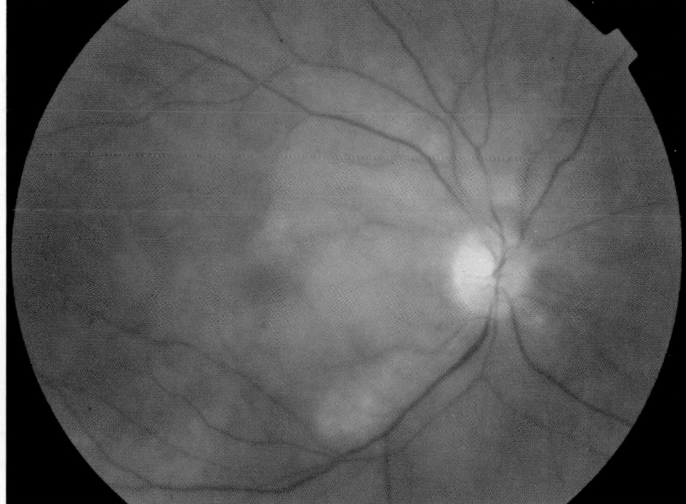

FIGURE 331.1. A color fundus photograph of a patients right eye showing the classical appearance of a central retinal artery occlusion with diffuse retinal whitening sparing the fovea and the resultant cherry red spot.

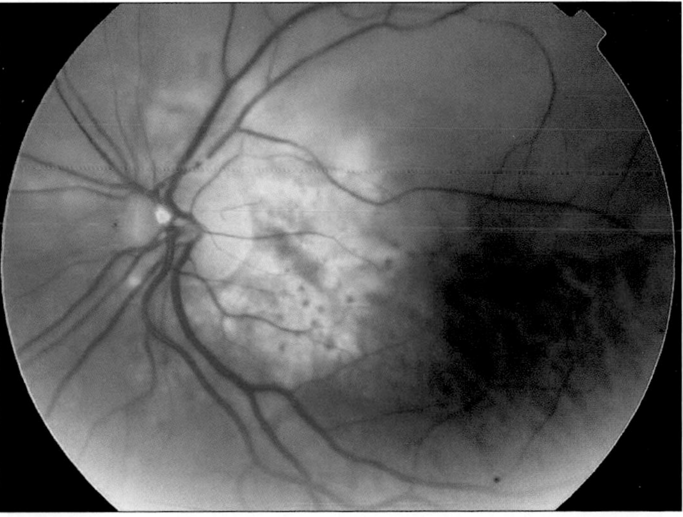

FIGURE 331.3. A color fundus photograph of a patients left eye showing a large Hollenhorst plaque within the central retinal artery resulting in a central retinal artery occlusion.

CRAO, prompt treatment is instituted. Laboratory studies may help determine the etiology of the occlusion but rarely affect the emergency room treatment.

- Obtain a CBC for baseline and check ESR and CRP to exclude an inflammatory endarteritis such as giant cell arteritis.
- Obtain fasting blood sugar, cholesterol, triglyceride and lipid panels to screen for atherosclerotic disease.
- Coagulopathy screen and blood cultures can identify more unusual causes.
- Arrange carotid Doppler ultrasound or magnetic resonance angiogram to evaluate for carotid disease.
- Echocardiogram and ECG (possibly a 24-hour ECG if paroxysmal atrial fibrillation is suspected) can be ordered for detection of structural abnormalities of the heart and arrhythmias.
- Electroretinogram (ERG) can serve to determine whether ophthalmic artery occlusion is present in addition to CRAO. In a pure CRAO, the B wave is lost as a result of inner retinal ischemia, but the A wave remains because the photoreceptors still function (intact choroidal circulation maintains oxygenation of the outer third of the retina). With ophthalmic artery occlusion or infarction of retinal and choroidal circulation from extraocular pressure, both the A and B waves of the ERG are lost.
- Fluorescein angiography may show a normal or delayed arm-to-retina circulation time. There may be slowing or even cessation of retinal arterial filling, corresponding to the site of occlusion. Increased arteriovenous transit time and attenuation of the vasculature are other features seen. With reperfusion, the fluorescein angiogram may return to normal despite persistently decreased vision.

Differential diagnosis

- Ophthalmic artery occlusion results in nonperfusion of the choroidal and retinal circulations. The presenting visual acuity is usually worse than that of CRAO, usually in the range of light perception to no light perception. Because of choroidal non-perfusion there usually is no cherry-red spot in the macula.
- A cherry-red spot is the most striking retinal lesion seen in the sphingolipidoses, a rare group of inherited metabolic disorders. Lipids are stored in the ganglion cells of the retina, giving a white appearance absent at the fovea. These disorders are usually seen bilaterally in the pediatric population and include Tay-Sachs disease and Niemann-Pick and Sandhoff disease. Their appearances may mimic CRAO but they are bilateral.

PROPHYLAXIS

The individual cause of an arterial occlusion often remains obscure but cardiovascular risk factors may be addressed to improve the patient's systemic condition and minimize the risk of ocular and non-ocular sequelae. These include smoking, hypertension, hypercholesterolemia, diabetes, coronary artery disease or history of stroke/TIA.

The iatrogenic causes can be anticipated, and surgical procedures should be altered to reduce the risk of occlusion. For example, after a scleral buckle is placed, the patency of the central retinal artery should be verified by indirect ophthalmoscopy.

TREATMENT

Systemic

Possible underlying causes of retinal artery occlusion are evaluated and treated directly.

- If temporal arteritis is the cause of the retinal artery occlusion, high-dose corticosteroids should be started to prevent visual loss in the fellow eye.
- Hemodynamically significant atherosclerotic carotid disease may be amenable to surgery such as carotid endarterectomy or may be treated by an antiplatelet regimen.
- Anticoagulation has a role to play in treating occlusion due to thrombophilia or other pro-coagulopathies such as in the antiphospholipid syndrome (probably an important cause of retinal vascular occlusion in young patients).

Ocular

In BRAO, most patients regain good vision; therefore, treatment is of questionable value, especially because no treatment is of proven therapeutic benefit.

With CRAO, prompt intervention, preferably within 100 minutes of the onset of symptoms, improves the chance for visual recovery and long term ocular prognosis. Complete occlusion for more than 6 hours probably produces irreversible retinal damage, but most clinicians still recommend treatment if the CRAO is of less than 24 hours' duration. The goal of the treatment is to restore blood flow and prevent irreversible retinal cell death by dislodging the emboli. Treatment modalities can be divided into medical and interventional.

Medical

- Acetazolamide 500 mg IV, to lower intraocular pressure relatively rapidly, thereby increasing the intravascular pressure gradient across the embolus and theoretically allowing dislodgment of any embolus downstream.
- Digital ocular massage to enhance aqueous humor outflow, followed by the abrupt release of pressure, increases the pressure gradient across the obstruction. This sudden change has the potential to mechanically dislodge the embolus.
- Hyperbaric oxygen, if instituted between 2 and 12 hours after onet, may be beneficial but transport to a chamber can waste precious time
- Hyperoxia during CRAO is associated with improved electroretinogram recovery in cats. It is probably worthwhile to start hyperoxia whilst other treatments are given.
- Carbogen, a mixture of 95% oxygen and 5% carbon dioxide, inhaled for 10 minutes every 2 hours for up to 48 hours, may induce retinal vasodilatation and increase oxygenation and retinal blood flow.

Surgical

- Anterior chamber paracentesis, using a 30-gauge needle to remove approximately 0.1 to 0.4 mL of aqueous humor, also abruptly lowers the intraocular pressure. The procedure may be carried out in the office at the slit lamp as long as aseptic technique is ensured.
- Local intraarterial fibrinolysis (LIF) by injection of urokinase or recombinant tissue plasminogen activator into the proximal part of the ophthalmic artery may result in significantly improved outcome compared with conservative treatment. Thrombolytics are ideally delivered directly into the ophthalmic artery by transfemoral catheterization in a

procedure usually performed by an interventional radiologist, to reduce the risk of systemic side effects such as hemorrhagic stroke. As with all treatments for CRAO it is important for LIF to be initiated within the first few hours of occlusion, before irreversible damage has occurred.

COMPLICATIONS

Approximately 18% of all patients with CRAO develop rubeosis iridis, which often results in rubeotic glaucoma. Other complications depend on the cause of the arterial occlusion. For example if an embolus caused the occlusion, then further emboli could affect the fellow eye or lead to a cerebrovascular accident. Temporal arteritis can swiftly lead to blinding involvement of the other eye, usually within the first 6 weeks of the first occlusion. Giant cell arteritis is a systemic condition that can affect numerous end organs.

COMMENTS

In patients with BRAO or CRAO, the search for an associated systemic disease is crucial regardless of the ocular presentation. In one study, the expected survival time for patients with CRAO was 5.5 years compared with 15.4 years for an age-matched control population. In another report, patients with retinal arterial emboli had a 56% mortality rate over 9 years compared with a 27% rate for age-matched control subjects without emboli.

While increased mortality secondary to fatal stroke has been shown in studies, the most common cause of death in this population is cardiovascular disease. A thorough medical workup can often lead to identification of underlying disorders. Clearly retinal arterial occlusion is a warning sign heralding the need for systemic evaluation and reduction of vasculopathic and cardiovascular risk factors. Expeditious treatment of these disorders may decrease the risk of complications and result in longer life expectancy.

REFERENCES

Augsburger JJ, Magargal LE: Visual prognosis following treatment of acute central retinal artery obstruction. Br J Ophthalmol 64:913–917, 1980.

Duker JS, Sivalingam A, Brown GC, et al: A prospective study of acute central retinal artery obstruction: The incidence of secondary ocular neovascularization. Arch Ophthalmol 109:339–342, 1991.

Ffytche TJ: A rationalization of treatment of central retinal artery occlusion. Trans Ophthalmol Soc UK 94:468 479, 1974.

Hayreh SS, Zimmerman MB, Kimura A, Sanon A: Central retinal artery occlusion. Retinal tolerance time. Exp Eye Research 78(3):723–736, 2004.

Schmidt D, Schulte-Monting J, Schumacher M: Prognosis of central retinal artery occlusion: local intraarterial fibrinolysis versus conservative treatment. Am J Neuroradiol. 23(8):1301–1307, 2002.

332 CENTRAL SEROUS CHORIORETINOPATHY 362.41

(Central Serous Retinopathy)

Christopher N. Singh, MD
Seattle, Washington
Peter N. Youssef, MD
Seattle, Washington
David A. Saperstein, MD
Seattle, Washington

ETIOLOGY/INCIDENCE

Central serous chorioretinopathy (CSC) is a disorder of the central macula. It is characterized by serous leakage from the choriocapillaris through the retinal pigment epithelium (RPE) leading to neurosensory retinal detachment (NSD) and occasionally RPE detachment. Hyperpermeability and leakage of the RPE and choriocapillaris can be demonstrated on fluorescein angiography (FA) and indocyanine green (ICG) angiography. The NSD can be visualized and quantitated using optical coherence tomography (OCT).

CSC typically affects people between the ages of 20 to 55 years old. There is a higher reported incidence among Caucasians, Hispanics and Asians, and a low occurrence rate in African Americans. Other risk factors, as described in retrospective studies, include male gender, corticosteroid use, pregnancy, 'type A' personality, psychological stress, and elevated levels of endogenous steroid, as in Cushing's syndrome. Some evidence also exists for uncontrolled hypertension, allergic respiratory disease, antibiotic use, systemic lupus erythematosis, end-stage renal disease, gastroesophageal reflux disease, and the use of psychiatric medications as additional risk factors.

COURSE/PROGNOSIS

Presenting symptoms include decreased visual acuity, metamorphopsia, micropsia, central color vision deficiency, central scotoma, decrease in contrast sensitivity and increasing hyperopia. Presenting visual acuity deficits are usually mild. Patients presenting with 20/20 vision usually maintain that level. Patients with an initial visual acuity of 20/30 or worse tend to gain one to two lines of Snellen visual acuity upon resolution of the NSD.

The majority of patients with this disease will have resolution of the NSD in two to four months without treatment. Often resolution of visual symptoms and return of visual acuity to baseline or near baseline are attained, but may lag behind resolution of the NSD. One-third to one-half of patients will have chronic or recurrent NSD. Chronic NSD for a period of greater than 4 months can lead to foveal atrophy, as demonstrated on OCT studies. Foveal atrophy in these cases corresponds to lower final best-corrected visual acuity, regardless of anatomic reattachment.

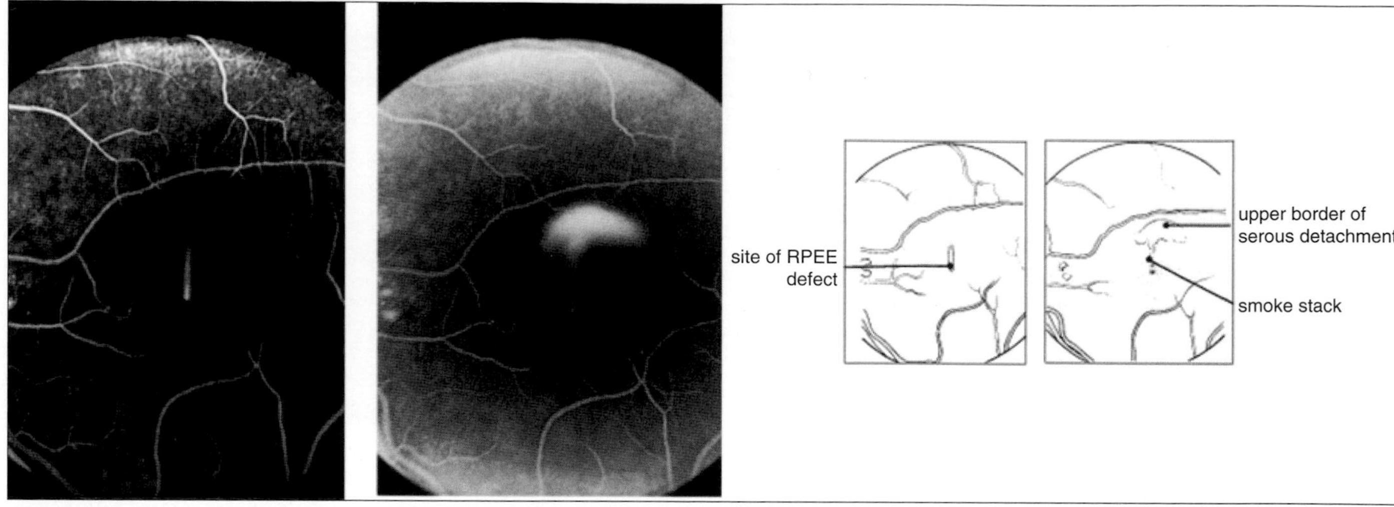

FIGURE 332.1. a) Fundus photograph of CSC, revealing a neurosensory detachment extending into macula. (b and c) Fluorescein angiography, revealing an expansile dot pattern, with an early and late phase, respectively. d) OCT of the same eye, revealing superior subretinal fluid extending to the fovea (From Spaltan et al. Atlas of Clinical Opthalmology, 3e, 2005).

DIAGNOSIS

Clinical signs and symptoms

Patients present with the aforementioned symptoms. In taking history, the clinician should probe for risk factors as described above. Fundoscopic exam typically reveals NSD without subretinal blood (Figure 332.1a). RPE atrophy at the site of detachment or elsewhere in the posterior pole is common evidence of recurrence. Chronic CSC findings also include subretinal yellowish fibrin deposits, cystoid macular edema and, rarely, choroidal neovascularization (CNV).

Laboratory findings

FA findings include patterns of hyperfluorescence within the area of NSD. These typically include an 'expansile dot' pattern in 62–72% of patients, a 'smokestack' pattern in 10–25% of patients, or diffuse hyperfluorescence without a definitive leakage point in a minority of patients (Figure 332.1b–c). FA is limited in its ability to visualize the choroidal circulation. ICG angiography has shown zonal hyperpermeability at the level of the choriocapillaris not detected by FA. This is suggestive of zonal hyperperfusion or hyperpermeability of the choriocapillaris as a contributing factor in the pathophysiology of this disease.

OCT is an effective method to diagnose and quantify neurosensory and RPE detachments as well as thinning of the foveal neurosensory retina, which may correlate to the duration of disease and final visual acuity measurements (Figure 332.1d). OCT may reduce the need for FA in the management of CSC.

Differential diagnosis

Other disease processes that may resemble CSC include age-related macular degeneration, stage one macular holes, idiopathic CNV, cystoid macular degeneration, optic nerve pits with serous macular detachment, polypoid choroidal vasculopathy, posterior scleritis and Harada's disease.

TREATMENT

Observation is recommended in most cases. Thermal laser is considered for patients who require immediate resolution of symptoms (a mean of 5 weeks vs. 23 weeks) or those with chronic or recurrent NSD. Extrafoveal areas of focal leakage are the best candidates for laser therapy. Laser treatment (vs. observation) does not improve the final visual outcome in patients with new onset CSC and can be associated with complications, including expanding scar formation and CNV.

Patients with sub- or extra- foveal fluorescein leakage are poor candidates for thermal laser photocoagulation. Verteporfin photodynamic therapy (PDT), directed to areas of choroidal hyperpermeability as demonstrated by ICG angiography, has been shown to be effective in a retrospective case series of chronic CSC.

REFERENCES

Gilbert CM, Owens SL, Smith PD, et al: Long-term follow-up of central serous chorioretinopathy. Br J Ophthalmol 68(11):815–20, 1984.

Haimovici R, Koh S, Gagnon DR, et al: Risk factors for central serous chorioretinopathy. Ophthalmology 111(2):244–249, 2004.

Matsunaga H, Nangoh K, Uyama M, et al: Occurrence of choroidal neovascularization following photocoagulation treatment for central serous retinopathy. Nippon Ganka Gakkai Zasshi 99:460–468, 1995.

Montero JA, Ruiz-Moreno JM: Optical coherence tomography characterization of idiopathic central serous chorioretinopathy. Br J Ophthalmol 89:562–564, 2005.

Ober MD, Yannuzzi LA, Do DV, et al: Photodynamic therapy for focal retinal pigment epithelial leaks secondary to central serous chorioretinopathy. Ophthalmology 112(12):2088–2094, 2005.

Watzke RC, Burton TC, Leaverton PE: Ruby laser photocoagulation therapy of central serous retinopathy. Trans Am Acad Ophthalmol Otolaryngol 78(2):OP205–OP211, 1974.

333 COATS' DISEASE 362.15
(Primary or Congenital Retinal Telangiectasia, Leber's Miliary Aneurysms)

Lihteh Wu, MD
San José, Costa Rica

In 1908, Coats described an idiopathic entity characterized by unilateral retinal vascular abnormalities with intraretinal and subretinal exudation. He further classified this entity into 3 groups. Group I had massive subretinal exudates but no visible retinal vascular abnormalities. Group II had massive subretinal exudates with retinal vascular abnormalities. Group III had massive exudates with arteriovenous malformations. Von Hippel later characterized Group III as a distinct entity: angiomatosis retinae. In 1912, Leber described a similar condition characterized by retinal aneurysms, hemorrhages and telangiectasia but without the massive subretinal exudates. This condition was named Leber's multiple miliary aneurysm disease. However, in 1915 Leber himself recognized that his disease was an earlier stage of the entity described by Coats. Reese confirmed this concept in 1956 by describing an eye that had Leber's multiple miliary aneurysms that developed the classic picture of Coats' disease with time.

ETIOLOGY/INCIDENCE

- Idiopathic primary retinal vascular abnormality leading to a loss of the blood–retina barrier with plasma leakage can result in severe lipemic retinal edema.
- Males are affected three times as often as females.
- Eighty percent of cases are unilateral.
- The disease is not inherited.
- The majority of patients are diagnosed before age 16 years; as many as 30% present after the age of 30 years.
- There is no racial or ethnic predilection.
- Coats' disease is not associated with any systemic disease.

COURSE/PROGNOSIS

- Pediatric patients often present with strabismus, painless loss of vision, or leukocoria. Adult patients usually complain of a painless loss of vision.
- Patients younger than 4 have a more explosive exudative response.
- Retinal vascular abnormalities lead to vascular leakage, severe retinal edema, and lipid exudation in the area of the abnormal retinal vessels.
- Lipid exudate may accumulate, creating a subretinal mass.
- An exudative retinal detachment may ensue and even progress to a total detachment.
- Vitreous hemorrhage occurs infrequently.
- Total retinal detachment may progress to a secondary glaucoma and to a blind painful eye requiring enucleation.
- Natural history is that of progression at variable rates.
- A minority of eyes stabilize and even regress spontaneously.
- Laser treatment can stabilize the disease or improve the visual outcome.

CLASSIFICATION

Stage 1: Retinal telangiectasia only.
Stage 2: Telangiectasia and exudation:
- A. Extrafoveal exudation.
- B. Foveal exudation.

Stage 3: Exudative retinal detachment:
- A. Subtotal detachment:
  - **1.** Extrafoveal.
  - **2.** Foveal.
- B. Total retinal detachment.

Stage 4: Total retinal detachment and glaucoma.
Stage 5: Advanced end-stage disease.

DIAGNOSIS

Clinical signs and symptoms

Funduscopic findings include retinal vascular abnormalities such as telangiectasia, vascular loops, beading, neovascularization, and focal or segmental aneurysmal dilatation of the retinal capillaries. These vascular abnormalities lead to retinal edema, retinal lipid exudation, and exudative retinal detachment (Figure 333.1).

Laboratory findings

Fluorescein angiography is useful in equivocal cases and can demonstrate large aneurysmal ('lightbulb') dilatation of the retinal vessels and variable leakage from the telangiectatic vessels. Capillary nonperfusion and other microvascular abnormalities may be present.

Differential diagnosis

- Retinoblastoma: the identification of calcium by either B-scan ultrasound or computed tomography is a strong indication that retinoblastoma is present.

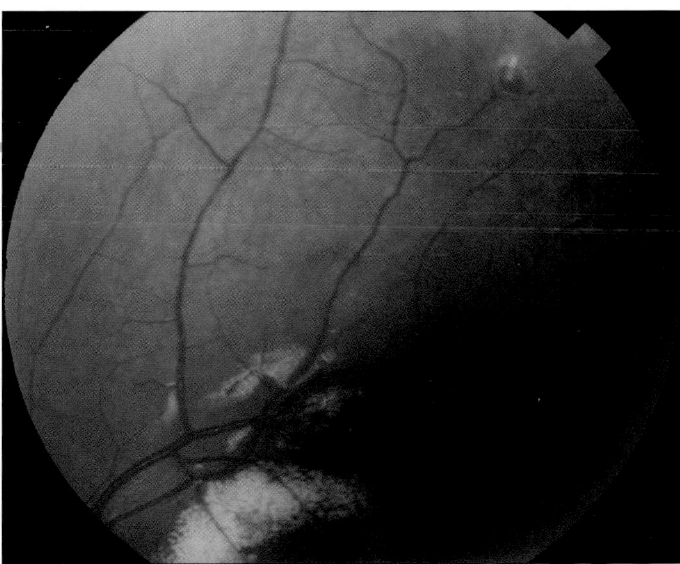

FIGURE 333.1. Note the dilated aneurysmal dilatation of the retinal vessel and the lipid exudation in the macular area.

- Persistent hyperplastic primary vitreous.
- Intraocular toxocariasis.
- Congenital cataract.
- Familial exudative vitreoretinopathy.
- Retinal detachment.
- Eales disease.
- Branch retinal vein occlusion with secondary vascular leakage.
- Parafoveal telangiectasia.
- Intraocular tumor with exudation.
- Retinal angiomatosis.

TREATMENT

The patient may be followed conservatively if the lesions are limited and do not threaten the macular area.

The goal of treatment is obliteration of the vascular abnormalities to stop the exudation. More than one session might be necessary. It is important to treat the entire area of abnormal blood vessels.

Laser photocoagulation

- Preferred method of treatment.
- Leaking lesions treated directly.
- Treat mildly to avoid an exudative reaction (Coats' response).
- Spot size of 200 to 500 µm.
- Duration of 0.2 to 0.5 second.
- Yellow or argon green dye.
- End point: spasm or whitening of the vascular anomalies.

Cryotherapy

- Useful when the retina is detached or lesions are far anterior.
- Double freeze-thaw technique.
- Treat directly on the abnormal vessels.

External drainage of the subretinal fluid

- Selected cases with bullous or total retinal detachments.
- With or without scleral buckle.
- Followed by laser photocoagulation or cryotherapy.

Vitrectomy

- Selected cases with bullous, total or tractional retinal detachments.

COMPLICATIONS

- Cystoid macular edema.
- Exudative retinal detachment.
- Neovascular glaucoma.
- Secondary angle-closure glaucoma.
- Iridocyclitis.
- Cataract.
- Phthisis bulbi.

REFERENCES

Coats G: Forms of retinal dysplasia with massive exudation. R Lond Ophthalmol Hosp Rep 17:440, 1908.

Kiratli H, Eldem B: Management of moderate to advanced Coats' disease. Ophthalmologica 212:19–22, 1998.

Shields JA, Shields CL, Honavar SG, Demirci H: Clinical variations and complications of Coats disease in 150 cases: the 2000 Sanford Gifford Memorial Lecture. Am J Ophthalmol 131:561–571, 2001.

Shields JA, Shields CL: Review: Coats disease: the 2001 LuEsther T. Mertz lecture. Retina 22:80–91, 2002.

Shields JA, Shields CL, Honavar SG, et al: Classification and management of Coats disease: the 2000 Proctor Lecture. Am J Ophthalmol 131:572–583, 2001.

334 DIFFUSE UNILATERAL SUBACUTE NEURORETINITIS 363.05

Geoffrey Emerson, MD, PhD
Portland, Oregon

Diffuse unilateral subacute neuroretinitis (DUSN) was first reported by Gass and Scelfo in 1978. The earliest described patients were otherwise healthy and presented with unilateral vision loss that often was severe and progressive. The ocular findings included vitritis, papillitis, arteriolar narrowing, and extensive retinal pigmentary change. The syndrome is now thought to be secondary to the presence of an intraretinal nematode. The ocular damage is believed to be secondary to the direct toxic effect of the worm and the ocular inflammatory reaction. Elimination of the nematode results in resolution of ocular inflammation and arrest of disease. Failure to eliminate the nematode results in progressive ocular destruction.

ETIOLOGY/INCIDENCE

Ocular larvae migrans of nematode origin have been associated with diffuse unilateral subacute neuroretinitis. A number of nematodes remain etiologic candidates in DUSN. *Toxocara canis* was the first worm to be considered, but more recently, *Baylisascaris* larvae, especially *B. procyonis*, which is found in raccoons, has been implicated. *Ancylostoma caninum*, *Strongyloides* spp. and *Brugia malayi* are also reported. Endemic areas of the United States for this disease include the southeast and Midwest. A heightened awareness of the disease has resulted in recent reports of DUSN in Canada, Brazil, Venezuela, the Caribbean, Senegal, and India. The nematode may persist in the fundus for up to 3 years; hence, the various sizes of the worm may be due to variations in its age. Evidence implicating multiple species is the finding that a larger worm is reported to predominate in the midwestern United States, whereas a smaller variety predominates in the southeastern United States. Despite the association, a worm is actually identified in only a minority of cases. It is the other clinical signs that usually lead to the diagnosis.

COURSE/PROGNOSIS

- Early characteristics include vision loss, mild vitritis, papillitis, and recurrent crops of gray-white lesions.
- Later characteristics include progressive visual loss, optic atrophy, and retinal vessel narrowing; diffuse pigment epithelial degeneration ('wipeout') may develop.
- Other clinical presentations include coarse clumping of subretinal pigment, which is occasionally arranged in a pattern suggesting 'worm tracks,' and scattered focal chorioretinal atrophic scars.

- Progressive changes in the structure and function of the eye continue as long as the worm remains viable. With continuance, an afferent pupillary defect may evolve.
- The end stage of this process may appear ophthalmoscopically similar to that of advanced cases of retinitis pigmentosa.

DIAGNOSIS

Laboratory findings

The history, fundus examination, and electrophysiologic findings may serve to distinguish DUSN from other entities.

- History:
  - Any patient with late or early signs of the neuroretinitis should be investigated for nematodes and questioned for exposure to raccoons or skunks, as well as for travel in endemic areas.
- Fundus examination:
  - When visualized, the intraocular nematodes are usually detected in the macular area. They range from 400 to 2000 μm in length; are white, often with a glistening sheen; and are gently tapered at both ends. Detailed biomicroscopy, fundus photography, and indocyanine green angiography may be required to locate smaller worms.
  - Associated fundus findings include the following: optic nerve: atrophy, edema, papillitis, vasculature: vascular narrowing.
  - Retina and retinal pigment epithelium: diffuse or focal atrophy, multifocal gray-white lesions (a nematode may be present).
  - Vitreous: vitritis (although inflammatory signs, particularly vitreous cells, are usually present in the early and late stages of the disease, they may be absent, even in an extensively damaged eye containing a viable nematode).
- Electroretinography may be normal in the early stages of the disease. B-wave depression, proportional to the extent of retinal involvement, with relative a-wave preservation is characteristic of latter stages. A completely extinguished electroretinographic signal, as may be observed in retinitis pigmentosa, is rare.
  - Electro-oculography is nonspecifically depressed in about half of patients tested.

Enzyme-linked immunosorbent assays specific for individual nematode species have been used in some cases.

Differential diagnosis

DUSN may be confused with a variety of entities depending on the stage of disease at the time of presentation:

- Early in the course: optic neuritis, pars planitis, acute posterior multifocal placoid pigment epitheliopathy, histoplasmosis, and toxoplasmosis.
- Later in the course: unilateral retinitis pigmentosa, post-traumatic retinal/choroidal injury, iron toxicity, and prior central retinal artery occlusion.

PROPHYLAXIS

Avoid endemic areas and suspect lower carnivores such as skunks and raccoons.

TREATMENT

Systemic

- Serial biomicroscopic examinations often fail to localize the nematode, which can be identified on average in only 25% of patients. Consequently, there has been an interest in the use of antihelmintic agents in the treatment of this syndrome.
- Viable worms and the progression of disease have been observed after treatment with both oral thiabendazole and oral ivermectin. Medical treatment may be most effective in patients in whom the inflammatory reaction both obscures the view of the nematode and facilitates penetration of the drug.
- A case series from Brazil demonstrates the efficacy and safety of oral albendazole (400 mg/day for 30 days) in the treatment of DUSN.
- Corticosteroid therapy has failed to demonstrate usefulness in limiting the progression of this syndrome.

Ocular

- No local or topical treatment has proved to be effective in control of the parasite or course of disease.

Surgical

- When the worm can be visualized, laser photocoagulation is the preferred treatment. This treatment is effective in destroying the nematode and in arresting the destructive process.
- Although photocoagulation of the parasite does not result in an augmented toxic reaction or inflammatory response, the damage and atrophic change that occurred before photocoagulation generally is not reversible.
- Both transscleral and transvitreal extractions of the parasite have been carried out. In view of the efficacy of direct photocoagulation, these techniques are best applied when laser facilities are unavailable or when attempting to retrieve an undamaged parasite for study.
- Cryoablation has been reported to destroy the nematode.

COMMENTS

The significance of the early consideration of DUSN in patients presenting with unilateral findings consistent with the syndrome is that early elimination of the parasite halts progression of the vision loss. Moreover, an opportunity to identify DUSN and to treat the patient with laser photocoagulation may be lost if a visible worm migrates and subsequently is able to elude detection. Failure to identify the nematode may result in therapy with anthelmintic agents that may be less effective.

The early condition should be considered a cause of treatable vision loss in the young and healthy. Recent increased awareness has resulted in its detection and treatment in patients in areas previously considered to be nonendemic. Signs and symptoms consistent with this condition should precipitate a directed history, detailed search of the fundus, and consideration of electroretinographic testing.

REFERENCES

Gass JD, Braunstein RA: Further observations concerning the diffuse unilateral subacute neuroretinitis syndrome. Arch Ophthalmol 101:1689–1697, 1983.

Gass JD, Gilbert WR, Jr, Guerry RK, Scelfo R: Diffuse unilateral subacute neuroretinitis. Ophthalmology 85:521–545, 1978.

Gass JD, Scelfo R: Diffuse unilateral subacute neuroretinitis. J R Soc Med 71:95–111, 1978.

Kazacos KR, Vestre WA, Kazacos EA, Raymond LA: Diffuse unilateral subacute neuroretinitis syndrome: probable cause. Arch Ophthalmol 102:967–968, 1984.

Oppenheim S, Rogell G, Peyser R: Diffuse unilateral subacute neuroretinitis. Ann Ophthalmol 17:336–338, 1985.

335 EALES DISEASE 379.23

(Angiopathia Retinae Juvenilis, Inflammatory Disease of the Retinal Veins, Primary Perivasculitis of the Retina, Retinal Vasculitis Associated with Tuberculoprotein Hypersensitivity)

Thomas S. Hwang, MD
Portland, Oregon
Michael L. Klein, MD
Portland, Oregon

Originally described as an entity characterized by recurrent vitreous hemorrhage, epistaxis, and constipation, Eales' disease is now understood as an idiopathic obliterative peripheral retinal vasculopathy with variable ocular inflammation.

ETIOLOGY/INCIDENCE

- The cause is unclear, although an association with exposure to tuberculosis, as well as frequent recovery of *Mycobacterium tuberculosis* DNA in affected patients' vitreous have been reported.
- Rare in North America and Western Europe, the entity is found commonly in India and portions of the Middle East.
- Typical age of presentation is 20 to 30 years, with a male predominance.

COURSE/PROGNOSIS

Many patients are asymptomatic in the early phase of the disease.

DIAGNOSIS

Clinical signs and symptoms

Patients most frequently present with unilateral vision loss related to vitreous hemorrhage or inflammation. Although bilateral involvement is the rule (80–90%), the condition is frequently asymmetric. Other symptoms may include floaters and photopsia. Although vestibuloauditory dysfunction has been reported in 17–48% of patients with Eales disease, this sign alone is neither necessary nor sufficient for the diagnosis. Other causes of retinal ischemia and vascular sheathing should be sought as this is a diagnosis of exclusion.

The hallmark of the disease is peripheral retinal nonperfusion. Intraretinal hemorrhages, vascular tortuosity, microvascular abnormalities, collateral vessels, and neovascularization are seen (Figure 335.1). Non-perfusion usually spares the macula allowing up to $^2/_3$ of patients to have vision better than or equal to 20/40. Some patients with Eales disease can develop branch vein occlusion and its related findings. Neovascular changes affect both the anterior and posterior segments. Rubeosis irides, neovascularization of the disc or peripheral neovascularization akin to sickle cell disease are all common. Neovascular glaucoma, traction retinal detachment and vitreous hemorrhage are possible sequelae.

Signs of inflammation are frequently present. Retinal vascular sheathing involving both arterioles and venules is most characteristic of this disease, although other signs, such as keratic precipitates, anterior chamber cells and flare, and vitreous debris are frequently present. Macular edema and epiretinal membrane are also common. Inflammation is rarely seen in the late stages of the disease.

Laboratory findings

Fluorescein angiography shows sharply demarcated areas of retinal nonperfusion. Vascular abnormalities such as telangiectatic vessels, shunt vessels and neovascularization, as well as leakage from sheathed vessels, are also seen.

Laboratory studies should be directed at ruling out other causes of retinal ischemia and ocular inflammation. In patients with potential risk, a screening test for tuberculosis may be considered.

Differential diagnosis

- Sickle cell disease.
- Diabetic retinopathy.
- Retinal vasculitis.
- Incontinentia pigmenti.
- Retinopathy of prematurity.
- Familial exudative vitreoretinopathy.
- Retinal venous occlusive disease.
- Pars planitis.
- Idiopathic hypereosinophilia.
- Idiopathic retinal vasculitis and neuroretinitis.
- Familial retinal arteriolar tortuosity and retinal hemorrhage.
- Sarcoidosis.

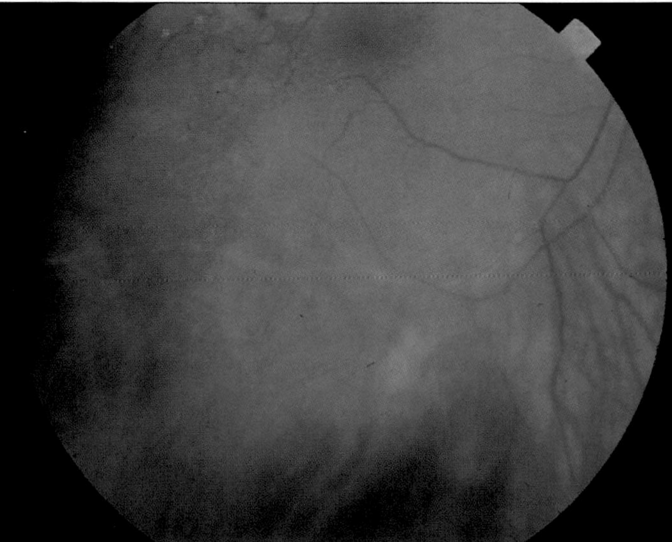

FIGURE 335.1. Eales disease.

PROPHYLAXIS

No effective preventative measures are known for this condition.

TREATMENT

Systemic

No clear benefit has been shown from systemic therapy, including high-dose corticosteroids.

Surgical

The mainstay of treatment for Eales disease is scatter photocoagulation of the ischemic retina. Neovascular tissue regresses readily with this treatment, but vigilance is required as larger areas of ischemia may develop, resulting in further neovascularization. Some patients will go on to have non-clearing or repeated vitreous hemorrhage, or other complications of neovascularization such as traction retinal detachment. Pars plana vitrectomy is effective in treating these complications.

COMMENTS

Although considered a distinct entity with characteristic clinical, funduscopic, and fluorescein angiographic findings, Eales disease remains a diagnosis of exclusion, and other retinal causes of inflammation and neovascularization must be excluded.

REFERENCES

Biswas J, Therese L, Madhavan HN: Use of polymerase chain reaction in detection of *Mycobacterium tyberculosis* complex DNA from vitreous samples of Eales' disease. Br J Ophthalmol 83(8):994, 1999.

Gass JDM: Macular dysfunction caused by retinal vascular diseases. In: Gass JDM, ed: Stereoscopic atlas of macular diseases diagnosis and treatment. vol. 1. St Louis, Mosby-Year Book, 1997:1:534–538.

Katz B, Wheeler D, Weinreib RN, et al: Eales' disease with central nervous system infarction. Ann Ophthalmol 23(12):460–463, 1991.

Renie WA, Murphy RP, Anderson KC, et al: The evaluation of patients with Eales' disease. Retina 3:243–248, 1983.

Smiddy WE, Isernhagen RD, Michels RG, et al: Vitrectomy for nondiabetic vitreous hemorrhage. Retinal and choroidal vascular disorders. Retina 8:88–95, 1988.

336 GYRATE ATROPHY OF THE CHOROID AND RETINA WITH HYPERORNITHINEMIA 363.57

(Ornithine-Δ-Aminotransferase Deficiency)

La-ongsri Atchaneeyasakul, MD
Bangkok, Thailand
Richard G. Weleber, MD
Portland, Oregon

ETIOLOGY/INCIDENCE

Gyrate atrophy of the choroid and retina is a rare, autosomal recessive, progressive dystrophy that is associated with hyperornithinemia and deficient activity of the mitochondrial matrix enzyme ornithine-Δ-aminotransferase (OAT), a pyridoxal phosphate-dependent enzyme required for the synthesis of proline from ornithine. Plasma, urine, spinal fluid, and aqueous humor levels of ornithine are 10 to 20 times higher than normal. The human *OAT* gene was mapped to chromosome 10q26, and multiple mutant alleles and compound heterozygotes have been described.

DIAGNOSIS

Clinical signs and symptoms

Ocular or periocular

- Choroid: atrophy.
- Iris: atrophy, loss of pigment.
- Lens: subcapsular cataracts (usually seen before the third decade of life).
- Optic nerve: pallor, peripapillary atrophy, astrocytic hamartoma of the optic disc.
- Retina: abnormal dark adaptometry, abnormal EOG, atrophy, epiretinal membrane, macular edema, retinal detachment, subnormal or nonrecordable ERG, traction schisis, vascular leakage and shunt vessels, vascular sheathing and attenuation.
- Vitreous: opacity, hemorrhage.
- Other: constriction of visual fields, decreased visual acuity, dyschromatopsia, moderate to high myopia.

Laboratory findings

The disease is characterized by circular patches of total vascular choroidal atrophy, which begin in the periphery in early childhood, enlarge and coalesce, and eventually extend toward the posterior pole. Constriction of the visual field, night blindness, cataracts (usually posterior subcapsular type), defective color vision, retinal vascular leakage, peripapillary atrophy, and macular changes develop as the disease progresses. Rarely, macular edema results. Myopia of a moderate to severe degree is frequent. Rhegmatogenous and nonrhegmatogenous retinal detachments have been described, along with the management. Legal blindness usually occurs in the fourth to fifth decade. Electroretinogram (ERG) responses and electro-oculogram (EOG) light-induced increases in the resting potential of the eye, as measured by the light-to-dark ratios, are consistently abnormal and eventually unrecordable by standard techniques. Studies in a mouse model suggested that retinal pigment epithelial cells are the initial site of pathologic changes. Seizures with or without abnormal electroencephalograms have been reported. Although the neuromuscular and electromyographic examinations are normal, eosinophilic subsarcolemmal deposits, which appear as tubular aggregates on electron microscopy, are seen on muscle biopsy. Skeletal muscle changes can also be demonstrated by computed tomography scanning and magnetic resonance imaging. They may be secondary to the inhibition of creatine synthesis by ornithine.

Parents who are carriers of this condition are normal clinically. Siblings may be affected and should be evaluated through the determination of serum ornithine levels and fundus examination because eye disease may be unrecognized. Prenatal diagnosis is possible by measuring OAT activity in cultured amniotic fluid cells or cultured chorionic villi. In families with a previous history of gyrate atrophy, the study of restriction fragment length polymorphism for OAT might be helpful for prenatal diagnosis and carrier detection.

At least two forms of gyrate atrophy with hyperornithinemia are known: a vitamin B_6-nonresponsive form and a slightly milder vitamin B_6-responsive form. Only a small percentage of patients with gyrate atrophy are vitamin B_6 responsive. E318K and A226V mutations in the *OAT* gene were among those mutations correlated with the vitamin B_6-responsive phonotype. There is an even milder form of total vascular atrophy of the peripheral choroid and retina resembling gyrate atrophy; these patients have normal serum ornithine levels and normal OAT activity in cultured skin fibroblasts.

TREATMENT

Systemic

Supplemental vitamin B_6

Supplemental pyridoxine in doses of 15 to 20 mg/day can result in more than 50% reduction in the serum ornithine level in vitamin B_6-responsive patients; large doses (600 to 750 mg/day) have produced mild short-term improvement in the ERG, EOG, and dark adaptometry in certain patients. However, chorioretinal atrophy has continued to progress at a slow rate despite partially reduced serum ornithine levels after vitamin B_6 administration. Because of the reported peripheral neuropathy that can occur with high-dose pyridoxine, we recommend only modest dietary supplementation for patients who have been proved biochemically to respond to vitamin B_6 with a reduction in serum or plasma ornithine levels.

Dietary restriction of arginine

Severe dietary arginine restriction can reduce the elevated serum ornithine levels in patients who do not respond biochemically to oral pyridoxine. Foods rich in arginine include chocolate, peanuts, almonds, and other nuts and seeds. Some patients have had short-term improvements or stabilization in visual acuity, ERG, visual field, color vision, and dark adaptometry after prolonged marked reduction of serum ornithine by dietary restriction of arginine. Some studies have documented the continual progression of atrophy of choroid and retina despite normal ornithine concentrations in children 3 to 4.5 years old. However, a recent study found that patients who adhered to an arginine-restricted diet sufficient to lower the plasma ornithine level below an average of 5.29 to 6.61 mg/dL (400–500 micromol/L) had slower mean rates of change of sequential electroretinography and visual field examinations.

Dietary supplementation with creatine

Oral supplementation with creatine (1.5 g/day) has been reported to reverse the muscle abnormalities but has no effect on the retina. Supplementary proline, a nonessential amino acid, has been suggested to possibly lessen the progression of the retinal lesions in some patients; however, this treatment has not been proved to be beneficial.

Gene therapy

In vitro studies of intraocular gene replacement therapy have been performed with adenovirus or retrovirus vectors carrying the OAT cDNA to transfer the gene into primary cultures of human retinal pigment epithelial cells.

Another possible therapeutic approach is the use of genetically manipulated human keratinocytes, which would be then transplanted into the gyrate atrophy patient as a 'metabolic sink' for reduction of ornithine accumulation. This concept may prove useful for several metabolic diseases.

Ocular

Optical correction of myopia is indicated. Occasionally, cataract extraction is warranted. Intraocular tamponade with silicone oil is mandatory for the treatment of rhegmatogenous retinal detachment in gyrate atrophy due to the lack of RPE resulting in ineffectiveness of laser photocoagulation.

COMPLICATIONS

Only approximately 5% of patients with gyrate atrophy respond clinically and biochemically to oral pyridoxine supplementation. Further studies will be necessary in these patients who do respond to determine whether the long-term course of the disease can be slowed or halted.

Vitamin B_6 is present in varying amounts in food and multiple vitamin preparations. At least one patient has been incorrectly considered to be a nonresponder because of failure to respond to dietary supplemental pyridoxine at a time when the patient was already receiving pyridoxine in multiple vitamin preparations sufficient to lower serum ornithine. Patients should be without any supplemental pyridoxine for several weeks before their biochemical responsiveness to oral vitamin B_6 is determined.

Severe dietary restriction of arginine requires an extremely low protein diet that is both unpalatable and potentially dangerous. Careful monitoring of the serum ammonia and nitrogen balance is essential, particularly in children.

Periodic documentation of retinal function over many years will be needed to determine stability or progression of the disease.

COMMENTS

One study showed the estimated odds for thyroid disease, which reflects the relative risk, in patients with gyrate atrophy to be almost 13 times that of normal volunteers ($P = 0.02$).

Recently, posterior chamber intraocular lens dislocation with the capsular bag was reported in a patient with gyrate atrophy several years after uneventful cataract surgery. This might be the result of capsule fibrosis leading to zonular disruption. Complete cortical cleanup in gyrate atrophy patients who have cataract extraction is recommended.

REFERENCES

Barrett DJ, Bateman JB, Sparkes RS, et al: Chromosome localization of human ornithine aminotransferase gene sequences to 10q26 and Xp11.2. Invest Ophthalmol Vis Sci 28:1037–1042, 1987.

Kaiser-Kupfer MI, Caruso RC, Valle D, Reed GF: Use of an arginine-restricted diet to slow progression of visual loss in patients with gyrate atrophy. Arch Ophthalmol 122:982–984, 2004.

Kennaway NG, Weleber RG, Buist NRM: Gyrate atrophy of choroid and retina: deficient activity of ornithine ketoacid aminotransferase in cultured skin fibroblasts. N Engl J Med 297:1180, 1977.

Weleber RG, Kennaway NG: Clinical trial of vitamin B_6 for gyrate atrophy of the choroid and retina. Ophthalmology 88:316–324, 1981.

Weleber RG, Kennaway NG, Buist NRM: Gyrate atrophy of the choroid and retina: approaches to therapy. Int Ophthalmol 4:23–32, 1981.

337 PERIPHERAL RETINAL BREAKS AND VITREORETINAL DEGENERATIVE DISORDERS 362.60

Charles P. Wilkinson, MD
Baltimore, Maryland

The peripheral retina is defined as the area of the retina that lies anterior to the vortex vein ampullae. Peripheral vitreoretinal degenerative disorders, including retinal breaks, vary in their importance (Figure 337.1). Some are caused or are related to the development of rhegmatogenous retinal detachment (RRD). At the other end of the spectrum is a group of incidental congenital or acquired entities that are of little importance other than their potential for being misdiagnosed. Lattice degeneration is the most important degenerative entity associated with RRD. Cystic retinal tufts are also visible sites of vitreoretinal adhesion and have some potential to be sites of later retinal tears. Retinal breaks are responsible for RRD, but most retinal breaks are not dangerous. Most of the other peripheral retinal abnormalities described in this chapter have little potential to cause RRD.

ETIOLOGY/INCIDENCE

Peripheral vitreoretinal degenerative disorders can be categorized as vitreoretinal, intraretinal, or chorioretinal. The presence of some type is almost ensured in all post-adolescent eyes. The goal is to identify conditions that may predispose to retinal break formation and subsequent retinal detachment. *Retinal breaks* include atrophic holes, operculated tears, horseshoe tears, and retinal dialyses.

Vitreoretinal disorders

Lattice degeneration occurs in approximately 8% of the population and is frequently bilateral. It is usually present by adolescence.

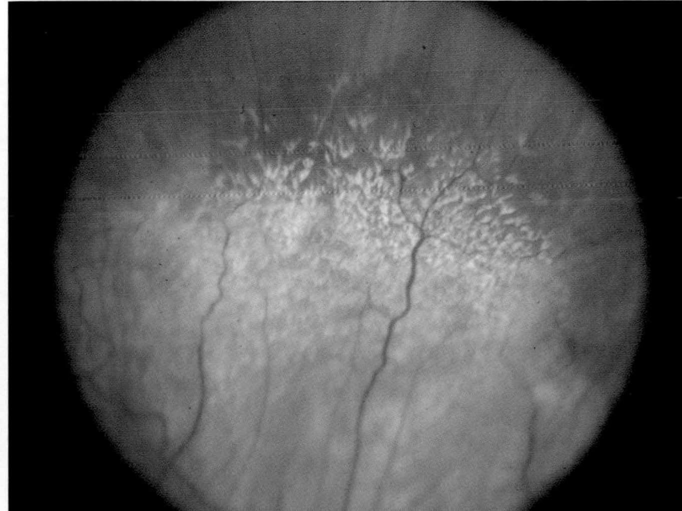

FIGURE 337.1. Peripheral retinal lattice degeneration.

Cystic retinal tufts are seen in approximately 5%, but they are usually unilateral. They are present at birth.

White-without-pressure occurs primarily in young, heavily pigmented patients.

Intraretinal disorders

Peripheral cystoid degeneration affects all eyes in patients older than 8 years.

Typical retinoschisis occurs in 4% to 8% of patients.

Chorioretinal disorders

Paving-stone degeneration occurs in roughly 30% of patients older than 50.

Reticular chorioretinal pigmentary degeneration of some degree increases with advancing age and is very common in the elderly.

Retinal breaks

Incidental retinal breaks are found in about 6% of eyes in both clinical and autopsy studies, and they become more common with advancing age. They usually do not cause RRD. In one large clinical series of incidental retinal breaks, horseshoe tears accounted for 10%, round holes with an operculum for 13%, and round holes without an operculum for approximately 77%.

COURSE/PROGNOSIS

Although lattice degeneration is seen in 30% of patients with retinal detachments, an overwhelming majority of patients with lattice degeneration do not develop retinal detachment. Approximately 20% of lattice lesions develop atrophic holes, but only approximately 2% of lattice lesions become sites of tractional horseshoe breaks. The odds of RRD associated with a cystic retinal tuft have been estimated at less than 0.3 %. A very small percentage of patients with retinoschisis may develop RRD. For the remainder of the patients with peripheral vitreoretinal disorders, the prognosis is usually benign.

Retinal breaks associated with persistent vitreoretinal traction are frequent causes of RRD. At least 50% of horseshoe tears that are associated with 'flashes and floaters' will progress to RRD. On the other hand, symptomatic operculated tears that are *not* associated with persistent vitreoretinal traction on the nearby retina are most unlikely to progress to RRD. Since atrophic holes occurring in lattice lesions are associated with possible vitreoretinal traction on the lattice, they occasionally progress to RRD, but atrophic holes unassociated with vitreoretinal traction are not such a threat. Similarly, asymptomatic horseshoe tears other than retinal dialyses rarely progress to RRD.

The usual sequence of events leading to RRD includes vitreous liquefaction leading to partial or complete posterior vitreous detachment (PVD) followed by the production of retinal tears at the sites of vitreoretinal adhesions. These adhesions may be visible, as with lattice lesions, or invisible. Traction on lattice lesions causes horseshoe tears along the lesion margins; RRD also occurs in association with traction on lattice lesions containing atrophic holes. Retinal detachment due to a retinal dialysis is usually discovered incidentally or following ocular trauma, and prophylactic therapy to prevent retinal dialysis is rarely considered.

DIAGNOSIS

Most peripheral vitreoretinal degenerative disorders and retinal breaks exhibit characteristic distinguishing features.

Vitreoretinal disorders

Lattice degeneration usually occurs as oval-shaped areas of retinal thinning that are primarily located parallel to the ora serrata; however, some lesions are radial and associated with larger blood vessels. Varying degrees of pigmentation are seen around the margins, and criss-crossed areas of sclerotic vessels and atrophic holes also may be present within the margins of the lesions. Scleral depression usually reveals localized vitreous liquefaction over the lesions, and vitreoretinal adhesions are always present at the margins.

Cystic retinal tufts appear as discrete, sharply circumscribed opaque white or gray lesions, usually in the equatorial zones. Pigment alterations in the base of the lesion are frequent, and there commonly are significant vitreous condensations attached to the surface of the tuft.

White without pressure refers to sharply demarcated geographic areas of relative whiteness appearing to lie at the inner surface of the peripheral retina. It is probably a reflex related to relative youth and pigmentation of the patient.

Intraretinal disorders

Peripheral typical cystoid degeneration appears as a multitude of tiny cysts within the far peripheral retina. It most commonly is seen inferior temporally but can sometimes be seen for 360 degrees. Temporally, it frequently appears as a grayish band of irregularly surfaced retina.

Typical retinoschisis occurs when cysts of cystoid degeneration enlarge to more than 1.5 mm mm in diameter. It most commonly is seen inferior temporally. A cyst-like structure that cannot be decompressed with scleral depression is its most likely appearance. It usually occurs first in the inferotemporal quadrant. If the inner layer of retina is sufficiently elevated, retinoschisis can mimic the appearance of RRD.

Chorioretinal disorders

Paving-stone degeneration consists of one or more well-demarcated yellowish-white lesions that primarily occur very anteriorly in the inferior quadrants. These represent areas of atrophic outer retina, retinal pigment epithelium, and inner choroid.

Reticular chorioretinal pigmentary degeneration is a net-like subretinal pigmentary change in the equatorial retina, associated with equatorial drusen. Associated intraretinal and perivascular pigment spicules are occasionally observed.

Retinal breaks

Retinal tears are due to vitreoretinal traction on vitreoretinal adhesions. Horseshoe tears appear as retinal defects associated with U- or V-shaped flaps, with the bases located at the anterior edge of the break and the flap pointing posteriorly. An operculated tear results from a horseshoe tear that has an avulsed flap.

Atrophic holes are round or oval-shaped dehiscences in the retina that are found in lattice lesions or in isolated areas of the peripheral retina. A retinal dialysis appears as a circumferential break or disinsertion of the retina at or within one disk diameter of the ora serrata.

TREATMENT

Most contemporary preventative therapies have been proposed to reduce the frequency of retinal tears at sites of *visible* vitreoretinal adhesive lesions or to prevent the accumulation of subretinal fluid around retinal breaks. Treatment has usually consisted of creation of chorioretinal adhesions, with lasers or cryotherapy, around visible focal degenerative lesions or retinal breaks. Others have proposed creating a peripheral ring of chorioretinal adhesions to prevent the development of tears at sites of both visible and invisible vitreoretinal adhesions. The results of treating visible vitreoretinal adhesions, such as lattice degeneration, to prevent retinal detachment have been evaluated by expert panels, and the American Academy of Ophthalmology (AAO) has published a 'Preferred Practice Pattern' (PPP) regarding prophylactic therapy.

In the American Academy of Ophthalmology Preferred Practice Patterns (AAO PPP), no prospective randomized trials of preventative therapy of any vitreoretinal lesions, including all types of retinal breaks, were identified. In cases of prior retinal detachment due to lattice degeneration, there was 'substantial' evidence that treating lattice lesions in the fellow eye was of limited value. However, the same evidence demonstrated that such treatment was of no value if the degree of myopia exceeded -6 diopters or if there were more than 6 clock-hours of lattice degeneration. Thus, prophylactic therapy appears to be of less value in higher-risk cases, and the best evidence also indicated that there was 'substantial' evidence that routine treatment of lattice degeneration in non-fellow eyes was of no benefit.

The major limitation in treating visible vitreoretinal adhesions is that subsequent retinal tears and detachments occur in areas that appear normal prior to PVD. To accomplish a goal of treating invisible adhesions, some authors have recommended the placement of chorioretinal burns over a 360-degree zone of peripheral retina extending from the equator to the ora serrata, and both laser and cryotherapy has been employed for this purpose. Good evidence that this form of therapy is effective is currently lacking.

COMMENTS

Focal abnormalities in the peripheral retina are encountered frequently, but most are of no significance. Although lattice degeneration and retinal breaks are clearly associated with RRD, evidence for the value of treating these lesions in asymptomatic patients is currently lacking. The best management strategies should include thorough discussions with patients regarding (1) the presence of entities that may predispose to RRD, (2) the critical importance of the onset of symptoms suggestive of PVD, and (3) the need for periodic examinations.

REFERENCES

American Academy of Ophthalmology: Preferred practice pattern. posterior vitreous detachment, retinal breaks, and lattice degeneration. San Francisco, American Academy of Ophthalmology, 2003.

Byer NE: Cystic retinal tufts and their relationship to retinal detachment, Arch Ophthalmol 99:1788–1790, 1981.

Byer NE: Long term natural history of lattice degeneration of the retina. Ophthalmology 96:1396–1402, 1989.

Byer NE: Prognosis of asymptomatic retinal breaks. Arch Ophthalmol 92:208–210, 1974.

Byer NE: The natural history of asymptomatic retinal breaks. Ophthalmology 89:1033–1039, 1982.

Davis MD: The natural history of retinal breaks. Arch Ophthalmol 92:183–194, 1974.

338 REFSUM'S DISEASE 356.3 (Heredopathia Atactica Polyneuritiformis, Phytanic Acid Oxidase Deficiency, Hereditary Motor and Sensory Neuropathy IV, HMSN IV)

La-ongsri Atchaneeyasakul, MD
Bangkok, Thailand
Richard G. Weleber, MD
Portland, Oregon

ETIOLOGY/INCIDENCE

Refsum's disease is a rare autosomal recessive disorder of lipid metabolism affecting mostly those of Scandinavian and Northern European descent. The deficiency of the peroxisomal enzyme phytanoyl-coenzyme A α-hydroxylase (PhyH), which catalyzes the a-oxidative process in phytanic acid catabolism, leads to the accumulation of the branched chain fatty acid phytanic acid in the serum and the tissues, with a predilection for adipose tissue, liver, and kidneys. The gene encoding PhyH (*PHYH* gene), located on chromosome 10p, has been identified, and different mutations have been demonstrated in patients with Refsum's disease. Recently, linkage analysis of patients diagnosed with Refsum's disease, but without mutations in *PHYH*, suggested a second locus on chromosome 6q22-24. This region includes the *PEX7* gene, which codes for the peroxin 7 receptor protein required for peroxisomal import of proteins containing a peroxisomal targeting signal type 2. The age of onset of this disease varies from the first to the fifth decade of life.

DIAGNOSIS

This syndrome is characterized by atypical retinitis pigmentosa, chronic polyneuropathy, and cerebellar signs. Other clinical findings include congestive heart failure, nerve deafness, and ichthyosiform skin lesions. Skeletal abnormalities have been described in some cases, including multiple epiphyseal dysplasia and shortening of the fourth metatarsals.

Clinical signs and symptoms

Although phytanic acid is stored in fatty tissues, symptoms of the disease are related to the concentration of phytanic acid in the blood rather than total body stores. The earliest symptom is almost invariably night blindness, which usually occurs before the age of 20. Electroretinogram responses are profoundly abnormal or nondetectable, although there is a report of mild retinal changes in an older patient. The disturbance in retinal pigmentation, which early in the disease is often limited to the periphery, may be granular, rather than 'bone-spicule.' Weakness in the extremities, unsteadiness of gait, and a history of chronic exacerbations and remissions are common. Complete external ophthalmoplegia and cataracts have been reported. Often, the diagnosis of Friedreich's ataxia is entertained; however, tendon reflexes that are initially undetectable may return weeks or months later. Invariably, cerebrospinal fluid shows an elevation in protein content without pleocytosis. Histologic study of the peripheral nerves shows thickening and hypertrophy around the nerve roots and degeneration of nuclei and fiber tracts in the brain stem. Ichthyosiform skin lesions may wax and wane with the rising and falling of the serum phytanic acid level. Impairment of renal function has also been reported. Impaired atrioventricular conduction, bundle-branch blocks, and cardiac arrhythmia may have contributed to the occasional occurrence of sudden death.

Ocular or periocular

- Cornea: epithelial and stromal edema, hypertrophy of the corneal nerves, reduced corneal sensation.
- Eyelids: ptosis.
- Lens: cataracts (usually posterior subcapsular).
- Optic nerve: partial demyelination, atrophy.
- Pupils: miosis, poor reaction to light and accommodation-convergence, poor response to cycloplegic and mydriatic drugs.
- Retina: lipid deposits in pigment epithelium with degeneration of overlying photoreceptors.
- Sclera: lipid deposits.
- Other: lipid deposits in the iris pigment epithelium and trabecular meshwork, glaucoma, visual field constriction, nystagmus, progressive external ophthalmoplegia.

TREATMENT

When untreated, the life expectancy is shortened.

Systemic

Dietary restriction of phytanic acid

Because phytanic acid is not metabolized in patients with Refsum's disease and the only source of phytanic acid in humans is dietary, restriction of oral intake of phytanic acid and, to a lesser extent, of phytol, which can be converted into phytanic acid, has been advised and found beneficial. Specifically, dietary intake of dairy products and fats and meats from ruminant animals, all of which contain phytanic acid, must be markedly curtailed. Caution should be observed to avoid starvation diets, as they can cause rapid mobilization of body stores of phytanic acid with a marked increase in the elevation of serum phytanic levels, acute toxicity, cardiac arrhythmias, and possible cardiac arrest.

Plasmapheresis

Plasmapheresis or plasma exchange is a useful treatment to lower plasma phytanic acid concentrations rapidly and has a definite role in the treatment of acute toxic states. Another procedure, called lipapheresis or cascade filtration, appears to be the treatment of choice to reduce plasma phytanic acid without the need for albumin replacement and also to reduce the loss of immunoglobulin.

Supportive

Carrier detection

Refsum's disease is an autosomal recessive genetic trait. Carriers with dietary loading may show elevated phytanic acid levels.

However, carrier detection is best determined by assay of phytanic acid a-oxidase activity in cultured skin fibroblasts.

Prenatal diagnosis

Because cultured amniocentesis cells show the enzyme activity, antenatal diagnosis of the affected or carrier state is theoretically possible.

COMMENTS

If started early, dietary restriction may prevent the development of neuromuscular and retinal changes. However, no conclusive evidence of improvement in cranial nerve and retinal function has been reported with dietary restriction or plasmapheresis. This lack of improvement may reflect the extent of irreversible damage to the retina. Early recognition and prompt treatment may forestall the development of these irreversible visual changes, although no improvement in the vision of patients with well-advanced disease should be expected. Because careful monitoring of diet and serum phytanic levels is required, these patients should be referred to tertiary medical centers for medical evaluation and therapy.

The diagnosis of Refsum disease might be delayed or misdiagnosed as Kearns-Sayre syndrome in a patient with the combined clinical features of ptosis, progressive external ophthalmoplegia, retinitis pigmentosa, and myocardiopathy. Such failure to make the correct diagnosis results in the delay in appropriate treatment.

Definite clinical and biochemical improvement has been reported with reduction of dietary phytanic acid and plasmapheresis. Muscle strength, tendon reflexes, sensory and motor nerve conduction, and certain objective tests of coordination have improved with treatment. The ichthyosiform rash and cardiac arrhythmias also clear as the serum phytanic acid decreases. One 39-year-old patient treated with dietary restriction over the past 13 years has shown only minimal progression of the visual findings during this period.

REFERENCES

Claridge KG, Gibberd FB, Sidey MC: Refsum disease: the presentation and ophthalmic aspects of Refsum disease in a series of 23 patients. Eye 6:371–375, 1992.

Gutsche HU, Siegmund JB, Hoppmann I: Lipapheresis: an immunoglobulin-sparing treatment for Refsum's disease. Acta Neurol Scand 94:190–193, 1996.

Jansen GA, Ofman R, FerdinanAusse S, et al: Refsum disease is caused by mutations in the phytanoyl-CoA hydroxylase gene. Nat Genet 17:190–193, 1997.

Jansen GA, Wanders RJ, Watkins PA, Mihalik SJ: Phytanoyl-coenzyme A hydroxylase deficiency: the enzyme defect in Refsum's disease. N Engl J Med 337:133–134, 1997.

339 RETINAL DETACHMENT 361.9

Graham Duguid, MD, BMedBiol, FRCS
London, UK

Retinal detachment is the separation of the neurosensory retina from the adjacent retinal pigment epithelium. Retinal detachments can be classified into three groups: rhegmatogenous, traction, and exudative. *Rhegmatogenous retinal detachments* are caused by the migration of vitreous cavity fluid through one or more holes or breaks in the retina. *Traction retinal detachments* are caused by the proliferation and contraction of fibrous or vascular scar tissue on the inner and / or outer surface of the retina. *Exudative retinal detachments* are caused by the leakage or production of fluid under the retina due to a diverse group of pathologic conditions. The successful treatment of retinal detachment is dependent on the identification of the underlying cause of the detachment. In complex cases, more than one pathologic mechanism may be present, such as a combined traction and rhegmatogenous retinal detachment in a patient with proliferative diabetic retinopathy.

ETIOLOGY

Rhegmatogenous retinal detachment

- This may occur with or without posterior vitreous detachment (PVD).
- A hole or tear develops in the retina.
- Retinal holes usually occur in an area of thinning such as retinal atrophy or lattice.
- Retinal tears are usually associated with posterior vitreous detachment and occur at an area of increased vitreo-retinal adhesion, often close to a retinal blood vessel.
- Attached vitreous gel can elevate the margin of the retinal tear.
- Fluid in the vitreous cavity migrates through the retinal defect and enters the potential space between the photoreceptor elements and the retinal pigment epithelium.
- The most important inherent predisposing factors are vitreous liquefaction, acute posterior vitreous detachment, abnormally firm vitreoretinal adhesion, lattice degeneration, cystic retinal tufts and myopia.

Traction retinal detachment

- The underlying disease process causes an inflammatory response affecting the posterior segment.
- Abnormal vitreous combines with breakdown of blood-retina barrier to initiate wound-healing response.
- Cells in the posterior segment migrate and proliferate.
- Proliferated cells attain critical mass and contract with a force exceeding the forces that maintain retinal attachment.
- The initiation of traction retinal detachment results in further inflammation and breakdown of the blood–retinal barrier, resulting in a vicious cycle that accelerates the detachment process.
- Alternatively, new blood vessels may grow from the retina onto the posterior hyaloid face, as in diabetic retinopathy or sickle-cell retinopathy.
- Traction may result anteroposteriorly from an incomplete posterior vitreous detachment or tangentially from contraction of the fibrovascular proliferation.

Exudative retinal detachment

- This results from the leakage or production of fluid in the subretinal space.
- Subretinal fluid usually originates from retinal or choroidal vasculature.
- There is a diverse spectrum of underlying pathology, including neoplasms, inflammatory disease, retinal vascular disease, and congenital disorders.

DIAGNOSIS

Clinical signs and symptoms

- The detailed history should include the present ocular symptoms, previous or concurrent ocular disease, and previous ocular trauma or surgery.
- Usually symptoms of floaters, photopsia and/or a peripheral visual field defect progressing centrally are described. The visual acuity may be reduced if the macula becomes involved.
- Past ophthalmic history should note any pre-exisiting eye disease, previous trauma or surgery. Any refractive error should be noted.
- A past medical history and review of systems, medications, and allergies should be included.
- The family history is important, especially with regard to the occurrence of retinal detachment in blood relatives.
- Comprehensive examination of *both* eyes should be done. Specific signs to be noted include, the visual acuity, the presence of a relative afferent pupil defect, the extent of any visual field defect, any intraocular inflammation, raised or lowered intraocular pressure, and the presence of any pigmented or white cells in the vitreous.
- A detailed evaluation of the retina using biomicroscopy and indirect ophthalmoscopy with scleral indentation is the most crucial portion of the examination.
- Critical features to identify during the retinal examination of the involved eye include the extent and topography of the retinal detachment, the type and location of all retinal breaks, presence of PVD, areas of persistent vitreoretinal traction, the presence and configuration of epiretinal membranes, the status of the optic nerve and macula, and any signs of conditions causing exudative retinal detachment.
- The retina of the fellow eye should be examined to look for PVD, asymptomatic retinal tears or detachments, lesions predisposing to rhegmatogenous detachments, proliferative retinopathy, or signs of systemic disease associated with exudative detachments.

Differential diagnosis

Rhegmatogenous retinal detachments

- There are convex surfaces and convex borders.
- Vitreous pigment cells are usually present (Schaffer's sign).
- The presence of a retinal break is diagnostic of a rhegmatogenous detachment, although occasionally the hole or holes cannot be identified before or during surgery.
- Alternating retinal bullae and folds oriented in a radial direction from the optic disk to the ora serrata are present.
- The topography and extent of the detachment usually predict the location of the retinal break or breaks.

Traction retinal detachments

- There usually are concave surfaces and some concave borders.
- The configuration, site, and extent of the detachment can be accounted for by the manifest vitreous traction.
- Fibrous (PVR) membranes or neovascularisation may be present.
- Retinal holes or vitreal pigment are absent unless combined rhegmatogenous and traction detachment.

Exudative retinal detachments

- There are convex surfaces and convex boundaries.
- The subretinal fluid typically shifts to the portion of the eye that is dependent (e.g. a patient may have poor vision on awakening after sleeping in the supine position because the subretinal fluid detaches the macula).
- No retinal breaks are observed.
- Signs of the causative underlying disease are usually apparent in the affected eye or, in the case of a systemic condition, in both eyes.

Retinoschisis

- Usually convex borders and surfaces, and inferotemporal or superotemporal in location. Retina appears very thin and may have multiple small holes or white spots on inner surface.
- Patient is often hypermetropic and very rarely myopic.
- Associated visual field defect is absolute (rather than relative in retinal detachment.)

Investigations

Ultrasonography

- Ultrasonography may show the presence or absence of retinal detachment in eyes with opaque media e.g. vitreous hemorrhage, may show the location of retinal tears, and may show the cause of exudative retinal detachment, e.g. neoplasms, choroidal effusions, scleritis.
- Doppler ultrasound may demonstrate retinal blood flow and be used to differentiate a retinal detachment from an incomplete vitreous detachment in vitreous hemorrhage.

Optical coherence tomography (OCT)

- OCT may differentiate a retinal detachment from a retinoschisis, but only if the lesion is fairly central (30°).

Fluorescein angiography

- This may be useful in eyes with suspected exudative detachments to identify leakage from the choroidal or retinal vasculature, and may show retinal or macular ischemia in eyes with traction detachments due to proliferative retinopathy or occlusive vascular disease.
- Macular ischemia carries a poor prognosis for the return of central visual function.

Electrophysiology

- The absence of a recordable response electroretinogram ERG to bright-flash stimulation may indicate severe occlusive retinal vascular disease or extensive retinal detachment, and implies a poor prognosis.
- A normal electroretinogram and absent visually evoked response suggest a lesion in the optic pathway (most often, the optic nerve).

Associations

Rhegmatogenous retinal detachment

- Accommodation spasm, including miotics.
- Myopia.
- Lattice degeneration.
- Cystic retinal tufts.
- Acute posterior vitreous detachment.
- Retinoschisis (senile or congenital X-linked).
- Trauma (surgical and nonsurgical).
- Marfan syndrome.
- Stickler syndrome.

- Wagner syndrome.
- Viral retinitis (acute retinal necrosis and cytomegalovirus retinitis).

Traction retinal detachment

- Proliferative diabetic retinopathy.
- Proliferative vitreoretinopathy.
- Hypertensive retinopathy.
- Sickle cell retinopathy.
- Retinopathy of prematurity.
- Penetrating trauma.
- Retinal vascular occlusive disease.

Exudative retinal detachment

- Choroidal malignant melanoma.
- Choroidal hemangioma.
- Choroidal metastasis.
- Retinoblastoma.
- Toxocariasis.
- Vogt–Koyanagi–Harada syndrome.
- Central serous chorioretinopathy.
- Posterior scleritis.
- Sympathetic ophthalmia.
- Coats disease.
- von Hippel–Lindau syndrome.
- Eales disease.
- Optic nerve pit.
- Morning glory syndrome.
- Familial exudative vitreo-retinopathy (FEVR).

PROPHYLAXIS

Rhegmatogenous retinal detachment

- Eyes with a previous posterior vitreous detachment have a lower risk of rhegmatogenous detachment than eyes without a posterior vitreous detachment, regardless of other risk factors.
- Patients should be educated to seek ophthalmologic attention within 24 hours if the symptoms of an acute posterior vitreous detachment occur.
- Prophylactic treatment usually involves creating a chorioretinal scar around the margins of a retinal break or subclinical small detachment to prevent the ingress of fluid into the subretinal space.
- A chorioretinal adhesion is most commonly created using laser photocoagulation delivered through a slit lamp or an indirect ophthalmoscope.
- Transconjunctival and transscleral cryotherapy are equally efficacious; occasionally, both laser therapy and cryotherapy are useful in the same eye. Cryotherapy is often useful if the retinal view is impeded by hemorrhage or cataract.
- Retinal breaks may be classified as 'asymptomatic' if found on routine examination or 'symptomatic' if detected when accompanied by symptoms.
- In addition to the presence of symptoms, risk factors such as aphakia or pseudophakia, myopia, family history of retinal detachment or retinal detachment in the fellow eye influence the decision to offer prophylactic treatment to a retinal lesion.
- Symptomatic acute retinal tears (horseshoe or u-tears) or dialyses are almost always treated prophylactically.
- Symptomatic eyes manifesting lattice degeneration with atrophic holes are now believed not to require prophylactic treatment, but may be followed depending on co-existing risk factors.
- Asymptomatic subclinical detachments are treated if there is a tear with persistent vitreoretinal traction or if the detachment extends posterior to the equator.
- Fellow eyes of patients with a prior rhegmatogenous detachment are considered for prophylactic treatment of lattice degeneration, asymptomatic breaks, subclinical detachments, and cystic retinal tufts particularly if the lesion is in the mirror-image position of the primary retinal break in the opposite eye with the retinal detachment.
- Fellow eyes of patients with non-traumatic giant retinal tears usually receive scatter or confluent peripheral panretinal photocoagulation.

Traction retinal detachment

- Prophylaxis depends on the underlying cause of traction detachment.
- Patients with proliferative diabetic retinopathy should undergo full panretinal laser photocoagulation.
- Patients with non-diabetic proliferative retinopathy, such as from a vascular occlusion or hypertensive retinopathy, should be considered for scatter laser photocoagulation treatment.
- The incidence of proliferative vitreoretinopathy may be reduced using anti-metabolite treatment at the time of vitrectomy surgery.

Exudative retinal detachment

- Prevention of exudative detachment usually involves appropriate identification and treatment of the underlying cause.

TREATMENT

Rhegmatogenous retinal detachment

- The main principles guiding the treatment of rhegmatogenous retinal detachments include identification and closure of the all retinal breaks by laser or cryo retinopexy, with internal or external tamponade, and relief of residual vitreoretinal traction. Subretinal fluid may be drained at the time of surgery or be allowed to be absorbed passively by the retinal pigment epithelium.
- The decision regarding the optimal treatment approach is dependent on multiple variables and must be made by the surgeon after a thorough discussion with the patient.

Pneumatic retinopexy

- This may be used as a primary outpatient office procedure for rhegmatogenous detachments with retinal breaks in the superior 3 clock-hours.
- Contraindications include lattice degeneration extending more than 3 clock-hours, active severe uveitis, significant vitreoretinal adhesions, inferior breaks with subretinal fluid, proliferative vitreoretinopathy worse than grade C2, and media opacities precluding adequate visualization of the entire fundus.
- Relative contraindications include pseudophakic eyes and eyes with advanced glaucoma.
- Excellent patient compliance with postoperative positioning is required.
- Anterior chamber paracentesis usually is performed initially.

- A gas bubble is injected through the pars plana into the midvitreous cavity with a 27- or 30-gauge 0.5-inch needle.
- 0.3 mL of air or perflurocarbon gases SF_6, C_2F_6, or C_3F_8 (100% concentration) depending on the size of the eye, the degree of vitreoretinal traction, and the size, location, and number of retinal breaks.
- It is critical to verify that the central retinal artery is perfused and light perception vision has returned after gas injection.
- If the central retinal artery is not patent within 1 minute, repeat the aqueous paracentesis.
- Cryotherapy may be applied to the area surrounding the retinal break or breaks just before the gas injection.
- Alternatively, cryotherapy or laser photocoagulation may be used to create a chorioretinal adhesion 1 or 2 days after gas injection.
- In addition to treating the retinal breaks, scatter panretinal laser photocoagulation may be performed once the retina has reattached.
- Approximately 80% of all primary retinal detachments meet the criteria for pneumatic retinopexy.
- The overall anatomic success rate is approximately 70%.
- The complications of pneumatic retinopexy include new or missed retinal breaks, increased intraocular pressure, vitreous hemorrhage, subretinal gas, gas in the anterior hyaloid space, subconjunctival gas, cataract, vitreous incarceration, endophthalmitis, proliferative vitreoretinopathy, delayed reabsorption of subretinal fluid, cystoid macular edema, and extension of the detachment into the macula.

Scleral buckling

- This may require local or general anesthesia.
- It involves dissection of the conjunctiva and Tenon's capsule to expose sclera.
- All retinal breaks must be localized and marked.
- Cryotherapy is applied to surround all breaks.
- The scleral explant is sutured to the sclera over each break.
- Patency of the central retinal artery is ensured after the buckle sutures are tied.
- Buckling material may be oriented radially or circumferentially.
- Radial buckles are used for large horseshoe tears to minimize fishmouth phenomenon or for posterior retinal breaks.
- A circumferential buckle may be segmental or encircle the globe. Encircling buckles create permanent indents but segmental ones tend to fade after 3 months.
- A segmental circumferential buckle is used for localized detachments with small breaks, localized detachments without identifiable breaks, detachments with minimal subretinal fluid, detachments of any size if the breaks are clustered within 2 clock-hours, retinal dialysis, or eyes with glaucoma (to preserve the conjunctiva for possible filtering surgery).
- Encircling circumferential buckles are relatively indicated in aphakic or pseudophakic eyes, with multiple breaks in multiple quadrants, for vitreoretinal pathology (e.g. lattice degeneration) in multiple quadrants, for extensive detachment without an identifiable break, for high myopia, or for the presence of significant proliferative vitreoretinopathy.
- External drainage of subretinal fluid is not necessary in 90% of cases.
- Occasionally, an intravitreal gas bubble may be injected to tamponade the retinal breaks internally.
- The overall anatomic success rate is approximately 90%.
- The complications of scleral buckling include scleral rupture or perforation, choroidal or retinal perforation, cystoid macular edema, vitreous hemorrhage, subretinal hemorrhage, serous or hemorrhagic choroidal detachment, retinal incarceration in the drainage site, exposure or infection of the buckle, intrusion of the buckle, endophthalmitis, anterior segment ischemia, persistent subretinal fluid, proliferative vitreoretinopathy, change in refractive error, and strabismus.

Pars plana vitrectomy

- Vitrectomy is indicated in an increasing proportion of retinal detachments including patients with giant retinal tears, unusual or multiple large breaks, posterior breaks or macular holes, coexisting vitreous hemorrhage or other significant media opacities, pseudophakic or aphakic eyes, and proliferative vitreoretinopathy requiring membrane peel.
- Most surgeons use a three-port system in which sclerotomy incisions are made through the pars plana 3.0 to 4.0 mm posterior to the limbus.
- The inferotemporal sclerotomy is usually used for an infusion line, and the two superior sclerotomies are used for hand-held instruments and light sources.
- The vitreous is resected to the level of the vitreous base for 360°, with special attention paid to the meticulous removal of vitreous attached to the edges of all breaks and visible areas of abnormally firm vitreoretinal adhesion.
- Transcleral cryotherapy may be applied to the retinal breaks before drainage of shallow subretinal fluid.
- Alternatively, transcleral cryotherapy or laser treatment with an endoscopic probe or the indirect ophthalmoscopic delivery system can be performed after complete drainage of the subretinal fluid.
- Subretinal fluid is drained internally during a simultaneous air-fluid exchange through a preexisting retinal break or by creating a posterior drainage retinotomy (preferably in the superonasal quadrant). An external transcleral drain is also possible.
- Air is then exchanged for either gas SF_6, C_2F_6, or C_3F_8 or silicone oil to provide internal tamponade of the retina whilst chorioretinal adhesion forms at the retinopexy.
- Heavy perfluorocarbon liquids may be a useful surgical adjunct during vitrectomy, especially for unrolling the flap of a giant retinal tear, in cases with a co-existing retinal traction detachment, for flattening detachments associated with posterior breaks, or for searching for small breaks not identifiable on initial internal search.
- Heavy silicone oil may provide inferior tamponade and may be left in the eye indefinitely if necessary.
- A scleral explant may be used in conjunction with vitrectomy.
- The anatomic success rate is approximately 90% after one operation.
- Complications of vitrectomy include cataract, transiently increased intraocular pressure, vitreous hemorrhage, subretinal hemorrhage, subretinal air or gas, subretinal perfluorocarbon liquid, retained perfluorocarbon liquid, endophthalmitis, failure of retinal reattachment, iatrogenic retinal breaks, proliferative vitreoretinopathy, macular pucker, cystoid macular edema, and serous or hemorrhagic choroidal detachment.

Traction retinal detachment

- Treatment of traction retinal detachments usually requires vitrectomy with or without scleral buckling, to relieve all retinal traction.
- An encircling scleral buckle may be used to relieve residual anterior traction and provide permanent support for peripheral retinal breaks.
- Peripheral traction detachments may be observed initially, until they extend posterior to the equator or develop a rhegmatogenous component.
- Epiretinal membranes require peeling, but fibrovascular membranes require segmentation and/or delamination in addition to hemostasis.
- Significant fibrotic subretinal membranes may occur in patients with proliferative vitreoretinopathy; and may be segmented or removed via a retinotomy.
- If significant vitreoretinal traction exists in the far periphery, e.g. anterior loop syndrome in PVR or anterior hyaloidal proliferation in diabetics, relief by anterior dissection, with lensectomy if necessary, may be required.
- All pre-existing or iatrogenic retinal breaks must be identified, relieved of residual vitreoretinal traction, and treated with retinopexy.
- Heavy perfluorocarbon liquids may be used to enhance identification of the epiretinal membranes, as a 'soft surgical tool' to provide retinal countertraction during membrane dissection, or to reattach the retina before gas or silicone oil instillation.
- Internal tamponade usually requires longer-acting C_3F_8 gas or silicone oil.
- Internal tamponade is not required if there is no retinal break (e.g. diabetic traction detachment without retinal breaks at the conclusion of surgery).
- The anatomic success rate varies to some degree according to the underlying disease process, but it is in the range of 90%.

Exudative retinal detachment

- The treatment is directed toward controlling or eradicating the underlying cause of the exudative detachment.
- Intraocular tumors may be treated with external beam radiation, radioactive plaque brachytherapy, chemotherapy, transscleral resection, thermal ablation, or enucleation.
- Inflammatory diseases such as Vogt–Koyanagi–Harada syndrome, posterior scleritis, and sympathetic ophthalmia are treated with corticosteroids or immunosuppressive medications such as cyclosporin A.
- Vascular diseases such as Coats or Eales disease may be treated with laser photocoagulation or cryotherapy.
- Central serous chorioretinopathy is usually observed initially and may be considered for focal laser photocoagulation if leakage persists for longer than 6 months or recurs at a later time.

COMMENTS

The timing of surgery depends on several variables, including the type of retinal detachment, the status of the macula, and the general medical condition of the patient.

For rhegmatogenous detachments, surgery should be performed at the earliest opportunity usually within 24 hours if the macula is imminently threatened.

Surgery may be delayed for up to 1 week if a rhegmatogenous detachment is in the periphery and does not have features that suggest rapid progression (bullous fluid, large tears, or superior tears).

If the macula has become detached a few days before the patient's presentation, surgery is usually performed at the earliest elective opportunity within 1 week.

If the macula has been detached for more than 1 week, the surgery may be scheduled electively in 1 to 2 weeks.

Because many traction detachments are slowly progressive, surgery may be scheduled electively.

Preoperative panretinal laser photocoagulation may be useful in some cases of diabetic traction detachments to arrest the proliferative process and help secure the surrounding retina.

In some cases of proliferative vitreoretinopathy, it may be advantageous to defer surgery for several weeks to allow the membranes to 'mature' and thus render them easier to remove.

Postoperative care includes the appropriate positioning of the patient with internal retinal tamponade, topical antibiotics, topical anti-inflammatory medications, topical cycloplegic agents, control of intraocular pressure, and pain and nausea management.

Patients with intravitreal gas are restricted from ground travel above 4000 feet elevation and airplane travel until the gas reabsorbs. A 10pc gas bubble will double the intraocular pressure at cabin altitude (approximately 6000 feet above sea level).

Should unexpected general anesthesia be required whilst gas remains in the eye, the anesthetist should be informed and anesthesia avoiding use of nitrous oxide can be planned to avoid sight-threatening increase in intraocular pressure.

REFERENCES

Abrams GW, Azen SP, McCuen BW, II, et al (for the Silicone Oil Study Group): Vitrectomy with silicone oil or long-acting gas in eyes with severe proliferative vitreoretinopathy: results of additional and long-term follow-up: Silicone Study Report 11. Arch Ophthalmol 115:335–344, 1997.

Green SN, Yarian DL, Masciulli L, et al: Office repair of retinal detachment using a Lincoff temporary balloon buckle. Ophthalmology 103:1804–1810, 1996.

Hakin KN, Lavin MJ, Leaver PK: Primary vitrectomy for rhegmatogenous retinal detachment. Graefes Arch Clin Exp Ophthalmol 231:344–346, 1993.

Han DP, Murphy ML, Mieler WF: A modified en bloc excision technique during vitrectomy for diabetic traction retinal detachment: results and complications. Ophthalmology 101:803–808, 1994.

Hilton GF, McClean EB, Brinton DA: American Academy of Ophthalmology: the repair of rhegmatogenous retinal detachments. Ophthalmology 103:1313–1324, 1996.

Kirsch LS: Retina. In: Roy FH: Ocular differential diagnosis. 6th edn. Baltimore, Williams & Wilkins, 1997:485–582.

Michels RG: Scleral buckling methods for rhegmatogenous retinal detachment. Retina 6:1–49, 1986.

Mills MD, et al: Ophthalmology 108(1):40–44, 2001.

Peyman GA, Schulman JA, Sullivan B: Perfluorocarbons in ophthalmology. Surv Ophthalmol 39:375–395, 1995.

Ryan SJ: Traction retinal detachment: XLIX Edward Jackson Memorial Lecture. Am J Ophthalmol 115:1–20, 1993.

Tornambe PE, Hilton GF, The Pneumatic Retinopexy Study Group: Pneumatic retinopexy: a two-year follow-up study of the multicenter trial comparing pneumatic retinopexy with scleral buckling. Ophthalmology 98:1115–1123, 1991.

Wilkinson CP, Rice TA: Michels Retinal Detachment. 2nd edn. St Louis, Mosby-Year Book, 1997:471–594.

340 RETINAL VENOUS OBSTRUCTION 362.30

Thomas K. Schlesinger, MD, PhD
Portland, Oregon
Christina J. Flaxel, MD
Portland, Oregon

Retinal vein occlusion is the second most frequent retinovascular disorder encountered in clinical practice.

ETIOLOGY

This entity occurs when there is an occlusion at the level of either the branch or central retinal venous system, causing a reduction in venous return. Patients typically present with acute, painless visual loss and should be followed for the development of retinal or iris neovascularization or macular edema.

Retinal arteries and veins, when adjacent, share an adventitial sheath. It is believed that chronic hypertension produces increasing thickness of the muscular arterial walls, leading to compression of the adjacent vein, creating turbulence. This results in the formation of a thrombus, located at the lamina in ischemic central retinal vein occlusion (CRVO) and at an arteriovenous crossing in branch retinal vein occlusion (BRVO). Other possible causes for retinal vein occlusion include hypercoagulable states, diabetes mellitus, chronic open-angle glaucoma, and prothrombotic states.

COURSE/PROGNOSIS

CRVO can be clinically classified as ischemic or nonischemic. Although 30% of non-ischemic CRVO cases progress to ischemic CRVO within 3 years, this clinical classification has important prognostic implications because nonischemic CRVO has a much more benign course. Visual loss in nonischemic CRVO is variable, with macular edema the major cause of reduced vision. Ischemic CRVO may lead to profound visual loss from macular edema or ischemia, hemorrhage, or neovascular glaucoma.

BRVO has a variable visual prognosis. Poor vision can be due to macular edema or ischemia, vitreous hemorrhage associated with posterior segment neovascularization, or epiretinal membrane.

DIAGNOSIS

Clinical signs and symptoms

Patients typically present with visual loss or metamorphopsia, although BRVO may be asymptomatic if it does not involve the macula. The presence of numerous 'flame-shaped' intraretinal hemorrhages is the hallmark of the disease. Nerve fiber layer infarcts are common, and these together with the hemorrhages give the classic 'blood and thunder' appearance of an acute CRVO. Retinal veins may be dilated and tortuous, and there may be evidence of disk swelling or macular edema. Clinical classification of this entity is made on the basis of the distribution of the retinal hemorrhages. CRVO involves all four quadrants, while BRVO is segmental. Neovascularization of the retina or disk may occur in BRVO. Posterior segment neovascularization is uncommon in CRVO, but neovascularization of the iris or angle often complicates ischemic CRVO.

Laboratory findings

Fluorescein angiography may be useful in distinguishing nonischemic from ischemic vein occlusion, documenting the presence of macular edema, or demonstrating macular ischemia. Nonischemic CRVO is defined as having less than 10 disk diameters of capillary non-perfusion, while nonischemic BRVO has less than 5. Furthermore, this modality can be used to confirm the presence of retinal, disk, or iris neovascularization.

Optical coherence tomography (OCT) has emerged as a powerful test to assess macular edema, its progression or regression, and its response to treatment.

Differential diagnosis

- Ocular ischemic syndrome.
- Diabetic retinopathy.
- Vasculitis.

TREATMENT

Although anticoagulation, surgical adventitial sheathotomy (BRVO), radial optic neurotomy (CRVO), and creation of a chorioretinal anastomosis have been suggested to treat selected cases, no therapy for reversing a retinal vein occlusion has been proved beneficial by a controlled study. Intravitreal injection of triamcinolone acetonide for macular edema has become popular, numerous cases and series have been reported, but controlled trials are lacking. Some evidence suggests intravitreal injection of vascular endothelial growth factor (VEGF) inhibitors may stabilize or improve visual acuity in selected CRVO cases.

Laser therapy has been proved beneficial for treating complications arising from retinal vein occlusion.

Central vein occlusion study

- Multicenter, randomized clinical trial that demonstrated panretinal laser photocoagulation caused regression of iris or angle neovascularization.
- Failed to demonstrate a beneficial effect of grid laser therapy for the treatment of macular edema in patients with CRVO.

Branch retinal vein study

- Multicenter randomized clinical trial that demonstrated the benefit of grid laser treatment for persistent macular edema in patients with worse than 20/40 vision.
- Demonstrated the efficacy of sectoral scatter laser photocoagulation for proliferative retinopathy associated with BRVO.

Laser photocoagulation guidelines

Branch retinal vein occlusion

- Persistent macular edema:
  - A fluorescein angiogram is obtained to confirm macular edema. There should be significant clearing of hemorrhage to adequately assess macular edema.
  - Treatment is offered to patients with macular edema without significant loss of macular perfusion, who have worse than 20/40 vision and who have had sufficient

time to allow for spontaneous improvement (4 months).
    - Treatment (argon green, 100-µm spot size, 0.1-second duration, to create a mild burn) is applied to the area of edema from the arcades to the edge of the foveal avascular zone.
- Retinal neovascularization:
    - Retinal neovascularization, with or without vitreous hemorrhage, is an indication for sectoral laser photocoagulation.
    - Laser energy (argon green laser, 200-µm spot size, 0.1-second duration, with burns being applied two burn widths apart, to create a moderately intense burn) is applied to the area affected by the vein occlusion.

Central retinal vein occlusion

- Baseline examination includes iris and gonioscopic examination to rule out the presence of neovascularization.
- Patients should be followed monthly for the development of iris or angle neovascularization for 6 months, then less frequently.
- If either iris or angle neovascularization develops, panretinal photocoagulation is performed using using 200- to 500-µm spot size burns of 0.1-second duration to create moderately intense burns.
- If persistent corneal edema is present with neovascular glaucoma, indirect laser photocoagulation or retinal cryotherapy may be necessary.

COMPLICATIONS

- Macular edema.
- Retinal neovascularization.
- Iris neovascularization.
- Vitreous hemorrhage.
- Neovascular glaucoma.
- Epiretinal membrane.

COMMENTS

Retinal vein occlusion is a common retinovascular entity that may be complicated by macular edema or ocular neovascularization. Laser therapy has been proved beneficial in treating macular edema and retinal neovascularization in the setting of BRVO and for the regression of anterior segment neovascularization in CRVO. Intravitreal triamcinolone decreases macular edema caused by venous occlusion, but its exact place in the therapeutic progression is not clear. VEGF inhibitors may provide an additional weapon in treating venous occlusion, but more study is necessary.

REFERENCES

Branch Retinal Vein Occlusion Study Group: Argon laser photocoagulation for macular edema in branch retinal vein occlusion. Am J Ophthalmol 98:271–282, 1984.

Branch Retinal Vein Occlusion Study Group: Argon laser photocoagulation for prevention of neovascularization and vitreous hemorrhage in branch retinal vein occlusion. Arch Ophthalmol 104:34–41, 1986.

Green WR, Chan CC, Hutchins GM, et al: Central retinal vein occlusion: a prospective histological study of 29 eyes in 28 cases. Trans Am Ophthalmol Soc 89:371–422, 1981.

Heyreh SS: Classification of central retinal vein occlusion. Ophthalmol 90:458–474, 1983.

Iturralde D, Spaide RF, Meyerle CB, et al: Intravitreal bevacizumab (avastin) treatment of macular edema in central retinal vein occlusion. A short term study. Retina 26(3):279–284, 2006.

Jonas JB: Intravitreal triamcinolone acetonide for treatment of intraocular oedematous and neovascular diseases. Acta Ophthalmologica Scandinavica 83(6):645–663, 2005.

The Central Retinal Vein Occlusion Study Group: Evaluation of grid pattern photocoagulation for macular edema in central vein occlusion: The Central Retinal Vein Occlusion Study Group M Report. Ophthalmology 102:1425–1433, 1995.

The Central Vein Occlusion Study Group: Natural history and clinical management of central retinal vein occlusion. Arch Ophthalmol 115:486–491, 1997.

The Eye Disease Case-Control Study Group: Risk factors for central retinal vein occlusion. Arch Ophthalmol 114:545–554, 1996.

Zhao J, Sastry SM, Sperduto RD, et al: Arteriovenous crossing patterns in branch retinal vein occlusion: The Eye Disease Case-Control Study Group. Ophthalmology 100:423–428, 1993.

341 RETINITIS PIGMENTOSA 362.74

Saul C. Merin, MD
Jerusalem, Israel

ETIOLOGY/INCIDENCE

Retinitis pigmentosa (RP) is an inherited, progressive disease of the retina characterized by early and diffuse functional retinal abnormalities, a subnormal or 'extinct' (nonrecordable) electroretinogram, early involvement of the retinal pigment epithelium and visual receptors, and an outcome of severely impaired vision or blindness. It is conceivable that in both humans and animals, the primary event in most cases of retinitis pigmentosa is the loss of photoreceptors by apoptosis, a programmed cell death.

Retinitis pigmentosa may occur as an isolated ocular disease, may be linked to another affected organ such as the ear or kidney, or may be part of a systemic disease. It occurs in virtually every race and population in the world. The recorded incidence varies from 1 in 2000 to 1 in 7000, with an incidence of approximately 1 in 4000 in most populations. Males are affected more often than females.

In most patients, the inherited nature of the disease is manifested by additional members of the family being similarly affected, by consanguinity of the parents, or by some signs of the disease in the female carrier. Any one of three modes of monogenic transmission may transmit RP through many different genes and mutations. By 2004, at least 12 autosomal dominant genes, 21 autosomal recessive genes and 5 X-chromosome linked genes were identified and delineated as causing retinitis pigmentosa.

COURSE/PROGNOSIS

The symptoms of retinitis pigmentosa usually become apparent during the second decade of life though they are sometimes present in early childhood or may occur much later, in the third to fifth decade. Night blindness is usually the earliest symptom,

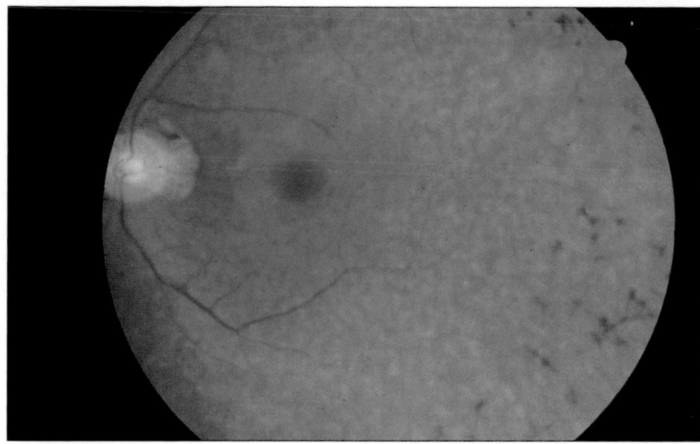

FIGURE 341.1. Typical fundus manifestation of retinitis pigmentosa. Note pigmentary stippling, pale dots, attenuated retinal arteries and bone corpuscular pigmentation more peripheral.

followed by progressive loss of peripheral visual fields. Often central vision is involved early due to cystoid macular edema or atrophic maculopathy. Before the involvement of central vision, the patient may be aware of the deterioration of color vision. The progression of morphologic changes of the fundus depends on the genetic entity and varies in different types of retinitis pigmentosa (Figure 341.1).

In some cases, visual loss may be rapid, unexpectedly causing severe reduction in visual acuity. This occurs especially in the autosomal recessive and X-linked forms. The autosomal dominant form is usually milder. Forty-two percent of patients have good visual acuity at 60 years of age. The average 'half-life' for visual fields is approximately 5 to 7 years.

DIAGNOSIS

The diagnosis of retinitis pigmentosa is based on the typical symptoms, such as night blindness and abnormalities of the visual fields, together with the typical ocular manifestations. The diagnosis is confirmed with electroretinography.

Clinical signs and symptoms

Ocular

- Choroid: disappearance of choriocapillaries and, later, loss of larger choroidal vessels.
- Optic nerve: waxy-pale (late).
- Retina: attenuated arteries, depigmentation of pigment epithelium, fine pigmentary stippling and pale-gray dots, retinal thinning, vascular pigmentary sheathing, bone corpuscular pigmentation, reduction in blood flow, cystoid macular edema, atrophic maculopathy, epiretinal membrane.
- Vitreous: cells, pigment, abnormal or broken fibers and floaters.
- Lens: early development of posterior subcapsular cataract.

Associated retinitis pigmentosa

Retinitis pigmentosa may be associated with a variety of disease entities, such as various lipid disorders, mucopolysaccharidoses, spinocerebellar degenerations, and other seemingly unrelated conditions. The association with retinitis pigmentosa is for the most part not understood. In some, treatment of the underlying systemic disease may benefit the ocular disability, so the proper diagnosis must be established.

- In Refsum's disease, the restriction of dietary intake of phytol and phytanic acid, together with periodic plasmapheresis, has been shown to be beneficial in arresting progression of the retinal dystrophy.
- In abetalipoproteinemia (Bassen–Kornzweig syndrome), combined vitamin A and vitamin E therapy is efficient in arresting the visual deterioration, including the electroretinographic progressive reduction.

TREATMENT

There is no cure for retinitis pigmentosa, but certain conditions can be specifically treated, and there are indications for possible ways to reduce progression of the disease. In addition, new avenues of research raise hope for a future cure.

Systemic

- Acetazolamide (Diamox) 125 mg twice daily or 125 mg three times daily has been successfully used to improve central vision in patients with macular edema associated with retinitis pigmentosa. It was also reported that with prolonged use of this medication, a progressive increase in extrafoveal retinal sensitivity was noted.
- Methazolamide has been used instead of acetazolamide but is less effective.
- Vitamin A palmitate 15,000 IU/day was effective in slowing the rate of decline of retinal function, as measured with cone electroretinography, in a proportion of patients. The study has been performed in 600 patients who were followed up for 6 years. Vitamin A supplement is not given to patients with liver disease, and liver function blood tests should be performed before administration and at intervals later. Vitamin A should not be used in pregnancy.
  - Docosahexaenoic acid (DHA) supplementation by capsules, 600 mg twice a day slowed the course of RP for two years in a subgroup of patients who simultaneously started treatment with both vitamin A and DHA.
  - A dietary benefit of omega-3 rich food became recently evident. One or two weekly intakes of omega-3 rich fish, such as salmon, tuna, mackerel, herring or sardines resulted in an average 40%–50% slower annual loss of visual field. This could achieve a gain of almost two decades of visual preservation.

Ocular

- Recommendations based on theoretic and clinical considerations suggest that patients with retinitis pigmentosa wear dark sunglasses for outdoor use, especially in bright sunlight. The addition of side shields to the dark sunglasses is helpful in further restricting the amount of sunlight that reaches the eye. Special sunglasses that reduce considerably (more than 75%) the total transmission of light and cut out the lower wavelengths of light and the ultraviolet rays are produced by several manufacturers and are commercially available. Almost all patients fitted with such glasses report subjective visual improvement, mainly through enhanced contrasts; however, objective measurements confirmed such an improvement in only a proportion of patients.
- The correction of associated refractive errors and the use of low-vision aids may help improve central vision. Optical devices may be used to widen the visual fields in patients

with good central vision and narrow visual fields; these include properly designed Fresnel lenses. An image intensifier may be used to improve vision in the darkness. Early clinical trials have been encouraging. A wide-field high-intensity lantern was useful and practical for night mobility.

- Dorzolamide eye drops t.i.d. were found to improve the visual acuity of some patients with cystoid macular edema, but acetazolamide was found to be more effective. These drops can be used in patients who cannot take acetazolamide due to side effects.

Surgical

- Patients with advanced retinitis pigmentosa often have a posterior subcapsular cataract. Even when the electroretinogram is very low or extinct, such patients may benefit from cataract extraction if the macular function is still preserved. In such cases, the best preoperative test is the visual evoked potential; its presence indicates good macular function. An ultraviolet-shielded intraocular lens should be implanted.
- Some patients with retinitis pigmentosa develop telangiectatic capillaries in the retina, followed by extensive intraretinal and subretinal leakage similar to that of Coats' disease and neovascularization on the disk and elsewhere. Panretinal photocoagulation by laser was found to be effective in reducing the complications from this condition, especially recurrent intravitreal hemorrhage.
- Grid laser therapy has been used to reduce visual loss associated with cystoid macular edema, which is frequently found in patients with retinitis pigmentosa. Its beneficial effect has not yet been confirmed.

Experimental

- Three investigational approaches may lead to future therapies and possible cure for RP. First, the transplantation of neural retinal cells from 14- to 16-week-old human fetuses injected into the recipient's subretinal space, or the transplantation of sheets of retinal pigment epithelial cells (RPE transplants) has been experimentally performed on patients with retinitis pigmentosa. Despite evidence that the implanted cells are functioning, no visual improvement has occurred.
- The use of gene therapy, through the transfer of corrective functional genes into ocular tissue or systemically by link to virus, is being investigated in animal studies.
- Artificial retina or retinal prosthesis is the term used for an electronic device surgically inserted in front of or behind the retina. The artificial retina is intended to take over the function of the RP retina, at least in the central part of it.

Genetic counseling

- Genetic counseling should be provided. The probability of an affected person to have affected children depends on the mode of inheritance and this information can be used for counseling if the genetic type is known. In sporadic cases, the risk of having affected children depends on the severity of the disease in the affected parent, the gender, the prevalence of the various types of retinitis pigmentosa in the family population, and unknown factors.
- The identification of the involved gene and the associated mutation can be of great help in determining the prognosis and severity of the disease in a particular individual or in his or her descendants.

COMMENTS

Many drugs, operations, and bizarre procedures for the treatment of retinitis pigmentosa have been suggested, including the use of anticoagulants, xanthinol niacinate, and other vasodilators; RNA; retrobulbar injections of hyaluronidase and acid phosphates; and even the subconjunctival injection of peat distillate. The transplantation of human placenta, which has been practiced for many years, continues to be used by some. The surgical transplantation of strips of extraocular muscles has been suggested to improve choroidal blood flow. It has been reported that patients responded favorably to ultrasonography and acupuncture; however, reliable evidence of the success of any of these treatments is not available.

ENCAD is a hydrolysate of yeast RNA that was used extensively in the former Soviet Union for the treatment of hereditary retinal degenerations including retinitis pigmentosa. Several studies have not shown a benefit of this treatment.

Retinitis pigmentosa is a serious disease that may gradually progress to blindness, so many patients desperately seek a 'wonder drug' to cure them. The number of attempted medications and procedures to 'treat' retinitis pigmentosa is more numerous than those mentioned here. In recent years, some patients with retinitis pigmentosa have gone to Cuba for a remedy. They were treated with electric stimulation, ozonation of blood, and undefined ocular surgery. Two studies, one performed in the United States and one performed in Norway, on patients treated in Cuba showed that such treatment was of no benefit and could worsen the situation.

Vitamin E supplementation was routinely administered to patients with retinitis pigmentosa by some physicians. The results of a clinical study in which 400 IU/day was administered and an experimental in vitro study indicated that this supplementation may have a negative effect on the course of the disease, so the use of vitamin E seems to be ill-advised.

REFERENCES

Adler R: Mechanisms of photoreceptor death in retinal degenerations: from the cell biology of the 1990s to the ophthalmology of the 21st century? Arch Ophthalmol 114:79–83, 1996.

Berson EL, Rosner B, Sandberg MA, et al: A randomized trial of vitamin A and vitamin E supplementation for retinitis pigmentosa. Arch Ophthalmol 111:761–772, 1993.

Berson EL, Rosner B, Sandberg MA, et al: Clinical trial of docosahexaenoic acid in patients with retinitis pigmentosa receiving vitamin A treatment. Arch Ophthalmol 122(9):1297–1305, 2004.

Bok D: Retinal transplantation and gene therapy: present realities and future possibilities. Invest Ophthalmol Vis Sci 34:473–476, 1993.

Chen JC, Fitzke FW, Bird AC: Long-term effect of acetazolamide in a patient with retinitis pigmentosa. Invest Ophthalmol Vis Sci 31:1914–1918, 1990.

Del Cerro M, Das T, Reddy VL, et al: Human fetal neural retinal cell transplantation in retinitis pigmentosa. Vis Res 35(suppl):S140, 1995.

Dryja TP, McGee TL, Hahn LB, et al: Mutations within the rhodopsin gene in patients with autosomal dominant retinitis pigmentosa. N Engl J Med 323:1302–1307, 1990.

Litchfield TM, Whiteley SJ, Lund RD: Transplantation of retinal pigment epithelial, photoreceptor, and other cells as treatment for retinal degeneration. Exp Eye Res 64:655–666, 1997.

Merin S, Auerbach E: Retinitis pigmentosa. Surv Ophthalmol 20:303–346, 1976.

342 RETINOPATHY OF PREMATURITY 362.21

Earl A. Palmer, MD, FAAP
Portland, Oregon

ETIOLOGY/INCIDENCE

Retinopathy of prematurity (ROP) is a maturational disorder of retinal blood vessels that occurs in premature infants. Its incidence varies inversely with gestational age, and ROP affects $^{2}/_{3}$ of infants born weighing less than 1251 g. Although oxygen in excess of need can cause vaso-obliteration in the immature peripheral retina, other factors likely also play a causative role. Presumably in response to peripheral retina ischemia, neovascularization later develops just posterior to the junction of vascularized and nonvascularized retina.

COURSE/PROGNOSIS

ROP is detected best 4 to 6 weeks after birth and usually involutes spontaneously. Treatment is available if it progresses. In some cases, complications such as vitreous hemorrhage, fibrous proliferation, and retinal detachment supervene during the neovascular phase and lead to irreversible scarring. Cicatricial sequellae may range from mild dragging of the retina compatible with good visual acuity to total retinal detachment, retrolental mass of fibrovascular tissue, anterior chamber collapse, corneal opacity, and phthisis bulbi. Although these findings are generally apparent in the first year of life, retinal detachment may occur as a later sequel of severe ROP throughout childhood and adolescence.

DIAGNOSIS

Clinical signs and symptoms

Ocular or periocular

- Iris:
  - Proliferative phase: persistence of tunica vasculosa lentis, vascular engorgement, poor response to mydriatics;
  - Involutional and cicatricial phases: anterior or posterior synechiae.
- Optic nerve: pallor, in severe cases; enlarged cup sometimes associated with periventricular leukomalacia.
- Retina: detachment, 'dragged' appearance, folds, attenuated vessels, dilated vessels, vascular tortuosity, hemorrhage, neovascularization, pigmentary changes, retrolental mass.
- Vitreous: haze, hemorrhage, organization, traction.
- Other: myopia, anisometropia, strabismus, amblyopia, altered angle kappa, shallow anterior chamber, band keratopathy, glaucoma, cataract, leukocoria, microphthalmos, phthisis.

TREATMENT

Systemic

Augmented supplementation of inspired oxygen once ROP develops does not significantly alter its course. Research efforts continue to seek the optimal oxygen regimen for prematurely born children.

Supportive

Because prematurity is recognized as the most important cause of ROP, prevention of ROP largely depends on public health measures designed to reduce the incidence of premature birth. Restricting light to the faces and eyes of infants may be restful, but has not been found to alter the likelihood of severe ROP.

Premature infants weighing less than 1500 g at birth, or deemed otherwise at special risk by a neonatologist, should be examined for ROP at 4 to 6 weeks of age. Infants showing ROP and those in whom vascularization of the peripheral retina is incomplete should be examined again at an interval depending on examination findings. Patients with zone I ROP or stage 3 ROP in zone II generally should be reexamined at least weekly, and other patients are seen every 2 weeks. There is considerable variation from case to case as to the significance of stage 2 or 3 ROP. Variables include: degree of prematurity, zone of vessels, clock hour extent, rate of progression, race (lower risk among Afro-Americans), and degree of oxygen dependency. Because of this, a mandatory rigid examination schedule is somewhat impractical. For most premies, examinations every week or two suffice. For a few, more frequent examination is necessary.

For examination, the binocular indirect ophthalmoscope should be used after dilation of the pupils with phenylephrine (1% to 2.5%) combined with either cyclopentolate (0.2% to 0.5%) or tropicamide (0.5% to 1.0%). A lid speculum is generally used, and the sclera is gently depressed as necessary. After involution of ROP, children with cicatricial fundus changes should be followed throughout life, particularly during childhood and adolescence, to help prevent further visual loss due to amblyopia, retinal detachment, or angle-closure glaucoma.

Ocular

No medication is known to be effective in preventing or treating ROP. Topical corticosteroids may be helpful in controlling secondary glaucoma if it occurs, and must be used judiciously due to systemic absorption.

Surgical

In 1988 cryotherapy was reported to decrease the risk of severe visual loss by approximately 20%, when applied to the peripheral nonvascularized zone of eyes with 'threshold' ROP (zone I or II, stage 3 'plus'; 5 to 8 clock-hours). Within the following decade indirect ophthalmoscopically delivered laser photocoagulation was found to yield at least equivalent results, with greater ease of application, particularly in zone 1 disease.

In December, 2003, the results of the Early Treatment for ROP study showed significant benefit from earlier intervention in high risk eyes that were likely to eventually reach the traditional threshold of disease known to benefit from cryotherapy. Essentially, eyes with plus disease may be treated, with the possible exception of zone III ROP. Also, zone I ROP at stage 3 is treated even in the absence of plus disease, and zone II stage 1 could be observed even in the presence of plus disease. The definition of plus disease relies on a published standard photograph (Figure 342.1), and has been used in the major multicenter ROP clinical trials. Otherwise, there is considerable inter-examiner variation in making this diagnosis.

For eyes in which retinal detachment has developed despite laser or cryotherapy, optimal management remains controversial. Indications for scleral buckling for partial but progressive

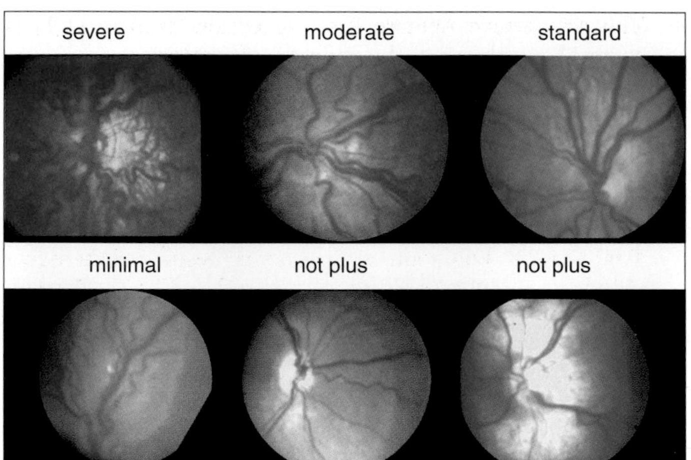

FIGURE 342.1. Plus disease is a subjective determination. At least 4 major clinical trials have employed the standard photo shown here (upper right), originally picked for the CRYO-ROP study, as the depiction of the minimum necessary degree of dilatation and tortuosity needed to officially qualify as plus disease. Recently the term 'pre-plus' was introduced (reference) to describe what is shown here in the two examples as 'not plus.' (Adapted from STOP-ROP Multicenter Study Group: Supplemental therapeutic oxygen for prethreshold retinopathy of prematurity (STOP-ROP), a randomized, controlled trial. I: Primary outcomes. Pediatrics 105(2):295–310, 2000.)

traction detachment from ROP remain subject to individual specialists' interpretation. In eyes with tractional/exudative total retinal detachment, microsurgical vitrectomy with or without lensectomy and/or scleral buckling, usually applied between 3 and 12 months of age, have been successful in reattaching the retina in many cases. Even among eyes with initial anatomic success, however, visual results usually are disappointing.

Still today, no matter what is done, some infants go blind from this disease.

PRECAUTIONS

Since topical medications may cause adverse systemic side effects in premature infants, 10% phenylephrine and 1% cyclopentolate should not be used. (See Supportive above.) Because absorption and systemic toxic effects of ocular medications occur mainly through the nasal mucosa, excess solution should be wiped away promptly.

Ophthalmoscopic examinations are both disturbing and potentially hazardous to the critically ill infant. However, the consequences of unrecognized and untreated high risk ROP are extremely severe. Because ROP progresses to 'threshold' for treatment at an average of 37 weeks' postconceptional (postmenstrual) age, it is extremely important that examinations be carried out before this. *It is advised that examinations begin at 31 weeks postmenstrual age or at 4 weeks from birth, whichever comes first.* In particularly ill infants, if the neonatologist directs that the examination should be delayed until the infant has stabilized, this information should be explicitly stated in the medical record. In scheduling subsequent examinations during the preterm period, the examiner should err on the side of caution. If in doubt about zoning or staging, the next interval should be planned according to the worse scenario. Examinations must not be discontinued until the retinopathy has unequivocally involuted and the retina has finished vascularizing to the ora serrata at least on the nasal side. If ROP remains unresolved at the time of discharge or transfer, it is imperative that the chain of indicated examinations continue unbroken in the outpatient setting.

COMMENTS

The identification of affected infants leads to timely diagnosis and treatment. Their families should learn about ROP and its potential complications from the physicians providing care. Follow-up throughout childhood permits the detection of further complications that threaten visual loss.

Not all cases of proliferative vascular retinopathy in infancy and childhood are ROP. Other etiologic factors should be considered, particularly in infants born weighing more than 1500 g; examples include Norrie's disease, familial exudative vitreoretinopathy, and incontinentia pigmenti.

REFERENCES

Cryotherapy for Retinopathy of Prematurity Cooperative Group: Fifteen-year outcomes following threshold retinopathy of prematurity: final results from the Multicenter Trial of Cryotherapy for Retinopathy of Prematurity. Arch Ophthalmol 123:311–318, 2005.

Early Treatment for Retinopathy of Prematurity Cooperative Group: Revised indications for the treatment of retinopathy of prematurity: results of the early treatment for retinopathy of prematurity randomized trial. Arch Ophthalmol 121:1684–1694, 2003.

Reynolds JD, Dobson V, Quinn GE, et al: Evidence-based screening criteria for retinopathy of prematurity. Arch Ophthalmol 120:1470–1476, 2002.

An International Committee for the Classification of Retinopathy of Prematurity: The International Classification of Retinopathy of Prematurity Revisited. *Arch Ophthalmol* 123:991–999, 2005.

STOP-ROP Multicenter Study Group: Supplemental therapeutic oxygen for prethreshold retinopathy of prematurity (STOP-ROP), a randomized, controlled trial. I: primary outcomes. Pediatrics 105(2):295–310, 2000.

343 SUBRETINAL NEOVASCULAR MEMBRANES 362.16 *(Choroidal Neovascularization, Subretinal Neovascularization)*

M. Vaughn Emerson, MD
Portland, Oregon

ETIOLOGY/INCIDENCE

Subretinal neovascularization (SRN), refers to the presence of blood vessels in the subretinal space. The origin of these blood vessels can be the retinal circulation, but is more commonly the choroidal circulation, with vessels extending through a defect in Bruch's membrane or around Bruch's membrane at the margin of the optic disc. These membranes are therefore commonly referred to as choroidal neovascularization (CNV). Although SRN can occur anywhere in the posterior pole, it most commonly presents in the macula or peripapillary retina.

The most common underlying etiology is age-related macular degeneration (AMD), although several other ocular disorders have been linked to SRN, including but not limited to presumed ocular histoplasmosis syndrome, choroidal scars (in multifocal choroiditis or laser scars), choroidal ruptures, angioid streaks, myopia, lacquer cracks, choroidal nevus, optic nerve head drusen, or other optic nerve head anomalies. Idiopathic SRN is not uncommon.

COURSE/PROGNOSIS

Initially, SRN causes visual disturbance with a serous or hemorrhagic retinal detachment. Treatment-related or spontaneous regression of the SRN leads to disciform scar formation and visual acuity is dependent on the extent of tissue destruction and the particular area of involved retina, retinal pigmented epithelium, and underlying choroid.

DIAGNOSIS

Clinical signs and symptoms

- Gray or pigmented subretinal lesions can be subfoveal, juxtafoveal, extrafoveal, peripapillary, or peripheral.
- Subretinal bleeding is common and frequently outlines the SRN in a circular pattern.
- In some cases, very large subretinal hemorrhages occur, which can be mistaken for malignant melanoma of the choroid.
- Lipid exudation and serous fluid often accompany the SRN.
- Common symptoms include metamorphopsia and central or cecocentral scotomata.

Laboratory findings

- Fluorescein angiography may assist in confirming the diagnosis, guiding laser therapy, and determining the efficacy of treatment modalities.
- Optical coherence tomography has recently been employed more frequently in the initial diagnosis and monitoring of therapy. Optical coherence tomography commonly demonstrates retinal thickening with cystoid spaces, subretinal fluid, and subretinal hyperreflectivity, demonstrating the SRN.
- Indocyanine green angiography may be of use in cases in which subretinal hemorrhage or fluid blocks fluorescein.

Differential diagnosis

Central serous chorioretinopathy, vitelliform detachment due to basal laminar drusen or pattern dystrophy, choroidal melanoma or other tumor.

Prophylaxis

- Micronutrient supplementation, as studied in the Age-related Eye Disease Study (AREDS), yields a 25% risk reduction in progression to advanced AMD (CNV or geographic atrophy) and a 19% risk reduction in moderate vision loss over five years in patients with non-neovascular AMD with at least 1 large (>125 μm) druse or extensive medium-sized drusen. The AREDS formula includes vitamin A 25,000 IU (as beta carotene), vitamin C 500 mg, vitamin E 400 IU, zinc oxide 80 mg, and cupric oxide 2 mg. Some studies suggest a theoretical benefit to lutein dietary supplementation, although this has not been demonstrated with the same systematic rigor as the AREDS formula.
- The Anecortave Acetate Risk Reduction Trial (AART) is currently evaluating the efficacy of posterior sub-Tenon injection of anecortave acetate in the prevention of wet macular degeneration in eyes with drusen and pigment clumping.
- Argon laser treatment of drusen is currently being evaluated following promising results of two pilot studies. The Complications of Age-related Macular Degeneration Prevention Trial (CAPT) will soon publish 6-year results of the effect of light grid and focal laser to eyes with = 10 large drusen.

TREATMENT

Systemic

No systemic therapy has been demonstrated to be effective in the treatment of SRN. Squalamine, an aminosterol with anti-angiogeneic properties and relatively low systemic toxicity, and combretastatin A-4 Phosphate (CA4P), an antimitotic agent with both antitubulin and antivascular properties, are undergoing clinical evaluation as intravenous anti-SRN therapies.

Intravenous interferon alfa-2a, thalidomide, steroids, plasmapheresis, and many other medications and strategies have been used in an attempt to inhibit the neovascular activity in SRN. Although many agents have shown promise in pilot studies, these systemic therapies have not been shown to be effective in randomized clinical trials.

Medical

- Laser photocoagulation, as studied in the Macular Photocoagulation Study (MPS) significantly decreases vision loss at 5 years for extrafoveal, juxtafoveal, and subfoveal SRN due to AMD, histoplasmosis, and idiopathic membranes when compared to observation. Most surgeons do not treat subfoveal lesions because of the risk of immediate loss of six or more lines of vision. The recurrence rate can be as high as 78% in cases of juxtafoveal SRN, usually extending into the fovea. However, laser photocoagulation remains the treatment of choice for patients with extrafoveal or peripapillary SRN, with the alternative of observation in some cases.
- Photodynamic therapy (PDT), approved by the FDA in 2000 for the treatment of predominantly classic CNV associated with AMD, ocular histoplasmosis, and myopia, involves an intravenous injection of verteporfin (Visudyne, Novartis) followed by photoactivation of the dye with a 689 nm wavelength laser. Treatment is repeated every three months, as necessary, based on angiographic leakage. This treatment has been demonstrated to reduce vision loss (defined by = 15 ETDRS letters) in patients with predominantly classic CNV, and is most effective in patients with no occult component. PDT is not used within 200 μm of the optic nerve, and the maximum treatable lesion size is 5400 μm in greatest linear diameter.
- Photodynamic therapy is currently commonly used in combination with intravitreal steroid injections, although this regimen has yet to be supported by a randomized, controlled clinical trial. The Visudyne with Intravitreal Triamcinolone Acetonide (VisTA) trial may clarify which patients may benefit from this treatment combination.
- Macugen (pegaptanib, Eyetech) is a single-stranded RNA molecule that binds vascular endothelial growth factor (VEGF), which was FDA-approved for the treatment of neovascular AMD in 2005. When repeated every 6 weeks, Macugen decreases the rate of moderate vision loss by one-

third. These results are similar to those of PDT in the prevention of SRN-associated vision loss at 2 years.

- Phase III studies of monthly injections of another anti-VEGF agent, Lucentis (ranibizumab, Genentech), a humanized anti-VEGF antibody fragment, are ongoing. However, 1-year results have demonstrated a treatment benefit over PDT and = 15 ETDRS-letter improvement in vision in 25–34% of patients. Avastin (Bevacizumab, Genentech), an anti-VEGF antibody has also been used intravenously and intravitreally with anecdotally positive results.
- Randomized clinical trials of low-dose radiation to SRN in AMD have shown no benefit.

Surgical

- The Submacular Surgery Trial (SST) demonstrated no benefit to surgery over observation on visual acuity with the removal of SRN and evacuation of subretinal hemorrhage. Because the quality of life assessment was slightly better in patients undergoing surgery, submacular surgery may be of use in select cases.
- Neither macular translocation surgery nor the implantation of miniature intraocular telescopes has been studied in a randomized, controlled fashion, although each may be of benefit in select cases.
- Stem cell and retinal pigmented epithelium transplantation and gene therapy are other investigational treatments.

COMPLICATIONS

The introduction of intravitreal administration of pharmaceuticals has increased the rate of ocular complications, including endophthalmitis, retinal detachment, cataract, and glaucoma. As use of these therapies become more widespread, the occurrence of adverse events will increase, particularly when compounded over multiple injections. Nor are laser photocoagulation and PDT without complications, including inadvertent laser burns, absolute scotomas, retina pigmented epithelial rips, and choroidal nonperfusion.

COMMENTS

With the recent explosion of research concerning the prevention and treatment of SRN, particularly in association with AMD, treatment recommendations for SRN are evolving more rapidly than ever. It is important to tailor management to each individual case, with a thorough discussion of the treatment options, risks and benefits.

REFERENCES

Age-related Eye Disease Study Research Group. A randomized, placebo-controlled, clinical trial of high-dose supplementation with vitamins C and E, beta carotene, and zinc for age-related macular degeneration and vision loss: AREDS report no. 8. Arch Ophthalmol 119:1417–1436, 2001.

Bressler NM, Bressler SB, Gragouds ES: Clinical characteristics of choroidal neovascular membranes. Arch Ophthalmol 105:209–213, 1987.

Gragoudas ES, Adamis AP, Cunningham ET, et al: Pegaptanib for neovascular age-related macular degeneration. N Engl J Med 351:2805–2816, 2004.

Macular Photocoagulation Study Group. Laser photocoagulation of subfoveal neovascular lesions of age-related macular degeneration: updated findings from two clinical trials. Arch Ophthalmol 111:1200–1209, 1993.

Miller J, Chung CY, Kim RY, MARINA Study Group: Randomized, controlled phase III study of ranibizumab (*Lucentis*) for minimally classic or occult neovascular age-related macular degeneration. Program and abstracts of the American Society of Retina Specialists 23rd Annual Meeting. Montreal, Canada, July 16–20, 2005.

Submacular Surgery Trials (SST) Research Group. Surgery for subfoveal choroidal neovascularization in age-related macular degeneration: ophthalmic findings: SST report no. 11. Ophthalmology 111:1967–1980, 2004.

344 WHITE DOT SYNDROMES 363.15

(Acute Posterior Multifocal Placoid Pigment Epitheliopathy, Birdshot Chorioretinopathy, Multifocal Choroiditis and Panuveitis, Multiple Evanescent White Dot Syndrome, Presumed Ocular Histoplasmosis Syndrome, Punctate Inner Choroidopathy, Retinal Pigment Epitheliitis, Serpiginous Choroiditis, Subretinal Fibrosis and Uveitis)

Lyndell L. Lim, MD
East Melbourne, Australia
Eric B. Suhler, MD
Portland, Oregon

The term *white dot syndrome* refers to acquired diseases that cause inflammation and multifocal lesions at the level of the outer retina, retinal pigment epithelium (RPE), and inner choroid. Nine separate diseases are commonly included in this category, associated with many acronyms. New variations or related inflammatory conditions are constantly being added in the literature, such as *acute zonal occult outer retinitis* and *unilateral acute idiopathic maculopathy*. Many argue whether some of these separate conditions are simply different manifestations of the same unidentified inflammatory insult. Nevertheless, until a unifying mechanism is identified for all of these diseases, it helps to consider the white dot syndromes as individual entities, if only to simplify diagnosis and prognosis. The white dot syndromes definitely must be distinguished from the numerous other causes of 'white dots' in the fundus, such as vascular problems like cotton-wool spots or degenerative changes such as Stargardt's disease, drusen, or cobblestone degeneration. The acute, multifocal, inflammatory nature of these nine entities usually makes this distinction simple.

The entities included in this article are retinal pigment epitheliitis (RPE-itis), multiple evanescent white dot syndrome (MEWDS), acute posterior multifocal placoid pigment epitheliopathy (APMPPE), serpiginous choroiditis, presumed ocular histoplasmosis syndrome (POHS), punctate inner choroidopathy (PIC), multifocal choroiditis and panuveitis (MCP), subretinal fibrosis and uveitis (SFU), and birdshot (or vitiliginous) chorioretinopathy.

Retinal pigment epitheliitis (RPE-itis; formerly known as Krill disease)

ETIOLOGY/INCIDENCE

- RPE-itis occurs primarily in otherwise healthy patients in the third decade of life.
- This is thought to involve focal inflammation at the level of the RPE with surrounding RPE edema.
- A viral precipitant has been postulated, but none has been identified.

COURSE/PROGNOSIS

- There is usually a unilateral mild decrease in vision at presentation. Symptoms usually resolve in 6 to 12 weeks with little or no sequelae. There has been one case report of a choroidal neovascular membrane (CNVM).

DIAGNOSIS

- There usually are 2–4 clusters of dark-gray spots surrounded by a hypopigmented halo.
- Fluorescein angiography may be normal, or the halo may become more hyperfluorescent with time. Fluorescein lesions have been described as 'honeycomb' or 'target' shaped.

TREATMENT

- No treatment is required.

Multiple evanescent white dot syndrome

ETIOLOGY/INCIDENCE

- MEWDS occurs in younger patients, with a female preponderance.
- Patients often describe an antecedent (4 weeks) viral illness, and this entity is thought to represent a postviral RPE inflammation with secondary retinal and photoreceptor changes.
- Vision is usually moderately decreased, in the 20/40 to 20/200 range.

COURSE/PROGNOSIS

- The prognosis is excellent, and most patients recover. There usually is some mild subjective decrease in visual function that persists, and the enlarged blind spot may take months to resolve.
- Recurrences are unusual; the development of a CNVM has been reported but is rare.

DIAGNOSIS

Patients usually complain of photopsias, scotomata, and decreased vision, with examination revealing multiple soft, gray-white spots in the posterior pole and midperiphery. These dots can be very faint and are seen best in the midperiphery. There usually is a small amount of posterior vitreous cells. The fovea of the involved eye also demonstrates a peculiar and almost pathognomonic orangish granular appearance; often, this is the only physical finding to explain the patient's symptoms, particularly if the white spots have faded markedly.

Both the symptoms and findings are usually (80%) unilateral; however, a few spots are often seen in the fellow eye on close examination.

The white dots usually last approximately 3 weeks and then fade; however, the patient may have an enlarged blind spot on perimetry that lasts longer.

Fundus fluorescein angiogram features include early hyperfluorescence of the dots with late staining, with each spot appearing as a cluster of smaller dots arranged in a wreath-like pattern. Electroretinogram findings are typically a decreased A wave and early receptor potential.

A presumptive diagnosis of this entity can therefore often be made in patients presenting with a big blind spot syndrome, a small number of posterior vitreous cells, and an orangish granularity of the fovea even if the prominent white lesions are no longer present.

TREATMENT

No treatment is required for this entity. Recovery of visual acuity is typically excellent; however, subjective visual dysfunction and an enlarged blind spot may persist for some time. A choroidal neovascular membrane is a result of MEWDS on rare occasions.

Acute posterior multifocal placoid pigment epitheliopathy

ETIOLOGY/INCIDENCE

APMPPE usually affects patients in the third decade of life. About one-third of patients report an antecedent viral syndrome, and this condition may represent some sort of postviral hypersensitivity process.

The pathology is thought to be a choroidal microvasculitis with choroidal lobule closure and secondary RPE changes.

COURSE/PROGNOSIS

Patients usually present with a fairly rapidly progressive decrease in vision, the severity of which depends on whether lesions are present directly under the fovea. Involvement is also usually bilateral, with the second eye being involved in days to weeks.

Symptoms usually resolve in 1 to 2 months and the prognosis is generally good, with most patients recovering 20/30 vision or better, although the vision may be much worse if there is extensive subfoveal scarring. Even with good visual return, there may be lingering metamorphopsia or scotomata. Recurrences and secondary CNVM are rare.

DIAGNOSIS

Classically, there are large yellow-white creamy infiltrates at the level of the RPE and inner choroids (Figure 344.1). The

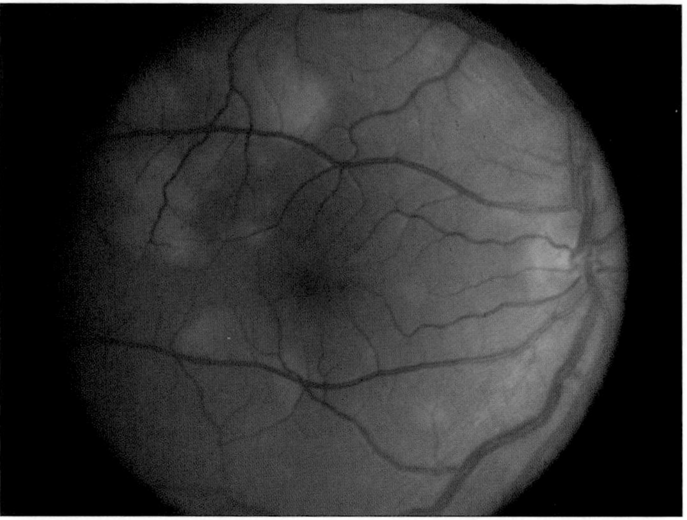

FIGURE 344.1. Color fundus photo of the right eye demonstrating the classic creamy white lesions seen in APMPPE.

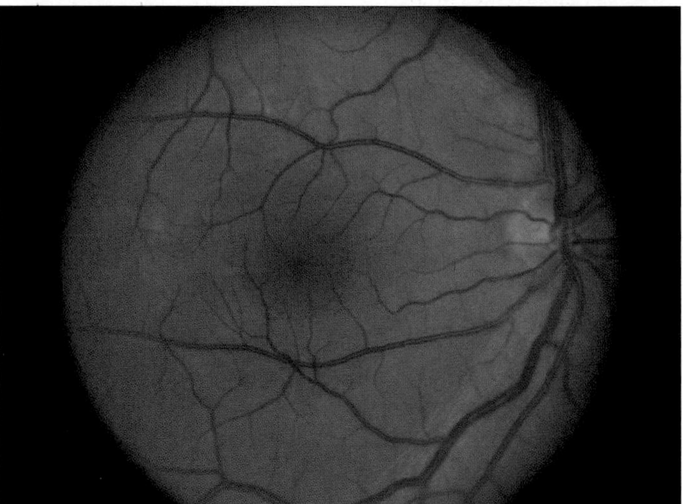

FIGURE 344.2. Color fundus photo of the same eye shown in Figure 344.1 several weeks later showing complete resolution of the acute creamy lesions with residual pigmentary changes at the level of the RPE.

infiltrates may form one large central lesion. This disease is remarkable for the rate at which pigment changes develop; they usually begin in 1–2 weeks, and variations in pigment reaction can occur on almost a daily basis (Figure 344.2).

Several associated ocular findings have been noted, including papillitis, serous retinal detachment, retinal vasculitis, macular edema, superficial retinal hemorrhages, corneal infiltrates, and episcleritis. There usually are few anterior chamber or vitreous cells.

Fluorescein angiography of these creamy lesions shows a classic early hypofluorescence and late hyperfluorescence with leakage.

TREATMENT

APMPPE usually resolves without the need for treatment. Some believe that severe vision loss or significant vitreous cells merit the use of corticosteroids. Others routinely treat all patients with corticosteroids and believe that this therapy provides more rapid regression. There are no controlled studies to support either of these approaches. Patients with severe or complicated cases require systemic investigations (see below).

COMPLICATIONS

Of note, this syndrome is the only white dot syndrome that has been associated with death; there have been case reports of death from associated cerebral vasculitis. Other systemic associations include systemic vasculidities such as Wegener's granulomatosis, acute nephritis, thyroiditis, hearing changes, erythema nodosum, headache, and cerebrospinal fluid pleocytosis. Most patients do not have these systemic associations; however, if a patient complains of a particularly severe headache or neurologic symptoms, he or she should be referred for appropriate workup.

Serpiginous choroiditis

ETIOLOGY/INCIDENCE

- The average age is in the fifth decade, which is somewhat older than for most of the other white dot diseases.
- There is no clear racial or sexual predisposition and no known systemic association.
- The disease usually starts at the disk and spreads centripetally with recurrent episodes of inflammation. The active areas are gray-white and usually occur at the edge of previous atrophy. The active edge may remain active for weeks to months, gradually resolving to RPE mottling and atrophy. Twenty percent of patients may have isolated macular lesions as the initial site of involvement. Multifocal noncontiguous recurrences can also occur. Focal phlebitis and retinal neovascularization have been described on rare occasions.

COURSE/PROGNOSIS

The course is characterized by recurrences at intervals ranging from weeks to years. Progression may be asymptomatic if the macula is not involved, and this may explain why these patients present at older ages than patients with other white dot syndromes. CNVMs occur in up to 25% of patients. Early serpiginous choroiditis may be difficult to differentiate from other focal inflammations, such as toxoplasmosis, APMPPE, or idiopathic peripapillary CNVMs. Usually, the diagnosis becomes clear as the patient is followed and the disease recurs. In general, the prognosis is fair, with useful vision preserved in at least one eye. The prognosis can be very poor if foveal involvement or a CNVM develops.

DIAGNOSIS

- Patients present with blurred vision, floaters, or both.
- Histopathology shows aggregates of lymphocytes in the choroid, presumably causing focal choriocapillaris and RPE damage.
- The fluorescein angiogram is characteristic, with the atrophic areas showing staining along the edge where functional

choriocapillaris exists. The acute lesions are similar to APMPPE lesions with early hypofluorescence and late hyperfluorescence.

TREATMENT

Because this entity has a tendency to be recurrent and destructive, many authorities are more aggressive in treating it; however, the recurrent nature of the disease and tendency of the lesions to spontaneously resolve make the assessment of treatment efficacy difficult. Acute exacerbations may respond to local injections or oral administration of corticosteroids (see General therapeutic approach), but for management of chronic disease, immunosuppression is often required. There is no consensus on the ideal immunosuppressive regimen, with case series advocating triple agent immunosuppression with cyclosporin A and an antimetabolite, alkylating agents such as cyclophosphamide or chlorambucil, or high-dose intravenous steroids. Patients requiring immunosuppressive therapy generally have vision-threatening disease and should be referred to a tertiary care center.

Presumed ocular histoplasmosis syndrome

ETIOLOGY/INCIDENCE

- *Histoplasma capsulatum* is found in the valleys of rivers such as the Mississippi and Ohio at a latitude between 45 degrees north and 45 degrees south. In these areas approximately 90% of the people are skin-test positive, yet only 1.6% to 2.6% will have the discrete chorioretinal scars known as histospots.
- The ocular disease can present in any decade but is more common in the fourth decade.

COURSE/PROGNOSIS

- The primary histoplasmosis infection is usually benign and often consists of flu symptoms or cough lasting 2 days to 2 weeks. The organism invades the lungs and then disseminates, especially to the reticuloendothelial system, leaving multiple focal calcified granulomas.

DIAGNOSIS

A multifocal choroidal inflammation develops but it is not associated with manifest vitreous or anterior chamber inflammation, distinguishing it from the multifocal choroiditis and panuveitis syndrome (MCP). Otherwise, typical disease with vitreous inflammation is sometimes referred to as 'pseudo-POHS.'

Presumably, the organism is killed but leaves behind residual nests of stimulated, immunoreactive cells. Either there is a chronic low level of smoldering inflammation or some precipitate causes a nest of cells to flare up, resulting in local exudation (an active histo spot). This flare-up may cause further scarring or stimulate neovascularization with subsequent disciform scar formation.

The initial multifocal inflammation that occurs with disease dissemination is asymptomatic, which is why acute multifocal ocular histoplasmosis is not seen (unless the patient has fulminant disseminated disease, as often occurs in the immunosuppressed patient). It may be that because primary infections are usually acquired in childhood, the acute inflammation is less likely to be noticed. The patient becomes symptomatic not due to the peripheral scars but rather due to scars present in the posterior pole (see complications, below).

TREATMENT

It is very important to monitor the patient closely for the development of a CNVM (see Complications, below). Any patient with symptomatic histoplasmosis must be assumed to have a neovascular membrane until proved otherwise. The Macular Photocoagulation Study has clearly demonstrated the benefit of laser treatment for extrafoveal CNVMs in patients with POHS. For subfoveal or juxtafoveal CNVMs, several small case series have suggested a benefit with verteporfin photodynamic therapy.

Once the diagnosis of POHS has been made on clinical grounds, the patient should therefore have continuous Amsler grid monitoring at home. If a CNVM develops, laser treatment should be performed if the membrane does not involve the center of the fovea. If the patient seems to be having an inflammatory exacerbation of a histo spot, the corticosteroid regimen discussed (see General therapeutic approach) usually proves to be effective in controlling the flare-up. Sub-Tenon injection of steroids may also be useful. This type of patient must be monitored closely for the development of a CNVM.

COMPLICATIONS

There are two mechanisms by which POHS scars can cause visual loss:

- The most common complication is the development of a CNVM in the area of the prior histospot at the macula. This can cause disciform scarring and loss of central vision if not treated with laser photocoagulation or verteporfin photodynamic therapy.
- Another possibility is that the recurrent inflammation adjacent to a macular scar may generate a small amount of subretinal fluid, leading to symptomatic decreased vision in the absence of a full-blown neovascular membrane. This type of inflammatory reaction may respond well to systemic or local steroids or resolve over time without treatment.

Punctate inner choroidopathy

ETIOLOGY/INCIDENCE

- Almost all patients with PIC are myopic women in the third decade of life.

COURSE/PROGNOSIS

Symptoms usually decrease after approximately 1 month, although patients can have mild blurred vision and photopsias for a longer time. The spots evolve to atrophic scars very similar to those seen with POHS. Diagnostic tests for histoplasmosis, however, are generally negative.

The prognosis is usually excellent, with almost all patients returning to 20/20 visual acuity unless there is a subfoveal lesion. The initial disease usually does not recur, although some patients have photopsias for years; however, 40% of these patients develop a CNVM from the parafoveal scars in approximately 3–12 months. These CNVMs respond well to laser treatment. Patientswith subfoveal CNVMs may benefit from verteporfin photodynamic therapy but have a more guarded prognosis.

DIAGNOSIS

Patients usually present with symptoms of decreased vision, scotomata, and photopsias.

These symptoms are usually unilateral, but the findings are generally bilateral, albeit asymmetric.

Examination usually reveals small gray-yellow spots, of 0.1 to 0.2 disk diameter, in the posterior pole and periphery. Serous elevations can develop over the spots. The eyes are quiet with few or no anterior chamber or vitreous cells.

TREATMENT

This entity is usually self-limited and does not require treatment. As with the other multifocal choroidopathies, there is danger of a CNVM occurring later; as a result, these patients require continuous monitoring with the Amsler grid.

Multifocal choroiditis and panuveitis (MCP)

ETIOLOGY/INCIDENCE

There is a female preponderance with an average age of onset of about 33.

COURSE/PROGNOSIS

Approximately one-third of patients may develop a CNVM. This disease can be recurrent, with either new spots developing, or simply recurrent inflammation in the eye, without any change in the number of spots.

The prognosis is fair if inflammation can be controlled. The development of a CNVM results in a more guarded prognosis and is the leading cause of visual loss in patients with this disease.

DIAGNOSIS

Unlike POHS and PIC, MCP has a tendency to have more vitreous inflammation, more leakage from spots, and more recurrences. Patients usually complain of floaters and blurred vision, but they may also note photopsias and visual field defects. The initial vision loss ranges from mild to severe, depending on the amount of cystoid macular edema or the presence of a CNVM.

About half of the patients will have at least a mild anterior chamber reaction; 90% to 100% of patients have a significant number of inflammatory cells in the vitreous, which distinguishes this entity from POHS and PIC. Approximately one-third of patients may also have peripapillary pigment changes; there often are many more lesions than are present in POHS or PIC. More lesions are often seen in the nasal fundus. A peripapillary 'napkin ring' of fibrosis may also develop and is thought to be a characteristic finding in this disease.

Acute lesions are grayish-yellow infiltrates at the level of the RPE and inner choroid, whereas old lesions tend to be punched out like those seen in POHS. It is not uncommon for patients to have both acute, symptomatic spots and old, quiet scars.

Fluorescein angiography of very acute lesions shows early hypofluorescence. Both acute and semiacute lesions show late staining. Old punched-out scars may act as window defects. Disk staining and cystoid macular edema may also be present.

TREATMENT

Because this entity tends to be recurrent and more severe, these patients are more likely to require systemic immunosuppression, initially with corticosteroids, with recurrent or aggressive cases treated with chronic immunosuppression with agents such as cyclosporin A or antimetabolites. Visual field testing should be part of the management of these patients because they may have diffuse visual dysfunction without an obvious change in the number or activity of spots. They also require continuous Amsler grid monitoring for the development of a CNVM. Most clinicians attempt laser photocoagulation if the CNVM is extrafoveal. Photodynamic therapy has also shown some promise in treating subfoveal and juxtafoveal CNVM secondary to inflammatory disease such as MCP.

Progressive subretinal fibrosis and uveitis

ETIOLOGY/INCIDENCE

- This is the most severe of the multifocal choroidopathies.
- Patients are usually women in their 20s.
- No etiologic agent has been identified.

COURSE/PROGNOSIS

Patients present with an acute, progressive decrease in vision. The disease is bilateral but often asymmetric. It is common for the second eye to become involved months after initial disease onset.

The prognosis is poor. The vision often drops to counting fingers or hand motions over months to years. Recurrent episodes of the multifocal choroiditis stage may occur. The fibrosis stage usually progresses to a certain point and then stops. In its end stage, this entity must be distinguished from other causes of subretinal fibrosis, such as a CNVM, retinal detachment, or old inflammatory scarring (Figure 344.3).

DIAGNOSIS

- Patients develop extensive subretinal fibrosis that results in marked visual loss.
- One-third of patients have an anterior chamber reaction, and most have mild vitreous cells.

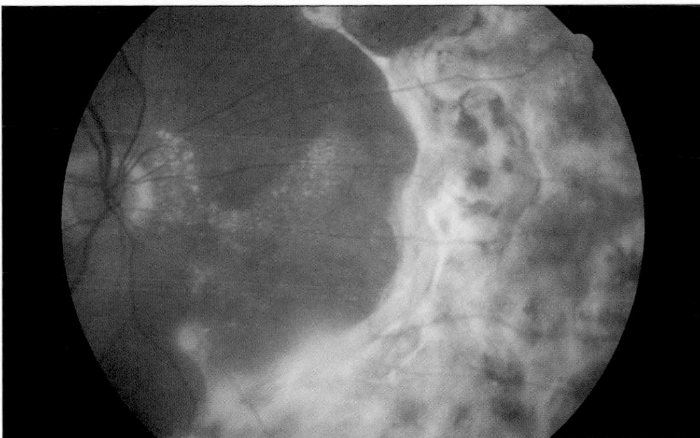

FIGURE 344.3. Advanced progressive subretinal fibrosis and uveitis affecting the right eye. Extensive subretinal fibrosis can be seen affecting the nasal portion of the eye.

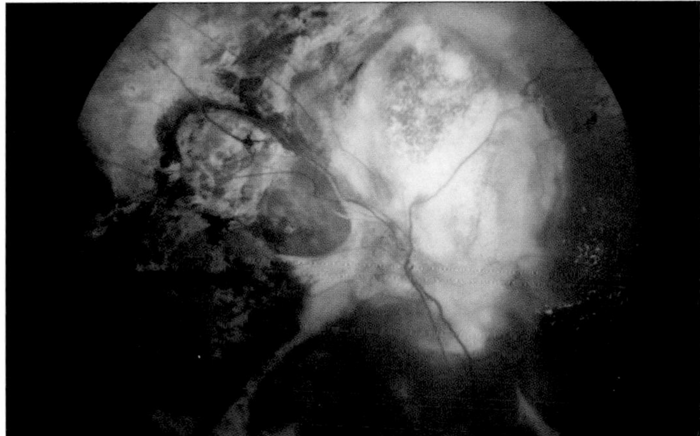

FIGURE 344.4. End stage progressive subretinal fibrosis and uveitis of the left eye with extensive posterior pole and peripheral involvement.

- The disease starts as a posterior to midperipheral multifocal choroiditis with 0.1- to 0.5-disk diameter whitish lesions in the RPE and inner choroid. Many small lesions are often clustered in the posterior pole between the temporal vascular arcades.
- With follow-up, some of the initial dots disappear, but others develop progressive fibrotic extensions that coalesce and spread under the posterior pole (Figures 344.4 and 344.5). These fibrotic bands are usually nonpigmented. A CNVM may also develop, but the appearance is not classic, and they seem to be only a small part of the overall fibrotic response.

TREATMENT

Patients with this disease have a very poor prognosis. Many have severe visual loss in both eyes despite treatment. Some investigators have been able to prevent severe visual loss with the aggressive use of corticosteroids and other systemic immunosuppressive agents to decrease scarring before the fibrosis becomes fully developed.

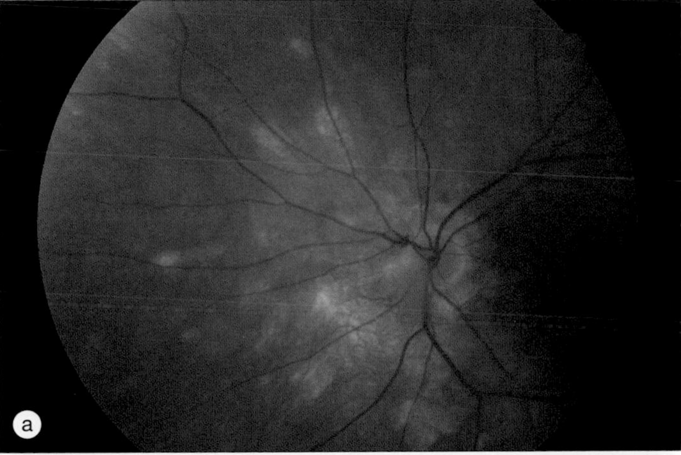

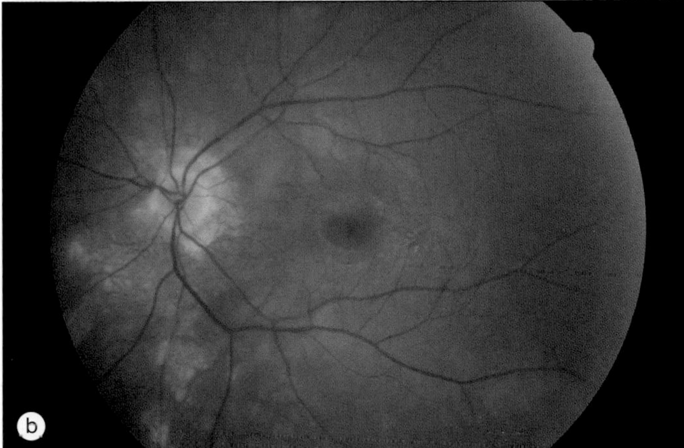

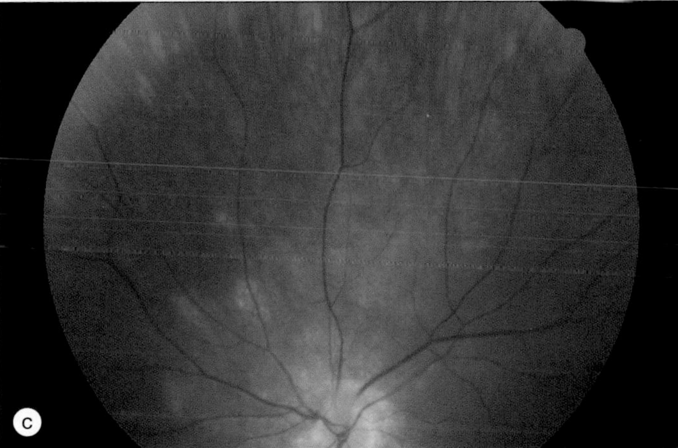

FIGURE 344.5. (a–c) Color fundal photographs of the left eye demonstrating classic birdshot chorioretinopathy lesions emanating from the optic disk.

Birdshot chorioretinopathy

ETIOLOGY/INCIDENCE

- Patients tend to be older, and there is a slight female preponderance. It is rare in nonwhites.
- This disease has an extremely high association with HLA-29. More than 95% of patients with the disease have this allele.

COURSE/PROGNOSIS

Overall, these patients tend to have a slowly and relentlessly progressive loss of vision over a long period of time (i.e. years). Often, this loss is detectable on electrophysiologic testing (e.g. ERG and dark adaptation) and visual field monitoring long before a drop in visual acuity is seen.

The most common cause of vision loss is cystoid macular edema, which occurs in up to 50% of patients, with associated vitreal haze often present. Other less common complications include optic nerve edema and atrophy, epiretinal membranes, CNVM and retinal vasculitis resulting in neovascularization and vitreal hemorrhage.

DIAGNOSIS

- Patients present with floaters and blurred vision. They may develop problems with nyctalopia and decreased color vision in later stages.
- The vision is usually mildly decreased. The disease is almost always bilateral but can be asymmetric.
- Most patients have vitreous cells and haze; anterior segment inflammation is not a common feature and if present, it is mild.
- The lesions are 0.25 to 1 disk diameter and are usually oval. They may be very subtle, particularly in blond fundi, and may be more readily apparent with the indirect ophthalmoscope than with high diopter lenses. The lesions are most often found around the disk and nasal periphery. They appear to radiate outward from the disk into the periphery (Figure 344.5). The macula is not usually involved with the lesions.
- The lesions usually do not develop pigmentation, in comparison to many other entities that may also cause multifocal lesions. The lesions themselves are usually less visible on fluorescein angiography than on color photography, due to their deep level in the choroid and minimal interference with the RPE and choriocapillaris.

TREATMENT

The decision regarding when to start treatment in these patients is still a subject of some debate. Previously, some authors felt that treatment should be reserved for flare-ups or late complications that significantly decrease vision. However, severe deficits on ERG and visual field testing may occur well in advance of a drop in visual acuity, leading others to advocate the commencement of treatment as soon as such abnormalities are detected. Therefore, regular ERGs and visual field examinations may be useful for monitoring early disease progression.

Corticosteroids, either orally or as periocular or intravitreal injections, are generally the mainstay of treatment for severe exacerbations or complications such as cystoid macular edema. More recently, the use of cyclosporin A has been advocated for long term therapy to stabilize the course of this disease and maintain visual acuity. The use of other immunosuppressives, including antimetabolites and biologic therapies, has also been reported to be useful.

Differential diagnosis

Disseminated infection

When entertaining the diagnosis of one of the white dot syndromes, it is of paramount importance to ensure that the patient does not have a disseminated infection that is causing a multifocal choroiditis. In general, patients with a white dot syndrome are healthy, although in some cases there may be an antecedent viral infection. Patients who are sick, debilitated, or immunosuppressed should raise concern for another etiology, such as an endogenous endophthalmitis or systemic infectious disease. A careful review of systems looking for evidence of systemic disease is mandatory in these patients, and patients with suspicious symptoms may need to be referred for a medical evaluation. Multifocal infections, such as bacterial sepsis, *Mycobacteria* infection, syphilis, Lyme disease, fungal infections, and pneumocystis, must be considered depending on the clinical situation. In general, multifocal infectious entities have much more fluffy lesions with denser vitreous debris than any of the white dot syndromes. Most infectious causes also have a much more fulminant course than the more indolent white dot syndromes. As in all ocular inflammatory diseases, the history is of paramount importance in guiding the medical workup for potential masquerades. One test that should always be ordered is an FTA-Abs to exclude syphilis, the classic masquerading infectious disease.

Autoimmune diseases

Certain autoimmune diseases should be considered in the differential diagnosis of white dot syndromes. Sarcoidosis may present with a panuveitis simulating multifocal choroiditis or primarily posterior disease similar to birdshot. In cases where there is a high suspicion for sarcoidosis, a high resolution chest CT should be performed, as this modality has been shown to detect pulmonary sarcoidosis that can be missed on chest X-ray. In such cases, a tissue diagnosis via a transbronchial biopsy may be considered. Other tests that may be useful include serum angiotensin converting enzyme (ACE) levels, pulmonary function testing with measurement of carbon monoxide diffusion capacity (PFTs with DLCO), conjunctival or lacrimal gland biopsy, and/or a gallium scan.

Most of the other systemic autoimmune diseases that can affect the posterior part of the eye, such as Behçet's disease or systemic vasculitis, do not present as multifocal choroidopathies. Instead, these entities usually present with diffuse intraocular inflammation and retinal vasculitis. As a result, unless the patient has a very suggestive history, laboratory tests to evaluate for these entities are not done. A patient's complete blood cell count and chemistry profile are often checked, not so much as a diagnostic maneuver but rather to assess their general medical status, particularly if immunosuppressive therapy is considered. Purified protein derivative skin testing is included, more to define the patient's tuberculosis (TB) status before immunosuppression than to look for a TB-associated multifocal choroiditis, which would be unusual in an otherwise healthy patient. If the diagnosis of birdshot choroidopathy is entertained, testing for HLA-A29 should be done. If the patient presents with an appearance that is typical for one of the milder white dot syndromes (e.g. MEWDS), it may not be necessary to perform any laboratory testing.

Diffuse unilateral subacute neuroretinitis and toxoplasmosis

Two other local ocular entities must be kept in mind. Diffuse unilateral subacute neuroretinitis occurs when certain nematodes enter the subretinal space. Patients have severe visual loss in only one eye with scattered whitish lesions that ultimately form marked pigment changes associated with optic atrophy. Any patient with such a clinical picture should be carefully inspected for the presence of a small worm in the subretinal space, and fluorescein angiography will often reveal pathognomonic diffuse hyperfluorescent lesions in areas of previous worm tracks. Toxoplasmosis is another disease that may present with one or more small outer retinal white lesions (punctate outer retinal toxoplasmosis). These are unilateral in immunocompetent patients, and there usually is evidence of previous scarring from toxoplasmosis. A toxoplasmosis titer may be helpful, and treatment for this entity may be necessary if lesions threaten the optic nerve, macula, or retinal vasculature.

Masquerade processes

Finally, masquerade processes such as ocular lymphoma, metastatic disease, and choroidal lymphoproliferative diseases may present as a multifocal process. They often have larger, more mass-like lesions that differ from the smaller lesions of the white dot syndromes. Usually the ultrasound examination, the systemic status, or a lack of response to treatment will suggest this type of process.

Observation

Once the clinician is satisfied that the patient has one of the idiopathic white dot syndromes rather than a systemic disease, differentiation is usually fairly simple and depends largely on the clinical appearance and degree of severity. Sometimes a period of observation is required for all the clinical manifestations of the disease to become apparent. For instance, both PIC and MCP can present initially as a multifocal process. With follow-up, MCP usually demonstrates more intraocular inflammation and tends to be recurrent and to require immunosuppression. Serpiginous choroiditis may also be problematic initially, particularly if it starts in one localized area and the characteristic pattern of scarring is not present. The diagnosis usually becomes apparent with follow-up as recurrent, gradual spread of the inflammation occurs.

GENERAL THERAPEUTIC APPROACH

Although there are a number of white dot syndromes, the overall therapeutic approach is very similar. Basically, if there is little inflammation and the vision is not markedly decreased, no treatment is required. If there is more inflammation or more significant visual loss, immunosuppression may be necessary, usually with depot or oral corticosteroids. Those entities that have a high risk of a CNVM, such as POHS, PIC, and MCP, require continuous monitoring with the Amsler grid and laser or photodynamic treatment if necessary. More chronic diseases, such as birdshot or MCP, have the potential to damage peripheral vision, and this parameter should also be monitored.

More specific guidelines for therapy include the use of topical steroids and cycloplegics if there is significant anterior chamber reaction. If the decision to use systemic corticosteroids has been made, the patient should be started on a dosage of 0.5 to 1 mg/kg (usually 60 to 80 mg) daily of prednisone or its equivalent. The patient should be seen in 1 to 2 weeks. The steroids can be gradually tapered depending on the clinical response. Depending on severity, flare-ups may require a return to the initial dose or simply going back to the lowest dose at which inflammation was controlled. However, long term high dose (= 10mg/day) oral prednisone will almost always result in severe side effects and therefore patients who are unable to be weaned below this dose without flares should be referred for commencement of a steroid sparing agent. If the patient is not a steroid responder, posterior sub-Tenon's injections of 20 to 40 mg triamcinolone acetonide may be useful for disease exacerbations.

COMMENTS

A few important points must be kept in mind when treating patients with the white dot syndromes. It is very important to use both the clinical history and physical examination to eliminate a systemic infectious cause for a multifocal choroiditis; only then can the clinician be assured that immunosuppressive treatment can be performed safely. Any multifocal process that progresses despite presumably appropriate treatment requires reevaluation for an infectious cause. A lymphoproliferative process must be considered, particularly if there appear to be masses or deposits in the subretinal or sub-RPE space, or in the presence of suspicious systemic (especially neurologic) symptoms.

In disease processes such as MCP, SRF, serpiginous choroiditis, and birdshot choroidopathy, early recognition is important due to their more chronic and sometimes aggressive courses, often requiring systemic immunosuppression.

One must constantly reassess the risks and benefits of the therapy in these entities. If continuous treatment is found to be required, strong consideration should be given to the use of immunosuppressive agents such as cyclosporin A to prevent complications from chronic steroid use. Consultation with a uveitis expert, or an internist or rheumatologist, should be obtained to assist with this.

Finally, the patient must be warned about the late development of a neovascular membrane, particularly if the patient has one of the multifocal choroidopathies (POHS, PIC, MCP, SFU) or serpiginous choroidopathy. If a subfoveal membrane develops, many investigators believe that surgical removal may be beneficial, although controlled studies are lacking.

REFERENCES

Brown J, Folk JC, Reddy CV, et al: Visual prognosis of multifocal choroiditis, punctate inner choroidopathy, and the diffuse subretinal fibrosis syndrome. Ophthalmology 103:1100–1105, 1996.

Cantrill HL, Folk JC: Multifocal choroiditis associated with progressive subretinal fibrosis. Am J Ophthalmol 101:170–180, 1986.

Comu S, Verstraeten T, Rinkoff JS, et al: Neurological manifestations of acute posterior multifocal placoid pigment epitheliopathy. Stroke 27:996–1001, 1996.

Dreyer RF, Gass JDM: Multifocal choroiditis and panuveitis. Arch Ophthalmol 102:1776–1784, 1984.

Folk JC, Pulido JS, Wolf ME: White dot chorioretinal inflammatory syndromes. Focal points. American Academy of Ophthalmology: December 1990.

Gass JDM: Stereoscopic atlas of macular diseases. St Louis, CV Mosby, 1997.

Hooper PL, Kaplan HJ: Triple-agent immunosuppression in serpiginous choroiditis. Ophthalmology 98:944–952, 1991.

Mamalis N, Daily MJ: Multiple evanescent white dot syndrome. Ophthalmology 94:1209–1212, 1987.

Priem HA, Oosterhuis JA: Birdshot chorioretinopathy: Clinical characteristics and evolution. Br J Ophthalmol 72:646–659, 1988.

Rosenfeld PJ, Saperstein DA, Bressler NM, et al: Verteporfin in ocular histoplasmosis study group. Photodynamic therapy with verteporfin in ocular histoplasmosis: uncontrolled, open-label 2-year study. Ophthalmology 111(9):1725–1733, 2004.

Watzke RC, Packer AJ, Folk JC, et al: Punctate inner choroidopathy. Am J Ophthalmol 98:572–584, 1984.

SECTION

31 Sclera

345 EPISCLERITIS 379.00

Peter G. Watson, MA, MBBChir, FRCS, FRCOphth, DO
Cambridge, England

Episcleritis is a benign, recurrent, self-limiting inflammation of the highly vascularized episclera which is closely attached to the underlying sclera and the mobile Tenon's capsule. It is contiguous with the fascial coats of the extraocular muscles. As neither the conjunctiva above nor the sclera below is involved in the inflammatory process, episcleritis does not threaten the vision or anatomical integrity of the eye.

The etiology of episcleral disease is unknown, but with the exception of children below 12 years of age, almost all patients who have an associated systemic disease – often gout, rosacea or connective tissue disorder are in the older age group, whereas those who have evidence of hypersensitivity reactions or migraine are in the younger group. Episcleritis with onset before puberty usually ceases at puberty; episcleritis starting before the menopause usually ceases with menopause. However, no hormonal abnormalities have ever been demonstrated. There is no genetic predisposition to episcleritis.

Clinically there are two ill defined and overlapping groups of patients. The first group is younger, between 13 months and 60 years old. These patients have an acute onset and a rapid benign course with recurrences over a period of 1 month to 3 years. The second group of patients, age 40 to 80, have less severe inflammation but a much longer course. More than half of patients with episcleritis have intermittent attacks that usually continue for 3 to 6 years, although some patients have had attacks for as long as been known to go on for up to 30 years.

The onset is sudden and unpredictable and may or may not be accompanied by pain or discomfort. The pain is localized to the eye and does not radiate to the face or jaw. Attacks last between 7 to 10 days, whether treated or not, and have a strong tendency to recur either at the same site or elsewhere in the same or opposite eye.

DIAGNOSIS

Episcleritis may be simple (diffuse) or nodular. Simple episcleritis accounts for 75% of cases, nodular episcleritis for the remainder. Both varieties are twice as common in women as men.

Clinical signs and symptoms

In simple episcleritis the onset is sudden. Pateints report discomfort, a pricking sensation, and some swelling around the eyes. The affected eye can be intensely red and watery but there is never any purulent discharge. The inflammation may cover part of the anterior episclera or the whole globe. Involvement of the posterior episclera and muscle fascia may result in minor transient diplopia.

In nodular episcleritis the inflammation remains localised to one place and recurrences are generally at the same location. The onset is less acute and resolution is slower in nodular disease. Some of the nodules can be very large but there are no residual structural abnormalities in the episcleral tissue or the sclera.

In both simple and nodular episcleritis, anterior segment angiography reveals a very rapid circulation time with transudation of fluid resulting from increased permeability of vessels.

In those patients who develop episcleritis as a result of migraine there is temporary localised vascular closure of pre capillary arterioles. In all varieties the vascular pattern remains normal and does not become distorted or rearranged as in scleral disease.

The diagnosis of episcleritis is through the history and the clinical observation of the depth and extent of the inflammation. No specific laboratory investigations are available. Seven percent of patients have hyperuricemia even in the absence of clinical gout and 15% have serological indicators of connective tissue disease. Episcleritis may be the first sign of a systemic connective tissue disorder. Children under the age of 12 years with episcleritis have a high incidence of systemic disease or viral infection.

TREATMENT

As episcleritis is self limiting and causes no permanent damage to the eye it does not usually require treatment. However, treatment is appropriate on the first attack or if the inflammation or discomfort is particularly severe. Therapy reduces patient discomfort but does not affect the duration of the inflammation.

First attack of episcleritis

A careful history is required to rule out the possibility of any intercurrent disease. If any is present, including migraine, this should be treated appropriately, immediately and vigorously. Vigorous, focused treatment at this stage often eliminates recurrences.

In the active phase of inflammation (within 48 hours of onset) offer topical prednisolone 0.5% administered every 30 minutes during the day and on waking at night. The dose is then reduced to 4 times daily for 2 days, twice the next day and once daily for the next 2 days. If prednisolone treatment is introduced the therapy should continue over the full course. If withdrawn early, rebound inflammation frequently occurs.

If the episcleritis is first seen after 48 hours no treatment other than cold artificial tears and cold compresses should be prescribed.

Recurrent episcleritis

Treat initially with cold compresses and artificial tears. However, if the inflammation is severe and disabling a systemic NSAID should be prescribed such as flubiprofen 100 mg 3 times a day, or its equivalent. COX II inhibitors do not appear to be as effective as NSAIDs, but as patients responses can be idiosyncratic, different preparations should be tried as some patients will respond to one compound but not another.

PRECAUTIONS

Long term, continuous local corticosteroid therapy should not be administered because of the danger of inducing cataract and glaucoma.

REFERENCES

Foster CS, Sainz de la Maza M: The sclera. New York, Springer-Verlag, 1993.

Read RW, Weiss AG, Sherry D: Episcleritis in childhood. Ophthalmology 106:2377–2379, 1999.

Watson PG, Hayreh SS: Scleritis and episcleritis. Br J Ophthalmol 60:163–191, 1976.

Watson PG, Hazleman BL, Pavesio C, Green WR: The sclera and systemic disorders. 2nd edn. New York, Butterworth-Heinemann, 2004.

346 SCLERAL STAPHYLOMAS AND DEHISCENCES 379.11

Bishara M. Faris, MD, FACS
Worcester, Massachusetts
H. Mackenzie Freeman, MD
Boston, Massachusetts

Localized weakening of the sclera may lead to formation of a thin oval or elliptic area through which the choroid is visible. When flat and meridionally oriented, such areas are termed *scleral dehiscences*; they are referred to as *staphylomas* when they are bulging.

ETIOLOGY/INCIDENCE

Staphylomas may be congenital or acquired. They are classified as anterior or posterior, depending on their relationship to the equator of the eye.

- *Posterior staphylomas* are found in patients with myopia of great than -8 diopters (D) as well as in patients with the connective tissue disorders of Ehlers–Danlos and Marfan syndromes.
- *Anterior staphylomas* are common operative findings among patients with nontraumatic rhegmatogenous retinal detachment, with a reported incidence of 14%. Less commonly, they occur in eyes with increased intraocular pressure and recurrent necrotizing scleritis and after deep scleral resection for episcleral malignancies. Anterior staphylomas also have been reported after subconjunctival injections of corticosteroids and in patients with neurofibromatosis and sarcoidosis.

COURSE/PROGNOSIS

Staphylomas may progress with patient age. The progression of posterior staphylomas causes increasing chorioretinal degeneration and breaks in Bruch's membrane, which may result in subsequent growth of neovascular membranes and subretinal bleeding.

Posterior staphylomas may contribute to the development of macular hole formation and retinal detachment.

DIAGNOSIS

- *Anterior staphylomas* are seen through the bulbar conjunctiva as areas of bluish discoloration of the thin sclera.
- *Posterior staphylomas* can be seen best with indirect ophthalmoscopy. The thinned sclera bulges posteriorly and is lined by a thin and atrophic choroid. The size and location of these lesions can be accurately determined using ophthalmic B-scan ultrasound and computed tomography (CT) scan.

PROPHYLAXIS

Rupture of the globe may complicate scleral dehiscences and staphylomas. Extraocular muscles in the large staphylomatous globes are commonly thin. During strabismus surgery on such eyes and when scleral bites are taken, scleral perforation may result.

Scleral perforation may also occur when local anesthetics are administered to eyeballs with staphylomas in preparation for intra- or extraocular surgery. Hence, periocular infiltration is mandatory in patients with posterior staphylomas and retrobulbar infiltration in patients with anterior staphylomas.

In planning for retinal detachment surgery, that a history of staphyloma in one eye should alert the surgeon to the possibility of its occurrence in the fellow eye.

TREATMENT

Supportive

A sustained elevation of intraocular pressure, especially in children, may result in formation of anterior scleral dehiscences or staphyloma, so lowering pressure by carbonic anhydrase inhibitors, adrenergics, beta-adrenergic blocking agents, alpha agonists, prostaglandins, or miotics is in order. Forceful rubbing of the eyeballs produces a marked elevation in pressure and should be avoided.

Surgical

During surgery for retinal detachment

When dehiscences and staphylomas are discovered in the area to be buckled during retinal detachment surgery, certain operative precautions should be taken to prevent accidental rupture of the globe. In localizing the retinal breaks, the indentation should be performed using a cotton-tipped applicator rather than a metal electrode. The blunt edges of the implant should extend over thin scleral zones and end on healthy sclera. When applying cryoapplications, the cryoprobe tip should be applied gently and should not be removed until it has completely thawed. Premature probe movements may rupture the sclera.

The assistant surgeon has an important role to play during surgery. Gentle exposure of the globe prevents sudden increases in intraocular pressure and subsequent rupture of the globe. It may be safer to detach more rectus muscles to obtain good exposure of the surgical field than to resort to forceful exposure.

The use of intravenous acetazolamide and mannitol to lower the intraocular pressure and minimize the risk of globe rupture is advised in all cases, unless there is a medical contraindication. Paracentesis may be used as a last resort when intravenous medications fail to lower the eye pressure adequately.

Our recommended procedure is pars plana vitrectomy, internal drainage with endophotocoagulation, and air-gas exchange.

During surgery for episcleral malignancies

Scleral resection is done whenever there is evidence of scleral involvement. Deep resections involving two-thirds or more of the scleral thickness may predispose a patient to the formation of dehiscences and staphylomas. In such cases, it is wise to cover the resected zones with a preserved scleral graft or an autogenous pretibial periosteal patch graft.

Surgical reinforcement of posterior staphylomas using donor sclera, silicone rubber, or fascia lata has been performed in countries outside the United States. No controlled studies have been made to document the benefits of such procedures.

COMMENTS

Anterior scleral staphylomas are most often located in the superior temporal quadrants. Hence, these quadrants should be avoided when subconjunctival injections of antibiotics and corticosteroids are indicated. Preoperative inspection of these quadrants is mandatory when retinal detachment occurs in myopic eyes. When staphylomas are encountered during retinal detachment surgery, they can be the site of rupture of the globe unless specific operative measures are taken.

REFERENCES

Coroneo MT, Beaumont JT, Hollows FC: Scleral reinforcement in the treatment of pathologic myopia. Aust N Z J Ophthalmol 16:317–320, 1988.

Faris B, Freeman HM, Schepens CL: Scleral dehiscences, anterior staphyloma and retinal detachments-Part 1: incidence and pathogenesis. Trans Am Acad Ophthalmol Otolaryngol 79:851–853, 1975.

Freeman HM, Schepens CL, Faris B: Scleral dehiscences, anterior staphyloma, and retinal detachment-Part 2: surgical management. Trans Am Acad Ophthalmol Otolaryngol 79:854–857, 1975.

Ripandelli G, Parisi V, Friberg TR, et al: Retinal detachment associated with macular hole in high myopia: using the vitreous anatomy to optimize the surgical approach. Ophthalmology 111(4):726–31, 2004.

Sasoh M, Yoshida S, Ito Y, et al: Macular buckling for retinal detachment due to macular hole in highly myopic eyes with posterior staphyloma. Retina 20(5):445–449, 2000.

347 SCLERITIS 379.00

Sinan Tatlipinar, MD
Baltimore, Maryland
Ozge Ilhan-Sarac, MD
Baltimore, Maryland
Esen Karamürsel Akpek, MD
Baltimore, Maryland

Scleritis is an inflammatory disorder of the sclera and deep episclera often associated with vision-threatening ocular complications. Approximately 40% to 50% of patients with scleritis have an identifiable underlying disease. Importantly, scleritis can be the initial manifestation of these disorders. Morbidity in patients with scleritis is primarily based on vasculitis and microangiopathy, suggesting that it is part of an immune complex reaction caused by the interaction of genetic, environmental and endogenous factors. Early diagnosis of scleritis and the underlying disease and the initiation of appropriate systemic therapy can control the progression of the active vasculitic process. Without treatment, the disease course is generally destructive and potentially life threatening. Therefore, it is essential to understand the exact nature of the disease.

EPIDEMIOLOGY/INCIDENCE

Current estimates suggests that the prevalence of scleritis ranges from 0.08% to 4% in the general population. However, the disease may be more common than is currently recognized because of misdiagnoses. Scleritis is generally a disease of middle-aged populations, with a peak of presentation in the fifth decade (age range 11 to 87 years). Most series report a slight female predilection, with a female to male ratio of approximately 1.6 : 1. There is no known racial or geographical predisposition.

COURSE/PROGNOSIS

Scleritis is classified based on the site of pathology and severity of inflammation (Box 347.1). This classification is a useful predictor of the disease course and prognosis as well as a guide to therapy. Scleritis is traditionally divided into anterior (94%) and posterior (6%) types (Box 347.1). Depending on clinical appearance, anterior scleritis is further divided into subtypes such as diffuse, nodular, necrotizing (necrotizing with inflammation) and scleromalacia perforans (necrotizing without inflammation).

Diffuse anterior scleritis is the most common type of scleritis, followed by, in order of frequency: nodular, necrotizing with inflammation, posterior scleritis, and scleromalacia perforans.

The type of scleritis and the severity of inflammation are largely related to the underlying systemic disease. Patients with Wegener's granulomatosis are more likely to have necrotizing scleritis with peripheral corneal involvement, whereas patients with seronegative spondyloarthropathies tend to have more benign inflammation. Patients with rheumatoid arthritis or relapsing polychondritis usually have disease of intermediate severity.

BOX 347.1 – Clinical classification of scleritis

Scleritis
Anterior
Diffuse
Nodular
Necrotizing
With inflammation (necrotizing)
Without inflammation (scleromalacia perforans)
Posterior

DIAGNOSIS

Clinical signs and symptoms

Patients with anterior scleritis complain of a gradual onset of deep eye pain radiating to temple, jaw, and sinuses with associated redness, tenderness, lacrimation, and photophobia. Redness is intense with a violaceous hue and may be localized in one sector or the entire sclera. Approximately 34 to 50% of patients have bilateral scleritis.

In diffuse anterior scleritis, the redness is generalized all over the anterior sclera. Slit-lamp examination reveals distortion, tortuosity and congestion of the superficial and deep episcleral plexi with loss of the normal radial pattern (Figure 347.1). When the inflammation disappears, the sclera may appear bluish, mainly because of rearrangement of the collagen fibers, at times with associated thinning.

In the nodular type of anterior scleritis, the hyperemia is localized to one or more areas over scleral nodules that are immobile and extremely tender to touch. Slit-lamp examination reveals congestion and tortuosity of the superficial and deep episcleral plexi overlying the nodules, which are usually localized in the interpalpebral region close to the limbus (Figure 347.2).

Necrotizing scleritis is the most severe and destructive form of scleritis. Patients have more severe pain, which can be provoked by minimal touch to the scalp. On slit-lamp examination white avascular areas surrounded by swelling of the sclera and abnormally congested episcleral vessels can be seen. Without appropriate treatment, these lesions may progress to perforation.

Scleromalacia perforans usually does not cause pain, redness, or clinically apparent inflammation. Yellow or grayish anterior scleral nodules that gradually develop a necrotic slough or sequestrum, eventually separating from the underlying sclera and leaving the choroid bare or covered only by a thin layer of conjunctiva are the characteristic findings of this disorder. Slit-lamp examination reveals a reduction in the size and number of the episcleral vessels surrounding the sequestrum, giving a porcelain-like appearance.

Patients with posterior scleritis often present with pain, redness, chemosis, lid edema, lid retraction, proptosis and, most importantly, decreased vision. Exudative retinal detachment, choroidal folds, subretinal mass, vitreitis, disc edema, macular edema, and annular ciliochoroidal detachment may be present. Posterior scleritis is often associated with anterior scleritis. The absence of anterior scleritis makes the diagnosis difficult.

Laboratory findings

Fluorescein angiography of the anterior segment can be used in the diagnosis and reveals early leakage into the extravascular space and venular obstruction. In necrotizing scleritis, arteriolar beading, non-perfused areas and increased transition time and distortion of normal radial pattern of episcleral vessels may be detected. Indocyanine green angiography is also useful, particularly to differentiate episcleritis from scleritis. These two tests provide different and complementary information because each dye has different leakage patterns caused by the difference in optical and chemical properties, and each detects areas of damage not clinically visible.

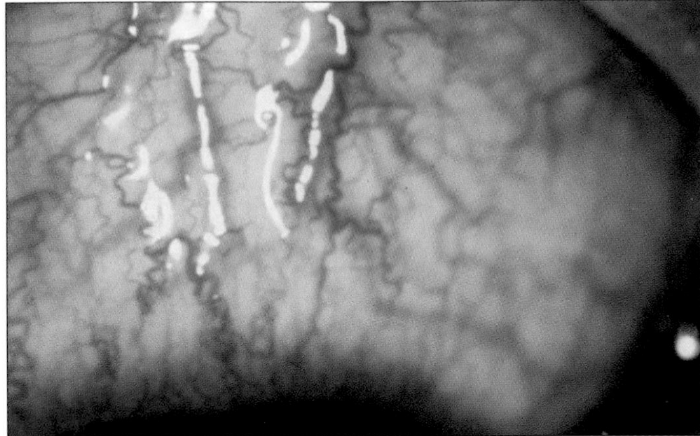

FIGURE 347.1. Diffuse anterior scleritis with violaceous hue of the underlying sclera and tortuosity of the vasculature.

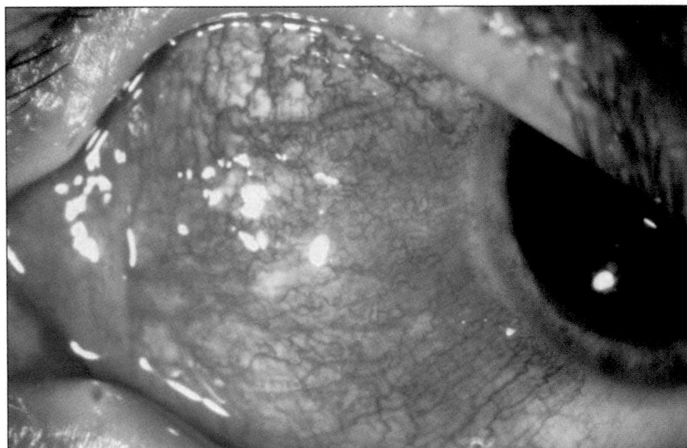

FIGURE 347.2. A nasal scleral nodule with loss of normal radial pattern of vessels.

B-scan ultrasonography is the most useful test in the diagnosis of posterior scleritis. Increased thickness of the sclera and choroid, separation of the posterior surface of the sclera from the episclera, the presence of retinal or choroidal detachments, and swelling of the disc are common findings. Fundus fluorescein angiography is also helpful in the diagnosis of posterior scleritis to detect serous retinal detachment, choroidal folds, retinal striae, and disc and macular edema.

The presence of microangiopathy in most scleritis specimens suggests an underlying Type III hypersensitivity reaction in which the vascular injury is the result of antigen-antibody conjugation within and outside of the vessel wall, with subsequent activation of complement, attraction of neutrophils and fibrinoid necrosis of vessels and surrounding tissue. The antigen is usually the aberrant expression of the HLA-DR on scleral fibroblasts, induced by interferon gamma. Persistent immunologic injury may lead to a chronic response (a type IV hypersensitivity) mediated by epithelioid cells, macrophages, multinucleated giant cells, and mainly Th1 lymphocytes. This activated immune network, if not treated, leads to scleral destruction.

Differential diagnosis

Diagnosis of scleritis is a clinical one. A painful, intense deep bluish redness or violaceous hue of the sclera is the main sign of anterior scleritis. This is best detected under natural daylight or on penlight examination. Areas of scleral thinning or early necrosis can also be detected with daylight examination. Slit-lamp examination with red-free light reveals edema of the sclera and congestion of deep episcleral plexus. White diffuse illumination helps detect abnormal vessels, avascular or necrotic areas, and scleral thinning. The congested deep episcleral vessels are typically not blanched with topically applied 10% phenylephrine.

Approximately half of patients with scleritis have an associated medical condition. A rheumatic disease is seen in about 30–40% of patients. Rheumatoid arthritis (RA) is the most common systemic condition associated with scleritis, seen in 10 to 33% of patients. The majority of these patients (80%) carry a diagnosis of RA at the time of presentation with scleritis. Scleromalacia perforans is almost exclusively associated with rheumatoid arthritis. Systemic vasculitis is the second most common medical condition. About 50% of patients with vasculitis-associated scleritis have Wegener's granulomatosis. Most importantly, scleritis is the presenting or only clinical finding in a significant proportion of these patients. Systemic lupus erythematosus, relapsing polychondritis, and inflammatory bowel disease are some of the other common rheumatic diseases associated with scleritis.

An infectious etiology, such as herpes zoster, herpes simplex, tuberculosis, syphilis, and Lyme disease, is seen in about 5 to 10% of patients. Herpes zoster is by far the most commonly associated infectious disease.

All patients with scleritis should undergo a diagnostic workup, based on a careful review of systems, for proper treatment and assessment of prognosis.

Scleritis must be differentiated from both diffuse and nodular episcleritis. Patients with episcleritis do not commonly complain about pain. The eye appears salmon pink to fiery red but not bluish or violaceous and the sclera is not edematous. White diffuse illumination helps detect the depth of the inflammation to differentiate these two disorders. Since the edema and congestion are both localized in superficial episcleral plexus in episcleritis, topically applied 10% phenylephrine blanches the hyperemia, in contrast with scleritis.

Scleral hyaline plaque in elderly people, between the cornea and the insertion of the lateral or medial rectus muscles sometimes can simulate necrotizing scleritis without inflammation. But unlike the findings in scleromalacia perforans the overlying conjunctiva is healthy in these cases.

Posterior scleritis must be differentiated from uveal effusion syndrome, Vogt–Koyanagi–Harada disease and central serous retinopathy. Choroidal melanoma, uveal metastatic tumors, and choroidal hemangioma must be excluded when the patient appears to have a subretinal mass. CT and MRI scans are especially important in these cases.

Systemic vasculitides are the main entities to be considered in the differential diagnosis of scleritis. Therefore, all patients with scleritis should be evaluated carefully for a vasculitic process. Wegener's granulomatosis is the most common of these and appears to be the underlying etiology in approximately half of cases of vasculitis-associated scleritis. Anti-neutrophil cytoplasmic antibody (ANCA) (cytoplasmic: c-ANCA and perinuclear: p-ANCA), a circulating autoantibody against intracytoplasmic extranuclear components of neutrophils, is nearly always present in Wegener's granulamotosis. More importantly, patients with scleritis, positive ANCA results, but no clinical evidence of systemic vasculitis will usually have refractory inflammation, and may need to be treated as for Wegener's granulamatosis.

TREATMENT

Systemic

The treatment of scleritis always requires systemic therapy based on the type of scleritis, severity of inflammation, and course of the underlying systemic disease. In patients with diffuse or nodular scleritis, oral non-steroidal anti-inflammatory drug (NSAID) therapy (indomethacin sustained-release 75 mg q12h, naproxen sodium 375–500 mg q12h) is the initial choice, unless the underlying disease is a known vasculitic disorder. Response to therapy may not be seen until up to 2–3 weeks after commencement of NSAIDs. If the first NSAID is found to be ineffective, another can be tried, up to a maximum of three. Generally patients require a one-year course of therapy before attempting to taper and discontinue the medication. For unresponsive cases and posterior scleritis, oral steroids (prednisone 1 mg/kg/day, up to 60 mg total daily dose) should be considered. With the improvement of clinical findings, the dose can be tapered gradually and the therapy discontinued while maintaining remission with NSAIDs.

Intravenous pulse corticosteroid therapy (methylprednisolone, 1 g/day for 3 consecutive days) followed by oral steroids can be used for refractory cases. Adjunctive preseptal, periorbital and subconjunctival long-acting steroid injections (such as triamcinolone acetonide) have also been reported to be effective in small case series on patients with non-necrotizing scleritis. However, extreme caution should be exercised with these injections as progression to necrosis and perforation can occur. In cases of therapeutic failure of steroids, immunomodulatory drugs such as oral methotrexate (7.5–25 mg once a week), mycophenolate mofetil (1 g/twice daily), azathioprine (2–3 mg/kg/day), cyclosporin A (2.5–5 mg/kg/day) or cyclophosphamide (2–3 mg/kg/day), may be considered as third-line therapy. Oral corticosteroids should be combined with immunosuppressives during the first 3–4 weeks of the treatment as the response to immunosuppressive therapy may take up to 6 weeks. After the first month of treatment steroids should be tapered slowly and discontinued.

Immunosuppressive therapy as initial treatment is required for definitively diagnosed systemic vasculitic disease, necrotizing scleritis, and/or progressive destructive ocular inflammation especially involving the cornea. Cyclophosphamide is the first choice in these patients and may be given as a single daily oral dose (2–3 mg/kg/day) or as intravenous pulse therapy (750 mg/m^2 of body surface) in patients with vision threatening conditions. In cases of therapeutic failure, plasmapheresis may be considered.

Although clinicians' experience is limited as yet, the recent introduction of new immunomodulatory agents has expanded the treatment options, particularly for refractory cases. Daclizumab (1 mg/kg IV) is a newly introduced monoclonal antibody that exerts its effect by binding to the alpha subunit (CD25) of the human interleukin (IL)-2 receptor on the surface of activated lymphocytes, thus preventing the binding of IL-2.

Anti-IL-2 receptor therapy is an effective therapeutic approach for disorders with a predominant Th1 profile. Infliximab (3–10 mg/kg given as intravenous infusion followed with additional similar doses at 2 and 6 weeks after the first infusion, and every 8 weeks thereafter) and etanercept (50 mg per week given as two 25 mg subcutaneous injections at separate sites) are tumor necrosis factor alpha (TNF-α) blockers.

Medical

In patients with infectious scleritis surgical debridement of the infected tissues, systemic, topical and subconjunctival antibiotic treatments are required. Treatment is needed for six or more weeks. In active stages of the disease corticosteroid and immunosuppressive treatments are contraindicated.

Surgical

In cases of extreme scleral thinning or perforation reinforcement is required. Donor sclera, fascia lata, periosteum, split-thickness dermis, aortic tissue, or artificial materials such as Gore-Tex can be used for this purpose. To maintain the integrity of the globe this tectonic surgery should always be accompanied with systemic immunosuppressive therapy.

COMPLICATIONS

Ocular complications are not uncommon and are more frequently seen with necrotizing scleritis. Corneal complications are the most frequent, and include peripheral corneal thinning, peripheral ulcerative keratitis, stromal keratitis, and sclerosing keratitis. Peripheral ulcerative keratitis is the most severe form of corneal involvement. It is usually associated with necrotizing scleritis and if not treated may lead to perforation. Stromal keratitis is the extension of the inflammation into the cornea that can lead to sclerocornea. Uveitis is seen in about one-third of patients. It is more frequently anterior and occurs later during the course of the inflammation. Posterior uveitis is relatively rare and usually appears in patients with posterior scleritis. Increased intraocular pressure can develop due to the uveitis and scleral edema. Open angle glaucoma, angle closure glaucoma and neovascular glaucoma may occur. Cataracts can also develop due to prolonged inflammation secondary to long-term steroid treatment.

REFERENCES

Akpek EK, Thorne JE, Qazi FA, et al: Evaluation of patients with scleritis for systemic disease. Ophthalmology 111:501–506, 2004.

Akpek EK, Uy HS, Christen W, et al: Severity of episcleritis and systemic disease association. Ophthalmology 106:729–731, 1999.

Hernandez-Illas M, Tozman E, Fulcher SFA, et al: Recombinant human tumor necrosis factor receptor Fc fusion protein (Etanercept): experience as a therapy for sight threatening scleritis and sterile corneal ulceration. Eye Contact Lens 30:2–5, 2004.

Legmann A, Foster CS: Noninfectious necrotizing scleritis. Int Ophthalmol Clin 36:73–80, 1996.

Murphy CC, Ayliffe WH, Booth A, et al: Tumor necrosis a blockade with infliximab for refractory uveitis and scleritis. Ophthalmology 111:352–356, 2004.

Watson PG, Young RD: Scleral structure, organization and disease. A review. Exp Eye Res 78:609–623, 2004.

348 SCLEROMALACIA PERFORANS 379.04

Gregory J. McCormick, MD
Rochester, New York
James V. Aquavella, MD
Rochester, New York

ETIOLOGY

The term *scleromalacia perforans* was coined by van der Hoeve in 1934 to describe a rare form of scleritis that occurs mainly in postmenopausal women with long-standing polyarticular rheumatoid arthritis. The condition also occurs as a sequela of ocular carcinoma in acquired immune deficiency syndrome (AIDS) and in predisposed patients following a latent period after ocular surgery with or without intraoperative antimetabolite application.

COURSE/PROGNOSIS

The principal feature is the formation of multiple areas of deep scleral ulceration that coalesce to reveal the underlying uveal tissue. The condition is of insidious onset and is typically painless and characterized by a lack of clinical signs of inflammation. Yellowish necrotic lesions appear in the anterior sclera between the limbus and the equator ultimately resulting in sequestration of necrotic tissue, scleral thinning, and a characteristic bluish hue. Tissue loss apparently follows occlusion of smaller episcleral capillaries with pathology characterized as immune complex-mediated vasculitis. Although the overlying conjunctiva may be thinned, spontaneous perforation and anterior staphyloma formation are rare and are usually associated with glaucoma. However, these eyes are at high risk from the occurrence of even minor trauma (Figure 348.1).

DIAGNOSIS

The diagnosis is made by identifying a necrotizing anterior scleritis in the absence of significant pain or objective signs of

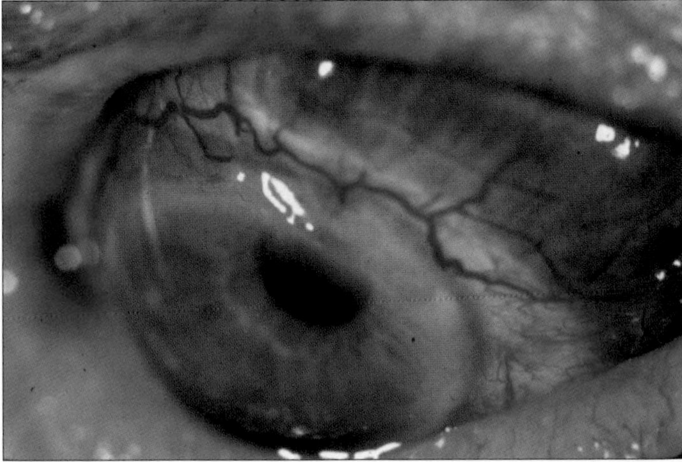

FIGURE 348.1. Scleromalacia perforans with scleral thinning, anterior staphyloma and characteristic engorged overlying vessels.

inflammation. Although the number of lesions varies, they can coalesce into large areas of scleral necrosis. Associated findings may include uveitis, secondary glaucoma, cataract, and perforation. All of the lesions share the same pathologic features. A history of rheumatoid arthritis and the presence of rheumatoid nodules in other parts of the body are common in this patient population.

Clinical signs and symptoms

Ocular or periocular

- Cornea: aseptic necrosis, pannus, ulceration.
- Extraocular muscles: limitation of motion, tendonitis.
- Sclera: episcleritis, scleritis, anterior staphyloma.
- Other: cataract, retinal vasculitis, secondary glaucoma, uveitis.

TREATMENT

Ocular

Although the clinical appearance is non-inflammatory, the underlying cause is believed to be inflammatory in nature and therefore the mainstay of treatment is immunomodulatory and is reserved for patients with symptoms, progressive disease or complications. Topical prednisolone and prednisone, typically 100 to 250 mg daily, in combination with other anti-inflammatory agents such as phenylbutazone or cytotoxic agents (cyclosphamide), may be helpful. Low-dose cyclosporin A (5 mg/kg per day) has been reported to be effective in conjunction with a minimum controlling systemic steroid dosage. Intensive anti-inflammatory therapy seems to produce rapid resolution and may prevent progression of lesions. Patients with scleromalacia perforans often suffer from rheumatoid arthritis, so a comprehensive medical approach is indicated. Nonsteroidal anti-inflammatory drugs have not been proven to be of value. Once the inflammatory process has been stabilized, steroids should be slowly tapered over a period of several weeks.

Surgical

Surgical techniques are directed towards reinforcing areas of thinned sclera, anterior staphyloma or perforation. Free or rotational scleral autografts have been used with success in treating some lesions. Larger areas of thinning have been repaired with preserved sclera, fascia lata from the lateral thigh, cadaveric aorta, periosteum from the anterior tibial crest, tarsus, dura mater, preserved pericardium, and split thickness dermis. The surgeon should be careful not to rupture the choroid during the placement of the graft. Intraoperative cautery of prolapsing areas has been repored to safely shrink tissue without evidence of fundus abnormalities 6 months after grafting surgery. It is important for the grafts to be covered totally by sliding or free conjunctival grafts when possible. Larger grafts have been successfully epithelialized after being covered with buccal mucous membrane and more recently with amniotic membrane transplantation (Figure 348.2).

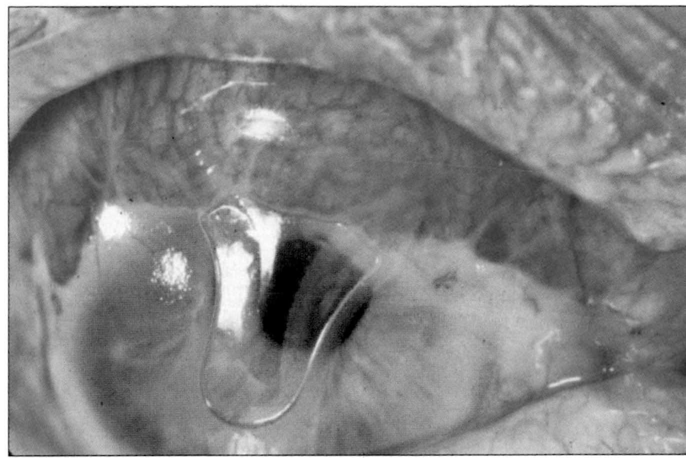

FIGURE 348.2. Postoperative appearance after placement of periosteal graft and hydrophilic bandage contact lens.

COMPLICATIONS

Careful observation after initiating systemic immunosuppressive therapy is important in view of the known deleterious effects of these drugs. Periocular injections of corticosteroids are absolutely contraindicated. When surgical therapy is undertaken, the surgeon should be aware of the potential for recurrence. Finally, it is important to differentiate true scleromalacia perforans from other forms of scleral necrosis secondary to inflammatory conditions in which patients are more symptomatic.

COMMENTS

Scleromalacia perforans, although uncommon, poses a major management problem. If the patient is asymptomatic in the absence of complications, it may be that no therapy is necessary. Once a decision to intervene has been made, comprehensive medical therapy with both topical and systemic corticosteroids, often accompanied by immunosuppressive drugs, must be instituted. If these measures fail, surgical modalities using overlying grafts with various materials may have to be considered.

REFERENCES

Bick MW: Surgical treatment of scleromalacia perforans. Arch Ophthalmol 61:907–917, 1959.

Breslin CW, Katz JI, Kaufman HE: Surgical management of necrotizing scleritis. Arch Ophthalmol 95:2038–2040, 1977.

Hakin KN, Ham J, Lightman SL: Use of cyclosporin in the management of steroid-dependent non-necrotizing scleritis. Br J Ophthalmol 75:340–341, 1991.

Watson PG, Hazleman BL: The sclera and systemic disorders. Philadelphia, WB Saunders, 1976.

Watson PG: The nature and the treatment of scleral inflammation. Trans Ophthalmol Soc UK 102:257–281, 1982.

SECTION

32 Vitreous

349 FAMILIAL EXUDATIVE VITREORETINOPATHY 743.51
(Criswick–Schepens Syndrome)

Alexander P. Hunyor, MBBS, FRANZCO, FRACS
Sydney, Australia
Joseph E. Robertson, Jr., MD
Portland, Oregon

Familial exudative vitreoretinopathy (FEVR) is a hereditary abnormality characterized by abnormal vascularization of the peripheral retina, which may appear strikingly similar to retinopathy of prematurity (ROP). Ocular involvement is bilateral and often symmetric. The condition was first described in 1969 by Criswick and Schepens. Also formerly known as autosomal dominant exudative vitreoretinopathy, this condition has now been described in X-linked recessive and autosomal recessive forms. It is an important cause of retinal detachment in younger patients, especially in the Japanese population.

ETIOLOGY

- Autosomal dominant inheritance.
  - Most common (and classically described) form.
  - High penetrance and highly variable expressivity.
  - 3 loci identified:
    - EVR1 — chromosome 11q, FZD4 gene mutation
    - EVR3 — chromosome 11p
    - EVR4 — chromosome 11q, LRP5 gene mutation.
- X-linked recessive inheritance.
  - Locus: EVR2 — chromosome Xp11.4.
  - More severe form, due to mutation of the Norrie disease gene, NDP.
- Autosomal recessive inheritance.
  - One recessive EVR4 mutation in LRP5 has been described.

COURSE/PROGNOSIS

Findings generally remain stable once adulthood is reached. Disease progression with visual loss is uncommon after age 20, although patients are at risk of late rhegmatogenous retinal detachment.

DIAGNOSIS

Classification

Various classification schemes have been proposed to describe the clinical course and angiographic findings in FEVR. Most recently, a staging scheme similar to that for ROP has been suggested by Pendergast and Trese.

Clinical signs and symptoms

Symptomatic patients usually present in childhood with strabismus or reduced visual acuity due to retinal fold or detachment. Clinical appearance may simulate that in ROP, but there is rarely a history of low birth weight. Patients with milder forms of FEVR are commonly asymptomatic and have good visual acuity. Findings include peripheral avascular zones that are usually temporal and wedge-shaped but may be more extensive; vasodilatation and arteriovenous anastomosis; abnormal vitreoretinal adhesion; and a V-shaped area of chorioretinal degeneration corresponding to the avascular zone. The peripheral avascular zone usually persists without regression or neovascular complications, in contradistinction to ROP, in which the peripheral retina vascularizes as the disease regresses.

In more advanced cases, patients may develop retinal neovascularization, intraretinal and subretinal hemorrhage and exudate, and fibrovascular membranes that can lead to cicatricial complications similar to those of ROP. These include retinal (falciform) folds; tractional, rhegmatogenous, or combined retinal detachments; and macular ectopia. Patients may present with advanced retinal detachment complicated by neovascular glaucoma, band keratopathy, or even phthisis bulbi.

Other findings may include:

- Myopia;
- White-with-pressure and white-without-pressure, cystoid degeneration, and retinoschisis;
- Cystoid macular edema, epiretinal membrane;
- Vitreous hemorrhage is relatively uncommon;
- Isolated intraretinal deposits may be the only clinical manifestation.

Diagnosis is based on the spectrum of clinical features listed previously, in combination with:

- History of familial tendency;
- No history of prematurity, low birth weight, or supplemental oxygen therapy.

Detailed family history and examination of relatives, who are often asymptomatic, is essential for correct diagnosis and proper genetic counseling.

Laboratory findings

Fluorescein angiography, concentrating on the temporal periphery, may demonstrate capillary nonperfusion. This can be a useful diagnostic adjunct, particularly in patients with subtle retinal findings. Genetic testing for EVR mutations is available in some centers.

Differential diagnosis

ROP may be ophthalmoscopically indistinguishable from FEVR, hence the importance of neonatal and family history.

Other causes of peripheral retinal vascular abnormality with neovascularization: sickle cell retinopathy, Eales disease, autosomal dominant neovascular inflammatory vitreoretinopathy.

- Other causes of disk dragging, macular heterotopia, retinal fold: Norrie's disease, combined hamartoma of retinal pigment epithelium and retina, posterior persistent hyperplastic primary vitreous, retinal dysplasia, congenital retinal fold, congenital toxoplasmosis.
- Other causes of peripheral retinal exudation/fibrovascular proliferation: Coats' disease, toxocariasis, retinal angiomatosis, pars planitis, incontinentia pigmenti.

TREATMENT

Genetic counseling is indicated for all affected patients, regardless of degree of clinical manifestation. Although most patients who have severe visual loss as a result of this disorder have developed it by the end of the second decade of life, all affected individuals have an ongoing increased risk of retinal detachment and deserve long-term follow-up. Accurate refraction, and consideration of amblyopia therapy in the pediatric age group, are important.

Surgical

- Ablation of the peripheral avascular zone (with laser photocoagulation or cryotherapy) is indicated if there is active extraretinal vascularization or subretinal exudation threatening the macula. The value of prophylactic ablation in milder cases remains to be established.
- Scleral buckling, vitrectomy, or both may be required in the management of retinal detachments associated with FEVR.
- Vitrectomy, with lens preservation where possible, is used when it is anticipated that:
  - Scleral buckling alone cannot adequately relieve vitreoretinal traction to allow retinal reattachment;
  - Dense vitreous hemorrhage accompanies the retinal detachment; or
  - Posterior retinal breaks or advanced proliferative vitreoretinopathy are present.
- In patients old enough to report symptoms, prophylactic treatment of symptomatic retinal tears with laser photocoagulation or cryotherapy may be possible.

COMPLICATIONS

- Retinal detachment: exudative, tractional, rhegmatogenous, or combined mechanism.
- Retinal folds, macular ectopia, disk dragging, strabismus.
- Chronic retinal detachment may be complicated by band keratopathy, rubeosis, neovascular glaucoma, cataract, and ultimately, phthisis bulbi.

COMMENTS

Rather than a true vitreoretinopathy, FEVR appears to be a developmental abnormality involving premature arrest of peripheral retinal vascularization, especially in the temporal retina. The major threat to vision is retinal detachment, but visual loss may also result from macular ectopia, epiretinal membrane, cystoid macular edema, retinal folds, and amblyopia. Pathologic progression of FEVR, regardless of disease stage, is not inevitable. Active progression with visual loss is uncommon after 20 years of age, although late rhegmatogenous retinal detachment is a significant complication. The genetic implications of the diagnosis of FEVR, and the importance of family history and the screening of relatives, cannot be overemphasized.

REFERENCES

Criswick VG, Schepens CL: Familial exudative vitreoretinopathy. Am J Ophthalmol 68:578, 1969.

Glazer LC, Maguire A, Blumenkranz MS, et al: Improved surgical treatment of familial exudative vitreoretinopathy in children. Am J Ophthalmol 120:471–479, 1995.

Pendergast SD, Trese MT: Familial exudative vitreoretinopathy: results of surgical management. Ophthalmology 105:1015–1023, 1998.

Toomes C, Bottomley HM, Jackson RM, et al: Mutations in LRP5 or FZD4 underlie the common familial exudative vitreoretinopathy locus on chromosome 11q. Am J Hum Genet 74:721–730, 2004.

Van Nouhuys CE: Dominant exudative vitreoretinopathy and other vascular developmental disorders of the peripheral retina. Doc Ophthalmol 54(1–4):1–414, 1982.

350 PERSISTENT HYPERPLASTIC PRIMARY VITREOUS 743.51 *(Persistent Fetal Vasculature)*

James H. Antoszyk, MD
Charlotte, North Carolina
Andrew Antoszyk, MD
Charlotte, North Carolina

ETIOLOGY/INCIDENCE

Persistent hyperplastic primary vitreous (PHPV) is a congenital ocular disorder with the potential to affect the eye's anterior and posterior anatomy. This condition typically occurs in full-term infants and usually is identified within the first 3 months of life because of leukocoria, microphthalmos, and strabismus. It can be classified into three different anatomic typesanterior, intermediate, and posterior-each with its own associated pathologic features and prognosis. The majority of patients have the intermediate form with abnormalities in both the anterior and posterior segments.

Classically, PHPV affects only one eye, although bilateral involvement has been reported in 2.4% to 17% of cases. Patients in whom both eyes are affected frequently have accompanying systemic abnormalities, such as polydactyly, microcephaly, and cleft palate and lip, as well as central nervous system abnormalities.

In most instances, a specific cause has not been identified, although bilateral cases may occasionally be associated with trisomy 13, X-linked recessive mutations, and autosomal recessive mutations.

The incidence of the disorder has not been established.

COURSE/PROGNOSIS

The child's lens is usually clear initially. With time, disruption of the lens capsule and fibrovascular ingrowth occurs, with progressive lenticular opacification and swelling and a secondary shallowing of the anterior chamber. Typically, glaucoma develops in advanced cases; it may result from either open- or closed-angle mechanisms. Several factors contribute to closure of the anterior chamber angle, including peripheral anterior synechiae, anterior displacement of the iris-lens diaphragm, lens swelling, and seclusion of the pupil. Open-angle glaucoma has been attributed to chronic uveitis and intraocular hemorrhage. Spontaneous hemorrhage into the vitreous, lens, and anterior or posterior chamber may originate from either abnormal iris vessels or the retrolental tissue. These processes may result in a blind, painful eye if surgical intervention does not take place.

Early surgical treatment has been recommended to prevent the progressive changes that result in blindness, phthisis, and globe loss. It has been recommended that the treatment for this condition be determined by (1) evidence of visual function, (2) clinical progression, and (3) the absence of severe optic nerve or retinal involvement, intractable amblyopia, or phthisis.

DIAGNOSIS

PHPV can be divided into anterior, intermediate, and posterior anatomic types on the basis of findings on clinical examination supplemented with ancillary studies. Visual function is evaluated with pupillary responsiveness, visual evoked response, and electroretinography, whereas the posterior segment can be assessed with ophthalmoscopy, ultrasonography, computed tomography, and magnetic resonance imaging.

Anterior PHPV occurs with incomplete reabsorption of the tunica vasculosa lentis (17%). Clinically, it is associated with:

- Engorged radial iris vessels;
- Microcornea (diameter <10 mm);
- Various degrees of persistence of the tunica vasculosa;
- Mittendorf dot to dense retrolental vascularized membrane;
- Elongated ciliary processes;
- Shallowing of the anterior chamber;
- Microphthalmos;
- Progressive cataract.

Posterior PHPV results from incomplete regression of the primary vitreous, particularly the hyaloid vessel remnants (25%). It is associated with:

- Complex vitreous membranes with secondary retinal changes.

Small whitish membranes overlying the optic nervehead (Bergmeister's papillae) to large peripapillary and posterior pole membranes with secondary membranes.

- Traction retinal detachment.

Intermediate PHPV combines features of both anterior and posterior PHPV (58%) (Figure 350.1).

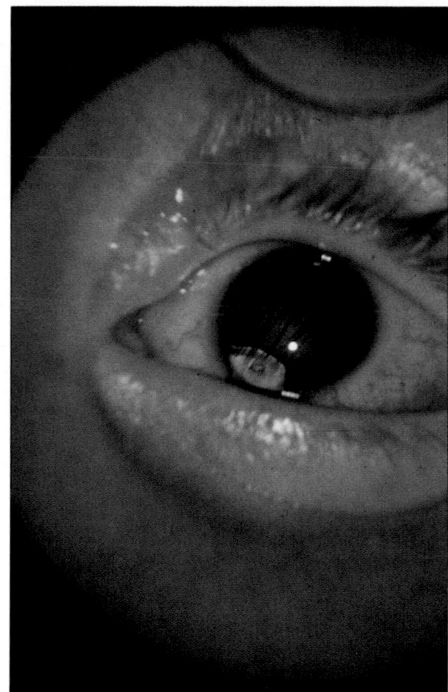

FIGURE 350.1. Persistent hyperplastic primary vitreous.

Differential diagnosis

- Leukocoria in children.
- Retinoblastoma.
- Congenital cataract.
- Retrolental fibroplasia.
- Parasitic endophthalmitis.
- Norrie's disease.
- Incontinentia pigmenti.

TREATMENT

Medical

- Good visual results in children with visually significant monocular structural abnormalities have been reported; the treatment issues are similar to those with monocular congenital cataracts. Effective surgical treatment and treatment for amblyopia must be instituted for both groups during the critical period for maturation of the central nervous system; the best results occur when treatment is initiated within the first 2 months of life.
- Early surgery must be complemented by early optical correction and occlusion therapy, usually within 2 weeks of surgery. Both extended-wear (Silisoft) and gas-permeable hard contact lenses have been used. Frequent lens changes are required because of the eyes' dynamic growth. Intraocular lens implantation has been reported as potentially beneficial for the management of patients with unilateral involvement.
- Amblyopia therapy is initiated in conjunction with the optical correction. Several part-time patching regimens have been developed. The visual development is monitored with the binocular fixation pattern response, and frequent postoperative visits are required.

Surgical

A posterior transciliary approach is used to access the peripheral lens remnants, vitreous base, and posterior vitreous cavity, facilitating membrane dissection in eyes with extensive proliferation. In situations in which the retina is drawn anteriorly over the pars plicata or into a retrolental mass, the translimbal approach is preferable and less hazardous. In either instance, a detailed examination under anesthesia is required, as are ancillary studies, if necessary, to determine the most efficacious approach. If pathology is primarily anterior in location an anterior approach can be performed with the goal of preserving enough capsular support to permit placement of an intraocular lens. The following is an outline for the posterior approach.

- After the induction of general anesthesia, limbal conjunctival periotomies are developed under microscopic control at the 10 and 2 o'clock positions and inferotemporally.
- A 20 gauge microvitreoretinal (MVR) blade is introduced posterior to clear cornea infertemporally, and a 20 gauge self retaining anterior chamber maintainer is inserted into the anterior chamber for infusion of the irrigating solution (balanced salt solution [BSS] with 1 : 1000 epinephrine HCl [0.3 mL/500 mL BSS]).
- With poor pupillary dilation, the pupil can be enlarged with the vitreous cutter or, preferably, with flexible iris retractors.
- Sclerotomies are created at 10 o'clock and 2 o'clock, 1 to 2 mm posterior to the limbus.
- A vitreous cutter and an end gripping microforceps (DORC) are inserted and the anterior capsule, lens nucleus and cortex are removed. The peripheral lenticular and capsular remnants can be visualized with indentation if required.
- The posterior capsule and retrolental membrane are evaluated for a clear zone between the membrane and the ciliary processes. An opening is made in this area with a MVR blade or automated scissors, and the membrane-capsule complex is dissected from the ciliary processes for a full 360 degrees. If a clear zone is not identified, an opening is made in the central portion of the membrane and this surgical plane is maintained peripherally to the ciliary processes. Complete removal of the membrane-capsule complex is preferred if technically feasible.
- The separated membrane-capsule complex is removed with the vitrector. Increasing the intraocular pressure (raising the infusion bottle height), unimanual bipolar diathermy, or adding low-dose thrombin (100 units/mL) to the infusion fluid can control intraoperative bleeding from the ciliary processes.
- If the pathologic process is anterior in location, an anterior vitrectomy is performed with a wide field viewing system (BIOM), vitrector and fiberoptic endoilluminator. If the hyaloid artery is present and cut, the remnant is cauterized to prevent bleeding.
- In the presence of either bilateral involvement or a mild tractional retinal detachment of the posterior pole, a complete vitrectomy should be performed. Epiretinal membranes are stripped, delaminated, or segmented using bimanual technique and combination-function instruments. Xenon light sources provide excellent illumination for dual function instruments.
- The retina is examined with indirect ophthalmoscopy and scleral indentation and if significant peripheral traction remains or retinal breaks are identified, an encircling element such as a 41 or 240 band is placed to support the vitreous base. The band ends are secured with a Watzke sleeve, and the band is tightened to achieve a moderately high and broad buckle.
- Retinal tears and dialysis are treated with external cryopexy or laser photocoagulation. Extended intraocular tamponade is achieved by infusing silicone oil.
- The sclerotomies, limbal incisions, and periotomies are closed with 8-0 vicryl suture, and subconjunctival injections of cefazolin (25 mg) and dexamethasone (4 mg) are given. A patch and shield are placed after a drop of atropine (1 %) is instilled.

COMPLICATIONS

Technical alternatives and pitfalls

- Peripheral retinal and vitreous base prolapsed through the sclerotomy, retinal holes, and retinal dialysis have all been reported with the posterior approach to PHPV. These complications have been attributed to both abnormal anterior retinal insertion and thick vitreous gel.
- In instances in which an anterior approach is required, the surgical technique is similar, although only two limbal incision sites are used.
- Other technical alternatives for the management of these patients include primary sector iridectomy and simple lensectomy. To prevent secondary papillary complications, primary peripheral iridectomy, pupilloplasty, lensectomy, anterior membranectomy, and anterior vitrectomy have been advocated.
- The postoperative complications are similar to those of congenital cataract surgery and have included amblyopia, glaucoma, retinal detachment, secondary pupillary membranes, endophthalmitis and phthisis.

COMMENTS

Since Reese's original description, most investigators have considered the visual prognosis to be dismal, even when early surgery is performed to salvage the eye. This premise has been questioned because an enucleation is infrequently required for either treated or untreated eyes. However, surgical intervention has not uniformly averted the development of intractable glaucoma and phthisis.

Several recent retrospective studies have reported improved outcomes, with up to 19% of the patients having 20/200 vision, even in the presence of microphthalmos. These results must be judged in light of the risk of surgical complications, amblyopia treatment failure, and treatment noncompliance.

REFERENCES

Anteby I, Cohen E, Karshai I, et al: Unilateral persistent hyperplastic primary vitreous: course and outcome. J AAPOS 2:92–99, 2002.

Haddad R, Font RL, Reeser F: Persistent hyperplastic primary vitreous: a clinicopathologic study of 62 cases and review of the literature. Surv Ophthalmol 23:123–134, 1978.

Reese AJ: Persistent hyperplastic primary vitreous. Trans Am Acad Ophthalmol Otol 59:271–284, 1955.

Scott WE: Treatment of congenital cataracts and persistent hyperplastic primary vitreous. Trans New Orleans Acad Ophthalmol 34:461–477, 1986.

Stark WJ, Lindsey PS, Fagadau WR, et al: Persistent hyperplastic primary vitreous: surgical treatment. Ophthalmology 90:452–457, 1983.

351 PROLIFERATIVE VITREORETINOPATHY 379.29

Steve Charles, MD

Memphis, Tennessee

ETIOLOGY

Proliferative vitreoretinopathy (PVR) is a reparative process initiated by full- or partial-thickness retinal breaks, retinopexy, or other types of retinal damage. Loss of contact inhibition causes the surrounding glial or retinal pigment epithelial cells to migrate to both surfaces of the retina and proliferate. These cells then migrate farther and cover the posterior surface of the detached posterior hyaloid face. Fibronectin-lined, coated pits serve as attachments of retinal pigment epithelial or glial cells to collagen fibers and other components of the extracellular matrix. The migration/contraction mechanism causes tangential force on the retina, resulting in multiple starfolds and fixed folds. Similarly, the vitreous collagen matrix contracts because of a similar hypocellular process.

DIAGNOSIS

Clinical signs and symptoms

Ocular or periocular

- Retina: epiretinal membranes, fixed folds, starfolds, subretinal placoid or dendritic proliferation.
- Vitreous: condensation, contraction, pigmentation, and posterior vitreous detachment.
- Other: visual loss.

TREATMENT

Surgical

- The *surgical objective* is to enable the retina to conform to the retinal pigment epithelium. In cases of moderate starfolds without static vitreous traction, scleral buckling without vitreous surgery is indicated. Minimal retinopexy to the breaks should be used to avoid inflammation and further proliferation. Re-treatment of the retinal pigment epithelium and multiple rows of retinopexy should be avoided to reduce recurrent PVR and inflammation. Post-reattachment retinopexy helps to reduce retinal pigment epithelium and glial cell proliferation as well as inflammation and increased vascular permeability but it requires a vitrectomy approach. Laser endophotocoagulation causes less PVR than does cryotherapy but it can only be used with vitrectomy.
- A broad, moderately high, *360-degree encircling buckle* with a smooth contour should be used. This is best achieved with a silicone explant and two or three mattress sutures per quadrant. The posterior scleral bites should be single, long, and circumferential and as posterior as possible to avoid damage to the vortex veins. The anterior bites should be limbus-parallel and placed in the scleral condensations at the muscle ring representing the external landmark of the ora. Sutures of 5-0 monofilament nylon are preferred to Mersilene sutures because the former can be tied without the help of an assistant and do not slip. The ends must be cut on the knot to avoid protrusion through the conjunctiva. The broad buckle extends back to the thicker, stronger, untreated retina and to the ora to prevent anterior leakage. Complete or near-complete drainage of subretinal fluid (SRF), preferably using a direct needle drainage method, is required to achieve reattachment and create space for the large buckle. Vitrectomy in aphakic eyes or anterior chamber paracentesis in phakic or pseudophakic eyes may be necessary to achieve volume requirements. Air or, preferably, expandable C3F8 gas injection 'seals' the retinal breaks via surface tension and allows restoration of a trans-retinal pressure gradient and more complete drainage of SRF. Because air (or gas) causes attachment of the anterior retina and posterior displacement of SRF, transscleral drainage of SRF should be performed very posteriorly if done after air (or gas) injection to avoid retinal incarceration in the drainage site.
- *Vitreous surgery* should be performed when it is anticipated that scleral buckling alone cannot compensate for vitreous traction and periretinal membrane contraction sufficiently to reattach the retina. In most instances, the lens should be removed with trans-pars plana lensectomy or preferably with intraocular lens implantation. Phaco to permit better release of the anterior traction and for decompartmentalization, which may reduce recurrent proliferative vitreoretinopathy. Endocapsular lensectomy with the aspirating phacofragmenter and linear (proportional) suction should be used if there is any substantial inflammation or any reason to avoid phaco. The anterior and posterior portions of the vitreous cortex are usually in contact, resulting in a frontal plane configuration. This frontal plane component should be removed first, preferably with the vitreous cutter and minimal, linear suction. The anterior PVR radial traction then should be resected with the vitreous cutter, if sufficient distance exists between the anterior attachment at the pars plana and the posterior attachment of this former peripheral cortical vitreous to the retina at the equator. A 25-, 23-, or 20-gauge delamination scissors are required in many instances to resect this anterior loop.
- The *epiretinal membrane* can be peeled away from the retina when it is minimally adherent. End-opening, 25G DSP forceps or conformal forceps are used for inside-out peeling of epiretinal membranes; picks, needles and forceps with one blade under the epiretinal membrane cause more trauma to the retina. In cases of stronger adherence, it is better to perform segmentation or delamination using fine curved scissors with blades essentially parallel to the retina. Segmentation of the epiretinal membrane in the center of a starfold and between each fold releases the tangential traction. If the membrane is dense and well developed, it can be delaminated from the retinal surface using both scissor blades between the retina and membrane. The goal is to release sufficient tangential traction to allow retinal conformation to the retinal pigment epithelium with minimal damage to the retina, not removing all membranes.
- *Subretinal membranes* can be segmented or removed with forceps if they are creating sufficient contour change in the retina to prevent reattachment. This can be accomplished through a pre-existing retinal break, or a retinotomy can be created for this purpose, using the closed forceps to push through the retina. Large retinotomies are not required for subretinal surgery and they do unnecessary damage to the retina.
- *Internal drainage* of SRF should precede fluid-air exchange to enable removal of all posterior SRF through preexisting peripheral retinal breaks. Drainage retinotomies are used if the peripheral breaks can be easily accessed for internal drainage. Use of internal drainage often reduces the need for perfluoroctane except in cases of giant breaks without PVR. Internal drainage of SRF through a tapered, angulated cannula placed through a convenient retinal break and held near the retinal pigment epithelium allows a feasibility test for intraoperative retinal attachment. The appearance of subretinal air indicates the failure to release all tangential forces on the retina and the need for further forceps membrane peeling, segmentation, delamination, retinectomy, or scleral buckling. It may also indicate inoperability.

If internal drainage of SRF and fluid-air exchange with continued internal drainage of SRF results in subretinal air, incremental retinectomy with the vitreous cutter can be effective to release tangential forces on the retina. Retinectomy is also indicated when the retina is incarcerated in a wound or previous drain site and when dense membranes are strongly adherent over broad areas of atrophic retina. Air-gas exchange or air-silicone exchange should be performed after internal drainage of SRF, fluid-air exchange, and laser endophotocoagulation. Confluent, moderate-intensity endolaser should be used around breaks. Laser retinopexy in rows and panretinal laser photocoagulation (PRP) should be avoided to reduce tissue damage. Laser indirect ophthalmoscopy is not necessary in vitreous surgery and may cause corneal and iris damage as well as light-scatter-mediated macular damage.

- *Air (gas) surface tension management* should be used in all cases requiring vitrectomy because the viscosity of the vitreous is significantly reduced, preventing the retinal pigment epithelial pump from maintaining a transretinal pressure gradient. Subsequent air-gas exchange allows creation of a total fill of the vitreous space without hypotony or multiple small bubbles. Using an 18% concentration of C_3F_8 has been shown to produce better outcomes than 25% SF_6 because the bubble lasts longer than 3 weeks instead of 1 week. Concentrations greater than these are not used because expansion would cause elevation of intraocular pressure with a total fill. The gas is injected through the infusion cannula, preferably using a power gas injector. Fluid egress is accomplished through an extrusion cannula positioned through the retinal break, near the retinal pigment epithelium, and is controlled by a foot-operated linear suction system.

Surface tension management with highly purified silicone oil (1000 centistokes) is preferable to the use of gas for most advanced or recurrent cases of PVR. If a posterior chamber lens is in place, it will maintain the silicone posteriorly, preventing corneal contact and subacute angle-closure glaucoma. If the eye is phakic, endocapsular lensectomy or phaco should be utilized, as cataract formation universally follows extended periods of silicone oil usage. An Ando inferior iridectomy should be used in all aphakic eyes to prevent silicone pupillary block. The capsule should be removed with diamond-coated forceps to prevent fibrosis at the iridectomy site and the development of cyclitic membranes and hypotony. Viscoelastics, blood, and inflammation increase emulsification of the silicone oil and should be avoided, if possible. Aphakic patients who have received silicone treatment are instructed to avoid prolonged supine positioning to reduce the incidence of subacute angle-closure glaucoma and corneal contact. The author removes silicone oil in about 10% of cases and is opposed to performing multiple procedures just to enable silicone removal, especially in older and pseudophakic patients. Silicone is used for rhegmatogenous confinement and facilitates stabilization of inferior and peripheral retinal detachments. Silicone should be removed only if all breaks are sealed by retinopexy.

- *Scleral buckling* using a 9-mm-wide, 360-degree silicone explant imbricated flush with the surface of the globe and sutured end-to-end is used in most cases. It is a mistake to think of PVR as a localized disease and to buckle only the abnormal-appearing areas. An encircling band is required. Care should be taken to avoid muscle removal or damage to the vortex veins, especially during buckle revision.

PRECAUTIONS

- Vitreous (periretinal membrane) surgery should be done when it is apparent that conventional scleral buckling alone will not be effective and the eye has minimal inflammation and 'mature' epiretinal membranes.
- Inside-out forceps membrane peeling with diamond-coated or conformal forceps is superior to other membrane peeling methods.
- Laser retinopexy should not used only around retinal breaks, not in PRP fashion.
- Subconjunctival steroids decrease the release of fibrin and reduce proliferation and therefore should be used in all cases without steroid glaucoma. Systemic steroids should never be used in these cases because of systemic side effects.

COMMENTS

The above techniques have approximately a 95% intraoperative anatomic success rate, with 75% long-term anatomic success and a 50% long-term visual success rate. Visual acuities are better than 5/200 in the author's series. With the possibility of bilateral visual loss in PVR, it is mandatory to consider this procedure with its greater success rate and 0.5- to 1.5-hour operating time to retain an eye with ambulatory vision.

Antiproliferative drugs, radiation therapy, and intraocular steroids have not been proven effective against PVR.

REFERENCES

Abrams GW, Ryan SJ, Lai MY, et al: Vitrectomy with silicone oil or long-acting gas in eyes with severe proliferative vitreoretinopathy: results of additional and long-term follow-up. Silicone Study Report 11. Arch Ophthalmol 115:335–344, 1997.

Campochiaro PA: Pathogenic mechanism in proliferative vitreoretinopathy. Arch Ophthalmol 115:237–241, 1997.

Charteris DG: Proliferative vitreoretinopathy: pathobiology, surgical management, and adjunctive treatment. Br J Ophthalmol 79:953–960, 1995.

van Horn DL, Aaberg TM, Machemer R, et al: Glial cell proliferation in human retinal detachment with massive periretinal proliferation. Am J Ophthalmol 84:383–393, 1977.

352 VITREOUS HEMORRHAGE 379.23

Irvin L. Handelman, MD
Portland, Oregon

Vitreous hemorrhage is a common cause of profound visual loss. Understanding the pathogenesis and etiology is important in its successful management. Current therapy has two components: prophylaxis and vitreous surgery.

ETIOLOGY/INCIDENCE

Blood enters the vitreous from ruptured vessels derived from the retina or uveal tract. From the retinal circulation there are both proliferative and nonproliferative retinopathies. Traction

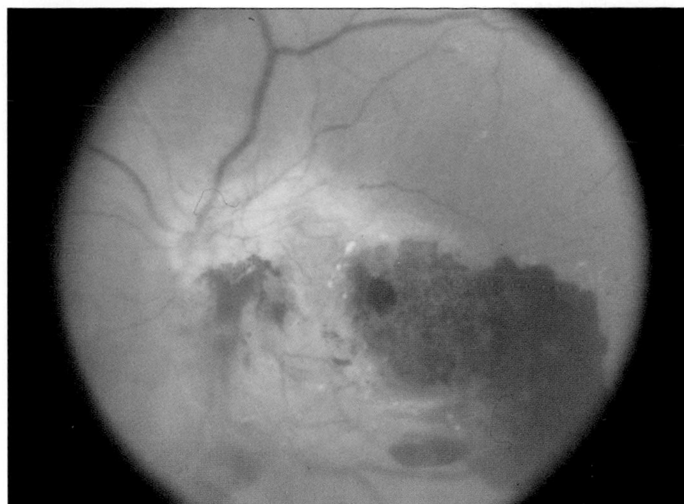

FIGURE 352.1. Vitreous hemorrhage in proliferative diabetic retinopathy.

on the retina as seen with a rhegmatogenous retinal detachment represents another type of causation. Trauma to the retina and choroid can be either perforating or contusional. Bleeding from the uveal tract as seen in age-related macular degeneration can also lead to significant vitreous hemorrhages. This type of ocular hemorrhage is relatively rare and may occur in about 7 out of 100,000 individuals in the general population. The most common causes, which represent at least 75% of the hemorrhages, include proliferative diabetic retinopathy, retinal tear and detachment, branch retinal vein occlusion, and posterior vitreous detachment without retinal tears (Figure 352.1).

COMMON CAUSES OF VITREOUS HEMORRHAGE

Retinal vascular

Proliferation of new vessels

- Proliferative diabetic retinopathy.
- Branch retinal vein occlusion.
- Retinopathy of prematurity.
- Carotid artery insufficiency.
- Retinal vasculitis and uveitis.
- Sickle cell disease.
- Eales' disease.

Nonproliferative

- Central retinal vein occlusion.
- Acquired arterial macroaneurysm.
- Terson's syndrome (intracranial hemorrhage).
- Valsalva phenomenon.

Traction on retinal vessels

- Retinal break or tear.
- Rhegmatogenous retinal detachment.
- Posterior vitreous detachment.

Trauma

- Contusion (commotio retinae).
- Penetrating injury.
- Shaken-baby syndrome.

Uveal tract

- Choroidal neovascularization associated with macular degeneration.
- Hyphema.
- Malignant melanoma.

COURSE/PROGNOSIS

Since the vitreous is avascular, hemorrhage within it tends to reabsorb slowly. However, the rate of reabsorption depends upon the amount of hemorrhage and status of the vitreous gel. Small hemorrhages through which the retina can usually be visualized without too much difficulty generally reabsorb more or less completely within a relatively short period of time. In the presence of advanced vitreous syneresis or posterior vitreous detachment, blood reabsorbs more quickly unless there have been recurrent hemorrhages over a number of months. Subhyaloid hemorrhages are very slow to reabsorb and can often, especially in the presence of diseased retinal vessels, predispose to the formation of fibrous membranes. Even after clearing of vitreous blood in the visual axis, some hemorrhagic membranes may remain in the inferior periphery of the eye for months or years.

The underlying pathology often correlates with the course of vitreous bleeding. The Diabetic Retinopathy Vitrectomy study demonstrated that dense vitreous hemorrhages, especially in type I diabetics, have a high risk of producing complex fibrovascular membranes if the blood is not removed either naturally or surgically within one to two months; in older, type II diabetics on the other hand, the vitreous hemorrhage may remain in the eye without as high a risk of causing tractional complications. In the presence of a retinal tear or rhegmatogenous detachment, extensive hemorrhage in the vitreous is thought to predispose to increasing traction and formation of fibrous membranes, which can cause further tractional complications. Vitreous blood can obscure visualization of peripheral retinal pathology and create significant difficulty in treating these problems. Bleeding from a posterior vitreous detachment without breaks carries a favorable prognosis since it usually resolves spontaneously and rarely requires a vitrectomy.

The long-term prognosis often relates to the quantity of vitreous hemorrhage and integrity of the retina and uveal tract. In general when the retina can be visualized through the vitreous hemorrhage, there is a high likelihood of spontaneous reabsorption of the blood without surgical intervention. However, eyes with hemorrhage obscuring significant portions of the inferior retina may need to be closely monitored for many months to watch for retinal tears that could be hidden under the hemorrhage. If the retina is very ischemic or chronically detached, even removal of the hemorrhage may create little improvement in visual function. Hypotony and anterior segment neovascularization are often grave prognostic signs indicating the presence of severe posterior segment pathology. Infrequently ghost cell glaucoma can result from a vitreous hemorrhage.

DIAGNOSIS

A complete history and comprehensive examination are critical to establish the cause of the vitreous hemorrhage. Of special importance are slit lamp biomicroscopy and indirect ophthalmoscopy with scleral depression. The patient often will report sudden onset of floaters, which may be described as cobwebs or multiple mobile, dot-like floaters. The presence of photopsia often points to a tractional etiology such as a retinal tear or detachment. In addition, sectoral visual field loss may indicate a retinal detachment or branch retinal vein occlusion. In all but rare cases of proliferative diabetic retinopathy, the diagnosis of diabetes mellitus has been well documented. In some cases, such as sickle cell disease and retinal vasculitis, pertinent laboratory findings may help to establish the diagnosis. Consumption of aspirin for its platelet-inhibition properties probably carries little increased risk for vitreous hemorrhage, and this has been established in the Early Treatment of Diabetic Retinopathy study. The risk of other platelet inhibitors and anticoagulants in causing vitreous hemorrhage is controversial.

B-scan ultrasonography can be an invaluable aid in evaluating dense vitreous hemorrhages. This test can document the presence and location of a retinal detachment and sometimes a retinal tear. In the proliferative retinopathies, ultrasound examination can localize and quantify traction on the retina. Visualization of a posterior vitreous detachment is helpful, for example, in following patients with a vitreous hemorrhage since it usually carries a good prognosis unless there is a coexistent retinal tear.

In some individuals sequential ultrasound examinations may be needed to monitor a nonclearing vitreous hemorrhage.

Bedrest with elevation of the head has been advocated to aid in settling and clearing of vitreous hemorrhage. This technique is of uncertain value since normal eye movements tend to disperse blood throughout the eye. However, in some cases settling of the vitreous hemorrhage may allow visualization of a superior retinal break and allow its treatment; similarly increased visualization of the superior retina may facilitate panretinal photocoagulation in cases of proliferative diabetic retinopathy.

PROPHYLAXIS

Treatment of the underlying pathology often will prevent visually significant vitreous hemorrhages.

In most eyes with neovascularization of the optic disc or retina, there is significant underlying ischemia, and most of these eyes will benefit from scatter or panretinal laser photocoagulation. Depending upon the etiology, this is applied to the retinal midperiphery and periphery in all quadrants; however, in cases of segmental pathology, this treatment is restricted to the appropriate area of the retina.

In proliferative diabetic retinopathy the presence of even a small vitreous hemorrhage is associated with a high risk of severe visual loss, and panretinal photocoagulation is indicated to decrease this risk. The value of this technique was definitively demonstrated in the Diabetic Retinopathy study. Generally laser treatment is applied with a green wavelength either at the slit lamp using a contact lens or with the indirect ophthalmoscope; however, other wavelengths, especially red and infrared, also are effective. In general 1200 to 2000 burns are scattered over one to four sessions. Usually only topical anesthesia is required; however, in some cases retrobulbar anesthesia will facilitate complete treatment. The endpoint of panretinal photocoagulation is regression of the neovascularization. Although rarely used, panretinal cryoablation probably is also effective.

Ischemic branch retinal vein occlusions can develop neovascularization of the optic disc and retina as a late development. In general scatter photocoagulation applied to the affected quadrant will, in most cases, produce regression of the new vessels and prevent further bleeding. Other than applying treatment to a more limited area of the retina, the technique is the same as used in proliferative diabetic retinopathy.

In retinopathy of prematurity, threshold disease can lead to vitreous hemorrhages and retinal detachments. Cryotherapy was initially determined to be effective in stimulating regression of neovascularization. More recently a relatively confluent laser photocoagulation technique applied to the retinal periphery has been used and led to successful involution of new vessels in many cases.

A hemorrhage associated with a symptomatic retinal tear can be caused either from a coexistent posterior vitreous detachment or rupture of a bridging retinal vessel. Appropriate laser photocoagulation or cryotherapy applied around the retinal break can minimize the risk of a retinal detachment. The vitreous hemorrhage, if not severe, will usually clear spontaneously.

However, in a few retinal tears there is an avulsed retinal vessel which may bleed into the vitreous following adequate prophylactic treatment; in some of these cases, if the vitreous is sufficiently clear, the avulsed vessel can be directly treated with laser photocoagulation.

Pneumatic retinopexy is a minimally invasive technique which can be used to manage selected retinal detachments that can be associated with vitreous bleeding; in this technique an intravitreal injection of a long-acting gas tamponade, such as sulfur hexafluoride, combined with laser photocoagulation or cryotherapy can seal retinal breaks, repair the detachment, and minimize the risk of additional bleeding. Repair of retinal detachments by scleral buckling techniques can be accomplished in the presence of mild to moderate vitreous hemorrhages with little risk of complications; usually successful repair of the retinal detachment will decrease the risk of recurrent bleeding.

VITREOUS SURGERY

A vitrectomy will be needed for nonclearing, severe vitreous hemorrhages or for eyes in which there are recurrent hemorrhages of moderate severity. In general a three-port pars plana vitrectomy is the usual approach. Depending upon the underlying pathology, there may be special intraoperative techniques to gain a successful outcome. Recently a sutureless vitrectomy technique has been developed using 25-gauge instrumentation, and this can lead to shorter operating times and faster postoperative rehabilitation.

In the case of rhegmatogenous retinal detachments, the presence of extensive hemorrhage requires a vitrectomy. Currently most surgeons would also employ some degree of a scleral buckling technique. However, at the present time there is some movement away from scleral buckling when a vitrectomy is required for management of a retinal detachment with or without vitreous hemorrhage. This surgery is usually combined with laser photocoagulation and intravitreal gas or silicone oil. Contusional or perforating injuries associated with dense vitreous hemorrhages usually should be managed with vitrectomy within one to two weeks because of a high risk of retinal detachment.

In proliferative diabetic retinopathy the timing of vitrectomy depends to some extent upon the age of the patient. In general, severe vitreous hemorrhages in the younger, type I diabetics are operated on within about one month of onset of the bleeding if there is no spontaneous clearing. In type II diabetics there is somewhat less urgency because of slower progression of neovascular and fibrovascular proliferation; however, generally these eyes are operated on within two to three months if the hemorrhage is severe. It is of great importance to remove fibrovascular membranes with the vitreous cutter or scissors. In most diabetic eyes without traction detachments of the macula, vitreous surgery can usually restore useful vision including macular function. However, in these cases the visual outcome is always limited by the extent of retinal vascular damage from diabetes.

Dense vitreous hemorrhages can develop in eyes with age-related macular degeneration, and most of these have significant, disciform scars. Nevertheless vitrectomy may be helpful in restoring useful peripheral vision in many cases.

There is no currently available medical or ocular treatment for vitreous hemorrhages. However, research using various enzymes, such as hyaluronidase, injected into the vitreous has shown promise in clearing vitreous hemorrhages. Current studies are beginning to evaluate the use of vascular endothelial growth factor inhibitors, such as pegaptanib (Macugen) and bevacizumab, injected into the vitreous to stimulate regression of neovascularization.

Complications of vitreous surgery include cataract development, glaucoma, and retinal detachment. These problems can usually be managed medically or with additional surgery.

Neovascular glaucoma can complicate eyes with ischemic retinopathy before or after a vitrectomy. In addition, depending upon the underlying pathology, there is at least a small risk of recurrent bleeding following a vitrectomy despite removal of or cautery applied to posterior segment neovascularization.

REFERENCES

Coats DK, Miller AM, McCreery KMB, et al: Involution of threshold retinopathy of prematurity after diode laser photocoagulation. Ophthalmology 111:1894–1898, 2004.

Eller AW: Diagnosis and management of vitreous hemorrhage: American Academy of Ophthalmology Focal Points 18:1–8, 2000.

Ibarra MS, Hermel M, Premer JL, Hassan TS: Longer-term outcomes of transconjunctival sutureless 25-gauge vitrectomy. Am J Ophthalmol 139:831–836, 2005.

Kupperman BD, Thomas EL, de Smet MD, Grillone LR, for the Vitrase for Vitreous Hemorrhage Study Groups: Pooled efficacy results from two multinational randomized controlled clinical trials of a single intravitreal injection of highly purified ovine hyaluronidase (Vitrase®) for the management of vitreous hemorrhage. Am J Ophthalmol 140:573–584, 2005.

Sarrafizadeh RH, Hassan TS, Ruby AJ, et al: Incidence of retinal detachment and visual outcome in eyes presenting with posterior vitreous separation and dense fundus-obscuring vitreous hemorrhage. Ophthalmology 108:2273–2278, 2001.

353 VITREOUS WICK SYNDROME 379.26

James P. Bolling, MD
Jacksonville, Florida

ETIOLOGY

The vitreous wick syndrome occurs when vitreous is incarcerated in a corneal or corneoscleral incision; this creates a 'wick' to the external ocular surface. Vitreous wick may be more common in the age of intravitreal injections and no-stitch vitrectomy. Vitreous loss or incarceration (wick) usually occurs:

- In the setting of unrecognized rupture in the posterior capsule; or
- After inadequate vitrectomy following recognized posterior capsule rupture;
- After intravitreal injection of steroids or other pharmacologic agents;
- After a laceration of the sclera when the edges of the wound are not completely cleaned of vitreous.

A vitreous wick can produce a noninfectious ocular inflammation with entrapment of vitreous, distortion of the pupil and release of mediators of inflammation. This in turn may result in cystoid macular edema. The anterior traction may extend to the vitreous base, causing retinal breaks or detachment. The vitreous incarcerated in the wound may serve as a stent and delay would closure increasing the risk of endophthalmitis.

DIAGNOSIS

Clinical signs and symptoms

- Anterior chamber cells and flare.
- Hypopyon.
- Strand(s) of vitreous in anterior chamber.
- Distorted pupil.
- Dilated iris vessels.
- Cells in vitreous.
- Degenerative vitreous changes and membranes.
- Cystoid macular edema.
- Retinal tears or detachment.
- Endophthalmitis.

TREATMENT

Ocular

Treatment varies, depending on the complications of the vitreous wick. Sometimes the vitreous incarceration in the wound may not be apparent until after completion of the surgery; if this is the case and no wound leak is present, no therapy need be given, although the patient should be followed closely in the immediate postoperative period.

If cystoid macular edema develops and abnormal inflammation is present, medical therapy should first be attempted.

- Topical prednisolone acetate drops can be tried for 2 weeks.

If no improvement is seen:

- Sub-Tenon's injections of triamcinolone acetate may be used;
- Topical nonsteroidal anti-inflammatory drugs may also be tried;
- Oral acetazolamide also has been shown to be effective in reducing cystoid macular edema.

Surgical

If the primary situation involves wound leak, this may be recognized at the conclusion of surgery. It can then be repaired by:

- 'Sponge vitrectomy,' lifting the vitreous strand at the wound with a small cellulose surgical sponge and cutting it with scissors; or

- Using the vitreous cutter to aspirate over the wound with the cutter on.

If these methods are not effective in releasing all of the vitreous from the wound, it may be necessary to:
- Reopen the incision and clean the vitreous from the wound edges;
- Make a second incision away from the site of incarceration, permitting the vitreous strand(s) to be severed with an iris sweep or vitreous cutter.

Occasionally, the wound leak is the primary problem, carrying prolapsed vitreous forward to lodge in the wound. If this is the case, securely suturing the wound closed should prevent recurrent prolapse. If all these measures are not adequate, it may be necessary to perform:
- An anterior vitrectomy.

All cataract surgeons should be prepared to perform an anterior vitrectomy at the time of routine cataract surgery.

Sometimes the vitreous entrapped in the wound is not recognized until well after surgery; if symptoms of endophthalmitis are present (sudden onset of pain, vision loss, hypopyon, and vitreous inflammation):
- Immediate vitreous tap should be performed; and
- Systemic (oral, intravenous, or both) antibiotics should be started as soon as possible.

If endophthalmitis has compromised the patient's vision to the level of light perception:
- A vitrectomy is indicated.

During a posterior vitrectomy, the wick can sometimes be released by aspirating immediately behind the implant.

Depending on the lapse of time since the original surgery:
- An anterior chamber incision may be necessary to pull a fibrin plaque off the surface of the implant, using a bent needle; sometimes the vitreous can also be engaged in this manner.

If manipulation of the wound and anterior chamber is not completely successful in removing the vitreous from the anterior structures:
- A pars plana vitrectomy may be necessary.

In fact, this is usually the situation because in most cases, the vitreous is adherent not only to the wound but also to the back of the iris, the capsule and the implant.

COMMENTS

In many cases, cataract surgery is now performed without any sutures to close the wound; vitrectomy surgery is also being performed without sutures. This may result in more patient comfort and less astigmatism postoperatively. Unfortunately, if the unsutured wound is leaking, vitreous may readily become lodged in the wound and endophthalmitis may be more common. It is important to check the wound carefully for leaks and securely close them when necessary.

REFERENCES

Chen SD, Mohammed Q, Bowling B, Patel CK: Vitreous wick syndrome-a potential cause of endophthalmitis after intravitreal injection of triamcinolone through the pars plana. Am J Ophthalmol 137(6):1159–1160, 2004.

Endophthalmitis Vitrectomy Study Group: Results of the Endophthalmitis Vitrectomy Study: a randomized trial of immediate vitrectomy and of intravenous antibiotics for the treatment of postoperative bacterial endophthalmitis. Arch Ophthalmol 113:1479–1496, 1995.

Nelson DB, Donnenfeld ED, Perry HD: Sterile endophthalmitis after sutureless cataract surgery. Ophthalmology 99:1655–1657, 1992.

Ruiz RS, Teeters VS: The vitreous wick syndrome: a late complication following cataract extraction. Am J Ophthalmol 70:483–490, 1970.

Turkalj JW, Carlson AN, Manos JP, Apple DJ: Is the sutureless cataract incision a valve for bacterial inoculation? J Cataract Refract Surg 21:472–476, 1995.

Venkatesh P, Verma L, Tewari H: Posterior vitreous wick syndrome: a potential cause of endophthalmitis following vitreo-retinal surgery. Medical Hyothesis 58(6):513–515, 2002.

Whitcup SM, Csaky KG, Podgor MJ, et al: A randomized, masked cross-over trial of acetazolamide for cystoid macular edema in patients with uveitis. Ophthalmology 103:1054–1062, 1996.

Index

'vs' indicates the differential diagnosis of various conditions.

D

E

H

J

K

L

M

Index

O

P

Q

R

S

T

W

X

Y

Z